HIGH-YIELD IMAGING

Gastrointestinal

HIGH-YIELD IMAGING

Gastrointestinal

EDITORS

Richard M. Gore, MD
Professor of Radiology
University of Chicago
Chief, Gastrointestinal Radiology Section
NorthShore University Health System
Evanston, Illinois

Marc S. Levine, MD
Professor of Radiology
Advisory Dean
University of Pennsylvania School of Medicine
Chief, Gastrointestinal Radiology Section
University of Pennsylvania Medical Center
Philadelphia, Pennsylvania

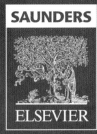

SAUNDERS

ELSEVIER

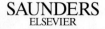

1600 John F. Kennedy Blvd.
Ste 1800
Philadelphia, PA 19103-2899

HIGH-YIELD IMAGING: GASTROINTESTINAL   ISBN: 978-1-4160-5544-0

Notice

Knowledge and best practice in this field are constantly changing. As new research and experience
broaden our knowledge, changes in practice, treatment and drug therapy may become necessary
or appropriate. Readers are advised to check the most current information provided (i) on
procedures featured or (ii) by the manufacturer of each product to be administered, to verify the
recommended dose or formula, the method and duration of administration, and contraindications.
It is the responsibility of the practitioner, relying on his or her own experience and knowledge of
the patient, to make diagnoses, to determine dosages and the best treatment for each individual
patient, and to take all appropriate safety precautions. To the fullest extent of the law, neither
the publisher nor the authors assume any liability for any injury and/or damage to persons or
property arising out of or related to any use of the material contained in this book.

The Publisher

Library of Congress Cataloging-in-Publication Data
Gore, Richard M.
   High-yield imaging. Gastrointestinal / Richard M. Gore, Marc S. Levine. — 1st ed.
      p. ; cm.
   ISBN 978-1-4160-5544-0
   1. Gastrointestinal system—Imaging—Handbooks, manuals, etc. I. Levine, Marc S. II. Title.
III. Title: Gastrointestinal.
   [DNLM: 1. Gastrointestinal Diseases—radiography. WI 141 G666h 2010]
   RC804.D52G67 2010
   616.3'307572—dc22   2009041680

Acquisitions Editor: Rebecca Gaertner
Developmental Editor: Timothy C. Maxwell
Publishing Services Manager: Tina Rebane
Production Manager: Amy L. Cannon
Design Direction: Steve Stave

Working together to grow
libraries in developing countries

www.elsevier.com | www.bookaid.org | www.sabre.org

ELSEVIER   BOOK AID International   Sabre Foundation

Printed in China

Last digit is the print number: 9 8 7 6 5 4 3 2 1

For Margaret and our children,
Diana, Elizabeth, and George

Richard M. Gore

To my beautiful wife Deborah
you had me at hello

Marc S. Levine

Preface

Patients with abdominal and pelvic disease often present with a perplexing constellation of radiographic findings demonstrated on a variety of different imaging examinations. This imaging conundrum occurs on a daily basis and in the setting of increasingly busy workloads. The harried radiologist has scant time to interpret and report confusing imaging findings on abdominal imaging studies, much less review the literature or perform a rushed "Google" search to facilitate the diagnostic interpretation of such cases. As a result, these diagnostic dilemmas can become forgotten enigmas, as the radiologist moves on quickly to the next case.

The purpose of *High-Yield Imaging: Gastrointestinal* as one of several teaching tools in the ongoing series of High-Yield texts from Elsevier is to provide user-friendly, hardcopy and web-based resources that the practicing radiologist can use to quickly and easily confirm a suspected diagnosis or generate a reasonable differential when the diagnosis is in doubt. The text has been organized into a series of topics on virtually every pathologic condition affecting the gastrointestinal tract, including the hollow organs (pharynx, esophagus, stomach, duodenum, small bowel, colon, and rectum), solid viscera (gallbladder and biliary tract, liver, pancreas, and spleen), and peritoneal cavity (peritoneum, retroperitoneum, mesentery, omentum, and abdominal wall).

Each topic contains brief, concise sections on the anatomic findings, clinical presentation, incidence/ prevalence/epidemiology, imaging findings, and differential diagnosis, as well as a brief synopsis of what the referring physician needs to know. Each section is formatted as a bulleted list for rapid extraction of the relevant clinical information and imaging features of the disease by the reader. Each topic also contains several pertinent radiographs to illustrate the important imaging features. We believe this format is extremely user friendly, enabling the practicing radiologist to approach the text in a "hit and run" style for maximum information with a minimum of effort in order to better diagnose challenging cases without disrupting a busy clinical schedule.

The guiding principle of this resource is to illustrate and integrate the spectrum of abnormalities seen on all abdominal imaging studies, including conventional radiography, single-contrast and double-contrast barium studies, cholangiography, multidetector CT, ultrasonography, MRI, PET, PET/CT, and angiography.

We believe we have achieved our goal of creating a concise, well-illustrated, practical text on gastrointestinal/ abdominal imaging for the busy radiologist, but, of course, we welcome your input.

Richard M. Gore, MD
Marc S. Levine, MD

Acknowledgments

We wish to gratefully acknowledge the following colleagues whose outstanding contributions to the third edition of *Textbook of Gastrointestinal Radiology* (Elsevier, 2008) formed the basis for many of the topics included in this text. Some of their figures from the third edition of *Textbook of Gastrointestinal Radiology* were also used in this work.

Contributors

Samuel Nathan Adler, MD
Stephen R. Baker, MD, MPHIL
Aparna Balachandran, MD
Dennis M. Balfe, MD
Emil J. Balthazar, MD
Stuart A. Barnard, MB, BS, MA, MRCS, FRCR
Clive Bartram, MD, FRCS, FRCP, FRCR
Genevieve L. Bennett, MD
Jonathan W. Berlin, MD, MBA
George S. Bissett III, MD
Peyman Borghei, MD
James L. Buck, MD
Carina L. Butler, MD
Marc A. Camacho, MD, MS
Dina F. Caroline, MD, PHD
Caroline W.T. Carrico, MD
Richard I. Chen, MD
Byung Ihn Choi, MD
Howard B. Chrisman, MD
Peter I. Cooperberg, MDCM, FRCPC, FACR
Abraham H. Dachman, MD
Susan Delaney, MD, FRCPC
Gerald D. Dodd III, MD
Ronald L. Eisenberg, MD
Sukru Mehmet Erturk, MD, PHD
Sandra K. Fernbach, MD
Julia R. Fielding, MD
Elliot K. Fishman, MD
Frans-Thomas Fork, MD, PHD
Martin C. Freund, MD
Ann S. Fulcher, MD
Emma E. Furth, MD
Helena Gabriel, MD
Ana Maria GACA, MD
Gabriela Gayer, MD
Gary G. Ghahremani, MD, FACR
Seth N. Glick, MD
Margaret D. Gore, MD
Richard M. Gore, MD
Nicholas C. Gourtsoyiannis, MD
David Hahn, MD

Robert A. Halvorsen, MD, FACR
Nancy A. Hammond, MD
Marjorie Hertz, MD
Frederick L. Hoff, MD
Caroline L. Hollingsworth, MD, MPH
Karen M. Horton, MD
Jill E. Jacobs, MD
Werner R. Jaschke, MD, PHD
Bruce R. Javors, MD
Bronwyn Jones, MD, FRACP, FRCR
Mannudeep K. Kalra, MD
Ana L. Keppke, MD
Stanley Taeson Kim, MD
Michael L. Kochman, MD, FACP
John C. Lapps, MD
Thomas C. Lauenstein, MD
Igor Laufer, MD
Jeong Min Lee, MD
Kang Hoon Lee, MD
Marc S. Levine, MD
Russell N. Low, MD
Michael Macari, MD
Robert L. MacCarty, MD, FACR
Dean D.T. Maglinte, MD, FACR
Charles S. Marn, MD
Gabriele Masselli, MD
Alan H. Maurer, MD
Joseph Patrick Mazzie, DO
Alec J. Megibow, MD, MPH, FACR
Uday K. Mehta, MD
James M. Messmer, MD, MED
Morton A. Meyers, MD, FACR, FACG
Frank H. Miller, MD
Koenraad J. Mortele, MD
Karen A. Mourtzikos, MD
Saravanan Namasivayam, MD, DNB, DHA
Vamsi R. Narra, MD, FRCR
Rendon C. Nelson, MD
Albert A. Nemcek, JR., MD
Geraldine Mogavero Newmark, MD
Paul Nikolaidis, MD

David J. Ott, MD
Nickolas Papanikolaou, PHD
Erik K. Paulson, MD
F. Scott Pereles, MD
Christine M. Peterson, MD
Vikram A. Rao, MD
Richard D. Redvanly, MD
Pablo R. Ros, MD, MPH
Stephen E. Rubesin, MD
Sanjay Saini, MD
Riad Salem, MD, MBA
Kumaresan Sandrasegaran, MD
Kent T. Sato, MD
Christopher D. Scheirey, MD
Francis J. Scholz, MD
Ali Shirkhoda, MD
Paul M. Silverman, MD
Stuart G. Silverman, MD
Jovitas Skucas, MD
William C. Small, MD, PHD
Claire H. Smith, MD, FACR
Robert H. Smith, MD
Sat Somers, MBCHB, FRCPC, FFRRCSI
Allison L. Summers, MD
Rajeev Suri, MD
Richard A. Szucs, MD
Mark Talamonti, MD
Andrew J. Taylor, MD
Ruedi F. Thoeni, MD
William Moreau Thompson, MD
Ranista Tongdee, MD
Mitchell E. Tublin, MD
Mary Ann Turner, MD
Sean M. Tutton, MD, FSIR
Robert L. Vogelzang, MD
Patrick M. Vos, MD
Daphna Weinstein, MD
Noel N. Williams, MD
Stephanie R. Wilson, MD
Ellen L. Wolf, MD
Vahid Yaghmai, MD, MS
Silaja Yitta, MD
Rivka Zissin, MD

Contents

General Radiologic Principles

Part 1 **ULTRASONOGRAPHY OF THE HOLLOW VISCUS**

Mural Masses of the Gut

DEFINITION: Intramural masses affecting the gastrointestinal tract are frequently solid or complex.

IMAGING

Ultrasound
Findings
- Frequently solid or complex
- With ulceration, pockets of gas often are seen within mass, and typically show bright echogenicity with a distal ring-down artifact.
- Complex masses with both cystic and solid components
- Hypoechoic and possibly suggestive sonographically of a cyst or fluid collection

Utility
- Excellent means of assessing gastrointestinal tract diseases, notably those that produce mural abnormality or abnormality of adjacent soft tissues

PATHOLOGY

- Gut wall thickening is the dominant feature.
- Complex masses occur with both cystic and solid components.
- With ulceration, pockets of gas are often seen within mass.
- Intramural masses affecting the gastrointestinal tract are frequently solid or complex.
- Pathologic considerations for gut wall masses include lymphoma, mesenchymal tumors, gut metastases, and adenocarcinoma with local tumor extension.

DIAGNOSTIC PEARLS

- Masses are often large at the time of presentation.
- Central necrosis frequently results in complex masses with both cystic and solid components.

DIFFERENTIAL DIAGNOSIS

- Bowel ischemia
- Bowel infection
- Bowel inflammation

Suggested Readings

Derchi LE, Bandereali A, Bossi MC, et al: Sonographic appearance of gastric lymphoma. *J Ultrasound Med* 3:251-256, 1984.
Fleischer AC, Muhletaler CA, James AE Jr: Sonographic assessment of the bowel wall. *AJR Am J Roentgenol* 136:887-891, 1981.
Heyder N, Kaarmann H, Giedi J: Experimental investigations into the possibility of differentiating early from invasive carcinoma of the stomach by means of ultrasound. *Endoscopy* 19:228-232, 1987.
Kaftori JK, Aharon M, Kleinhaus U: Sonographic features of gastrointestinal leiomyosarcoma. *J Clin Ultrasound* 9:11-15, 1981.
Muradali D, Burns PN, Pron G, et al: Improved retroperitoneal and gastrointestinal sonography using oral contrast agents in a porcine model. *AJR Am J Roentgenol* 171:475-481, 1998.
Puylaert JBCM: Acute appendicitis: US evaluation using graded compression. *Radiology* 158:355-360, 1986.
Wilson SR: Gastrointestinal tract sonography. In Rumack C, Wilson SR, Charboneau JW (eds): *Diagnostic Ultrasound*, 3rd ed. St. Louis, Mosby, 2005, pp 269-320.

WHAT THE REFERRING PHYSICIAN NEEDS TO KNOW
- Intramural masses affecting the gastrointestinal tract are frequently solid or complex.
- If these masses are large, their origin may not always be obvious.
- Gastrointestinal tumors should be considered if intraperitoneal or retroperitoneal masses are identified that do not arise from the abdominal solid organs.
- A mural mass should be assessed for ulceration and mass morphology.

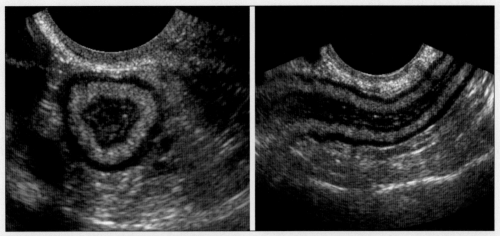

Figure 1. Normal gut signature: terminal ileum. Sonograms in a patient with mild gut thickening from Crohn disease. Muscle is black or hypoechoic on the sonogram, whereas submucosa and the superficial mucosa are hyperechoic. (*From Wilson SR: Gastrointestinal tract sonography. In Rumack C, Wilson SR, Charboneau JW [eds]: Diagnostic Ultrasound, 3rd ed. St. Louis, Mosby, 2005, pp 269-320.*)

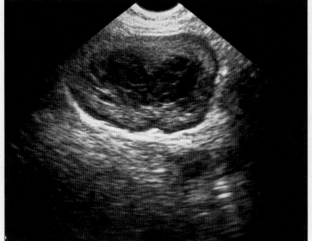

Figure 2. Gastrointestinal stromal tumor (GIST) shows as intraperitoneal mass with a highly complex nature typical of this pathologic process. (*From Wilson SR: Gastrointestinal tract sonography. In Rumack C, Wilson SR, Charboneau JW [eds]: Diagnostic Ultrasound, 3rd ed. St. Louis, Mosby, 2005, pp 269-320.*)

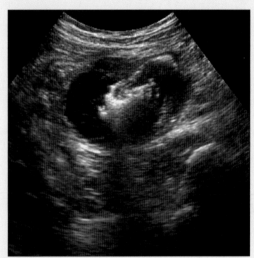

Figure 3. Lymphoma of the cecum suggests a pseudokidney morphology. The gut wall is thickened and extremely hypoechoic consistent with this diagnosis.

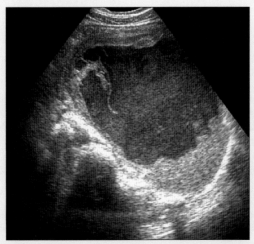

Figure 4. GIST shows as intraperitoneal mass with a highly complex nature typical of this pathologic process. (*From Wilson SR: Gastrointestinal tract sonography. In Rumack C, Wilson SR, Charboneau JW [eds]: Diagnostic Ultrasound, 3rd ed. St. Louis, Mosby, 2005, pp 269-320.*)

Mural Thickening of the Gut

DEFINITION: Gut wall thickening, with the central echogenicity representing the lumen of the gut and the hypoechoic rim representing the thickened gut wall.

ANATOMIC FINDINGS

Intestine
- Noncompressible mass trapped between transducer anteriorly and body wall musculature posteriorly

Terminal Ileum
- Loop is uniformly thickened.
- Stratification of normal gut wall layers is partially preserved.

IMAGING

Ultrasound
Findings
- Benign thickening: diffuse, symmetric, with some preservation of the gut wall layers
- *Pseudokidney* or *target sign*
- Malignant thickening: focal, asymmetric, and without preservation of gut wall stratification
- Doppler ultrasound can show vascularity of bowel wall or mass.

Utility
- Excellent means of assessing gastrointestinal tract diseases, notably those that produce mural abnormality or abnormality of adjacent soft tissues

CLINICAL PRESENTATION
- Abdominal pain
- Diarrhea
- Blood in stool
- Weight loss

DIFFERENTIAL DIAGNOSIS
- Crohn disease (gastrointestinal)
- Inflammatory bowel disease
- Gastrointestinal neoplasms

DIAGNOSTIC PEARLS
- Benign thickening: diffuse, symmetric, with some preservation of the gut wall layers
- *Pseudokidney* or *target sign*
- Malignant thickening: focal, asymmetric, and without preservation of gut wall stratification

PATHOLOGY
- Gut wall thickening is the dominant feature.
- Malignant thickening is focal, asymmetric, and is without preservation of gut wall stratification.
- Benign thickening is diffuse and symmetric, with some preservation of the gut wall layers.
- Pathologic considerations for thickened gut include inflammatory, neoplastic, and edematous diseases of the gut wall.

Suggested Readings

Bluth EL, Merritt CRB, Sullivan MA: Ultrasonic evaluation of the stomach, small bowel, and colon. *Radiology* 133:677-680, 1979.
Downey DB, Wilson SR: Pseudomembranous colitis: Sonographic features. *Radiology* 180:61-64, 1991.
Fleischer AC, Muhletaler CA, James AE Jr: Sonographic assessment of the bowel wall. *AJR Am J Roentgenol* 136:887-891, 1981.
Heyder N, Kaarmann H, Giedl J: Experimental investigations into the possibility of differentiating early from invasive carcinoma of the stomach by means of ultrasound. *Endoscopy* 19:228-232, 1987.
Khaw KT, Yeoman LJ, Saverymuttu SH, et al: Ultrasonic patterns in inflammatory bowel disease. *Clin Radiol* 43:171-175, 1991.
Lutz H, Petzoldt R: Ultrasonic patterns of space occupying lesions of the stomach and intestine. *Ultrasound Med Biol* 2:129-131, 1976.
Muradali D, Burns PN, Pron G, et al: Improved retroperitoneal and gastrointestinal sonography using oral contrast agents in a porcine model. *AJR Am J Roentgenol* 171:475-481, 1998.
Parente F, Greco S, Molteni M, et al: Imaging inflammatory bowel disease using bowel ultrasound. *Eur J Gastroenterol Hepatol* 17:283-291, 2005.
Pauls S, Gabelmann A, Schmidt SA, et al: Evaluating bowel wall vascularity in Crohn's disease: A comparison of dynamic MRI and wideband harmonic contrast-enhanced low MI ultrasound. *Eur Radiol* 16:2410-2417, 2006.

WHAT THE REFERRING PHYSICIAN NEEDS TO KNOW
- Physician should document the location, length, number of segments involved, gut wall layer preservation or destruction, symmetric or asymmetric pattern, and external gut surface appearance.
- Pathologic considerations for thickened gut include inflammatory, neoplastic, and edematous diseases of the gut wall.
- Sonographic features of gut wall thickening are not always specific.
- The clinical picture should be considered in conjunction with the sonographic abnormalities.

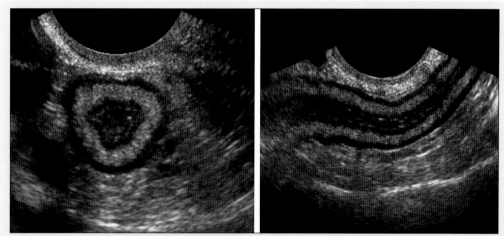

Figure 1. Normal gut signature: terminal ileum. Sonograms in a patient with mild gut thickening from Crohn disease. Muscle is black or hypoechoic on the sonogram, while submucosa and the superficial mucosa are hyperechoic. (*From Wilson SR: Gastrointestinal tract sonography. In Rumack C, Wilson SR, Charboneau JW [eds]:* Diagnostic Ultrasound, *3rd ed. St. Louis, Mosby, 2005, pp 269-320.*)

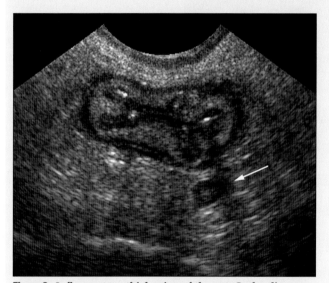

Figure 2. Inflammatory thickening of the gut: Crohn disease. Cross-section. Sonogram shows a uniformly thickened loop of terminal ileum. Stratification of the normal gut wall layers is partially preserved. An arrow marks a perienteric lymph node. (*From Wilson SR: Gastrointestinal tract sonography. In Rumack C, Wilson SR, Charboneau JW [eds]:* Diagnostic Ultrasound, *3rd ed. St. Louis, Mosby, 2005, pp 269-320.*)

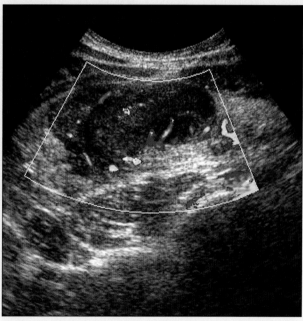

Figure 3. Malignant neoplasm of the bowel. Color Doppler image shows vascularity within the mass.

Puylaert JBCM: Acute appendicitis: US evaluation using graded compression. *Radiology* 158:355-360, 1986.

Robotti D, Cammarota T, Debani P, et al: Activity of Crohn's disease: Value of color-power-Doppler and contrast-enhanced ultrasonography. *Abdom Imaging* 29:648-652, 2004.

Wilson SR, Wilson SR: Gastrointestinal tract sonography. In Rumack C, Charboneau JW (eds): *Diagnostic Ultrasound*, 3rd ed. St. Louis, Mosby, 2005, pp 269-320.

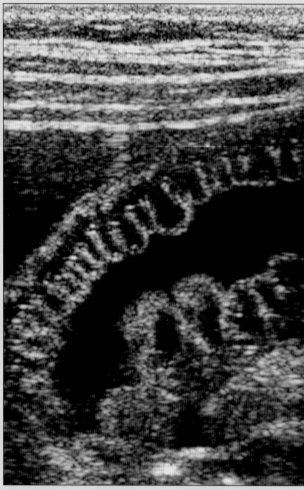

Figure 4. Edematous valvulae conniventes. This appearance is usually encountered in patients with vasculitis or venous thrombosis. (*From Wilson SR: Gastrointestinal tract sonography. In Rumack C, Wilson SR, Charboneau JW [eds]:* Diagnostic Ultrasound, *3rd ed. St. Louis, Mosby, 2005, pp 269-320.*)

Part 2

MAGNETIC RESONANCE ANGIOGRAPHY OF THE MESENTERIC VASCULATURE

Median Arcuate Ligament Syndrome

DEFINITION: Compression of celiac artery by median arcuate ligament resulting in intestinal ischemia.

ANATOMIC FINDINGS

Celiac Artery
- Externally compressed by median arcuate ligament

IMAGING

Interventional Radiology
Findings
- Extrinsic impression and narrowing of celiac artery

Utility
- Gold standard

MR Angiography
Findings
- Extrinsic impression and narrowing of celiac artery, often with poststenotic dilatation

Utility
- Procedure is a noninvasive vascular imaging technique that is being used with increasing frequency as an alternative to conventional catheter angiography.
- High-resolution images are provided within a short imaging time.
- Sensitivity of 100% and specificity of 87% in the overall detection of visceral artery stenosis have been reported.
- MR angiography should be performed at end-inspiration in patients with suspected intestinal ischemia.

CT
Findings
- Sagittal reformatted CT commonly shows extrinsic compression of the celiac artery by the median arcuate ligament, but only a small minority of these patients are symptomatic.

CLINICAL PRESENTATION

- Postprandial pain
- Abdominal bruit

DIAGNOSTIC PEARLS

- Postprandial pain
- Abdominal bruit
- External compression of celiac artery at end-inspiration on MR angiographic study

DIFFERENTIAL DIAGNOSIS

- Superior mesenteric artery syndrome
- Mesenteric ischemia
- Peptic ulcer disease
- Gastric hypomotility

PATHOLOGY

- Median arcuate ligament compresses the celiac artery resulting in intestinal ischemia.

INCIDENCE/PREVALENCE AND EPIDEMIOLOGY

- Occurs in 12.5% to 49.7% of patients

Suggested Readings

Bron KM, Redman HC: Splanchnic artery stenosis and occlusion: Incidence, arteriographic and clinical manifestations. *Radiology* 92:323-328, 1969.

Lee VS, Morgan JN, Tan AG, et al: Celiac artery compression by the median arcuate ligament: A pitfall of end-expiratory MR imaging. *Radiology* 228:437-442, 2003.

Reilly LM, Ammar AD, Stoney RJ, et al: Late results following operative repair for celiac artery compression syndrome. *J Vasc Surg* 2:79-91, 1985.

Szilagyi DE, Rian RL, Elliott JP, et al: The celiac artery compression syndrome: Does it exist? *Surgery* 72:849-863, 1972.

WHAT THE REFERRING PHYSICIAN NEEDS TO KNOW
- MR angiography should be performed at end-inspiration in patients with suspected ischemia.
- MR angiographic findings should be correlated with clinical history and physical examination.

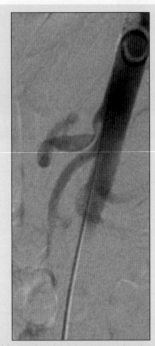

Figure 1. Sagittal maximal-intensity projection MR angiographic image of the abdominal aorta in a patient with postprandial abdominal pain and bruit on auscultation. Conventional angiography demonstrates extrinsic impression and severe narrowing of celiac axis from median arcuate ligament compression.

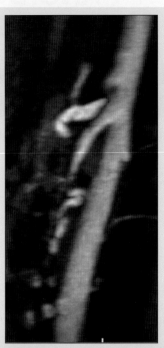

Figure 2. Sagittal maximal-intensity projection MR angiographic image of the abdominal aorta in a patient with postprandial abdominal pain and bruit on auscultation. Sagittal maximal-intensity projection MR angiography images of abdominal aorta demonstrating extrinsic impression and severe narrowing of celiac axis from median arcuate ligament compression.

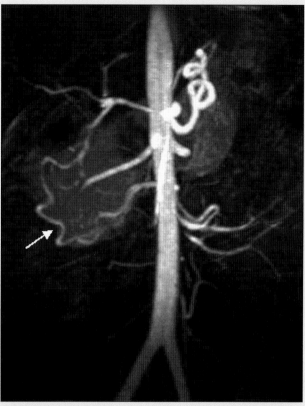

Figure 3. **Sagittal maximal-intensity projection MR angiographic image of the abdominal aorta in a patient with postprandial abdominal pain and bruit on auscultation.** Coronal maximal-intensity projection MR angiographic image of abdominal aorta demonstrating extrinsic impression and severe narrowing of celiac axis from median arcuate ligament compression. Note also the distal reconstitution of revascularization of the common hepatic artery and its distal branches from the superior mesenteric artery via enlarged gastroduodenal artery *(arrow)*.

Mesenteric Ischemia

DEFINITION: A gradual occlusive process in mesentery typically caused by atherosclerotic changes of the splanchnic arteries.

ANATOMIC FINDINGS

Splanchnic Arteries
- Atherosclerosis
- Development of extensive arterial collateral vessels

IMAGING

Interventional Radiology
Findings
- Significant stenosis in two or three of three main mesenteric vessels

Utility
- Gold standard

MR Angiography
Findings
- Stenoses in two or three of three main mesenteric vessels
- Diminished postprandial flow augmentation in the diseased patient

Utility
- This noninvasive vascular imaging technique is being used with increasing frequency as an alternative to conventional catheter angiography.
- Contrast-enhanced three-dimensional MR angiography provides anatomic information similar to conventional angiography.
- High-resolution images are provided within a short imaging time.
- Sensitivity of 100% and specificity of 87% overall for detection of visceral artery stenosis
- Accuracy is lower in evaluation of small peripheral branches.
- MR flow quantification using cine phase-contrast MRI allows functional evaluation and quantification of mesenteric vascular flow.
- Greatest difference in flow rates between normal and diseased patients achieved when measurements are made 30 minutes postprandial.

CT Angiography
Findings
- Stenosis of celiac, superior mesenteric, and/or inferior mesenteric arteries

DIAGNOSTIC PEARLS
- Demonstration of significant stenosis in two or three of the three main mesenteric vessels
- Diminished postprandial flow augmentation in MR flow quantification using phase-contrast MRI
- Development of extensive collateral vessels

Utility
- Useful in showing stenosis and secondary signs of ischemia in the bowel

CLINICAL PRESENTATION
- Postprandial abdominal pain
- Weight loss
- Food avoidance
- Gastrointestinal hemorrhage
- Can be asymptomatic

PATHOLOGY
- Gradual occlusive process occurs in splanchnic arteries.
- Bowels are still viable, but blood supply is inadequate to support metabolic and functional demands.
- Extensive arterial collateral vessels develop over time.

Suggested Readings

Burkart DJ, Johnson CD, Reading CC, et al: MR measurements of mesenteric venous flow: Prospective evaluation in healthy volunteers and patients with suspected chronic mesenteric ischemia. *Radiology* 194:801-806, 1995.

Li KC, Whitney WS, McDonnell CH, et al: Chronic mesenteric ischemia: Evaluation with phase-contrast cine-MR imaging. *Radiology* 190:175-179, 1994.

Meaney JF, Prince MR, Nostrant TT, et al: Gadolinium-enhanced MR angiography of visceral arteries in patients with suspected chronic mesenteric ischemia. *J Magn Reson Imaging* 7:171-176, 1997.

Moawad J, Gewertz BL: Chronic mesenteric ischemia: Clinical presentation and diagnosis. *Surg Clin North Am* 77:357-369, 1997.

WHAT THE REFERRING PHYSICIAN NEEDS TO KNOW
- Because of the collateral vessels, significant stenosis of major mesenteric vessels can be seen in asymptomatic patients.

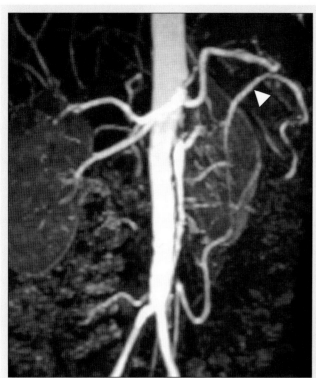

Figure 1. Chronic abdominal pain with atherosclerotic changes and arterial occlusion. Coronal maximal-intensity projection image of abdominal aorta in a 65-year-old man with chronic abdominal pain demonstrates atherosclerotic changes of abdominal aorta and segmental occlusion at the origin of superior mesenteric artery. Note that the distal part of superior mesenteric artery is revascularized by collaterals arising from the left marginal artery *(arrowhead)*.

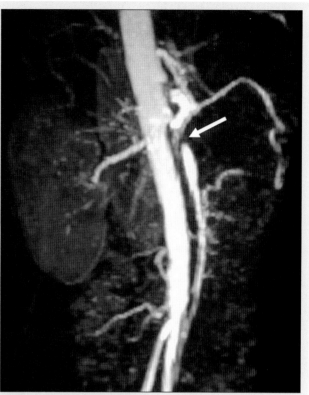

Figure 2. Chronic abdominal pain with atherosclerotic changes and arterial occlusion. Sagittal maximal-intensity projection image of abdominal aorta in a 65-year-old man with chronic abdominal pain demonstrates atherosclerotic changes of the abdominal aorta and segmental occlusion at the origin of the superior mesenteric artery *(arrow)*.

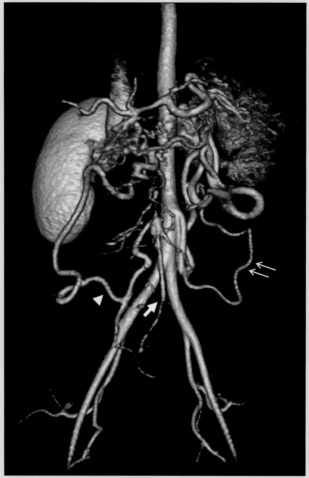

Figure 3. **Three-dimensional, shaded-surface display image in a 35-year-old woman with Takayasu arteritis showing segmental occlusion of the superior mesenteric artery.** The distal superior mesenteric artery *(arrow)* is reconstituted via collaterals from the right marginal artery *(arrowhead)*, left marginal artery *(double arrows)*, and gastroduodenal artery.

Vascular Invasion by Tumor

DEFINITION: Involvement of vasculature by tumor.

IMAGING

Interventional Radiology
Findings
- Tumor invasion

Utility
- Gold standard

MR Angiography
Findings
- Tumor invasion of vessel
- Contrast enhancement in tumor thrombus

Utility
- Contrast-enhanced three-dimensional MR angiography is a valuable tool for evaluating vascular involvement by hepatocellular carcinoma, pancreatobiliary cancers, and hepatic metastases.
- High-resolution images are provided within a short imaging time.
- Contrast-enhanced MR portography is excellent for evaluating tumor invasion of portal vein.
- Used to differentiate bland thrombus from tumor thrombus

CT Angiography
Findings
- Tumor invasion of vessel

Utility
- Better shows bowel consequences of vascular invasion than MR angiography

DIFFERENTIAL DIAGNOSIS

- Bland thrombus
- Arteritis

DIAGNOSTIC PEARLS

- Contrast enhancement in tumor thrombus is shown.
- Contrast-enhanced three-dimensional MR angiography is a valuable tool for evaluating vascular involvement by tumor.
- Contrast-enhanced MR portography is excellent for evaluating tumor invasion of portal vein.

PATHOLOGY

- Invasion of vasculature by a tumor from hepatocellular carcinoma, pancreatobiliary cancers, and hepatic metastases

Suggested Readings

Maki JH, Chenevert TL, Prince MR: Contrast-enhanced MR angiography. *Abdom Imaging* 23:469-484, 1998.

Meaney JF: Non-invasive evaluation of the visceral arteries with magnetic resonance angiography. *Eur Radiol* 9:1267-1276, 1999.

Shirkhoda A, Konez O, Shetty AN, et al: Mesenteric circulation: Three-dimensional MR angiography with a gadolinium-enhanced multiecho gradient-echo technique. *Radiology* 202:257-261, 1997.

WHAT THE REFERRING PHYSICIAN NEEDS TO KNOW

- Contrast-enhanced three-dimensional MR angiography is a valuable tool for evaluating vascular involvement by tumor.
- Contrast enhancement in tumor thrombus is shown.
- Contrast-enhanced MR portography is excellent for evaluating tumor invasion of portal vein.

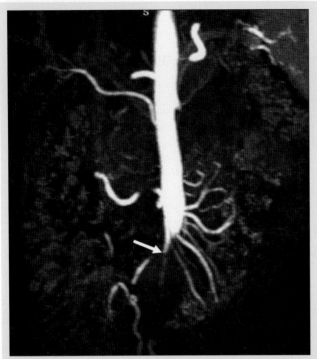

Figure 1. Subvolumetric maximal-intensity projection reconstruction demonstrates severe narrowing of the distal superior mesenteric artery *(arrow)*.

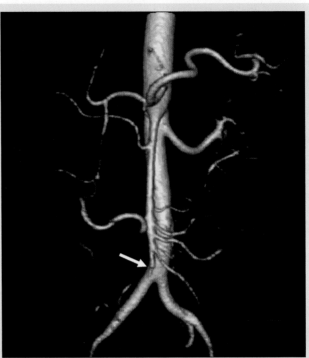

Figure 2. Three-dimensional shaded-surface display (SSD) of subtracted MR angiography data demonstrates severe narrowing of the distal superior mesenteric artery *(arrow)*; however, the image does not demonstrate streak of contrast through encasing tumor because it is eliminated or segmented during postprocessing.

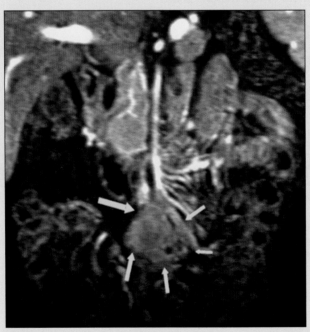

Figure 3. Source nonsubtraction delayed MR angiographic image demonstrates tumor encasing the distal superior mesenteric artery and venous branches *(arrows)*.

Visceral Artery Aneurysm

DEFINITION: Aneurysm of visceral arteries.

IMAGING

Interventional Radiography
Findings
- Aneurysm

Utility
- Gold standard
- Invasive

MR Angiography
Findings
- Aneurysm

Utility
- Procedure is noninvasive.
- High-resolution images within a short imaging time are provided.
- If test bolus technique shows aneurysm, estimated contrast arrival time should be timed to include the distal part of aneurysm.
- Potential pitfall is the presence of thrombosis in aneurysm, which can be prevented by looking at the source images.

CT Angiography
Findings
- Aneurysm

Utility
- This technique nicely depicts the aneurysm and its relationship to the gut.

CLINICAL PRESENTATION

- Hemorrhage
- Hypotension
- Abdominal pain

DIAGNOSTIC PEARLS

- Arteries involved include the splenic artery, hepatic artery, superior mesenteric, celiac, gastric and gastroepiploic, ileocolic, and pancreatoduodenal arteries.
- Aneurysms are seen on interventional radiography and MR angiography.

PATHOLOGY

- Dilatation of vessels can lead to rupture, resulting in life-threatening hemorrhage.
- Hepatic artery pseudoaneurysms occur owing to percutaneous and therapeutic biliary procedures.

INCIDENCE/PREVALENCE AND EPIDEMIOLOGY

- Incidence is uncommon.
- Splenic artery is most commonly affected.
- Incidence of hepatic artery pseudoaneurysm is increasing.
- Other commonly affected vessels, in decreasing order, include superior mesenteric, celiac, gastric and gastroepiploic, ileocolic, and pancreatoduodenal arteries.

Suggested Readings

Carr SC, Pearce WH, Vogelzang RL: Current management of visceral artery aneurysms. *Surgery* 120:627-634, 1996.
Grego FG, Lepidi S, Ragazzi R, et al: Visceral artery aneurysms: A single center experience. *Cardiovasc Surg* 11:19-25, 2003.
Zelenock GB, Stanley JC: Splanchnic artery aneurysms. In Rutherford RB (ed): *Vascular Surgery,* 5th ed. Philadelphia, WB Saunders, 2000, pp 1369-1382.

WHAT THE REFERRING PHYSICIAN NEEDS TO KNOW

- Reviewing MR angiography or multiplanar reformat (MPR) imaging prevents thrombosed aneurysm from being overlooked.

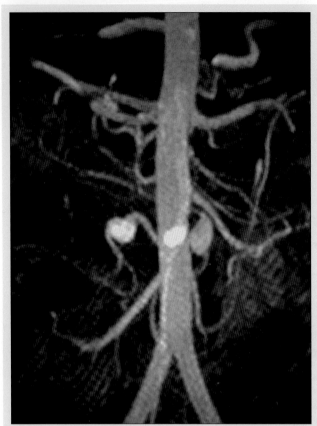

Figure 1. Superior mesenteric artery aneurysms. Coronal maximal-intensity projection image of contrast-enhanced abdominal MR angiography in an 18-year-old man with duodenal hemorrhage reveals multiple aneurysms involving branches of superior mesenteric artery.

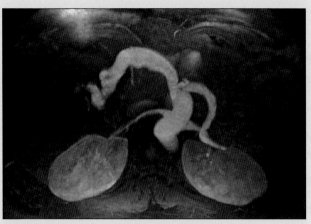

Figure 2. Celiac artery and hepatic artery aneurysms. Axial maximal-intensity projection MR angiographic image demonstrates fusiform dilatation of celiac trunk and hepatic artery.

Abdominal Radiographs

Part 3

GAS AND SOFT TISSUE ABNORMALITIES

Abdominal Radiographs: Pneumoperitoneum, Pneumatosis, Pneumobilia, and Portal Venous Gas

DEFINITION: Abnormal intra-abdominal gas patterns include pneumoperitoneum (free intraperitoneal air), pneumatosis (intestinal wall gas), pneumobilia (bile duct gas), and portal venous gas.

ANATOMIC FINDINGS

Peritoneal Cavity
- Free intraperitoneal gas

Gastrointestinal Tract
- Intramural wall gas collection

Pancreaticobiliary System
- Bile duct gas
- Biliary-enteric fistula

Portal Vein
- Gas in portal veins

IMAGING

Radiography
Findings
- Pneumoperitoneum on supine abdominal radiographs: Rigler's sign with gas on both sides of bowel wall, lucency in right upper quadrant, visualized diaphragmatic undersurface
- Other signs of pneumoperitoneum: lucency above lesser curvature of stomach, *football sign,* and gas outlining intraperitoneal ligaments, including the falciform ligament

DIAGNOSTIC PEARLS

- Pneumoperitoneum: Rigler's sign, lucency in right upper quadrant, visualized diaphragmatic undersurface
- Pneumatosis: clustered, bubbly extraluminal or thin, linear intramural gas collections
- Pneumobilia: thin, branched, tubular areas of lucency in the central portion of liver
- Portal venous gas: thin, branching, tubular areas of lucency in the liver periphery, extending almost to the liver surface

- Pneumatosis: clustered, bubbly extraluminal or thin, linear intramural gas collections
- Pneumobilia: thin, branched, tubular areas of lucency in central portion of liver
- Portal venous gas: thin, branching, tubular areas of lucency in liver periphery, extending almost to liver surface

Utility
- Using proper technique, upright chest radiograph can detect as little as 1 mL of air beneath diaphragms.
- Upright chest radiographs and CT are equally sensitive in detecting small amounts of free intraperitoneal air.
- Whenever horizontal beam views cannot be obtained, supine abdominal radiographs can be used.

WHAT THE REFERRING PHYSICIAN NEEDS TO KNOW

- Upright chest radiograph and CT are equally sensitive tools for detecting small amounts of free intraperitoneal air.
- Pneumoperitoneum is an important diagnosis in acutely ill patients, given that it usually indicates perforated viscus.
- In the setting of ischemic bowel disease, the combination of pneumatosis and portomesenteric venous gas almost always indicates bowel infarction.
- Most common cause of pneumobilia is surgically created biliary-enteric fistula.
- Finding of portal venous gas should lead to careful search for gas in wall of bowel as a result of intestinal infarction.
- Most important differential diagnosis in pneumobilia is presence of portal venous gas.
- Differentiate between benign and serious causes of extraluminal gas collections in abdomen by looking for signs of underlying disease.

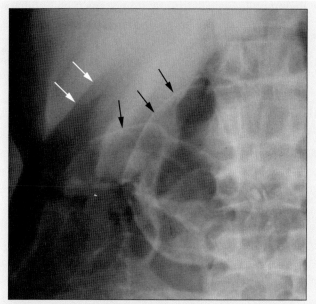

Figure 1. Pneumoperitoneum with Rigler's sign. A close-up view of the right upper quadrant in a patient with massive pneumoperitoneum shows a sharp liver edge *(white arrows)* with air outlining both sides of the bowel wall *(black arrows)*.

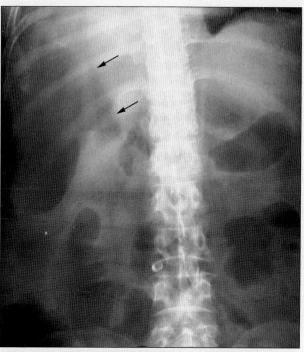

Figure 2. Other signs of pneumoperitoneum on supine abdominal radiographs. Increased radiolucency is seen in the right upper quadrant *(arrows)*. This finding is due to air interposed between the anterior abdominal wall and the liver.

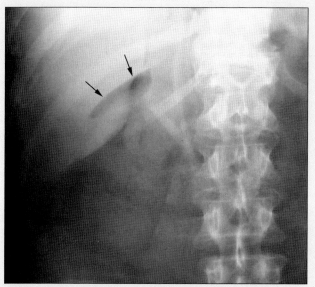

Figure 3. Other signs of pneumoperitoneum on supine abdominal radiographs. Air collecting in Morison pouch outlines the inferior border of the liver *(arrows)*.

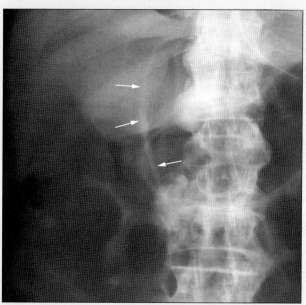

Figure 4. Other signs of pneumoperitoneum on supine abdominal radiographs. Air outlines the falciform ligament *(arrows)*.

CT

Findings

- Pneumoperitoneum: visualization of extraluminal gas in peritoneal cavity
- Pneumatosis: bubbly, extraluminal or thin, linear streaks of intramural gas collections
- Pneumobilia: thin, branched, tubular areas of lucency in central portion of liver
- Portal venous gas: thin, branching, tubular areas of lucency in liver periphery, extending almost to liver surface

Utility

- Upright chest radiographs and CT are equally sensitive in detecting small amounts of free intraperitoneal air.
- CT is useful for detection of pneumatosis due to bowel ischemia or infarction.

Ultrasound-Doppler

Findings

- Gas in portal vein

Utility

- Used to detect portal vein gas in immediate postoperative period after liver transplantation

CLINICAL PRESENTATION

- The presence of pneumoperitoneum usually indicates an acute abdominal emergency in patients with peritoneal signs and symptoms.
- The presence of portal venous gas indicates a poor prognosis in patients with bowel ischemia or infection.

DIFFERENTIAL DIAGNOSIS

- Emphysematous gastritis
- Periportal fat

PATHOLOGY

- Presence of free intraperitoneal air usually indicates perforated viscus in patient with acute peritoneal signs and symptoms, but causes are varied, including pelvic examination and sexual intercourse.

- Pneumobilia usually results from some type of biliary-enteric communication or fistula.
- Intraluminal intestinal air can breach damaged mucosa and reach portal venous system via hematogenous route.

INCIDENCE/PREVALENCE AND EPIDEMIOLOGY

- Most common cause of pneumobilia is surgically created biliary-enteric fistula.

Suggested Readings

Balthazar EJ, Gurkin S: Cholecystoenteric fistulas: Significance and radiographic diagnosis. *Am J Gastroenterol* 65:168-173, 1976.

Kernagis LY, Levine MS, Jacobs JE: Pneumatosis intestinalis in patients with ischemia: Correlation of CT finding with viability of the bowel. *AJR Am J Roentgenol* 180:733-736, 2003.

Levine MS, Scheiner JD, Rubesin SE, et al: Diagnosis of pneumoperitoneum on supine abdominal radiographs. *AJR Am J Roentgenol* 156:731-735, 1991.

Miller RE, Becker GJ, Slabaugh RA: Detection of pneumoperitoneum: Optimum body position and respiratory phase. *AJR Am J Roentgenol* 135:487-490, 1980.

Miller RE, Nelson SW: The roentgenological demonstration of tiny amounts of free intraperitoneal gas: Experimental and clinical studies. *Am J Roentgenol Radium Ther Nucl Med* 112:574-585, 1971.

Mindelzun R, McCort JJ: Hepatic and perihepatic radiolucencies. *Radiol Clin North Am* 18:221-238, 1980.

Pear BL: Pneumatosis intestinalis: A review. *Radiology* 207:13-19, 1998.

Sisk PB: Gas in the portal venous system. *Radiology* 77:103-107, 1981.

Stapakis JC, Thickman D: Diagnosis of pneumoperitoneum: Abdominal CT vs. upright chest film. *J Comput Assist Tomogr* 16:713-716, 1992.

Wiesner W, Koenraad J, Mortele JN, et al: Pneumatosis intestinalis and portomesenteric venous gas in intestinal ischemia. *AJR Am J Roentgenol* 177:1319-1323, 2003.

Woodring JH, Heiser MJ: Detection of pneumoperitoneum on chest radiographs: Comparison of upright lateral and posteroanterior projections. *AJR Am J Roentgenol* 165:45-47, 1995.

Abdominal Radiographs: Soft Tissue Abnormalities and Ascites

DEFINITION: Soft tissue abnormalities on abdominal radiographs include changes in organ size and contour as well as inflammation and the presence of intraperitoneal fluid.

ANATOMIC FINDINGS

Liver
- Decrease or increase in size with displacement of adjacent structures

Spleen
- Increase in size with displacement of adjacent structures

Kidneys
- Increase in size
- Contour distortion

Peritoneal Cavity
- Intraperitoneal fluid accumulation

IMAGING
Radiography
Findings
- Hepatomegaly: displacement of hepatic flexure and transverse colon inferiorly, leftward displacement of stomach
- Small liver: right kidney higher than left, stomach displaced upward and to right, and duodenal bulb displaced upward
- Splenomegaly: extension of splenic tip inferiorly below twelfth rib, displacement of stomach medially
- Obliteration of psoas muscle and preperitoneal fat planes outlining internal oblique, external oblique, and transversalis muscles seen in appendicitis
- Ascites: obliteration of inferior liver edge, widening of distance between flank stripe and ascending colon, fluid accumulation in pelvis
- Helmer's sign of ascites: medial displacement of lateral liver edge
- Other signs of ascites: bowel loop separation, ground-glass appearance, centrally located bowel loops with bulging flanks

Utility
- Radiography is one of the first diagnostic tools used.
- Only large amounts of ascites can be identified on abdominal radiographs.

DIAGNOSTIC PEARLS

- Hepatomegaly: displacement of hepatic flexure and transverse colon inferiorly, leftward displacement of stomach
- Splenomegaly: extension of splenic tip inferiorly below twelfth rib and displacement of stomach medially
- Obliteration of fat planes (seen in inflammation)
- Ascites: obliteration of inferior liver edge, widening of distance between flank stripe and ascending colon, and fluid accumulation in pelvis

- Obliteration of fat planes is an important but nonspecific sign of inflammation.

CT
Findings
- Peri-organ fluid accumulation

Utility
- CT has reduced emphasis on diagnostic utility of abdominal radiographs in ascites.

Ultrasound
Findings
- Peri-organ fluid accumulation

Utility
- Ultrasound has reduced emphasis on diagnostic utility of abdominal radiographs in ascites.

CLINICAL PRESENTATION

- Abdominal distention
- Bloating
- Palpable abdominal mass

PATHOLOGY

- Ascites may be caused by cirrhosis or malignancy.
- Surrounding inflammation may cause fat to become edematous so it approximates soft-tissue density, thus obliterating contiguous planes.

WHAT THE REFERRING PHYSICIAN NEEDS TO KNOW

- Inferior tip of spleen can be seen on abdominal radiographs in 44% of patients without splenomegaly.
- Renal enlargement does not displace intra-abdominal organs owing to its retroperitoneal location.
- Only large amounts of ascites can be detected on abdominal radiographs.

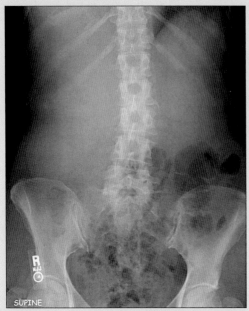

Figure 1. Hepatomegaly. Marked hepatic enlargement causes increased soft-tissue density over the upper abdomen and displacement of bowel inferiorly.

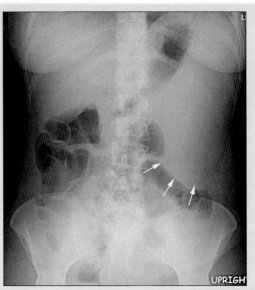

Figure 2. Splenomegaly. Abdominal radiograph demonstrates marked splenic enlargement *(arrows)* with displacement of bowel inferiorly.

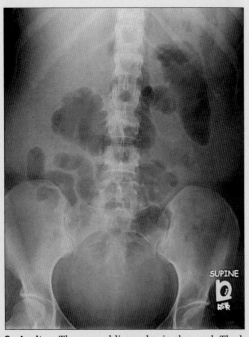

Figure 3. Ascites. The normal liver edge is obscured. The bowel loops are centrally located in the abdomen, and separation of bowel loops is seen.

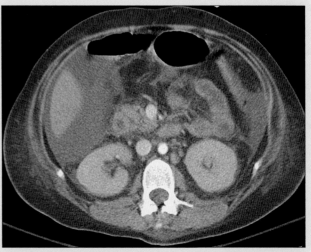

Figure 4. Ascites. CT in the same patient as in Figure 3 confirms the presence of perihepatic ascites.

Suggested Readings

Brogdon BG, Cros NE: Observations on the "normal" spleen. *Radiology* 72:412-414, 1959.

Gelfand DW: The liver: Plain film diagnosis. *Semin Roentgenol* 10:177-185, 1975.

Moell H: Size of the normal kidneys. *Acta Radiol* 46:640, 1956.

Pfahler GE: Measurement of the liver by means of roentgen rays based upon a study of 502 subjects. *AJR Am J Roentgenol* 16: 558-564, 1926.

Part 4 ABDOMINAL CALCIFICATIONS

Abdominal Radiographs: Abdominal Calcifications

DEFINITION: Abdominal calcifications may occur in the walls of blood vessels or other conduits, the lumina of hollow structures, and the solid substance of viscera or neoplasms.

ANATOMIC FINDINGS

Pancreaticobiliary System
- Biliary calculi are usually oval or rounded, whereas gallstones are often faceted, with smooth margins.
- Pancreatic stones often have jagged edges.
- Gallstones are often multiple and are frequently laminated.
- Gallbladder wall calcification has a marginal arcuate configuration.
- Multiple calcifications crossing mid-line of upper abdomen are characteristic of pancreatic lithiasis.

Gastrointestinal Tract
- Appendicoliths appear as a single or tight grouping of laminated calcifications in the right lower quadrant.

Urinary Tract
- Ureteral concretions often have jagged edges, but urinary bladder concretions usually have smooth margins.
- Stones in renal pelvis and ureters have a range of specific appearances and are oriented along course of urinary tract.

Female Genital System
- Ossification may occur in ovarian teratomas or cysts.
- Uterine leiomyomas are the most common calcified solid masses in the female pelvis.

Abdominal Wall
- Abdominal scars may calcify, particularly after gastric surgery or suprapubic bladder catheterization.

Blood Vessels
- Marginal branching pattern observed at bifurcation of abdominal aorta or in intrarenal arteries
- Calcification of uterine artery characterized by horizontal or slightly undulating linear opacity or by series of curvilinear, string-like densities
- Cystic calcification most commonly occurs in abdominal aortic aneurysms.
- Transverse orientation and conduit morphologic features indicate calcification of renal artery.

Abdominopelvic Lymph Nodes
- Calcified mesenteric lymph nodes lie along oblique path extending from the left mid-abdomen to the right lower quadrant.

IMAGING

Radiography
Findings
- Concretions: faint to bright opacities of various shapes depending on location; uninterrupted edge without lucent gaps; lamination, central lucency
- Conduit wall calcifications: ring-like or parallel linear opacities depending on vessel orientation; often with lucent gaps
- Calcification of narrow-caliber vessels produces string-like appearance.
- Cystic calcifications: smooth, arcuate, typically incomplete rim of radiopacity in wall of cyst; larger diameter than conduits
- Solid calcification: nongeometric inner architecture and irregular, often with incomplete margin
- Solid masses: mottled densities with scattered radiolucencies on calcified background (typical of calcified mesenteric lymph nodes)
- Leiomyomas: whorled configuration with incomplete bands and arcs of calcification or numerous flocculent densities superimposed on a radiolucent background

Utility
- Lateral margin of transverse process of lumbar vertebra can mimic calcification in renal artery.
- Systematic evaluation of morphologic features, location, and mobility of abnormal opacity usually narrows diagnostic considerations.

WHAT THE REFERRING PHYSICIAN NEEDS TO KNOW
- In many cases, pattern of calcium deposition is the most informative and distinctive radiographic finding.
- Systematic evaluation of morphologic features, location, and mobility of abnormal opacity usually narrows diagnostic considerations to just several likely possibilities.
- In many instances, appearance of radiographic abdominal calcification provides sufficient information for unequivocal diagnosis without need for additional examinations.

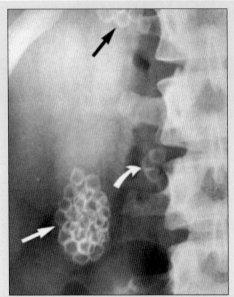

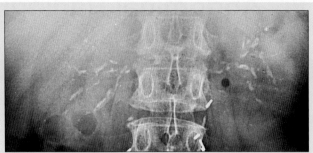

Figure 2. Calcification of the renal arteries and their intrarenal branches. These opacities have the typical configuration of conduit wall calcification.

Figure 1. **Biliary stones.** Numerous stones are seen in the gallbladder *(straight white arrow)*, cystic duct *(black arrow)*, and common bile duct *(curved white arrow)*. Note how the stones have faceted margins.

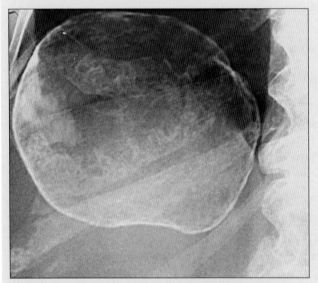

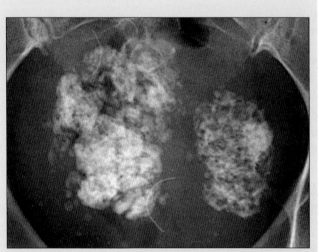

Figure 4. Two calcified uterine fibroids are manifested by areas of flocculent calcification in the pelvis.

Figure 3. Large *Echinococcus* cyst in the liver. Note how the calcified wall of the cyst is flattened inferiorly.

CLINICAL PRESENTATION

- Abdominal pain
- Biliary or renal colic
- Signs or symptoms of appendicitis
- Abdominal or pelvic mass

PATHOLOGY

- Metastatic calcification: hypercalcemia and elevated pH cause extracellular precipitation of calcium salts.
- Dystrophic calcification caused by trauma, ischemia, infarction, or other pathologic processes resulting in calcium deposition
- Concretions: precipitates from solution inside vessel or hollow viscus, often containing central nidus of insoluble substance, inflammatory collection, or thrombus
- Mucin-producing adenocarcinomas of gastrointestinal tract possess glycoprotein similar in chemical configuration to cartilage, which shares affinity for calcium aggregation.

INCIDENCE/PREVALENCE AND EPIDEMIOLOGY

- Stomach and kidneys are most frequent sites of metastatic calcification.
- Common cause of radiographically detectable metastatic calcification is chronic renal failure with secondary hyperparathyroidism.

- Calcified mesenteric lymph nodes are usually found in middle-aged or elderly individuals previously infected by tuberculosis.
- Uterine leiomyomas are most common calcified solid masses in female pelvis.

Suggested Readings

Hilbish TF, Bartter FC: Roentgen findings in abnormal deposition of calcium in tissues. *Am J Roentgenol Radium Ther Nucl Med* 87:1128-1139, 1962.

Kutarna A: A contribution to the problem of calcifications in malignant tumors: A case of late calcified retroperitoneal metastasis of an ovarian carcinoma. *Neoplasma* 11:633-642, 1964.

Steinbach HL: Identification of pelvic masses by phlebolith displacement. *Am J Roentgenol Radium Ther Nucl Med* 83:1063-1066, 1960.

Widmann BF, Ostrum AW, Fried H: Practical aspects of calcification and ossification in the various body tissues. *Radiology* 30:598-609, 1938.

Pharynx

Part 5

STRUCTURAL ABNORMALITIES OF THE PHARYNX

Pouches and Diverticula

DEFINITION: Pharyngeal outpouchings (congenital or acquired).

IMAGING

Radiography
Findings
- Lateral pharyngeal pouch: transient, hemispheric, contrast-filled lateral hypopharyngeal wall protrusions below hyoid bone and above calcified thyroid cartilage edge
- Lateral pharyngeal diverticula: persistent, variable-size, barium-filled sacs connected by narrow neck to bulging lateral hypopharyngeal wall
- Laryngocele: air-filled sac above and lateral to ala of thyroid cartilage and anterior to epiglottic plate (These structures do not fill with barium on pharyngography.)
- Branchial cleft vestiges arise from tonsillar or piriform fossae or from lower piriform sinus to neck fascia (sinus) or skin (fistulas).
- Zenker diverticulum: posterior bulging of distal pharyngeal wall above anteriorly protruding pharyngoesophageal segment
- Killian-Jamieson diverticula: small, round to ovoid, smooth-surfaced outpouchings below level of cricopharyngeal muscle and anterior to esophagus

Utility
- Barium pharyngography
- Plain-film neck radiographs for laryngoceles

CT
Findings
- Laryngocele: mass filled with air or fluid, or both, in paralaryngeal space (External laryngocele extends through thyrohyoid membrane.)
- Branchial cleft cyst: noninfected cysts are smooth, thin-walled masses with homogeneous water core; infected cysts have a thickened wall.

DIAGNOSTIC PEARLS
- Lateral pharyngeal pouch: transient, hemispheric, contrast-filled lateral hypopharyngeal wall protrusions below the hyoid bone and above the calcified thyroid cartilage edge
- Lateral pharyngeal diverticula: persistent, variable-size, barium-filled sacs connected by narrow neck to bulging lateral hypopharyngeal wall
- Laryngocele: air-filled sac above and lateral to the ala of thyroid cartilage and anterior to epiglottic plate that does not fill with barium on pharyngograms
- Branchial cleft vestiges arise from tonsillar or piriform fossae or from lower piriform sinus to neck fascia (sinus) or skin (fistulas).
- Zenker diverticulum: posterior bulging of distal pharyngeal wall above anteriorly protruding pharyngoesophageal segment
- Killian-Jamieson diverticula: small, round to ovoid, smooth-surfaced outpouchings below the level of cricopharyngeal muscle and anterior to esophagus

CLINICAL PRESENTATION
- Lateral pharyngeal pouches and diverticula usually cause no symptoms.
- When present, symptoms include dysphagia, choking, regurgitation of undigested food, and overflow aspiration.
- Patients with Zenker diverticulum usually exhibit dysphagia, regurgitation of undigested food, halitosis, choking, hoarseness, or neck mass.
- Patients with external or mixed laryngoceles may have compressible lateral neck masses.

WHAT THE REFERRING PHYSICIAN NEEDS TO KNOW
- Pharyngeal pouches and diverticula carry a risk of overflow aspiration, which can be documented on barium swallow.
- Complications of Zenker diverticulum include bronchitis, bronchiectasis, lung abscess, diverticulitis, ulceration, fistula formation, and carcinoma.
- Any change in character of dysphagia or bloody discharge in patient known to have Zenker diverticulum should suggest a complication.
- Irregularity of contour of Zenker diverticulum on barium studies should suggest an inflammatory or neoplastic complication.

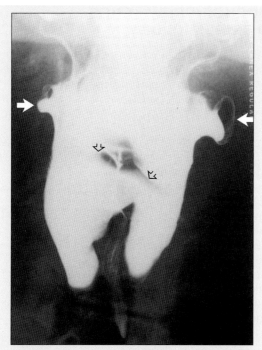

Figure 1. Lateral pharyngeal pouches. Frontal view of the pharynx during swallowing shows right and left lateral pharyngeal pouches *(white arrows)* protruding through the region of the thyrohyoid membrane. The epiglottis has slightly asymmetric tilt *(open arrows)*. (*From Rubesin SE: Pharyngeal morphology. In Ekberg O [ed]: Radiology of the Pharynx and Oesophagus. Berlin, Springer, 2004, pp 51-77.*)

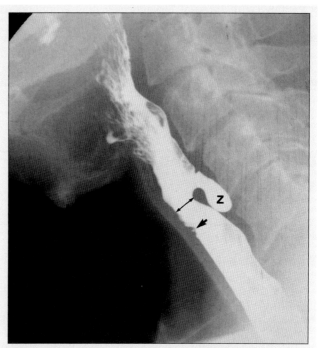

Figure 2. Zenker diverticulum during swallowing. The relationship between the mouth of the Zenker diverticulum (Z) and a prominent cricopharyngeus is demonstrated. Most of the bolus has passed through the pharynx. The pharynx and larynx have continued to rise (approximately 3 mm), and the anterior wall of the trachea has been pulled forward slightly. The pharyngoesophageal segment is open *(double arrow)*. Redundant mucosa is seen in the postcricoid region *(arrow)*. Opening of the pharyngoesophageal segment depends on elevation and anterior movement of the larynx as well as the pressure of the bolus as a result of gravity, tongue base thrust, and constrictor muscle contraction.

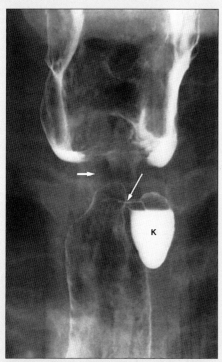

Figure 3. Killian-Jamieson diverticulum. Frontal view of the pharynx shows a barium-filled sac (K) to the left of the cervical esophagus. The neck of the diverticulum *(long arrow)* is below the level of the cricopharyngeal muscle *(short arrow)*. (*From Rubesin SE: Pharynx. In Laufer I, Levine MS [eds]: Double Contrast Gastrointestinal Radiology, 2nd ed. Philadelphia, WB Saunders, 1992.*)

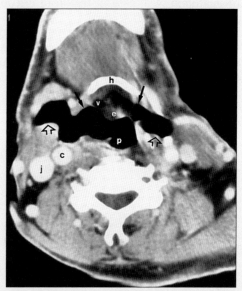

Figure 4. Right and left mixed laryngoceles. Axial CT scan at the level of the hyoid bone (h) shows air-filled sacs that extend through the thyrohyoid membrane and are anterior to the carotid artery (c) and jugular vein (j). The internal component *(solid arrows)* of the mixed laryngocele is in the paralaryngeal space. The external component *(open arrows)* of the laryngoceles is indicated. (*e, Epiglottis; p, pharynx; v, vallecula.*)

- Patients with internal laryngoceles may complain of hoarseness, dysphagia, or choking.
- Most patients with Killian-Jamieson diverticula are asymptomatic, but some may complain of dysphagia or regurgitation.
- Branchial cysts are painless or fluctuant masses in upper neck along upper third of anterior border of sternocleidomastoid.

DIFFERENTIAL DIAGNOSIS

- Benign tumors (pharynx)

PATHOLOGY

- Increased intrapharyngeal pressure is a common mechanism for acquired pharyngeal pouches and diverticula causing wall protrusion beyond normal pharyngeal contour in areas unsupported by muscle layers.
- Laryngocele is a saccular dilatation of the appendix of the laryngeal ventricle composed of ciliated pseudostratified columnar epithelium and loose areolar connective tissue.
- Pharyngeal diverticulum is a protrusion of nonkeratinizing squamous mucosa originating in the pharynx.
- Persistence of branchial pouches or clefts results in formation of sinus tracts or cysts.
- Unilocular cyst is lined by keratinizing stratified squamous epithelium and filled with desquamated keratinaceous debris with surrounding lymphoid tissue.
- Zenker diverticulum (posterior hypopharyngeal diverticulum) is an acquired mucosal herniation through area of anatomic weakness in region of cricopharyngeal muscle (Killian dehiscence).
- Killian-Jamieson diverticulum (lateral cervical esophageal diverticulum) is a transient or persistent protrusion of anterolateral cervical esophagus into Killian-Jamieson space.

INCIDENCE/PREVALENCE AND EPIDEMIOLOGY

- Laryngeal diverticula and laryngoceles are common in wind instrument players, glass blowers, and persons with severe sneezing episodes.
- Lateral pharyngeal pouches are extremely common and are usually bilateral; they frequency increase with age.
- Laryngoceles are common between 50 and 70 years of age; 20% of cases are bilateral, and 15% are associated with laryngeal neoplasms.
- Branchial clefts or pouches usually occur between 10 and 40 years of age.
- Zenker diverticulum is usually found in elderly patients.
- Fifteen percent of patients with laryngoceles have associated laryngeal neoplasms.
- Carcinoma arises in less than 1% of all patients with Zenker diverticulum but is usually fatal.

Suggested Readings
Bachman AL, Seaman WB, Macken KL: Lateral pharyngeal diverticula. *Radiology* 91:774-782, 1968.
Glazer HS, Mauro MA, Aronberg DJ, et al: Computed tomography of laryngoceles. *AJR Am J Roentgenol* 40:549-552, 1983.
Knuff TE, Benjamin SB, Castell DO: Pharyngoesophageal (Zenker's) diverticulum: A reappraisal. *Gastroenterology* 82:734-736, 1982.
Lindell MM, Jing BS, Fischer EP, et al: Laryngocele. *AJR Am J Roentgenol* 131:259-262, 1978.
Maran AG, Buchanan DR: Branchial cysts, sinuses and fistulae. *Clin Otolaryngol Allied Sci* 77-92, 1978.
Norris CW: Pharyngoceles of the hypopharynx. *Laryngoscope* 89:1788-1807, 1979.
Perrott JW: Anatomical aspects of hypopharyngeal diverticula. *Aust N Z J Surg* 31:307-317, 1962.
Rubesin SE, Levine MS: Killian-Jamieson diverticula: Radiographic findings in 16 patients. *AJR Am J Roentgenol* 177:85-89, 2001.

Pharyngeal and Cervical Esophageal Webs

DEFINITION: Webs are thin mucosal folds most frequently located along anterior wall of lower hypopharynx and proximal cervical esophagus and are usually composed of normal epithelium and lamina propria.

ANATOMIC FINDINGS

Pharynx
- Some webs are present in valleculae or the lower piriform sinus.
- Shelf-like filling defects along anterior wall of hypopharynx

Cervical Esophagus
- Shelf-like filling defects along anterior wall of cervical esophagus

IMAGING

Fluoroscopy
Findings
- Webs appear radiographically as 1- to 2-mm-wide, shelf-like filling defects along anterior wall of hypopharynx or cervical esophagus.
- Webs may protrude to various depths into esophageal lumen.
- Webs may extend laterally and occasionally may extend circumferentially.
- Circumferential webs appear as ring-like shelves in cervical esophagus.
- Partial obstruction is suggested by a jet phenomenon or by dilatation of esophagus or pharynx proximal to web.

Utility
- Dynamic pharyngeal examination reveals higher percentage of webs than do spot images alone.
- Better demonstration of webs is also achieved with use of large boluses of barium.
- Webs may be confused with redundant mucosa in anterior wall of hypopharynx at the level of cricoid cartilage (postcricoid defect).

DIAGNOSTIC PEARLS
- Webs appear radiographically as 1- to 2-mm-wide, shelf-like filling defects along anterior wall of hypopharynx or cervical esophagus.
- Webs may extend laterally and occasionally may extend circumferentially.
- Webs may protrude to various depths into esophageal lumen.

- Webs should not be confused with prominent cricopharyngeal muscle.

CLINICAL PRESENTATION
- Dysphagia may occur if web significantly compromises lumen.
- Most patients with cervical esophageal webs are asymptomatic.

DIFFERENTIAL DIAGNOSIS
- Schatzki ring (gastroesophageal junction)
- Ring-like peptic stricture (esophagus)

PATHOLOGY
- Webs are usually composed of normal epithelium and lamina propria.
- Some webs show inflammatory changes.
- Vallecular and piriform sinus webs are composed of mucosa, lamina propria, and underlying blood vessels; these webs are thought to be normal variants.

WHAT THE REFERRING PHYSICIAN NEEDS TO KNOW
- Dynamic examination reveals higher percentage of webs than do spot images alone.
- Better demonstration of webs is also achieved with use of large boluses of barium.
- Webs may be confused with redundant mucosa on the anterior wall of hypopharynx at the level of cricoid cartilage (postcricoid defect).
- Webs may be confused with a prominent cricopharyngeal muscle, seen as a round, broad-based protrusion from posterior pharyngeal wall at the level of pharyngoesophageal segment.
- With severe luminal narrowing, dysphagia may result, especially in patients with circumferential cervical esophageal webs.
- Etiology and clinical significance of webs are controversial.

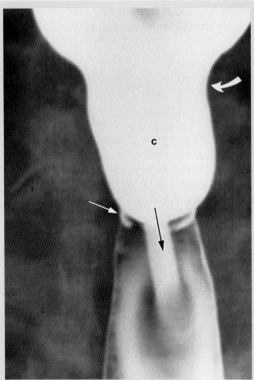

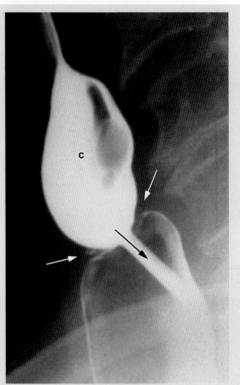

Figure 1. **Partially obstructing cervical esophageal web.** Frontal view shows a circumferential, radiolucent ring *(straight white arrow)* in the proximal cervical esophagus. Partial obstruction is suggested by a jet phenomenon *(black arrow)*, with barium spurting through the ring, and by mild dilatation of the proximal cervical esophagus (c). Cricopharyngeal level is identified *(curved arrow)*. *(From Rubesin SE: Pharynx. In Laufer I, Levine MS [eds]: Double Contrast Gastrointestinal Radiology, 2nd ed. Philadelphia, WB Saunders, 1992.)*

Figure 2. **Partially obstructing cervical esophageal web.** Lateral view from the same patient as in Figure 1 shows a circumferential, radiolucent ring *(straight white arrows)* in the proximal cervical esophagus. Partial obstruction is suggested by a jet phenomenon *(black arrow)*, with barium spurting through the ring, and by mild dilatation of the proximal cervical esophagus (c). *(From Rubesin SE: Pharynx. In Laufer I, Levine MS [eds]: Double Contrast Gastrointestinal Radiology, 2nd ed. Philadelphia, WB Saunders, 1992.)*

INCIDENCE/PREVALENCE AND EPIDEMIOLOGY

- Webs are seen as isolated findings in 3% to 8% of patients undergoing upper gastrointestinal barium studies.
- In one autopsy series, 16% of patients had incidental cervical esophageal webs.
- Some webs are associated with diseases that cause inflammation and scarring, such as epidermolysis bullosa dystrophica and benign mucous membrane pemphigoid.
- Some cervical esophageal webs may be associated with gastroesophageal reflux.

Suggested Readings

Clements JL, Cox GW, Torres WE, et al: Cervical esophageal webs—a roentgen-anatomic correlation. *Am J Roentgenol Radium Ther Nucl Med* 121:221-231, 1974.
Ekberg O: Cervical oesophageal webs in patients with dysphagia. *Clin Radiol* 32:633-641, 1981.
Ekberg O, Nylander G: Webs and web-like formations in the pharynx and cervical esophagus. *Diagn Imaging* 52:10-18, 1983.
Nosher JL, Campbell WL, Seaman WB: The clinical significance of cervical esophageal and hypopharyngeal webs. *Radiology* 117:45-47, 1975.
Weaver JW, Kaude JV, Hamlin DJ: Webs of the lower esophagus: A complication of gastroesophageal reflux? *AJR Am J Roentgenol* 142:289-292, 1984.

Inflammatory Lesions

DEFINITION: Inflammatory lesions of the pharynx may be acute or chronic conditions caused by infection or caustic substance exposure.

ANATOMIC FINDINGS

Pharynx
- Inflammatory disorders of pharynx or gastroesophageal reflux can alter pharyngeal elevation.
- Lymphoid hyperplasia can be coarsely nodular, asymmetrically distributed, or mass-like.

Larynx
- Inflammatory disorders of pharynx or gastroesophageal reflux can alter epiglottic tilt and closure of vocal cords.

IMAGING

Radiography
Findings
- Acute pharyngitis: normal findings on pharyngograms or evidence of nonspecific lymphoid hyperplasia of palatine or lingual tonsils
- Acute epiglottitis: smooth enlargement of epiglottis and aryepiglottic folds
- Lymphoid hyperplasia: multiple smooth, round or ovoid nodules are symmetrically distributed over base of tongue on frontal radiographs.
- Lymphoid hyperplasia: base of tongue sometimes nodular on lateral radiographs
- Double-contrast examination of pharynx may show plaques of *Candida* pharyngitis or ulcers of herpes pharyngitis, particularly in patients with acquired immunodeficiency syndrome.
- Lye ingestion: severe ulceration with subsequent scarring causing distorted pharyngeal contours
- With severe ulceration, amputation of uvula and tip of epiglottis may be observed.

Utility
- Plain-film radiographic diagnosis of acute epiglottitis is important because manipulation may exacerbate edema and respiratory distress.
- Barium studies are contraindicated in acute epiglottitis because they may exacerbate edema, triggering acute respiratory arrest.
- Barium studies of pharynx are of limited value in patients with acute sore throat.

DIAGNOSTIC PEARLS

- Acute epiglottitis: smooth enlargement of epiglottis and aryepiglottic folds
- Lymphoid hyperplasia: multiple smooth, round or ovoid nodules that are symmetrically distributed over base of tongue on frontal radiographs
- Asymmetrically distributed coarse nodularity or mass must be viewed with suspicion; endoscopy and MRI may help to rule out malignancy.

- With chronic sore throat, barium studies may help determine whether underlying gastroesophageal reflux or reflux esophagitis is present.

CLINICAL PRESENTATION

- Throat discomfort, globus sensation, and dysphagia
- Severe stridor and sore throat in adults

DIFFERENTIAL DIAGNOSIS

- Pharyngeal lymphoma
- Pharyngeal carcinoma

PATHOLOGY

- Hypertrophy of lingual tonsil frequently occurs as compensatory response after tonsillectomy or as a nonspecific response to allergies or repeated infection.

INCIDENCE/PREVALENCE AND EPIDEMIOLOGY

- Acute epiglottitis usually affects children between 3 and 6 years of age but is occasionally seen in adults.
- Pharyngeal inflammation and ulceration may be seen in patients with Behçet syndrome, Stevens-Johnson syndrome, Reiter syndrome, epidermolysis bullosa, or bullous pemphigoid.
- Hypertrophy of lingual tonsil frequently occurs after puberty.

WHAT THE REFERRING PHYSICIAN NEEDS TO KNOW

- Inflammation-induced dysmotility may result in laryngeal penetration and stasis.
- Asymmetrically distributed coarse nodularity or mass at base of tongue must be viewed with suspicion; endoscopy and MRI may help rule out malignancy.

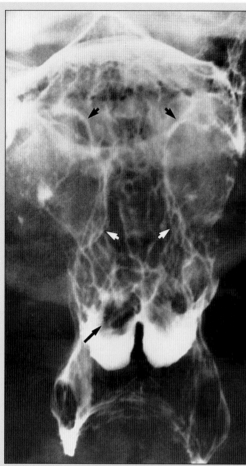

Figure 1. Lymphoid hyperplasia of palatine tonsils and tongue base in young patient with chronic sore throat. Frontal view of pharynx shows moderate nodularity of tongue base *(long arrow)* and bilateral, symmetric enlargement of palatine tonsils *(short arrows)*.

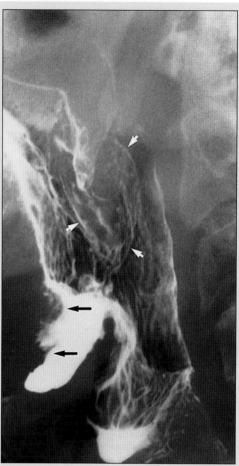

Figure 2. Lateral view of pharynx from same patient as in Figure 1 shows moderate nodularity of tongue base *(long arrows)* and bilateral, symmetric enlargement of palatine tonsils *(short arrows)*.

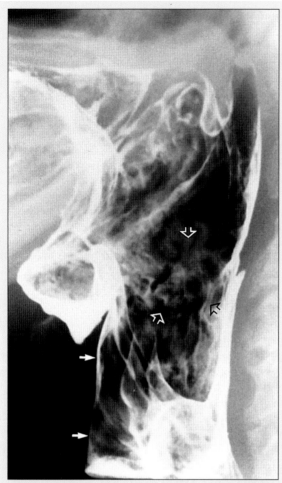

Figure 3. *Candida* **pharyngitis.** Lateral view of pharynx shows well-circumscribed plaques *(open arrows)* at level of epiglottis. Note laryngeal vestibule penetration *(solid arrows)* resulting from abnormal pharyngeal motility associated with this inflammatory pharyngitis. *(From Rubesin SE: Pharynx. In Laufer I, Levine MS [eds]: Double Contrast Gastrointestinal Radiology, 2nd ed. Philadelphia, WB Saunders, 1992.)*

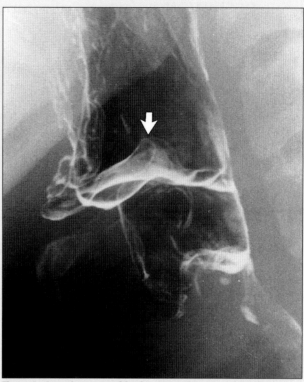

Figure 4. Scarring caused by lye ingestion. On a lateral view, the tip of epiglottis *(arrow)* appears truncated.

Suggested Readings

Agha FP, Francis IR, Ellis CN: Esophageal involvement in epidermolysis bullosa dystrophica: Clinical and roentgenographic manifestations. *Gastrointest Radiol* 8:111-117, 1983.

Balfe DM, Heiken JP: Contrast evaluation of structural lesions of the pharynx. *Curr Probl Diagn Radiol* 15:73-160, 1986.

Bosma JF, Gravkowski EA, Tryostad CW: Chronic ulcerative pharyngitis. *Arch Otolaryngol* 87:85-96, 1968.

Gromet M, Homer MJ, Carter BL: Lymphoid hyperplasia at the base of the tongue. *Radiology* 144:825-828, 1982.

Harris RD, Berdon WE, Baker DH: Roentgen diagnosis of acute epiglottis in the adult. *J Can Assoc Radiol* 21:270-272, 1970.

Kabakian HA, Dahmash MS: Pharyngoesophageal manifestations of epidermolysis bullosa. *Clin Radiol* 29:91-94, 1978.

Rubesin SE, Glick SN: The tailored double-contrast pharyngogram. *Crit Rev Diagn Imaging* 28:133-179, 1988.

Scott JC, Jones B, Eisele DW, et al: Caustic ingestion injuries of the upper aerodigestive tract. *Laryngoscope* 102:1-8, 1992.

Benign Tumors

DEFINITION: Nonmalignant lesions found in the pharynx.

ANATOMIC FINDINGS

Pharynx
- Retention cysts and granular cell tumors are common benign tumors at base of tongue.
- Ectopic thyroid tissue and thyroglossal duct cysts may also occur at tongue base.
- Benign tumors arising from minor mucoserous salivary glands are usually seen in oropharynx, in soft palate, or base of tongue.

Larynx
- Tumor-like lesions most commonly involving aryepiglottic folds are retention cysts and saccular cysts.
- Laryngeal involvement in neurofibromatosis most frequently affects the region of arytenoid cartilage and aryepiglottic folds.
- Chondromas usually arise from posterior lamina of cricoid cartilage.

IMAGING

Radiography
Findings
- Smooth, round, sharply circumscribed mass en face; hemispheric line with abrupt angulation in profile.
Utility
- Double-contrast pharyngography

CT
Findings
- Smooth, round, sharply circumscribed mass en face; hemispheric line with abrupt angulation in profile

CLINICAL PRESENTATION

- Benign tumors at base of tongue may cause no symptoms or may cause throat irritation or dysphagia.
- Aryepiglottic fold nodules or mass lesions may cause dysphonia or respiratory symptoms such as stridor.

DIAGNOSTIC PEARLS

- Barium studies may reveal smooth, round, sharply circumscribed mass en face and a hemispheric line with abrupt angulation in profile.
- Most common benign lesions are retention cysts of valleculae or aryepiglottic folds.

- Epiglottic and aryepiglottic fold tumors may also cause dysphagia, coughing, or choking because of laryngeal penetration.
- Rarely, pedunculated lesions may be coughed up into the mouth or may cause sudden death from asphyxiation.

PATHOLOGY

- Retention cysts are lined by squamous epithelium and filled with desquamated squamous debris.
- Saccular cysts of aryepiglottic folds arise from mucus-secreting glands of appendix of laryngeal ventricle and are filled with mucoid secretions.
- Benign cartilaginous tumors involving pharynx (chondromas) usually arise from posterior lamina of cricoid cartilage.

INCIDENCE/PREVALENCE AND EPIDEMIOLOGY

- Most common benign lesions are retention cysts of valleculae and aryepiglottic folds.
- Retention cysts and granular cell tumors are the most common benign tumors of tongue base.
- Tumor-like lesions that most commonly involve aryepiglottic folds are retention cysts and saccular cysts.
- Laryngeal involvement in neurofibromatosis (von Recklinghausen disease) is rare.
- Ectopic thyroid tissue and thyroglossal duct cysts are rare.

WHAT THE REFERRING PHYSICIAN NEEDS TO KNOW
- Regardless of underlying histologic characteristics of benign tumors, the radiologic appearance is similar.
- Benign nature of these lesions should be confirmed by endoscopic examination.
- Submucosal masses are sometimes missed at endoscopy.

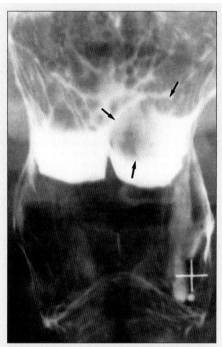

Figure 1. Retention cyst at base of tongue. Frontal view shows a faint, radiolucent filling defect in barium pool *(arrows)* in left vallecula. *(From Rubesin SE, Laufer I: Pictorial review: Principles of double contrast pharyngography. Dysphagia 6:170-178, 1991.)*

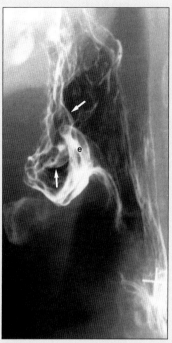

Figure 2. Retention cyst at base of tongue. Lateral view from same patient as in Figure 1 shows a smooth-surfaced hemispheric mass *(arrows)* protruding posteriorly from the base of tongue. Mass is partially obscured by epiglottic tip (e). *(From Rubesin SE, Laufer I: Pictorial review: Principles of double contrast pharyngography. Dysphagia 6:170-178, 1991.)*

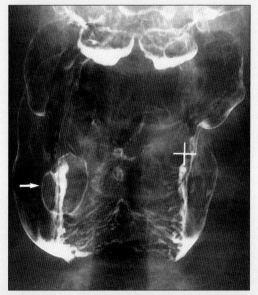

Figure 3. Retention cyst in mucosa overlying the muscular process of right arytenoid cartilage. A smooth-surfaced, well-circumscribed mass is seen in the region of mucosa overlying muscular process of right arytenoid cartilage *(arrow)*. This 2.5-cm mass was not detected on endoscopy. After repeat endoscopic examination confirmed the presence of lesion, surgery was performed, and pathologic evaluation revealed a retention cyst lined by squamous epithelium. *(Reprinted with permission from Rubesin SE, Glick SN: The tailored double-contrast pharyngogram. Crit Rev Diagn Imaging 28:133-179, 1988. Copyright CRC Press, Inc. Boca Raton, FL.)*

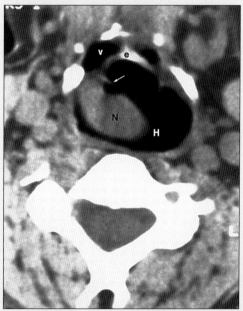

Figure 4. Neurofibroma of right aryepiglottic fold. A 41-year-old man with known neurofibromatosis came to emergency department complaining of work-related neck pain and mild inspiratory stridor. CT scan shows a smooth-surfaced mass (N) protruding into hypopharynx (H). Arrow indicates uppermost portion of aryepiglottic fold. (*e*, Epiglottis; *v*, vallecula.)

- True soft-tissue tumors of aryepiglottic folds, such as lipomas, neurofibromas, hamartomas, granular cell tumors, and oncocytomas, are rare.
- Nonepithelial tumors arising from supporting tissues of pharynx are rare.
- Pedunculated, polypoid lesions (e.g., papilloma or fibrovascular polyp) are rarely seen.

Suggested Readings

Bachman AL: Benign, non-neoplastic conditions of the larynx and pharynx. *Radiol Clin North Am* 16:273-290, 1978.

Chang-Lo M: Laryngeal involvement in Von Recklinghausen's disease. *Laryngoscope* 87:435-442, 1977.

DiBartolomeo JR, Olsen AR: Pedunculated lipoma of the epiglottis. *Arch Otolaryngol* 98:55-57, 1973.

Hyams VJ, Rabuzzi DD: Cartilaginous tumors of the larynx. *Laryngoscope* 80:755-767, 1970.

Mansson T, Wilske J, Kindblom L-G: Lipoma of the hypopharynx: A case report and a review of the literature. *J Laryngol Otol* 92:1037-1043, 1978.

Patterson HC, Dickerson GR, Pilch BZ, et al: Hamartoma of the hypopharynx. *Arch Otolaryngol* 107:767-772, 1981.

Semenkovich JW, Balfe DM, Weyman PJ, et al: Barium pharyngography: Comparison of single and double contrast. *AJR Am J Roentgenol* 144:715-720, 1985.

Woodfield C, Levine MS, Rubesin SE, et al: Pharyngeal retention cysts: Radiographic findings in seven patients. *AJR Am J Roentgenol* 184:793-796, 2005.

Malignant Tumors

DEFINITION: Malignant tumors of pharynx primarily include squamous cell carcinoma and lymphoma.

ANATOMIC FINDINGS

Palatine Tonsil
- Squamous cell carcinoma of palatine tonsil is the most common malignant tumor arising in the pharynx.
- Well-differentiated tumors are usually exophytic.
- Tonsillar tumors may spread to the soft palate, base of tongue, and posterior pharyngeal wall.
- Approximately 50% of patients develop cervical lymph node metastases.
- Most frequent pharyngeal location of lymphoma is palatine tonsil (40%-60% of patients).
- Pharyngeal lymphomas are lobulated masses obliterating surface landmarks, similar in appearance to hyperplastic palatine tonsils.

Base of Tongue
- Exophytic lesions appear as polypoid masses projecting into the oropharyngeal airspace.
- Nodules of tumor may spread to the palatine tonsil, valleculae, or pharyngoepiglottic folds.
- Deeply infiltrating submucosal lesions may occasionally be manifested by subtle, asymmetric enlargement of the tongue base.
- Small or predominantly submucosal lesions may be hidden in the vallecula or glossotonsillar recess.
- Lymphoma is also common in this region.

Supraglottic Region
- Exophytic lesions are more common than endophytic lesions.
- Ulcerative lesions may deeply penetrate the tongue and valleculae, invading the pre-epiglottic space.
- These tumors may spread laterally to pharyngoepiglottic folds and lateral pharyngeal walls.

Piriform Sinus
- Advanced lesions are typically seen as bulky exophytic masses.
- Medial wall tumors may infiltrate the aryepiglottic fold, arytenoid and cricoid cartilages, and paraglottic space.
- Tumors involving lateral wall may infiltrate the thyrohyoid membrane, thyroid cartilage, and soft tissues of neck.
- Early lesions may appear as subtle areas of mucosal irregularity.

DIAGNOSTIC PEARLS
- Intraluminal mass
- Mucosal irregularity
- Loss of normal distensibility of pharynx

Posterior Pharyngeal Wall
- Large, fungating lesions are usually greater than 5 cm in length.
- These lesions may spread vertically into nasopharynx and cervical esophagus.
- Approximately 50% of patients have jugular or retropharyngeal lymphatic metastases at the time of diagnosis.

Postcricoid Area
- Postcricoid carcinomas appear as annular, infiltrating lesions that may extend into the lower hypopharynx or cervical esophagus.
- Cartilaginous tumors: Smooth-surfaced masses are usually seen in posterior lamina of cricoid cartilage, distorting the lower hypopharynx and pharyngoesophageal segment.

Soft Palate
- Obliteration of contour is typically seen.
- Minor salivary gland tumors of the pharynx are most commonly found in the soft palate.
- Palatal salivary gland tumors may spread to the tongue, submandibular gland, lingual and hypoglossal nerves, and mandible.

IMAGING

Radiography
Findings
- Intraluminal mass: luminal contour obliteration, barium-coated lines protruding into air column, focal area of increased radiopacity, filling defect in barium pool
- Mucosal irregularity: abnormal barium collections resulting from surface ulceration; lobulated, finely nodular, or granular surface texture
- Asymmetric distensibility: flattening of pharyngeal contour

WHAT THE REFERRING PHYSICIAN NEEDS TO KNOW
- Multiple primary lesions of oral cavity, pharynx, esophagus, and lung are seen in more than 20% of patients.
- Important goal of preoperative imaging for squamous cell carcinoma of the pharynx is to rule out synchronous primary esophageal cancer.
- Cross-sectional imaging study is examination of choice for showing spread of tumor.

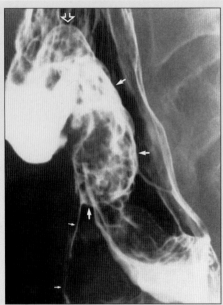

Figure 1. Polypoid squamous cell carcinoma of the epiglottis.
Lateral view shows a bulbous, enlarged epiglottic tip *(open arrow)* and a large epiglottic mass *(large solid arrows)* extending down the aryepiglottic fold and along the anterior wall of the laryngeal vestibule. The lower portion of the laryngeal vestibule *(small solid arrows)* is not involved by tumor. *(From Rubesin SE: Pharynx. In Laufer I, Levine MS [eds]: Double Contrast Gastrointestinal Radiology, 2nd ed. Philadelphia, WB Saunders, 1992.)*

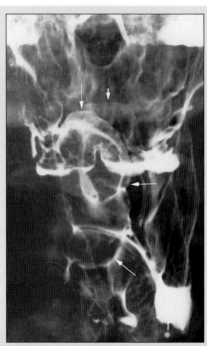

Figure 2. Squamous cell carcinoma of the lateral wall of the right piriform sinus. Frontal view shows obliteration of the right lateral wall of the piriform sinus. Note the large, polypoid mass *(long arrows)* protruding into the hypopharynx. The tip of the epiglottis *(short arrow)* is spared. *(Reprinted with permission from Rubesin SE, Glick SN: The tailored double-contrast pharyngogram. Crit Rev Diagn Imaging 28:133-179, 1988. Copyright CRC Press, Inc. Boca Raton, FL.)*

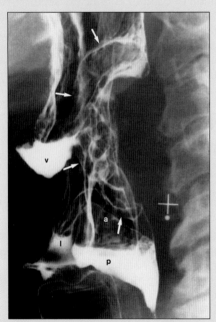

Figure 3. Squamous cell carcinoma of the posterior pharyngeal wall. Lateral spot image of the pharynx shows a large fungating mass *(arrows)* on the posterior pharyngeal wall, extending from the level of the uvula to the level of the muscular processes of the arytenoid cartilages (a). Note evidence of pharyngeal dysfunction with pooling of barium in the valleculae (v), piriform sinus (p), and laryngeal vestibule (l). *(Reprinted with permission from Rubesin SE, Glick SN: The tailored double-contrast pharyngogram. Crit Rev Diagn Imaging 28:133-179, 1988. Copyright CRC Press, Inc. Boca Raton, FL.)*

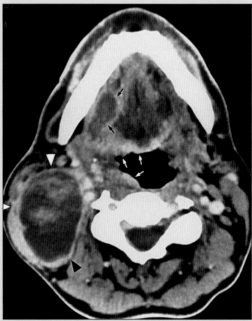

Figure 4. Deeply infiltrating squamous cell carcinoma of the base of the tongue. CT scan through the base of the tongue shows asymmetry of the tongue base and lateral pharyngeal wall *(white arrows),* with a peripherally enhanced mass also invading the sublingual space *(black arrows).* A large, centrally necrotic cervical lymph node metastasis *(arrowheads)* is identified.

- Cartilaginous tumors: smooth-surfaced mass usually seen in posterior lamina of cricoid cartilage, with stippled calcification centrally or peripherally

Utility
- Initial diagnostic pharyngography for patients with pharyngeal symptoms or palpable neck mass
- In patients with known pharyngeal cancer, pharyngography is of value in planning proper workup and therapy.
- Barium study also useful for ruling out synchronous cancers in the esophagus and coexisting structural lesions.
- Barium study can show size, extent, and inferior limit of pharyngeal tumors and degree of functional impairment.
- Barium examination can show areas behind bulky tumors that are difficult to visualize by endoscopy.
- Barium studies allow detection of more than 95% of structural lesions below the pharyngoesophageal fold.
- Nasopharyngeal squamous cell carcinoma: Barium studies can be used to evaluate nasal regurgitation, voice changes, and synchronous lesions.

CT
Findings
- Intraluminal mass, mucosal irregularity, asymmetric distensibility
- Plaque-like lesions, ulcerations, infiltrative lesions

Utility
- Cross-sectional imaging study is examination of choice for showing spread of tumor.
- CT may occasionally reveal lesions (typically submucosal masses) not visible even with modern endoscopes.

MRI
Findings
- Intraluminal mass, mucosal irregularity, asymmetric distensibility
- Plaque-like lesions, ulcerations, infiltrative lesions

Utility
- Cross-sectional imaging study is examination of choice for showing spread of tumor.
- MRI may occasionally reveal lesions (typically submucosal masses) that are not visible even with modern endoscopes.
- MRI is method of choice for evaluating tumors of nasopharynx.
- Carefully search for spread to nasal cavity, sinuses, and cranial base, especially for cranial nerve involvement.

Fluoroscopy
Findings
- Intraluminal mass: luminal contour obliteration, barium-coated lines protruding into air column, focal area of increased radiopacity, filling defect in barium pool
- Asymmetric distensibility: flattening of pharyngeal contour
- Postcricoid carcinomas: annular lesions

Utility
- Tumors are best shown with video recordings and rapid-sequence spot images during swallowing while pharyngoesophageal segment is distended with barium.

CLINICAL PRESENTATION
- Symptoms are usually of short duration (less than 4 months) and include sore throat, dysphagia, and odynophagia.
- Hoarseness occurs primarily in patients with laryngeal carcinoma, supraglottic carcinoma, or carcinoma of medial piriform sinus.
- Referred earache or hearing loss may occur when tumors block the eustachian tube.
- Some patients are asymptomatic but have a palpable neck mass.

DIFFERENTIAL DIAGNOSIS
- Tonsillar hyperplasia

PATHOLOGY
- Most carcinomas are keratinizing squamous cell carcinomas occurring as exophytic, infiltrative, or ulcerative lesions.
- Many nasopharyngeal squamous cell cancers are undifferentiated tumors with reactive lymphoid stroma.
- Alcohol, smoking, poor ventilation, nasal balms, ingested carcinogens, and Epstein-Barr virus have been implicated as causative factors of nasopharyngeal carcinoma.
- Squamous cell carcinoma of posterior pharyngeal wall is most frequently associated with synchronous or metachronous malignant lesions.
- Almost all pharyngeal lymphomas are non-Hodgkin type, arising from Waldeyer's ring (i.e., adenoids, palatine tonsils, and lingual tonsil).
- Minor salivary gland malignancy arises from minor mucoserous salivary glands located deep to epithelial layer of pharynx.
- Common salivary gland malignancies are adenoid cystic carcinoma, solid adenocarcinoma, and mucoepidermoid carcinoma.

INCIDENCE/PREVALENCE AND EPIDEMIOLOGY
- Squamous cell carcinomas of head and neck (tongue, pharynx, and larynx) constitute 5% of all cancers in the United States.
- Most patients with squamous cell carcinoma are 50 to 70 years of age.
- Almost all patients (more than 95%) are moderate to heavy abusers of alcohol and tobacco.

- Squamous cell carcinomas represent 90% of malignant lesions of oropharynx and hypopharynx.
- Pharyngeal lymphomas represent approximately 10% of malignant pharyngeal tumors.
- Most patients with pharyngeal lymphoma are in fifth to sixth decades of life.
- Minor salivary gland tumors constitute 20% of all salivary gland tumors; 65% to 88% of minor salivary gland tumors are malignant.

Suggested Readings

Apter AJ, Levine MS, Glick SN: Carcinomas of the base of the tongue: Diagnosis using double-contrast radiography of the pharynx. *Radiology* 151:123-126, 1984.

Carpenter RJ III, DeSanto LW, Devine KD, et al: Cancer of the hypopharynx. *Arch Otolaryngol* 102:716-721, 1976.

Goldstein HM, Zornoza J: Association of squamous cell carcinoma of the head and neck with cancer of the esophagus. *AJR Am J Roentgenol* 131:791-794, 1978.

Kassel E, Keller A, Kuchorczyk W: MRI of the floor of the mouth, tongue and orohypopharynx. *Radiol Clin North Am* 27:331-351, 1989.

Levine MS, Rubesin SE, Ott DJ: Update on esophageal radiology. *AJR Am J Roentgenol* 155:933-941, 1990.

Rubesin SE, Laufer I: Pictorial review: Principles of double contrast pharyngography. *Dysphagia* 6:170-178, 1991.

Semenkovich JW, Balfe DM, Weyman PJ, et al: Barium pharyngography: Comparison of single and double contrast. *AJR Am J Roentgenol* 144:715-720, 1985.

Thompson WM, Oddson TA, Kelvin F, et al: Synchronous and metachronous squamous cell carcinoma of the head, neck, and esophagus. *Gastrointest Radiol* 3:123-127, 1978.

Vogl T, Dresel S, Bilaniuk LT, et al: Tumors of the nasopharynx and adjacent areas: MR imaging with Gd-DTPA. *AJNR Am J Neuroradiol* 11:187-194, 1990.

Esophagus

Part 6

MOTILITY DISORDERS OF THE ESOPHAGUS

Primary Achalasia

DEFINITION: Achalasia is characterized by aperistalsis and lower esophageal sphincter (LES) dysfunction.

ANATOMIC FINDINGS

Esophagus
- Smooth, tapered, beak-like narrowing at level of esophageal hiatus
- Markedly dilated and tortuous esophagus above hiatus

IMAGING

Radiography
Findings
- Primary peristalsis is absent on all swallows.
- Lower end of esophagus has smooth, tapered, beak-like appearance at level of esophageal hiatus.
- Esophagus may become markedly dilated and tortuous, producing a sigmoid appearance.
- Food, secretions, and barium are retained in dilated esophagus.
- Massive esophageal dilatation may be seen even on chest radiographs.
Utility
- Fluoroscopic examination is adequate to evaluate esophageal motility, but motion-recording techniques may be used.
- Patient is placed in the prone right anterior oblique position, then swallows barium for adequate evaluation of esophageal peristalsis and LES relaxation.
- Rapid, repetitive swallowing does not assess primary esophageal peristalsis but distends esophagus maximally for structural evaluation.
- Presence of carcinoma at esophagogastric junction may simulate achalasia.
- Radiographic evaluation after treatment is helpful in detecting complications.

Nuclear Medicine
Utility
- Aids in diagnosis and management of patients with achalasia
- Radionuclide transit and emptying studies are particularly helpful for quantifying esophageal retention before and after therapy.

DIAGNOSTIC PEARLS

- Characterized manometrically by absence of primary peristalsis, elevated or normal resting LES pressures, and incomplete or absent LES relaxation
- Radiographically, primary peristalsis is absent on all swallows observed.
- Lower end of esophagus appears smooth, tapered, beak-like at level of esophageal hiatus.

CLINICAL PRESENTATION

- Long-standing dysphagia
- Chest pain
- Regurgitation

DIFFERENTIAL DIAGNOSIS

- Secondary achalasia
- Diffuse esophageal spasm with LES dysfunction

PATHOLOGY

- Cause of achalasia is unknown, but histologic lesions have been found in the dorsal motor nucleus of vagus, vagal trunks, and myenteric ganglia of esophagus.
- Achalasia appears to be a neurogenic disorder.
- Ganglionic cells are decreased in number.
- Manometric findings include absent primary peristalsis, elevated or normal resting LES pressures, and incomplete or absent LES relaxation.

INCIDENCE/PREVALENCE AND EPIDEMIOLOGY

- Incidence: occurs during middle decades of life and equally in both sexes
- Risk of carcinoma is 9 to 28 times greater than that of general population in patients with long-standing achalasia

---

WHAT THE REFERRING PHYSICIAN NEEDS TO KNOW

- Treatment involves pneumatic dilatation, laparoscopic myotomy, or botulinum toxin injection.
- Complications such as reflux esophagitis and peptic strictures may be prevented by performing *loose* fundoplication wrap with laparoscopic myotomy.
- Radiographic evaluation after pneumatic dilatation is helpful in detecting serious complications such as perforation.

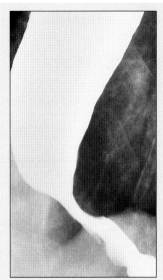

Figure 1. Achalasia. Close-up view shows smooth, beak-like tapering at lower end of the esophagus caused by LES dysfunction.

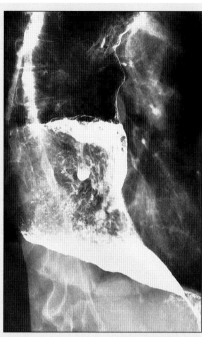

Figure 2. Advanced achalasia. Markedly dilated esophagus with retained secretions and food.

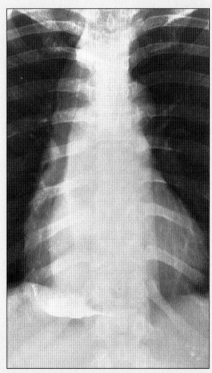

Figure 3. Advanced achalasia. Double contour of right mediastinal border seen in a patient with advanced achalasia. The outer border represents a dilated esophagus projecting beyond the shadows of the aorta and heart. A small amount of retained barium is present in the distal esophagus.

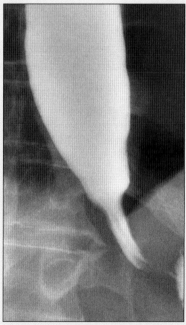

Figure 4. Secondary achalasia or pseudoachalasia. Smooth narrowing of the esophagogastric junction simulating achalasia. This patient had a scirrhous carcinoma of the proximal stomach invading the distal esophagus. (*From Ott DJ: Radiologic evaluation of esophageal dysphagia.* Curr Probl Diagn Radiol *17:1-33, 1988.*)

Suggested Readings

Goldenberg SP, Burrell M, Fette GG, et al: Classic and vigorous achalasia: A comparison of manometric, radiographic, and clinical findings. *Gastroenterology* 101:743-748, 1991.

Ott DJ, Donati D, Wu WC, et al: Radiographic evaluation of achalasia immediately after pneumatic dilatation with the Rigiflex dilator. *Gastrointest Radiol* 16:279-282, 1991.

Vaezi MF, Richter JE: Diagnosis and management of achalasia. *Am J Gastroenterol* 94:3406-3412, 1999.

West RL, Hirsch DP, Bartelsman JF, et al: Long term results of pneumatic dilation in achalasia followed for more than 5 years. *Am J Gastroenterol* 97:1346-1351, 2002.

Diffuse Esophageal Spasm

DEFINITION: An uncommon esophageal motility disorder characterized by chest pain.

ANATOMIC FINDINGS

Esophageal Smooth Muscle
- Thickened

IMAGING

Radiography
Findings
- Primary peristalsis present in cervical esophagus but intermittently absent in thoracic esophagus
- Nonperistaltic contractions of varying severity replace the disrupted primary wave.
- Lumen-obliterating nonperistaltic contractions may produce a *corkscrew* or *rosary bead* appearance.
- *Beak-like* narrowing of distal esophagus due to incomplete opening of lower esophageal sphincter (LES) in more than 50% of patients
- Wall thickness of 2 cm or more

Utility
- Radiographic features of diffuse esophageal spasm (DES) reflect manometric findings.
- Radiographic findings in DES can be nonspecific so correlation with clinical symptoms and esophageal manometry is sometimes required.
- Thickening of esophageal wall is best estimated along right border of the esophagus where the wall is close to pleural reflection line.

CT
Utility
- Wall thickness can be measured directly.

Ultrasound
Utility
- Endoscopic ultrasound can directly measure wall thickness.

CLINICAL PRESENTATION

- Chest pain
- Dysphagia

DIAGNOSTIC PEARLS

- Manometric studies show simultaneous contractions on more than 10% of wet swallows and intermittently normal primary peristalsis.
- Diagnosis of DES is based on clinical, radiographic, and manometric findings.
- Classic *corkscrew* or *rosary bead* appearance of DES seen in minority of patients

DIFFERENTIAL DIAGNOSIS

- Presbyesophagus
- Vigorous achalasia
- Other esophageal motility disorders

PATHOLOGY

- May be related to varying degrees of neurogenic damage
- Involves smooth-muscle portion of esophagus
- Repetitive or prolonged contractions, high-amplitude contractions, and frequent spontaneous contractions

INCIDENCE/PREVALENCE AND EPIDEMIOLOGY

- Uncommon

Suggested Readings

Chen YM, Ott DJ, Hewson EG, et al: Diffuse esophageal spasm: Radiographic and manometric correlation. *Radiology* 170:807-810, 1989.

Henderson RD, Ryder D, Marryatt G: Extended esophageal myotomy and short total fundoplication hernia repair in diffuse esophageal spasm: Five-year review in 34 patients. *Ann Thorac Surg* 43:25-31, 1987.

Mittal RK, Kassab G, Puckett JL, Liu J: Hypertrophy of the muscularis propria of the lower esophageal sphincter and the body of the esophagus in patients with primary motility disorders of the esophagus. *Am J Gastroenterol* 98:1705-1712, 2003.

Prabhakar A, Levine MS, Rubesin S, et al: Relationship between diffuse esophageal spasm and lower esophageal sphincter dysfunction on barium studies and manometry in 14 patients. *AJR Am J Roentgenol* 183:409-413, 2004.

WHAT THE REFERRING PHYSICIAN NEEDS TO KNOW

- Radiation of pain to the shoulder or back may simulate angina and may even be relieved by nitroglycerin.

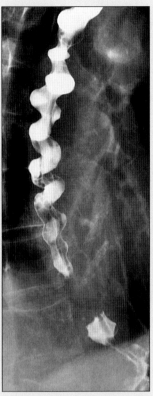

Figure 1. Diffuse esophageal spasm. This patient has typical *corkscrew* or *rosary bead* appearance of diffuse esophageal spasm. (*From Levine MS, Rubesin SE, Ott DJ: Update on esophageal radiology.* AJR Am J Roentgenol *155:933-941, 1990, © by American Roentgen Ray Society.*)

Other Esophageal Motility Disorders

DEFINITION: Esophageal motility disorders can be categorized into the following groups: inadequate lower esophageal sphincter (LES) relaxation, uncoordinated contraction, and hypercontraction or hypocontraction.

ANATOMIC FINDINGS

Esophagus
- Hypocontraction
- Hypercontraction

Lower Esophageal Sphincter
- Incompetent

IMAGING

Radiography
Findings
- Esophageal motility may appear normal on barium studies in patients with nutcracker esophagus or hypertensive LES.
- Disruption of primary peristalsis with multiple non-peristaltic contractions in nonspecific esophageal motility disorder
- Signs include absent esophageal smooth-muscle peristalsis, presence of hiatal hernia, and findings related to reflux esophagitis and peptic strictures in patients with scleroderma involving esophagus.
- Diabetic with peripheral neuropathy; barium studies may show decreased primary peristalsis with increased nonperistaltic contractions, mild esophageal dilatation, and hiatal hernia with gastroesophageal reflux.
- Findings similar to primary achalasia are seen in Chagas disease and intestinal pseudo-obstruction.

Utility
- Multiple, discrete barium swallows are critical for proper radiologic assessment of esophageal function if results are to correlate well with esophageal manometry.
- Nutcracker esophagus and hypertensive LES are not diagnosed radiographically.
- Observation of five barium swallows improves radiologic detection of nonspecific esophageal motility disorders.
- Radiographic sensitivity in patients with recurrent chest pain is only 36%.

CLINICAL PRESENTATION
- Dysphagia
- Chest pain

DIAGNOSTIC PEARLS
- Manometric diagnosis of nutcracker esophagus requires peristaltic contractions with average amplitudes greater than 180 mm Hg.
- Manometric diagnosis of hypertensive LES requires a resting LES pressure greater than 40 mm Hg.
- Manometric features of scleroderma include decreased or absent resting LES pressure and weakened or absent peristalsis in the lower two thirds of the esophagus.
- Manometric criteria for presbyesophagus include decreased frequency of normal peristalsis, increased frequency of nonperistaltic contractions, and, less commonly, incomplete LES relaxation.
- Nonspecific esophageal motility disorder has absence of peristalsis on 20% or more of wet swallows, low-amplitude peristalsis, prolonged duration of peristalsis, repetitive or triple-peaked contractions, and/or incomplete LES relaxation.

DIFFERENTIAL DIAGNOSIS
- Primary and secondary achalasia (esophagus)
- Diffuse esophageal spasm

PATHOLOGY
- Normal peristalsis with distal contractions of abnormally high amplitude and prolonged duration in nutcracker esophagus
- Nutcracker esophagus characterized by peristaltic contractions with average amplitudes greater than 180 mm Hg
- Nonspecific esophageal motility disorder characterized by absence of peristalsis or low-amplitude peristalsis, prolonged duration of peristalsis, repetitive or triple-peaked contractions, and/or incomplete LES relaxation
- Presbyesophagus characterized by decreased frequency of normal peristalsis, increased frequency of nonperistaltic contractions, and, less commonly, incomplete LES relaxation

WHAT THE REFERRING PHYSICIAN NEEDS TO KNOW
- Recurrent chest pain is not a reliable indicator of esophageal motility disorders, and cardiac disease must first be excluded.

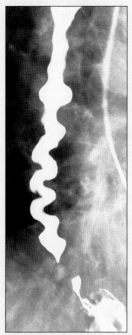

Figure 1. Nonperistaltic contractions in the esophagus.
Barium study of an 89-year-old man with dysphagia but no
chest pain. Diffuse *curling* of the esophagus is present because
of simultaneous nonperistaltic contractions. A nonspecific
esophageal motility disorder was diagnosed on manometric
examination. (*From Ott DJ: Radiologic evaluation of esophageal
dysphagia.* Curr Probl Diagn Radiol *17:1-33, 1988.*)

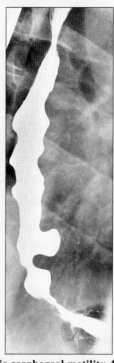

Figure 2. Nonspecific esophageal motility disorder. This
asymptomatic patient had simultaneous nonperistaltic
contractions. Primary peristalsis was disrupted intermittently
at fluoroscopy. Nonspecific esophageal motility disorder was
diagnosed by manometry. (*From Levine MS, Rubesin SE, Ott DJ:
Update on esophageal radiology.* AJR Am J Roentgenol *155:933-941,
1990, © by American Roentgen Ray Society.*)

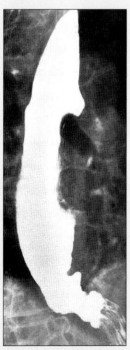

Figure 3. Esophageal involvement by scleroderma. This patient
has a dilated esophagus and patulous esophagogastric junction.
Aperistalsis was noted at fluoroscopy.

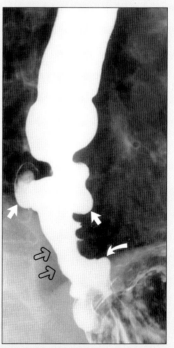

Figure 4. Esophageal involvement by scleroderma. This patient
with scleroderma has developed a peptic stricture *(open arrows)*
as a complication of reflux disease. Also note a small hiatal
hernia *(curved arrow)* and sacculations *(straight arrows)* in the
distal esophagus above the level of the stricture.

- Collagen vascular disease characterized by systemic involvement with immunologic and inflammatory changes in connective tissue
- Scleroderma involving esophagus characterized by decreased or absent resting LES pressures and weakened or absent peristalsis in lower two thirds of esophagus

INCIDENCE/PREVALENCE AND EPIDEMIOLOGY

- Esophageal dysmotility is common in alcoholics.

Suggested Readings

Campbell WL, Schultz JC: Specificity and sensitivity of esophageal motor abnormality in systemic sclerosis (scleroderma) and related diseases: A cineradiographic study. *Gastrointest Radiol* 11:218-222, 1986.

Chobanian SJ, Curtis DJ, Benjamin SB, et al: Radiology of the nutcracker esophagus. *J Clin Gastroenterol* 8:230-232, 1986.

Hsu JJ, O'Connor MK, Kang YW, Kim CH: Nonspecific motor disorder of the esophagus: A real disorder or a manometric curiosity? *Gastroenterology* 104:1281-1284, 1993.

Ott DJ: Motility disorders of the esophagus. *Radiol Clin North Am* 32:1117-1134, 1994.

Pilhall M, Borjesson M, Rolny P, Mannheimer C: Diagnosis of nutcracker esophagus, segmental or diffuse hypertensive patterns, and clinical characteristics. *Dig Dis Sci* 47:1381-1388, 2002.

Ren J, Shaker R, Kusano M, et al: Effect of aging on the secondary esophageal peristalsis: Presbyesophagus revisited. *Am J Physiol* 268:G772-G779, 1995.

Wo JM: Esophageal involvement in systemic diseases. In Castell DO, Richter RE (eds): *The Esophagus*, 4th ed. Philadelphia, Lippincott Williams & Wilkins, 2004, pp 611-633.

Part 7

GASTROESOPHAGEAL REFLUX DISEASE

Reflux Esophagitis

DEFINITION: Inflammation of distal esophageal mucosa secondary to gastroesophageal reflux disease.

IMAGING

Radiography
Findings
- Abnormal esophageal motility and gastroesophageal reflux
- Finely nodular or granular appearance of mucosa in distal esophagus
- Occasionally, plaque-like lesions caused by exudates and pseudomembranes, mimicking appearance of *Candida* esophagitis
- Distal esophageal ulcers: variously sized and shaped collections of barium, often with surrounding edematous mucosa, radiating folds, and distortion of adjacent wall
- Grossly irregular esophageal contour, with serrated or spiculated margins, wall thickening, deeper ulcers, and decreased distensibility in advanced disease
- Thickened longitudinal folds caused by submucosal edema
- Thickened transverse folds
- Inflammatory esophagogastric polyp seen as smooth protuberance atop prominent mucosal fold in distal esophagus

Utility
- Double-contrast esophagography is much more sensitive than single-contrast esophagography for detecting reflux esophagitis.
- Procedure should be performed as biphasic examination with upright double-contrast and prone single-contrast views to optimize diagnostic value.
- Technical artifacts may simulate disease.
- Flow artifact (too much barium coating mucosa) may obscure disease.

CLINICAL PRESENTATION

- Classic symptoms: heartburn, indigestion, substernal chest pain, and regurgitation
- Some patients may have epigastric pain or right upper quadrant pain, mimicking peptic ulcer disease or cholecystitis.

DIFFERENTIAL DIAGNOSIS

- Barrett esophagus
- *Candida* esophagitis

DIAGNOSTIC PEARLS

- Abnormal esophageal motility and gastroesophageal reflux
- Ulcers on posterior wall of distal esophagus
- Continuous area of disease extending proximally from gastroesophageal junction

- Herpes esophagitis
- Drug-induced esophagitis
- Glycogenic acanthosis (esophagus)
- Crohn disease (esophagus)

PATHOLOGY

- Peptic acid reflux causes mucosal damage.
- Inflammatory cells accumulate in lamina propria.
- Ulceration and stricture formation may develop.
- Inflammation of distal esophageal mucosa secondary to reflux disease

INCIDENCE/PREVALENCE AND EPIDEMIOLOGY

- Gastroesophageal reflux disease (GERD) is the most common inflammatory disease of the esophagus.
- Abnormal reflux is seen in asthma and scleroderma.

Suggested Readings

Chen YM, Ott DJ, Gelfand DW, et al: Multiphasic examination of the esophagogastric region for strictures, rings, and hiatal hernia: Evaluation of the individual techniques. *Gastrointest Radiol* 10:311-316, 1985.

Creteur V, Thoeni RF, Federle MP, et al: The role of single- and double-contrast radiography in the diagnosis of reflux esophagitis. *Radiology* 147:71-75, 1983.

Dibble C, Levine MS, Rubesin SE, et al: Detection of reflux esophagitis on double-contrast esophagrams and endoscopy using the histologic findings as the gold standard. *Abdom Imaging* 29:421-425, 2004.

Kressel HY, Glick SN, Laufer I, et al: Radiologic features of esophagitis. *Gastrointest Radiol* 6:103-108, 1981.

Laufer I: Radiology of esophagitis. *Radiol Clin North Am* 20:687-699, 1982.

Ott DJ, Wu WC, Gelfand DW: Reflux esophagitis revisited: Prospective analysis of radiologic accuracy. *Gastrointest Radiol* 6:1-7, 1981.

WHAT THE REFERRING PHYSICIAN NEEDS TO KNOW
- Endoscopy is most definitive diagnostic test, but double-contrast esophagography is useful for showing wide spectrum of morphologic abnormalities in reflux esophagitis.

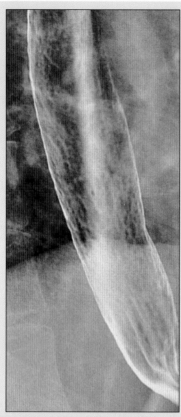

Figure 1. Reflux esophagitis with a granular mucosa. A finely nodular or granular appearance of the mucosa extends proximally from the gastroesophageal junction as a continuous area of disease. (*From Levine MS, Rubesin SE: Diseases of the esophagus: Diagnosis with esophagography.* Radiology *237:414-427, 2005.*)

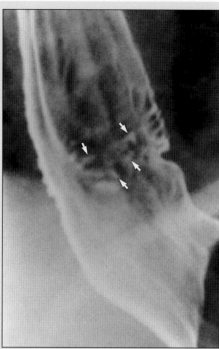

Figure 2. Reflux esophagitis with superficial ulceration. Multiple tiny ulcers *(arrows)* are seen en face in the distal esophagus near the gastroesophageal junction. Note radiating folds and puckering of the adjacent esophageal wall.

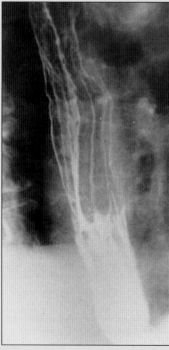

Figure 3. Reflux esophagitis with thickened longitudinal folds. (*From Levine MS:* Radiology of the Esophagus. *Philadelphia, WB Saunders, 1989.*)

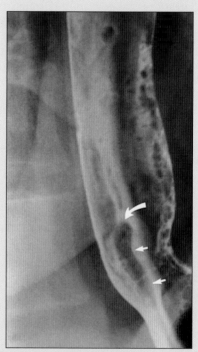

Figure 4. Inflammatory esophagogastric polyp. A prominent fold *(straight arrows)* is seen arising at the cardia and extending into the distal esophagus as a smooth, polypoid protuberance *(curved arrow)*. This appearance is characteristic of inflammatory polyps. (*From Levine MS:* Radiology of the Esophagus. *Philadelphia, WB Saunders, 1989.*)

Scarring from Reflux Esophagitis

DEFINITION: Scarring of distal esophagus secondary to reflux disease.

IMAGING

Radiography

Findings

- Subtle scarring from reflux esophagitis is manifested by slight flattening or puckering of esophageal wall or radiating folds, or both.
- Focal outpouching or sacculation of distal esophagus caused by asymmetric scarring from reflux esophagitis must be differentiated from wide-mouthed outpouchings in scleroderma.
- Fixed transverse folds are seen, producing a characteristic *stepladder* appearance because of pooling of barium between folds.
- Unlike feline esophagus, transverse folds in stepladder esophagus are 2 to 5 mm thick, do not extend more than halfway across esophagus, are few in number, and are not obliterated by esophageal distention.
- Concentric peptic stricture is seen as tapered segment of narrowing in distal esophagus.
- Ring-like peptic stricture is seen at gastroesophageal junction, with slightly tapered borders and a length of only 0.4 to 1.0 cm.

Utility

- Biphasic examination with upright double-contrast and prone single-contrast views is used to optimize detection of peptic strictures.
- Continuous drinking of low-density barium in the prone position can detect mild strictures not visible on upright double-contrast images.
- Barium studies may even detect strictures missed at endoscopy.

CLINICAL PRESENTATION

- Slowly progressive dysphagia for solids (followed by liquids)
- History of long-standing reflux symptoms

DIFFERENTIAL DIAGNOSIS

- Schatzki ring
- Esophageal adenocarcinoma
- Achalasia

DIAGNOSTIC PEARLS

- Fixed transverse folds
- Smooth, tapered area of concentric narrowing or ring-like narrowing
- Associated with hiatal hernia

PATHOLOGY

- Long-standing reflux disease that results in scar formation
- Circumferential narrowing of distal esophagus
- Outward ballooning or sacculation of esophageal wall between areas of fibrosis
- Longitudinal shortening and subsequent hernia formation in almost all patients with peptic strictures

INCIDENCE/PREVALENCE AND EPIDEMIOLOGY

- Gastroesophageal reflux disease (GERD) is most common inflammatory disease of esophagus.
- 10% to 20% of patients with reflux esophagitis develop peptic strictures.

Suggested Readings

Chen YM, Ott DJ, Gelfand DW, et al: Multiphasic examination of the esophagogastric region for strictures, rings, and hiatal hernia: Evaluation of the individual techniques. *Gastrointest Radiol* 10:311-316, 1985.

Gupta S, Levine MS, Rubesin SE, et al: Usefulness of barium studies for differentiating benign and malignant strictures of the esophagus. *AJR Am J Roentgenol* 180:737-744, 2003.

Luedtke P, Levine MS, Rubesin SE, et al: Radiologic diagnosis of benign esophageal strictures: A pattern approach. *Radiographics* 23:897-909, 2003.

WHAT THE REFERRING PHYSICIAN NEEDS TO KNOW

- Any suspicious radiographic features in region of stricture warrant endoscopy and biopsy to rule out carcinoma.

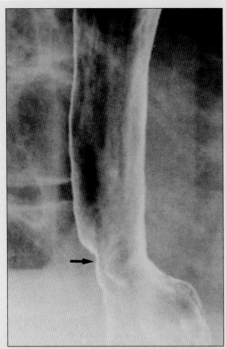

Figure 1. Mild peptic scarring in the distal esophagus. Note slight flattening and puckering of the distal esophagus *(arrow)* with radiating folds in this region as a result of scarring from reflux esophagitis.

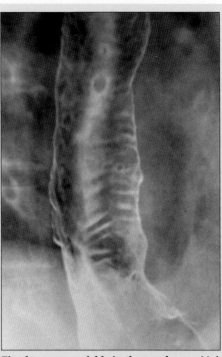

Figure 2. Fixed transverse folds in the esophagus. Multiple transverse folds in the distal esophagus produce a *stepladder* appearance caused by longitudinal scarring from reflux esophagitis. (*From Levine MS, Goldstein HM: Fixed transverse folds in the esophagus: A sign of reflux esophagitis. AJR Am J Roentgenol 143:275-278, 1984, © by American Roentgen Ray Society.*)

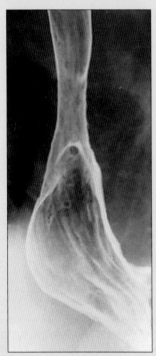

Figure 3. Peptic stricture. A concentric area of smooth, tapered narrowing is seen in the distal esophagus above a hiatal hernia, the classic appearance of a peptic stricture. (*From Levine MS: Radiology of the Esophagus. Philadelphia, WB Saunders, 1989.*)

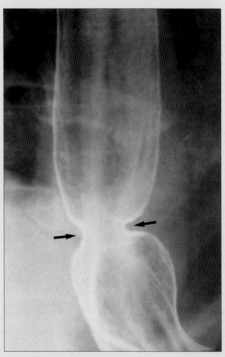

Figure 4. Ring-like peptic stricture. Note a ring-like stricture *(arrows)* in the distal esophagus above a hiatal hernia. Although this stricture can be mistaken for a Schatzki ring, it has a greater vertical height and more tapered borders than does a true Schatzki ring. (*From Luedtke P, Levine MS, Rubesin SE, et al: Radiologic diagnosis of benign esophageal strictures: A pattern approach. RadioGraphics 23:897-909, 2003.*)

Barrett Esophagus

DEFINITION: Columnar metaplasia of the distal esophagus above gastroesophageal junction secondary to reflux disease.

ANATOMIC FINDINGS

Esophagus
- Long-segment Barrett esophagus is a zone of columnar metaplasia that extends more than 3 cm from gastroesophageal junction.
- Short-segment Barrett esophagus is a zone of columnar metaplasia that extends 3 cm or less from gastroesophageal junction.

IMAGING

Radiography
Findings
- Classic finding is a mid-esophageal stricture or ulcer or reticular pattern associated with sliding hiatal hernia or gastroesophageal reflux.
- Strictures appear as ring-like constrictions or tapered areas of narrowing.
- Ulcer craters are relatively deep and occur at a discrete distance from the gastroesophageal junction.
- Early strictures are seen as subtle contour abnormalities with focal indentations or gently sloping concavities.
- Reticular pattern of innumerable tiny, barium-filled grooves or crevices often adjacent to distal aspect of mid-esophageal stricture
- Patient may show associated radiographic signs of reflux disease, such as peptic strictures.
Utility
- Double-contrast esophagography findings help determine which patients require endoscopy based on Gilchrist criteria.
- Short-segment disease may have normal esophagus on double-contrast esophagography.
- Similar strictures are caused by caustic ingestion and radiation.

DIAGNOSTIC PEARLS
- Classic finding of mid-esophageal stricture or ulcer
- Reticular pattern of innumerable tiny, barium-filled grooves often adjacent to the distal aspect of mid-esophageal stricture
- Associated radiologic signs of reflux disease

CLINICAL PRESENTATION
- Condition may produce reflux symptoms or dysphagia.
- Many patients are asymptomatic.

DIFFERENTIAL DIAGNOSIS
- Reflux esophagitis
- *Candida* esophagitis
- Caustic esophagitis
- Radiation esophagitis
- Adenocarcinoma (esophagus)
- Squamous cell carcinoma (esophagus)
- Idiopathic eosinophilic esophagitis
- Drug-induced esophagitis
- Benign mucous membrane pemphigoid involving the esophagus
- Epidermolysis bullosa dystrophica involving the esophagus

PATHOLOGY
- Long-standing reflux disease leads to columnar metaplasia of squamous epithelium in esophagus.

WHAT THE REFERRING PHYSICIAN NEEDS TO KNOW
- Endoscopy and biopsy are required for definitive diagnosis.
- Findings of mid-esophageal stricture, ulcer, or reticular mucosal pattern warrant endoscopy because of high risk of Barrett esophagus.
- Barrett esophagus is unlikely on double-contrast esophagography in absence of esophagitis, strictures, or other morphologic abnormalities in the esophagus.
- Endoscopic surveillance every 2 to 3 years is advocated to detect dysplastic changes leading to adenocarcinoma.
- Endoscopy without biopsy has sensitivity of greater than 90%.
- Double-contrast esophagography is a useful screening examination for Barrett esophagus to determine the relative need for endoscopy and biopsy in patients with reflux symptoms.
- When mid-esophageal strictures are detected on esophagography, caustic ingestion and radiation injury can be differentiated from Barrett esophagus based on history and clinical presentation.

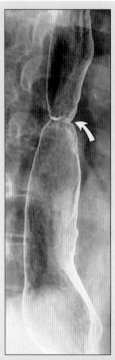

Figure 1. Barrett esophagus with mid-esophageal stricture. There is a ring-like constriction *(arrow)* in the mid-esophagus. In the presence of a hiatal hernia and gastroesophageal reflux, a mid-esophageal stricture should be strongly suggestive of Barrett esophagus. (*From Levine MS:* Radiology of the Esophagus. *Philadelphia, WB Saunders, 1989.*)

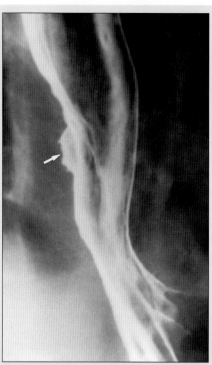

Figure 2. Barrett esophagus with a high ulcer. The relatively deep ulcer crater *(arrow)* is at a greater distance from the gastroesophageal junction than expected for uncomplicated reflux esophagitis. In the presence of a hiatal hernia and gastroesophageal reflux, a high ulcer should be strongly suggestive of Barrett esophagus. (*From Levine MS:* Radiology of the Esophagus. *Philadelphia, WB Saunders, 1989.*)

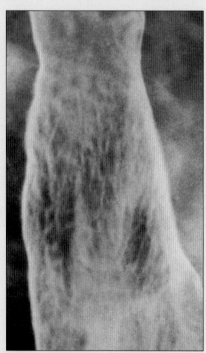

Figure 3. Barrett esophagus with a reticular mucosal pattern. A mild stricture is present in the mid-esophagus with a distinctive reticular pattern of the mucosa extending distally from the stricture. (*From Levine MS, Kressel HY, Caroline DF, et al: Barrett esophagus: Reticular pattern of the mucosa.* Radiology 147:663-667, 1983.)

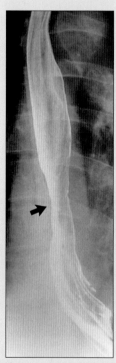

Figure 4. Barrett esophagus with a distal stricture. A concentric area of narrowing *(arrow)* in the distal esophagus is seen above a hiatal hernia. An ordinary peptic stricture without Barrett esophagus can produce identical findings. (*From Levine MS:* Radiology of the Esophagus. *Philadelphia, WB Saunders, 1989.*)

- A velvety, pinkish red columnar mucosa is produced, which extends above the lower esophageal sphincter or an endoscopically identified hiatal hernia.
- Intestinal metaplasia on esophageal endoscopic biopsy specimens is a major prerequisite for the histopathologic diagnosis of Barrett esophagus.
- Intestinal metaplasia is characterized by goblet cells with acidic mucin, enterocyte differentiation, and brush border formation.

INCIDENCE/PREVALENCE AND EPIDEMIOLOGY

- Mean age is 55 to 60 years.
- Male to female ratio is 2:1.
- More common in whites than blacks
- Prevalence in patients with reflux esophagitis is approximately 10%.
- Most cases are undiagnosed because of the absence of esophageal symptoms.
- Short-segment disease more common than long-segment disease.
- Long-segment disease is more likely to develop dysplasia.

Suggested Readings

Agha FP: Radiologic diagnosis of Barrett's esophagus. Critical analysis of 65 cases. *Gastrointest Radiol* 11:123-130, 1986.

Chen YM, Gelfand DW, Ott DJ, et al: Barrett esophagus as an extension of severe esophagitis: Analysis of radiologic signs in 29 cases. *AJR Am J Roentgenol* 145:275-281, 1985.

Gilchrist AM, Levine MS, Carr RF, et al: Barrett's esophagus: Diagnosis by double-contrast esophagography. *AJR Am J Roentgenol* 150:97-102, 1988.

Glick SN: Barium studies in patients with Barrett's esophagus: Importance of focal areas of esophageal deformity. *AJR Am J Roentgenol* 163:65-67, 1994.

Spechler SJ: Barrett's esophagus. *N Engl J Med* 346:836-842, 2002.

Yamamoto AJ, Levine MS, Katzka DA, et al: Short-segment Barrett's esophagus: Findings on double-contrast esophagography in 20 patients. *AJR Am J Roentgenol* 176:1173-1178, 2001.

Part 8

INFECTIOUS ESOPHAGITIS

Candida Esophagitis

DEFINITION: Esophageal infection by *Candida* organisms.

IMAGING

Radiography
Findings
- Discrete plaque-like lesions separated by normal mucosa in linear or irregular pattern
- Finely nodular or granular appearance
- *Snakeskin* or cobblestone appearance
- Grossly irregular or *shaggy* contour with severe candidiasis in patients with acquired immunodeficiency syndrome (AIDS)
- One or more deep ulcers superimposed on background of diffuse plaque formation
- Other unusual findings include intramural tracks (*double-barreled* esophagus) and polypoid lesions caused by balls of mycelia.
- *Candida* esophagitis may lead to foamy esophagus in patients with achalasia or scleroderma.

Utility
- Single-contrast esophagography is an unreliable technique for diagnosis.
- Double-contrast esophagography has a sensitivity of approximately 90% for detecting this condition.

CLINICAL PRESENTATION

- Acute onset of dysphagia or odynophagia characterized by intense substernal pain or burning during swallowing
- Nonspecific findings (e.g., chest pain, epigastric pain, or upper gastrointestinal bleeding)
- Occasional patients may be asymptomatic

DIAGNOSTIC PEARLS

- Discrete plaque-like lesions separated by normal mucosa in linear or irregular pattern
- Finely nodular or granular appearance
- *Snakeskin* appearance or cobblestone appearance
- One or more deep ulcers superimposed on background of diffuse plaque formation
- Other unusual findings: intramural track or *double-barreled* esophagus and polypoid balls of mycelia

DIFFERENTIAL DIAGNOSIS

- Glycogenic acanthosis
- Superficial spreading carcinoma
- Reticular pattern of Barrett esophagus
- Reflux esophagitis

PATHOLOGY

- *Candida albicans,* a commensal inhabitant of pharynx, is almost always offending organism.
- Downward spread of fungus to esophagus is the presumed cause.
- Local esophageal stasis contributes to *Candida* colonization.

WHAT THE REFERRING PHYSICIAN NEEDS TO KNOW

- Only 50% of patients with *Candida* esophagitis have fungal lesions in oropharynx.
- *Candida* esophagitis may be difficult to differentiate from viral esophagitis on clinical grounds.
- Esophagus may simultaneously be colonized by fungal and viral organisms.
- Mucosal plaques or nodules may also be caused by reflux esophagitis, glycogenic acanthosis, and superficial spreading carcinoma but with different radiographic findings and clinical history.
- Presence of multiple discrete plaque-like lesions or shaggy esophagus is virtually diagnostic of *Candida* esophagitis on barium studies.
- Presence of budding yeast cells, hyphae, and pseudohyphae on endoscopic biopsy specimens is diagnostic of *Candida* esophagitis.
- Characteristic endoscopic appearance of *Candida* esophagitis consists of patchy, white plaques covering a friable, erythematous mucosa.

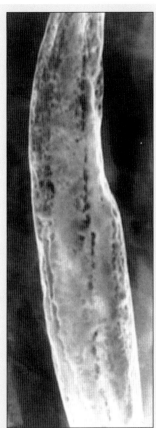

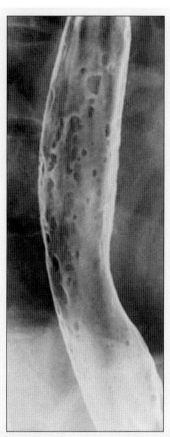

Figure 1. *Candida* **esophagitis with discrete plaques.**
Multiple plaque-like lesions are present in the esophagus. The
plaques have a characteristic appearance with discrete borders
and a predominantly longitudinal orientation. (*From Levine
MS, Macones AJ, Laufer I:* Candida *esophagitis: Accuracy of
radiographic diagnosis.* Radiology *154:581-587, 1985.*)

Figure 2. *Candida* **esophagitis with discrete plaques.** In
this patient, the plaques have a more irregular configuration.
However, they are still seen as discrete lesions separated by
normal mucosa. (*From Levine MS, Macones AJ, Laufer I:* Candida
esophagitis: Accuracy of radiographic diagnosis. Radiology *154:
581-587, 1985.*)

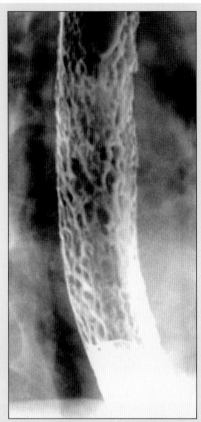

Figure 3. *Candida* **esophagitis with a cobblestone appearance.** Confluent involvement of the mucosa is recognized by innumerable round, oval, and polygonal plaques. (*From Levine MS: Radiology of the Esophagus. Philadelphia, WB Saunders, 1989.*)

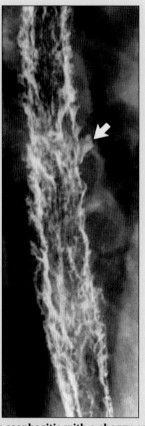

Figure 4. *Candida* **esophagitis with a shaggy esophagus.** The esophagus has a grossly irregular contour as a result of multiple plaques and pseudomembranes with trapping of barium between these lesions. A deep area of ulceration *(arrow)* is also seen. This patient had AIDS. (*From Levine MS, Woldenberg R, Herlinger H, et al: Opportunistic esophagitis in AIDS: Radiographic diagnosis. Radiology 165:815-820, 1987.*)

INCIDENCE/PREVALENCE AND EPIDEMIOLOGY

- Occurs primarily in patients who are immunocompromised or have localized esophageal stasis
- Particularly prevalent with AIDS, occurring in 15% to 20% of patients with this disease
- Candidiasis is the most common cause of infectious esophagitis.

Suggested Readings

Agha FP: Candidiasis-induced esophageal strictures. *Gastrointest Radiol* 9:283-286, 1984.

Baehr PH, McDonald GB: Esophageal infections: Risk factors, presentation, diagnosis, and treatment. *Gastroenterology* 106:509-532, 1994.

Barbaro G, Barbarini G, Calderon W, et al: Fluconazole versus itraconazole for *Candida* esophagitis in acquired immunodeficiency syndrome. *Gastroenterology* 111:1169-1177, 1996.

Beauchamp JM, Nice CM, Belanger MA, et al: Esophageal intramural pseudodiverticulosis. *Radiology* 113:273-276, 1974.

Brayko CM, Kozavek RA, Sanowski RA, et al: Type I herpes simplex esophagitis with concomitant esophageal moniliasis. *J Clin Gastroenterol* 4:351-355, 1982.

Farman J, Tivitian A, Rosenthal LE, et al: Focal esophageal candidiasis in acquired immunodeficiency syndrome (AIDS). *Gastrointest Radiol* 11:213-217, 1986.

Friedman HM, Gluckman SJ: Infections of the esophagus. In Cohen S, Soloway RD (eds): *Diseases of the Esophagus*. New York, Churchill Livingstone, 1982, pp 277-286.

Gefter WB, Laufer I, Edell S, et al: Candidiasis in the obstructed esophagus. *Radiology* 138:25-28, 1981.

Glick SN: Barium studies in patients with *Candida* esophagitis: Pseudo-ulcerations simulating viral esophagitis. *AJR Am J Roentgenol* 163:349-352, 1994.

Levine MS, Macones AJ, Laufer I: *Candida* esophagitis: Accuracy of radiographic diagnosis. *Radiology* 154:581-587, 1985.

Levine MS, Woldenberg R, Herlinger H, et al: Opportunistic esophagitis in AIDS: Radiographic findings. *Radiology* 165:815-820, 1987.

Herpes Esophagitis

DEFINITION: Infectious esophagitis caused by herpesvirus.

IMAGING

Radiography

Findings
- Ulcers appear as multiple small (< 1 cm), superficial ulcers in upper or mid-esophagus without plaque formation.
- Ulcers are punctate, linear, ring-like, or stellate and are often surrounded by radiolucent mounds of edema.
- Extensive ulceration, plaque formation, or combination of ulcers and plaques occurs in more advanced disease.
- Otherwise healthy patients with herpes esophagitis may have innumerable tiny ulcers that tend to be clustered together in the mid-esophagus.

Utility
- Ulcers are visible on double-contrast esophagography in more than 50% of endoscopically proven cases.
- Advanced cases may be indistinguishable from *Candida* esophagitis.

CLINICAL PRESENTATION

- Acute odynophagia occurs with severe substernal chest pain during swallowing.
- Occasionally signs or symptoms of upper gastrointestinal bleeding occur.
- Condition is usually self-limited, but symptoms resolve when treated with antiviral agents (e.g., acyclovir).
- Although vast majority of patients are immunocompromised, otherwise healthy individuals with herpes esophagitis may exhibit a 3- to 10-day influenza-like prodrome characterized by fever, sore throat, upper respiratory tract infection, and myalgias.
- Otherwise healthy patients with herpes esophagitis usually have a history of recent exposure to sexual partners with herpetic lesions on lips or buccal mucosa.

DIFFERENTIAL DIAGNOSIS

- Drug-induced esophagitis
- Cytomegalovirus esophagitis
- Human immunodeficiency virus esophagitis
- Reflux esophagitis

DIAGNOSTIC PEARLS

- Signs include multiple small (< 1 cm), superficial ulcers in the upper esophagus or mid-esophagus without plaque formation.
- Ulcers are punctate, linear, ring-like, or stellate and are often surrounded by radiolucent mounds of edema.
- Extensive ulceration, plaque formation, or combination of ulcers and plaques occur in more advanced disease.
- Innumerable tiny ulcers tend to be clustered together in the mid-esophagus in otherwise healthy patients.
- Histologic finding of Cowdry type A intranuclear inclusions in intact epithelial cells adjacent to ulcers is virtually pathognomonic of herpes.

- *Candida* esophagitis
- Radiation esophagitis
- Crohn disease (esophagitis)

PATHOLOGY

- Condition is caused by herpes simplex virus type 1 (DNA core virus) in immunocompromised patients.
- Histologic finding of Cowdry type A intranuclear inclusions in intact epithelial cells adjacent to ulcers is pathognomonic of herpes.
- Diagnosis of herpes esophagitis can also be confirmed by positive viral cultures from esophagus or by direct immunofluorescence staining for the herpes simplex antigen.

INCIDENCE/PREVALENCE AND EPIDEMIOLOGY

- Otherwise healthy patients are typically sexually active young men.
- Herpes esophagitis more commonly occurs in patients who are immunocompromised.

WHAT THE REFERRING PHYSICIAN NEEDS TO KNOW

- Radiographic finding of multiple small, discrete ulcers in upper or middle esophagus should be highly suggestive of herpes esophagitis in immunocompromised patient with odynophagia.
- Histologic finding of Cowdry type A intranuclear inclusions in intact epithelial cells adjacent to ulcers is virtually pathognomonic of herpes.
- Diagnosis of herpes esophagitis can also be confirmed by positive viral cultures from esophagus or by direct immunofluorescence staining for herpes simplex antigen.

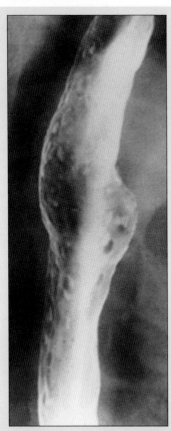

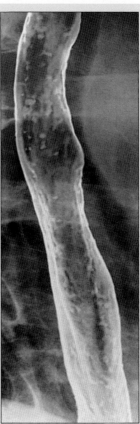

Figure 1. Herpes esophagitis with discrete ulcers. Multiple discrete, superficial ulcers are seen in the mid-esophagus. Many of the ulcers are surrounded by radiolucent mounds of edema. (*From Levine MS: Radiology of esophagitis: A pattern approach.* Radiology *179:1-7, 1991.*)

Figure 2. Herpes esophagitis with discrete ulcers. Multiple discrete, superficial ulcers are seen in the mid-esophagus. Many of the ulcers are surrounded by radiolucent mounds of edema. (*Courtesy of Harvey M. Goldstein, MD, San Antonio, TX.*)

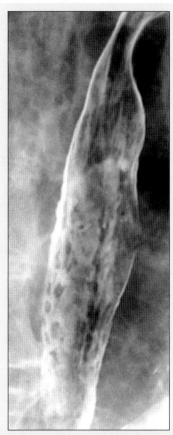

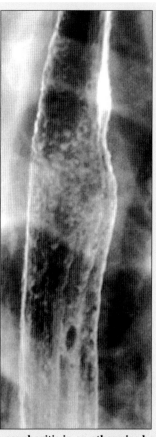

Figure 3. Herpes esophagitis. Multiple plaque-like lesions are seen in the mid-esophagus, mimicking the appearance of candidiasis. (*From Levine MS, Laufer I, Kressel HY, et al: Herpes esophagitis. AJR Am J Roentgenol 136:863-866, 1981; © by American Roentgen Ray Society.*)

Figure 4. Herpes esophagitis in an otherwise healthy patient. Multiple punctate and linear areas of ulceration are seen in the mid-esophagus below the level of the left main bronchus. This appearance is characteristic of herpes esophagitis in immunocompetent patients. (*From DeGaeta L, Levine MS, Guglielmi GE, et al: Herpes esophagitis in an otherwise healthy patient. AJR Am J Roentgenol 144:1205-1206, 1985; © by American Roentgen Ray Society.*)

Suggested Readings

Depew WT, Prentice RS, Beck IT, et al: Herpes simplex ulcerative esophagitis in a healthy subject. *Am J Gastroenterol* 68:381-385, 1977.

Deshmukh M, Shah R, McCallum RW: Experience with herpes esophagitis in otherwise healthy patients. *Am J Gastroenterol* 79:173-176, 1984.

Desigan G, Schneider RP: Herpes simplex esophagitis in healthy adults. *South Med J* 78:1135-1137, 1985.

Fishbein PG, Tuthill R, Kressel HY, et al: Herpes simplex esophagitis: A cause of upper gastrointestinal bleeding. *Dig Dis Sci* 24:540-544, 1979.

Friedman HM, Gluckman SJ: Infections of the esophagus. In Cohen S, Soloway RD (eds): *Diseases of the Esophagus.* New York, Churchill Livingstone, 1982, pp 277-286.

Klotz DA, Silverman L: Herpes virus esophagitis, consistent with herpes simplex, visualized endoscopically. *Gastrointest Endosc* 21:71-73, 1974.

Levine MS, Laufer I, Kressel HY, et al: Herpes esophagitis. *AJR Am J Roentgenol* 136:863-866, 1981.

Levine MS, Loevner LA, Saul SH, et al: Herpes esophagitis: Sensitivity of double-contrast esophagography. *AJR Am J Roentgenol* 151: 57-62, 1988.

Levine MS, Macones AJ, Laufer I: *Candida* esophagitis: Accuracy of radiographic diagnosis. *Radiology* 154:581-587, 1985.

Levine MS, Woldenberg R, Herlinger H, et al: Opportunistic esophagitis in AIDS: Radiographic diagnosis. *Radiology* 165:815-820, 1987.

Cytomegalovirus Esophagitis

DEFINITION: Infectious esophagitis caused by cytomegalovirus (CMV).

IMAGING

Radiography
Findings
- Discrete, superficial ulcers that are indistinguishable from those of herpes esophagitis
- More commonly, one or more giant (greater than 1 cm in size), flat ulcers in distal or mid-esophagus
- Ulcers are seen as ovoid, elongated, or diamond-shaped collections of barium surrounded by radiolucent rim of edematous mucosa.
- Human immunodeficiency virus (HIV) esophagitis may also be recognized by one or more giant ulcers indistinguishable from those in CMV esophagitis.

Utility
- Double-contrast esophagography

CLINICAL PRESENTATION

- Severe odynophagia
- Dysphagia

DIFFERENTIAL DIAGNOSIS

- Herpes esophagitis
- HIV esophagitis
- Drug-induced esophagitis

PATHOLOGY

- CMV belongs to a group of herpesviruses that cause infectious esophagitis in patients with acquired immunodeficiency syndrome (AIDS).
- Characteristic microscopic features include intranuclear inclusions and small cytoplasmic inclusions in endothelial cells or fibroblasts at base of ulcers.

INCIDENCE/PREVALENCE AND EPIDEMIOLOGY

- CMV is rare in immunocompromised states other than AIDS.

DIAGNOSTIC PEARLS

- Some patients have discrete, superficial ulcers indistinguishable from those in herpes esophagitis.
- More commonly, there are one or more giant (> 1 cm), flat ulcers in middle or distal esophagus.
- Ulcers are ovoid, elongated, or diamond-shaped collections of barium surrounded by radiolucent rim of edematous mucosa.
- Characteristic microscopic features include intranuclear inclusions and small cytoplasmic inclusions in endothelial cells or fibroblasts at base of ulcers.
- Endoscopic biopsy is necessary for definitive diagnosis.

Suggested Readings

Baehr PH, McDonald GB: Esophageal infections: Risk factors, presentation, diagnosis, and treatment. *Gastroenterology* 106:509-532, 1994.

Balthazar EJ, Megibow AJ, Hulnick DH: Cytomegalovirus esophagitis and gastritis in AIDS. *AJR Am J Roentgenol* 144:1201-1204, 1985.

Balthazar EJ, Megibow AJ, Hulnick D, et al: Cytomegalovirus esophagitis in AIDS: Radiographic features in 16 patients. *AJR Am J Roentgenol* 149:919-923, 1987.

Frager DH, Frager JD, Brandt LJ, et al: Gastrointestinal complications of AIDS: Radiologic features. *Radiology* 158:597-603, 1986.

Levine MS, Woldenberg R, Herlinger H, et al: Opportunistic esophagitis in AIDS: Radiographic diagnosis. *Radiology* 165:815-820, 1987.

Teixidor HS, Honig CL, Norsoph E, et al: Cytomegalovirus infection of the alimentary canal: Radiologic findings with pathologic correlation. *Radiology* 163:317-323, 1987.

Wilcox CM, Diehl DL, Cello JP, et al: Cytomegalovirus esophagitis in patients with AIDS: A clinical, endoscopic, and pathologic correlation. *Ann Intern Med* 113:589-593, 1990.

WHAT THE REFERRING PHYSICIAN NEEDS TO KNOW

- HIV may cause giant esophageal ulcers indistinguishable from CMV ulcers on esophagography.
- Endoscopy and biopsy are therefore required to differentiate CMV esophagitis from HIV esophagitis before treating these patients.
- If biopsy specimens or viral cultures are positive for CMV, treatment can be initiated with potent antiviral agents.

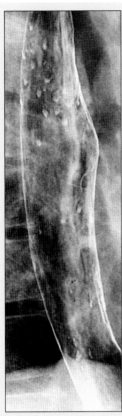

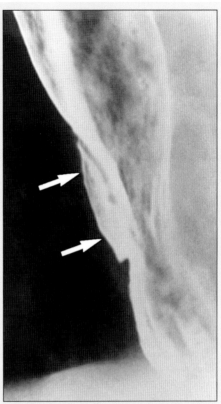

Figure 1. Cytomegalovirus esophagitis. Multiple discrete, superficial ulcers are seen in the mid-esophagus. Herpes esophagitis can produce identical radiographic findings. (*From Levine MS: Radiology of the Esophagus. Philadelphia, WB Saunders, 1989.*)

Figure 2. Cytomegalovirus esophagitis. A giant, relatively flat ulcer *(arrows)* is seen in profile in the distal esophagus. (*Courtesy of Sidney W. Nelson, MD, Seattle, WA.*)

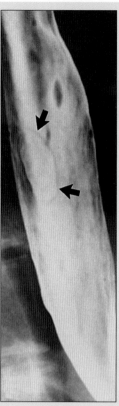

Figure 3. Cytomegalovirus esophagitis. A large, ovoid ulcer *(arrows)* is seen en face. Note the thin radiolucent rim of edema surrounding the ulcer. Because herpetic ulcers rarely become this large, the presence of one or more giant esophageal ulcers should raise the possibility of cytomegalovirus esophagitis in patients with AIDS. However, HIV esophagitis can produce identical findings. Endoscopy and biopsy are therefore required for a definitive diagnosis before treating these patients. (*Courtesy of Kyunghee C. Cho, MD, Newark, NJ.*)

Human Immunodeficiency Virus Esophagitis

DEFINITION: Esophageal lesions caused by human immunodeficiency virus (HIV) infection.

IMAGING

Radiography
Findings
- Ulcers appear as one or more giant (> 1 cm in size), flat ulcers in middle or distal esophagus, sometimes associated with small, satellite ulcers.
- Ulcers are ovoid, elongated, or diamond-shaped collections of barium surrounded by radiolucent rim of edema.
- HIV ulcers are indistinguishable from giant ulcers in cytomegalovirus (CMV) esophagitis.

Utility
- Double-contrast esophagography

CLINICAL PRESENTATION

- Acute onset of odynophagia or dysphagia, sometimes so severe that affected individuals are unable to swallow their saliva.
- Occasionally, hematemesis or other signs of upper gastrointestinal bleeding develop.
- HIV ulcers occur at or soon after seroconversion or, more commonly, when patient develops clinically overt acquired immunodeficiency syndrome (AIDS).
- Some patients have associated ulcers in soft palate and oropharynx, as well as characteristic maculopapular rash on face, trunk, and upper extremities.

DIFFERENTIAL DIAGNOSIS

- CMV esophagitis
- Kaposi sarcoma
- Tuberculous esophagitis
- Nasogastric intubation
- Endoscopic sclerotherapy
- Drug-induced esophagitis

DIAGNOSTIC PEARLS

- Acute onset of severe odynophagia or dysphagia
- Associated with maculopapular rash involving face, trunk, and upper extremities in patients with AIDS
- One or more giant (> 1 cm), flat ulcers in the mid-esophagus or distal esophagus, sometimes associated with small, satellite ulcers
- Imaging findings indistinguishable from those of CMV esophagitis

PATHOLOGY

- Electron microscopy of biopsy specimens has demonstrated viral particles with morphologic features of HIV.
- HIV ulcers in the esophagus may be associated with oropharyngeal or soft palate ulcers.
- Affected individuals may have characteristic maculopapular rash involving face, trunk, and upper extremities.

INCIDENCE/PREVALENCE AND EPIDEMIOLOGY

- Condition occurs in HIV-positive patients at or soon after seroconversion or, more commonly, in those with full-blown AIDS.

Suggested Readings

Bach MC, Howell DA, Valenti AJ, et al: Aphthous ulceration of the gastrointestinal tract in patients with the acquired immunodeficiency syndrome (AIDS). *Ann Intern Med* 112:465-466, 1990.

Bach MC, Valenti AJ, Howell DA, et al: Odynophagia from aphthous ulcers of the pharynx and esophagus in the acquired immunodeficiency syndrome (AIDS). *Ann Intern Med* 109:338-339, 1988.

Baehr PH, McDonald GB: Esophageal infections: Risk factors, presentation, diagnosis, and treatment. *Gastroenterology* 106:509-532, 1994.

Frager D, Kotler DP, Baer J: Idiopathic esophageal ulceration in the acquired immunodeficiency syndrome: Radiologic reappraisal in 10 patients. *Abdom Imaging* 19:2-5, 1994.

Sor S, Levine MS, Kowalski TE, et al: Giant ulcers of the esophagus in patients with human immunodeficiency virus: Clinical, radiographic, and pathologic findings. *Radiology* 1994:447-451, 1995.

WHAT THE REFERRING PHYSICIAN NEEDS TO KNOW

- HIV esophagitis is primarily a diagnosis of exclusion.
- In contrast to CMV ulcers, HIV ulcers may heal spontaneously or may respond to treatment with oral steroids (without need for potentially toxic agents such as ganciclovir).
- Endoscopic biopsies, brushings, and cultures are required to differentiate HIV ulcers from CMV ulcers so appropriate treatment can be initiated.
- HIV esophagitis rarely may be associated with the development of esophagoesophageal or esophagogastric fistulas or focal perforation into the mediastinum.
- Other considerations in differential diagnosis include tuberculous esophagitis, nasogastric intubation, endoscopic sclerotherapy, and drug-induced esophagitis, which can usually be excluded by history and clinical presentation.

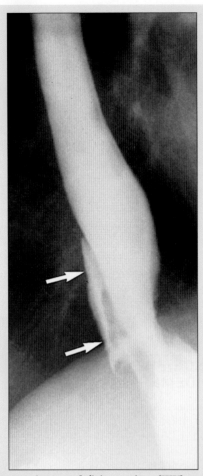

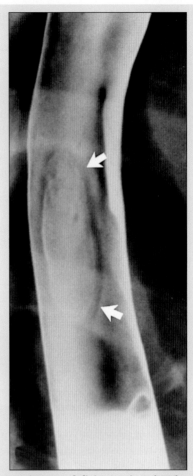

Figure 1. Human immunodeficiency virus (HIV) esophagitis. A giant, relatively flat ulcer (*arrows*) is seen in profile in the distal esophagus. This patient was HIV positive. The ulcer is indistinguishable from CMV ulcers. However, endoscopic biopsy specimens, brushings, and cultures were negative for CMV in this patient. (*From Levine MS, Loercher G, Katzka DA, et al: Giant, human immunodeficiency virus-related ulcers in the esophagus.* Radiology *180:323-326, 1991.*)

Figure 2. Human immunodeficiency virus (HIV) esophagitis. In an HIV-positive patient, a large ovoid ulcer *(arrows)* is seen en face with a thin surrounding rim of edema. The ulcer is indistinguishable from CMV ulcers. However, endoscopic biopsy specimens, brushings, and cultures were negative for CMV in this patient. (*From Levine MS, Loercher G, Katzka DA, et al: Giant, human immunodeficiency virus-related ulcers in the esophagus.* Radiology *180:323-326, 1991.*)

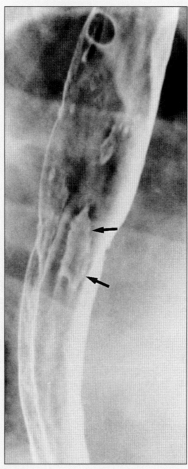

Figure 3. **Human immunodeficiency virus (HIV) esophagitis.** In a third patient, a diamond-shaped ulcer *(arrows)* is seen in the mid-esophagus with a cluster of small satellite ulcers. The ulcer is indistinguishable from CMV ulcers. However, endoscopic biopsy specimens, brushings, and cultures were negative for CMV in this patient. (*From Levine MS, Loercher G, Katzka DA, et al: Giant, human immunodeficiency virus-related ulcers in the esophagus.* Radiology *180:323-326, 1991.*)

Tuberculous Esophagitis

DEFINITION: Esophagitis caused by tubercle bacilli.

IMAGING

Radiography
Findings
- Extrinsic involvement includes compression, displacement, or narrowing of esophagus.
- Caseating nodes may cause ulceration, sinus tracks into mediastinum or tracheobronchial tree, strictures, or traction diverticula.
- Intrinsic involvement includes mucosal irregularity, ulcers, plaques, fistulas, and, eventually, strictures.
- Rarely, esophageal tuberculosis can lead to intramural abscess seen on esophagography as smooth submucosal mass.

Utility
- Esophagography
- Similar findings to those seen in Crohn disease, trauma, radiation esophagitis, esophageal carcinoma, but without pulmonary and mediastinal findings seen in tuberculosis

CT
Findings
- Well-marginated cystic mass with enhancing rim

CLINICAL PRESENTATION

- May be asymptomatic or present with dysphagia, odynophagia, or chest pain

DIFFERENTIAL DIAGNOSIS

- Caustic esophagitis
- Radiation esophagitis
- Crohn disease (esophagus)
- Human immunodeficiency virus esophagitis

PATHOLOGY

- *Mycobacterium tuberculosis* and *Mycobacterium avium-intracellulare* may cause esophageal tuberculosis by hematogenous seeding or swallowing of sputum with tubercle bacilli.

DIAGNOSTIC PEARLS

- Extrinsic involvement is manifested by compression, displacement, or narrowing of the esophagus.
- Caseating nodes may cause ulceration, sinus tracks into mediastinum or tracheobronchial tree, and strictures or traction diverticula.
- Intrinsic involvement is manifested by mucosal irregularity, ulcers, plaques, fistulas, and, eventually, strictures.
- Condition is associated with advanced tuberculosis in lungs or mediastinum.

INCIDENCE/PREVALENCE AND EPIDEMIOLOGY

- Extremely uncommon
- Usually associated with advanced tuberculosis in lungs or mediastinum

Suggested Readings

de Silva R, Stoopack PM, Raufman JP: Esophageal fistulas associated with mycobacterial infection in patients at risk for AIDS. *Radiology* 175:449-453, 1990.

Goodman P, Pinero SS, Rance RM, et al: Mycobacterial esophagitis in AIDS. *Gastrointest Radiol* 14:103-105, 1989.

Kim HG: Esophageal tuberculosis manifesting as submucosal abscess. *AJR Am J Roentgenol* 180:1482-1483, 2003.

Ramakantan R, Shah P: Tuberculous fistulas of the pharynx and esophagus. *Gastrointest Radiol* 15:145-147, 1990.

Savage PE, Grundy A: Oesophageal tuberculosis: An unusual cause of dysphagia. *Br J Radiol* 57:1153-1155, 1984.

Williford ME, Thompson WM, Hamilton JD, et al: Esophageal tuberculosis: Findings on barium swallow and computed tomography. *Gastrointest Radiol* 8:119-124, 1983.

WHAT THE REFERRING PHYSICIAN NEEDS TO KNOW

- Similar findings may be demonstrated in patients with Crohn disease, trauma, radiation, or caustic ingestion.
- Diagnosis may be confirmed by presence of tubercle bacilli or caseating granulomas on endoscopic biopsy specimens.

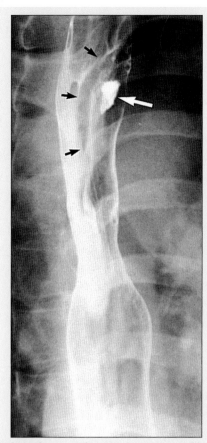

Figure 1. Tuberculous esophagitis. Compression *(black arrows)* of the upper thoracic esophagus occurs with associated ulceration *(white arrow)* as a result of caseating tuberculous nodes that have eroded into the esophagus. *(Courtesy of Alan Grundy, MD, London, England.)*

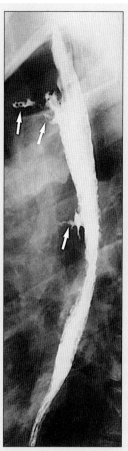

Figure 2. Tuberculous esophagitis in a patient with acquired immunodeficiency syndrome. Diffuse esophagitis with several deep sinus tracks *(arrows)* occurs and extends anteriorly from the esophagus into the mediastinum. *(From Goodman P, Pinero SS, Rance RM, et al: Mycobacterial esophagitis in AIDS. Gastrointest Radiol 14:103-105, 1989.)*

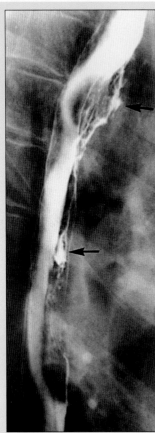

Figure 3. **Tuberculous esophagitis.** The initial esophagogram shows two areas of irregular ulceration (*arrows*) in the mid-esophagus caused by proven tuberculous esophagitis. (*From Savage PE, Grundy A: Oesophageal tuberculosis: An unusual cause of dysphagia. Br J Radiol 57:1153-1155, 1984.*)

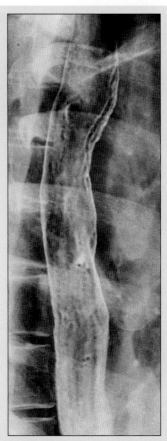

Figure 4. **Tuberculous esophagitis.** Another esophagogram in the same patient as in Figure 3 after 6 months of antituberculous therapy shows healing of ulcers. (*From Savage PE, Grundy A: Oesophageal tuberculosis: An unusual cause of dysphagia. Br J Radiol 57:1153-1155, 1984.*)

Drug-Induced Esophagitis

DEFINITION: Injury to esophagus after ingestion of medication.

IMAGING

Radiography

Findings

- Solitary ulcer, several discrete ulcers, or multiple small ulcers on normal background mucosa
- Ulcers seen en face as punctate, linear, ovoid, stellate, or serpiginous collections of barium on esophageal mucosa or in profile as shallow depressions
- Because of associated edema and inflammation, considerable mass effect surrounding a large ulcer can mimic the appearance of an ulcerated carcinoma.
- Giant, relatively flat ulcers that are several centimeters or more in length
- Healing ulcers may lead to development of smooth, re-epithelialized depressions mistaken for active ulcer craters.
- Severe ulcerative esophagitis and stricture formation in mid- or distal esophagus

Utility

- Double-contrast esophagography is a useful technique for detecting shallow ulcers that cannot easily be recognized on single-contrast studies.
- Follow-up esophagogram 7 to 10 days after withdrawal of offending agent may show dramatic healing of ulcers.

CLINICAL PRESENTATION

- Patient exhibits odynophagia (painful swallowing) or unremitting chest pain accentuated by swallowing.
- Other patients may show signs or symptoms of upper gastrointestinal bleeding.
- Symptoms usually develop within several hours to days after taking medication.
- Symptoms resolve rapidly after withdrawal of offending agent; patients may become asymptomatic within 7 to 10 days after stopping medication.
- Occasionally, patients may have progressive dysphagia because of development of strictures.

DIAGNOSTIC PEARLS

- Solitary ulcer, several discrete ulcers, or multiple small ulcers on normal background mucosa
- Punctate, linear, ovoid, stellate, or serpiginous collections of barium on esophageal mucosa
- Ulcers resolve rapidly after withdrawal of offending agent.

DIFFERENTIAL DIAGNOSIS

- Herpes esophagitis
- Cytomegalovirus esophagitis
- Reflux esophagitis
- Crohn disease (esophagitis)
- Caustic esophagitis
- Human immunodeficiency virus esophagitis
- Radiation esophagitis

PATHOLOGY

- Medications that are implicated most frequently include tetracycline, doxycycline, potassium chloride, quinidine, aspirin, other nonsteroidal anti-inflammatory drugs (NSAIDs), and alendronate sodium.
- Prolonged retention of medication may result from esophageal compression by an enlarged heart.
- Occurs in patients with abnormal motility or preexisting strictures that delay transit of pills from esophagus
- Focal contact esophagitis with ulceration of adjacent mucosa by dissolving pills

INCIDENCE/PREVALENCE AND EPIDEMIOLOGY

- Tetracycline and doxycycline, two widely used antibiotics, account for approximately 50% of reported cases of drug-induced esophagitis.

WHAT THE REFERRING PHYSICIAN NEEDS TO KNOW

- Diagnosis should be considered only when a definite temporal relationship exists between ingestion of offending medication and the onset of esophagitis.
- Correct diagnosis can usually be suggested based on the clinical history.
- Possibility of drug-induced stricture should be suspected in patients with cardiomegaly and history of taking potassium chloride or quinidine.

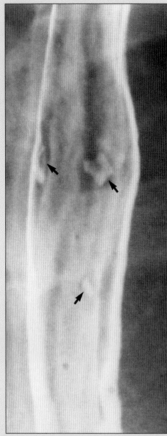

Figure 1. Drug-induced esophagitis with superficial ulcers.
Several discrete ulcers *(arrows)* are seen in the mid-esophagus
on a normal background mucosa. The largest ulcer has a stellate
configuration. The patient was taking tetracycline. (*From Levine
MS:* Radiology of the Esophagus. *Philadelphia, WB Saunders,
1989.*)

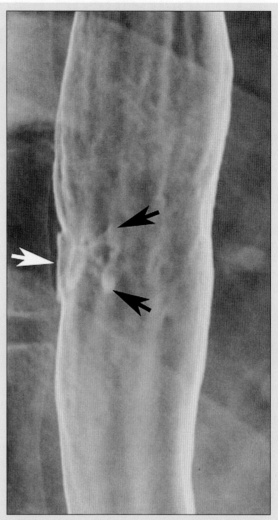

Figure 2. Drug-induced esophagitis with superficial ulcers.
This patient has a flat ulcer *(white arrow)* on the right lateral
wall of the mid-esophagus with a cluster of small ulcers *(black
arrows)* abutting the larger ulcer. The patient was taking
ibuprofen.

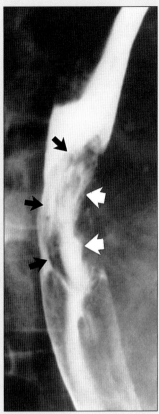

Figure 3. **Giant esophageal ulcer caused by potassium chloride.** A giant ulcer *(white arrows)* is seen in the mid-esophagus with an associated area of mass effect *(black arrows)* as a result of a surrounding mound of edema. This lesion could be mistaken for an ulcerated carcinoma.

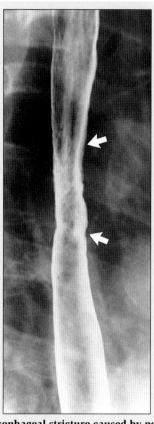

Figure 4. **Mid-esophageal stricture caused by potassium chloride.** A mid-esophageal stricture *(arrows)* is seen in a patient who had been taking slow-release potassium chloride tablets. The stricture has relatively tapered borders. (*From Levine MS:* Radiology of the Esophagus. *Philadelphia, WB Saunders, 1989.*)

Suggested Readings

Agha FP, Wilson JAP, Nostrand TT: Medication-induced esophagitis. *Gastrointest Radiol* 11:7-11, 1986.

Bonavina L, DeMeester TR, McChesney L, et al: Drug-induced esophageal strictures. *Ann Surg* 206:173-183, 1987.

Bova JG, Dutton NE, Goldstein HM, et al: Medication-induced esophagitis: Diagnosis by double-contrast esophagography. *AJR Am J Roentgenol* 148:731-732, 1987.

Coates AG, Nostrand TT, Wilson JAP, et al: Esophagitis caused by nonsteroidal antiinflammatory medication. *South Med J* 79:1094-1097, 1986.

Colina RE, Smith M, Kikendall JW, et al: A new probable increasing cause of esophageal ulceration: Alendronate. *Am J Gastroenterol* 92:704-706, 1997.

de Groen PC, Lubbe DF, Hirsch LJ, et al: Esophagitis associated with the use of alendronate. *N Engl J Med* 335:1016-1021, 1996.

Enzenauer RW, Bass JW, McDonnell JT: Esophageal ulceration associated with oral theophylline. *N Engl J Med* 310:261, 1984.

Heller SR, Fellows IW, Ogilvie AL, et al: Non-steroidal anti-inflammatory drugs and benign oesophageal stricture. *BMJ* 285:167-168, 1982.

Kikendall JW, Friedman AC, Oyewole MA, et al: Pill-induced esophageal injury: Case reports and review of the medical literature. *Dig Dis Sci* 28:174-182, 1983.

Lanza FL, Hunt RH, Thomson ABR, et al: Endoscopic comparison of esophageal and gastroduodenal effects of risedronate and alendronate in postmenopausal women. *Gastroenterology* 119:631-638, 2000.

Levine MS: Drug-induced disorders of the esophagus. *Abdom Imaging* 24:3-8, 1999.

Levine MS, Borislow SM, Rubesin SE, et al: Esophageal stricture caused by a Motrin tablet (ibuprofen). *Abdom Imaging* 19:6-7, 1994.

Levine MS, Loercher G, Katzka DA, et al: Giant, human immunodeficiency virus–related ulcers in the esophagus. *Radiology* 180:323-326, 1991.

Levine MS, Rothstein RD, Laufer I: Giant esophageal ulcer due to Clinoril. *AJR Am J Roentgenol* 156:955-956, 1991.

Ravich WJ, Kashima H, Donner MW: Drug-induced esophagitis simulating esophageal carcinoma. *Dysphagia* 1:13-18, 1986.

Ryan JM, Kelsey P, Ryan BM, et al: Alendronate-induced esophagitis: Case report of a recently recognized form of severe esophagitis with esophageal stricture—radiographic features. *AJR Am J Roentgenol* 206:389-391, 1998.

Semble EL, Wu WC, Castell DO: Nonsteroidal antiinflammatory drugs and esophageal injury. *Semin Arthritis Rheum* 19:99-109, 1989.

Shortsleeve MJ, Levine MS: Herpes esophagitis in otherwise healthy patients: Clinical and radiographic findings. *Radiology* 182:859-861, 1992.

Sugawa C, Takekuma Y, Lucas CE, et al: Bleeding esophageal ulcers caused by NSAIDs. *Surg Endosc* 11:143-146, 1997.

Radiation Esophagitis

DEFINITION: Self-limited esophagitis caused by radiation therapy.

IMAGING

Radiography
Findings
- Distinctive granular appearance of mucosa and decreased distensibility resulting from edema and inflammation of irradiated segment
- Multiple discrete ulcers within known radiation portal
- With severe disease, grossly irregular esophagus, with serrated contour caused by larger ulcers, and mucosal sloughing
- Radiation-induced strictures seen as smooth, tapered areas of narrowing in upper or mid-esophagus within preexisting radiation portal

Utility
- Double-contrast esophagography
- Esophagography used primarily to detect strictures or other signs of chronic radiation injury
- If esophageal-airway fistula is suspected, use barium sulfate because water-soluble contrast agent in the airway causes severe pulmonary edema.

CT
Utility
- CT can be used to differentiate radiation stricture from recurrent tumor in mediastinum.

CLINICAL PRESENTATION

- Patient exhibits self-limited esophagitis with acute onset of substernal burning, odynophagia, or dysphagia 1 to 3 weeks after onset of radiation therapy.
- Symptoms subside within 24 to 48 hours but may occasionally persist for several weeks.
- Chronic radiation injury to the esophagus may cause dysphagia within several months after completion of radiation therapy.
- Dysphagia may result from abnormal esophageal motility or, less commonly, from the development of strictures.
- Occasionally, severe radiation injury may lead to life-threatening complications such as an esophageal-airway fistula or esophageal perforation.
- Abnormal esophageal motility may develop 4 to 8 weeks after completion of radiation therapy.

DIAGNOSTIC PEARLS

- Self-limited esophagitis
- Multiple small, discrete ulcers within known radiation portal

DIFFERENTIAL DIAGNOSIS

- *Candida* esophagitis
- Cytomegalovirus esophagitis
- Herpes esophagitis
- Human immunodeficiency virus esophagitis
- Recurrent mediastinal tumor encasing esophagus

PATHOLOGY

- Total doses of 45 to 60 Gy may lead to severe esophagitis with irreversible damage and stricture formation.
- Smaller doses (20-45 Gy) may cause self-limited esophagitis without permanent sequelae.
- Chronic radiation esophagitis: Progressive submucosal scarring and fibrosis can lead to development of esophageal strictures 4 to 8 months after completion of radiation therapy.
- If radiation dose is more than 60 Gy, esophageal strictures may develop within 3 to 4 months.
- Tracheoesophageal and esophagobronchial fistulas are potentially life-threatening complications of mediastinal irradiation.
- Fistulas are usually caused by radiation necrosis, with erosion of tumor into esophagus and adjacent airway.
- Most frequent site of fistula formation is left main bronchus, which crosses esophagus at level of fourth or fifth thoracic vertebra.

Suggested Readings

Collazzo LA, Levine MS, Rubesin SE, et al: Acute radiation esophagitis: Radiographic findings. *AJR Am J Roentgenol* 169:1067-1070, 1997.

Goldstein HM, Rogers LF, Fletcher GH, et al: Radiological manifestations of radiation-induced injury to the normal upper gastrointestinal tract. *Radiology* 117:135-140, 1975.

Lepke RA, Libshitz HI: Radiation-induced injury of the esophagus. *Radiology* 148:375-378, 1983.

Northway MG, Libshitz HI, West JJ, et al: The opossum as an animal model for studying radiation esophagitis. *Radiology* 131:731-735, 1979.

WHAT THE REFERRING PHYSICIAN NEEDS TO KNOW

- Acute radiation esophagitis is treated empirically with viscous lidocaine and analgesics.
- Radiologic or endoscopic examinations are not often performed in this setting, given that the condition is usually self-limited.
- Esophagography is more important for patients who develop dysphagia months after completion of radiation therapy.

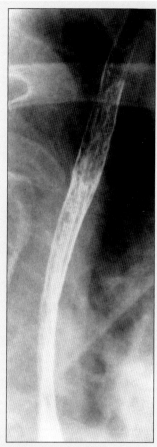

Figure 1. Acute radiation esophagitis. The mucosa has a granular appearance in the upper thoracic esophagus. Also note decreased distensibility of the irradiated segment. The patient had acute odynophagia 3 weeks after undergoing mediastinal irradiation for bronchogenic carcinoma.

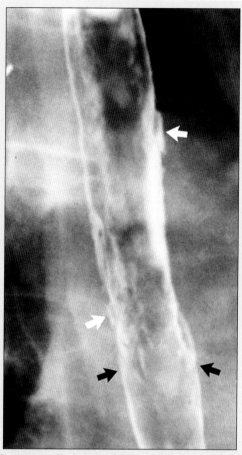

Figure 2. Acute radiation esophagitis. Multiple superficial ulcers are seen en face and in profile *(white arrows)* in the mid-esophagus. The area of ulceration has a relatively abrupt inferior demarcation *(black arrows)*, which corresponds to the lower border of the radiation portal. This patient had undergone mediastinal irradiation for bronchogenic carcinoma several weeks earlier. (*From Levine MS:* Radiology of the Esophagus. *Philadelphia, WB Saunders, 1989.*)

Phillips TL, Ross G: Time-dose relationships in the mouse esophagus. *Radiology* 113:435-440, 1974.

Roswit B: Complications of radiation therapy: The alimentary tract. *Semin Roentgenol* 9:51-63, 1974.

Rubin P: The radiographic expression of radiotherapeutic injury: An overview. *Semin Roentgenol* 9:5-13, 1974.

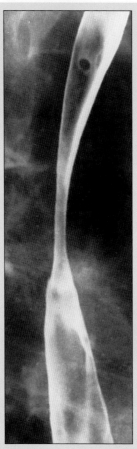

Figure 3. **Acute radiation esophagitis with subsequent stricture formation.** Another esophagogram from the same patient as in Figure 1. This esophagogram, taken 6 months later because of recurrent dysphagia, shows a smooth, tapered stricture within the radiation portal.

Caustic Esophagitis

DEFINITION: Injury to esophagus caused by ingestion of alkali, acids, ammonium chloride, phenols, silver nitrate, and a variety of other common household products.

IMAGING

Radiography

Findings

- Dilated, gas-filled esophagus or, if esophageal perforation has occurred, mediastinal widening, pneumomediastinum, or pleural effusions; pneumoperitoneum in severe injury
- Abnormal esophageal motility with poor primary peristalsis, nonperistaltic contractions, diffuse esophageal spasm, or dilated, atonic esophagus
- Multiple shallow, irregular ulcers
- Diffusely narrowed esophagus with grossly irregular contour because of marked edema, spasm, and ulceration
- Double-barreled appearance, with linear or streaky collections in esophageal wall
- One or more smooth or irregular strictures in upper or middle esophagus, often with eccentric areas of sacculation because of asymmetric scarring
- Severe scarring of entire thoracic esophagus with thread-like, filiform appearance highly suggestive of caustic stricture

Utility

- Chest and abdominal radiographs should be obtained routinely in patients who have ingested caustic agents.
- Perform water-soluble contrast study in patients with suspected esophageal or gastric perforation to document presence of leak.
- Water-soluble contrast agents are used because barium in the mediastinum causes mediastinal fibrosis, and barium in peritoneal cavity causes severe peritonitis.
- If evidence of esophageal or gastric perforation is not found, barium should be given for a more detailed examination.
- Esophagography is used to determine degree and extent of stricture formation and to gauge response to treatment.

DIAGNOSTIC PEARLS

- Endoscopy is performed within 24 hours of caustic ingestion to assess extent and severity of esophageal injury
- Double-barreled appearance
- Strictures

- Endoscopy is performed within 24 hours of caustic ingestion to assess extent and severity of esophageal injury.

CLINICAL PRESENTATION

- Rapid onset of intense odynophagia, chest pain, drooling, vomiting, or hematemesis
- Severe substernal pain, fever, and shock usually indicate esophageal perforation and mediastinitis.
- Associated gastric perforation may lead to development of peritonitis.
- Latent period of several weeks (if patient survives acute illness) during which the patient is no longer symptomatic
- Severe dysphagia resulting from progressive stricture formation 1 to 3 months after initial injury

DIFFERENTIAL DIAGNOSIS

- Reflux esophagitis
- Drug-induced esophagitis
- Radiation esophagitis
- Herpes esophagitis
- Human immunodeficiency virus esophagitis
- Idiopathic esophagitis
- Tuberculous esophagitis

WHAT THE REFERRING PHYSICIAN NEEDS TO KNOW

- Subsequent cicatrization and fibrosis may lead to development of diffuse or segmental strictures in esophagus 1 to 3 months after acute injury.
- Liquid corrosives may be swallowed rapidly; therefore caustic esophagitis often occurs without associated pharyngeal injury.
- Direct visualization of esophagus is required to confirm the diagnosis.
- Treatment of caustic esophagitis is generally aimed at preventing stricture formation.
- Diagnosis of caustic esophagitis is usually apparent from the clinical history.
- Endoscopy within 24 hours of caustic ingestion is recommended to assess the extent and severity of esophageal injury.

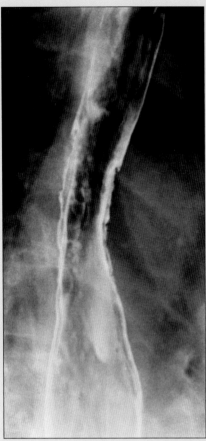

Figure 1. Acute caustic esophagitis. Multiple shallow, irregular ulcers are seen en face and in profile in the mid-esophagus. This patient had swallowed concentrated potassium hydroxide in a suicide attempt. (*From Levine MS:* Radiology of the Esophagus. *Philadelphia, WB Saunders, 1989.*)

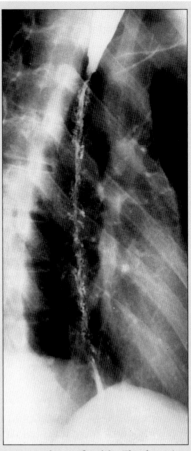

Figure 2. Severe caustic esophagitis. The thoracic esophagus is diffusely narrowed and has a grossly irregular contour with extensive ulceration due to ingestion of concentrated sodium hydroxide (liquid lye). (*From Levine MS:* Radiology of the Esophagus. *Philadelphia, WB Saunders, 1989.*)

PATHOLOGY

- Caused by ingestion of alkali, acids, ammonium chloride, phenols, silver nitrate, and a variety of other common household products
- Children usually ingest these corrosive substances accidentally, whereas adults take them intentionally to commit suicide.
- Liquid lye (concentrated sodium hydroxide) causes severe esophageal injury by liquefaction necrosis, and acids cause tissue damage by coagulative necrosis.
- Three pathologic phases of injury: (1) acute necrotic phase, (2) ulceration-granulation phase, and (3) final phase of cicatrization and scarring.
- Acute cellular necrosis phase begins immediately, lasts 1 to 4 days, and is accompanied by intense inflammatory reaction in surrounding tissues.
- Ulceration-granulation phase occurs 3 to 5 days after ingestion and produces edema, ulceration, and sloughing of necrotic mucosa.
- Cicatrization phase begins 3 to 4 weeks after ingestion and may lead to severe scarring and stricture formation in the esophagus.

INCIDENCE/PREVALENCE AND EPIDEMIOLOGY

- Caustic esophagitis leads to stricture formation in 10% to 40% of patients.
- Patients with lye strictures have significantly increased risk of developing esophageal carcinoma 20 to 40 years after initial caustic injury.

Suggested Readings

Appelqvist P, Salmo M: Lye corrosion carcinoma of the esophagus: A review of 63 cases. *Cancer* 45:2655-2685, 1980.

Cardona JC, Daly JF: Current management of corrosive esophagitis: An evaluation of results in 239 cases. *Ann Otol* 80:521-527, 1971.

Citron BP, Pincus IJ, Geokas MC, et al: Chemical trauma of the esophagus and stomach. *Surg Clin North Am* 48:1303-1311, 1968.

Dantas RO, Mamede RCM: Esophageal motility in patients with esophageal caustic injury. *Am J Gastroenterol* 91:1157-1161, 1996.

Franken EA: Caustic damage of the gastrointestinal tract: Roentgen features. *AJR Am J Roentgenol* 118:77-85, 1973.

Goldman LP, Weigert JM: Corrosive substance ingestion: A review. *Am J Gastroenterol* 79:85-90, 1984.

Guelrud M, Arocha M: Motor function abnormalities in acute caustic esophagitis. *J Clin Gastroenterol* 2:247-250, 1980.

Hopkins RA, Postlethwait RW: Caustic burns and carcinoma of the esophagus. *Ann Surg* 194:146-148, 1981.

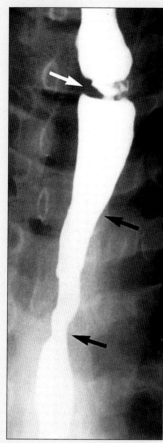

Figure 3. Lye strictures. A long, tapered stricture *(black arrows)* is seen in the upper thoracic esophagus. Another short, asymmetric stricture *(white arrow)* is seen more proximally at the thoracic inlet. The presence of one or more segmental strictures in the cervical or thoracic esophagus is characteristic of caustic injury. (*From Levine MS:* Radiology of the Esophagus. *Philadelphia, WB Saunders, 1989.*)

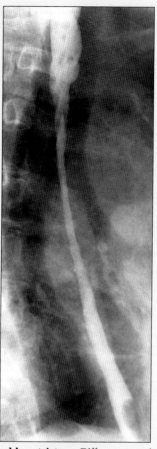

Figure 4. Advanced lye stricture. Diffuse narrowing of the thoracic esophagus is seen as a result of extensive scarring and fibrosis in this patient with lye stricture. This appearance should suggest caustic injury because other conditions are rarely associated with such severe esophageal narrowing. (*From Levine MS:* Radiology of the Esophagus. *Philadelphia, WB Saunders, 1989.*)

Kirsh MM, Ritter F: Caustic ingestion and subsequent damage to the oropharyngeal and digestive passages. *Ann Thorac Surg* 21:74-82, 1976.

Leape LL, Ashcraft KW, Scarpelli DG, et al: Hazard to health: Liquid lye. *N Engl J Med* 284:587-591, 1971.

Martel W: Radiologic features of esophagogastritis secondary to extremely caustic agents. *Radiology* 103:31-36, 1972.

Moody FG, Garrett JM: Esophageal achalasia following lye ingestion. *Ann Surg* 170:775-784, 1969.

Muhletaler CA, Gerlock AJ, de Soto L, et al: Acid corrosive esophagitis: Radiographic findings. *AJR Am J Roentgenol* 134:1137-1140, 1980.

Neimark S, Rogers AI: Chemical injury of the esophagus. In Berk JA (ed): *Bockus Gastroenterology,* 4th ed. Philadelphia, WB Saunders, 1985, pp 769-776.

Webb WR, Koutras P, Ecker RR: An evaluation of steroids and antibiotics in caustic burns of the esophagus. *Ann Thorac Surg* 9:95-102, 1970.

Idiopathic Eosinophilic Esophagitis

DEFINITION: Increased number of intraepithelial eosinophils (more than 20 per high-power field) on endoscopic biopsy specimens from esophagus.

IMAGING

Radiography
Findings
- Development of one or more segmental strictures in the upper esophagus, mid-esophagus, or, less commonly, distal esophagus
- Distinctive ring-like indentations, resulting in ringed esophagus
- Multiple, closely spaced, concentric rings traversing stricture
- Diffuse esophageal narrowing, resulting in *small-caliber* esophagus
- Abnormal motility with increased frequency of nonperistaltic contractions or even an achalasia-like syndrome
- Small, sessile eosinophilic polyps in the esophagus (rare)

Utility
- Esophagography

CLINICAL PRESENTATION
- Long-standing dysphagia and recurrent food impactions in young men

DIFFERENTIAL DIAGNOSIS
- Congenital esophageal stenosis
- Barrett esophagus
- Caustic stricture
- Drug-induced stricture
- Radiation stricture
- Feline esophagus

PATHOLOGY
- Characterized by increased number of intraepithelial eosinophils (> 20 per high-power field) on endoscopic biopsy specimens from esophagus
- Etiology is uncertain; may develop as result of inflammatory response to ingested food allergens

DIAGNOSTIC PEARLS
- Increased number of intraepithelial eosinophils (> 20 per high-power field) on endoscopic biopsy specimens from esophagus
- Ringed esophagus
- Diffuse esophageal narrowing, resulting in a *small-caliber* esophagus

- Muscular layers of esophageal wall are involved, sometimes resulting in development of strictures.
- Affected individuals may have atopic history and peripheral eosinophilia, sometimes associated with eosinophilic infiltration of stomach and small bowel.
- Frequently occurs as isolated condition in the absence of other allergic manifestations or gastrointestinal disease.

Suggested Readings

Arora AS, Perrault J, Smyrk TC: Topical corticosteroid treatment of dysphagia due to eosinophilic esophagitis in adults. *Mayo Clin Proc* 78:830-835, 2003.

Attwood SE, Smyrk TC, DeMeester TR, et al: Esophageal eosinophilia with dysphagia: A distinct clinicopathologic syndrome. *Dig Dis Sci* 38:109-116, 1993.

Bousvaros A, Antonioli DA, Winter HS: Ringed esophagus: An association with esophagitis. *Am J Gastroenterol* 87:1187-1190, 1992.

Croese J, Fairley SK, Masson JW, et al: Clinical and endoscopic features of eosinophilic esophagitis in adults. *Gastrointest Endosc* 58:516-522, 2003.

Feczko PJ, Halpert RD, Zonca M: Radiographic abnormalities in eosinophilic esophagitis. *Gastrointest Radiol* 10:321-324, 1985.

Fox VL, Nurko S, Furuta GT: Eosinophilic esophagitis: It's not just kid's stuff. *Gastrointest Endosc* 56:260-270, 2000.

Khan S, Orenstein SR, Di Lorenzo C, et al: Eosinophilic esophagitis: Strictures, impactions, dysphagia. *Dig Dis Sci* 48:22-29, 2003.

Landres RT, Kuster GGR, Strum WB: Eosinophilic esophagitis in a patient with vigorous achalasia. *Gastroenterology* 74:1298-1301, 1978.

Liacouras CA, Wenner WJ, Brown K, et al: Primary eosinophilic esophagitis in children: Successful treatment with oral corticosteroids. *J Pediatr Gastroenterol Nutr* 26:380-385, 1998.

Markowitz JE, Liacouras CA: Eosinophilic esophagitis. *Gastroenterol Clin North Am* 32:949-966, 2003.

Markowitz JE, Spergel JM, Ruchelli E, et al: Elemental diet is an effective treatment for eosinophilic esophagitis in children and adolescents. *Am J Gastroenterol* 98:777-782, 2003.

Matzinger MA, Daneman A: Esophageal involvement in eosinophilic gastroenteritis. *Pediatr Radiol* 13:35-38, 1983.

WHAT THE REFERRING PHYSICIAN NEEDS TO KNOW
- Most patients are treated with antiallergy therapy, oral or inhaled steroids, and elemental diets, with varying degrees of success.
- Patients with strictures causing intractable dysphagia may undergo endoscopic dilatation procedures with transient relief of dysphagia; multiple dilatation procedures are therefore required in most cases.

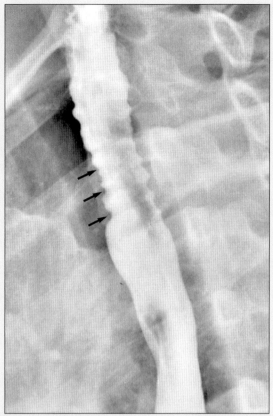

Figure 1. Eosinophilic esophagitis with a ringed esophagus.
A moderately long stricture is seen in the upper thoracic esophagus, with multiple distinctive ring-like indentations *(arrows)* in the region of the stricture. *(From Zimmerman SL, Levine MS, Rubesin SE, et al: Idiopathic eosinophilic esophagitis in adults: The ringed esophagus. Radiology 236:159-165, 2005.)*

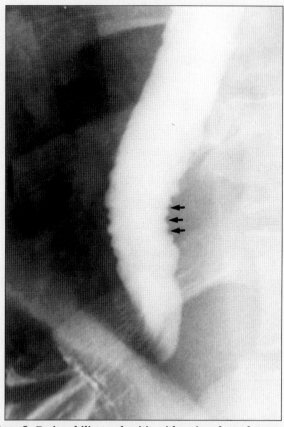

Figure 2. Eosinophilic esophagitis with a ringed esophagus.
A mild stricture is seen in the distal esophagus with multiple ring-like constrictions *(arrows)* in the region of the stricture. *(From Zimmerman SL, Levine MS, Rubesin SE, et al: Idiopathic eosinophilic esophagitis in adults: The ringed esophagus. Radiology 236:159-165, 2005.)*

Munitiz V, Martinez de Haro LF, Ortiz A, et al: Primary eosinophilic esophagitis. *Dis Esoph* 16:165-168, 2003.

Orenstein SR, Shalaby TM, Di Lorenzo C, et al: The spectrum of pediatric eosinophilic esophagitis beyond infancy: A clinical series of 30 children. *Am J Gastroenterol* 95:1422-1430, 2000.

Picus D, Frank PH: Eosinophilic esophagitis. *AJR Am J Roentgenol* 136:1001-1003, 1981.

Siafakas CG, Ryan CK, Brown MR, et al: Multiple esophageal rings: An association with eosinophilic esophagitis. *Am J Gastroenterol* 95:1572-1575, 2000.

Vasilopoulos S, Murphy P, Auerbach A, et al: The small-caliber esophagus: An unappreciated cause of dysphagia for solids in patients with eosinophilic esophagitis. *Gastrointest Endosc* 55:99-106, 2002.

Vitellas KM, Bennett WF, Bova JG, et al: Idiopathic eosinophilic esophagitis. *Radiology* 186:789-793, 1993.

Walsh SV, Antonioli DA, Goldman H, et al: Allergic esophagitis in children: A clinicopathological entity. *Am J Surg Pathol* 23:390-396, 1999.

Zimmerman SL, Levine MS, Rubesin SE, et al: Idiopathic eosinophilic espophagitis in adults: The ringed esophagus. *Radiology* 236:159-165, 2005.

Other Esophagitides

DEFINITION: Different diseases that cause esophagitis.

IMAGING

Radiography

Findings

- Aphthoid ulcers in Crohn disease seen as punctate, slit-like, or ring-like collections of barium surrounded by radiolucent halos of edematous mucosa
- Advanced Crohn disease characterized by thickened folds, pseudomembranes, *cobblestone* appearance, transverse or longitudinal intramural tracks, and fistulas
- Bullous skin diseases involving the esophagus characterized by small, nodular filling defects in the esophagus or extensive bulla formation with diffusely serrated or spiculated esophageal contour
- Alkaline reflux esophagitis characterized by mucosal nodularity, thickened folds, and ulceration of the distal esophagus above esophagojejunal anastomosis
- Scarring from nasogastric intubation, alkaline reflux esophagitis, and Zollinger-Ellison syndrome characterized by the development of unusually long, rapidly progressive strictures in the distal esophagus
- Scarring from benign mucous membrane pemphigoid and epidermolysis bullosa dystrophica associated with the development of high strictures in the esophagus
- Scarring from residual glutaraldehyde on endoscopic equipment associated with the development of long strictures in thoracic esophagus resembling lye strictures

Utility

- Double-contrast esophagography important for detecting aphthoid ulcers
- Esophagography

CLINICAL PRESENTATION

- Dysphagia or odynophagia
- Chest pain, heartburn, or upper gastrointestinal bleeding
- Regurgitation of bile in alkaline reflux disease
- Hematemesis in chronic graft-versus-host disease

DIFFERENTIAL DIAGNOSIS

- Esophageal intramural pseudodiverticulosis
- Other causes of esophagitis

DIAGNOSTIC PEARLS

- Aphthoid ulcers in Crohn disease seen as punctate, slit-like, or ring-like collections of barium surrounded by radiolucent halos of edematous mucosa
- *Cobblestone* appearance in advanced Crohn disease
- Long strictures in distal esophagus in patients with nasogastric intubation, alkaline reflux esophagitis, and Zollinger-Ellison syndrome
- Flask-shaped outpouchings in esophageal intramural pseudodiverticulosis

PATHOLOGY

- Epidermolysis bullosa is a rare hereditary skin disease in which minimal trauma causes separation of epidermis and dermis, with subsequent bulla formation.
- Pemphigoid is a dermatologic disease characterized by chronic, recurrent bullous eruptions of skin and mucous membranes.
- Erythema multiforme is a hypersensitivity reaction characterized by maculopapular or bullous rash that usually develops during the first three decades of life.
- Nasogastric intubation has been recognized as an unusual cause of esophagitis and stricture formation.
- Alkaline reflux esophagitis is an unusual condition caused by reflux of bile and pancreatic secretions into the esophagus after total or partial gastrectomy.
- Acute alcohol-induced esophagitis is an acute, transient form of esophagitis occurring after an alcoholic binge.
- Behçet disease is a multisystem disorder characterized by nonspecific vasculitis, with resulting skin lesions, arthritis, colitis, thrombophlebitis, and, rarely, encephalitis.

INCIDENCE/PREVALENCE AND EPIDEMIOLOGY

- Benign mucous membrane pemphigoid usually occurs in middle-aged patients and is twice as common in women as in men.

WHAT THE REFERRING PHYSICIAN NEEDS TO KNOW

- Definitive diagnosis of esophageal Crohn disease requires histologic confirmation.
- Absence of definitive histologic findings should not preclude a diagnosis of Crohn disease if clinical and radiographic findings are suggestive of this condition.
- Endoscopy should be avoided in patients with known or suspected epidermolysis bullosa dystrophica involving esophagus because of the risk of further traumatizing an already fragile mucosa.

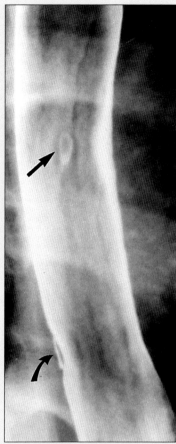

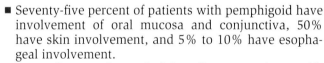

Figure 1. Esophageal Crohn disease with aphthoid ulcers.
Discrete, widely separated aphthoid ulcers are seen en face
(straight arrow) and in profile *(curved arrow)* as a result of early
esophageal involvement by Crohn disease. *(From Gohel V,
Long BW, Richter G: Aphthous ulcers in the esophagus with Crohn
colitis. AJR Am J Roentgenol 137:872-873, 1981, © by American
Roentgen Ray Society.)*

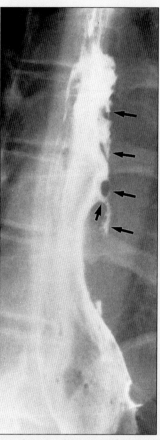

Figure 2. Esophageal Crohn disease with intramural tracks.
Longitudinal *(long arrows)* and transverse *(short arrow)* tracks
are seen in the distal third of the esophagus resulting from
transmural involvement by Crohn disease. *(Courtesy of Peter J.
Feczko, MD, Royal Oak, MI.)*

- Seventy-five percent of patients with pemphigoid have involvement of oral mucosa and conjunctiva, 50% have skin involvement, and 5% to 10% have esophageal involvement.
- Depending on the underlying disease, patients with esophageal involvement by chronic graft-versus-host disease have 5-year survival rates of 60% to 80% after marrow transplantation.

Suggested Readings

Canon CL, Levine MS, Cherukuri R, et al: Intramural tracking: A feature of esophageal intramural pseudodiverticulosis. AJR Am J Roentgenol 175:371-374, 2000.
Carucci LR, Levine MS, Rubesin SE: Diffuse esophageal stricture caused by erythema multiforme major. AJR Am J Roentgenol 180:749-750, 2003.
Chung SY, Ha HK, Kim JH, et al: Radiologic findings of Behçet syndrome involving the gastrointestinal tract. RadioGraphics 21:911-926, 2001.
Karasick S, Mapp E, Karasick D: Esophageal involvement in benign mucous membrane pemphigoid. J Can Assoc Radiol 32:247-248, 1981.
Levine MS, Fisher AR, Rubesin SE, et al: Complications after total gastrectomy and esophagojejunostomy: Radiologic evaluation. AJR Am J Roentgenol 157:1189-1194, 1991.
McDonald GB, Shulman HM, Sullivan KM, et al: Intestinal and hepatic complications of human bone marrow transplantation: II. Gastroenterology 90:770-784, 1986.
McDonald GB, Sullivan KM, Plumley TF: Radiographic features of esophageal involvement in chronic graft-vs.-host disease. AJR Am J Roentgenol 142:501-506, 1984.
McDonald GB, Sullivan KM, Schuffler MD, et al: Esophageal abnormalities in chronic graft-vs.-host disease in humans. Gastroenterology 890:914-921, 1981.
Minocha A, Mandanas RA, Kida M, et al: Bullous esophagitis due to chronic graft-versus-host disease. Am J Gastroenterol 92:529-530, 1997.
Mori S, Yoshihira A, Kawamura H, et al: Esophageal involvement in Behçet's disease. Am J Gastroenterol 78:548-553, 1983.
Naylor MF, MacCarty RL, Rogers RS: Barium studies in esophageal cicatricial pemphigoid. Abdom Imaging 20:97-100, 1995.
O'Riordan D, Levine MS, Laufer I: Acute alcoholic esophagitis. J Can Assoc Radiol 37:54-55, 1986.
Peters ME, Gourley G, Mann FA: Esophageal stricture and web secondary to Stevens-Johnson syndrome. Pediatr Radiol 13:290-291, 1983.
Rosenberg HK, Serota FT, Hock P, et al: Radiographic features of gastrointestinal graft-vs.-host disease. Radiology 138:371-374, 1981.
Salo J, Kivilaakso E: Failure of long limb Roux-en-Y reconstruction to prevent alkaline reflux esophagitis after total gastrectomy. Endoscopy 22:65-67, 1990.
Sandvik AK, Halvorsen TB: Barrett's esophagus after total gastrectomy. J Clin Gastroenterol 10:587-588, 1988.

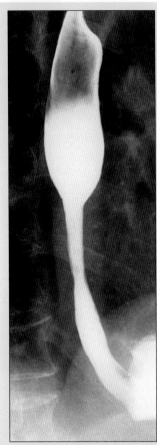

Figure 3. Rapidly progressive stricture caused by nasogastric intubation. Esophagogram 3 weeks after removal of nasogastric tube shows an unusually long, rapidly progressive stricture with marked narrowing of the distal esophagus. (*Courtesy of Vijay Gohel, MD, Philadelphia, PA.*)

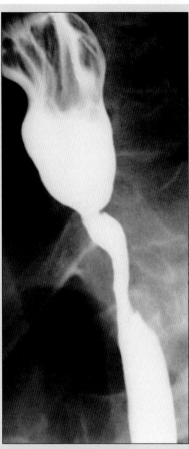

Figure 4. Benign mucous membrane pemphigoid with a high esophageal stricture. A long, asymmetric stricture is seen in the cervical and upper thoracic esophagus. (*Courtesy of John A. Bonavita, MD, Philadelphia, PA.*)

Stampien TM, Schwartz RA: Erythema multiforme. *Am Fam Physician* 46:1171-1176, 1992.

Tan YM, Goh KL: Esophageal stricture as a late complication of Stevens-Johnson syndrome. *Gastrointest Endosc* 50:566-568, 1999.

Weinstein T, Valderrama E, Pettei M, et al: Esophageal Crohn's disease: Medical management and correlation between clinical, endoscopic, and histologic features. *Inflamm Bowel Dis* 3:79-83, 1997.

Wong WL, Entwisle K, Pemberton J: Gastrointestinal manifestations in the Hallopeau-Siemens variant of recessive dystrophic epidermolysis bullosa. *Br J Radiol* 66:788-793, 1993.

Esophageal Intramural Pseudodiverticulosis

DEFINITION: Dilated excretory ducts of deep mucous glands in esophagus.

IMAGING

Radiography

Findings
- Innumerable, tiny (1- to 4-mm), flask-shaped outpouchings in longitudinal rows parallel to long axis of esophagus
- Pseudodiverticula viewed in profile may seem to be "floating" or "levitating" outside esophageal wall without apparent communication with lumen.
- Bridging may sometimes occur between adjacent pseudodiverticula, resulting in discrete intramural tracks.
- Condition is often associated with strictures in mid-esophagus or, more commonly, distal esophagus (i.e., peptic strictures).
- Localized extravasation of contrast material into mediastinum from perforated pseudodiverticulum

Utility
- Dilated excretory duct orifices are extremely difficult to visualize with endoscopy.
- Esophagography is more sensitive than endoscopy for detecting these structures.

CT

Findings
- Marked thickening of esophageal wall, diffuse irregularity of lumen, and intramural gas collections
- Periesophageal inflammatory mass with or without associated collections of gas

CLINICAL PRESENTATION

- Intermittent or slowly progressive dysphagia due to high prevalence of associated strictures
- Perforation of esophageal intramural pseudodiverticulum that results in diverticulitis with development of periesophageal inflammatory mass or abscess in mediastinum

DIAGNOSTIC PEARLS

- Flask-shaped outpouchings in longitudinal rows parallel to long axis of the esophagus
- Tiny collections "floating" outside wall of esophagus
- Discrete intramural tracks

- Chest pain, fever, leukocytosis, or other signs of mediastinitis in patients with diverticulitis

DIFFERENTIAL DIAGNOSIS

- Diverticula (esophagus)
- Ulcers (esophagus)

PATHOLOGY

- Pathologic studies have shown that esophageal intramural pseudodiverticula represent dilated excretory ducts of deep mucous glands in esophagus.
- Ductal dilatation results from plugging and obstruction of duct by thick, viscous mucous, inflammatory material, and desquamated epithelium.
- Bridging may occur between adjacent pseudodiverticula, resulting in discrete intramural tracks.

INCIDENCE/PREVALENCE AND EPIDEMIOLOGY

- *Candida albicans* has been cultured from the esophagus in small percentage of patients.
- Endoscopic or histologic evidence of esophagitis is seen in 80% to 90% of patients with esophageal intramural pseudodiverticulosis.

WHAT THE REFERRING PHYSICIAN NEEDS TO KNOW

- Treatment is usually directed toward the underlying stricture because pseudodiverticula themselves rarely cause symptoms.
- Mechanical dilatation of strictures produces dramatic clinical response in almost all patients.
- Strictures associated with pseudodiverticulosis are not always benign; therefore cases should be evaluated individually for radiographic signs of malignancy.
- Esophageal perforation by ruptured pseudodiverticula are more likely to heal with conservative medical treatment than other types of esophageal perforations.
- Failure to visualize the pseudodiverticula may result from ductal obstruction by inflammatory material or debris that prevents barium from entering ducts.
- Long tracks can be mistaken for large ulcers or extraluminal esophageal dissection or perforation.
- Condition must be differentiated from true diverticula, ulcers, or extraluminal collections associated with intramural esophageal dissection or perforation.

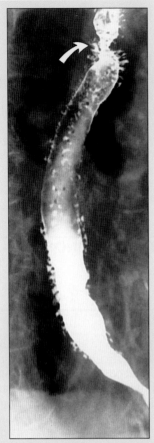

Figure 1. **Esophageal intramural pseudodiverticulosis with high stricture.** The pseudodiverticula appear as characteristic outpouchings in longitudinal rows parallel to the long axis of the esophagus. Associated stricture *(arrow)* is seen in the upper thoracic esophagus. (*From Levine MS:* Radiology of the Esophagus. *Philadelphia, WB Saunders, 1989.*)

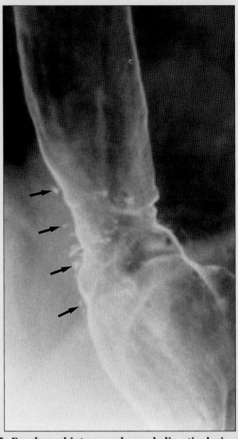

Figure 2. **Esophageal intramural pseudodiverticulosis with a peptic stricture.** When viewed en face, the pseudodiverticula can be mistaken for tiny ulcers. When viewed in profile, however, the pseudodiverticula *(arrows)* do not appear to communicate with the esophageal lumen. This characteristic feature helps differentiate these structures from ulcers. Narrowing and deformity of the distal esophagus are also seen as a result of an associated peptic stricture. (*From Levine MS:* Radiology of the Esophagus. *Philadelphia, WB Saunders, 1989.*)

- Ninety percent of cases have associated strictures, mostly in distal esophagus, with focal cluster of pseudodiverticula in region of peptic stricture.
- Condition usually occurs in elderly patients and is slightly more common in men than women.
- Twenty percent of affected individuals are diabetics, and 15% are alcoholics.

Suggested Readings

Abrams LJ, Levine MS, Laufer I: Esophageal peridiverticulitis: An unusual complication of esophageal intramural pseudodiverticulosis. *Eur J Radiol* 19:139-141, 1995.

Beauchamp JM, Nice CM, Belanger MA, et al: Esophageal intramural pseudodiverticulosis. *Radiology* 113:273-276, 1974.

Boyd RM, Bogoch A, Greig JH, et al: Esophageal intramural pseudodiverticulosis. *Radiology* 113:267-270, 1974.

Bruhlmann WF, Zollikofer CL, Maranta E, et al: Intramural pseudodiverticulosis of the esophagus: Report of seven cases and literature review. *Gastrointest Radiol* 6:199-208, 1981.

Castillo S, Aburashed A, Kimmelman J, et al: Diffuse intramural esophageal pseudodiverticulosis. *Gastroenterology* 72:541-545, 1977.

Cho SR, Sanders MM, Turner MA, et al: Esophageal intramural pseudodiverticulosis. *Gastrointest Radiol* 6:9-16, 1981.

Flora KD, Gordon MD, Lieberman D, et al: Esophageal intramural pseudodiverticulosis. *Dig Dis* 15:113-119, 1997.

Graham DY, Goyal RK, Sparkman J, et al: Diffuse intramural esophageal diverticulosis. *Gastroenterology* 68:781-785, 1975.

Hammon JW, Rice RP, Postlethwait RW, et al: Esophageal intramural diverticulosis. *Ann Thorac Surg* 17:260-267, 1974.

Kim S, Choi C, Groskin SA: Esophageal intramural pseudodiverticulitis. *Radiology* 173:418-419, 1989.

Levine MS, Moolten DN, Herlinger H, et al: Esophageal intramural pseudodiverticulosis: A reevaluation. *AJR Am J Roentgenol* 147:1165-1170, 1986.

Medeiros LJ, Doos WG, Balogh K: Esophageal intramural pseudodiverticulosis: A report of two cases with analysis of similar, less extensive changes in "normal" autopsy esophagi. *Hum Pathol* 19:928-931, 1988.

Mendl K, McKay JM, Tanner CH: Intramural diverticulosis of the oesophagus and Rokitansky-Aschoff sinuses in the gallbladder. *Br J Radiol* 33:496-501, 1960.

Pearlberg JL, Sandler MA, Madrazo BL: Computed tomographic features of esophageal intramural pseudodiverticulosis. *Radiology* 147:189-190, 1983.

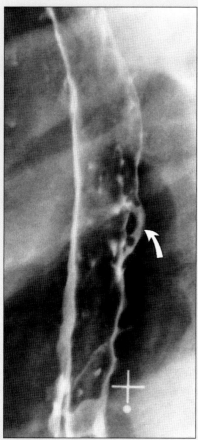

Figure 3. Esophageal intramural pseudodiverticulosis with an intramural track. This track *(arrow)* is caused by bridging of adjacent pseudodiverticula. Other pseudodiverticula seen en face can be mistaken for shallow ulcers. *(Courtesy of Stephen E. Rubesin, MD, Philadelphia, PA.)*

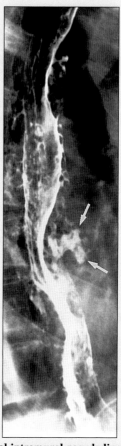

Figure 4. Esophageal intramural pseudodiverticulosis with associated diverticulitis. Note the large, irregular, extraluminal barium collection *(arrows)*, presumably caused by a sealed-off perforation of a pseudodiverticulum. *(Courtesy of Peter J. Feczko, MD, Royal Oak, MI.)*

Plavsic BM, Chen MYM, Gelfand DW, et al: Intramural pseudodiverticulosis of the esophagus detected on barium esophagograms: Increased prevalence in patients with esophageal carcinoma. *AJR Am J Roentgenol* 165:1381-1385, 1995.

Sabanathan S, Salama FD, Morgan WE: Oesophageal intramural pseudodiverticulosis. *Thorax* 40:849-857, 1985.

Troupin RH: Intramural esophageal diverticulosis and moniliasis. *AJR Am J Roentgenol* 104:613-616, 1968.

Umlas J, Sakhuja R: The pathology of esophageal intramural pseudodiverticulosis. *Am J Clin Pathol* 65:314-320, 1976.

Wightman AJA, Wright EA: Intramural esophageal diverticulosis: A correlation of radiological and pathological findings. *Br J Radiol* 47:496-498, 1974.

Part 10

BENIGN TUMORS OF THE ESOPHAGUS

Glycogenic Acanthosis

DEFINITION: Benign condition of unknown cause in which accumulation of cytoplasmic glycogen occurs in the squamous epithelium of the esophagus.

IMAGING

Radiography
Findings
- Multiple small, rounded nodules or plaques in middle or, less commonly, distal third of esophagus

Utility
- Barium esophagography

CLINICAL PRESENTATION

- Affected individuals are almost always asymptomatic.

DIFFERENTIAL DIAGNOSIS

- Reflux esophagitis
- *Candida* esophagitis
- Esophageal papillomatosis
- Leukoplakia (esophagus)
- Superficial spreading carcinoma (esophagus)

PATHOLOGY

- Unknown etiology
- Accumulation of cytoplasmic glycogen in squamous epithelium of esophagus
- White mucosal plaques or nodules, ranging from 2 to 15 mm in size
- Histologically, hyperplasia of squamous epithelial cells resulting from increased cytoplasmic glycogen
- Degenerative, age-related phenomenon

DIAGNOSTIC PEARLS

- Multiple small, rounded nodules or plaques in the middle or, less commonly, distal third of the esophagus
- Accumulation of cytoplasmic glycogen in the squamous epithelium of the esophagus
- Hyperplasia of squamous epithelial cells resulting from increased cytoplasmic glycogen
- The nodules or plaques in glycogenic acanthosis may be indistinguishable from those in *Candida* esophagitis, but patients with glycogenic acanthosis are usually elderly individuals who are asymptomatic, whereas patients with esophageal candidiasis are immunocompromsed and present with odynophagia or dysphagia.

INCIDENCE/PREVALENCE AND EPIDEMIOLOGY

- Common condition at endoscopy with prevalence of 3% to 15%
- Usually found in patients older than 60 years of age

Suggested Readings
Bender MD, Allison J, Cuartas F, et al: Glycogenic acanthosis of the esophagus: A form of benign epithelial hyperplasia. *Gastroenterology* 65:373-380, 1973.
Berliner L, Redmond P, Horowitz L, et al: Glycogen plaques (glycogenic acanthosis) of the esophagus. *Radiology* 141:607-610, 1981.
Ghahremani GG, Rushovich AM: Glycogenic acanthosis of the esophagus: Radiographic and pathologic features. *Gastrointest Radiol* 9:93-98, 1984.

WHAT THE REFERRING PHYSICIAN NEEDS TO KNOW

- Definitive diagnosis is made by demonstrating characteristic glycogen-rich epithelial cells on biopsy specimens stained with periodic acid-Schiff material.
- Endoscopy usually not required in asymptomatic patients with this condition on barium esophagography.

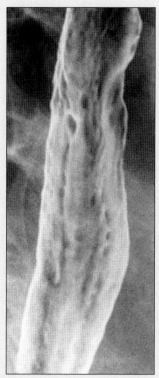

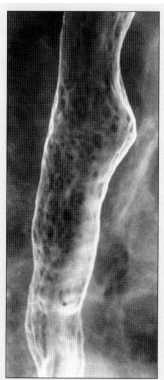

Figure 1. In this patient, glycogenic acanthosis is manifested by multiple small plaques and nodules in the mid-esophagus. The lesions tend to have a rounded appearance. *Candida* esophagitis can produce similar findings, but patients with glycogenic acanthosis are almost always asymptomatic.

Figure 2. In this patient, glycogenic acanthosis is manifested by multiple small plaques and nodules in the mid-esophagus. The lesions tend to have a rounded appearance. *Candida* esophagitis can produce similar findings, but patients with glycogenic acanthosis are almost always asymptomatic.

Glick SN, Teplick SK, Goldstein J, et al: Glycogenic acanthosis of the esophagus. *AJR Am J Roentgenol* 139:683-688, 1982.

Rose D, Furth EE, Rubesin SE. Glycogenic acanthosis. *AJR Am J Roentgenol* 164:96, 1995.

Rywlin AM, Ortega R: Glycogenic acanthosis of the esophagus. *Arch Pathol* 90:439-443, 1970.

Stern Z, Sharon P, Ligumsky M, et al: Glycogenic acanthosis of the esophagus: A benign but confusing endoscopic lesion. *Am J Gastroenterol* 74:261-263, 1980.

Vadva MD, Triadafilopoulos G: Glycogenic acanthosis of the esophagus and gastroesophageal reflux. *J Clin Gastroenterol* 17:79-83, 1993.

Leiomyoma

DEFINITION: Benign esophageal tumors consisting histologically of intersecting bands of smooth muscle and fibrous tissue in a well-defined capsule.

IMAGING

Radiography
Findings
- Mediastinal mass on chest radiographs
- Possible amorphous or punctate areas of calcification
- Discrete submucosal masses (ranging from 2 to 8 cm in size) on barium studies
- Round or ovoid filling defects sharply outlined by barium on each side when viewed en face
- Smooth surface and slightly obtuse borders with adjacent esophageal wall when viewed in profile
- Rounded filling defect in esophagus, with splitting of barium around lesion when viewed en face
- Larger leiomyomas may indent lumen, causing esophagus to appear narrowed in tangential projections but stretched and widened en face

Utility
- Chest radiographs
- Barium studies

CT
Findings
- Homogeneous soft-tissue mass
Utility
- Differentiates submucosal tumor from mediastinal mass compressing esophagus

CLINICAL PRESENTATION

- Most patients are asymptomatic.
- If leiomyoma indents lumen, it may cause intermittent, slowly worsening dysphagia or, less commonly, substernal discomfort, vomiting, or weight loss.
- Tumors rarely may ulcerate, but upper gastrointestinal bleeding is extremely uncommon.
- Symptoms may be present for several years before patients seek medical attention.
- Rarely, patients may show signs and symptoms of acute esophageal obstruction.

DIAGNOSTIC PEARLS

- Discrete submucosal masses, ranging from 2 to 8 cm in size
- Smooth surface and slightly obtuse borders when viewed in profile
- Rounded filling defect in the esophagus, with splitting of barium around the lesion when viewed en face
- Homogeneous soft-tissue masses on CT

DIFFERENTIAL DIAGNOSIS

- Other benign mesenchymal tumors (esophagus)
- Duplication cyst (esophagus)
- Submucosally infiltrating carcinoma (esophagus)

PATHOLOGY

- Tumors consist histologically of intersecting bands of smooth muscle and fibrous tissue in a well-defined capsule.
- Discrete submucosal masses, ranging from 2 to 8 cm in size
- Tumors may have an exophytic, intraluminal, or circumferential pattern of growth.
- Most leiomyomas in esophagus occur as solitary lesions, but multiple leiomyomas are present in 3% to 4% of patients.
- Esophageal leiomyomas have also been documented in patients with hypertrophic osteoarthropathy.

INCIDENCE/PREVALENCE AND EPIDEMIOLOGY

- These tumors represent more than 50% of all benign esophageal tumors.
- Sixty percent are located in the distal third of the esophagus, 30% in the middle third, and 10% in the proximal third.

WHAT THE REFERRING PHYSICIAN NEEDS TO KNOW

- Granular cell tumors, lipomas, hemangiomas, fibromas, and neurofibromas may produce identical radiographic findings.
- Leiomyomas have also been documented in patients with hypertrophic osteoarthropathy.
- Treatment of choice for symptomatic patients is surgical enucleation of tumor.
- Occasionally, larger lesions may necessitate more extensive esophageal resection.
- Presence of calcified esophageal mass is highly suggestive of a leiomyoma, given that calcification almost never occurs in other benign or malignant esophageal tumors.

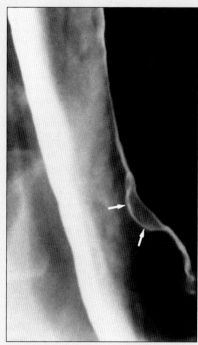

Figure 1. Esophageal leiomyoma. The lesion *(arrows)* has a smooth surface *(etched in white)* and slightly obtuse borders characteristic of submucosal masses.

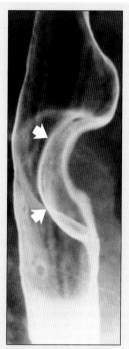

Figure 2. Esophageal leiomyoma. The lesion *(arrows)* has a smooth surface *(etched in white)* and slightly obtuse borders characteristic of submucosal masses.

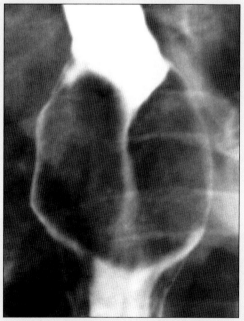

Figure 3. Esophageal leiomyoma. En face view shows a smooth, rounded filling defect in the esophagus, with splitting of barium around the lesion. The esophagus appears widened at this level. *(Courtesy of Marc P. Banner, MD, Philadelphia, PA.)*

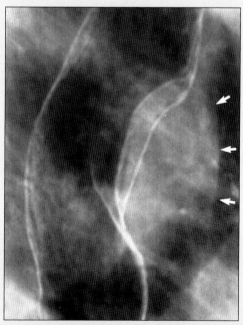

Figure 4. Esophageal leiomyoma. Tangential view from same examination as in Figure 3 reveals the characteristic features of a submucosal lesion. The outer margin of the leiomyoma is seen as a soft tissue shadow *(arrows)* abutting the lung. *(Courtesy of Marc P. Banner, MD, Philadelphia, PA.)*

Suggested Readings

Attah EB, Hajdu SI: Benign and malignant tumors of the esophagus at autopsy. *J Thorac Cardiovasc Surg* 5:396-404, 1968.

Barriero F, Seco JL, Molina J, et al: Giant esophageal leiomyoma with secondary megaesophagus. *Surgery* 7:436-439, 1976.

Ghahremani GG, Meyers MA, Port RB: Calcified primary tumors of the gastrointestinal tract. *Gastrointest Radiol* 2:331-339, 1978.

Glanz I, Grunebaum M: The radiological approach to leiomyoma of the oesophagus with a long-term follow-up. *Clin Radiol* 28:197-200, 1977.

Godard JE, McCranie D: Multiple leiomyomas of the esophagus. *AJR* 117:259-262, 1973.

Goldstein HM, Zornoza J, Hopens T: Intrinsic diseases of the adult esophagus: Benign and malignant tumors. *Semin Roentgenol* 16:183-197, 1981.

Griff LC, Cooper J: Leiomyoma of the esophagus presenting as a mediastinal mass. *AJR* 101:472-481, 1967.

Gutman E: Posterior mediastinal calcification due to esophageal leiomyoma. *Gastroenterology* 63:665-666, 1972.

Itai Y, Shimazu H: Leiomyosarcoma of the oesophagus with dense calcification. *Br J Radiol* 51:469-471, 1978.

Megibow AJ, Balthazar EJ, Hulnick DH, et al: CT evaluation of gastrointestinal leiomyomas and leiomyosarcomas. *AJR* 144:727-731, 1985.

Orchard JL, Peternel WW, Arena S: Remarkably large, benign esophageal tumor: Difficulties in diagnosis. *Dig Dis* 22:266-269, 1977.

Plachta A: Benign tumors of the esophagus: Review of literature and report of 99 cases. *Am J Gastroenterol* 38:639-652, 1962.

Rubin RA, Lichtenstein GR, Morris JB: Acute esophageal obstruction: A unique presentation of a giant intramural esophageal leiomyoma. *Am J Gastroenterol* 87:1669-1671, 1992.

Schapiro RL, Sandrock AR: Esophagogastric and vulvar leiomyomatosis: A new radiologic syndrome. *J Can Assoc Radiol* 24:184-187, 1973.

Schatzki R, Hawes LE: The roentgenological appearance of extramucosal tumors of the esophagus: Analysis of intramural extramucosal lesions of the gastrointestinal tract in general. *AJR* 48:1-15, 1942.

Schnug GE: Leiomyoma of the cardioesophageal junction. *Arch Surg* 65:342-346, 1952.

Seremetis MG, Lyons WS, DeGuzman VC, et al: Leiomyomata of the esophagus: An analysis of 838 cases. *Cancer* 38:2166-2177, 1976.

Shaffer HA: Multiple leiomyomas of the esophagus. *Radiology* 118:29-34, 1976.

Totten RS, Stout AP, Humphreys GH, et al: Benign tumors and cysts of the esophagus. *J Thorac Surg* 25:606-622, 1953.

Tsuzuki T, Kakegawa T, Arimori M, et al: Giant leiomyoma of the esophagus and cardia weighing more than 1,000 grams. *Chest* 60:396-399, 1971.

Ullal SR: Hypertrophic osteoarthropathy and leiomyoma of the esophagus. *Am J Surg* 123:356-358, 1972.

Wahlen T, Astedt B: Familial occurrence of coexisting leiomyomas of vulva and oesophagus. *Acta Obstet Gynecol Scand* 44:197-203, 1965.

Fibrovascular Polyp

DEFINITION: Rare, benign, tumor-like lesions characterized by the development of pedunculated, intraluminal masses that can grow to gigantic size in the esophagus.

ANATOMIC FINDINGS

Esophagus
- Pedunculated, intraluminal masses that can grow to gigantic size

IMAGING

Radiography
Findings
- Right-sided superior mediastinal mass and anterior tracheal bowing on chest radiographs
- Smooth, expansile, sausage-shaped intraluminal mass arising in cervical esophagus and extending into upper or middle third of thoracic esophagus on barium studies
- Varying degrees of lobulation are sometimes present.

Utility
- Barium esophagography

CT
Findings
- Expansile mass in thoracic esophagus with thin rim of contrast material surrounding lesion
- Fat-density lesion that expands lumen of esophagus if composed predominantly of adipose tissue
- Homogeneous lesion with focal areas of fat density juxtaposed with areas of soft-tissue density if composed of varying amounts of adipose and fibrovascular tissue
- Centrally located feeding artery within the polyp that may show contrast enhancement

Utility
- Spectrum of CT findings depends on amounts of adipose and fibrovascular tissue in lesions.

MRI
Findings
- High signal intensity on T1-weighted MRI

CLINICAL PRESENTATION

- Long-standing dysphagia that slowly progresses over a period of years
- Wheezing or inspiratory stridor if polyp compresses trachea

DIAGNOSTIC PEARLS

- Pedunculated, intraluminal masses that can grow to gigantic sizes
- Smooth, expansile, sausage-shaped intraluminal masses that arise in the cervical esophagus and extend into the upper or middle third of the thoracic esophagus
- Fat-density lesions that expand the lumen of the esophagus on CT
- Heterogeneous lesions with focal areas of fat density juxtaposed with areas of soft-tissue density on CT

- Regurgitation of a fleshy mass into pharynx or mouth
- Potentially life-threatening situation because such lesions have rarely been known to occlude larynx, causing asphyxia and sudden death

DIFFERENTIAL DIAGNOSIS

- Extrinsic impressions (esophagus)
- Spindle cell carcinoma (esophagus)
- Malignant melanoma (esophagus)
- Giant, coalescent air bubbles

Suggested Readings

Avezzano EA, Fleischer DE, Merida MA, et al: Giant fibrovascular polyps of the esophagus. *Am J Gastroenterol* 85:299-302, 1990.

Burrell M, Toffler R: Fibrovascular polyp of the esophagus. *Am J Dig Dis* 18:714-718, 1973.

Carter MM, Kulkarni MV: Giant fibrovascular polyp of the esophagus. *Gastrointest Radiol* 9:301-303, 1984.

Cochet B, Hohl P, Sans M, et al: Asphyxia caused by laryngeal impaction of an esophageal polyp. *Arch Otolaryngol* 106:176-178, 1980.

Kim TS, Song SY, Han J, et al: Giant fibrovascular polyp of the esophagus: CT findings. *Abdom Imaging* 20:653-655, 2005.

Lawrence SP, Larsen BR, Stacy CC, et al: Echoendosonographic and histologic correlation of a fibrovascular polyp of the esophagus. *Gastrointest Endosc* 40:81-84, 1994.

LeBlanc J, Carrier G, Ferland S, et al: Fibrovascular polyp of the esophagus with computed tomographic and pathological correlation. *Can Assoc Radiol J* 41:87-89, 1990.

Levine MS, Buck JL, Pantongrag-Brown L, et al: Fibrovascular polyps of the esophagus: Clinical, radiographic, and pathologic findings in 16 patients. *AJR AM J Roentgenol* 166:781-787, 1996.

WHAT THE REFERRING PHYSICIAN NEEDS TO KNOW

- Malignant degeneration is extremely rare.
- Removal of lesions is recommended because of progressive, debilitating nature of symptoms and risk of asphyxia and sudden death.
- Small fibrovascular polyps may be resected endoscopically, but large tumors should be removed surgically.
- Condition can be mistaken on barium studies for giant, coalescent air bubbles, extrinsic masses compressing esophagus, or other polypoid intraluminal tumors.

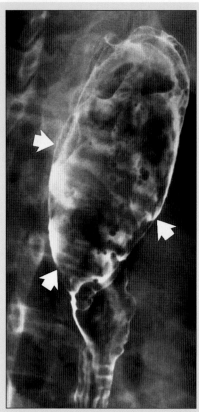

Figure 1. **Barium study shows a smooth, sausage-shaped mass** *(arrows)* **expanding the lumen of the upper thoracic esophagus.** This lesion has the classic appearance of a fibrovascular polyp. (*From Levine MS, Buck JL, Pantongrag-Brown L, et al: Fibrovascular polyps of the esophagus: Clinical, radiographic, and pathologic findings in 16 patients. AJR Am J Roentgenol 166:781-787, 1996, © by American Roentgen Ray Society.*)

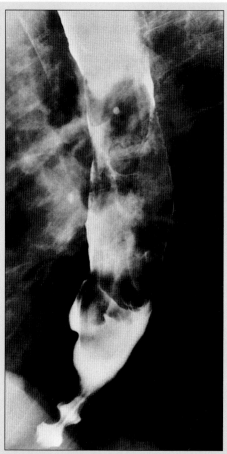

Figure 2. **Barium study shows an expansile mass extending into the distal thoracic esophagus.** In contrast to the polyp in Figure 1, this lesion has a lobulated contour, so it can be mistaken for a malignant esophageal tumor. (*From Levine MS, Buck JL, Pantongrag-Brown L, et al: Fibrovascular polyps of the esophagus: Clinical, radiographic, and pathologic findings in 16 patients. AJR Am J Roentgenol 166:781-787, 1996, © by American Roentgen Ray Society.*)

Lolley D, Razzuk MA, Urschel HC: Giant fibrovascular polyp of the esophagus. *Ann Thorac Surg* 22:383-385, 1976.

Patel J, Kieffer RW, Martin M, et al: Giant fibrovascular polyp of the esophagus. *Gastroenterology* 87:953-956, 1984.

Timmons B, Sedwitz JL, Oller DW: Benign fibrovascular polyp of the esophagus. *South Med J* 84:1370-1372, 1991.

Walters NA, Coral A: Fibrovascular polyp of the oesophagus: The appearances on computed tomography. *Br J Radiol* 61:641-643, 1988.

Watanabe H, Jass JR, Sobin LH: *World Health Organization: Histological Typing of Oesophageal and Gastric Tumours*, 2nd ed. Berlin, Springer-Verlag, 1990.

Whitman GJ, Borkowski GP: Giant fibrovascular polyp of the esophagus: CT and MR findings. *AJR Am J Roentgenol* 152:518-520, 1989.

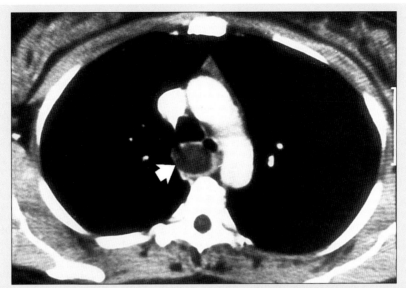

Figure 3. Expansile mass *(arrow)* in the thoracic esophagus with a thin rim of contrast material surrounding the fibrovascular polyp on CT. The fat density of the lesion is caused by an abundance of adipose tissue. *(From Levine MS, Buck JL, Pantongrag-Brown L, et al: Fibrovascular polyps of the esophagus: Clinical, radiographic, and pathologic findings in 16 patients. AJR Am J Roentgenol 166:781-787, 1996, © by American Roentgen Ray Society.)*

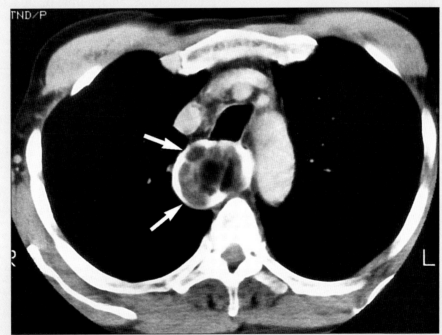

Figure 4. CT scan shows an expansile mass *(arrows)* in the esophagus with intraluminal contrast material surrounding the fibrovascular polyp on CT. In this case, note the heterogeneous appearance of the polyp with areas of fat juxtaposed with areas of soft-tissue density. *(From Levine MS, Buck JL, Pantongrag-Brown L, et al: Fibrovascular polyps of the esophagus: Clinical, radiographic, and pathologic findings in 16 patients. AJR Am J Roentgenol 166:781-787, 1996, © by American Roentgen Ray Society.)*

Other Benign Tumors

DEFINITION: Esophageal tumors that have no malignant potential.

IMAGING

Fluoroscopy
Findings
- Papillomas: small (< 1 cm), sessile polyps with a smooth or slightly lobulated contour
- Esophageal adenomas: sessile or pedunculated polyps in esophagus arising in setting of Barrett esophagus
- Esophageal leiomyomatosis: smooth, tapered narrowing of distal esophagus, with decreased or absent esophageal peristalsis
- Idiopathic muscular hypertrophy of the esophagus: *corkscrew* appearance with multiple lumen-obliterating nonperistaltic contractions
- Granular cell tumors: small, round or oval submucosal masses in the middle or distal third of esophagus
- Lipoma: discrete submucosal mass or, more commonly, pedunculated, intraluminal mass
- Hamartomas in Cowden disease: innumerable tiny hamartomatous polyps in esophagus, producing a diffusely nodular mucosa on double-contrast images

Utility
- Double-contrast esophagography
- Endoscopy should be performed to exclude an early esophageal cancer when a papilloma is suspected on barium studies.

CT
Findings
- Leiomyomatosis; marked circumferential thickening of distal esophageal wall
- Lipoma in esophagus may be diagnosed by characteristic fat density on CT

CLINICAL PRESENTATION
- Most lesions are small and cause no symptoms.
- Occasionally, these lesions may cause dysphagia, bleeding, or other symptoms.

PATHOLOGY
- Most lesions are small and have no malignant potential.
- Depending on the site of origin, benign tumors may be classified as mucosal or submucosal lesions.

DIAGNOSTIC PEARLS
- Sessile or pedunculated polyps in the esophagus
- Leiomyomatosis causes marked circumferential thickening of distal esophageal wall.
- Idiopathic muscular hypertrophy of the esophagus produces *corkscrew* appearance with multiple lumen-obliterating, nonperistaltic contractions

- Esophageal leiomyomatosis is a rare, benign condition in which neoplastic smooth-muscle proliferation causes marked circumferential thickening of esophageal wall, particularly in distal esophagus.
- Leiomyomatosis is found predominantly in children and young adults with long-standing dysphagia.
- Idiopathic muscular hypertrophy is characterized by non-neoplastic thickening of smooth muscle in esophageal wall, possibly in response to severe esophageal spasm.
- Most granular cell tumors in esophagus occur as solitary lesions, ranging from 0.5 to 2.0 cm in diameter.
- Most vascular tumors in esophagus are solitary cavernous hemangiomas.

INCIDENCE/PREVALENCE AND EPIDEMIOLOGY
- Benign tumors of the esophagus constitute only about 20% of all esophageal neoplasms.
- Squamous papillomas are uncommon benign tumors, accounting for less than 5% of all esophageal neoplasms.
- Esophagus is least common site of involvement by lipomas and vascular tumors in gastrointestinal tract.

Suggested Readings

Montesi A, Alessandro P, Graziani L, et al: Small benign tumors of the esophagus: Radiological diagnosis with double-contrast examination. *Gastrointest Radiol* 8:207-212, 1983.
Plachta A: Benign tumors of the esophagus: Review of literature and report of 99 cases. *Am J Gastroenterol* 38:639-652, 1962.

WHAT THE REFERRING PHYSICIAN NEEDS TO KNOW
- Benign tumors of the esophagus are usually discovered fortuitously on radiologic or endoscopic examinations.
- In symptomatic patients, endoscopic or surgical removal may be required.
- Treatment of choice for symptomatic patients with granular cell tumors is local excision.
- With esophageal hemangiomas, the treatment of choice is surgical enucleation because of the risk of significant upper gastrointestinal bleeding.

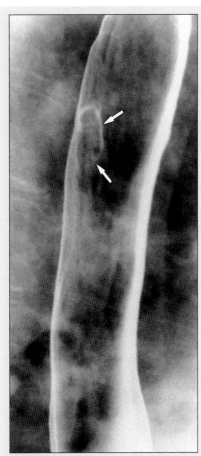

Figure 1. Papilloma. The lesion appears as a sessile, slightly lobulated polyp *(arrows)* in the mid-esophagus. An early esophageal carcinoma can produce similar findings.

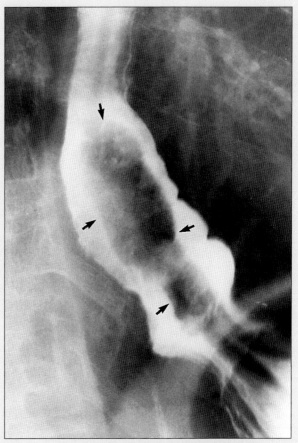

Figure 2. Adenomatous polyp in Barrett esophagus. The polyp *(arrows)* originates at the gastroesophageal junction and extends into the distal esophagus above a hiatal hernia. Although this lesion can be mistaken for an inflammatory esophagogastric polyp, it is larger and more lobulated than most inflammatory polyps. The resected specimen contained a solitary focus of adenocarcinoma. *(From Levine MS, Caroline D, Thompson JJ, et al: Adenocarcinoma of the esophagus: Relationship to Barrett mucosa. Radiology 150:305-309, 1984.)*

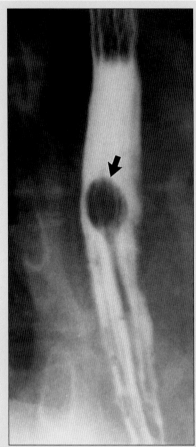

Figure 3. Granular cell tumor. A smooth submucosal mass *(arrow)* is seen in the mid-esophagus. This lesion cannot be differentiated from other, more common submucosal lesions in the esophagus, such as leiomyomas. (*From Levine MS:* Radiology of the Esophagus. *Philadelphia, WB Saunders, 1989.*)

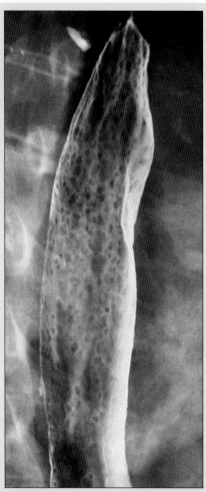

Figure 4. Cowden disease with multiple hamartomatous polyps in the esophagus. The lesions appear as tiny, nodular elevations on the mucosa. (*Courtesy of Stephen W. Trenkner, MD, Minneapolis, MN.*)

Part 11

CARCINOMA OF THE ESOPHAGUS

Squamous Cell Carcinoma

DEFINITION: Malignant tumor of esophagus with histologic features of squamous cell carcinoma.

ANATOMIC FINDINGS

Esophagus
- Infiltrating, polypoid, ulcerative, or varicoid lesions in the upper or middle third of esophagus; less common in distal third
- Tracheoesophageal or esophagobronchial fistulas relatively common with advanced lesions

Lymph Nodes
- Metastatic implants may spread through submucosal lymphatics.
- Segmental lymph node involvement is common.
- May have *jump metastases* to neck, as well as mediastinal, celiac, and upper abdominal lymph nodes

Stomach
- Solitary submucosal mass in fundus due to subdiaphragmatic spread of tumor via lymphatics

IMAGING

Radiography
Findings
- Chest radiographs may reveal mediastinal widening; hilar, retrohilar, or retrocardiac mass; anterior tracheal bowing; or thickened retrotracheal stripe.
- Early cancers may be seen on double-contrast esophagograms as plaque-like lesions or as small, sessile polyps.
- Other early cancers may be manifested by focal irregularity, nodularity, or ulceration of mucosa.
- Superficial spreading carcinoma may produce a short or long area of confluent nodularity or granularity of mucosa.
- Advanced esophageal carcinomas may appear as infiltrating, polypoid, ulcerative, or varicoid lesions.
- Infiltrating lesions cause narrowing and constriction of lumen with irregular mucosa and shelf-like or tapered borders.

DIAGNOSTIC PEARLS

- Upper or middle third of esophagus is usually involved.
- Early cancers are seen as plaque-like lesions, small, sessile polyps, or superficial spreading lesions.
- Advanced carcinomas most commonly appear on barium studies as infiltrating lesions with narrowing and constriction of lumen, irregular mucosa, and shelf-like borders.

- Submucosal spread of the tumor may occasionally be recognized by a smooth, tapered stricture that resembles a benign stricture.
- Polypoid carcinomas are lobulated or fungating intraluminal masses, usually greater than 3.5 cm in size, often with associated ulceration.
- Primary ulcerative carcinomas manifested by giant meniscoid ulcer surrounded by thick, irregular rind of tumor
- Varicoid carcinomas manifested by multiple submucosal defects resembling varices due to submucosal spread of tumor

Utility
- Abnormal chest radiographs are seen in nearly 50% of all patients with advanced disease.
- Double-contrast esophagography is the best radiologic technique for detecting early esophageal cancer.
- Relatively large intraluminal early cancers are difficult to distinguish from advanced carcinomas.
- Varicoid carcinomas can usually be differentiated from esophageal varices at fluoroscopy.
- When esophageal-airway fistula is suspected, barium rather than water-soluble contrast agent should be used.

WHAT THE REFERRING PHYSICIAN NEEDS TO KNOW
- Periodic surveillance is advocated for patients with known predisposing conditions.
- Early detection is possible and results in better prognosis.
- Most cases are advanced lesions at time of clinical presentation and are associated with a poor prognosis.
- Endoscopy is not routinely warranted in patients who have normal barium studies.
- All suspicious lesions on barium studies should prompt endoscopy with multiple biopsies for a definitive diagnosis.

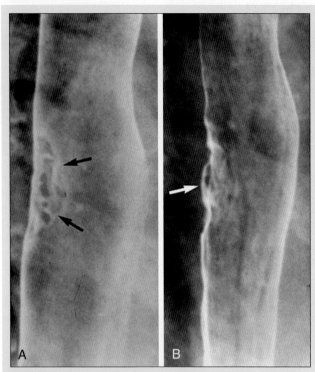

Figure 1. Early esophageal cancer. Oblique (**A**) and tangential (**B**) views reveal a characteristic plaque-like lesion containing a central area of ulceration *(arrows).* (From Laufer I, Levine MS (eds): Double Contrast Gastrointestinal Radiology, 2nd ed. Philadelphia, WB Saunders, 1992.)

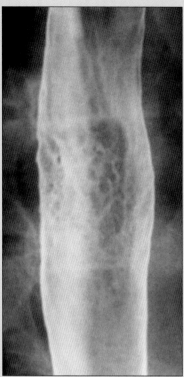

Figure 2. Superficial spreading carcinoma. Note the focal nodularity in the mid-esophagus as a result of tiny, coalescent nodules and plaques. (*From Levine MS:* Radiology of the Esophagus. *Philadelphia, WB Saunders, 1989.*)

CLINICAL PRESENTATION

- Patients typically present with recent onset of dysphagia and weight loss.
- Localizing esophageal symptoms are not always present.
- Patients may also complain of substernal chest pain unrelated to swallowing, hoarseness, or paroxysmal cough on swallowing if tumor erodes into tracheobronchial tree.
- Other symptoms include anorexia, weight loss, guaiac-positive stool, and iron-deficiency anemia caused by occult gastrointestinal bleeding.
- Recurrent or suddenly worsening dysphagia in patients with known predisposing condition is an ominous finding.

DIFFERENTIAL DIAGNOSIS

- Adenocarcinoma (esophagus)
- Spindle cell carcinoma (esophagus)
- Malignant melanoma (esophagus)
- Leiomyosarcoma (esophagus)
- Varices (esophagus)
- Benign esophageal ulcers
- Squamous papilloma

PATHOLOGY

- Tumors appear grossly as infiltrating, polypoid, ulcerative, or varicoid lesions; infiltrating lesions are the most common type.
- Most patients have advanced, unresectable tumors at the time of diagnosis.
- Cause is exposure to carcinogens (e.g., tobacco, alcohol) and a variety of predisposing conditions.
- Early esophageal cancer is confined to mucosa or submucosa without lymphatic involvement.
- Growth of tumor may result in areas of necrosis and ulceration.
- Extratumoral spread occurs through lymphatics and bloodstream, with a marked tendency to invade contiguous structures in neck or chest.
- Most common sites of metastases are lungs, liver, adrenals, kidneys, pancreas, peritoneum, and bones.

INCIDENCE/PREVALENCE AND EPIDEMIOLOGY

- One percent of all cancers and 7% of those in gastrointestinal tract arise in the esophagus.
- Fifty percent of esophageal cancers are squamous cell carcinomas, and 50% are adenocarcinomas.

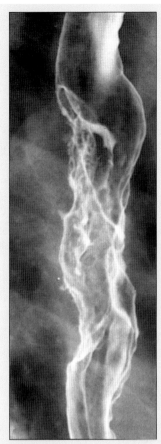

Figure 3. Advanced esophageal carcinoma seen as infiltrating lesion with irregular luminal narrowing and shelf-like borders in mid-esophagus. (*From Levine MS:* Radiology of the Esophagus. *Philadelphia, WB Saunders, 1989.*)

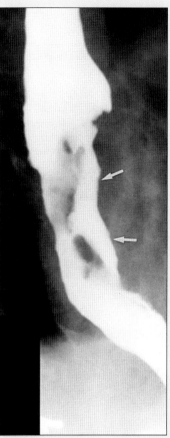

Figure 4. Advanced esophageal carcinoma seen as ulcerative lesion with a large, meniscoid ulcer (*arrows*) and a thick, irregular radiolucent rind of tumor. (*From Levine MS:* Radiology of the Esophagus. *Philadelphia, WB Saunders, 1989.*)

- Disease occurs predominantly in elderly men, with a peak incidence between 65 and 74 years of age.
- Male-to-female ratio is nearly 4:1.
- Major risk factors are tobacco and alcohol consumption.
- Risk is increased in patients with achalasia, lye strictures, or tylosis.

Suggested Readings

Japanese Society for Esophageal Diseases: Guidelines for the clinical and pathologic studies on carcinoma of the esophagus. *Jpn J Surg* 6:69-78, 1976.

Koehler RE, Moss AA, Margulis AR: Early radiographic manifestations of carcinoma of the esophagus. *Radiology* 119:1-5, 1976.

Levine MS, Chu P, Furth EE, et al: Carcinoma of the esophagus and esophagogastric junction: Sensitivity of radiographic diagnosis. *AJR Am J Roentgenol* 168:1423-1426, 1997.

Livstone EM, Skinner DB: Tumors of the esophagus. In Berk JE (ed): *Gastroenterology.* Philadelphia, WB Saunders, 1985, pp 818-850.

Sato T, Sakai Y, Kajita A, et al: Radiographic microstructures of early esophageal carcinoma: Correlation of specimen radiography with pathologic findings and clinical radiography. *Gastrointest Radiol* 11:12-19, 1986.

Yamada A: Radiologic assessment of resectability and prognosis in esophageal carcinoma. *Gastrointest Radiol* 4:213-218, 1979.

Zornoza J, Lindell MM: Radiologic evaluation of small esophageal carcinoma. *Gastrointest Radiol* 5:107-111, 1980.

Adenocarcinoma

DEFINITION: Malignant tumor of esophagus with histologic features of adenocarcinoma.

ANATOMIC FINDINGS

Esophagus
- Infiltrating, polypoid, ulcerative, or varicoid lesions
- Located in distal or, less commonly, middle third of esophagus
- Involve a longer vertical segment of esophagus than most squamous cell carcinomas

Stomach
- Frequent subdiaphragmatic spread to gastric cardia or fundus (unlike squamous cell carcinoma)

IMAGING

Radiography
Findings
- Chest radiographs may show mediastinal widening; hilar, retrohilar, or retrocardiac mass; anterior tracheal bowing; and widened retrotracheal stripe.
- Early cancers are seen as plaque-like lesions or as small, sessile, or pedunculated polyps.
- Localized area of flattening or stiffening in one wall of a peptic stricture may be only sign of early, developing adenocarcinoma.
- Superficial spreading carcinoma may produce an area of confluent nodularity or granularity of mucosa.
- Advanced esophageal carcinomas may appear as infiltrating, polypoid, ulcerative, or varicoid lesions.
- Smooth submucosal mass is occasionally seen.
- Gastric involvement may be manifested by polypoid or ulcerated mass or distortion of normal anatomic landmarks at cardia, with irregular areas of ulceration but no discrete mass.

Utility
- Abnormal chest radiographs occur in nearly 50% of all patients with advanced disease.
- Double-contrast esophagography is the best radiologic technique for diagnosing early esophageal cancer.
- Barium studies are used for differentiating benign and malignant strictures and varicoid tumors from esophageal varices.

DIAGNOSTIC PEARLS
- Infiltrative, polypoid, ulcerative, or varicoid lesions
- Usually involves long segment of distal third of esophagus
- Clinical or radiologic evidence of reflux disease
- Frequent spread to gastric cardia or fundus

CLINICAL PRESENTATION
- Recent onset of dysphagia and weight loss
- Possible long-standing reflux symptoms caused by underlying reflux disease
- Gastrointestinal bleeding, odynophagia, low-grade anemia, and chest pain

DIFFERENTIAL DIAGNOSIS
- Squamous cell carcinoma (esophagus)
- Spindle cell carcinoma (esophagus)
- Malignant melanoma (esophagus)
- Gastric carcinoma invading esophagus
- Varices (esophagus)
- Benign esophageal ulcers
- Squamous papilloma

PATHOLOGY
- Columnar metaplasia (Barrett esophagus) caused by long-standing gastroesophageal reflux and reflux esophagitis
- Progressively severe epithelial dysplasia that eventually leads to malignant degeneration

INCIDENCE/PREVALENCE AND EPIDEMIOLOGY
- One percent of all cancers and 7% of those in the gastrointestinal tract arise in the esophagus.
- Predominantly a disease of elderly men.

WHAT THE REFERRING PHYSICIAN NEEDS TO KNOW
- Most esophageal adenocarcinomas are advanced, unresectable tumors at time of diagnosis.
- Endoscopic surveillance of patients with Barrett esophagus does not necessarily decrease mortality rates from esophageal adenocarcinoma.

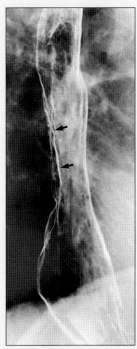

Figure 1. **Early adenocarcinoma in Barrett esophagus.** Note the relatively long peptic stricture in the distal esophagus with slight flattening and stiffening of one wall of the stricture *(arrows)*. Surgery revealed an intramucosal adenocarcinoma arising in Barrett esophagus. *(From Levine MS, Caroline D, Thompson JJ, et al: Adenocarcinoma of the esophagus: Relationship to Barrett mucosa.* Radiology *150:305-309, 1984.)*

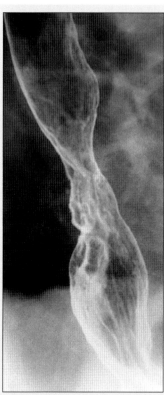

Figure 2. **Advanced adenocarcinoma in Barrett esophagus.** Seen as infiltrating lesion causing irregular luminal narrowing of distal esophagus above a hiatal hernia.

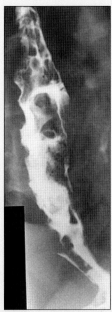

Figure 3. **Advanced adenocarcinoma in Barrett esophagus.** This lesion is seen as varicoid lesion with multiple submucosal defects in distal esophagus, mimicking the appearance of varices on a simple image. *(From Levine MS, Caroline D, Thompson JJ, et al: Adenocarcinoma of the esophagus: Relationship to Barrett mucosa.* Radiology *150:305-309, 1984.)*

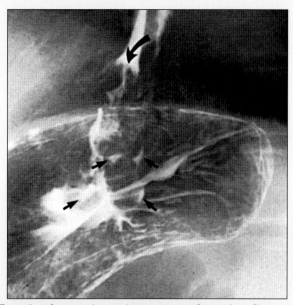

Figure 4. **Adenocarcinoma in Barrett esophagus invading the stomach.** Double-contrast view of the gastric fundus shows obliteration of the normal anatomic landmarks at the cardia with irregular areas of ulceration *(straight arrows)*. Also note tumor involving the distal esophagus *(curved arrow)*. At surgery, this patient had a primary adenocarcinoma arising in Barrett mucosa with secondary gastric involvement. *(From Levine MS, Caroline D, Thompson JJ, et al: Adenocarcinoma of the esophagus: Relationship to Barrett mucosa.* Radiology *150:305-309,1984.)*

- Male-to-female ratio is nearly 4:1.
- Peak incidence is between 65 and 74 years of age.
- Fifty percent of esophageal cancers are adenocarcinomas.
- Almost all (95%-100%) primary esophageal adenocarcinomas arise on background of Barrett mucosa.
- Patients with Barrett esophagus have 30 to 40 times greater risk of developing esophageal carcinoma than the general population.

Suggested Readings

Agha FP: Barrett carcinoma of the esophagus: Clinical and radiographic analysis of 34 cases. *AJR Am J Roentgenol* 145:41-46, 1985.

Bosch A, Frias Z, Caldwell WL: Adenocarcinoma of the esophagus. *Cancer* 43:1557-1561, 1979.

Bytzer P, Christensen PB, Damkier P, et al: Adenocarcinoma of the esophagus and Barrett's esophagus: A population-based study. *Am J Gastroenterol* 94:86-91, 1999.

Engelman RM, Scialla AV: Carcinoma of the esophagus presenting radiologically as a benign lesion. *Dis Chest* 53:652-655, 1968.

Keen SJ: Dodd GD, Smith JL. Adenocarcinoma arising in Barrett's esophagus: Pathologic and radiologic features. *Mt Sinai J Med* 51:442-450, 1984.

Levine MS, Caroline D, Thompson JJ, et al: Adenocarcinoma of the esophagus: Relationship to Barrett mucosa. *Radiology* 150:305-309, 1984.

Livstone EM, Skinner DB: Tumors of the esophagus. In Berk JE (ed): *Gastroenterology*. Philadelphia, WB Saunders, 1985, pp 818-850.

Staging of Esophageal Carcinoma

DEFINITION: Staging of esophageal neoplasms.

ANATOMIC FINDINGS

Esophagus
- Infiltrating, polypoid, ulcerative, or varicoid tumors

Lymph Nodes
- Metastases are found above and below or adjacent to primary tumor.
- Distal esophageal cancers usually have upper abdominal lymph node involvement.

IMAGING

Radiography
Utility
- Radiography is used as a tool for diagnosis rather than for staging of esophageal cancer.

CT
Findings
- Enlarged lymph nodes
- Bowing or indentation of posterior wall of trachea or bronchus indicates invasion by tumor.
- Tumor extending to posterior surface of heart with no intervening fat plane and bulging into left atrial lumen indicates pericardial invasion.
- Tumor that obliterates more than one fourth of circumferential aortic fat plane (> 90 degrees) indicates aortic invasion. (If tumor obliterates less than 45 degrees of circumference, then no aortic invasion; if tumor obliterates 45 to 90 degrees, CT findings are indeterminant for aortic invasion.)
- Patients with distant metastases to lungs, bones, liver, or other structures have a much worse prognosis.

Utility
- CT is initial test for esophageal cancer staging.
- Intravenous contrast material is administered whenever possible for identification of hepatic and lymph node metastases.
- Scan should include upper abdomen as well as thorax.
- Major CT criteria include local invasion of mediastinum, regional lymph node involvement, and distant metastases.
- CT is more accurate for predicting upper abdominal lymph node metastases than mediastinal lymph node metastases.

DIAGNOSTIC PEARLS
- Esophageal tumor
- Lymph node metastases
- Direct invasion of contiguous structures
- Distant metastases

Ultrasound
Findings
- Tumor seen as hypoechogenic mass causing disruption or widening of layers of esophageal wall
- Excellent differentiation of T2 tumors (confined to wall) from T3 tumors (extending beyond wall into periesophageal fat)
- Hypoechoic foci are secondary to mediastinal lymph node involvement.
- Abnormal lymph nodes have diameter larger than 5 mm or a short-to-long ratio of greater than 50%.

Utility
- Endoscopic ultrasound (EUS) is used for staging if CT is negative or indeterminant for local invasion or distant metastases.
- 20% to 45% of advanced esophageal cancers cause severe intraluminal narrowing that prevents passage of ultrasound probe.
- Ultrasound is limited in evaluating T4 tumors.
- Accuracy can be increased by transesophageal EUS-guided fine-needle aspiration cytology of peritumoral mediastinal lymph nodes.
- Used to detect cervical lymph node metastases for tumors located in upper esophagus
- Further investigation is needed to determine whether ultrasonography of neck should be performed routinely.

Positron-Emission Tomography (PET)
Findings
- Esophageal tumors and metastases are areas with avid fluorodeoxyglucose (FDG) uptake.

Utility
- Used to detect local invasion or distant metastases not recognized on CT or EUS.

WHAT THE REFERRING PHYSICIAN NEEDS TO KNOW
- Most cases are advanced at the time of clinical presentation and are associated with poor prognosis.
- Combination of CT, EUS, and PET is advocated for staging.
- Stage is used to determine appropriate treatment modalities.

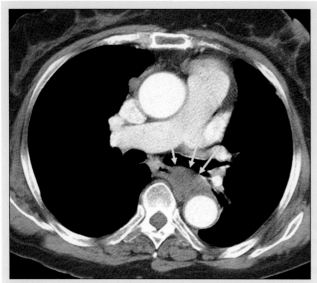

Figure 1. Bronchial invasion by esophageal carcinoma.
CT scan shows esophageal tumor bowing and displacing the
posterior wall *(arrows)* of the left main bronchus. This finding is
diagnostic of bronchial invasion.

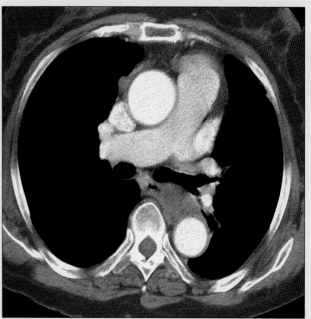

Figure 2. Aortic invasion by esophageal carcinoma. CT scan
shows greater than 90 degrees of contact between the esophageal
tumor and aorta without intervening fat planes. This is a useful
CT criterion for predicting aortic invasion.

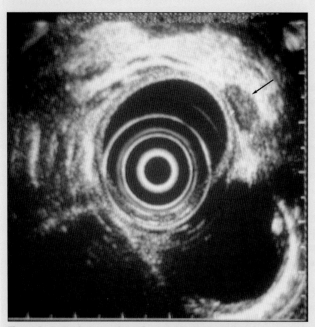

**Figure 3. EUS showing lymph node metastasis from
esophageal carcinoma.** The enlarged node is characterized by a
hypoechoic focus *(arrow)*.

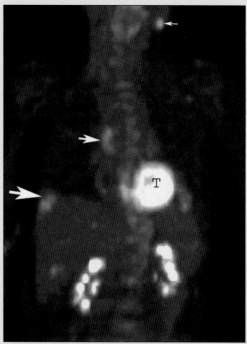

Figure 4. Value of PET for showing metastases. Coronal PET
image shows marked uptake of radionuclide in distal esophageal
tumor (T). However, uptake also occurs in metastases to the
liver *(large arrow)*, mediastinum *(medium arrow)*, and left
cervical lymph node *(small arrow)*. The PET scan has therefore
dramatically altered the staging of this patient's disease.

CLINICAL PRESENTATION

- Persistent substernal chest pain unrelated to swallowing is a sign of advanced esophageal carcinoma invading the mediastinum.
- Paroxysmal coughing on swallowing is a sign of tumor invading airway with a tracheoesophageal or esophagobronchial fistula.
- Other symptoms include anorexia, weight loss, and signs of occult gastrointestinal bleeding.

INCIDENCE/PREVALENCE AND EPIDEMIOLOGY

- One percent of all cancers and 7% of those in the gastrointestinal tract arise in esophagus.
- Disease occurs predominantly in elderly men.
- Male-to-female ratio is nearly 4:1.
- Peak incidence is between 65 and 74 years of age.
- Major risk factors are tobacco and alcohol consumption for squamous cell carcinoma and Barrett esophagus for adenocarcinoma.

Suggested Readings

Doldi SB, Lattuada E, Zappa MA, et al: Ultrasonographic evaluation of the cervical lymph nodes in preoperative staging of esophageal neoplasms. *Abdom Imaging* 23:275-277, 1998.

Griffith JF, Chanc ACW, Ahuja AT, et al: Neck ultrasound in staging squamous oesophageal carcinoma—a high yield technique. *Clin Radiol* 55:696-701, 2000.

Halvorsen RA, Magruder-Habib K, Foster W, et al: Esophageal cancer: Long-term follow-up of staging by computed tomography. *Radiology* 161:147-151, 1986.

Heidemann J, Schilling MK, Schmassmann A, et al: Accuracy of endoscopic ultrasonography in preoperative staging of esophageal carcinoma. *Dig Surg* 17:219-224, 2000.

Imdahl A, Hentschel M, Kleimaier M, et al: Impact of FDG-PET for staging of oesophageal cancer. *Langenbecks Arch Surg* 389:283-288, 2004.

Kato H, Miyazaki T, Nakajima M, et al: The incremental effect of positron emission tomography on diagnostic accuracy on the initial staging of esophageal cancer. *Cancer* 103:148-156, 2005.

Kelly S, Harris KM, Berry E, et al: A systematic review of the staging performance of endoscopic ultrasound in gastroesophageal carcinoma. *Gut* 49:534-539, 2001.

Koch J, Halvorsen RA, Thompson WM: Therapy hinges on staging in upper GI tract cancer. *Diagn Imaging* 15:74-81, 1993.

Lightdale CJ, Kulkarni KG: Role of endoscopic ultrasonography in the staging and follow-up of esophageal cancer. *J Clin Oncol* 23:4483-4489, 2005.

Picus D, Balfe DM, Koehler RE, et al: Computed tomography in the staging of esophageal carcinoma. *Radiology* 146:433-438, 1983.

Savides TJ: EUS FNA staging of esophageal cancer [editorial]: *Gastroenterology* 125:1883-1886, 2003.

Thompson WM, Halvorsen RA, Foster WL, et al: Computed tomography for staging esophageal and gastroesophageal cancer: Reevaluation. *AJR Am J Roentgenol* 141:951-958, 1983.

Part 12

OTHER MALIGNANT TUMORS OF THE ESOPHAGUS

Metastases to the Esophagus

DEFINITION: Esophageal involvement by metastatic tumor.

IMAGING

Radiography
Findings
- Smooth or slightly irregular defect with gently sloping, obtuse borders and a contiguous soft-tissue mass, with serrated, scalloped, or nodular contour
- Circumferential narrowing of esophagus with mass effect, nodularity, ulceration, or obstruction
- Carcinoma of gastric cardia or fundus; polypoid mass extending from the fundus into distal esophagus or irregular distal esophageal narrowing without a discrete mass
- Distortion or obliteration of normal anatomic landmarks at the cardia with subtle areas of nodularity, mass effect, or ulceration
- Smooth, slightly lobulated extrinsic indentation at or below the carina with irregular contour and ulceration and, if circumferential invasion exists, concentric narrowing with surrounding soft-tissue mass
- Short, eccentric strictures with intact overlying mucosa and smooth, tapered margins

Utility
- Gastric cardia and fundus should be evaluated radiographically to determine the presence of associated gastric involvement in patients with distal esophageal tumors.
- Meticulous double-contrast examination of fundus is essential to rule out an underlying carcinoma of cardia.

CT
Findings
- Esophageal compression by mediastinal lymphadenopathy

Utility
- Shows extent and location of adenopathy in mediastinum
- Differentiates recurrent tumor from radiation stricture by showing a mediastinal mass or lymphadenopathy in region of stricture

CLINICAL PRESENTATION
- Dysphagia and weight loss

DIAGNOSTIC PEARLS
- Mass with irregular, serrated, or nodular contour associated with angulated, tethered folds or ulceration
- Usually appears on barium studies as short, eccentric strictures (most frequently in the middle third of the esophagus) with intact overlying mucosa and smooth, tapered margins
- Circumferential narrowing of the esophagus with mass effect, nodularity, ulceration, or even obstruction

DIFFERENTIAL DIAGNOSIS
- Idiopathic eosinophilic esophagitis
- Radiation stricture

PATHOLOGY
- Direct invasion by primary malignant tumors of the stomach, lung, and neck
- Contiguous involvement of tumor-containing lymph nodes in mediastinum
- Hematogenous metastases from breast cancer or other malignant tumor

INCIDENCE/PREVALENCE AND EPIDEMIOLOGY
- Found in less than 5% of patients dying of carcinoma
- Carcinoma of stomach accounts for approximately 50% of all esophageal metastases.
- Esophagus is involved by contiguous spread of malignant tumors in neck, such as laryngeal, pharyngeal, and thyroid carcinomas.
- Hematogenous metastases are rare, mostly caused by breast carcinoma.

WHAT THE REFERRING PHYSICIAN NEEDS TO KNOW
- Presence of esophageal metastases usually indicates a poor prognosis.
- When dysphagia occurs, these patients usually have widespread metastatic disease.

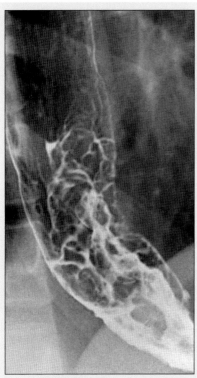

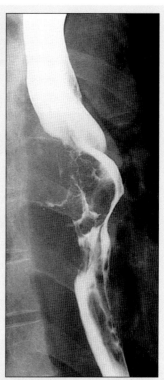

Figure 1. Direct esophageal invasion by gastric carcinoma. Double-contrast esophagogram shows a polypoid lesion in the distal esophagus that extends inferiorly to the gastroesophageal junction. (*From Levine MS:* Radiology of the Esophagus. *Philadelphia, WB Saunders, 1989.*)

Figure 2. Esophageal involvement by mediastinal lymphadenopathy from carcinoma of the cervix. Eccentric mass effect on the mid-esophagus with an irregular contour and areas of ulceration caused by esophageal invasion by tumor in adjacent subcarinal nodes. (*From Levine MS:* Radiology of the Esophagus. *Philadelphia, WB Saunders, 1989.*)

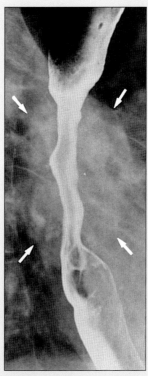

Figure 3. Circumferential esophageal involvement by metastatic breast cancer in the mediastinum. A smooth, tapered area of narrowing is seen in the mid-esophagus. However, a surrounding soft-tissue mass *(arrows)* in the mediastinum suggests esophageal involvement by lymphadenopathy. (*From Levine MS:* Radiology of the Esophagus. *Philadelphia, WB Saunders, 1989.*)

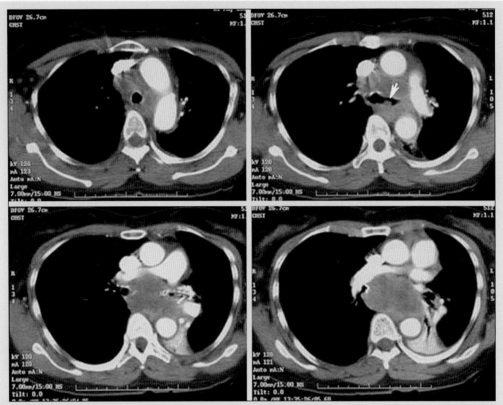

Figure 4. Esophageal compression by mediastinal lymphadenopathy from carcinoma of the lung. CT scan shows bulky mediastinal and subcarinal adenopathy compressing the esophagus. An endobronchial lesion *(arrow)* is also seen in the left main bronchus near the carina. Patient was found to have a small cell carcinoma of the lung. *(Courtesy of Vincent Low, MD, Perth, Australia.)*

■ Breast cancer may have late-onset metastases to esophagus, with average interval of 8 years from time of diagnosis.

Suggested Readings

Agha FP: Secondary neoplasms of the esophagus. *Gastrointest Radiol* 12:187-193, 1987.

Anderson MF, Harell GS: Secondary esophageal tumors. *AJR Am J Roentgenol* 135:1243-1246, 1980.

Balthazar EJ, Goldfine S, Davidian NM: Carcinoma of the esophago-gastric junction. *Am J Gastroenterol* 74:237-243, 1980.

Fisher MS: Metastasis to the esophagus. *Gastrointest Radiol* 1:249-251, 1976.

Secondary Achalasia

DEFINITION: Absent esophageal peristalsis and a hypertensive lower esophageal sphincter that fails to relax normally in response to deglutition.

IMAGING

Radiography
Findings
- Absent peristalsis in body of esophagus
- Smooth, tapered narrowing of distal esophagus with bird-beak configuration
- Asymmetric or eccentric narrowing, abrupt transitions, rigidity, and mucosal nodularity or ulceration
- Length of narrowed segment can extend 3.5 cm or more above gastroesophageal junction
- Associated evidence of tumor in gastric cardia and fundus

Utility
- Double-contrast studies can better detect less advanced lesions

CT
Findings
- Asymmetric esophageal wall thickening, soft-tissue mass at the cardia, or mediastinal adenopathy in patients with secondary achalasia

Utility
- Helps differentiate primary from secondary achalasia
- Identifies site of primary tumor in patients with secondary achalasia caused by remote tumors

CLINICAL PRESENTATION

- Recent onset of dysphagia and weight loss in patients over 60 years of age is characteristic of secondary achalasia.

DIFFERENTIAL DIAGNOSIS

- Primary achalasia (esophagus)
- Other esophageal motility disorders

PATHOLOGY

- May be caused by tumor directly invading myenteric plexus in the wall of the distal esophagus and gastroesophageal junction or by tumor in the vagus nerve or dorsal motor nucleus of the brainstem

DIAGNOSTIC PEARLS

- *Bird-beak* configuration at or just above gastroesophageal junction
- Length of narrowed segment may extend 3.5 cm or more above gastroesophageal junction.
- Most patients are older than 60 years of age, and the duration of symptoms is usually less than 6 months.

- May occur as a paraneoplastic phenomenon caused by circulating tumor products that alter esophageal motor function
- Malignant neuroendocrine tumors express a variety of neural antigens that initiate an autoimmune response with circulating antibodies (anti-Hu antibodies), causing neural degeneration.

INCIDENCE/PREVALENCE AND EPIDEMIOLOGY

- Mainly affects persons older than 60 years of age
- Malignancy-induced secondary achalasia accounts for only 2% to 4% of all patients with findings of achalasia.
- Seventy-five percent of cases are caused by carcinoma of the gastric cardia or fundus.

Suggested Readings

McCallum RW: Esophageal achalasia secondary to gastric carcinoma: Report of a case and review of the literature. Am J Gastroenterol 71:24-29, 1979.

Parkman HP, Cohen S: Malignancy-induced secondary achalasia. Dysphagia 8:292-296, 1993.

Rabushka LS, Fishman EK, Kuhlman JE: CT evaluation of achalasia. J Comput Assist Tomogr 15:434-439, 1991.

Simeone J, Burrell M, Toffler R: Esophageal aperistalsis secondary to metastatic invasion of the myenteric plexus. AJR Am J Roentgenol 27:862-864, 1976.

Tucker HJ, Snape WJ, Cohen SC: Achalasia secondary to carcinoma: Manometric and clinical features. Ann Intern Med 89:315-318, 1978.

Woodfield CA, Levine MS, Rubesin SE, et al: Diagnosis of primary versus secondary achalasia: Reassessment of clinical and radiographic criteria. AJR Am J Roentgenol 175:727-731, 2000.

WHAT THE REFERRING PHYSICIAN NEEDS TO KNOW

- Condition often necessitates exploratory laparotomy or other treatment for widespread metastatic disease.
- An underlying malignant tumor should be suspected whenever secondary achalasia is diagnosed.

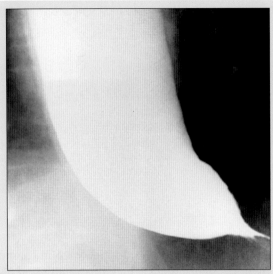

Figure 1. Secondary achalasia caused by gastric carcinoma. Smooth, tapered narrowing of the distal esophagus produces a characteristic *bird-beak* appearance typically associated with primary achalasia.

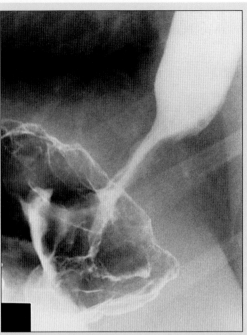

Figure 2. Secondary achalasia caused by carcinoma of the gastric cardia. Smooth, tapered narrowing of the distal esophagus, but the narrowed segment extends a considerable distance from the gastroesophageal junction (a finding not often seen in patients with primary achalasia). Also note how the tumor causes marked nodularity of the gastric fundus with obliteration of the normal anatomic landmarks at the cardia. (*From Levine MS:* Radiology of the Esophagus. *Philadelphia, WB Saunders, 1989.*)

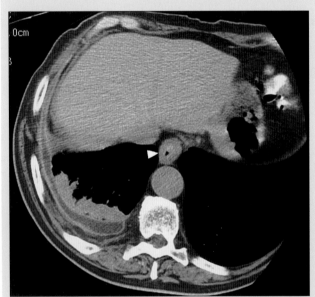

Figure 3. Secondary achalasia on CT. Note marked thickening of the esophageal wall *(arrowhead)* in the distal esophagus at the level where beak-like narrowing was seen on a prior barium study (not shown).

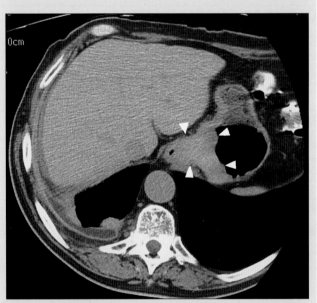

Figure 4. Secondary achalasia on CT. This scan more caudally shows an asymmetric soft-tissue mass *(arrowheads)* at the gastroesophageal junction protruding into the gas-filled fundus. The patient had a carcinoma of the cardia causing secondary achalasia.

Spindle Cell Carcinoma

DEFINITION: Malignant polypoid epithelial tumors of esophagus containing both carcinomatous and sarcomatous elements.

IMAGING

Radiography
Findings
- Large polyploid intraluminal mass dilates or expands esophagus without causing obstruction (primary malignant melanoma of esophagus may produce identical radiographic findings).
- Barium may form a dome over intraluminal portion of tumor, producing a cupola effect.
- Broad-based or narrow pedicle is occasionally seen.

Utility
- Esophagography

CT
Findings
- Bulky soft-tissue mass expanding lumen of esophagus

CLINICAL PRESENTATION
- Dysphagia
- Weight loss

DIFFERENTIAL DIAGNOSIS
- Primary malignant melanoma of the esophagus
- Adenocarcinoma (esophagus)
- Squamous cell carcinoma (esophagus)

PATHOLOGY
- Tumor contains both carcinomatous and sarcomatous elements; both elements can metastasize to regional lymph nodes or distant structures.
- Produces varying degrees of anaplastic spindle cell metaplasia of carcinomatous portion of tumor

DIAGNOSTIC PEARLS
- Produces a large polyploid intraluminal mass that expands or dilates esophagus without causing obstruction
- Tends to be located in the middle or distal third of esophagus
- Definitive diagnosis of spindle cell carcinoma can be made only on histologic grounds.

- Tumors are usually polyploid lesions, but some can be infiltrating or annular lesions indistinguishable from squamous cell carcinomas.

INCIDENCE/PREVALENCE AND EPIDEMIOLOGY
- Accounts for only 0.5% to 1.5% of all esophageal neoplasms
- Usually affects elderly men with a history of cigarette smoking or alcohol consumption
- Fifty percent of patients with spindle cell carcinoma have metastatic disease.
- Five-year survival rate is only 2% to 8%.

Suggested Readings

Agha FP, Keren DF: Spindle-cell squamous carcinoma of the esophagus: A tumor with biphasic morphology. *AJR Am J Roentgenol* 145:541-545, 1985.

Halvorsen RA, Foster WL, Williford ME, et al: Pseudosarcoma of the esophagus: Barium swallow and CT findings. *J Can Assoc Radiol* 34:278-281, 1983.

Martin MR, Kahn LB: So-called pseudosarcoma of the esophagus: Nodal metastases of the spindle cell element. *Arch Pathol Lab Med* 101:604-609, 1977.

Postlethwait RW, Wechsler AS, Shelburne JD: Pseudosarcoma of the esophagus. *Ann Thorac Surg* 19:198-205, 1975.

Talbert JL, Cantrell JR: Clinical and pathological characteristics of carcinosarcoma of the esophagus. *J Thorac Cardiovasc Surg* 45: 1-12, 1963.

WHAT THE REFERRING PHYSICIAN NEEDS TO KNOW
- Fifty percent of patients with spindle cell carcinoma have metastatic disease at time of diagnosis.
- Overall 5-year survival rate is only 2% to 8%.

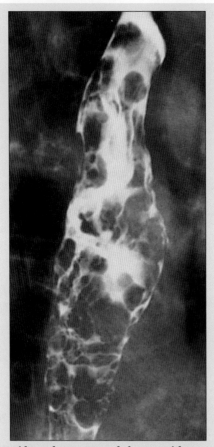

Figure 1. Long polypoid intraluminal mass in mid-esophagus expands lumen without causing obstruction. This appearance is typical of spindle cell carcinoma but can also be seen with primary malignant melanoma of esophagus. (*From Laufer I, Levine MS [eds]:* Double-Contrast Gastrointestinal Radiology, *2nd ed. Philadelphia, WB Saunders, 1992.*)

Leiomyosarcoma

DEFINITION: Rare low-grade malignant tumor characterized by slow growth and late metastases.

ANATOMIC FINDINGS

Esophagus
- Luminal narrowing
- Mass

IMAGING

Radiography
Findings
- Mediastinal mass on chest radiographs with dense calcification in tumor
- Large, lobulated intramural mass containing areas of ulceration or tracking
- Polypoid, expansile intraluminal mass in esophagus

Utility
- Same features on barium studies as malignant gastrointestinal stromal tumors in the stomach and small bowel

CT
Findings
- Heterogeneous mass containing large exophytic components, central areas of low density, and extraluminal gas or contrast material within tumor

Utility
- Same features on CT as malignant gastrointestinal stromal tumors elsewhere in the gastrointestinal tract.

MRI
Findings
- Esophageal mass isointense with skeletal muscle on T1-weighted images and hyperintense on T2-weighted images
- Central signal void caused by extraluminal gas within tumor

Ultrasound
Findings
- Well-defined hyperechoic mass arising from muscular layer of esophageal wall

Utility
- Endoscopic sonography

DIAGNOSTIC PEARLS
- Large exophytic components are recognized on chest radiographs as mediastinal masses.
- Barium studies show large, lobulated intramural masses containing areas of ulceration or tracking.
- CT shows heterogeneous masses containing large exophytic components, central areas of low density, and extraluminal gas or contrast material within the tumor.

Interventional Radiology
Findings
- Hypervascular mass with tumor vessels, dilated vascular channels, and venous lakes
- Early venous drainage

CLINICAL PRESENTATION
- Dysphagia is present for a longer interval than in most patients with malignant esophageal tumors.
- Gastrointestinal bleeding is common with ulcerated lesions.

DIFFERENTIAL DIAGNOSIS
- Esophageal invasion by tumor in mediastinum
- Malignant melanoma (esophagus)
- Spindle cell carcinoma (esophagus)

PATHOLOGY
- Low-grade malignant tumors that arise de novo in esophagus and are characterized by slow growth and late metastases
- Usual location is in the distal two thirds of esophagus.
- Spread is by direct extension to the pleura, pericardium, diaphragm, and stomach, or by hematogenous dissemination of tumor to the liver, lungs, and bones.

WHAT THE REFERRING PHYSICIAN NEEDS TO KNOW
- Prognosis is better than for squamous cell carcinomas, with 5-year survival rates approaching 35%.
- An esophagectomy or esophagogastrectomy is the treatment of choice.
- Lesions can also be palliated by radiation therapy in nonsurgical candidates.

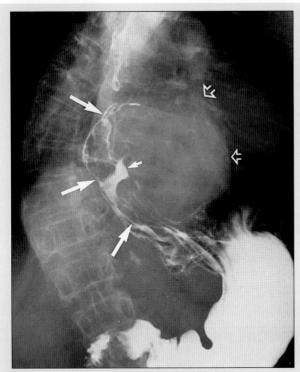

Figure 1. Esophageal leiomyosarcoma. Barium study shows giant intramural mass *(large arrows)* with bulky exophytic component in mediastinum *(open arrows)*. Note relatively small central ulcer *(small arrow)* within the lesion. (*From Levine MS, Buck JL, Pantongrag-Brown L, et al: Leiomyosarcoma of the esophagus: Radiographic findings in 10 patients. AJR Am J Roentgenol 167:27-32, 1996, © by American Roentgen Ray Society.*)

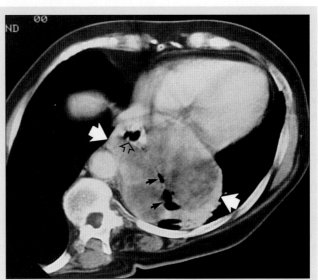

Figure 2. Esophageal leiomyosarcoma. CT scan shows heterogeneous mass *(white arrows)* in the left side of mediastinum with central areas of low density. Note extraluminal collections of gas *(solid black arrows)* within the lesion that are separate from esophageal lumen *(open black arrow)*. (*From Levine MS, Buck JL, Pantongrag-Brown L, et al: Leiomyosarcoma of the esophagus: Radiographic findings in 10 patients. AJR Am J Roentgenol 167:27-32, 1996, © by American Roentgen Ray Society.*)

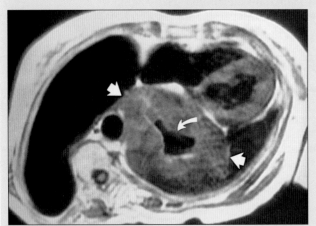

Figure 3. Esophageal leiomyosarcoma. T1-weighted MR image shows mass *(straight arrows)* in the left side of mediastinum. Note how the mass is isointense with skeletal muscle. Also note a focal area of signal void *(curved arrow)* caused by extraluminal gas within tumor. (*From Levine MS, Buck JL, Pantongrag-Brown L, et al: Leiomyosarcoma of the esophagus: Radiographic findings in 10 patients. AJR Am J Roentgenol 167:27-32, 1996, © by American Roentgen Ray Society.*)

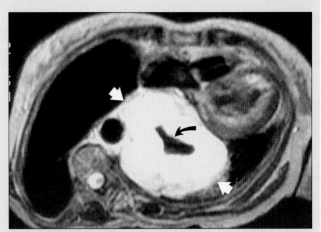

Figure 4. Esophageal leiomyosarcoma. T2-weighted MR image shows how the lesion *(straight arrows)* is markedly hyperintense relative to skeletal muscle. Note the focal area of signal void *(curved arrow)* caused by extraluminal gas within tumor. (*From Levine MS, Buck JL, Pantongrag-Brown L, et al: Leiomyosarcoma of the esophagus: Radiographic findings in 10 patients. AJR Am J Roentgenol 167:27-32, 1996, © by American Roentgen Ray Society.*)

INCIDENCE/PREVALENCE AND EPIDEMIOLOGY

- Found in middle-aged or elderly patients
- More common in men than in women
- Rare malignant tumor of esophagus

Suggested Readings

Athanasoulis CA, Aral IM: Leiomyosarcoma of the esophagus. *Gastroenterology* 54:271-274, 1968.

Choh JH, Khazei AH, Ihm HJ: Leiomyosarcoma of the esophagus: Report of a case and review of the literature. *J Surg Oncol* 32:223-226, 1986.

Koga H, Iida M, Suekane H, et al: Rapidly growing esophageal leiomyosarcoma: Case report and review of the literature. *Abdom Imaging* 20:15-19, 1995.

Ohnishi T, Yoshioka H, Ishida O: MR imaging of gastrointestinal leiomyosarcoma. *Radiat Med* 9:114-117, 1991.

Patel SR, Anandarao N: Leiomyosarcoma of the esophagus. *N Y State J Med* 90:371-372, 1990.

Weinstein EC, Kim YS, Young GJ, et al: Leiomyosarcoma of the esophagus. *Milit Med* 4:206-209, 1988.

Malignant Melanoma

DEFINITION: Rare but aggressive tumors that develop because of malignant degeneration of preexisting melanocytes in esophageal mucosa.

IMAGING

Radiography
Findings
- Bulky, polypoid intraluminal mass that expands the esophagus without causing obstruction. (Major consideration in differential diagnosis is spindle cell carcinoma, which produces identical radiographic findings.)

Utility
- Esophageal melanomas have strikingly similar findings on barium studies.

CT
Findings
- Large soft-tissue mass expanding the esophagus

CLINICAL PRESENTATION

- Dysphagia
- Weight loss

DIFFERENTIAL DIAGNOSIS

- Spindle cell carcinoma (esophagus)
- Adenocarcinoma (esophagus)
- Squamous cell carcinoma (esophagus)
- Leiomyosarcoma (esophagus)
- Fibrovascular polyp (esophagus)

PATHOLOGY

- Tumor is a rare but aggressive type that develops as a result of malignant degeneration of preexisting melanocytes in esophageal mucosa.
- Tendency is to grow intraluminally along longitudinal axis of esophagus, producing a polypoid mass that widens lumen as it enlarges.

DIAGNOSTIC PEARLS

- Barium studies show bulky, polypoid intraluminal masses that expand esophagus without causing obstruction.
- Most masses are located in lower half of the esophagus.
- Tendency is to grow intraluminally along longitudinal axis of esophagus, producing a polypoid mass that widens the lumen as it enlarges.

INCIDENCE/PREVALENCE AND EPIDEMIOLOGY

- Rare, accounting for less than 1% of all malignant esophageal neoplasms
- Usually diagnosed in elderly adults
- Ten times more common than metastatic melanoma involving esophagus
- Five-year survival rate of less than 5%
- Average overall survival of only 10 to 13 months from time of diagnosis
- Mostly located in lower half of esophagus

Suggested Readings

Chalkiadakis G, Wihlm JM, Morand G, et al: Primary malignant melanoma of the esophagus. *Ann Thorac Surg* 39:472-475, 1985.

Dela Pava S, Nigogosyan G, Pickren JW, et al: Melanosis of the esophagus. *Cancer* 16:48-50, 1963.

Sabanathan S, Eng J, Pradhan GN: Primary malignant melanoma of the esophagus. *Am J Gastroenterol* 84:1475-1481, 1989.

Tateishi R, Taniguchi H, Wada A, et al: Argyrophil cells and melanocytes in esophageal mucosa. *Arch Pathol* 98:87-89, 1974.

Yoo CC, Levine MS, McLarney JK, et al: Primary malignant melanoma of the esophagus: Radiographic findings in seven patients. *Radiology* 209:455-459, 1998.

WHAT THE REFERRING PHYSICIAN NEEDS TO KNOW

- Average overall survival is only 10 to 13 months from time of diagnosis.
- Treatment of primary esophageal melanoma is surgical; an extensive esophageal resection is required.

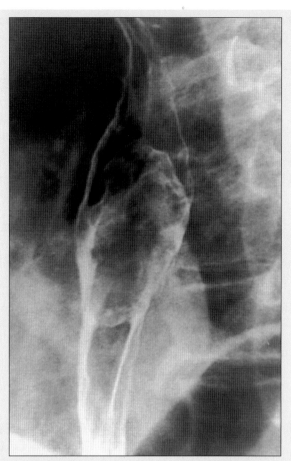

Figure 1. Primary malignant melanoma of the esophagus. Polypoid mass expanding lumen of distal esophagus. This lesion cannot be distinguished from spindle cell carcinoma or other rare malignant tumors of the esophagus. (*From Yoo CC, Levine MS, McLarney JK, et al: Primary malignant melanoma of the esophagus: Radiographic findings in seven patients. Radiology 209: 455-459, 1998.*)

Other Malignant Tumors

DEFINITION: Secondary involvement of esophagus by malignant tumors such as lymphoma, leukemia, Kaposi sarcoma, small cell carcinoma, and other tumors.

IMAGING

Radiography
Findings
- Irregular areas of narrowing seen in lymphoma and leukemia
- Lymphoma; smooth indentation and obtuse, gently sloping borders, diffuse esophageal narrowing, or infiltrating stricture
- Small submucosal nodules seen in lymphoma, Kaposi sarcoma, and leukemia
- Polypoid mass in esophagus seen in lymphoma, Kaposi sarcoma, small cell carcinoma, chondrosarcoma, synovial sarcoma, and, rarely, leukemia
- Small cell carcinomas manifested by fungating masses containing areas of ulceration or cavitation, or smoothly marginated, sessile, centrally ulcerated masses

Utility
- Esophagography
- Follow-up contrast studies after chemotherapy and radiation therapy

CT
Findings
- Extensive mediastinal adenopathy compressing the esophagus in mediastinal lymphoma
- Leukemia with esophageal wall thickening (possible)

Utility
- Assessing extent of disease in mediastinum

CLINICAL PRESENTATION
- Dysphagia
- Weight loss

DIFFERENTIAL DIAGNOSIS
- Esophageal carcinoma
- Varices

DIAGNOSTIC PEARLS
- Diffuse esophageal narrowing and strictures or smooth extrinsic indentation
- Small submucosal nodules in lymphoma, Kaposi sarcoma, or small cell carcinoma
- Polypoid masses in lymphoma, Kaposi sarcoma, small cell carcinoma, chondrosarcoma, synovial sarcoma, and, rarely, leukemia

PATHOLOGY
- Direct invasion of esophagus by lymphomatous nodes in mediastinum
- Contiguous spread from gastric fundus
- Synchronous development of lymphoma in the wall of the esophagus
- Kaposi sarcoma: multifocal neoplasm of reticuloendothelial system
- Small cell carcinoma derived from argyrophilic or Kulchitsky cells of neuroectodermal origin

INCIDENCE/PREVALENCE AND EPIDEMIOLOGY
- Esophagus is the least common site of gastrointestinal involvement by lymphoma; only 1% of cases.
- Both non-Hodgkin and, less commonly, Hodgkin lymphoma may involve the esophagus.
- More aggressive form of Kaposi sarcoma is occasionally seen in patients with acquired immunodeficiency syndrome (AIDS).
- More than 30% of patients with AIDS in United States have Kaposi sarcoma.
- Fifty percent of patients with Kaposi sarcoma have gastrointestinal involvement, but the esophagus is rarely involved.

WHAT THE REFERRING PHYSICIAN NEEDS TO KNOW
- When esophageal lymphoma is suspected, endoscopy should be performed, with deep esophageal biopsy specimens to confirm diagnosis.
- False-negative biopsy specimens in lymphoma have been reported in 25% to 35% of cases because of patchy nature of disease and sampling error.
- Kaposi sarcoma should be suspected when discrete esophageal lesions are found in patients with AIDS who have associated skin lesions.
- With small cell carcinoma, surgery is recommended primarily for palliation.
- Multimodality approach with combination chemotherapy and radiation therapy is advocated for small cell carcinoma to improve patient survival.
- Leukemic deposits in esophagus may undergo marked regression after radiation therapy.
- Esophageal symptoms may be palliated by mediastinal irradiation, but overall prognosis for the patient's leukemia is unchanged.

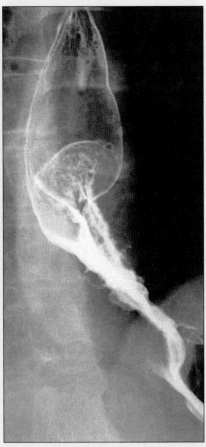

Figure 1. Primary AIDS-related non-Hodgkin lymphoma of the esophagus. Irregular, ulcerated area of narrowing with a shelf-like proximal border in distal thoracic esophagus. This lesion is indistinguishable from an advanced esophageal carcinoma. (*Courtesy of Jackie Brown, MD, Vancouver, British Columbia, Canada.*)

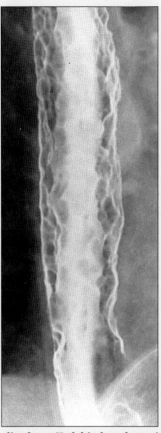

Figure 2. Generalized non-Hodgkin lymphoma involving the esophagus. Double-contrast image of the distal thoracic esophagus reveals innumerable 3- to 10-mm submucosal nodules extending from the thoracic inlet to the gastroesophageal junction. This appearance might initially be mistaken for varices, but the diffuse distribution and discrete margins of the lesions allow them to be differentiated from varices. (*From Levine MS, Sunshine AG, Reynolds JC, et al: Diffuse nodularity in esophageal lymphoma. AJR Am J Roentgenol 145:1218-1220, 1985, © by American Roentgen Ray Society.*)

- In small cell carcinoma, the average survival is 6 months or less from the time of diagnosis.
- Esophageal involvement by leukemia is reported at autopsy in 2% to 13% of patients.

Suggested Readings

Agha FP, Schnitzer B: Esophageal involvement in lymphoma. *Am J Gastroenterol* 80:412-416, 1985.

Attar BM, Levendoglu HA, Rhee H: Small cell carcinoma of the esophagus. *Dig Dis Sci* 35:145-152, 1990.

Beyer KI, Marshall JB, Diaz-Arias AA, et al: Primary small-cell carcinoma of the esophagus: Report of 11 cases and review of the literature. *J Clin Gastroenterol* 13:135-141, 1995.

Carnovale RL, Goldstein HM, Zornoza J, et al: Radiologic manifestations of esophageal lymphoma. *AJR Am J Roentgenol* 128:751-754, 1977.

Caruso RD, Berk RN: Lymphoma of the esophagus. *Radiology* 95: 381-382, 1970.

Coppens E, Nakadi IE, Nagy N, et al: Primary Hodgkin's lymphoma of the esophagus. *AJR Am J Roentgenol* 180:1135-1137, 2003.

Friedman SL, Wright TL, Altman DF: Gastrointestinal Kaposi's sarcoma in patients with acquired immunodeficiency syndrome: Endoscopic and autopsy findings. *Gastroenterology* 89:102-108, 1985.

Gollub MJ, Prowda JC: Primary melanoma of the esophagus: Radiologic and clinical findings in six patients. *Radiology* 213:97-100, 1999.

Hussein AM, Feun LG, Sridhar KS, et al: Combination chemotherapy and radiation therapy for small-cell carcinoma of the esophagus. *Am J Clin Oncol* 13:369-373, 1990.

Law SYK, Fok M, Lam KY, et al: Small cell carcinoma of the esophagus. *Cancer* 73:2894-2899, 1994.

Levine MS, Pantongrag-Brown L, Buck JL, et al: Small-cell carcinoma of the esophagus: Radiographic findings. *Radiology* 199:703-705, 1996.

Levine MS, Rubesin SE, Pantongrag-Brown L, et al: Non-Hodgkin's lymphoma of the gastrointestinal tract: Radiographic findings. *AJR Am J Roentgenol* 168:165-172, 1997.

Radin DR: Primary esophageal lymphoma in AIDS. *Abdom Imaging* 18:223-224, 1993.

Rose HS, Balthazar EJ, Megibow AJ, et al: Alimentary tract involvement in Kaposi sarcoma: Radiographic and endoscopic findings in 25 homosexual men. *AJR Am J Roentgenol* 139:661-666, 1982.

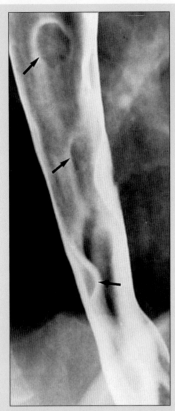

Figure 3. Kaposi sarcoma involving the esophagus. Multiple submucosal masses *(arrows)* are seen in the esophagus. This patient had additional submucosal lesions elsewhere in the gastrointestinal tract. *(Courtesy of Robert A. Goren, MD, Philadelphia, PA.)*

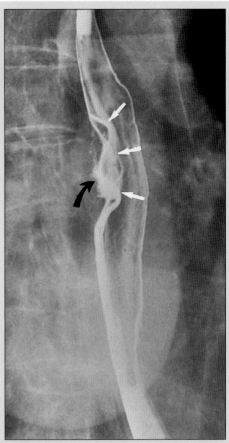

Figure 4. Small cell carcinoma of the esophagus. Smoothly marginated, sessile mass *(white arrows)* containing a relatively flat central area of ulceration *(black arrow)* on the right posterolateral wall of the mid-esophagus below the level of the carina. *(From Levine MS, Pantongrag-Brown L, Buck JL, et al: Small-cell carcinoma of the esophagus: Radiographic findings. Radiology 199:703-705, 1996.)*

Rosenberg SA, Diamond HD, Jaslowitz B, et al: Lymphosarcoma: A review of 1,269 cases. *Medicine (Baltimore)* 40:31-84, 1961.

Sabate JM, Franquet T, Palmer J, et al: AIDS-related primary esophageal lymphoma. *Abdom Imaging* 22:11-13, 1997.

Thompson BC, Feczko PJ, Mezwa DG: Dysphagia caused by acute leukemic infiltration of the esophagus [letter]. *AJR Am J Roentgenol* 155:654, 1990.

Umerah BC: Kaposi sarcoma of the oesophagus. *Br J Radiol* 53: 807-808, 1980.

Wall SD, Friedman SL, Margulis AR: Gastrointestinal Kaposi's sarcoma in AIDS: Radiographic manifestations. *J Clin Gastroenterol* 6:165-171, 1984.

Zornoza J, Dodd GD: Lymphoma of the gastrointestinal tract. *Semin Roentgenol* 15:272-287, 1980.

Part 13

MISCELLANEOUS ABNORMALITIES OF THE ESOPHAGUS

Mallory-Weiss Tears and Hematomas

DEFINITION: A linear mucosal laceration at or near the gastric cardia caused by a sudden rapid increase in intraesophageal pressure.

IMAGING

Radiography
Findings
- Mallory-Weiss tear: longitudinally oriented, linear 1-4 cm collection of barium in the distal esophagus at or slightly above the gastroesophageal junction
- Indistinguishable from a linear ulcer in the distal esophagus caused by reflux esophagitis
- Esophageal hematoma: solitary, ovoid or elongated submucosal mass in the distal esophagus
- *Double-barreled* appearance resulting from intramural dissection of barium

Utility
- Double-contrast or single-contrast esophagography

CT
Findings
- Esophageal hematoma: eccentric, well-defined intramural mass, sometimes with a tubular appearance, extending a considerable distance along the longitudinal axis of the esophagus
- Acute or subacute hematoma: hyperdense areas may be present within the lesion.

CLINICAL PRESENTATION

- Massive hematemesis occurs with Mallory-Weiss tears, but most tears heal spontaneously within 48-72 hours; thus, bleeding is usually self-limited.
- Patients with esophageal hematomas usually complain of sudden onset of severe retrosternal chest pain, dysphagia, or hematemesis.
- Most esophageal hematomas resolve spontaneously within 1-2 weeks.

DIAGNOSTIC PEARLS

- *Double-barreled* appearance
- Sudden intraesophageal pressure increase from one or more violent retching episodes or vomiting

DIFFERENTIAL DIAGNOSIS

- Crohn disease
- *Candida* esophagitis
- Tuberculous esophagitis
- Linear ulcer

PATHOLOGY

- Affected patients have a sudden increase in intraesophageal pressure from one or more violent episodes of retching or vomiting after an alcoholic binge or protracted vomiting.
- Also caused by prolonged hiccupping or coughing, seizures, straining at stool, childbirth, or blunt abdominal trauma or by direct laceration of mucosa by advancing endoscope or by sharp foreign body in the esophagus
- Esophageal hematomas are caused by a mucosal laceration or tear in the distal esophagus or by blunt trauma to the chest or abdomen.
- Tear is occluded by edema or blood clot; continued hemorrhage leads to progressive submucosal dissection of blood, producing intramural hematoma.
- Spontaneous hematomas develop in patients with impaired hemostasis because of thrombocytopenia, bleeding disorders, or anticoagulation.

WHAT THE REFERRING PHYSICIAN NEEDS TO KNOW
- Ninety-five percent of Mallory-Weiss tears are diagnosed by endoscopy.
- Selective intra-arterial infusion of vasopressin, transcatheter embolization, endoscopic electrocoagulation, or surgical repair of tear may be required to control bleeding.
- Esophageal hematomas usually resolve spontaneously within 1-2 weeks on conservative treatment with nasogastric suction, antibiotics, and intravenous fluids.

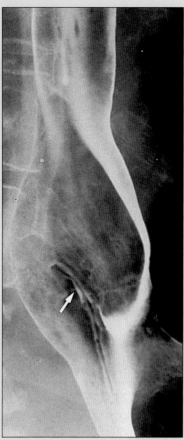

Figure 1. Mallory-Weiss tear. A linear collection of barium *(arrow)* is visible in the distal esophagus just above the gastroesophageal junction. Although a linear ulcer from reflux esophagitis can produce a similar appearance, the correct diagnosis was suggested by the clinical history. *(Courtesy of Harvey M. Goldstein, MD, San Antonio, TX.)*

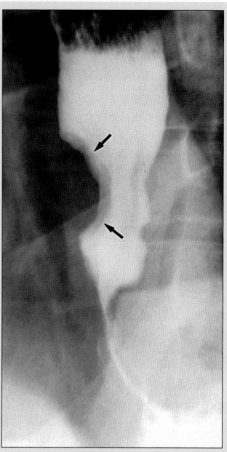

Figure 2. Esophageal hematoma. Note the smooth submucosal mass *(arrows)* in the distal esophagus. The hematoma was caused by a pneumatic dilation procedure for achalasia. The esophagus is narrowed below the hematoma because of the patient's underlying achalasia. *(From Levine MS:* Radiology of the Esophagus. *Philadelphia, WB Saunders, 1989.)*

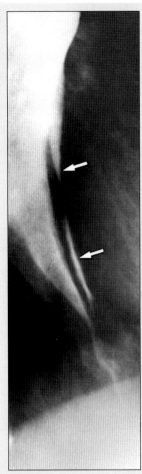

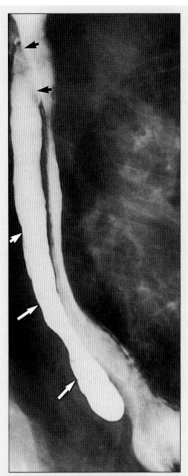

Figure 3. Example of intramural dissection with a double-barreled esophagus. The longitudinal intramural track *(white arrows)* is separated from the esophageal lumen by a radiolucent mucosal stripe. Patient had traumatic dissection that occurred during esophageal instrumentation.

Figure 4. Example of intramural dissection with a double-barreled esophagus. The longitudinal intramural track *(white arrows)* is separated from the esophageal lumen by a radiolucent mucosal stripe. Patient had traumatic dissection that occurred during esophageal instrumentation. The site of the laceration *(black arrows)* is well seen.

- Spontaneous hematomas typically spare the distal esophagus and occur at multiple sites.

INCIDENCE/PREVALENCE AND EPIDEMIOLOGY

- Mallory-Weiss tears account for 5%-10% of all cases of acute upper gastrointestinal bleeding.
- Mallory-Weiss tears are associated with overall mortality rate of only approximately 3%.

Suggested Readings

Andress M: Submucosal haematoma of the oesophagus due to anticoagulant therapy. *Acta Radiol Diagn* 11:216-219, 1971.

Ansari A: Mallory-Weiss syndrome: Revisited. *Am J Gastroenterol* 64:460-466, 1975.

Ashman FC, Hill MC, Saba GP, et al: Esophageal hematoma associated with thrombocytopenia. *Gastrointest Radiol* 3:115-118, 1978.

Baker RW, Spiro AH, Trnka YM: Mallory-Weiss tear complicating upper endoscopy. *Gastroenterology* 82:140-142, 1982.

Bradley JL, Han SY: Intramural hematoma (incomplete perforation) of the esophagus associated with esophageal dilatation. *Radiology* 130:59-62, 1979.

Bubrick MP, Lundeen JW, Onstad GR, et al: Mallory-Weiss syndrome: Analysis of fifty-nine cases. *Surgery* 88:400-405, 1980.

Carsen GM, Casarella WJ, Spiegel RM: Transcatheter embolization for treatment of Mallory-Weiss tears of the esophagogastric junction. *Radiology* 128:309-313, 1978.

Chen P, Lebowitz R, Lewicki AM: Spontaneous hematoma of the esophagus. *Radiology* 100:281-282, 1971.

Clark RA: Intraarterial vasopressin infusion for treatment of Mallory-Weiss tears of the esophagogastric junction. *AJR Am J Roentgenol* 133:449-451, 1979.

Dallemand S, Amorosa JK, Morris DW, et al: Intramural hematomas of the esophagus. *Gastrointest Radiol* 8:7-9, 1983.

Demos TC, Okrent DH, Studlo JD, et al: Spontaneous esophageal hematoma diagnosed by computed tomography. *J Comp Assist Tomogr* 10:133-135, 1986.

de Vries RA, Kremer-Schneider MME, Otten MH: Intramural hematoma of the esophagus caused by minor head injury 6 hours previously. *Gastrointest Radiol* 16:283-285, 1991.

Foster DN, Miloszewski K, Losowsky MS: Diagnosis of Mallory-Weiss lesions: A common cause of upper gastrointestinal bleeding. *Lancet* 2:483-485, 1976.

Graham DV, Schwartz JT: The spectrum of the Mallory-Weiss tear. *Medicine (Baltimore)* 57:307-318, 1977.

Harris JM, DiPalma JA: Clinical significance of Mallory-Weiss tears. *Am J Gastroenterol* 88:2056-2058, 1993.

Hastings PR, Peters KW, Cohn I: Mallory-Weiss syndrome: Review of 69 cases. *Am J Surg* 142:560-562, 1981.

Herbetko J, Delany D, Ogilvie BC, et al: Spontaneous intramural haematoma of the oesophagus: Appearance on computed tomography. *Clin Radiol* 44:327-328, 1991.

Hunter TB, Protell RL, Horsley WW: Food laceration of the esophagus: The taco tear. *AJR Am J Roentgenol* 140:503-504, 1983.

Joffe N, Millan VG: Postemetic dissecting intramural hematoma of the esophagus. *Radiology* 95:379-380, 1970.

Knaver CM: Mallory-Weiss syndrome: Characterization of 75 Mallory-Weiss lacerations in 528 patients with upper gastrointestinal hemorrhage. *Gastroenterology* 71:5-8, 1976.

Lowman RM, Goldman R, Stern H: The roentgen aspects of intramural dissection of the esophagus. *Radiology* 93:1329-1331, 1969.

Meulman N, Evans J, Watson A: Spontaneous intramural haematoma of the oesophagus: A report of three cases and review of the literature. *Aust N Z J Surg* 64:190-193, 1994.

Papp JP: Electrocoagulation of actively bleeding Mallory-Weiss tears. *Gastrointest Endosc* 26:128-130, 1980.

Pellicano A, Watier A, Gentile J: Spontaneous double-barreled esophagus. *J Clin Gastroenterol* 9:149-154, 1987.

Penston JG, Boyd EJ, Wormsley KG: Mallory-Weiss tears occurring during endoscopy: Report of four cases. *Endoscopy* 24:262-265, 1992.

Shay SS, Berendson RA, Johnson LF: Esophageal hematoma: Four new cases, a review, and proposed etiology. *Dig Dis Sci* 26:1019-1024, 1981.

Steenbergen WV, Fevery J, Broeckaert L, et al: Intramural hematoma of the esophagus: Unusual complication of variceal sclerotherapy. *Gastrointest Radiol* 9:293-295, 1984.

Perforation

DEFINITION: Penetrating or blunt injury or a sudden, rapid increase in intraluminal esophageal pressure, causing perforation of the esophagus.

IMAGING

Radiography

Findings
- Subcutaneous emphysema or retropharyngeal gas may be visible within 1 hour after a pharyngeal or cervical esophageal perforation.
- Widening of prevertebral space, anterior deviation of trachea, retropharyngeal abscess containing mottled gas or a single air-fluid level
- Mediastinal widening, pneumomediastinum
- Subcutaneous emphysema in neck, hydropneumothorax
- Distal esophageal perforations: sympathetic left pleural effusion or atelectasis in basilar segments of left lung
- Extravasation of contrast medium from esophagus into the neck or mediastinum

Utility
- Fluoroscopic esophagography is the study of choice for suspected esophageal perforation.
- When the initial study with water-soluble contrast agent fails to show a leak, the examination should be repeated with barium to demonstrate subtle leaks that might be missed with a water-soluble contrast agent.

CT

Findings
- Extraluminal gas in mediastinum should be highly suggestive of esophageal perforation
- Mediastinal, pleural, and pericardial fluid collections

Utility
- Useful for determining extent of extraluminal gas and fluid in the mediastinum and for monitoring patients who are treated nonoperatively
- Often cannot locate the exact site of perforation
- Helical CT esophagography with dilute low-osmolar contrast medium is a better technique than conventional CT for showing site of perforation.

DIAGNOSTIC PEARLS

- Extraluminal gas in the mediastinum
- Mediastinal, pleural, and pericardial fluid collections
- Widening of the prevertebral space, anterior deviation of trachea, and a retropharyngeal abscess containing mottled gas or a single air-fluid level

CLINICAL PRESENTATION

- Cervical esophageal perforations: neck pain, dysphagia, fever, or subcutaneous emphysema
- Thoracic esophageal perforation: classic triad of vomiting, severe substernal chest pain, and subcutaneous emphysema of the chest wall and neck
- Epigastric pain or atypical chest pain referred to the left shoulder or back

PATHOLOGY

- Most endoscopic perforations involve the piriform sinus or posterior wall of the hypopharynx or cervical esophagus.
- Presence of cervical osteophytes or pharyngeal diverticulum increases the risk of perforation.
- Thoracic esophageal perforations usually result from endoscopic injury at or above esophageal strictures or from other therapeutic procedures.
- Perforation may also occur after esophageal surgery, most frequently at the site of a ruptured anastomosis.
- Other causes include foreign-body obstructions with transmural inflammation and pressure necrosis and accidental or intentional ingestion of caustic agents.
- Penetrating or blunt injuries to the esophagus: the neck lacks bony protection afforded by the thorax; such perforations usually involve the cervical esophagus.

WHAT THE REFERRING PHYSICIAN NEEDS TO KNOW

- Early diagnosis of esophageal perforation is important because of the need for prompt surgical intervention in most cases.
- Most cervical esophageal perforations heal with conservative medical treatment, but larger perforations may require cervical mediastinotomy and open drainage to prevent abscess formation.
- Thoracic esophageal perforation can be mistaken for a variety of acute abdominal or cardiothoracic conditions.
- Signs or symptoms of esophageal perforation can also be masked by treatment with steroids.
- Thoracic esophageal perforations usually require an immediate thoracotomy (with surgical closure of perforation and mediastinal drainage) because of the high mortality if untreated.

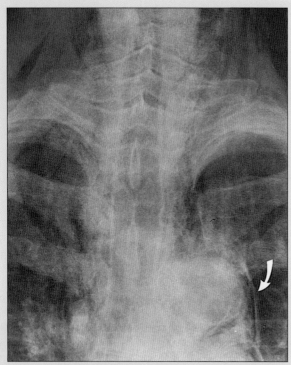

Figure 1. Cervical esophageal perforation by traumatic endoscopy. Close-up view from a posteroanterior chest radiograph obtained several hours after the procedure shows extensive subcutaneous emphysema in the neck and associated pneumomediastinum *(arrow).* (*From Levine MS:* Radiology of the Esophagus. *Philadelphia, WB Saunders, 1989.*)

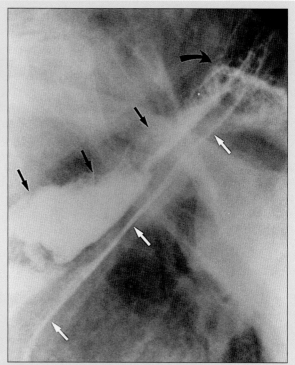

Figure 2. Cervical esophageal perforation by traumatic endoscopy. Same patient as in Figure 1. Study using water-soluble contrast medium in a steep oblique projection reveals a cervical esophageal perforation *(curved black arrow)* with contrast medium extending inferiorly in the mediastinum *(straight black arrows)* behind the esophagus *(white arrows).* (*From Levine MS:* Radiology of the Esophagus. *Philadelphia, WB Saunders, 1989.*)

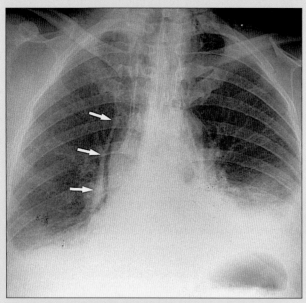

Figure 3. Spontaneous esophageal perforation or Boerhaave syndrome. Posteroanterior chest radiograph shows a right-sided pneumomediastinum *(arrows)* and a left pleural effusion. These findings are highly suggestive of spontaneous esophageal perforation in a patient (particularly an alcoholic) with severe retching or vomiting. (*Courtesy of Seth N. Glick, MD, Philadelphia, PA.*)

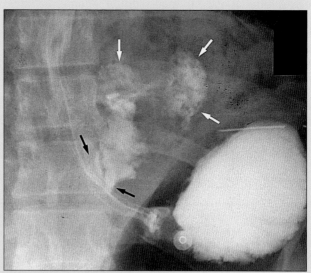

Figure 4. Spontaneous esophageal perforation or Boerhaave syndrome. Same patient as in Figure 3. Subsequent study using water-soluble contrast medium confirms the presence of a localized perforation of the left lateral wall of the distal esophagus *(black arrows),* with extension of the leak laterally and superiorly in the mediastinum *(white arrows).* (*Courtesy of Seth N. Glick, MD, Philadelphia, PA.*)

- Sudden, rapid increase in intraluminal esophageal pressure causes full-thickness perforation of normal esophageal tissue (Boerhaave syndrome), most commonly on the left lateral wall of the distal esophagus just above the gastroesophageal junction.

INCIDENCE/PREVALENCE AND EPIDEMIOLOGY

- Esophageal perforation is most serious and rapidly fatal type of perforation in the gastrointestinal tract.
- Untreated thoracic esophageal perforations have a mortality rate of nearly 100% because of fulminant mediastinitis that occurs after esophageal rupture.
- Endoscopic procedures are responsible for up to 75% of all esophageal perforations.
- Esophageal perforation occurs in approximately 1 in 3000 patients who undergo endoscopic examinations with modern fiberoptic instruments.
- Cervical esophageal perforation: overall mortality rate is less than 15%, which is a better prognosis than thoracic esophageal perforations.
- Overall mortality rate for all patients with thoracic esophageal perforation is approximately 25%.

Suggested Readings

Backer CL, LoCicero J, Hartz RS, et al: Computed tomography in patients with esophageal perforation. *Chest* 98:1078-1080, 1990.

Baron TH: Expandable metal stents for the treatment of cancerous obstruction of the gastrointestinal tract. *N Engl J Med* 344:1681-1687, 2001.

Berry BE, Ochsner JL: Perforation of the esophagus: A 30 year review. *J Thorac Cardiovasc Surg* 65:1-7, 1973.

Bradham RR, deSaussure C, Lemel AL: Spontaneous perforation of the cervical esophagus. *Arch Surg* 111:284-285, 1976.

Brick SH, Caroline DF, Lev-Toaff AS, et al: Esophageal disruption: Evaluation with iohexol esophagography. *Radiology* 169:141-143, 1988.

Buecker A, Wein BB, Neuerburg JM, et al: Esophageal perforation: Comparison of use of aqueous and barium-containing contrast media. *Radiology* 202:683-686, 1997.

Campbell TC, Andrews JL, Neptune WB: Spontaneous rupture of the esophagus (Boerhaave's syndrome). *JAMA* 235:526-528, 1976.

Chiu CL, Gambach RR: Hypaque pulmonary edema: A case report. *Radiology* 111:91-92, 1974.

Dodds WJ, Stewart ET, Vlymen WJ: Appropriate contrast media for evaluation of esophageal disruption. *Radiology* 144:439-441, 1982.

Fadoo F, Ruiz DE, Dawn SK, et al: Helical CT esophagography for the evaluation of suspected esophageal perforation or rupture. *AJR* 182:1177-1179, 2004.

Foley MJ, Ghahremani GG, Rogers LF: Reappraisal of contrast media used to detect upper gastrointestinal perforations. *Radiology* 144:231-237, 1982.

Foster JH, Jolly PC, Sawyers JL, et al: Esophageal perforation: Diagnosis and treatment. *Ann Surg* 161:701-709, 1965.

Ghahremani GG, Turner MA, Port RB: Iatrogenic intubation injuries of the upper gastrointestinal tract in adults. *Gastrointest Radiol* 5:1-10, 1980.

Gollub MJ, Bains MS: Barium sulfate: A new (old) contrast agent for diagnosis of postoperative esophageal leaks. *Radiology* 202:360-362, 1997.

Han SY, McElvein RB, Aldrete JS, et al: Perforation of the esophagus: Correlation of site and cause with plain film findings. *AJR Am J Roentgenol* 145:537-540, 1985.

Han SY, Tishler JM: Perforation of the abdominal segment of the esophagus. *AJR* 143:751-754, 1984.

Healy ME, Mindelzun RE: Lesser sac pneumoperitoneum secondary to perforation of the intraabdominal esophagus. *AJR Am J Roentgenol* 142:325-326, 1984.

Herbetko J, Delany D, Ogilvie BC, et al: Spontaneous intramural haematoma of the oesophagus: Appearance on computed tomography. *Clin Radiol* 44:327-328, 1991.

Isserow JA, Levine MS, Rubesin SE: Spontaneous perforation of the cervical esophagus after an alcoholic binge. *Can Assoc Radiol J* 49:241-243, 1998.

James AE, Montali RJ, Chaffee V, et al: Barium or Gastrografin: Which contrast media for diagnosis of esophageal tears. *Gastroenterology* 68:1103-1113, 1975.

Janjua KJ: Boerhaave's syndrome. *Postgrad Med J* 73:265-270, 1997.

Klygis LM, Jutabha R, McCrohan MB, et al: Esophageal perforations masked by steroids. *Abdom Imaging* 18:10-12, 1993.

Levine MS: What is the best oral contrast material to use for the fluoroscopic diagnosis of esophageal rupture? *AJR Am J Roentgenol* 162:1243, 1994.

Love L, Berkow AE: Trauma to the esophagus. *Gastrointest Radiol* 2:305-321, 1978.

Maglinte DDT, Edwards MC: Spontaneous closure of esophageal tear in Boerhaave's syndrome. *Gastrointest Radiol* 4:223-225, 1979.

Meyers MA, Ghahremani GG: Complications of fiberoptic endoscopy: I. Esophagoscopy and gastroscopy. *Radiology* 115:293-300, 1975.

O'Connell ND: Spontaneous rupture of the esophagus. *AJR* 99:186-203, 1967.

Parkin GJS: The radiology of perforated esophagus. *Clin Radiol* 24:324-332, 1973.

Pasricha PJ, Fleischer DE, Kalloo AN: Endoscopic perforations of the upper digestive tract: A review of their pathogenesis, prevention, and management. *Gastroenterology* 106:787-802, 1994.

Phillips LG, Cunningham J: Esophageal perforation. *Radiol Clin North Am* 22:607-613, 1984.

Polsky S, Kerstein MD: Pharyngo-esophageal perforation due to blunt trauma. *Am Surg* 61:994-996, 1995.

Rogers LF, Puig W, Dooley BN, et al: Diagnostic considerations in mediastinal emphysema: A pathophysiologic approach to Boerhaave's syndrome and spontaneous pneumomediastinum. *AJR Am J Roentgenol* 115:495-511, 1972.

Rubesin SE, Levine MS: Radiologic diagnosis of gastrointestinal perforation. *Radiol Clin North Am* 41:1095-1115, 2003.

Swanson JO, Levine MS, Redfern RO, et al: Usefulness of high-density barium for detection of leaks after esophagogastrectomy, total gastrectomy, and total laryngectomy. *AJR Am J Roentgenol* 181:415-420, 2003.

Tanomkiat W, Galassi W: Barium sulfate as contrast medium for evaluation of postoperative anastomotic leaks. *Acta Radiol* 41:482-485, 2000.

Vessal K, Montali RJ, Larson SM, et al: Evaluation of barium and Gastrografin as contrast media for the diagnosis of esophageal ruptures or complications. *AJR Am J Roentgenol* 123:307-319, 1975.

White CS, Templeton PA, Attar S: Esophageal perforation: CT findings. *AJR Am J Roentgenol* 160:767-770, 1993.

Wychulis AR, Fontana RS, Payne WS: Instrumental perforations of the esophagus. *Dis Chest* 55:184-189, 1969.

Foreign-Body Impactions in the Esophagus

DEFINITION: Foreign-body impactions in adults are usually caused by fish bones or other animal bones or unchewed boluses of meat. Bones tend to lodge in the pharynx near the level of the cricopharyngeus, whereas meat usually lodges in the distal esophagus near the gastroesophageal junction.

IMAGING

Radiography
Findings
- Animal or fish bones seen as linear filling defects in the vallecula, piriform sinus, or cricopharyngeal region
- Food impaction seen as a polypoid filling defect in the esophagus, with irregular meniscus resulting from barium outlining the superior border of impacted food bolus
- Food impactions often caused by underlying ring or stricture

Utility
- Neck and chest anteroposterior and lateral radiographs may demonstrate bones or other radiopaque foreign bodies in pharynx or esophagus.
- Lateral radiographs are more helpful than frontal radiographs in identifying the animal or fish bones lodged in the pharynx or cervical esophagus because of the overlying cervical spine on frontal radiographs.
- Barium swallow is used to determine whether a foreign body is present and whether it is causing the obstruction.
- Cotton balls or marshmallows soaked in barium are helpful for demonstrating small foreign bodies in the pharynx or esophagus.
- Esophagography may demonstrate the site of impaction and extravasation of contrast medium into the mediastinum in cases of esophageal perforation at the site of impaction.

CLINICAL PRESENTATION

- Animal or fish bones: pharyngeal dysphagia or sensation of foreign body is felt in the throat.
- Meat bolus impactions create sudden onset of substernal chest pain, odynophagia, or dysphagia.

DIAGNOSTIC PEARLS

- Linear filling defects in the vallecula, piriform sinus, or cricopharyngeal region
- Polypoid filling defect in the esophagus

- Esophageal perforation occurs in less than 1% of all patients with foreign-body impactions.
- Development of mediastinitis may lead to sudden, rapid clinical deterioration, manifested by chest pain, sepsis, and shock.

DIFFERENTIAL DIAGNOSIS

- Obstructing esophageal carcinoma, but correct diagnosis almost always suggested by the clinical presentation

PATHOLOGY

- Foreign-body impactions in adults are usually caused by animal or fish bones or unchewed boluses of meat.
- Bones usually lodge in the pharynx near the level of the cricopharyngeus, whereas meat usually lodges in the distal esophagus near the gastroesophageal junction.
- Meat impactions are often caused by underlying esophageal rings or strictures.
- Unchewed meat bolus can lodge above the gastroesophageal junction or pathologic area of narrowing such as a Schatzki ring or peptic stricture.
- Perforation results from transmural esophageal inflammation and subsequent pressure necrosis at the site of impaction.

WHAT THE REFERRING PHYSICIAN NEEDS TO KNOW

- Foreign bodies in the esophagus pass spontaneously in 80%-90% of cases; the remaining 10%-20% require some form of therapeutic intervention.
- Impacted foreign bodies are removed by endoscopy or by use of wire-basket or Foley catheter balloon under fluoroscopic guidance.
- Intravenous glucagon may facilitate passage of impacted food in the distal esophagus by relaxing the lower esophageal sphincter.
- Administration of gas-forming agents is advocated to distend the esophagus above the obstructing food bolus and facilitate passage of bolus into the stomach.
- Gas-forming agents should not be used if the obstruction is present longer than 24 hours, as such agents may cause esophageal perforation.
- Combination of glucagon, effervescent agent, and water appears to be an effective technique for relieving esophageal food impactions, with a 70% success rate.
- Follow-up esophagogram should be performed to rule out Schatzki ring or peptic stricture as the cause of the impaction.

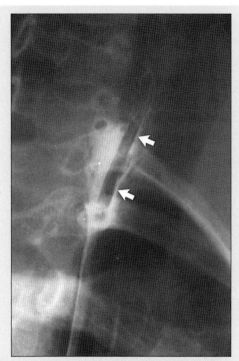

Figure 1. **Turkey bone in the cervical esophagus.** Barium swallow reveals a linear filling defect *(arrows)* resulting from a bone lodged in the cervical esophagus just below the cricopharyngeus. *(From Levine MS:* Radiology of the Esophagus. *Philadelphia, WB Saunders, 1989.)*

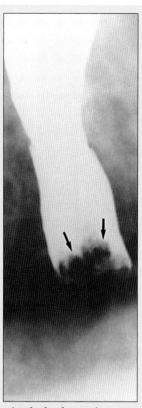

Figure 2. **Distal foreign-body obstruction caused by an underlying Schatzki ring.** Esophagogram shows barium outlining the superior border of an impacted bolus of meat *(arrows)* in the distal esophagus, with complete obstruction at this level.

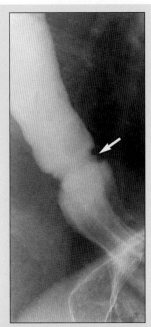

Figure 3. **Distal foreign-body obstruction caused by an underlying Schatzki ring.** Esophagogram after endoscopic removal of an impacted meat bolus shows an underlying Schatzki ring *(arrow)* as the cause of the impaction shown in Figure 1.

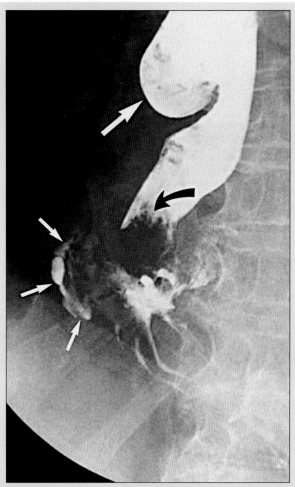

Figure 4. **Foreign-body obstruction with associated perforation.** A polypoid defect *(black arrow)* is present in the distal esophagus as a result of an esophageal food impaction. In addition, note extravasation of contrast medium into a focal collection *(small white arrows)* in the mediastinum, indicating perforation. Also note the large diverticulum *(large white arrow)* in the mid-esophagus. This perforation occurred within 6 hours of the onset of impaction. (*From Gougoutas C, Levine MS, Laufer I: Esophageal food impaction with early perforation. AJR Am J Roentgenol 171:427-428, 1998, © by American Roentgen Ray Society.*)

■ Risk of perforation increases substantially if the impaction persists more than 24 hours.
■ Impacted foreign body can erode through the esophageal wall, producing aortoesophageal, esophagobronchial, or esophagopericardial fistula.

INCIDENCE/PREVALENCE AND EPIDEMIOLOGY

■ Eighty percent of all pharyngeal or esophageal foreign-body impactions occur in children and are accidental or intentional.
■ Animal or fish bones or unchewed boluses of meat are the usual causes in adults.

Suggested Readings

Barber GB, Peppercorn MA, Ehrlich C, et al: Esophageal foreign body perforation. *Am J Gastroenterol* 79:509-511, 1984.

Ferrucci JT, Long JA: Radiologic treatment of esophageal food impaction using intravenous glucagon. *Radiology* 125:25-28, 1977.

Ginsberg GG: Management of ingested foreign objects and food bolus impactions. *Gastrointest Endosc* 41:33-38, 1995.

Giordano A, Adams G, Boies L, et al: Current management of esophageal foreign bodies. *Arch Otolaryngol* 107:249-251, 1981.

Gougoutas C, Levine MS, Laufer I: Esophageal food impaction with early perforation. *AJR Am J Roentgenol* 171:427-428, 1998.

Harned RK, Strain JD, Hay TC, et al: Esophageal foreign bodies: Safety and efficacy of Foley catheter extraction of coins. *AJR Am J Roentgenol* 168:443-446, 1997.

Hogan WJ, Dodds WJ, Hoke SE, et al: Effect of glucagon on esophageal motor function. *Gastroenterology* 69:160-165, 1975.

Kaszar-Seibert DJ, Korn WT, Bindman DJ, et al: Treatment of acute esophageal food impaction with a combination of glucagon, effervescent agent, and water. *AJR Am J Roentgenol* 154:533-534, 1990.

Macpherson RI, Hill JG, Othersen HB, et al: Esophageal foreign bodies in children: Diagnosis, treatment, and complications. *AJR Am J Roentgenol* 166:919-924, 1996.

Nandi P, Ong GB: Foreign bodies in the oesophagus: Review of 2,394 cases. *Br J Surg* 65:5-9, 1978.

Rice BT, Spiegel PK, Dombrowski PJ: Acute esophageal food impaction treated by gas-forming agents. *Radiology* 146:299-301, 1983.

Robbins MI, Shortsleeve MJ: Treatment of acute esophageal food impaction with glucagon, an effervescent agent, and water. *AJR Am J Roentgenol* 162:325-328, 1994.

Shaffer HA, Alford BA, de Lange EE, et al: Basket extraction of esophageal foreign bodies. *AJR Am J Roentgenol* 147:1010-1013, 1986.

Smith JC, Janower ML, Geiger AH: Use of glucagon and gas-forming agents in acute esophageal food impaction. *Radiology* 159:567-568, 1986.

Trenkner SW, Maglinte DDT, Lehman GA, et al: Esophageal food impaction: Treatment with glucagon. *Radiology* 149:401-403, 1983.

Underberg-Davis S, Levine MS: Giant thoracic osteophyte causing esophageal food impaction. *AJR Am J Roentgenol* 157:319-320, 1991.

Webb WA: Management of foreign bodies of the upper gastrointestinal tract. *Gastroenterology* 94:204-216, 1988.

Fistulas

DEFINITION: Fistulas are miscellaneous abnormalities of the esophagus characterized by communication between the esophagus and the airway, pleura, aorta, or pericardium.

IMAGING

Radiography

Findings
- Esophagopleural fistula: pleural effusion, pneumothorax, or hydropneumothorax
- Esophagopericardial fistula: pneumopericardium or hydropneumopericardium
- Extrinsic compression or displacement of the esophagus by aneurysm in patients with aortoesophageal fistula
- Extravasation of contrast medium from the esophagus outlining coiled springs of graft in an eroded aortic graft
- Esophagopericardial fistula confirmed by showing the fistulous track or by gross filling of the pericardial sac with contrast medium

Utility
- Esophagography
- Use water-soluble contrast agents to confirm the presence of an esophagopleural fistula and determine its site of origin.
- Esophagography with water-soluble contrast agents may reveal an esophagopleural fistula at the site of esophageal ballooning or thinning.
- Use barium to confirm the presence of an esophageal-airway fistula and determine its site of origin.

CT

Findings
- Esophagopleural fistula at the site of esophageal ballooning or thinning

Utility
- For demonstrating small collections of contrast agent, gas, or fluid in the pleural space

DIAGNOSTIC PEARLS
- Extravasation of contrast medium from esophagus outlining coiled springs of graft in an eroded aortic graft
- Esophagopericardial fistula is confirmed by demonstrating the fistulous track or by gross filling of the pericardial sac with contrast medium.
- Paroxysmal coughing after ingestion of liquids should suggest esophageal-airway fistula.

Interventional Radiology

Findings
- Extravasation of contrast medium from the aorta into the esophagus by aortography confirms presence of aortoesophageal fistula

Utility
- Origin of fistulous track is often occluded by thrombus; aortography may fail to delineate the fistula in these patients.

CLINICAL PRESENTATION
- Esophageal-airway fistulas: paroxysmal coughing after ingestion of liquids, recurrent pneumonitis, hemoptysis, and productive cough with food particles in the sputum
- Esophagopleural fistulas: nonspecific findings, including chest pain, fever, dysphagia, dyspnea, or foul-smelling regurgitations

WHAT THE REFERRING PHYSICIAN NEEDS TO KNOW
- Esophageal-airway fistulas may be difficult to differentiate from recurrent tracheobronchial aspiration on clinical grounds.
- When esophageal-airway fistulas are suspected, radiologic examination should be performed with barium rather than water-soluble contrast agents, which are hypertonic and draw fluid into the lungs, sometimes causing severe pulmonary edema.
- Most fistulas are readily demonstrated on barium studies, arising within advanced, infiltrating esophageal carcinomas.
- Initial swallow should be performed in lateral projection to differentiate the fistula from aspiration.
- Recovery of ingested methylene blue in fluid aspirated during thoracentesis confirms the presence of an esophagopleural fistula.
- Aortoesophageal fistulas should be suspected in patients with arterial hematemesis and a large atherosclerotic aneurysm of the descending thoracic aorta on radiographs.

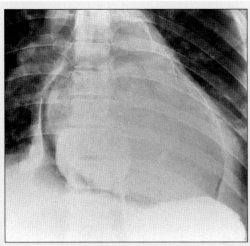

Figure 1. **Esophagopericardial fistula caused by a perforated ulcer associated with severe reflux esophagitis.** Posteroanterior chest radiograph after oral administration of water-soluble contrast medium reveals a pneumopericardium with free leakage of contrast medium into the pericardial space. Air and contrast medium outline the inner aspect of the pericardial sac. Also, contrast medium is seen faintly in a hiatal hernia. (*From Cyrlak D, Cohen AJ, Dana ER: Esophagopericardial fistula: Causes and radiographic features.* AJR Am J Roentgenol *141:177-179, 1983, © by American Roentgen Ray Society.*)

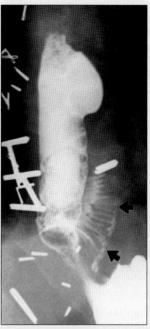

Figure 2. **Aortoesophageal fistula caused by an aortic aneurysm.** Esophagogram after placement of a Dacron aortic graft shows a recurrent aortoesophageal fistula with extravasated contrast medium from the esophagus outlining the aortic graft *(arrows)*. This fistula was caused by infection of the graft. (*From Baron RL, Koehler RE, Gutierrez FR, et al: Clinical and radiographic manifestations of aortoesophageal fistulas.* Radiology *141:599-605, 1981.*)

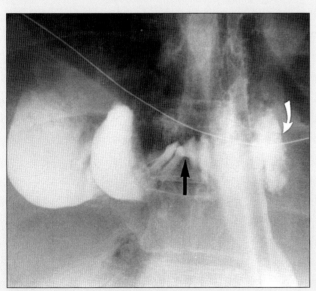

Figure 3. **Esophagopleural fistula caused by endoscopic sclerotherapy of esophageal varices.** Study using water-soluble contrast medium reveals an esophagopleural fistula *(black arrow)* with contrast medium extending laterally in the right pleural space. Note the extravasated contrast medium in the mediastinum *(white arrow)*. (*From Levine MS:* Radiology of the Esophagus. *Philadelphia, WB Saunders, 1989.*)

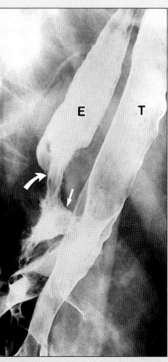

Figure 4. **Esophagobronchial fistula.** This fistula *(straight arrow)* was caused by an advanced, infiltrating esophageal carcinoma *(curved arrow)*. (E, Esophagus; T, trachea.) (*From Levine MS:* Radiology of the Esophagus. *Philadelphia, WB Saunders, 1989.*)

- Aortoesophageal fistula: episodes of arterial hematemesis, followed by symptom-free latent period, then a final episode of massive hematemesis, exsanguination, and death
- Esophagopericardial fistulas: rapid development of severe pericarditis or cardiac tamponade caused by leakage of esophageal contents into the pericardial sac

PATHOLOGY

- Esophageal-airway fistulas are caused by direct tracheobronchial tree invasion by advanced esophageal carcinoma after radiation therapy, esophageal instrumentation, endobronchial stents, trauma, or perforation.
- Esophagobronchial fistulas are also caused by tuberculosis, histoplasmosis, or other granulomatous diseases and are rarely congenital.
- Esophagopleural fistulas are usually caused by previous surgery, esophageal instrumentation, radiation, or advanced esophageal carcinoma directly invading the pleural space.
- When esophagopleural fistula is suspected, diagnosis can be confirmed by recovery of ingested methylene blue in fluid aspirated during thoracentesis.
- Aortoesophageal fistulas are rare but lethal as a result of intraesophageal rupture of atherosclerotic, syphilitic, or dissecting aneurysm of the descending thoracic aorta.
- Aortoesophageal fistulas are caused by a swallowed foreign body, esophageal carcinoma, infected aortic graft, or erosion of an endovascular stent into the esophagus.
- Esophagopericardial fistulas are rare and are caused by severe esophagitis, esophageal cancer, swallowed foreign bodies, or prior surgery.

INCIDENCE/PREVALENCE AND EPIDEMIOLOGY

- Tracheoesophageal or esophagobronchial fistulas have been reported in 5%-10% of patients with esophageal cancer.

- Nonoperative management of esophagopleural fistulas is associated with mortality rates approaching 100% versus mortality rates of 50% if surgically repaired.

Suggested Readings

Baron RL, Koehler RE, Gutierrez FR, et al: Clinical and radiographic manifestations of aortoesophageal fistulas. *Radiology* 141:599-605, 1981.

Cyrlak D, Cohen AJ, Dana ER: Esophagopericardial fistula: Causes and radiographic features. *AJR Am J Roentgenol* 141:177-179, 1983.

Fitzgerald RH, Bartles DM, Parker EF: Tracheoesophageal fistulas secondary to carcinoma of the esophagus. *J Thorac Cardiovasc Surg* 82:194-197, 1981.

Hollander JE, Quick G: Aortoesophageal fistula: A comprehensive review of the literature. *Am J Med* 91:279-287, 1991.

Khawaja FI, Varindani MK: Aortoesophageal fistula: Review of clinical, radiographic and endoscopic features. *J Clin Gastroenterol* 9:342-344, 1987.

Little AG, Ferguson MK, DeMeester TR, et al: Esophageal carcinoma with respiratory tract fistula. *Cancer* 53:1322-1328, 1984.

Liu PS, Levine MS, Torigian DA: Esophagopleural fistula secondary to esophageal wall ballooning and thinning after pneumonectomy: Findings on chest CT and esophagography. *AJR Am J Roentgenol* 186:1627-1629, 2006.

Massard G, Ducrocq X, Hentz JG, et al: Esophagopleural fistula: An early and long-term complication after pneumonectomy. *Ann Thorac Surg* 58:1437-1440, 1994.

Massard G, Wihlm JM: Early complications: Esophagopleural fistula. *Chest Surg Clin North Am* 9:617-631, 1999.

Seymour EQ: Aortoesophageal fistula as a complication of aortic prosthetic graft. *AJR Am J Roentgenol* 131:160-161, 1978.

Sheiner NM, LaChance C: Congenital esophagobronchial fistula in the adult. *Can J Surg* 23:489-491, 1980.

Spalding AR, Burney DP, Richie RE: Acquired benign bronchoesophageal fistulas in the adult. *Ann Thorac Surg* 28:378-383, 1979.

Vasquez RE, Landay M, Kilman WJ, et al: Benign esophagorespiratory fistulas in adults. *Radiology* 167:93-96, 1988.

Weschler RJ: CT of esophageal-pleural fistulae. *AJR Am J Roentgenol* 147:907-909, 1986.

Weschler RJ, Steiner RM, Goodman LR, et al: Iatrogenic esophageal-pleural fistula: Subtlety of diagnosis in the absence of mediastinitis. *Radiology* 144:239-243, 1982.

Diverticula

DEFINITION: Diverticula are outpouchings from the esophagus, which are classified as either traction or pulsion type.

ANATOMIC FINDINGS

Mid-esophagus
- Common location of traction diverticula
- Tented or triangular configuration

Distal Esophagus
- Common location of pulsion diverticula
- Called epiphrenic diverticulum if located within 10 cm of gastroesophageal junction

Pharyngoesophageal Junction
- Zenker diverticulum

IMAGING

Radiography
Findings
- Barium-filled outpouchings from the esophagus
- Recognized en face as ring shadows on double-contrast studies
- Pulsion diverticula: multiple outpouchings with rounded contour and wide neck, which remain filled with barium after esophagus collapses
- Traction diverticula: solitary outpouchings with tented or triangular configuration, which empty of barium when esophagus collapses
- Epiphrenic diverticulum: solitary diverticulum, most commonly arising from right side of distal esophagus on barium studies
- Epiphrenic diverticulum: soft-tissue mass on chest radiographs (often containing air-fluid level) that mimics hiatal hernia
Utility
- Barium esophagography

CLINICAL PRESENTATION

- Pulsion and traction diverticula are usually incidental findings in esophagus without clinical significance.
- Extremely large diverticula may cause symptoms.
- Patients with epiphrenic diverticula greater than 5 cm in diameter are more likely to be symptomatic.
- When an epiphrenic diverticulum fills with food, it may compress the true lumen of the esophagus, causing dysphagia.
- Food or fluid that accumulates within an epiphrenic diverticulum may be regurgitated into the esophagus, causing reflux symptoms, chest pain, and aspiration.
- Diverticula rarely may perforate into the mediastinum or form a fistula to the airway.

DIFFERENTIAL DIAGNOSIS

- Esophageal intramural pseudodiverticulosis
- Esophageal sacculations

PATHOLOGY

- Most common locations include the pharyngoesophageal junction (Zenker diverticulum), middle or distal third of the esophagus, and the most distal esophagus just above the gastroesophageal junction (epiphrenic diverticulum).
- A diverticulum is formed by pulsion (increased intraluminal esophageal pressure associated with esophageal dysmotility) or by traction (fibrosis in adjacent periesophageal tissues).
- Esophageal diverticula may be classified by their location or mechanism of formation.
- Pulsion diverticula are usually located in the middle or distal third of the esophagus and are associated with radiographic evidence of esophageal dysmotility.
- Traction diverticula are usually located in the mid-esophagus and have tented or triangular configuration as a result of scarring and retraction from surgery, radiation, or granulomatous disease in adjacent mediastinum.
- Traction diverticula are solitary outpouchings containing all layers of esophageal wall (including muscular layer); therefore they empty when the esophagus collapses.

WHAT THE REFERRING PHYSICIAN NEEDS TO KNOW

- Pulsion and traction diverticula are usually incidental findings in the esophagus without clinical significance.
- Development of symptoms appears to be related primarily to morphologic features of the diverticulum rather than to underlying esophageal dysmotility.
- Severe or intractable symptoms from epiphrenic diverticulum may necessitate surgical intervention, most commonly diverticulectomy and esophagomyotomy.

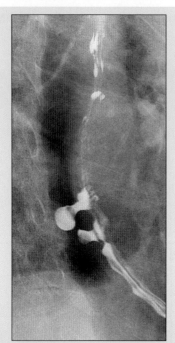

Figure 1. Pulsion diverticulum. In this patient, the pulsion diverticula remain filled after most of the barium has emptied from the esophagus by peristalsis. Note the rounded contour and wide necks of the diverticula. (*From Levine MS:* Radiology of the Esophagus. *Philadelphia, WB Saunders, 1989.*)

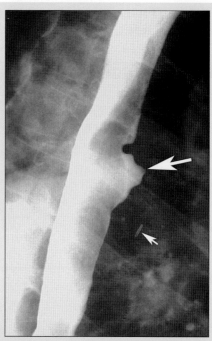

Figure 2. Traction diverticulum. The diverticulum has a pointed or triangular tip *(large arrow)* as a result of traction and volume loss in the adjacent mediastinum from prior surgery. A surgical clip *(small arrow)* is seen in the mediastinum. (*From Levine MS:* Radiology of the Esophagus. *Philadelphia, WB Saunders, 1989.*)

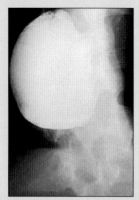

Figure 3. Large epiphrenic diverticulum. A barium study reveals a large epiphrenic diverticulum that remains filled with barium after the esophagus has emptied. (*From Levine MS:* Radiology of the Esophagus. *Philadelphia, WB Saunders, 1989.*)

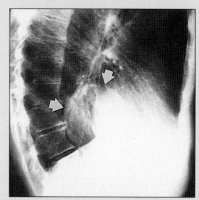

Figure 4. Large epiphrenic diverticulum. Lateral chest radiograph shows a soft-tissue mass *(arrows)*, mimicking the appearance of a hiatal hernia. (*From Levine MS:* Radiology of the Esophagus. *Philadelphia, WB Saunders, 1989.*)

- Epiphrenic diverticulum is located in the most distal esophagus and is a pulsion diverticulum, sometimes caused by diffuse esophageal spasm with markedly increased intraluminal esophageal pressures.

INCIDENCE/PREVALENCE AND EPIDEMIOLOGY

- Diffuse esophageal spasm is found in approximately 10% of patients with epiphrenic diverticula.

Suggested Readings

Altorki NK, Sunagawa M, Skinner DB: Thoracic esophageal diverticula: Why is operation necessary. *J Thorac Cardiovasc Surg* 105:260-264, 1993.

Benacci JC, Deschamps C, Trastek VF, et al: Epiphrenic diverticulum: Results of surgical treatment. *Ann Thorac Surg* 55:1109-1114, 1993.

Debas HT, Payne WS, Cameron AJ, et al: Physiopathology of lower esophageal diverticulum and its implications for treatment. *Surg Gynecol Obstet* 151:593-600, 1980.

Dodds WJ, Stef JJ, Hogan WJ, et al: Radial distribution of peristaltic pressure in normal subjects and patients with esophageal diverticulum. *Gastroenterology* 69:584-590, 1975.

Fasano NC, Levine MS, Rubesin SE, et al: Epiphrenic diverticulum: Clinical and radiographic findings in 27 patients. *Dysphagia* 18:9-15, 2003.

Kaye MD: Oesophageal motor dysfunction in patients with diverticula of the mid-thoracic oesophagus. *Thorax* 29:666-672, 1974.

Niv Y, Fraser G, Krugliak P: Gastroesophageal obstruction from food in an epiphrenic esophageal diverticulum. *J Clin Gastroenterol* 16:314-316, 1993.

Ectopic Gastric Mucosa

DEFINITION: Ectopic gastric mucosa is a common congenital anomaly seen as a shallow depression in the upper esophagus at or just above the thoracic inlet, hence the term inlet patch.

IMAGING

Radiography
Findings
- Shallow depression on the right lateral wall of the upper esophagus near the thoracic inlet with small indentations at the superior and inferior borders of the indentation

Utility
- Double-contrast esophagography
- Depression can be mistaken on barium studies for ulceration or even an intramural dissection.

CLINICAL PRESENTATION

- Most patients are asymptomatic.
- Affected individuals may occasionally develop dysphagia because of associated webs or strictures in the upper esophagus.

DIFFERENTIAL DIAGNOSIS

- Flat ulcer
- Intramural dissection

PATHOLOGY

- Common congenital anomaly
- Ectopic gastric mucosa almost always located in the upper esophagus at or just above the thoracic inlet, hence the term *inlet patch*

DIAGNOSTIC PEARLS

- Located in the upper esophagus at or just above the thoracic inlet, usually on the right
- Shallow depression with small indentations at its superior and inferior borders

INCIDENCE/PREVALENCE AND EPIDEMIOLOGY

- Incidence of 4%-10% at endoscopy

Suggested Readings

Jabbari M, Goresky CA, Lough J, et al: The inlet patch: Heterotopic gastric mucosa in the upper esophagus. *Gastroenterology* 89:352-356, 1985.

Lee J, Levine MS, Schultz CF: Ectopic gastric mucosa in the oesophagus mimicking ulceration. *Eur J Radiol* 31:197-200, 1997.

Takeji H, Ueno J, Nishitani H: Ectopic gastric mucosa in the upper esophagus: Prevalence and radiographic findings. *AJR Am J Roentgenol* 164:901-904, 1995.

Ueno J, Davis SW, Tanakami A, et al: Ectopic gastric mucosa in the upper esophagus: Detection and radiographic findings. *Radiology* 191:751-753, 1994.

WHAT THE REFERRING PHYSICIAN NEEDS TO KNOW

- Ectopic gastric mucosa has no relationship to gastroesophageal reflux disease or Barrett esophagus.
- Appearance and location of ectopic gastric mucosa are so characteristic that endoscopy is not warranted in asymptomatic patients with this finding on barium studies.

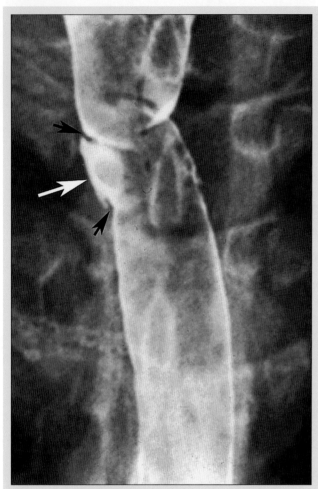

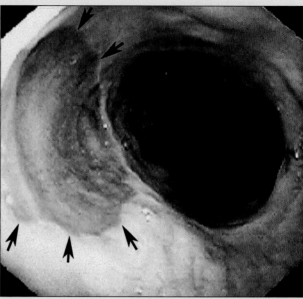

Figure 2. Endoscopy shows a reddish-brown epithelial-lined depression *(arrows)* in the upper esophagus characteristic of ectopic gastric mucosa. *(From Lee J, Levine MS, Shultz CF: Ectopic gastric mucosa in the oesophagus mimicking ulceration.* Eur J Radiol *31:97-200, 1997.)*

Figure 1. On the right lateral wall of the upper esophagus is a broad, flat depression *(white arrow)* near the thoracic inlet, with a pair of small indentations *(black arrows)* at both ends of the lesion. Although this lesion can be mistaken for an ulcer, it has the typical appearance and location of ectopic gastric mucosa in the esophagus. *(From Lee J, Levine MS, Shultz CF: Ectopic gastric mucosa in the oesophagus mimicking ulceration.* Eur J Radiol *31:97-200, 1997.)*

Congenital Esophageal Stenosis

DEFINITION: Congenital esophageal stenosis is a rare developmental anomaly caused by defective embryologic separation of the primitive foregut from the respiratory tract with sequestration of tracheobronchial precursor cells in the esophageal wall.

IMAGING

Radiography
Findings
- Smooth, tapered strictures in upper or mid-esophagus
- Multiple ring-like constrictions similar to those found in trachea

Utility
- Esophagography

CLINICAL PRESENTATION

- Patients with severe forms of congenital esophageal stenosis typically present during infancy with marked dysphagia and vomiting.
- Patients with milder forms (almost always men) have a long-standing history of intermittent dysphagia, chest pain, and occasional food impactions.

DIFFERENTIAL DIAGNOSIS

- Idiopathic eosinophilic esophagitis
- Feline esophagus

PATHOLOGY

- Congenital esophageal stenosis is a rare developmental anomaly caused by defective embryologic separation of the primitive foregut from the respiratory tract.
- Tracheobronchial precursor cells in the esophageal wall are sequestered.
- Infants may have a severe form of congenital esophageal stenosis associated with esophageal atresia or tracheoesophageal fistulas.
- Adults may have a mild form of disease characterized by esophageal strictures.

DIAGNOSTIC PEARLS

- Sequestration of tracheobronchial precursor cells in the esophageal wall
- Ring-like constrictions

- Ring-like indentations secondary to tracheobronchial rests (even cartilaginous rings) are present in the esophageal wall.

INCIDENCE/PREVALENCE AND EPIDEMIOLOGY

- All reported adults with this condition have been men.

Suggested Readings

Anderson LS, Shackelford GD, Mancilla-Jimenez R, et al: Cartilaginous esophageal ring: A cause of esophageal stenosis in infants and children. *Radiology* 108:665-666, 1973.

Katzka DA, Levine MS, Ginsberg GG, et al: Congenital esophageal stenosis in adults. *Am J Gastroenterol* 95:32-36, 2000.

McNally PR, Collier EH, Lopiano MC, et al: Congenital esophageal stenosis: A rare cause of food impaction in the adult. *Dig Dis Sci* 35:263-266, 1990.

McNally PR, Lemon JC, Goff JS, et al: Congenital esophageal stenosis presenting as noncardiac, esophageal chest pain. *Dig Dis Sci* 38:369-373, 1993.

Murphy SG, Yazbeck S, Russo P: Isolated congenital esophageal stenosis. *J Pediatr Surg* 30:1238-1241, 1995.

Oh CH, Levine MS, Katzka DA, et al: Congenital esophageal stenosis in adults: Clinical and radiographic findings in seven patients. *AJR Am J Roentgenol* 176:1179-1182, 2001.

Pokieser P, Schima W, Schober E, et al: Congenital esophageal stenosis in a 21-year-old man: Clinical and radiographic findings. *AJR Am J Roentgenol* 170:147-148, 1998.

Rose JS, Kassner EG, Jurgens KH, et al: Congenital esophageal strictures due to cartilaginous rings. *Br J Radiol* 48:16-18, 1975.

Yeung CK, Spitz L, Brereton RJ, et al: Congenital esophageal stenosis due to tracheobronchial remnants: A rare but important association with esophageal atresia. *J Pediatr Surg* 27:852-855, 1992.

WHAT THE REFERRING PHYSICIAN NEEDS TO KNOW
- Dysphagia is usually alleviated by endoscopic dilatation of strictures.
- Presence of esophageal stricture with distinctive ring-like constrictions should suggest congenital esophageal stenosis in the proper clinical setting.

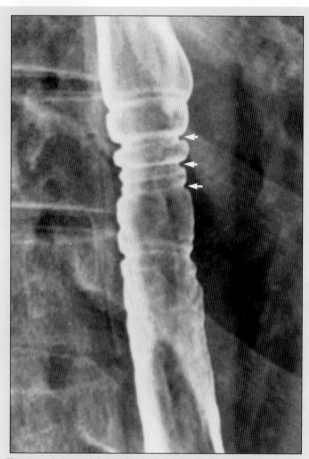

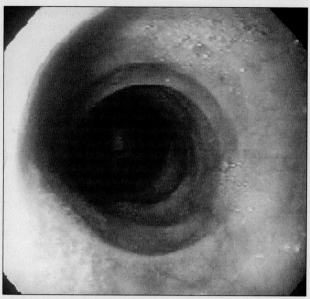

Figure 2. **Congenital esophageal stenosis.** Endoscopy shows ring-like indentations that resemble tracheal rings.

Figure 1. **Congenital esophageal stenosis.** Note area of mild narrowing in mid-esophagus with distinctive ring-like indentations *(arrows)* in region of the stricture. *(From Luedtke P, Levine MS, Rubesin SE, et al: Radiologic diagnosis of benign esophageal strictures: A pattern approach. RadioGraphics 23:897-909, 2003.)*

Extrinsic Impressions

DEFINITION: A variety of normal structures in the mediastinum, including the heart, aortic arch, and left main bronchus, may cause extrinsic impressions on the esophagus, whereas abnormal impressions are most commonly caused by the heart and great vessels, and esophageal deviation may be caused by pulmonary, pleural, or mediastinal scarring, with retraction of the esophagus toward the diseased hemithorax.

ANATOMIC FINDINGS

Esophagus
- If the esophagus is displaced or pushed by an extrinsic mass in the mediastinum (e.g., aneurysm, tumor, adenopathy), it will be narrower at the level of deviation than above or below the deviated segment.
- If the esophagus is retracted or pulled by pleuropulmonary scarring in the adjacent hemithorax (e.g., surgery, radiation, tuberculosis), it will be wider at the level of deviation than above or below the deviated segment.

IMAGING

Radiography
Findings
- Prominent right inferior supra-azygous recess causes smooth, gently sloping indentation on right posterolateral wall of the upper thoracic esophagus between the thoracic inlet and the aortic arch.
- Narrowed thoracic inlet causes extrinsic compression of the right side of the barium-filled esophagus without evidence of a mass.
- Tortuous or ectatic descending thoracic aorta causes a prominent impression on the right posterolateral wall of the distal esophagus near the esophageal hiatus of the diaphragm.
- Esophageal deviation may be caused by pulmonary, pleural, or mediastinal scarring, with widening and retraction of the esophagus toward the diseased hemithorax.

Utility
- Barium studies
- Chest radiographs confirm the presence of tuberculosis, radiation damage, or postsurgical changes, with signs of scarring and volume loss in the affected hemithorax.

CT
Findings
- Unusually, a prominent right inferior supra-azygous recess of the lung is indenting the upper esophagus.
- Thoracic inlet is narrowed, without evidence of a mass.

Utility
- Determines nature and extent of mass

DIAGNOSTIC PEARLS
- Normal structures in the mediastinum, including the heart, aortic arch, and left main bronchus, cause extrinsic impressions on the esophagus.
- When the esophagus is displaced or pushed by an extrinsic mass in the mediastinum, it is narrower at level of deviation than above or below the deviated segment.
- When the esophagus is retracted or pulled by pleuropulmonary scarring, it is wider at the level of deviation than above or below the deviated segment.

MRI
Utility
- Determines nature and extent of mass

CLINICAL PRESENTATION
- Dysphagia aortica: dysphagia resulting from compression of the distal esophagus by ectasia or aneurysm of the descending thoracic aorta
- Dysphagia lusoria: dysphagia resulting from compression of the mid-esophagus by congenital abnormalities of the great vessels, including an aberrant subclavian artery and double aortic arch.

PATHOLOGY
- Normal structures in mediastinum, including the heart, aortic arch, and left main bronchus, may cause extrinsic impressions on the esophagus.
- Abnormal impressions are most commonly caused by the heart and great vessels.
- Other causes include substernal thyroid goiter, mediastinal lymphadenopathy, and other benign or malignant neoplasms.

WHAT THE REFERRING PHYSICIAN NEEDS TO KNOW
- Physician must be able to determine whether the esophagus is pushed or pulled based on characteristic radiographic features.

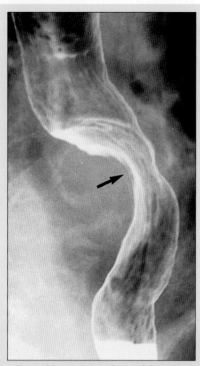

Figure 1. Esophageal impression *(arrow)* by an ectatic **descending thoracic aorta.** The esophagus is narrowed at the level of the deviation. (*From Levine MS, Gilchrist AM: Esophageal deviation: Pushed or pulled.* AJR Am J Roentgenol *149:513-514, 1987,* © *by American Roentgen Ray Society.*)

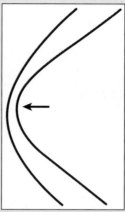

Figure 2. Pushed versus pulled esophagus. When the esophagus is displaced or pushed by an extrinsic mediastinal mass, it tends to be narrower at this level *(arrow)* than above or below the deviated segment. (*From Levine MS, Gilchrist AM: Esophageal deviation: Pushed or pulled.* AJR Am J Roentgenol *149:513-514, 1987,* © *by American Roentgen Ray Society.*)

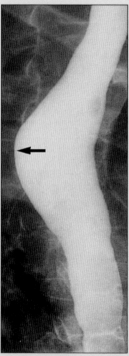

Figure 3. Esophageal retraction by pleuropulmonary scarring. The esophagus is deviated to the right *(arrow)* because of scarring and volume loss from right upper lobe tuberculosis. The esophagus is widened at the level of the deviation. This characteristic widening indicates retraction of the esophagus toward the side of pleuropulmonary scarring rather than displacement by a mass on the opposite side.

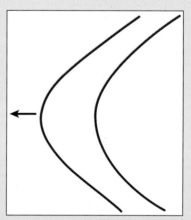

Figure 4. Pushed versus pulled esophagus. When the esophagus is retracted or pulled by pleuropulmonary scarring and volume loss, it tends to be wider at this level *(arrow)* than above or below the deviated segment. (*From Levine MS, Gilchrist AM: Esophageal deviation: Pushed or pulled.* AJR Am J Roentgenol *149:513-514, 1987,* © *by American Roentgen Ray Society.*)

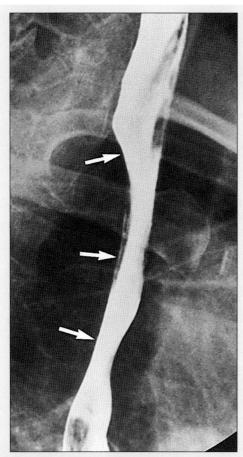

Figure 5. **Extrinsic impression on the esophagus by a prominent right inferior supra-azygous recess.** Note the smooth, gently sloping indentation *(arrows)* of the right posterolateral wall of the upper thoracic esophagus between the thoracic inlet and the aortic arch. (*From Sam JW, Levine MS, Miller WT: The right inferior supra-azygous recess: A cause of upper esophageal pseudomass on double-contrast esophagography. AJR Am J Roentgenol 171:1583-1586, 1998,* © *by American Roentgen Ray Society.*)

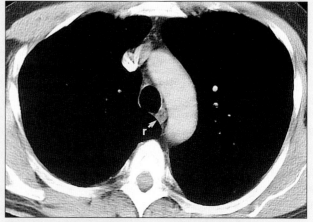

Figure 6. **Extrinsic impression on the esophagus by a prominent right inferior supra-azygous recess.** In the same patient as in Figure 5, CT of the chest shows a prominent right inferior supra-azygous recess (r) impinging on the right posterolateral wall of the upper esophagus *(arrow)*. (*From Sam JW, Levine MS, Miller WT: The right inferior supra-azygous recess: A cause of upper esophageal pseudomass on double-contrast esophagography. AJR Am J Roentgenol 171:1583-1586, 1998,* © *by American Roentgen Ray Society.*)

- Esophageal retraction resulting from pleuropulmonary scarring is usually detected as an incidental finding.
- Esophageal displacement by a mediastinal mass requires further investigation with CT or MRI to determine nature and extent of the mass.

Suggested Readings

Birholz JC, Ferrucci JT, Wyman SM: Roentgen features of dysphagia aortica. *Radiology* 111:93-96, 1974.

Levine MS, Gilchrist AM: Esophageal deviation: Pushed or pulled. *AJR Am J Roentgenol* 149:513-514, 1987.

Sam JW, Levine MS, Miller WT: The right inferior supraazygous recess: A cause of upper esophageal pseudomass on double-contrast esophagography. *AJR Am J Roentgenol* 171:1583-1586, 1998.

Esophageal Varices

DEFINITION: Esophageal varices are usually caused by portal hypertension or superior vena caval obstruction.

ANATOMIC FINDINGS

Esophagus
- Tortuous or serpiginous longitudinal filling defects on barium studies
- Thickened, lobulated, round, tubular, or serpentine structures with homogeneous enhancement on CT

Mediastinum
- Widening
- Lymphadenopathy

IMAGING

Radiography
Findings
- Tortuous or serpiginous longitudinal filling defects best seen in collapsed or partially collapsed esophagus
- Can easily be obscured on overly distended or collapsed views of the esophagus
- May be obliterated with esophageal distention
- Uphill varices: communicate with azygos venous system and superior vena cava
- Ligated varices: smooth, rounded filling defects in the distal esophagus indistinguishable from small polyps
- Idiopathic varix: solitary lesion seen as a smooth, slightly lobulated submucosal mass in the esophagus
Utility
- The barium study is performed with the patient in a recumbent position, using a high-density barium suspension/paste to increase adherence of barium to the esophageal mucosa.
- Mucosal relief views of collapsed esophagus are helpful for demonstrating varices.
- Esophagography is not considered a reliable technique for diagnosing esophageal varices.

DIAGNOSTIC PEARLS
- Tortuous or serpiginous longitudinal filling defects on barium studies
- Thickened, lobulated, round, tubular, or serpentine structures with homogeneous enhancement on CT

- Anticholinergic agents can improve visualization of varices by decreasing esophageal peristalsis.
- Venography may be performed to confirm the diagnosis and to determine the level and degree of stenosis or obstruction and extent of collateral circulation.
- Arteriograms may be performed to confirm the presence of uphill varices and to determine the nature and extent of underlying venous abnormalities.
- Esophagography has an overall sensitivity of 89% and an overall accuracy of 87% in detecting esophageal varices.

CT
Findings
- Bleeding into esophageal lumen
- Thickened, lobulated, round, tubular, or serpentine structures with homogeneous enhancement on CT
Utility
- Utility of multidetector CT (MDCT) in the diagnosis of active and occult sources of gastrointestinal hemorrhage has become accepted.
- Coronal and sagittal re-formations are helpful in demonstrating origin of hemorrhage.
- Unenhanced MDCT scan is initially obtained to detect intraluminal blood, followed by contrast-enhanced scan.
- MDCT may demonstrate coronary, paraumbilical, perisplenic, retrogastric, paraesophageal, omental, mesenteric, and abdominal wall varices in patients with portal hypertension.

WHAT THE REFERRING PHYSICIAN NEEDS TO KNOW
- Variceal bleeding requires more transfusions and emergency interventions and is associated with higher rates of rebleeding and death than bleeding from other sites.
- The primary diagnostic tool for upper gastrointestinal bleeding is endoscopy.
- When bleeding cannot be identified and controlled by endoscopy, MDCT or arteriography may help localize the bleeding source.
- Early endoscopy is mandatory in patients with cirrhosis.
- Treatment options include pharmacologic agents, endoscopic therapy, balloon tamponade, TIPS, surgical shunts, and liver transplantation.
- Endoscopic sclerotherapy is an alternative to surgery for controlling variceal bleeding and decreasing the risk of recurrent bleeding with fewer complications than surgery.
- In endoscopic sclerotherapy, mucosal sloughing at the injection sites may cause ulceration.

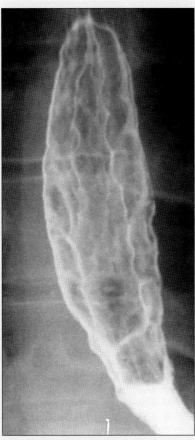

Figure 1. Uphill esophageal varices. Multiple varices are seen in the distal esophagus on a double-contrast esophagogram. Note how the varices are etched in white. (*From Levine MS:* Radiology of the Esophagus. *Philadelphia, WB Saunders, 1989.*)

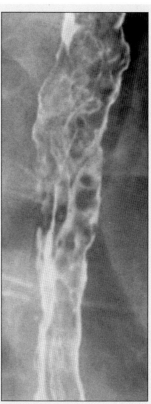

Figure 2. Downhill esophageal varices due to superior vena caval obstruction by bronchogenic carcinoma. Mucosal relief view of the esophagus shows prominent downhill varices in middle third of esophagus. (*From Levine MS:* Radiology of the Esophagus. *Philadelphia, WB Saunders, 1989.*)

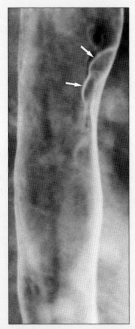

Figure 3. Idiopathic varix. There is a slightly lobulated, submucosal-appearing mass (*arrows*) indistinguishable from a leiomyoma or other submucosal tumor. (*Courtesy of Seth N. Glick, MD, Philadelphia, PA.*)

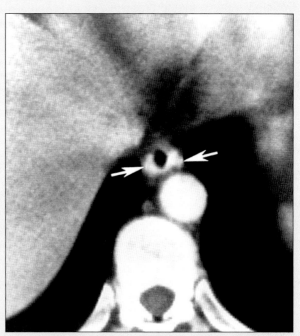

Figure 4. Esophageal varices: CT findings. CT during rapid infusion of intravenous contrast medium shows dense homogeneous enhancement of the varices (*arrows*). (*Courtesy of Robert A. Halvorsen, MD, San Francisco, CA.*)

Nuclear Medicine
Utility
- Radionuclide imaging has become accepted as the most sensitive, noninvasive study for detecting active gastrointestinal hemorrhage.
- Technetium Tc 99m-labeled red blood cell (Tc 99m-RBC) imaging is the method of choice because it allows monitoring of patients over a prolonged period.

Interventional Radiology
Findings
- Bleeding into esophageal lumen
Utility
- Angiography should be performed in patients with brisk upper gastrointestinal hemorrhage (if endoscopy is inconclusive) in anticipation of transcatheterization.
- Bleeding rate must exceed 0.5 mL/min to locate the site of hemorrhage.
- Scintigraphic studies should be performed before angiography to document active bleeding.

CLINICAL PRESENTATION
- Patients with major variceal hemorrhage may present with episodes of massive hematemesis or low-grade bleeding with melena, guaiac-positive stool, and iron-deficiency anemia.
- Hematochezia occurs in patients with massive hemorrhage (i.e., more than 1000 mL of blood).
- Symptoms of blood loss such as dyspnea, dizziness, or shock
- Aspiration of blood with nasogastric tube is diagnostic of an upper gastrointestinal bleeding source.
- Downhill varices should be suspected in patients with superior vena caval obstruction who develop signs of upper gastrointestinal bleeding.

DIFFERENTIAL DIAGNOSIS
- Esophagitis with thickened folds
- Varicoid carcinoma (esophagus)

PATHOLOGY
- The most common cause of portal hypertension and variceal bleeding worldwide is presinusoidal portal vein obstruction from schistosomiasis.

- In western countries, most patients with varices have underlying cirrhosis.
- Uphill varices result from changes in venous drainage of the esophagus caused by altered flow dynamics in patients with portal hypertension.
- Dilated esophageal veins secondary to obstruction of the superior vena cava are called downhill varices.
- Downhill varices are confined to the upper or middle third of the thoracic esophagus, whereas uphill varices are predominantly located in the distal third.
- Downhill varices may be caused by bronchogenic carcinoma, metastatic tumors, or lymphoma in the mediastinum or by benign causes of mediastinal fibrosis.
- Idiopathic varices are of unknown etiology and are thought to be caused by congenital weakness in venous channels of esophagus.

INCIDENCE/PREVALENCE AND EPIDEMIOLOGY
- Esophageal varices are found in 4% of all patients with upper gastrointestinal hemorrhage.
- Acute, massive upper gastrointestinal bleeding has an incidence of 40 to 150 episodes per 100,000 persons annually.
- Variceal bleeding is the most common cause of rapid upper gastrointestinal hemorrhage.
- First major upper gastrointestinal hemorrhage from esophageal varices has a 30%-50% mortality rate; almost two thirds of affected individuals die within 1 year.
- Variceal bleeding occurs in 25% to 35% of patients with cirrhosis, and as many as 30% of these hemorrhages are fatal.
- Thirty percent of patients who undergo sclerotherapy develop complications, including mild chemical esophagitis, ulceration, strictures, and esophageal perforation.

Suggested Readings
Howarth DM: The role of nuclear medicine in the detection of acute gastrointestinal bleeding. *Semin Nucl Med* 36:133-146, 2006.
Lin S, Rockey DC: Obscure gastrointestinal bleeding. *Gastroenterol Clin North Am* 34:679-698, 2005.
Manning-Dimmitt LL, Dimmitt SG, Wilson GR: Diagnosis of gastrointestinal bleeding in adults. *Am Fam Physician* 71:1339-1346, 2005.
Maurer AH: Gastrointestinal bleeding. In Murray IP, Ell PJ, (eds): *Nuclear Medicine in Clinical Diagnosis and Treatment.* New York, Churchill Livingstone, 1994, pp 47-54.

Part 14

ABNORMALITIES OF THE GASTROESOPHAGEAL JUNCTION

Normal Appearances of the Cardia (Including Lower Esophageal Rings)

DEFINITION: Intra-abdominal segment of esophagus terminates at the gastroesophageal junction or gastric cardia.

ANATOMIC FINDINGS

Gastric Cardia
- With a well-anchored cardia, protrusion of the distal esophagus into the fundus is seen as a circular elevation with four or five stellate folds radiating to a central point at the gastroesophageal junction (cardiac rosette).
- Folds are demarcated from the adjacent fundus by a curved *hooding fold* surrounding it laterally and superiorly.
- Cardiac rosette reflects a closed resting state of the lower esophageal sphincter.
- Rosette is transiently obliterated by relaxation during deglutition.
- With the cardia less firmly anchored, the cardiac rosette may be visible without an associated protrusion or circular elevation.
- With further ligamentous laxity, the cardia is characterized by a single undulant or crescentic line that crosses the area of the esophageal orifice.

Z-Line
- Seen on double-contrast esophagograms as a thin, radiolucent stripe in the distal esophagus with a characteristic zigzag appearance.
- Can occasionally be mistaken for superficial ulceration associated with reflux esophagitis, particularly if the esophagus is not completely distended
- An irregular, serrated line that demarcates the squamocolumnar mucosal junction

Lower Esophageal Mucosal Ring
- Lower esophageal mucosal ring is also known as the B-ring.
- Shown on barium studies as a thin, web-like area of narrowing at the gastroesophageal junction
- Has smooth, symmetric margins and a height of 2-4 mm

DIAGNOSTIC PEARLS
- Radiographic appearance of cardia depends on how firmly it is anchored to the esophageal hiatus.
- Z-line is seen as a thin, radiolucent stripe in the distal esophagus with zigzag appearance.
- Mucosal rings are thin, web-like areas of narrowing at the gastroesophageal junction.
- Muscular rings are transient broad, smooth areas of narrowing that change in caliber and configuration during fluoroscopy.

- The B-ring is fixed and reproducible if the esophagus above and hernia below are distended beyond the caliber of the ring.

Lower Esophageal Muscular Ring
- Lower esophageal muscular ring is also known as the A-ring.
- The A-ring is a relatively broad, smooth area of narrowing on esophagography that changes in caliber and configuration during fluoroscopy.
- Observed as a transient finding at fluoroscopy.

IMAGING

Radiography
Findings
- Circular elevation with four or five stellate folds
- Single undulant or crescentic line that crosses area of esophageal orifice
- Z-line: thin, radiolucent stripe in the distal esophagus with characteristic zigzag appearance
- Mucosal ring (B-ring): thin, web-like area of narrowing at the gastroesophageal junction

---

WHAT THE REFERRING PHYSICIAN NEEDS TO KNOW
- Radiographic appearance of the cardia depends on how firmly it is anchored by the surrounding phrenoesophageal membrane to the esophageal hiatus of the diaphragm.
- Ability to recognize normal appearances of the cardia improves dramatically with the use of double-contrast technique.
- Malignant lesions at the cardia are sometimes recognized only by distortion, effacement, or obliteration of normal landmarks.

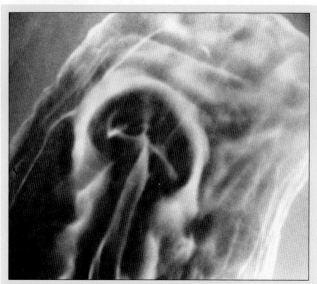

Figure 1. Normal appearances of the gastric cardia. This patient has a well-anchored cardia appearing as a circular protrusion with centrally radiating folds (i.e., the cardiac rosette). (*From Levine MS: Radiology of the Esophagus. Philadelphia, WB Saunders, 1989.*)

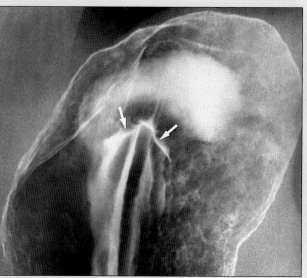

Figure 2. Normal appearances of the gastric cardia. Ligamentous laxity has resulted in obliteration of the cardiac rosette. Instead, this patient has a single crescentic line *(arrows)* at the cardia. (*From Levine MS:* Radiology of the Esophagus. *Philadelphia, WB Saunders, 1989.*)

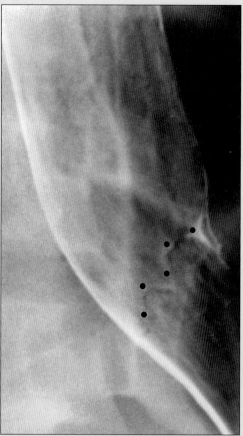

Figure 3. Z-line. The normal Z-line is seen as a thin, zigzagging, radiolucent stripe *(dots)* in the distal esophagus near the gastroesophageal junction. (*From Levine MS:* Radiology of the Esophagus. *Philadelphia, WB Saunders, 1989.*)

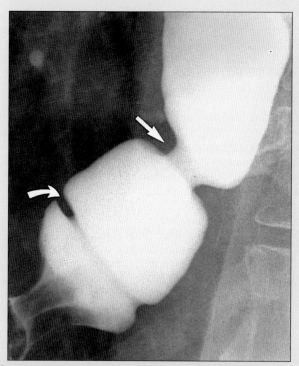

Figure 4. Lower esophageal rings. The mucosal ring, or B-ring, appears on a prone single-contrast view as a thin, web-like constriction *(curved arrow)* at the gastroesophageal junction above a small hiatal hernia, whereas the muscular ring, or A-ring, appears as a relatively broad area of narrowing *(straight arrow)* near the superior border of the esophageal vestibule. Unlike mucosal rings, which are fixed, reproducible structures, muscular rings are often seen as a transient finding at fluoroscopy. (*From Levine MS:* Radiology of the Esophagus. *Philadelphia, WB Saunders, 1989.*)

- Muscular ring (A-ring): broad, smooth, tapered area of narrowing above gastroesophageal junction

Utility

- Ability to recognize normal appearances of cardia improves dramatically with the use of double-contrast technique.
- Normal anatomic landmarks at the cardia are seen in more than 95% of double-contrast examinations.
- Single-contrast technique with the patient in the prone right anterior oblique position is best for demonstrating lower esophageal rings by permitting optimal distention of the distal esophagus.
- More than 50% of lower esophageal rings seen on prone single-contrast views of the esophagus are not visualized on upright double-contrast views.

DIFFERENTIAL DIAGNOSIS

- Schatzki ring (gastroesophageal junction)
- Reflux esophagitis

Suggested Readings

Dodds WJ: Current concepts of esophageal motor function: Clinical implications for radiology. *AJR Am J Roentgenol* 128:549-561, 1977.

Freeny PC: Double-contrast gastrography of the fundus and cardia: Normal landmarks and their pathologic changes. *AJR Am J Roentgenol* 133:481-487, 1979.

Friedland GW: Historical review of the changing concepts of lower esophageal anatomy: 430 B.C.–1977. *AJR Am J Roentgenol* 131:373-388, 1978.

Goyal RK, Glancy JJ, Spiro HM: Lower esophageal ring. *N Engl J Med* 282:1298-1305, 1970.

Herlinger H, Grossman R, Laufer I, et al: The gastric cardia in double-contrast study: Its dynamic image. *AJR Am J Roentgenol* 135:21-29, 1980.

Johnston JR, Griffin JC: Anatomic location of the lower esophageal ring. *Surgery* 61:528-534, 1967.

Ott DJ, Chen YM, Wu WC, et al: Radiographic and endoscopic sensitivity in detecting lower esophageal mucosal ring. *AJR Am J Roentgenol* 147:261-265, 1986.

Ott DJ, Gelfand DW, Wu WC, et al: Esophagogastric region and its rings. *AJR Am J Roentgenol* 142:281-287, 1984.

Schatzki R, Gary JE: The lower esophageal ring. *AJR Am J Roentgenol* 75:246-261, 1956.

Wolf BS, Heitmann P, Cohen BR: The inferior esophageal sphincter, the manometric high pressure zone and hiatal incompetence. *AJR Am J Roentgenol* 103:251-276, 1968.

Schatzki Ring (Gastroesophageal Junction)

DEFINITION: Narrow-caliber rings at gastroesophageal junction causing symptoms.

ANATOMIC FINDINGS

Gastroesophageal Junction
- Schatzki rings are thin (2-4 mm in height), weblike constrictions (<13 mm in diameter).
- Rings less than 13 mm in diameter almost always cause dysphagia.
- Rings between 13 and 20 mm in diameter sometimes cause dysphagia.
- Rings greater than 20 mm in diameter almost never cause dysphagia.

IMAGING

Radiography
Findings
- Rings are thin (2-4 mm in height), web-like constrictions (<13 mm in diameter) at the gastroesophageal junction.
- Rings are visualized on barium studies only if the lumen above and below the ring is distended beyond the caliber of the ring.
- Prone single-contrast views of the distal esophagus may demonstrate Schatzki rings that are not visible on upright double-contrast views.
- Overdistention of a hiatal hernia on prone views can result in overlap of the distal esophagus and hernia.
- This produces a double density of two superimposed, convex collections that prevents visualization of the Schatzki ring.
- Additional prone views of distal esophagus should be obtained when the hiatal hernia is less distended to allow visualization of the ring.

Utility
- Carefully performed biphasic esophagography is thought to be even more sensitive than endoscopy for detecting Schatzki rings.
- Overdistention of a hiatal hernia on a prone view prevents visualization of Schatzki rings.
- Additional prone views of distal esophagus should be obtained when the hiatal hernia is less distended to allow visualization of the rings.

DIAGNOSTIC PEARLS
- Rings are thin (2-4 mm in height), web-like constrictions (<13 mm in diameter) at the gastroesophageal junction.
- Hiatal hernia almost always observed below the level of the ring.
- Rings are visualized on barium studies only if the lumen above and below ring is distended beyond the caliber of the ring.

CLINICAL PRESENTATION
- Episodic dysphagia for solids, especially meat
- May have minimal dysphagia or be intermittently asymptomatic until a large bolus of meat lodges above the ring, causing esophageal food impaction (the *steakhouse syndrome*)

DIFFERENTIAL DIAGNOSIS
- Normal mucosal ring
- Ring-like peptic strictures

PATHOLOGY
- Rings of narrow-caliber at the gastroesophageal junction cause dysphagia.
- Pathogenesis of Schatzki rings is uncertain.
- Some authors favor a congenital origin, but rarity of symptoms before 50 years of age tends to refute this theory.
- Others believe that a Schatzki ring represents an annular, ring-like structure due to scarring from reflux esophagitis.

INCIDENCE/PREVALENCE AND EPIDEMIOLOGY
- Symptoms are rare before 50 years of age.

WHAT THE REFERRING PHYSICIAN NEEDS TO KNOW
- The term *Schatzki ring* should be reserved for symptomatic patients with narrow-caliber rings at the gastroesophageal junction.
- Rings are visualized on barium studies only if the lumen above and below ring is distended beyond the caliber of ring.
- Overdistention of hiatal hernias on prone views can result in the overlap phenonemon, preventing vizualization of ring.

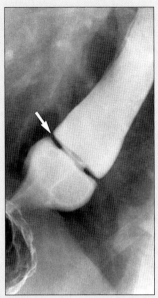

Figure 1. Schatzki ring seen only on prone single-contrast view of the esophagus. Prone single-contrast view shows ring *(arrow)* as a thin, web-like (<13 mm in diameter) constriction at the gastroesophageal junction above a hiatal hernia. Except for its smaller caliber, this ring has the same appearance and location as an asymptomatic mucosal ring. This patient had dysphagia.

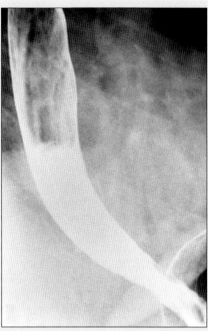

Figure 2. Schatzki ring on upright double-contrast view. This view from the same examination as in Figure 1 shows no evidence of the ring because of inadequate distention of the distal esophagus.

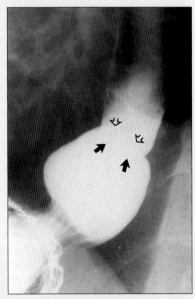

Figure 3. Overlap phenomenon obscuring the Schatzki ring. Prone single-contrast view of the distal esophagus shows a hiatal hernia without evidence of a lower esophageal ring. However, a double density can be found with two superimposed convex collections of barium caused by overlap of the distal end of the esophagus *(solid arrows)* and the proximal end of the hernia *(open arrows).* *(From Hsu WC, Levine MS, Rubesin SE: Overlap phenomenon: A potential pitfall in the radiographic detection of lower esophageal rings. AJR Am J Roentgenol 180, 745-747, 2003, © by American Roentgen Ray Society.)*

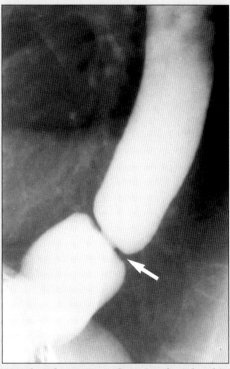

Figure 4. Overlap phenomenon obscuring the Schatzki ring. Repeat view from the same examination as in Figure 3 with less distention of the hernia shows a tight Schatzki ring *(arrow)* when the distal esophagus and adjacent hiatal hernia no longer overlap. *(From Hsu WC, Levine MS, Rubesin SE: Overlap phenomenon: A potential pitfall in the radiographic detection of lower esophageal rings. AJR Am J Roentgenol 180, 745-747, 2003, © by American Roentgen Ray Society.)*

Suggested Readings

Arvanitakis C: Lower esophageal ring: Endoscopic and therapeutic aspects. *Gastrointest Endosc* 24:17-18, 1977.

Burdick JS, Venu RP, Hogan WJ: Cutting the defiant lower esophageal ring. *Gastrointest Endosc* 39:616-619, 1993.

Chen YM, Gelfand DW, Ott DJ, et al: Natural progression of the lower esophageal mucosal ring. *Gastrointest Radiol* 12:93-98, 1987.

Desai DC, Rider JA, Puletti EJ, et al: Lower esophageal ring. *Gastrointest Endosc* 15:100-105, 1968.

DeVault KR: Lower esophageal (Schatzki's) ring: Pathogenesis, diagnosis and therapy. *Dig Dis* 14:323-329, 1996.

Friedland GW: Historical review of the changing concepts of lower esophageal anatomy: 430 B.C.–1977. *AJR Am J Roentgenol* 131:373-388, 1978.

Goyal RK, Glancy JJ, Spiro HM: Lower esophageal ring. *N Engl J Med* 282:1298-1305, 1970.

Gupta S, Levine MS, Rubesin SE, et al: Usefulness of barium studies for differentiating benign and malignant strictures of the esophagus. *AJR Am J Roentgenol* 180:737-744, 2003.

Hsu WC, Levine MS, Rubesin SE: Overlap phenomenon: A potential pitfall in the radiographic detection of lower esophageal rings. *AJR Am J Roentgenol* 180:745-747, 2003.

Marshall JB, Kretschmar JM, Diaz-Arias AA: Gastroesophageal reflux as a pathogenic factor in the development of symptomatic lower esophageal rings. *Arch Intern Med* 150:1669-1672, 1990.

Norton RA, King GD: "Steak house syndrome": The symptomatic lower esophageal ring. *Lahey Clin Found Bull* 13:55-59, 1963.

Pezzullo JC, Lewicki AM: Schatzki ring, statistically reexamined. *Radiology* 228:609-613, 2003.

Ott DJ, Chen YM, Wu WC, et al: Radiographic and endoscopic sensitivity in detecting lower esophageal mucosal ring. *AJR Am J Roentgenol* 147:261-265, 1986.

Scharschmidt BF, Watts HD: The lower esophageal ring and esophageal reflux. *Am J Gastroenterol* 69:544-549, 1978.

Schatzki R: The lower esophageal ring: Long term follow-up of symptomatic and asymptomatic rings. *AJR Am J Roentgenol* 90:805-810, 1963.

Schatzki R, Gary JE: Dysphagia due to a diaphragm-like localized narrowing in the lower esophagus ("lower esophageal ring"). *AJR Am J Roentgenol* 70:911-922, 1953.

Weaver JW, Kaude JV, Hamlin DJ: Webs of the lower esophagus: A complication of gastroesophageal reflux. *AJR Am J Roentgenol* 142:289-292, 1984.

Hiatal Hernias

DEFINITION: Portion of the stomach protruding above the diaphragm.

IMAGING

Radiography
Findings
- In axial hiatal hernias, the gastroesophageal junction is located above the esophageal hiatus of the diaphragm.
- A hiatal hernia may be diagnosed on prone single-contrast views when a mucosal ring is observed 2 cm or more above the diaphragmatic hiatus.
- In the absence of a definite mucosal ring, a hiatal hernia is also recognized by gastric folds within the hernia.
- In large hiatal hernias, the weight of the barium may cause the gastric fundus to droop inferiorly beneath the herniated gastric body, producing a distinctive radiographic appearance, also known as a *floppy fundus.*
- In paraesophageal hernias, the gastric fundus has herniated through the esophageal hiatus alongside the distal esophagus, whereas the cardia retains its normal position below the esophageal hiatus of the diaphragm.
- In mixed sliding-paraesophageal hernias, the cardia has also herniated above the diaphragm into the chest.

Utility
- Single-contrast views with the patient prone are more likely to demonstrate a hiatal hernia than double-contrast views with the patient upright.

CLINICAL PRESENTATION

- Controversy exists about relationship between an axial hiatal hernia and the subsequent development of gastroesophageal reflux and reflux esophagitis.
- In paraesophageal hernias, patients may be asymptomatic, and this type of hernia is rarely associated with gastroesophageal reflux or reflux esophagitis.
- As paraesophageal hernias enlarge, patients are at risk for serious complications, including obstruction, incarceration, strangulation, and infarction.

DIFFERENTIAL DIAGNOSIS

- Organoaxial gastric volvulus
- Mesenteroaxial gastric volvulus

DIAGNOSTIC PEARLS

- In axial hiatal hernias, the gastroesophageal junction is located above the esophageal hiatus of the diaphragm.
- In paraesophageal hernias, the gastric fundus has herniated through the esophageal hiatus alongside the distal esophagus, whereas the cardia retains a normal position.
- In mixed sliding-paraesophageal hernia, the cardia has also herniated above the diaphragm into the chest.

PATHOLOGY

- Hiatal hernias are classified either as axial hernias or as paraesophageal hernias.
- With aging, constant swallowing causes progressive wear and tear on the surrounding phrenoesophageal membrane.
- In axial hiatal hernias, eventual stretching or rupture of the phrenoesophageal membrane occurs, causing axial herniation of the stomach into the chest.
- In paraesophageal hernias, a portion of the stomach herniates through the esophageal hiatus alongside the distal esophagus, whereas the cardia retains a normal position below the esophageal hiatus of the diaphragm.

INCIDENCE/PREVALENCE AND EPIDEMIOLOGY

- Prevalence of axial hiatal hernias increases with age.
- Sixty percent of elderly people in the United States are found to have axial hiatal hernias on barium studies.
- Paraesophageal hernias comprise less than 5% of all hiatal hernias.

Suggested Readings

Dodds WJ: Esophagus and esophagogastric region. In Margulis AR, Burhenne HJ (eds): *Alimentary Tract Radiology*, 3rd ed. St. Louis, CV Mosby, 1983.

Dunn DB, Quick G: Incarcerated paraesophageal hernia. *Am J Emerg Med* 8:36-39, 1990.

Hill LD: Incarcerated paraesophageal hernia: A surgical emergency. *Am J Surg* 126:286-291, 1973.

Huang SY, Levine MS, Rubesin SE, et al: Large hiatal hernias with floppy fundus: Clinical and radiographic findings. *AJR Am J Roentgenol* 188:960-964, 2007.

WHAT THE REFERRING PHYSICIAN NEEDS TO KNOW

- Patients with axial hiatal hernias are often asymptomatic, although these hernias predispose affected individuals to reflux disease.
- Patients with paraesophageal hernias are at risk for serious complications related to strangulation or obstruction of hernias, but management is controversial if diagnosed in elderly adults or asymptomatic patients who are poor surgical candidates.

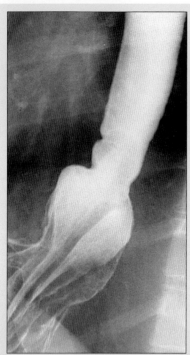

Figure 1. Sliding hiatal hernia. Gastric rugae are seen in a hiatal hernia on a prone, single-contrast view of the esophagus. (*From Levine MS:* Radiology of the Esophagus. *Philadelphia, WB Saunders, 1989.*)

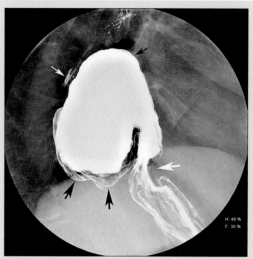

Figure 2. Large hiatal hernia with a floppy fundus. Supine oblique view shows a floppy fundus *(large black arrows)* inferior to the most superior portion of the gastric body *(small black arrow).* Note the narrowing of the stomach *(large white arrow)* where it traverses the diaphragm. (The small white arrow denotes the location of the gastroesophageal junction above the diaphragm.) (*From Huang SY, Levine MS, Rubesin SE, et al:* Large hiatal hernias with a floppy fundus. *AJR Am J Roentgenol 188:960-964, 2007, © by American Roentgen Ray Society.*)

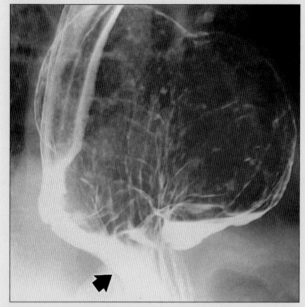

Figure 3. Paraesophageal hernia. The gastric fundus has herniated into the chest alongside the distal esophagus, but the gastric cardia *(arrow)* retains its normal position below the diaphragm. (*From Levine MS:* Radiology of the Esophagus. *Philadelphia, WB Saunders, 1989.*)

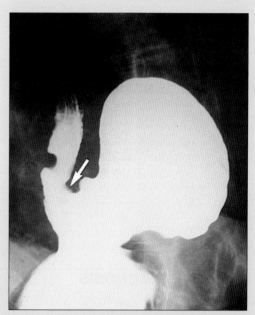

Figure 4. Mixed sliding-paraesophageal hernia. The gastric fundus has herniated into the chest alongside the distal esophagus. In this patient, however, the cardia *(arrow)* has also herniated above the diaphragm. These features are those of a mixed hernia.

Landreneau RJ, Hazelrigg SR, Johnson JA, et al: The giant paraesophageal hernia: A particularly morbid condition of the esophageal hiatus. *Mo Med* 87:884-888, 1990.

Landreneau RJ, Johnson JA, Marshall JB, et al: Clinical spectrum of paraesophageal herniation. *Dig Dis Sci* 37:537-544, 1992.

Shocket E, Neber J, Drosg RE: The acutely obstructed, incarcerated paraesophageal hiatal hernia. *Am J Surg* 108:805-810, 1964.

Skinner DB: Hernias (hiatal, traumatic, and congenital). In Berk JE (ed): *Bockus Gastroenterology,* 4th ed. Philadelphia, WB Saunders, 1985.

Vitelli CE, Jaffe BM, Kahng KU: Paraesophageal hernia. *NY State J Med* 89:654-657, 1989.

Wo JM, Branum GD, Hunter JG, et al: Clinical features of type III (mixed) paraesophageal hernia. *Am J Gastroenterol* 91:914-916, 1996.

Carcinoma of the Cardia

DEFINITION: Carcinoma of the gastric cardia.

IMAGING

Radiography

Findings

- Advanced tumors at the cardia may appear as obvious exophytic or infiltrating lesions in gastric fundus.
- Other adenocarcinomas are recognized only by subtle nodularity, mass effect, and ulceration with distortion, effacement, or obliteration of normal anatomic landmarks at the cardia.

Utility

- Abnormalities at cardia are difficult to demonstrate on conventional single-contrast barium studies.
- Double-contrast technique is essential for detecting these lesions at the earliest possible stage.

CLINICAL PRESENTATION

- Recent onset of dysphagia and weight loss
- Possible referred dysphagia to the suprasternal notch or even the pharynx

DIFFERENTIAL DIAGNOSIS

- Esophageal adenocarcinoma invading proximal stomach
- Lymphoma
- Esophagogastric prolapse

PATHOLOGY

- Advanced lesions at the cardia may appear as obvious exophytic or infiltrating lesions at the gastric fundus.
- Normal anatomic landmarks at the cardia may be obliterated and replaced by irregular areas of nodularity and ulceration as a result of the tumor arising in this location.

DIAGNOSTIC PEARLS

- Advanced lesions at the cardia may appear as obvious exophytic or infiltrating lesions in the gastric fundus.
- Other lesions are recognized only by subtle signs with distortion, effacement, or obliteration of normal anatomic landmarks.
- Double-contrast technique is essential for detecting these lesions at the earliest possible stage.

INCIDENCE/PREVALENCE AND EPIDEMIOLOGY

- Carcinoma of the cardia is increasing at faster rate than any other malignant tumor in the human body.
- Carcinoma of the cardia comprises as many as 40%-50% of all gastric carcinomas.
- Male-to-female ratio is 7:1.
- Small but significant percentage of cases occur in young patients (under 40 years of age).

Suggested Readings

Freeny PC: Double-contrast gastrography of the fundus and cardia: Normal landmarks and their pathologic changes. *AJR Am J Roentgenol* 133:481-487, 1979.

Freeny PC, Marks WM: Adenocarcinoma of the gastroesophageal junction: Barium and CT examination. *AJR Am J Roentgenol* 138:1077-1084, 1982.

Herlinger H, Grossman R, Laufer I, et al: The gastric cardia in double-contrast study: Its dynamic image. *AJR Am J Roentgenol* 135:21-29, 1980.

Levine MS, Laufer I, Thompson JJ: Carcinoma of the gastric cardia in young people. *AJR Am J Roentgenol* 140:69-72, 1983.

WHAT THE REFERRING PHYSICIAN NEEDS TO KNOW

- Advanced lesions at the cardia may appear as obvious exophytic or infiltrating lesions in the gastric fundus.
- Other lesions are recognized only by subtle nodularity, mass effect, or ulceration with distortion, effacement, or obliteration of normal anatomic landmarks at the cardia.
- Cardia and fundus should therefore be carefully evaluated in all patients with dysphagia in order to detect these lesions at the earliest possible stage.
- Radiologists should never be lulled into a false sense of security about the possibility of a malignancy based on the patient's age.

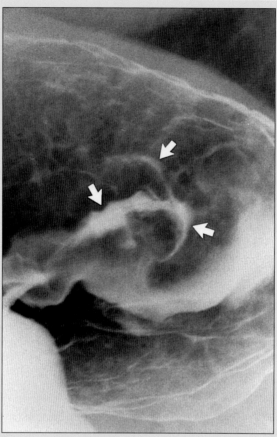

Figure 1. Carcinoma of the gastric cardia. The normal anatomic landmarks at the cardia have been obliterated and replaced by irregular areas of ulceration *(arrows)* as a result of the tumor in this region. (*From Levine MS:* Radiology of the Esophagus. *Philadelphia, WB Saunders, 1989.*)

Stomach and Duodenum

Gastric Ulcers

DEFINITION: Peptic ulcers in the stomach are one of the major causes of upper gastrointestinal bleeding.

ANATOMIC FINDINGS

Stomach
- Linear, rod-shaped, rectangular, serpiginous, or flame-shaped lesions
- Smooth, round or ovoid ulcer craters that project beyond contour of adjacent gastric wall

IMAGING

Radiography
Findings
- Classically round or ovoid collections of barium
- Linear, rod-shaped, rectangular, serpiginous, or flame shaped ulcers also seen
- Ulcers on the lesser curvature: smooth, round or ovoid craters that project beyond the contour of the adjacent gastric wall
- Ulcers on the posterior wall: craters fill with barium when patient is supine; often associated with radiating folds
- Ulcers on the greater curvature: intraluminal location caused by circular muscle spasm and retraction of the adjacent gastric wall
- Ulcers on the anterior wall: craters seen as ring shadows due to barium coating rim of nondependent ulcer. Craters fill with barium when patient is rotated into prone position.

Utility
- Double-contrast examination should be performed as a biphasic study.
- Ulcer detection is facilitated by the routine administration of 0.1 mg of glucagon intravenously to induce hypotonia.
- Flow technique can be used to better delineate shallow ulcers on the posterior wall of lesser curvature.
- Upright compression views are helpful for evaluating ulcers on the lesser curvature.
- Prone compression views of the gastric antrum and body should be obtained routinely to demonstrate anterior wall ulcers.

DIAGNOSTIC PEARLS
- Linear, rod-shaped, rectangular, serpiginous, or flame-shaped lesions
- Smooth, round or ovoid craters that project beyond the contour of the adjacent gastric wall
- Posterior wall ulcers: craters fill with barium when patient is supine.
- Anterior wall ulcers: craters seen as ring shadows when patient is supine due to barium coating rim of nondependent ulcers.
- Greater curvature ulcers are always located on distal half of greater curvature (when benign), and vast majority are caused by ingestion of aspirin or other nonsteroidal anti-inflammatory drugs (NSAIDs).

CLINICAL PRESENTATION
- Many patients experience epigastric pain: gnawing, aching, or burning discomfort between the xiphoid cartilage and the umbilicus (occurring less than 2 hours after meals) is classic.
- Other patients may have right upper quadrant, back, or chest pain.
- Bloating, belching, nausea, anorexia, and weight loss may occur.
- When ulcers on the posterior wall of the stomach penetrate into the pancreas, pain becomes more constant and radiates to the back.
- Gastric outlet obstruction causes postprandial nausea and vomiting.
- Major upper gastrointestinal hemorrhage may be manifested by hematemesis, melena, or rectal bleeding. Chronic, low-grade hemorrhage may be manifested by guaiac-positive stool or iron-deficiency anemia.

DIFFERENTIAL DIAGNOSIS
- Malignant gastric ulcers, carcinoma
- Malignant gastric ulcers, lymphoma

WHAT THE REFERRING PHYSICIAN NEEDS TO KNOW
- Most benign gastric ulcers are located on the lesser curvature or posterior wall of the gastric antrum or body.
- Almost all benign greater curvature gastric ulcers are caused by aspirin or other NSAIDs.
- Gastric ulcers that have an unequivocally benign appearance on double-contrast studies can be followed up by a repeat double-contrast study to document ulcer healing without need for endoscopy.

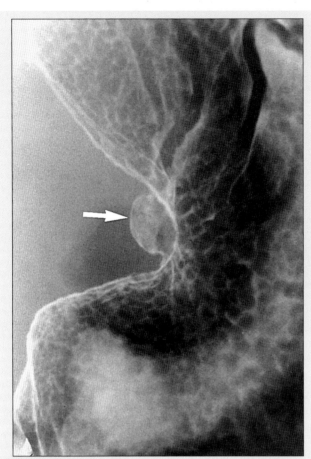

Figure 1. Lesser curvature ulcer. A smooth, round ulcer *(arrow)* is seen projecting beyond the lesser curvature. The radiating folds and enlarged areae gastricae in the adjacent mucosa are caused by surrounding edema and inflammation. *(From Levine MS, Creteur V, Kressel HY, et al: Benign gastric ulcer: Diagnosis and follow-up with double contrast radiography.* Radiology *164:9-13, 1987.)*

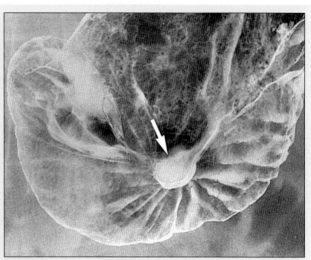

Figure 2. Posterior wall ulcer. A large ulcer *(arrow)* is present on the posterior wall of the stomach. Multiple folds are seen radiating to the edge of the ulcer crater. *(From Laufer I, Levine MS [eds]:* Double-Contrast Gastrointestinal Radiology, *2nd ed. Philadelphia, WB Saunders, 1992.)*

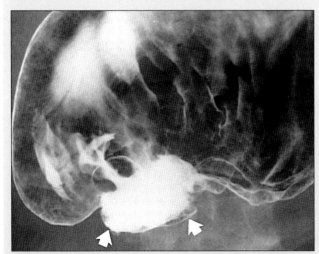

Figure 3. Giant greater curvature ulcer caused by aspirin. This large ulcer *(arrows)* on the greater curvature has an apparent intraluminal location and is associated with thickened, irregular folds and considerable mass effect from a surrounding mound of edema. *(From Laufer I, Levine MS [eds]:* Double-Contrast Gastrointestinal Radiology, *2nd ed. Philadelphia, WB Saunders, 1992.)*

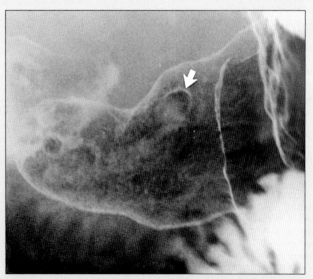

Figure 4. Partial ring shadow caused by an anterior wall ulcer. Supine double-contrast view shows a partial ring shadow *(arrow)* in the antrum.

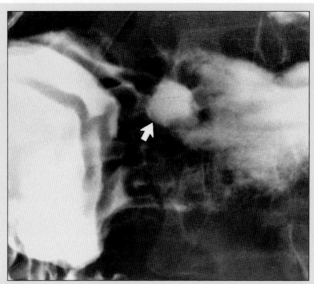

Figure 5. Partial ring shadow caused by an anterior wall ulcer. Prone compression view from same examination as in Figure 4 shows the anterior wall ulcer *(arrow)* filling with barium. (*From Levine MS, Rubesin SE, Herlinger H, et al: Double-contrast upper gastrointestinal examination: Technique and interpretation.* Radiology *168:593-602, 1988.*)

PATHOLOGY

- Gastric ulcers are characterized by seasonal variations, with a higher frequency of ulcers in the spring and autumn and a lower frequency in the summer.
- NSAIDs inhibit prostaglandin production by blocking formation of cyclooxygenase, leading to severe mucosal injury and ulceration.
- Most benign ulcers are located on the lesser curvature or the posterior wall of the antrum or body of the stomach.
- Gastric ulcer bleeding is caused by erosion of the ulcer into the wall of vessels.

INCIDENCE/PREVALENCE AND EPIDEMIOLOGY

- Gastric ulcers are associated with the use of alcohol, tobacco, and aspirin or other NSAIDs.
- They are found predominantly in patients older than 40 years of age, and gender distribution is equal.
- Prevalence of *Helicobacter pylori* has ranged from 60%-80% in patients with gastric ulcers.
- Prevalence of gastric ulcers in patients receiving regular treatment of NSAIDs has ranged from 15%-30%.

Suggested Readings

Howarth DM: The role of nuclear medicine in the detection of acute gastrointestinal bleeding. *Semin Nucl Med* 36:133-146, 2006.

Lin S, Rockey DC: Obscure gastrointestinal bleeding. *Gastroenterol Clin North Am* 34:679-698, 2005.

Manning-Dimmitt LL, Dimmitt SG, Wilson GR: Diagnosis of gastrointestinal bleeding in adults. *Am Fam Physician* 71:1339-1346, 2005.

Maurer AH: Gastrointestinal bleeding. In Murray IP, Ell PJ (eds): *Nuclear Medicine in Clinical Diagnosis and Treatment.* New York, Churchill Livingstone, 1994, pp 47–54.

Pyloric Channel Ulcers

DEFINITION: Peptic ulcer located in the pylorus.

ANATOMIC FINDINGS

Pylorus
- Pyloric channel ulcers are usually located on the lesser curvature of the pylorus or on the anterior wall of the pylorus.

IMAGING

Radiography
Findings
- Anterior wall ulcers appear as ring shadows on double-contrast views and fill with barium on prone compression views.
- Signs include marked edema and spasm of the pylorus and distal antrum, which can obscure ulcers.
- Ulcers have a fixed configuration in contrast to pseudodiverticula, which are likely to change in size and shape at fluoroscopy.

Utility
- Must be differentiated on barium studies from pseudodiverticula caused by scarring from a previous ulcer disease or surgical pyloroplasty.
- Presence of mucosal folds in the region of outpouching should also suggest a pseudodiverticulum.

CLINICAL PRESENTATION

- Localized epigastric pain characterized as gnawing, aching, or burning discomfort between the xiphoid cartilage and the umbilicus.
- Other symptoms include right upper quadrant, back, or chest pain, as well as bloating, belching, nausea, vomiting, anorexia, and weight loss.

DIAGNOSTIC PEARLS

- Anterior wall ulcers appear as ring shadows on double-contrast views; these are filled with barium on prone, upright compression views.
- Signs include marked edema and spasm of the pylorus and distal antrum, which can obscure ulcers.
- Ulcers have fixed configuration, in contrast to pseudodiverticula, which are likely to change in size and shape.

DIFFERENTIAL DIAGNOSIS

- Hypertrophic pyloric stenosis
- Gastric carcinoma
- Pseudodiverticulum

INCIDENCE/PREVALENCE AND EPIDEMIOLOGY

- Pyloric channel ulcers occur in adults with equal sex distribution.

Suggested Readings

Farack UM, Goresky CA, Jabbari M, et al: Double pylorus: A hypothesis concerning its pathogenesis. *Gastroenterology* 66:596-600, 1974.
Jamshidnejad J, Koehler RE, Narayan D: Double channel pylorus. *AJR Am J Roentgenol* 130:1047-1050, 1978.

WHAT THE REFERRING PHYSICIAN NEEDS TO KNOW

- Healing of pyloric channel ulcers may lead to narrowing, elongation, or angulation of the pylorus, sometimes associated with gastric outlet obstruction.
- Treated as a gastric ulcer in terms of the need for aggressive evaluation and follow-up to differentiate benign ulcers from ulcerated carcinomas.
- Differential diagnosis includes adult hypertrophic pyloric stenosis and pseudodiverticula secondary to scarring.

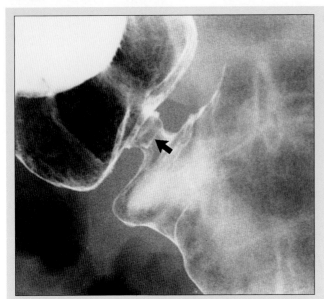

Figure 1. Pyloric channel ulcer. Initial double-contrast view with the patient in a supine position shows a partial ring shadow *(arrow)* in the region of the pylorus.

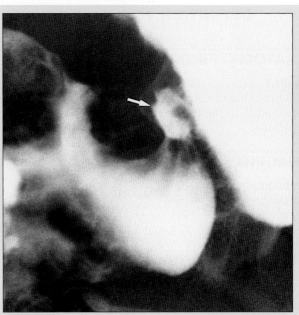

Figure 2. Pyloric channel ulcer (same patient as in Figure 1). Prone compression view shows barium filling an ulcer crater *(arrow)* on the anterior wall of the pyloric channel.

Duodenal Ulcers

DEFINITION: Peptic ulcers in the duodenum are almost always associated with *Helicobacter pylori* infection.

ANATOMIC FINDINGS

Duodenum
- Ninety percent of duodenal ulcers are located in the duodenal bulb.
- Fifty percent of duodenal ulcers are located on the anterior wall of the bulb.
- Ten percent of duodenal ulcers are located in the post-bulbar duodenum, usually the proximal descending duodenum above the papilla of Vater.

IMAGING

Fluoroscopy
Findings
- Duodenal ulcers are classically seen as round or ovoid collections of barium on the posterior wall of the duodenal bulb; linear ulcers may also be seen.
- Bulbar ulcers are visualized en face as discrete niches associated with radiating folds that converge centrally at the crater edge.
- Anterior wall ulcer may be seen on supine views as a ring shadow caused by barium coating the rim of the unfilled ulcer crater that fills on prone compression views.
- The size of the ulcer mound may be striking in relation to the central crater.
- Radiating folds and bulbar deformity may be the only signs of a postbulbar ulcer obscured by edema and spasm.
- Duodenal bulb deformity is caused by edema or by scarring from a previous ulcer.
- Large postbulbar ulcers may be associated with proximal and distal narrowing of the descending duodenum caused by marked amount of edema and spasm accompanying the ulcer craters.
- Giant duodenal ulcers have a fixed, unchanging configuration, in contrast to the changing appearance of the duodenal bulb.

Utility
- Double-contrast views with high-density barium and prone or upright compression views with low-density barium are employed.
- Prone compression views of duodenum should be obtained routinely to demonstrate anterior wall ulcers.

DIAGNOSTIC PEARLS
- Duodenal ulcers are classically seen as round or ovoid collections of barium, but linear ulcers may also be found.
- Bulbar ulcers may be visualized as discrete niches associated with radiating folds that converge centrally at the crater edge.
- Duodenal ulcers can be identified as source of bleeding on endoscopy, angiography, or red blood cell scans.
- Giant ulcer is fixed with unchanging configuration in contrast to the duodenal bulb.

- Major advantage of double-contrast technique is its ability to demonstrate small ulcers that are no more than several millimeters in diameter.
- Barium trapped in the crevices of the deformed bulb can mimic ulcer craters.

CLINICAL PRESENTATION
- Patients with duodenal ulcers are asymptomatic in 25%-50% of cases.
- Localized epigastric pain is characterized by gnawing, aching, or burning discomfort between the xiphoid cartilage and the umbilicus.
- Other patients may complain of right upper quadrant back or chest pain or of bloating, belching, nausea, vomiting, anorexia, or weight loss.
- Duodenal ulcer pain occurs 2-4 hours after meals and is more likely to awaken the patient at night.
- Some patients may initially show signs or symptoms caused by complications of ulcers, such as perforation, obstruction, and bleeding.
- Duodenal ulcers associated with edema, spasm, or scar formation may cause varying degrees of gastric outlet obstruction.
- Hematemesis or melena, hematochezia (massive hemorrhage > 1000 mL), dyspnea, dizziness, or shock may be present in patients with massive upper gastrointestinal bleeding.

WHAT THE REFERRING PHYSICIAN NEEDS TO KNOW
- When ulcers are detected on barium studies, patients can receive medical treatment without need for endoscopy.
- Major life-threatening complications include upper gastrointestinal bleeding, obstruction, and perforation.
- Postbulbar duodenal ulcers are more likely to be associated with upper gastrointestinal bleeding (particularly massive bleeding) than ulcers in the duodenal bulb.

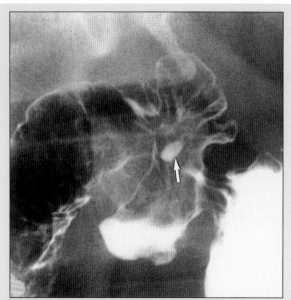

Figure 1. Duodenal ulcers. A small ulcer *(arrow)* is present in the central portion of the bulb. This ulcer is associated with radiating folds and bulbar deformity. Note how the crater fills with barium when patient is in a supine, semirecumbent position.

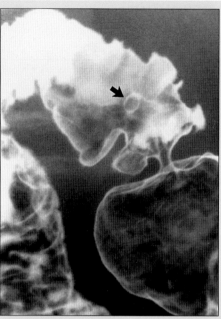

Figure 2. Ring shadow caused by an anterior wall duodenal ulcer. Supine oblique double-contrast view of the duodenum shows a ring shadow *(arrow)* in the bulb as a result of barium coating the rim of an unfilled ulcer on the nondependent surface. *(From Laufer I, Levine MS [eds]:* Double-Contrast Gastrointestinal Radiology, *2nd ed. Philadelphia, WB Saunders, 1992.)*

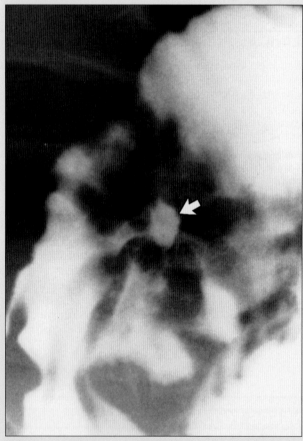

Figure 3. Ring shadow caused by an anterior wall duodenal ulcer. Prone compression view from the same examination as Figure 2 shows filling of the anterior wall ulcer *(arrow)*. Note the large, radiolucent mound of edema surrounding the ulcer. *(From Laufer I, Levine MS [eds]:* Double-Contrast Gastrointestinal Radiology, *2nd ed. Philadelphia, WB Saunders, 1992.)*

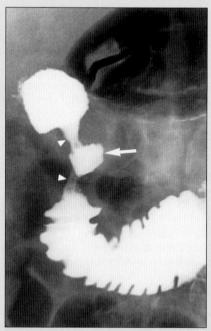

Figure 4. Large postbulbar duodenal ulcer. Patient with a large postbulbar ulcer *(arrow)* in the proximal descending duodenum. Note marked narrowing of the adjacent duodenum proximally and distally *(arrowheads)* as a result of severe edema and spasm accompanying the ulcer crater. *(From Carucci LR, Levine MS, Rubesin SE, et al: Upper gastrointestinal tract barium examination of postbulbar duodenal ulcers.* AJR Am J Roentgenol *182:927-930, 2004, © by American Roentgen Ray Society.)*

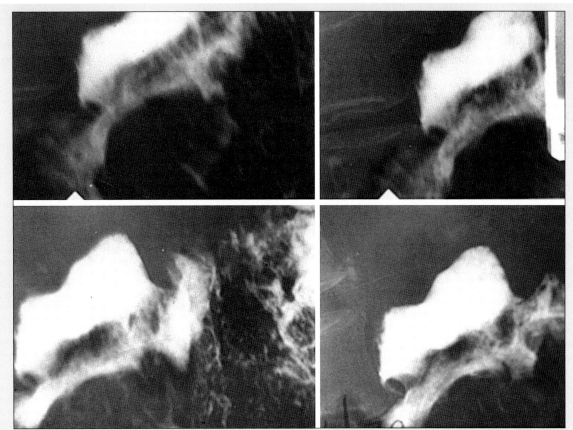

Figure 5. Giant duodenal ulcer. Four spot images of the bulb show a giant ulcer that has a constant size and shape. In contrast, the duodenal bulb usually has a changing appearance at fluoroscopy. Also note the large radiolucent band of edema adjacent to the ulcer.

DIFFERENTIAL DIAGNOSIS

- Duodenal diverticula (stomach and duodenum)
- Zollinger-Ellison syndrome (stomach and duodenum)
- Crohn disease (gastrointestinal)

PATHOLOGY

- Virulent cagA-positive strain of gram-negative, spiral bacillus *Helicobacter pylori* is a major causative factor.
- Pathogenesis is by a gastrin-mediated increase in gastric acid secretions and inhibition of normal physiologic mechanisms for controlling acid secretion.
- *H. pylori* causes gastric metaplasia at the borders of duodenal ulcers by infection of the metaplastic epithelium.
- Familial aggregation of ulcers is primarily hereditary.

INCIDENCE/PREVALENCE AND EPIDEMIOLOGY

- Duodenal ulcers occur in adults of all ages; gender distribution is equal; patients with upper gastrointestinal bleeding are significantly older and are more likely to be men than women.

- Duodenal ulcers have seasonal variations, with higher frequency of ulcers in the spring and autumn and lower frequency in the summer.
- Prevalence of *H. pylori* gastritis ranges from 95%-100% in patients with duodenal ulcers.
- Blood type O is associated with higher incidence of ulcers than other blood types.
- Duodenal ulcers may be seen in patients with genetic syndromes such as multiple endocrine neoplasia type 1, systemic mastocytosis, and tremor-nystagmus-ulcer syndrome.

Suggested Readings

Bonnevie O: Changing demographics of peptic ulcer disease. *Dig Dis Sci* 30(Suppl 11):85-145, 1985.
Carucci LR, Levine MS, Rubesin SE, et al: Upper gastrointestinal tract barium examination of postbulbar duodenal ulcers. *AJR Am J Roentgenol* 182:927-930, 2004.
Dunn JP, Etter LE: Inadequacy of the medical history in the diagnosis of duodenal ulcer. *N Engl J Med* 266:68-72, 1962.
Levine MS, Rubesin SE: The *Helicobacter pylori* revolution: Radiologic perspective. *Radiology* 195:593-596, 1995.
Pattison CP, Combs MK, Marshall BJ: *Helicobacter pylori* and peptic ulcer disease: Evolution to revolution to resolution. *AJR Am J Roentgenol* 168:1415-1420, 1997.
Tarpila S, Samloff IM, Pikkarainen P, et al: Endoscopic and clinical findings in first-degree relatives of duodenal ulcer patients and control subjects. *Scand J Gastroenterol* 17:503-506, 1982.
Yardley JH, Paull G: *Campylobacter pylori:* A newly recognized infectious agent in the gastrointestinal tract. *Am J Surg Pathol* 12(Suppl):89-99, 1988.

Zollinger-Ellison Syndrome and Peptic Ulcer Disease (Stomach and Duodenum)

DEFINITION: Life-threatening condition characterized by marked hypersecretion of gastric acid and a severe form of peptic ulcer disease resulting from high levels of gastrin in patients with underlying gastrinomas.

ANATOMIC FINDINGS

Gastrointestinal Tract
- Seventy-five percent of ulcers in Zollinger-Ellison syndrome are located in the stomach or duodenal bulb.
- Twenty-five percent of ulcers in Zollinger-Ellison syndrome are located in the postbulbar duodenum or proximal jejunum.

IMAGING

Radiography
Findings
- Markedly thickened folds in the fundus and body of the stomach are caused by gastrin-induced parietal cell hyperplasia.
- Duodenal and jejunal folds may have a thickened, edematous appearance caused by an enormous amount of gastric secretions entering the proximal small bowel.
- One or more ulcers are found in the stomach, duodenum, or proximal jejunum.
- Large volume of fluid is present in the stomach, duodenum, and proximal jejunum.

Utility
- Barium studies
- Large volume of fluid in the stomach, duodenum, and proximal jejunum dilutes barium and compromises mucosal coating by barium.
- Increased fluid in the upper gastrointestinal tract and one or more ulcers in unusual locations should strongly suggest Zollinger-Ellison syndrome.

CT
Utility
- Used for localization of gastrinoma

DIAGNOSTIC PEARLS
- One or more ulcers in the stomach, duodenum, or proximal jejunum
- Large volume of fluid in the stomach, duodenum, and proximal jejunum
- Duodenal and jejunal folds may have thickened, edematous appearance caused by an enormous amount of gastric secretions entering the proximal small bowel.
- Markedly thickened gastric folds in fundus and body of the stomach are caused by gastrin-induced parietal cell hyperplasia.

Nuclear Medicine
Utility
- Used for localization of gastrinoma

Interventional Radiology
Utility
- Used for localization of gastrinoma

CLINICAL PRESENTATION
- Ninety percent of patients have upper gastrointestinal tract ulcers (usually multiple) caused by gastric acid hypersection.
- Diarrhea is the second most common clinical finding.
- Other patients may have reflux symptoms or dysphagia caused by development of severe reflux esophagitis or peptic strictures.

WHAT THE REFERRING PHYSICIAN NEEDS TO KNOW
- This condition must be differentiated from *Helicobacter pylori* gastritis, hypertrophic gastritis, Ménétrier disease, and lymphoma.
- Thickened duodenal or jejunal folds may be caused by a host of inflammatory or infectious processes.
- When Zollinger-Ellison syndrome is suspected based on radiographic findings, a fasting serum gastrin level should be obtained for a more definitive diagnosis.
- Demonstration of hypergastrinemia and gastric acid hypersecretion in a patient with peptic ulcers, diarrhea, or other clinical features of gastrinoma is diagnostic of Zollinger-Ellison syndrome.
- A fasting serum gastrin level greater than 1000 pg/mL is diagnostic of Zollinger-Ellison syndrome.
- H_2-receptor antagonists and proton pump inhibitors are effective in suppressing acid secretion and promoting ulcer healing without surgery.
- CT, angiography, selective portal venous sampling for gastrin, or somatostatin scintigraphy may be used for localization of the gastrinoma.

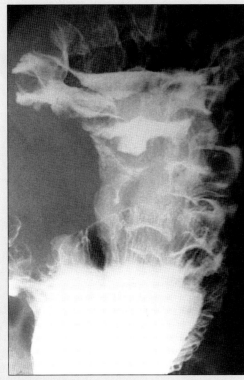

Figure 1. Zollinger-Ellison syndrome. Markedly thickened folds are seen in the gastric fundus and body. Also note how the barium is diluted by excessive fluid in the stomach.

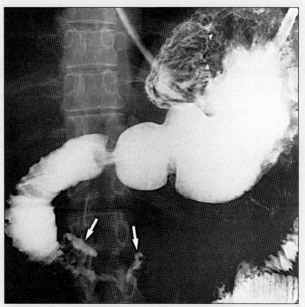

Figure 2. Zollinger-Ellison syndrome. Two discrete ulcers *(arrows)* are seen in the third and fourth portions of the duodenum. Ordinary peptic ulcers rarely occur distal to the papilla of Vater; thus ulcers in this location should suggest the possibility of Zollinger-Ellison syndrome. (*Courtesy of Stephen W. Trenkner, MD, Minneapolis, MN.*)

DIFFERENTIAL DIAGNOSIS

- *H. pylori* gastritis
- Hypertrophic gastritis
- Ménétrier disease (stomach and duodenum)
- Lymphoma (stomach and duodenum)
- Peptic ulcers

Pathology

- Multiple ulcers are caused by uncontrolled gastrin release from autonomously functioning non–beta islet cell tumors known as gastrinomas.
- Gastrinomas: 75% located in pancreas, 15% in duodenum, and 10% in extraintestinal locations
- Most gastrinomas are malignant; multiple tumors or metastases are found at the time of diagnosis in 30%-50% of patients.
- Twenty-five percent are genetically transmitted as part of a hereditary syndrome (multiple endocrine neoplasia type 1).
- The syndrome is characterized not only by pancreatic tumors, but also by parathyroid, pituitary, and adrenal tumors.

Suggested Readings

Cherner JA, Doppman JL, Norton JA, et al: Selective venous sampling for gastrin to localize gastrinomas: A prospective assessment. *Ann Intern Med* 105:841-847, 1986.

Del Valle J, Yamada T: Zollinger-Ellison syndrome. In Yamada T (ed): *Textbook of Gastroenterology.* Philadelphia, JB Lippincott, 1991, pp 1340-1352.

Gibril F, Reynolds JC, Doppman JL, et al: Somatostatin receptor scintigraphy: Its sensitivity compared with that of other imaging methods in detecting primary and metastatic gastrinomas: A prospective study. *Ann Intern Med* 125:26-34, 1996.

Maton PN, Miller DL, Doppman JL, et al: The role of selective angiography in the management of patients with Zollinger-Ellison syndrome. *Gastroenterology* 92:913-918, 1987.

Nelson SW, Lichtenstein JE: The Zollinger-Ellison syndrome. In Marshak RH (ed): *Radiology of the Stomach.* Philadelphia, WB Saunders, 1983, pp 334-381.

Wank SA, Doppman JL, Miller DL, et al: Prospective study of the ability of computerized axial tomography to localize gastrinomas in patients with Zollinger-Ellison syndrome. *Gastroenterology* 92:905-912, 1987.

Wolfe MM, Jensen RT: Zollinger-Ellison syndrome: Current concepts in diagnosis and management. *N Engl J Med* 317:1200-1209, 1987.

Zboralske FF, Amberg JR: Detection of the Zollinger-Ellison syndrome: The radiologist's responsibility. *Am J Roentgenol Radium Ther Nucl Med* 104:529-543, 1968.

Part 16

INFLAMMATORY CONDITIONS OF THE STOMACH AND DUODENUM

Erosive Gastritis

DEFINITION: Shallow epithelial defects in the stomach, most often caused by aspirin or other nonsteroidal anti-inflammatory drug (NSAID) ingestion.

IMAGING

Radiography
Findings
- Complete or varioliform erosions are seen as punctate or slit-like barium collections representing epithelial defects surrounded by radiolucent mounds of edema.
- May be characterized only by scalloped antral folds without definite visualization of erosions.
- Incomplete or flat erosions are seen as epithelial defects without surrounding mucosal elevation, appearing as linear streaks or dots of barium.
- NSAID-related erosions are sometimes seen as distinctive linear and serpiginous erosions clustered on or near greater curvature of stomach.
- Chronic NSAID ingestion may lead to relatively subtle flattening and deformity of the greater curvature of the distal antrum.
- Shallow ulcers may have iatrogenic causes such as endoscopic heater probe therapy.

Utility
- Double-contrast barium studies
- Erosions on the dependent or posterior wall may be better delineated by the use of flow technique.

CLINICAL PRESENTATION

- Patients may be asymptomatic or may present with dyspepsia, epigastric pain, or signs or symptoms of upper gastrointestinal bleeding.

DIFFERENTIAL DIAGNOSIS

- Centrally ulcerated submucosal masses (bull's-eye or target lesions)

PATHOLOGY

- Erosions are defined histologically as epithelial defects that do not penetrate beyond the muscularis mucosae.

DIAGNOSTIC PEARLS

- Punctate or slit-like barium collections representing epithelial defects surrounded by radiolucent mounds of edematous, elevated mucosa
- Linear streaks or dots of barium
- Distinctive linear and serpiginous erosions clustered on or near the greater curvature of the stomach are almost always caused by aspirin or other NSAIDs

- Aspirin and other NSAIDs are capable of disrupting the mucosal barrier in the stomach, causing erosive gastritis and gastric ulcers.
- Gastric erosions may form rapidly after ingestion of NSAIDs and may heal rapidly when these drugs are withdrawn.

INCIDENCE/PREVALENCE AND EPIDEMIOLOGY

- Erosive gastritis is a relatively frequent finding on double-contrast barium studies, with an overall prevalence of 0.5%-20% in the radiologic literature.
- Aspirin or other NSAIDs are thought to be the most common cause of erosive gastritis.
- Other causes include alcohol, stress, trauma, burns, Crohn disease, infection, and endoscopic heater probe therapy or other iatrogenic trauma.

Suggested Readings

Catalano D, Pagliari U: Gastroduodenal erosions: Radiological findings. *Gastrointest Radiol* 7:235-240, 1982.

Laveran-Stiebar RL, Laufer I, Levine MS: Greater curvature antral flattening: A radiologic sign of NSAID-related gastropathy. *Abdom Imaging* 19:295-297, 1994.

Levine MS, Verstandig A, Laufer I: Serpiginous gastric erosions caused by aspirin and other nonsteroidal anti-inflammatory drugs. *AJR Am J Roentgenol* 146:31-34, 1986.

McLean AM, Paul RE, Philipps E, et al: Chronic erosive gastritis—clinical and radiological features. *J Can Assoc Radiol* 33:158-162, 1982.

Rumerman J, Rubesin SE, Levine MS, et al: Gastric ulceration caused by heater probe coagulation. *Gastrointest Radiol* 13:200-202, 1988.

WHAT THE REFERRING PHYSICIAN NEEDS TO KNOW

- Not all patients with erosive gastritis are symptomatic.
- Clinical significance of gastric erosions demonstrated on radiologic or endoscopic examinations can be difficult to ascertain.
- Gastric erosions form rapidly after ingestion of aspirin or other NSAIDs and heal rapidly when these drugs are withdrawn.

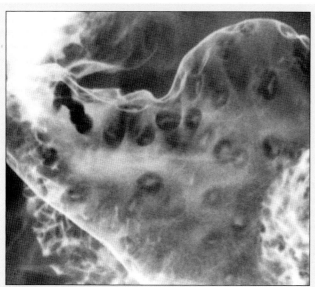

Figure 1. Erosive gastritis with varioliform erosions. Double-contrast barium study shows multiple varioliform erosions in the gastric antrum as tiny barium collections with surrounding halos of edematous mucosa. (*From Laufer I, Levine MS [eds]: Double-Contrast Gastrointestinal Radiology, 2nd ed. Philadelphia, WB Saunders, 1992.*)

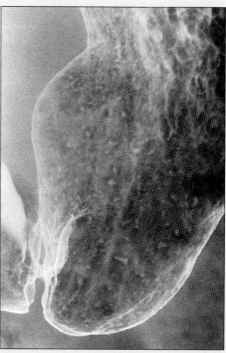

Figure 2. Erosive gastritis with incomplete erosions. Numerous linear and punctate erosions are seen in the gastric antrum and body. Many of the erosions are incomplete (i.e., they are not surrounded by mounds of edema).

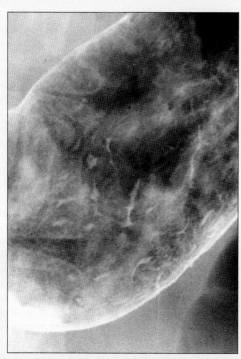

Figure 3. Erosive gastritis caused by a nonsteroidal anti-inflammatory drug (naproxen). Distinctive linear and serpiginous erosions are clustered in the body of the stomach near the greater curvature as a result of NSAID ingestion. The patient was taking naproxen. (*From Levine MS, Verstandig A, Laufer I: Serpiginous gastric erosions caused by aspirin and other nonsteroidal antiinflammatory drugs. AJR Am J Roentgenol 146:31-34, 1986, © by American Roentgen Ray Society.*)

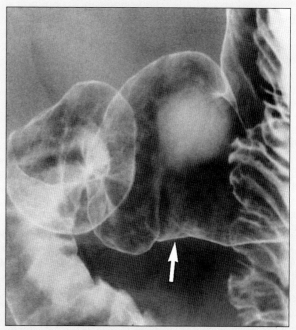

Figure 4. Antral flattening caused by NSAIDs. Note the flattening and deformity of the greater curvature of the distal antrum (*arrow*) caused by chronic aspirin therapy. This finding is characteristic of NSAID-related gastropathy.

Antral Gastritis

DEFINITION: Form of gastritis confined to gastric antrum.

ANATOMIC FINDINGS

Antrum of the Stomach
- Antral erosions
- Thickened, scalloped, or lobulated folds that are oriented longitudinally in the antrum
- Thickened transverse antral folds
- Crenulation or irregularity of lesser curvature of the distal antrum
- Single lobulated fold that arises on the lesser curvature of prepyloric antrum and extends into the pylorus or base of the duodenal bulb
- Fine transverse antral striations or striae, although this finding can also be seen as a normal variant

IMAGING

Radiography
Findings
- Thickened folds
- Antral erosions
- Crenulation of lesser curvature
- Mucosal nodularity, transverse antral striae
- Hypertrophied antral-pyloric fold
- Antral narrowing
Utility
- Thickened antral folds are the single most common sign of antral gastritis on double-contrast barium studies.

CLINICAL PRESENTATION

- Affected individuals may have dyspepsia, epigastric pain, or other symptoms indistinguishable from those of peptic ulcer disease.

DIFFERENTIAL DIAGNOSIS

- Gastric carcinoma
- Lymphoma (stomach)

DIAGNOSTIC PEARLS

- Thickened antral folds
- Crenulation or irregularity of the lesser curvature
- Mucosal nodularity and transverse antral striae
- Hypertrophied antral-pyloric fold

- Peptic ulcer disease
- Submucosally infiltrating carcinoma

PATHOLOGY

- Alcohol, tobacco, coffee, and *Helicobacter pylori* have been implicated in the development of antral gastritis.
- Form of gastritis that is confined to the gastric antrum
- Hypertrophied antral-pyloric fold is thought to develop as a sequela of chronic antral gastritis, often associated with other radiographic signs of gastritis.

Suggested Readings

Arora R, Levine MS, Harvey RT, et al: Hypertrophied antral-pyloric fold: Reassessment of radiographic findings in 40 patients. *Radiology* 213:347-351, 1999.
Cho KC, Gold BM, Printz DA: Multiple transverse folds in the gastric antrum. *Radiology* 64:339-341, 1987.
Dheer S, Levine MS, Redfern RO, et al: Radiographically diagnosed antral gastritis: Findings in patients with and without *Helicobacter pylori* infection. *Br J Radiol* 75:805-811, 2002.
Glick SN, Cavanaugh B, Teplick SK: The hypertrophied antral-pyloric fold. *AJR Am J Roentgenol* 145:547-549, 1985.
Lewis TD, Laufer I, Goodacre RL: Arteriovenous malformation of the stomach: Radiologic and endoscopic features. *Am J Dig Dis* 23:467-470, 1978.
Seymour EQ, Meredith HC: Antral and esophageal rimple: A normal variation. *Gastrointest Radiol* 3:147-149, 1978.
Turner CJ, Lipitz LR, Pastore RA: Antral gastritis. *Radiology* 113:305-312, 1974.

WHAT THE REFERRING PHYSICIAN NEEDS TO KNOW
- Affected individuals may exhibit dyspepsia, epigastric pain, or other symptoms indistinguishable from those of peptic ulcer disease.
- Alcohol, tobacco, coffee, and *Helicobacter pylori* have been implicated in the development of antral gastritis.
- Thickened antral folds are the single most common sign of antral gastritis on double-contrast barium studies.
- Treatment is generally aimed at suppressing acid production in the stomach.

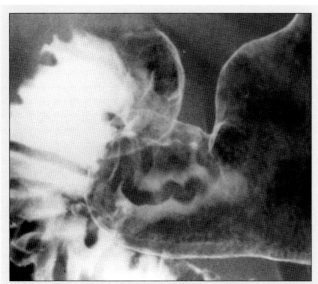

Figure 1. Antral gastritis. This patient has thickened, scalloped folds that are oriented longitudinally in the antrum.

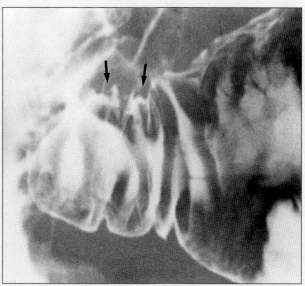

Figure 2. Antral gastritis. In this patient, note thickened transverse folds in the antrum with fine nodularity and crenulation of the adjacent lesser curvature *(arrows)*.

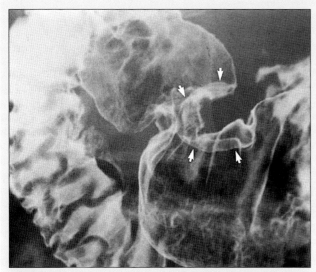

Figure 3. Antral gastritis with a hypertrophied antral-pyloric fold. A single lobulated fold *(arrows)* on the lesser curvature of the distal antrum extends through the pylorus into the base of the duodenal bulb. The characteristic appearance and location of this fold should differentiate it from a polypoid or plaque-like antral carcinoma.

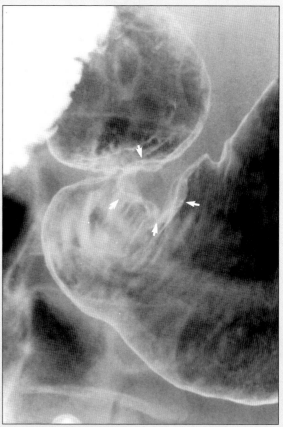

Figure 4. Antral gastritis with a hypertrophied antral-pyloric fold. A single lobulated fold *(arrows)* on the lesser curvature of the distal antrum extends through the pylorus into the base of the duodenal bulb. The characteristic appearance and location of this fold should differentiate it from a polypoid or plaque-like antral carcinoma.

Helicobacter pylori Gastritis

DEFINITION: Chronic active gastritis caused by *Helicobacter pylori* characterized by inflammation of the gastric mucosa.

IMAGING

Radiography
Findings
- Focally or diffusely thickened folds in gastric antrum, body, or fundus are often seen on barium studies.
- Some patients have a *polypoid* form of gastritis characterized by focally or diffusely thickened folds that are unusually large and lobulated, resembling the findings of hypertrophic gastritis, Ménétrier disease, or even gastric lymphoma.
- Enlarged areae gastricae (>3 mm in diameter) are seen in some patients.
- Enlarged lymphoid follicles are seen as innumerable tiny, round, frequently umbilicated nodules carpeting the mucosa of the gastric antrum or antrum and body.

Utility
- Double-contrast barium studies

CT
Finding
- Circumferential thickening of antrum or focal thickening of posterior gastric wall

CLINICAL PRESENTATION

- Most people with *H. pylori* are asymptomatic.
- Dyspepsia may be present.
- Epigastric pain may be present.

DIFFERENTIAL DIAGNOSIS

- Hypertrophic gastritis
- Ménétrier disease (stomach)
- Lymphoma
- Zollinger-Ellison syndrome (stomach)
- Portal hypertensive gastropathy (stomach)
- Low-grade gastric mucosa-associated lymphoid tissue (MALT) lymphoma

DIAGNOSTIC PEARLS

- *H.pylori* gastritis is the most common cause of diffuse or focal thickening of folds in the gastric antrum or body on double-contrast barium studies.
- Lymphoid hyperplasia is a potential marker for *H. pylori* gastritis even in the absence of other findings.
- In contrast to MALT lymphoma, the nodules of gastric lymphoid hyperplasia have more discrete borders, more uniform size, and frequent central umbilications.

PATHOLOGY

- *H. pylori* (formerly known as *Campylobacter pylori*) is a gram-negative bacillus and is the most common cause of chronic active gastritis.
- Clusters or clumps of the organism are found beneath the mucus layer on the surface epithelial cells or superficial foveolar cells in the stomach.
- *H. pylori* causes acute inflammatory reaction in the mucosa, with accumulation of neutrophils, plasma cells, and, eventually, lymphoid nodules.
- Gastric antrum is most common site of involvement, but proximal one half of the stomach or even the entire stomach may be involved.
- *H. pylori* is acquired by oral ingestion of bacterium and is mainly transmitted within families during early childhood.

INCIDENCE/PREVALENCE AND EPIDEMIOLOGY

- *H. pylori* is the most common cause of chronic active gastritis.
- *H. pylori* is a worldwide pathogen, being most common in developing countries.

WHAT THE REFERRING PHYSICIAN NEEDS TO KNOW

- *H. pylori* is associated with the development of gastric and duodenal ulcers, gastric carcinoma, and low-grade B-cell MALT lymphoma.
- The organism can be effectively eradicated from the stomach by treatment with a combination of antimicrobial agents and antisecretory agents.
- *H. pylori* can be accurately diagnosed at endoscopy based on histologic specimens, cultures, and rapid urease test.
- Highly accurate noninvasive tests such as a urea breath test and serologic tests also are widely available for detecting this infection.

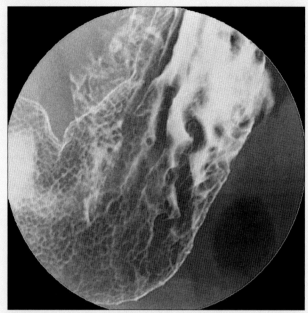

Figure 1. *H. pylori* **gastritis.** Thickened folds are seen in the body of the stomach and enlarged areae gastricae in the proximal antrum as a result of chronic infection by *H. pylori*. (*From Levine MS, Laufer I: The gastrointestinal tract: Dos and don'ts of digital imaging.* Radiology *207:311-316, 1998.*)

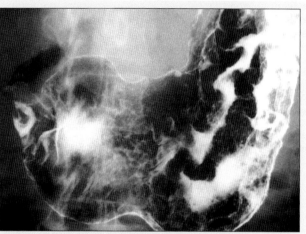

Figure 2. *H. pylori* **causing diffuse polypoid gastritis.** Markedly thickened, lobulated folds are seen in the gastric body. This appearance can be mistaken for severe hypertrophic gastritis, Ménétrier's disease, or lymphoma, but endoscopic biopsy specimens revealed *H. pylori* gastritis without evidence of tumor. (*From Sohn J, Levine MS, Furth EE, et al:* Helicobacter pylori *gastritis: Radiographic findings.* Radiology *195:763-767, 1995.*)

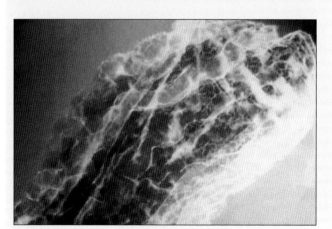

Figure 3. *H. pylori* **causing diffuse polypoid gastritis.** Markedly thickened, lobulated folds are seen in the gastric fundus. This appearance can be mistaken for severe hypertrophic gastritis, Ménétrier's disease, or lymphoma, but endoscopic biopsy specimens revealed *H. pylori* gastritis without evidence of tumor. (*From Sohn J, Levine MS, Furth EE, et al:* Helicobacter pylori *gastritis: Radiographic findings.* Radiology *195:763-767, 1995.*)

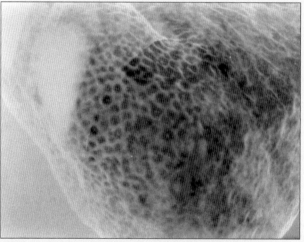

Figure 4. *H. pylori* **gastritis with lymphoid hyperplasia.** Enlarged lymphoid follicles are seen as innumerable tiny, round nodules that carpet the mucosa of the gastric antrum. Note how many of the nodules have central umbilications with punctate collections of barium seen en face in the lesions. (*From Torigian DA, Levine MS, Gill NS, et al: Lymphoid hyperplasia of the stomach: radiographic findings in five adult patients.* AJR Am J Roentgenol *177:71-75, 2001, © by American Roentgen Ray Society.*)

- In developed countries, *H. pylori* is more common in lower socioeconomic populations.
- Prevalence of *H. pylori* increases with age; more than 50% of Americans older than 60 years of age are infected.

Suggested Readings

Appelman HD: Gastritis: Terminology, etiology, and clinicopathological correlations: Another biased view. *Hum Pathol* 25:1006-1019, 1994.

Blum AL, Talley NJ, O'Morain C, et al: Lack of effect of treating *Helicobacter pylori* infection in patients with nonulcer dyspepsia. *N Engl J Med* 339:1875-1881, 1998.

Crocker JD, Bender GN: Antral nodularity, fold thickness, and narrowing: Signs on the upper gastrointestinal series that may indicate chronic active gastritis secondary to *Helicobacter pylori*. *Invest Radiol* 30:480-483, 1995.

Cutler AF, Havstad S, Ma CK, et al: Accuracy of invasive and noninvasive tests to diagnose *Helicobacter pylori* infection. *Gastroenterology* 109:136-141, 1995.

Dheer S, Levine MS, Redfern RO, et al: Radiographically diagnosed antral gastritis: Findings in patients with and without *Helicobacter pylori* infection. *Br J Radiol* 75:805-811, 2002.

Hopkins RJ: Current FDA-approved treatments for *Helicobacter pylori* and the FDA approval process. *Gastroenterology* 113:S126-S130, 1997.

International Update Conference on *Helicobacter pylori*: The Report of the Digestive Health Initiative International Update Conference on *Helicobacter pylori*. *Gastroenterology* 113:S4-S8, 1997.

Kuipers EJ, Uyterlinde AM, Pena AS, et al: Long-term sequelae of *Helicobacter pylori* gastritis. *Lancet* 345:1525-1528, 1995.

McColl K, Murray L, El-Omar E, et al: Symptomatic benefit from eradicating *Helicobacter pylori* infection in patients with nonulcer dyspepsia. *N Engl J Med* 339:1869-1874, 1998.

Mond DJ, Pochaczevsky R, Vernace F, et al: Can the radiologist recognize *Helicobacter pylori* gastritis? *J Clin Gastroenterol* 20:199-202, 1995.

Pattison CP, Combs MJ, Marshall BJ: *Helicobacter pylori* and peptic ulcer disease: Evolution to revolution to resolution. *AJR Am J Roentgenol* 168:1420-1450, 1997.

Rubesin SE, Furth EE, Levine MS: Gastritis from NSAIDs to *Helicobacter pylori*. *Abdom Imaging* 30:142-159, 2005.

Sohn J, Levine MS, Furth EE, et al: *Helicobacter pylori* gastritis: Radiographic findings. *Radiology* 195:763-767, 1995.

Suerbaum S, Michetti P: *Helicobacter pylori* infection. *N Engl J Med* 347:1175-1186, 2002.

Talley NJ, Vakil N, Ballard ED, et al: Absence of benefit of eradicating *Helicobacter pylori* in patients with nonulcer dyspepsia. *N Engl J Med* 341:1106-1111, 1999.

Thijs JC, van Zwet AA, Thijs WJ, et al: Diagnostic tests for *Helicobacter pylori*: A prospective evaluation of their accuracy, without selecting a single test as the gold standard. *Am J Gastroenterol* 91:2125-2129, 1996.

Torigian DA, Levine MS, Gill NS, et al: Lymphoid hyperplasia of the stomach: Radiographic findings in five adult patients. *AJR Am J Roentgenol* 177:71-75, 2001.

Urban BA, Fishman EK, Hruban RH: *Helicobacter pylori* gastritis mimicking gastric carcinoma at CT evaluation. *Radiology* 179:689-691, 1991.

Wyatt JI, Rathbone BJ: Immune response of the gastric mucosa to *Campylobacter pylori*. *Scand J Gastroenterol Suppl* 142:44-49, 1988.

Yoo CC, Levine MS, Furth EE, et al: Gastric mucosa-associated lymphoid tissue lymphoma: Radiographic findings in six patients. *Radiology* 208:239-243, 1998.

Hypertrophic Gastritis

DEFINITION: Gastropathy of uncertain pathogenesis characterized by marked glandular hyperplasia and increased secretion of acid.

IMAGING

Radiography
Findings
- Markedly thickened, lobulated folds, predominantly in the gastric fundus and body

Utility
- Barium studies

CLINICAL PRESENTATION

- Epigastric pain
- Nausea
- Vomiting
- Less frequently, signs or symptoms of upper gastrointestinal bleeding

DIFFERENTIAL DIAGNOSIS

- *Helicobacter pylori* gastritis
- Ménétrier disease (stomach)
- Lymphoma (stomach)
- Zollinger-Ellison syndrome (stomach)
- Eosinophilic gastritis
- Varices (stomach)

PATHOLOGY

- Hypertrophic hypersecretory gastropathy
- Condition is characterized by marked glandular hyperplasia and increased secretion of acid in the stomach.

DIAGNOSTIC PEARLS

- Characterized by marked glandular hyperplasia and increased secretion of acid in the stomach
- Markedly thickened, lobulated folds, predominantly in the gastric fundus and body as seen on barium studies

- Gastric folds may also be thickened because of edema and inflammation.
- Glandular hyperplasia may be caused by pituitary, hypothalamic, or vagal stimuli.

INCIDENCE/PREVALENCE AND EPIDEMIOLOGY

- Many cases of previously diagnosed hypertrophic gastritis have probably resulted from infection by *H. pylori*.

Suggested Readings

Balthazar EJ, Davidian MM: Hyperrugosity in gastric carcinoma: Radiographic, endoscopic, and pathologic features. *AJR Am J Roentgenol* 136:531-535, 1981.
Moghadam M, Gluckmann R, Eyler WR: The radiological assessment of gastric acid output. *Radiology* 89:888-895, 1967.
Press AJ: Practical significance of gastric rugal folds. *Am J Roentgenol Radium Ther Nucl Med* 125:172-183, 1975.
Stempien SJ, Dagradi AE, Reingold IM, et al: Hypertrophic hypersecretory gastropathy. *Am J Dig Dis* 9:471-493, 1964.
Tan DTD, Stempien SJ, Dagradi AE: The clinical spectrum of hypertrophic hypersecretory gastropathy. *Gastrointest Endosc* 18:69-73, 1971.

WHAT THE REFERRING PHYSICIAN NEEDS TO KNOW

- Treatment with antisecretory agents is usually recommended to suppress acid secretion in the stomach.
- *H. pylori* gastritis can be differentiated from hypertrophic gastritis by the urea breath test and serologic tests.
- Ménétrier disease should be suspected in patients who have normal or decreased acid secretion and protein-losing enteropathy.
- Lymphoma should be suspected when associated findings such as ulcers, masses, or bull's-eye lesions are present in the stomach.
- If radiographic findings are equivocal, endoscopy and biopsy may be required to rule out malignant tumor.

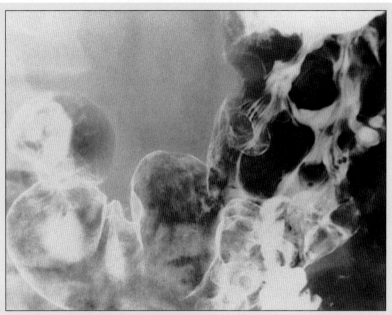

Figure 1. Hypertrophic gastritis. Thickened, lobulated folds are seen in the body of the stomach. The antrum appears normal. (*From Laufer I, Levine MS [eds]:* Double-Contrast Gastrointestinal Radiology, *2nd ed. Philadelphia, WB Saunders, 1992.*)

Ménétrier Disease

DEFINITION: Rare condition of unknown cause characterized by marked foveolar hyperplasia in the stomach, enlarged gastric rugae, hypochlorhydria, and hypoproteinemia.

IMAGING

Radiography
Findings
- Grossly thickened, lobulated folds in the fundus and body of the stomach with relative sparing of the antrum

Utility
- Barium studies
- Excessive mucus in stomach may dilute barium and compromise mucosal coating.

CT
Finding
- Markedly thickened gastric wall, with mass-like elevations representing giant, heaped-up folds protruding into the lumen

CLINICAL PRESENTATION

- Patients present with epigastric pain, nausea, vomiting, diarrhea, anorexia, weight loss, or peripheral edema.
- Most patients have a prolonged illness with intractable symptoms.

DIFFERENTIAL DIAGNOSIS

- *Helicobacter pylori* gastritis
- Lymphoma (stomach)
- Gastric carcinoma
- Zollinger-Ellison syndrome (stomach)
- Eosinophilic gastritis
- Hypertrophic gastritis
- Varices (stomach)

PATHOLOGY

- This rare condition of unknown cause is characterized by marked foveolar hyperplasia in the stomach, enlarged gastric rugae, hypochlorhydria, and hypoproteinemia.

DIAGNOSTIC PEARLS

- Classically manifested on barium studies by grossly thickened, lobulated folds in the gastric fundus and body with relative sparing of the antrum
- Diffuse thickening of the gastric folds in no way precludes the diagnosis.
- Stomach usually remains pliant and distensible.

- Mucosal thickening and hyperplasia occur as a result of cystic dilation and elongation of the gastric mucous glands associated with deepening of the foveolar pits.
- Gastric acid output is decreased or absent in approximately 75% of cases.
- Some patients have protein-losing enteropathy resulting from loss of protein from hyperplastic mucosa into the gastric lumen.
- Others have varying degrees of gastritis in either a patchy or diffuse distribution.

INCIDENCE/PREVALENCE AND EPIDEMIOLOGY

- Tends to occur in older patients
- More common in men than in women

Suggested Readings
Cutler AF, Havstad S, Ma CK, et al: Accuracy of invasive and noninvasive tests to diagnose *Helicobacter pylori* infection. *Gastroenterology* 109:136-141, 1995.

Fieber SS, Rickert RR: Hyperplastic gastropathy. *Am J Gastroenterol* 76:321-329, 1981.

Jarnum S, Jensen KB: Plasma protein turnover (albumin, transferrin, IgG, IgM) in Ménétrier's disease (giant hypertrophic gastritis): Evidence of non-selective protein loss. *Gut* 13:128-137, 1972.

Olmsted WW, Cooper PH, Madewell JE: Involvement of the gastric antrum in Ménétrier's disease. *AJR Am J Roentgenol* 126:524-529, 1976.

Reese DF, Hodgson JR, Dockerty MB: Giant hypertrophy of the gastric mucosa (Ménétrier's disease): A correlation of the roentgenographic, pathologic, and clinical findings. *Am J Roentgenol Radium Ther Nucl Med* 88:619-626, 1962.

WHAT THE REFERRING PHYSICIAN NEEDS TO KNOW

- Laboratory studies may reveal hypoalbuminemia resulting from protein-losing enteropathy or hypochlorhydria resulting from decreased acid secretion, or both.
- Rarely, development of gastric carcinoma has been described in patients with preexisting Ménétrier disease.
- Some patients have spontaneous remission of symptoms, and others respond to treatment with antisecretory agents, vagotomy, or antibiotics.
- Total gastrectomy may be required for patients who are unresponsive to medical therapy.
- When Ménétrier disease is suspected on barium studies or CT, full-thickness endoscopic biopsy specimens should be obtained for a definitive diagnosis.

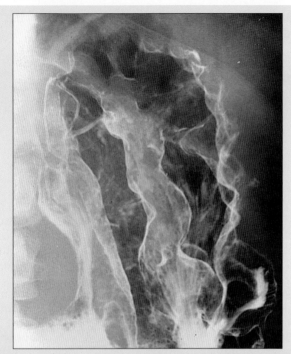

Figure 1. Ménétrier disease. Grossly thickened folds are present in the gastric fundus on a barium study. (*From Laufer I, Levine MS [eds]:* Double contrast gastrointestinal radiology, *ed 2, Philadelphia, 1992, WB Saunders.*)

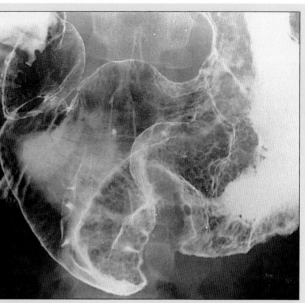

Figure 2. Ménétrier disease. In this patient, mass-like protrusions of the folds are seen on the greater curvature of the gastric body on a barium study. This appearance can be mistaken for a polypoid gastric carcinoma. The distal antrum is relatively spared.

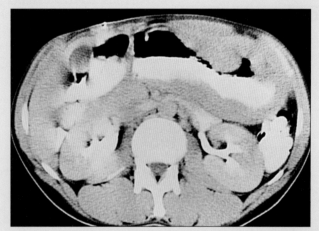

Figure 3. Ménétrier disease. In the patient shown in Fig. 2, a CT scan shows massive thickening of the gastric wall with mass-like protrusions into the lumen. Endoscopic biopsy specimens in this patient revealed typical pathologic findings of Ménétrier disease without evidence of tumor.

Rubin RG, Fink H: Giant hypertrophy of the gastric mucosa associated with carcinoma of the stomach. *Am J Gastroenterol* 47:379-388, 1967.

Scharschmidt BF: The natural history of hypertrophic gastropathy (Ménétrier's disease). *Am J Med* 63:644-652, 1977.

Searcy RM, Malagelada JR: Ménétrier's disease and idiopathic hypertrophic gastropathy. *Ann Intern Med* 100:560-565, 1984.

Williams SM, Harned RK, Settles RH: Adenocarcinoma of the stomach in association with Ménétrier's disease. *Gastrointest Radiol* 3: 387-390, 1978.

Wolfsen HC, Carpenter HA, Talley NJ: Ménétrier's disease: A form of hypertrophic gastropathy or gastritis? *Gastroenterology* 104: 1310-1319, 1993.

Atrophic Gastritis

DEFINITION: Characterized by atrophy of mucosal glands, loss of parietal and chief cells, thinning of mucosa, and, eventually, intestinal metaplasia.

ANATOMIC FINDINGS

Stomach
- Narrowed and tubular
- Decreased mucosal folds
- Atrophy of mucosal glands, loss of parietal and chief cells, thinning of mucosa, and, eventually, intestinal metaplasia

Areae Gastricae
- Areae gastricae may be small or absent.
- If focally enlarged, the possibility of intestinal metaplasia or even a superficial spreading carcinoma should be considered.

IMAGING

Radiography
Findings
- Narrowed, tubular stomach with decreased or absent mucosal folds and small or absent areae gastricae predominantly in the body and fundus
- Focal enlargement of areae gastricae should raise possibility of intestinal metaplasia or superficial spreading carcinoma.
Utility
- Confirmed by endoscopic biopsy

CLINICAL PRESENTATION

- Symptoms are rare.
- When associated with pernicious anemia, the condition may produce symptoms of long-standing vitamin-B_{12} deficiency.

DIFFERENTIAL DIAGNOSIS

- Peptic ulcer disease
- Scirrhous carcinoma of the stomach

DIAGNOSTIC PEARLS

- Narrowed, tubular stomach
- Decreased or absent mucosal folds, predominantly in the body and fundus
- Small or absent areae gastricae

PATHOLOGY

- Pathogenesis is unclear.
- Characterized pathologically by mucosal gland atrophy, loss of parietal and chief cells, thinning of mucosa, and, eventually, intestinal metaplasia
- Classified into types A and B atrophic gastritis, which have different histologic, immunologic, and secretory characteristics
- Type A atrophic gastritis is confined to the gastric fundus and body, with antral sparing.
- This type of gastritis is thought to result from immunologic injury and is usually associated with pernicious anemia.
- Type B atrophic gastritis involves the gastric antrum and is caused by mucosal injury from *Helicobacter pylori*, bile acids, or alcohol.

INCIDENCE/PREVALENCE AND EPIDEMIOLOGY

- More than 90% of patients with pernicious anemia have atrophic gastritis.
- Pernicious anemia is a disease of elderly adults, accounting for 50 out of 100,000 admissions in United States.
- Type B atrophic gastritis is more common than type A.

Suggested Readings

Asaka M, Takeda H, Sugiyama T, et al: What role does *Helicobacter pylori* play in gastric cancer? *Gastroenterology* 113:S56-S60, 1997.
Borch K: Epidemiologic, clinicopathologic, and economic aspects of gastroscopic screening of patients with pernicious anemia. *Scand J Gastroenterol* 21:21-30, 1986.

WHAT THE REFERRING PHYSICIAN NEEDS TO KNOW

- Ninety percent of patients with pernicious anemia have atrophic gastritis.
- Gastric lesions in pernicious anemia may antedate other abnormalities.
- Early diagnosis of atrophic gastritis may allow early treatment of pernicious anemia.
- Patients with atrophic gastritis and pernicious anemia have increased risk of developing gastric carcinoma.
- Patients with *H. pylori*-associated atrophic gastritis also have an increased risk of developing gastric carcinoma.

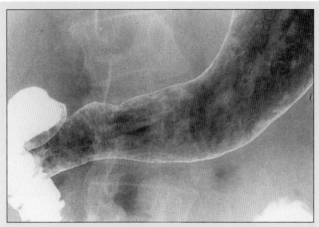

Figure 1. Atrophic gastritis. The stomach has a tubular configuration with decreased distensibility, a paucity of mucosal folds, and absence of discernible areae gastricae. These findings are characteristic of atrophic gastritis.

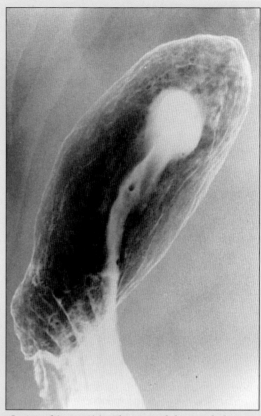

Figure 2. Atrophic gastritis. The stomach has a tubular configuration with decreased distensibility, a paucity of mucosal folds, and absence of discernible areae gastricae. These findings are characteristic of atrophic gastritis.

Cheli R, Santi L, Ciancamerla G, et al: A clinical and statistical follow-up study of atrophic gastritis. *Am J Dig Dis* 18:1061-1066, 1973.

Elsborg L, Mosbech J: Pernicious anaemia as a risk factor in gastric cancer. *Acta Med Scand* 206:315-318, 1979.

Furth EE, Rubesin SE, Levine MS: Pathologic primer on gastritis: An illustrated sum and substance. *Radiology* 197:693-698, 1995.

Jeffries GH, Sleisenger MH: Studies of parietal cell antibody in pernicious anemia. *J Clin Invest* 44:2021-2038, 1965.

Joske RA, Finckh ES, Wood IJ: Gastric biopsy: A study of 1,000 consecutive successful gastric biopsies. *Q J Med* 24:269-294, 1955.

Kuipers EJ, Klinkenberg-Knol EC, Vandenbroucke-Grauls JE, et al: Role of *Helicobacter pylori* in the pathogenesis of atrophic gastritis. *Scand J Gastroenterol Suppl* 223:28-34, 1997.

Laws JW, Pitman RG: The radiological features of pernicious anaemia. *Br J Radiol* 33:229-237, 1960.

Levine MS, Kong V, Rubesin SE, et al: Scirrhous carcinoma of the stomach: Radiologic and endoscopic diagnosis. *Radiology* 175:151-154, 1990.

Levine MS, Palman CL, Rubesin SE, et al: Atrophic gastritis in pernicious anemia: Diagnosis by double-contrast radiography. *Gastrointest Radiol* 14:215-219, 1989.

Mackintosh CE, Kreel L: Anatomy and radiology of the areae gastricae. *Gut* 18:855-864, 1977.

Maxfield DL, Boyd WC: Pernicious anemia: A review, an update, and an illustrative case. *J Am Osteopath Assoc* 2:133-142, 1983.

Siurala M, Lehtola J, Ihamaki T: Atrophic gastritis and its sequelae: Results of 19-23 years' follow-up examinations. *Scand J Gastroenterol* 9:441-446, 1974.

Sozzi M, Valentini M, Figura N, et al: Atrophic gastritis and intestinal metaplasia in *Helicobacter pylori* infection: The role of CagA status. *Am J Gastroenterol* 93:375-379, 1998.

Strickland RG, Mackay IR: A reappraisal of the nature and significance of chronic atrophic gastritis. *Am J Dig Dis* 18:426-440, 1973.

Granulomatous Conditions (Stomach and Duodenum)

DEFINITION: Diseases of the stomach and duodenum causing an inflammatory process resulting in the formation of granulomatous lesions.

ANATOMIC FINDINGS

Stomach
- Aphthoid ulcers
- Thickened, nodular folds
- Antral narrowing
- Filiform polyps

Duodenum
- Stricture formation
- Narrowing of lumen
- Ballooning or sacculation of wall between areas of fibrosis
- Megaduodenum in Crohn disease

IMAGING

Radiography
Crohn's Disease: Findings
- Aphthoid ulcers: punctate or slit-like collections of barium surrounded by radiolucent mounds of edema
- Ulcers and thickened, nodular folds
- Nodular or cobblestone mucosa in the gastric antrum or body
- *Ram's horn sign* of gastric Crohn disease
- Pseudo-Billroth I sign of gastroduodenal Crohn disease
- Filiform polyps, strictures, megaduodenum, and fistulas in Crohn disease
Other Granulomatous Diseases: Findings
- Syphilis: thick, irregular folds, ulcers, and narrowing
- Sarcoidosis: thick, irregular folds, ulcers, and narrowing
- Tuberculosis: ulcers and narrowing
Crohn Disease: Utility
- Barium studies
- Small-bowel follow-through or barium enema should be performed to determine presence of concomitant ileocolic disease when gastric involvement is suspected.

DIAGNOSTIC PEARLS
- *Ram's horn sign* of Crohn disease
- Pseudo-Billroth I sign of Crohn disease
- Megaduodenum of Crohn disease

CLINICAL PRESENTATION
- Often asymptomatic
- Nausea
- Vomiting
- Epigastric pain
- Weight loss
- Diarrhea
- Signs or symptoms of upper gastrointestinal bleeding

PATHOLOGY
- Inflammatory process results in the formation of granulomatous lesions that may lead to obstruction.
- Most patients with gastroduodenal Crohn disease have concomitant ileocolic disease.
- Sarcoidosis is a systemic granulomatous disease of unknown origin characterized pathologically by the presence of noncaseating granulomas.
- Most patients with gastric or duodenal tuberculosis are found to have generalized tuberculosis.
- Gastric syphilis confirmed by isolating *Treponema pallidum* on endoscopic biopsy specimens or by demonstrating typical spirochetes on darkfield microscopy.
- A variety of fungal diseases may rarely involve the stomach, including candidiasis, histoplasmosis, actinomycosis, and mucormycosis.

WHAT THE REFERRING PHYSICIAN NEEDS TO KNOW
- A surgical bypass procedure such as gastrojejunostomy or duodenojejunostomy may be required to alleviate the symptoms of gastric outlet obstruction.
- Endoscopic biopsy specimens are required for a definitive diagnosis.
- In patients with advanced Crohn disease, sulfasalazine or corticosteroids may effectively relieve epigastric pain or other upper gastrointestinal complaints.
- Possibility of gastric sarcoidosis should be suspected when chest radiographs reveal characteristic findings of sarcoidosis in the thorax.
- Individuals with syphilis usually have marked clinical response to antiluetic therapy if they are treated before substantial gastric scarring has occurred.
- When gastric involvement by Crohn disease is suggested on upper gastrointestinal studies, a small-bowel follow-through or barium enema should be performed.

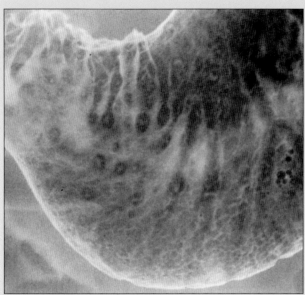

Figure 1. Early gastric Crohn disease with aphthoid ulcers. These lesions are indistinguishable from varioliform erosions in the stomach. This patient had typical findings of Crohn disease in the terminal ileum. (*Courtesy of Robert A. Goren, MD, Philadelphia, PA.*)

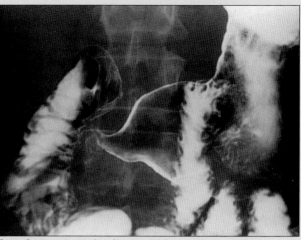

Figure 2. Gastric Crohn disease with antral narrowing. Smooth, funnel-shaped narrowing of the antrum is seen, resulting in the classic *ram's horn sign* of gastric Crohn disease. (*From Levine MS: Crohn's disease of the upper gastrointestinal tract.* Radiol Clin North Am *25:79-91, 1987.*)

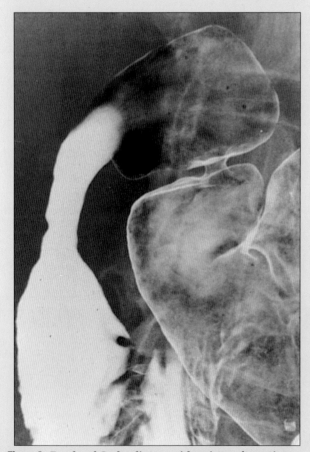

Figure 3. Duodenal Crohn disease with stricture formation. Smooth, tapered narrowing of the apical portion of the bulb and adjacent segment of the descending duodenum is seen. This appearance is characteristic of Crohn disease.

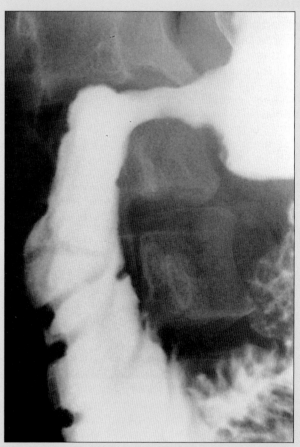

Figure 4. Gastroduodenal Crohn disease. Contiguous narrowing of the antrum and duodenum is seen, with obliteration of the normal anatomic landmarks at the pylorus. Because the antrum and duodenum merge together as a single tubular structure, this finding has been described as the pseudo-Billroth I sign of gastroduodenal Crohn disease. (*From Levine MS: Crohn's disease of the upper gastrointestinal tract.* Radiol Clin North Am *25:79-91, 1987.*)

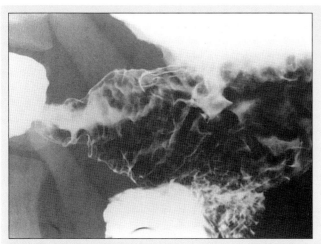

Figure 5. Gastric syphilis. Mucosal nodularity and thickened folds are seen in the antrum in this patient with proven gastric syphilis.

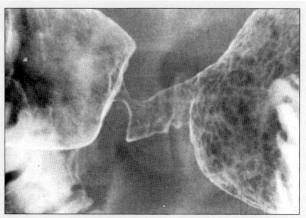

Figure 6. Gastric sarcoidosis. In this patient, more advanced gastric sarcoidosis is exhibited by marked antral narrowing and deformity. (*Courtesy of Seth N. Glick, MD, Philadelphia, PA.*)

INCIDENCE/PREVALENCE AND EPIDEMIOLOGY

- Signs of upper gastrointestinal involvement may be detected in more than 20% of patients with ileocolic Crohn disease.
- Noncaseating granulomas have been found in the stomach on mucosal biopsy specimens in 10% of patients with known sarcoidosis.
- Gastroduodenal involvement occurs in less than 0.5% of all patients with tuberculosis.
- Gastric and duodenal tuberculosis has been encountered with increased frequency in patients with acquired immunodeficiency syndrome, particularly those of Haitian origin.
- Gastric syphilis is a rare disease, occurring in less than 1% of all patients with secondary or tertiary syphilis.

Suggested Readings

Anai H, Okada Y, Okubo K, et al: Gastric syphilis simulating linitis plastica type of gastric cancer. *Gastrointest Endosc* 36:624-626, 1990.

Bellan L, Semelka R, Warren CPW: Sarcoidosis as a cause of linitis plastica. *Can Assoc Radiol J* 39:72-74, 1988.

Brody JM, Miller DK, Zeman RK, et al: Gastric tuberculosis: A manifestation of acquired immunodeficiency syndrome. *Radiology* 159:342-348, 1986.

Chinitz MA, Brandt LJ, Frank MS, et al: Symptomatic sarcoidosis of the stomach. *Dig Dis Sci* 30:682-688, 1985.

Cronan J, Burrell M, Trepeta R: Aphthoid ulcerations in gastric candidiasis. *Radiology* 134:607-611, 1980.

Farman J, Ramirez G, Rybak B, et al: Gastric sarcoidosis. *Abdom Imaging* 22:248-252, 1997.

Gray RR, Grosman H: Crohn's disease involving the proximal stomach. *Gastrointest Radiol* 10:43-45, 1985.

Gupta SK, Jain AK, Gupta JP, et al: Duodenal tuberculosis. *Clin Radiol* 39:159-161, 1988.

Jones BV, Lichtenstein JE: Gastric syphilis: Radiologic findings. *AJR Am J Roentgenol* 160:59-61, 1993.

Kelvin FM, Gedgaudas RK: Radiologic diagnosis of Crohn's disease (with emphasis on its early manifestations). *Crit Rev Diagn Imaging* 16:43-91, 1981.

Levine MS: Crohn's disease of the upper gastrointestinal tract. *Radiol Clin North Am* 25:79-91, 1987.

Levine MS, Ekberg O, Rubesin SE, et al: Gastrointestinal sarcoidosis: Radiographic findings. *AJR Am J Roentgenol* 153:293-295, 1989.

Misra D, Rai RR, Nundy S, et al: Duodenal tuberculosis presenting as bleeding peptic ulcer. *Am J Gastroenterol* 83:203-204, 1988.

Nair KV, Pai CG, Rajogopal KP, et al: Unusual presentations of duodenal tuberculosis. *Am J Gastroenterol* 86:756-760, 1991.

Patel M, Banerjee B, Block JG, et al: Gastric Crohn's disease complicated by adenocarcinoma of the stomach: Case report and review of the literature. *Am J Gastroenterol* 92:1368-1371, 1997.

Subei I, Attar B, Schmitt G, et al: Primary gastric tuberculosis. *Am J Gastroenterol* 82:769-772, 1987.

Thoeni RF, Margulis AR: Gastrointestinal tuberculosis. *Semin Roentgenol* 14:283-294, 1979.

Van Olmen G, Larmuseau MF, Geboes K, et al: Primary gastric actinomycosis. *Am J Gastroenterol* 79:512-516, 1984.

Wagtmans MJ, Verspaget HW, Lamers CB, et al: Clinical aspects of Crohn's disease of the upper gastrointestinal tract: A comparison with distal Crohn's disease. *Am J Gastroenterol* 92:1467-1470, 1997.

Other Infectious Gastritides

DEFINITION: Opportunistic infections caused by viral or protozoan agents in immunocompromised patients, producing an inflammatory reaction in the stomach and duodenum.

IMAGING

Radiography
Findings
- Cytomegalovirus (CMV) gastritis: mucosal nodularity, erosions, ulcers, thickened folds, and, in severe cases, irregular antral narrowing
- CMV duodenitis: luminal narrowing with thickened or effaced folds in proximal duodenum
- Cryptosporidiosis, toxoplasmosis, and strongyloidiasis: antral narrowing and rigidity, occasionally associated with one or more deep ulcers
- Strongyloidiasis: thickened or effaced mucosal folds, ulceration, and narrowing or dilation of the affected bowel
- Severe strongyloidiasis: *lead pipe* appearance with megaduodenum. Rarely, scarring of the duodenal wall permits reflux of barium into biliary tree via incompetent sphincter of Oddi.

Utility
- Barium studies

CT
Finding
- Narrowed antrum with marked thickening of gastric wall in cryptosporidiosis and toxoplasmosis

CLINICAL PRESENTATION

- CMV gastritis and duodenitis: severe abdominal pain or signs or symptoms of upper gastrointestinal bleeding
- Profuse secretory diarrhea in cryptosporidiosis
- Strongyloidiasis: abdominal pain, nausea and vomiting, diarrhea, malabsorption, or hypoalbuminemia; peripheral eosinophilia in 25%-35% of patients

DIFFERENTIAL DIAGNOSIS

- Zollinger-Ellison syndrome (stomach and duodenum)
- Celiac disease (small bowel)
- Tuberculosis (gastrointestinal)

DIAGNOSTIC PEARLS

- Antral narrowing and rigidity
- Affects immunocompromised patients, most notably those with acquired immunodeficiency syndrome (AIDS)
- Severe strongyloidiasis: *lead pipe* appearance with megaduodenum

PATHOLOGY

- This group of conditions is characterized by opportunistic infections caused by viral or protozoan agents in immunocompromised patients.
- CMV, a member of the herpesvirus group, is the most common viral pathogen affecting the gastrointestinal tract in patients with AIDS.
- *Cryptosporidium*, a protozoan, may infect the small bowel in patients with AIDS, causing profuse secretory diarrhea.
- *Toxoplasmosis:* presence of teardrop-shaped trophozoites in histologic specimens from stomach
- *Strongyloides stercoralis:* a parasite of worldwide distribution that causes infections of the stomach, duodenum, and proximal small bowel

INCIDENCE/PREVALENCE AND EPIDEMIOLOGY

- Affects immunocompromised patients, most notably those with AIDS
- Cases of strongyloidiasis are occasionally encountered in metropolitan areas of the United States in patients who have emigrated from areas of endemic infection.

Suggested Readings

Agel NM, Tanner P, Drury A, et al: Cytomegalovirus gastritis with perforation and gastrocolic fistula formation. *Histopathology* 18:165-168, 1991.

WHAT THE REFERRING PHYSICIAN NEEDS TO KNOW

- Treatment of CMV gastritis or duodenitis includes relatively toxic antiviral agents such as ganciclovir (associated with bone marrow suppression).
- When infectious gastritis is suspected based on the radiographic findings, biopsy specimens, brushings, or viral cultures should be obtained from the stomach for a more definitive diagnosis.
- CMV is confirmed by demonstrating characteristic inclusion bodies on endoscopic biopsy specimens or brushings or by obtaining positive cultures.
- Diagnosis of toxoplasmosis may be confirmed by the demonstration of teardrop-shaped trophozoites in histologic specimens from stomach.

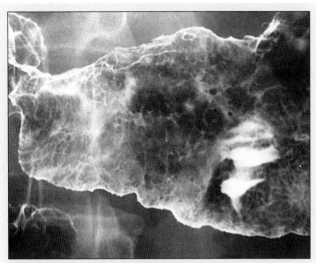

Figure 1. Cytomegalovirus gastritis. Mucosal nodularity and tiny ulcerations are seen in the gastric antrum. Note the irregular contour of the stomach. This patient had AIDS.

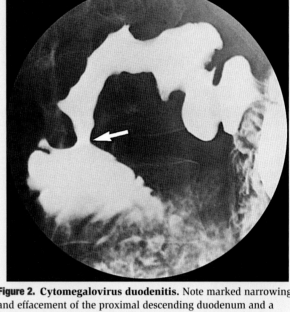

Figure 2. Cytomegalovirus duodenitis. Note marked narrowing and effacement of the proximal descending duodenum and a relatively abrupt transition (*arrow*) to the normal-appearing duodenum more distally. This patient had AIDS. (*From Mong A, Levine MS, Furth EE, et al: Cytomegalovirus duodenitis in an AIDS patient. AJR Am J Roentgenol 172:939-940, 1999, © by American Roentgen Ray Society.*)

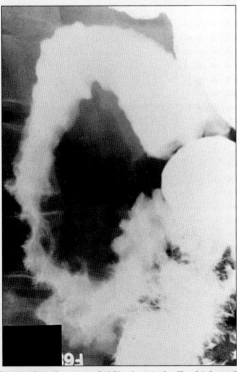

Figure 3. Duodenal strongyloidiasis. Markedly thickened, edematous folds are present in the duodenum. This patient had AIDS.

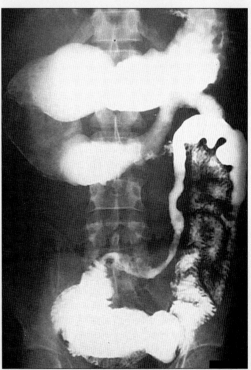

Figure 4. Duodenal strongyloidiasis. This patient with more advanced disease exhibits a markedly dilated duodenum (i.e., megaduodenum) with effaced mucosal folds. Also note the smooth, tubular appearance of the proximal jejunum, producing a *lead pipe* appearance. This patient had recently immigrated to the United States from an area where strongyloidiasis was endemic. (*Courtesy of Murray K. Dalinka, MD, Philadelphia, PA.*)

Alpert L, Miller M, Alpert E, et al: Gastric toxoplasmosis in acquired immunodeficiency syndrome: Antemortem diagnosis with histopathologic characterization. *Gastroenterology* 110:258-264, 1996.

Balthazar EJ, Megibow AJ, Hulnick DH: Cytomegalovirus esophagitis and gastritis in AIDS. *AJR Am J Roentgenol* 144:1201-1204, 1985.

Berk RN, Wall SD, McArdle CB, et al: Cryptosporidiosis of the stomach and small intestine in patients with AIDS. *AJR Am J Roentgenol* 143:549-554, 1984.

Berkman YM, Rabinowitz J: Gastrointestinal manifestations of strongyloidiasis. *Am J Roentgenol Radium Ther Nucl Med* 115:306-311, 1972.

Buhles WC, Mastre BJ, Tinker AJ, et al: Ganciclovir treatment of life- or sight-threatening cytomegalovirus infection: Experience in 314 immunocompromised patients. *Rev Infect Dis* 10(Suppl 3):S495-S506, 1988.

Dallemand S, Waxman M, Farman J: Radiological manifestations of *Strongyloides stercoralis*. *Gastrointest Radiol* 8:45-51, 1983.

Falcone S, Murphy BJ, Weinfeld A: Gastric manifestations of AIDS: Radiographic findings on upper gastrointestinal examination. *Gastrointest Radiol* 16:95-98, 1991.

Farman J, Lerner ME, Ng C, et al: Cytomegalovirus gastritis: Protean radiologic manifestations. *Gastrointest Radiol* 17:202-206, 1992.

Louisy CL, Barton CJ: The radiological diagnosis of *Strongyloides stercoralis* enteritis. *Radiology* 98:535-541, 1971.

Mong A, Levine MS, Furth EE, et al: Cytomegalovirus duodenitis in an AIDS patient. *AJR Am J Roentgenol* 172:939-940, 1999.

Rotterdam H, Tsang P: Gastrointestinal disease in the immunocompromised patient. *Hum Pathol* 25:1123-1140, 1994.

Smart PE, Weinfeld A, Thompson NE, et al: Toxoplasmosis of the stomach: A cause of antral narrowing. *Radiology* 174:369-370, 1990.

Soulen MC, Fishman EK, Scatarige JC, et al: Cryptosporidiosis of the gastric antrum: Detection using CT. *Radiology* 159:705-706, 1986.

Ventura G, Cauda R, Larocca LM, et al: Gastric cryptosporidiosis complicating HIV infection: Case report and review of the literature. *Eur J Gastroenterol Hepatol* 9:307-310, 1997.

Wilcox CM, Schwartz DA: Symptomatic CMV duodenitis. *J Clin Gastroenterol* 14:293-297, 1992.

Eosinophilic Gastritis

DEFINITION: Eosinophilic infiltration of the gastrointestinal tract, primarily the stomach and small bowel.

IMAGING

Radiography
Findings
- Mucosal nodularity, thickened folds, or narrowing and rigidity of the distal half of the stomach
- Occasionally, severe antral narrowing may cause gastric outlet obstruction.
- Diffuse thickening and nodularity of the small bowel folds are caused by associated eosinophilic enteritis.

Utility
- Barium studies
- When eosinophilic gastritis is suspected based on upper gastrointestinal examination, a small-bowel follow-through should be performed to look for concomitant disease in small bowel.

CLINICAL PRESENTATION

- Clinical symptoms are related to the site and extent of gastrointestinal involvement.
- Patients with gastric disease may have epigastric pain, nausea and vomiting, or, less frequently, signs or symptoms of upper gastrointestinal bleeding.

DIFFERENTIAL DIAGNOSIS

- *Helicobacter pylori* gastritis
- Hypertrophic gastritis
- Ménétrier disease (stomach)

PATHOLOGY

- Eosinophilic gastroenteritis is an unusual condition characterized by eosinophilic infiltration of the gastrointestinal tract, primarily the stomach and small bowel.

DIAGNOSTIC PEARLS

- Appearance on barium studies indistinguishable from that of other types of gastritis
- Eosinophilic gastritis should be considered in patients who have peripheral eosinophilia or history of allergic diseases.
- Correct diagnosis may be suggested by the clinical history and presentation.

- Eosinophilic gastroenteritis is a chronic, relapsing disease with intermittent exacerbations sometimes occurring after long asymptomatic intervals.
- Most patients with eosinophilic gastroenteritis have a peripheral eosinophilia ranging from 10%-80%.
- Approximately 50% of patients have a history of allergic diseases.
- Eosinophilic gastritis usually involves the antrum or antrum and body of the stomach.

INCIDENCE/PREVALENCE AND EPIDEMIOLOGY

- Fifty percent of patients with eosinophilic gastritis have a history of allergic diseases.

Suggested Readings
Balfe DM: General diagnosis case of the day. Eosinophilic gastritis. *AJR Am J Roentgenol* 152:1322, 1989.

Vitellas KM, Bennett WF, Bova JG, et al: Radiographic manifestations of eosinophilic gastroenteritis. *Abdom Imaging* 20:406-413, 1995.

WHAT THE REFERRING PHYSICIAN NEEDS TO KNOW
- Treatment with steroids often produces a dramatic clinical response.
- When eosinophilic gastritis is suspected based on the upper gastrointestinal barium study, a small-bowel follow-through should be performed to look for concomitant small-bowel disease.

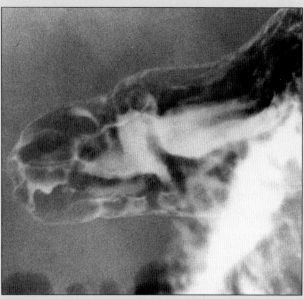

Figure 1. Eosinophilic gastritis. Thickened, nodular folds are seen in the gastric antrum. This appearance is indistinguishable from that of other types of antral gastritis. (*From Herlinger H, Maglinte D [eds]:* Clinical Radiology of the Small Intestine. *Philadelphia, WB Saunders, 1989.*)

Emphysematous Gastritis

DEFINITION: Rare type of phlegmonous gastritis in which gas is found in the gastric wall.

IMAGING

Radiography
Findings
- Multiple streaky, bubbly, or mottled collections of gas are seen in the wall of the stomach.
- Intraluminal gas collections have a constant relationship to the stomach with changes in position.
- Water-soluble contrast studies may be performed to confirm the extraluminal location of gas collections.
- Intramural dissection or extravasation of contrast material may be demonstrated.

Utility
- Water-soluble contrast studies

CT
Findings
- Small collections of gas in gastric wall may be detected.

Utility
- Gas collections not seen on abdominal radiographs may be detected.

CLINICAL PRESENTATION

- Patient may exhibit acute, fulminating illness characterized by severe abdominal pain, hematemesis, tachycardia, fever, and shock.

DIFFERENTIAL DIAGNOSIS

- Benign gastric emphysema

DIAGNOSTIC PEARLS

- Multiple streaks, bubbles, and collections of gas in the gastric wall
- Collections have a constant relationship with the stomach.
- Water-soluble contrast examination may show extraluminal location of gas.

PATHOLOGY

- Rare type of phlegmonous gastritis in which gas is found in the gastric wall because of infection by gas-forming organisms
- Usually caused by profound insults to stomach, such as caustic ingestion, gastroduodenal surgery, or gastric volvulus
- Subsequent ischemia or necrosis permits gas-forming organisms to enter the gastric wall.
- Offending organisms: *Escherichia coli, Proteus vulgaris, Clostridium perfringens,* and *Staphylococcus aureus*

Suggested Readings

Meyers HJ, Parker JJ: Emphysematous gastritis. *Radiology* 89:426-431, 1967.
Monteferrante M, Shimkin P: CT diagnosis of emphysematous gastritis. *AJR Am J Roentgenol* 153:191-192, 1989.
Nelson SW: Extraluminal gas collections due to diseases of the gastrointestinal tract. *Am J Roentgenol Radium Ther Nucl Med* 115:225-248, 1972.
Schorr S, Marcus M: Intramural gastric emphysema. *Br J Radiol* 35:641-644, 1962.

WHAT THE REFERRING PHYSICIAN NEEDS TO KNOW

- Profound insults to the stomach can cause ischemia or necrosis, allowing gas-forming organisms to enter the gastric wall.
- Supportive therapy with parenteral fluids and antibiotics should be initiated.
- Nasogastric tube should not be placed in the stomach because of the high risk of perforation.
- Despite intensive treatment, mortality rates as high as 60% have been reported.

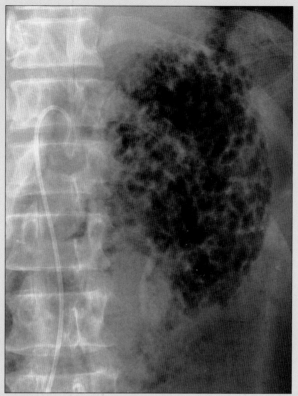

Figure 1. Emphysematous gastritis. Close-up view from an abdominal radiograph shows numerous mottled and bubbly collections of gas in the wall of the stomach. An attempted embolization of a gastric carcinoma led to gastric necrosis and subsequent infection by gas-forming organisms.

Caustic Injury (Stomach and Duodenum)

DEFINITION: Injury to the upper gastrointestinal tract, more commonly the stomach and duodenum, caused by accidental or intentional ingestion of caustic agents.

ANATOMIC FINDINGS

Stomach
- Sustains greatest degree of injury because pylorospasm delays entry of caustic agent into duodenum

Duodenum
- May be spared because of pylorospasm
- Severe injury characterized by thickened folds, spasm, atony, ulceration, and strictures

IMAGING

Radiography
Findings
- Acute phase of injury: thickened folds, ulceration, gastric atony, or mural defects resulting from edema and hemorrhage
- Fulminating cases: gastric necrosis with streaky, bubbly, or mottled collections of intramural gas unaffected by changes in patient's position
- Confined perforation with intramural dissection of contrast medium or loculated perigastric collections
- Free perforation into the peritoneal cavity and progressive narrowing and deformity of the antrum or antrum and body of the stomach
- Scarring characterized by a narrowed antrum with smooth, tubular configuration or irregular contour, mimicking the appearance of primary scirrhous carcinoma of the stomach
- Duodenal bulb and sweep may appear normal in patients with marked antral scarring
- Thickened folds, spasm, atony, ulceration, and, eventually, strictures in the duodenum anywhere from the bulb to the ligament of Treitz
Utility
- Barium studies

CT
Findings
- Absence of normally enhancing mucosa and remaining gastric wall

DIAGNOSTIC PEARLS
- Lesser curvature and distal antrum of stomach sustain greatest degree of injury, often with sparing of the duodenum.
- Thickened folds, ulceration, gastric atony, or mural defects may be present.

CLINICAL PRESENTATION
- Severe abdominal pain, nausea, vomiting, hematemesis, fever, and, eventually, shock

DIFFERENTIAL DIAGNOSIS
- Scarring from peptic ulcer disease, Crohn disease, or other causes
- Scirrhous gastric carcinoma

PATHOLOGY
- Accidental or intentional ingestion of caustic agents may lead to severe injury of the upper gastrointestinal tract.
- Stomach and duodenum are more likely to be damaged by strong acids such as hydrochloric, sulfuric, acetic, oxalic, carbolic, and nitric acid.
- Gastric and duodenal injury occurs in three phases: acute necrotic phase, ulceration-granulation phase, and final phase of intense cicatrization and scarring.
- Acute necrotic phase lasts 1-4 days after caustic ingestion.
- Ulceration-granulation phase lasts 5-28 days after caustic ingestion.
- Final phase of cicatrization and scarring lasts 3-4 weeks after caustic ingestion.
- Ingested caustic agents flow down the lesser curvature of the stomach into the antrum, causing severe pylorospasm that delays emptying into the duodenum.

WHAT THE REFERRING PHYSICIAN NEEDS TO KNOW
- In stable patients with no evidence of perforation, conservative treatment can be initiated with antibiotics, corticosteroids, and parenteral feedings.
- Gastroenterostomy or partial gastrectomy is required in patients with rapidly progressive gastric outlet obstruction because of antral scarring and fibrosis.
- Studies with water-soluble contrast agents are sometimes performed to assess the extent and severity of injury to the upper gastrointestinal tract after caustic ingestion.

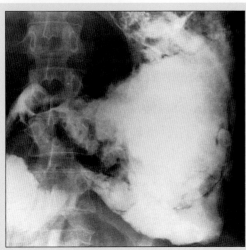

Figure 1. **Severe gastric injury caused by caustic ingestion.** Study with water-soluble contrast medium shows a grossly abnormal stomach with intramural dissection of contrast medium and numerous mural defects resulting from edema and hemorrhage after acid ingestion.

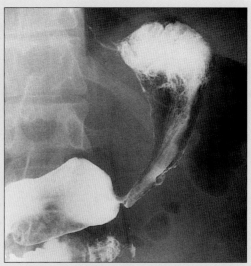

Figure 2. **Caustic scarring of the stomach.** Double-contrast study of the stomach shows marked antral narrowing and deformity as a result of scarring from previous lye ingestion. (*From Levine MS: Radiology of the Esophagus. Philadelphia, WB Saunders, 1989.*)

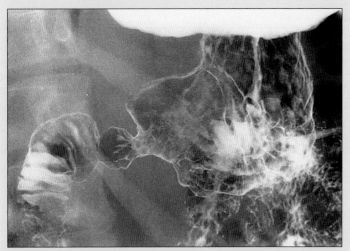

Figure 3. **Caustic scarring of the stomach.** Asymmetric narrowing and deformity of the distal antrum caused by scarring are noted as a result of previous acid ingestion. This appearance can be mistaken for a scirrhous carcinoma of the antrum. The duodenum appears normal.

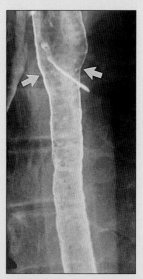

Figure 4. **Caustic scarring of the stomach and esophagus.** In this patient who had marked antral scarring, an esophagogram shows an associated stricture in the esophagus, extending distally from the carina *(arrows)* to the gastroesophageal junction. Aspirated barium is also present in both main bronchi. (*From Levine MS: Radiology of the Esophagus. Philadelphia, WB Saunders, 1989.*)

INCIDENCE/PREVALENCE AND EPIDEMIOLOGY

- Gastroduodenal injury occurs in 5%-10% of patients who ingest strong alkali.
- Approximately 20% of patients with antral scarring from caustic ingestion have associated esophageal scarring.

Suggested Readings

Citron BP, Pincus IJ, Geokas MC, et al: Chemical trauma of the esophagus and stomach. *Surg Clin North Am* 48:1303-1311, 1968.

Franken EA: Caustic damage of the gastrointestinal tract: Roentgen features. *Am J Roentgenol Radium Ther Nucl Med* 118:77-85, 1973.

Goldman LP, Weigert JM: Corrosive substance ingestion: A review. *Am J Gastroenterol* 79:85-90, 1984.

Kanne JP, Gunn M, Blackmore CC: Delayed gastric perforation resulting from hydrochloric acid ingestion. *AJR Am J Roentgenol* 185:682-683, 2005.

Kleinhaus U, Rosenberger A, Adler O: Early and late radiological features of damage to the stomach caused by acid ingestion. *Radiol Clin (Basel)* 46:26-37, 1977.

Levitt R, Stanley RJ, Wise L: Gastric bullae: An early roentgen finding in corrosive gastritis following alkali ingestion. *Radiology* 115:597-598, 1975.

Muhletaler CA, Gerlock AJ, de Soto L, et al: Gastroduodenal lesions of ingested acids: Radiographic findings. *AJR Am J Roentgenol* 135:1247-1252, 1980.

Poteshman NL: Corrosive gastritis due to hydrochloric acid ingestion. *Am J Roentgenol Radium Ther Nucl Med* 99:182-185, 1967.

Radiation Injury (Stomach and Duodenum)

DEFINITION: Inflammatory changes, scarring, or fibrosis after radiation exposure of 50 Gy or more to the abdomen.

IMAGING

Radiography

Findings
- Gastroparesis, spasm, thickened folds, or ulceration, predominantly involving the distal antrum and pyloric region and, occasionally, the duodenum
- Perforation of deep ulcers may result in acute peritonitis.

Utility
- Barium studies

CT

Findings
- Luminal narrowing with nonspecific gastric wall thickening and stranding in perigastric fat
- Narrowed antrum may have an irregular contour, simulating a scirrhous carcinoma of the stomach.

CLINICAL PRESENTATION

- Dyspepsia
- Epigastric pain
- Nausea
- Vomiting
- Signs and symptoms of upper gastrointestinal bleeding

DIFFERENTIAL DIAGNOSIS

- Peptic ulcer disease
- Crohn disease (stomach)
- Sarcoidosis (stomach)
- Syphilis (stomach)
- Tuberculosis (stomach)
- Caustic injury (stomach)

DIAGNOSTIC PEARLS

- Condition is characterized by acute gastroparesis, spasm, thickened folds, or ulceration, predominantly involving distal antrum and pylorus and, occasionally, the duodenum.
- Scarring may lead to development of antral or duodenal narrowing 6 months or more after completion of radiation therapy.
- Should be considered in patients who have received radiation therapy to the upper abdomen during the previous 12 months

PATHOLOGY

- Radiation doses of 50 Gy or more to upper abdomen may cause injury to the stomach and duodenum.
- Distal antrum and pyloric region are most commonly affected.
- Inflammatory changes occur 1-6 months after radiation therapy; scarring and fibrosis occur 6 months or more after treatment.

Suggested Readings

Capps GW, Fulcer AS, Szucs RA, et al: Imaging features of radiation-induced changes in the abdomen. *Radiographics* 17:1455-1473, 1997.

Goldstein HM, Rogers LF, Fletcher GH, et al: Radiological manifestations of radiation-induced injury to the normal upper gastrointestinal tract. *Radiology* 117:135-140, 1975.

Lane D: Irradiation gastritis simulating carcinoma. *Med J Aust* 2:576-577, 1970.

Roswit B, Malsky SJ, Reid CB: Severe radiation injuries of the stomach, small intestine, colon, and rectum. *Am J Roentgenol Radium Ther Nucl Med* 114:460-475, 1972.

WHAT THE REFERRING PHYSICIAN NEEDS TO KNOW

- Radiation injury to the stomach or duodenum should be considered in patients who have received radiation therapy to the upper abdomen during previous 12 months.

Floxuridine Toxicity

DEFINITION: Direct complication of arterial infusion of 5-floxuridine (5-FUDR) chemotherapy.

IMAGING

Radiography
Findings
- Gastroduodenal ulceration or severe gastritis or duodenitis with markedly thickened, edematous folds in the stomach or duodenum

Utility
- Barium studies

CLINICAL PRESENTATION

- Toxicity should be suspected in patients receiving hepatic artery infusion of 5-FUDR who develop intractable nausea, vomiting, epigastric pain, or upper gastrointestinal tract bleeding.

DIFFERENTIAL DIAGNOSIS

- Gastritis
- Duodenitis
- Peptic ulcer disease

PATHOLOGY

- 5-FUDR is the agent of choice for hepatic artery infusion chemotherapy in patients with unresectable liver metastases.
- Severe gastroduodenal toxicity may occur as a result of hepatic artery infusion of 5-FUDR via an external catheter system or an implantable pump.

DIAGNOSTIC PEARLS

- Gastroduodenal ulceration
- Markedly thickened, edematous folds in the stomach or duodenum
- Temporal relationship between 5-FUDR therapy and the onset of symptoms should suggest the correct diagnosis.

- Toxicity occurs because of direct infusion of 5-FUDR into the gastroduodenal and right gastric arteries, which supply the stomach and duodenum.
- With hepatic artery infusion of 5-FUDR via pumps, toxicity may still occur because of the development of small collateral channels.

INCIDENCE/PREVALENCE AND EPIDEMIOLOGY

- Gastroduodenal toxicity is an uncommon direct complication of 5-FUDR therapy for liver metastases.

Suggested Readings
Chuang VP, Wallace S, Stroehlein J, et al: Hepatic artery infusion chemotherapy: Gastroduodenal complications. *AJR Am J Roentgenol* 137:347-350, 1981.
Hiehle JF, Levine MS: Gastrointestinal toxicity of 5-FU and 5-FUDR: Radiographic findings. *Can Assoc Radiol J* 42:109-112, 1991.
Mann FA, Kubal WS, Ruzicka FF: Radiographic manifestations of gastrointestinal toxicity associated with intraarterial 5-fluorouracil infusion. *Radiographics* 2:329-339, 1982.

WHAT THE REFERRING PHYSICIAN NEEDS TO KNOW
- Temporal relationship between 5-FUDR therapy and onset of symptoms should suggest the correct diagnosis.
- Cessation of chemotherapy produces rapid clinical improvement in most cases.

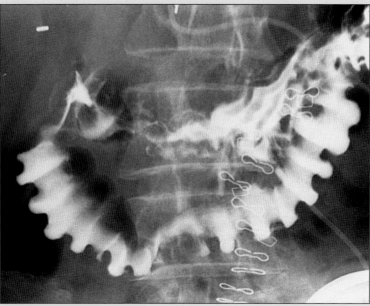

Figure 1. Severe duodenitis caused by 5-floxuridine (FUDR) toxicity. Barium study in a patient receiving 5-FUDR via a hepatic artery infusion pump shows markedly thickened, edematous folds in the duodenum to the level of the ligament of Treitz. (*Reprinted from Hiehle JF, Levine MS: Gastrointestinal toxicity of 5-FU and 5-FUDR: Radiographic findings. Can Assoc Radiol J 42:109-112, 1991. By permission of the publisher.*)

Duodenitis

DEFINITION: Inflammation of any part or the entirety of the duodenum.

ANATOMIC FINDINGS

Duodenum
- Spastic, irritable duodenal bulb
- Thickened mucosal folds in proximal duodenum

IMAGING

Radiography
Findings
- Spastic, irritable duodenal bulb or thickened, nodular folds in the proximal descending duodenum
- Mucosal nodules or nodular folds
- Diffuse coarsening of mucosal pattern of the bulb with lucent areas surrounded by barium-filled grooves
- Erosive duodenitis: incomplete erosions seen as tiny flecks of barium
- Erosive duodenitis: complete or varioliform erosions seen as central barium collections surrounded by radiolucent halos of edematous mucosa
- Underlying pancreatitis of the pancreatic head may also be characterized by thickened, spiculated duodenal folds, but this finding predominantly occurs on the medial border of the descending duodenum and is often associated with widening of duodenal sweep
- Celiac disease: small, hexagonal filling defects in the duodenal bulb, producing a distinctive mosaic pattern or *bubbly bulb*

Utility
- Barium studies
- May be present in patients who have no histologic or endoscopic evidence of inflammation
- Not considered a reliable radiologic diagnosis
- Normal mucosal pits in the duodenum can be mistaken for incomplete erosions.
- A confident diagnosis of erosive duodenitis can be made only when true varioliform erosions are demonstrated in the duodenum.

CT
Utility
- Useful when pancreatitis is suspected as the cause of the duodenitis

CLINICAL PRESENTATION

- Nonspecific upper gastrointestinal symptoms such as dyspepsia, epigastric pain, nausea, and fatty food intolerance

DIAGNOSTIC PEARLS

- Spastic duodenal bulb
- Thickened, nodular folds in proximal duodenum

- May be associated with signs or symptoms of upper gastrointestinal bleeding, such as hematemesis, melena, or guaiac-positive stool

DIFFERENTIAL DIAGNOSIS

- Crohn disease
- Caustic ingestion
- Radiation
- 5-FUDR toxicity
- Infectious conditions

PATHOLOGY

- Associated with gastric hyperacidity; it therefore has been postulated that duodenitis is part of the spectrum of peptic ulcer disease.
- Some patients with duodenitis have normal or decreased gastric acid secretion, so this condition may also occur as a distinct clinical entity.
- May also be caused by Crohn disease, caustic ingestion, radiation, 5-FUDR toxicity, and infectious conditions

Suggested Readings

Bova JG, Kamath V, Tio FO, et al: The normal mucosal surface pattern of the duodenal bulb: Radiologic-histologic correlation. *AJR Am J Roentgenol* 145:735-738, 1985.

Catalano D, Pagliari U: Gastroduodenal erosions: Radiological findings. *Gastrointest Radiol* 7:235-240, 1982.

Cheli R: Symptoms in chronic non-specific duodenitis. *Scand J Gastroenterol Suppl* 79:84-86, 1982.

Collen MJ, Loebenberg MJ: Basal gastric acid secretion in nonulcer dyspepsia with or without duodenitis. *Dig Dis Sci* 34:246-250, 1989.

Fraser GM, Pitman RG, Lawrie JH, et al: The significance of the radiological finding of coarse mucosal folds in the duodenum. *Lancet* 2(7367):979-982, 1964.

Gelfand DW, Dale WJ, Ott DJ, et al: Duodenitis: Endoscopic-radiologic correlation in 272 patients. *Radiology* 157:577-581, 1985.

Gelzayd EA, Biederman MA, Gelfand DW: Changing concepts of duodenitis. *Am J Gastroenterol* 64:213-216, 1975.

WHAT THE REFERRING PHYSICIAN NEEDS TO KNOW
- Duodenitis is not considered a reliable radiologic diagnosis.
- A confident diagnosis of erosive duodenitis can be made on double-contrast studies only when true varioliform erosions are demonstrated.

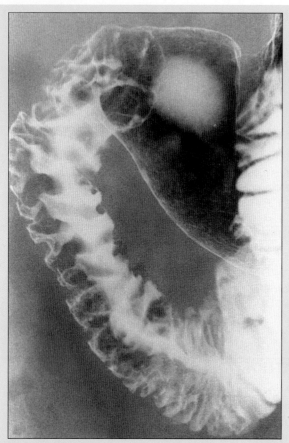

Figure 1. Duodenitis. Thickened, irregular folds are seen in the proximal duodenum.

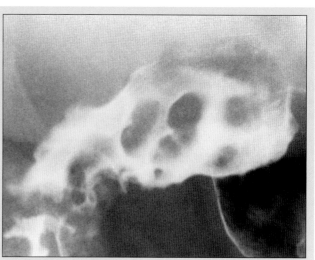

Figure 2. Duodenitis. In this patient, thickened folds and mucosal nodularity are present in the duodenal bulb.

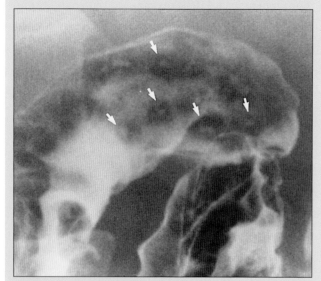

Figure 3. Erosive duodenitis. Varioliform erosions are seen in the duodenum as tiny flecks of barium surrounded by radiolucent mounds of edematous mucosa (*arrows*). (*From Levine MS, Rubesin SE, Herlinger H, et al: Double-contrast upper gastrointestinal examination: Technique and interpretation.* Radiology *168:593-602, 1988.*)

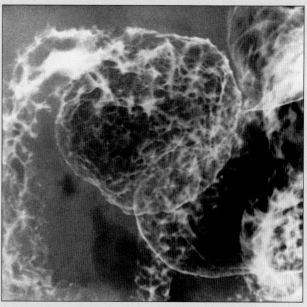

Figure 4. Celiac disease with a bubbly bulb. Multiple hexagonal filling defects are present in the duodenal bulb and thickened, irregular folds in the descending duodenum as a result of associated duodenitis. (*From Jones B, Bayless TM, Hamilton SR, et al: "Bubbly" duodenal bulb in celiac disease: Radiologic-pathologic correlation.* AJR Am J Roentgenol *142:119-122, 1984,* © *by American Roentgen Ray Society.*)

Gelzayd EA, Gelfand DW, Rinaldo JA: Nonspecific duodenitis: A distinct clinical entity. *Gastrointest Endosc* 19:131-133, 1973.

Glick SN, Gohel VK, Laufer I: Mucosal surface patterns of the duodenal bulb. *Radiology* 150:317-322, 1984.

Greenlaw R, Sheehan DG, DeLuca V, et al: Gastroduodenitis: A broader concept of peptic ulcer disease. *Dig Dis Sci* 25:660-662, 1980.

Jones B, Bayless TM, Hamilton SR, et al: "Bubbly" duodenal bulb in celiac disease: Radiologic-pathologic correlation. *AJR Am J Roentgenol* 142:119-122, 1984.

Levine MS, Turner D, Ekberg O, et al: Duodenitis: A reliable radiologic diagnosis? *Gastrointest Radiol* 16:99-103, 1991.

Marn CS, Gore RM, Ghahremani GG: Duodenal manifestations of nontropical sprue. *Gastrointest Radiol* 11:30-35, 1986.

Schweiger GD, Murray JA: Postbulbar duodenal ulceration and stenosis associated with celiac disease. *Abdom Imaging* 23:347-349, 1998.

Sircus W: Duodenitis: A clinical, endoscopic, and histopathologic study. *Q J Med* 56:593-600, 1985.

Thomson WO, Joffe SN, Robertson AG, et al: Is duodenitis a dyspeptic myth? *Lancet* 1(8023):1197-1198, 1977.

Wiener SN, Vertes V, Shapiro H: The upper gastrointestinal tract in patients undergoing chronic dialysis. *Radiology* 92:110-114, 1969.

Wyatt JI, Rathbone BJ, Dixon MF, et al: *Campylobacter pyloridis* and acid induced gastric metaplasia in the pathogenesis of duodenitis. *J Clin Pathol* 40:841-848, 1987.

Zukerman GR, Mills BA, Koehler RE, et al: Nodular duodenitis: Pathologic and clinical characteristics in patients with end-stage renal disease. *Dig Dis Sci* 11:1018-1024, 1983.

Part 17

BENIGN TUMORS OF THE STOMACH AND DUODENUM

Hyperplastic Polyps

DEFINITION: Hyperplastic polyps are benign elongated, branching, cystically dilated glandular structures.

ANATOMIC FINDINGS

Gastric Fundus and Body
- Multiple, small (less than 1 cm in size), rounded nodules in the gastric fundus or body

Duodenum
- Rarely found

IMAGING

Radiography
Findings
- Polyps are smooth, sessile, round or ovoid nodules, 5-10 mm in size.
- Multiple, small (less than 1 cm), rounded nodules are seen in the gastric fundus or body.
- Dependent surface: smooth, round filling defects are seen in the barium pool.
- Nondependent surface: ring shadows are etched in white because of barium trapped between the edge of the polyp and adjacent mucosa.
- Large polyps (2-6 cm in size) may appear as lobulated or pedunculated lesions.
- Giant hyperplastic polyp: conglomerate mass of hyperplastic polyps can be mistaken for polypoid gastric carcinoma.
- Rarely, pedunculated hyperplastic polyps in antrum may prolapse through the pylorus into the duodenum, causing gastric outlet obstruction.

Utility
- Double-contrast barium studies
- Hanging droplet of barium (*stalactite*) on a nondependent wall polyp can be mistaken for a central area of ulceration.
- Fluoroscopy shows the transient nature of hanging droplet.
- *See-through* artifacts mimic the appearance of anterior wall polyps on a single view, but location outside stomach is apparent on other projections.

DIAGNOSTIC PEARLS
- Small sessile nodules with a smooth dome-shaped contour
- Nondependent polyps appear as ring shadows etched in white.

CLINICAL PRESENTATION
- Most patients are asymptomatic; hyperplastic polyps are found incidentally on endoscopy.
- Polyps with friable or ulcerated surface may cause low-grade upper gastrointestinal bleeding.
- Pedunculated polyps in gastric antrum may prolapse through pylorus, causing intermittent symptoms of gastric outlet obstruction.

DIFFERENTIAL DIAGNOSIS
- Adenomatous polyps (stomach and duodenum)

PATHOLOGY
- Histology: elongated, branching, and cystically dilated glandular structures
- Gross appearance: one or more small, sessile nodules with smooth, dome-shaped contour
- Rarely undergo malignant degeneration

INCIDENCE/PREVALENCE AND EPIDEMIOLOGY
- Patients with hyperplastic polyps in the stomach found to have synchronous gastric carcinomas in 8%-28% cases.
- Multiple fundic gland polyps are typically found in middle-aged women.
- Fundic gland polyposis develops in approximately 40% of patients with familial adenomatous polyposis syndrome (FAPS).

WHAT THE REFERRING PHYSICIAN NEEDS TO KNOW
- Colonoscopy is recommended in patients with fundic gland polyposis to determine whether they have FAPS.
- Patients with hyperplastic polyps have an increased risk for harboring separate, coexisting gastric carcinomas.
- Polyps that are unusually large or lobulated should be evaluated by endoscopic biopsy or resected for a definitive diagnosis.

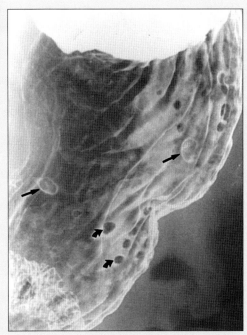

Figure 1. Multiple hyperplastic polyps. Polyps on the dependent surface or posterior wall appear as filling defects in the barium pool *(curved arrows)*, whereas polyps on the nondependent surface or anterior wall are etched in white *(straight arrows)*.

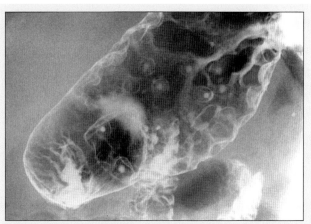

Figure 2. Multiple hyperplastic polyps. This patient has multiple anterior wall polyps (seen as ring shadows) containing hanging droplets of barium, or stalactites that could be mistaken for central areas of ulceration. *(From Laufer I, Levine MS [eds]: Double Contrast Gastrointestinal Radiology, 2nd ed. Philadelphia, WB Saunders, 1992.)*

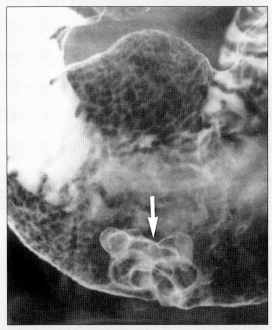

Figure 3. Atypical hyperplastic polyps. A conglomerate mass of hyperplastic polyps *(arrow)* is seen in the antrum in this patient. This lesion is quite lobulated and could be mistaken for a polypoid carcinoma.

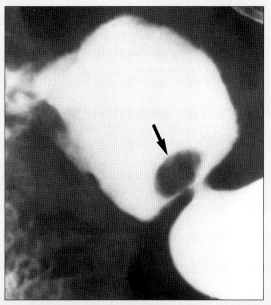

Figure 4. Prolapsed hyperplastic polyp. This patient has a pedunculated polyp *(arrow)* that has prolapsed from the antrum into the base of the duodenal bulb.

Suggested Readings

Good CA: Benign tumors of the stomach and duodenal bulb. *J Can Assoc Radiol* 16:92-104, 1965.

Gordon R, Laufer I, Kressel HY: Gastric polyps found on routine double-contrast examination of the stomach. *Radiology* 134:27-30, 1980.
Ochsner SF, Janetos GP: Benign tumors of the stomach. *JAMA* 191:881-887, 1965.

Adenomatous Polyps

DEFINITION: Benign lesions composed of dysplastic epithelium classified according to the glandular architecture; these lesions may undergo malignant degeneration via an adenoma-carcinoma sequence.

ANATOMIC FINDINGS

Stomach
- Most frequently located in antrum

Duodenum
- Smooth sessile lesions in the first and second portions of duodenum

IMAGING

Radiography
Findings
- Usually seen as solitary lesions larger than 1 cm in size
- *Mexican hat sign:* stalk of pedunculated lesions is seen en face as inner ring shadow overlying head of polyp as outer ring shadow.
- Multiple adenomatous polyps are sometimes found in the stomach or duodenum.
- Polyps are sessile or pedunculated and tend to be more lobulated than hyperplastic polyps.
- Lesions on the nondependent wall may be etched in white on double-contrast views.
- Hanging droplets of barium, or stalactites, on nondependent lesions can mimic the appearance of central ulcers.
- Adenomatous polyps versus hyperplastic polyps: hyperplastic polyps are almost always smaller than 1 cm, often multiple, and tend to have more proximal location in the upper body and fundus of the stomach.

DIAGNOSTIC PEARLS
- *Mexican hat sign:* stalk of pedunculated lesions is seen en face as inner ring shadow overlying head of polyp.
- Adenomatous polyps are usually solitary and larger than 1-2 cm in size.
- Adenomatous polyps are sessile or pedunculated and tend to be more lobulated than hyperplastic polyps.
- Endoscopic biopsy specimens should be obtained.

Utility
- Double-contrast barium studies
- Sessile adenomatous polyps can be mistaken for benign gastrointestinal stromal tumors or other submucosal lesions.
- Adenomatous polyps that are larger and more lobulated may be indistinguishable from polypoid gastric carcinomas.

CLINICAL PRESENTATION
- Gastric polyps may cause epigastric pain, bloating, upper gastrointestinal bleeding, or, rarely, gastric outlet obstruction.
- Duodenal polyps usually cause no symptoms and are detected as incidental findings.

WHAT THE REFERRING PHYSICIAN NEEDS TO KNOW
- Endoscopic biopsy specimens should be obtained for polyps larger than 1 cm in size.
- Adenomatous polyps should be resected because of the risk of malignant degeneration.
- Regardless of endoscopic findings, polyps larger than 2 cm in size should always be resected.
- If invasive carcinoma is present in resected specimen, a wedge resection of stomach or partial gastrectomy may be required.
- Detection of adenomatous polyp in stomach should lead to a careful search for other lesions.
- Sessile polyps in duodenum may be difficult to distinguish on barium studies from benign gastrointestinal stromal tumors, Brunner's gland hamartomas, or other submucosal masses.
- Other considerations in differential diagnosis for duodenal lesions include prolapsed antral mucosa, prolapsed antral lesion, and redundant mucosa at the superior duodenal flexure.

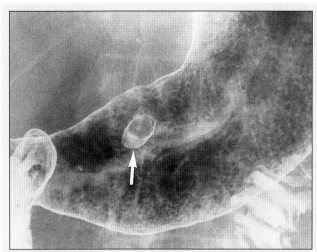

Figure 1. A sessile adenomatous polyp *(arrow)* is present in the antrum.

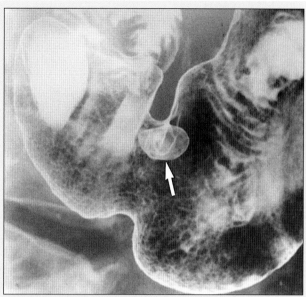

Figure 2. A pedunculated adenomatous polyp *(arrow)* is seen in the antrum. The stalk appears as an inner ring shadow overlying the head of the polyp, producing the *Mexican hat sign.* (*Courtesy of Dean D. T. Maglinte, MD, Indianapolis, IN.*)

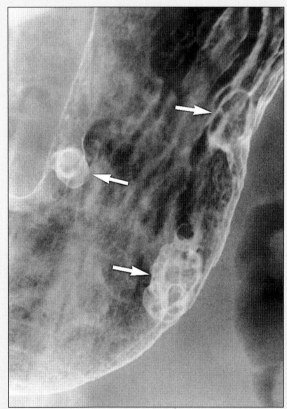

Figure 3. Multiple adenomatous polyps. These adenomatous polyps are larger and more lobulated than most hyperplastic polyps in the stomach. The most distal lesion on the greater curvature is indistinguishable from a polypoid carcinoma. (*From Laufer I, Levine MS [eds]:* Double Contrast Gastrointestinal Radiology, *2nd ed. Philadelphia, WB Saunders, 1992.*)

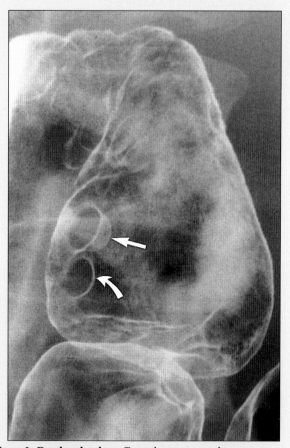

Figure 4. Duodenal polyps. Two adenomatous polyps are present in the duodenal bulb. The lower polyp is seen as a ring shadow *(curved arrow)* and the higher polyp as a bowler hat *(straight arrow)*. (*From Laufer I, Levine MS [eds]:* Double Contrast Gastrointestinal Radiology, *2nd ed. Philadelphia, WB Saunders, 1992.*)

- Duodenal polyps may occasionally cause low-grade upper gastrointestinal bleeding or obstructive jaundice if they obstruct papilla of Vater.

DIFFERENTIAL DIAGNOSIS

- Hyperplastic polyps (stomach and duodenum)
- Benign gastrointestinal stromal tumors
- Brunner's gland hyperplasia (duodenum)
- Flexural pseudolesions
- Prolapsed antral mucosa

PATHOLOGY

- Adenomatous polyps are composed of dysplastic epithelium.
- They are classified as tubular, villous, or tubulovillous adenomas, with the majority being tubular or mixed tubulovillous types.
- Malignant degeneration occurs via an adenoma-carcinoma sequence similar to that in colon.

INCIDENCE/PREVALENCE AND EPIDEMIOLOGY

- Adenomatous polyps constitute less than 20% of all gastric polyps.
- Invasive adenocarcinoma is present in 50% of resected adenomatous polyps larger than 2 cm in size.

- Adenomatous polyps are often found in the stomach in patients with chronic atrophic gastritis.
- As many as 30%-40% of patients with adenomatous polyps in the stomach are found to have coexisting gastric carcinomas.
- Duodenal polyps are much less common than gastric polyps, but most duodenal polyps are adenomatous.

Suggested Readings

Burrell M, Toffler R: Flexural pseudolesions of the duodenum. *Radiology* 120:313-315, 1976.

Deutschberger O, Tchertkoff V, Daino J, et al: Benign duodenal polyp: Review of the literature and report of a giant adenomatous polyp of the duodenal bulb. *Am J Gastroenterol* 38:75-84, 1962.

Feczko PJ, Halpert RD, Ackerman LV: Gastric polyps: Radiological evaluation and clinical significance. *Radiology 155*:581-584, 1985.

Ming S-C: The classification and significance of gastric polyps. In Yardly JH, Morson BC, Abell M (eds): *The Gastrointestinal Tract. International Academy of Pathology Monograph.* Baltimore, Williams & Wilkins, 1977, pp 149–175.

Nelson JA, Sheft DJ, Minagi H, et al: Duodenal pseudopolyp: The flexural fallacy. *Am J Roentgenol Radium Ther Nucl Med* 123: 262-267, 1975.

Tomasulo J: Gastric polyps: Histologic types and their relationship to gastric carcinoma. *Cancer* 27:1346-1355, 1971.

Villous Tumors

DEFINITION: Villous tumors are adenomatous polyps with predominantly villous elements, appearing grossly as polypoid masses with numerous frond-like projections and high malignant potential.

ANATOMIC FINDINGS

Stomach
- Equal distribution in the stomach

Duodenum
- Duodenal lesions tend to be located in the descending duodenum near the papilla of Vater.

IMAGING
Radiography
Finding
- Polypoid masses, ranging from 2-9 cm in size
- Reticular or *soap bubble* appearance with serrated, feathery margins is characteristic; this results from barium trapping in interstices of the lesion.
- Villous tumor versus bezoar: bezoars may also have *soap bubble* appearance but are freely mobile, whereas villous tumors have a fixed location in the stomach or duodenum.
- Villous tumor versus carcinoma or lymphoma: both may be seen as a bulky intraluminal mass, but carcinoma or lymphoma rarely produces a *soap bubble* appearance.

Utility
- Barium studies
- Duodenal lesions are best visualized on double-contrast studies with optimal distention of the descending duodenum.

CLINICAL PRESENTATION

- Signs and symptoms of upper gastrointestinal bleeding, including melena, guaiac-positive stool, and iron-deficiency anemia
- Villous tumors near the papilla of Vater may cause obstructive jaundice.
- Villous tumors in the stomach and duodenum rarely cause diarrhea or electrolyte depletion (unlike villous tumors in the colon).

DIAGNOSTIC PEARLS

- Reticular or *soap bubble* appearance with serrated, feathery margins is characteristic.
- Solitary polypoid mass ranging from 2-9 cm in size
- Located anywhere in the stomach or in descending duodenum, near the papilla of Vater

DIFFERENTIAL DIAGNOSIS

- Bezoar (stomach)
- Carcinoma (stomach and duodenum)
- Lymphoma (stomach and duodenum)

PATHOLOGY

- Polypoid masses with numerous frond-like projections
- Solitary lesions, ranging from 2-9 cm in size, but giant villous tumors occasionally as large as 15 cm in size

INCIDENCE/PREVALENCE AND EPIDEMIOLOGY

- Most patients with villous tumors in the stomach and duodenum are older than 50 years of age.
- The duodenum is the most commom extracolonic site of villous tumors in the gastrointestinal tract.

Suggested Readings

Gaitini O, Kleinhaus U, Munichor M, et al: Villous tumors of the stomach. *Gastrointest Radiol* 13:105-108, 1988.

Kutin ND, Ranson JHC, Gouge TH, et al: Villous tumors of the duodenum. *Ann Surg* 181:164-168, 1975.

Ring EJ, Ferucci JT, Eaton SB, et al: Villous adenoma of the duodenum. *Radiology* 104:45-48, 1972.

Schulten MF, Dyasu R, Beal JM: Villous adenoma of the duodenum: A case report and review of the literature. *Am J Surg* 132:90-96, 1976.

WHAT THE REFERRING PHYSICIAN NEEDS TO KNOW

- Villous tumors in the stomach and duodenum should be resected because of the high risk of malignant degeneration.
- Risk of malignancy is directly related to the size of the lesion.

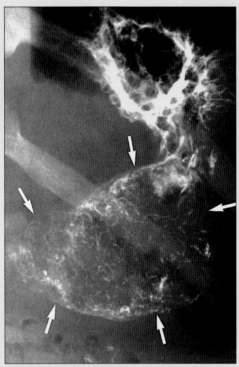

Figure 1. Villous tumor in stomach. A giant villous tumor *(arrows)* in the gastric antrum has a characteristic *soap bubble* appearance because of trapping of barium between the frond-like projections of the tumor. This lesion can be mistaken for a bezoar, but, unlike bezoars, it did not move with changes in the patient's position. *(Courtesy of Abraham Ghiatis, MD, San Antonio, TX.)*

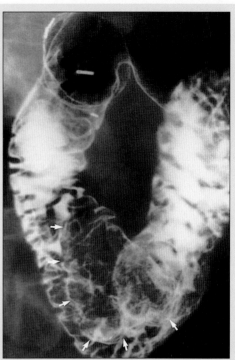

Figure 2. Villous tumor in the duodenum. This villous tumor appears as a polypoid mass *(arrows)* just below the level of the papilla. Note the characteristic reticular surface of the lesion. *(From Laufer I, Levine MS [eds]: Double Contrast Gastrointestinal Radiology, 2nd ed. Philadelphia, WB Saunders, 1992.)*

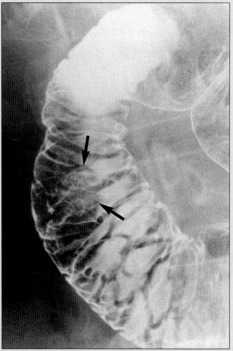

Figure 3. Villous tumor in the duodenum. In this patient, a more subtle villous tumor *(arrows)* is seen with optimal distention of the descending duodenum. Note the reticular surface of the lesion.

Polyposis Syndromes

DEFINITION: Syndromes with multiple polyps in the stomach and duodenum.

IMAGING

Radiography
Findings
- Multiple polypoid lesions of various size seen in stomach
- Barium studies show distinctive *whiskering* along the margins of the stomach because of trapping of barium between tiny mucosal excrescences in patients with Cronkhite-Canada syndrome.

Utility
- When accompanied by characteristic ectodermal findings, this appearance should be highly suggestive of Cronkhite-Canada syndrome.

CLINICAL PRESENTATION
- Epigastric pain
- Signs or symptoms of upper gastrointestinal bleeding

DIFFERENTIAL DIAGNOSIS
- Multiple hyperplastic polyps
- Lymphoma (stomach)

DIAGNOSTIC PEARLS
- Barium studies show distinctive *whiskering* along the margins of the stomach because of trapping of barium between tiny mucosal excrescences.
- Risk of gastric or duodenal carcinoma is increased.
- Ectodermal findings plus gastric polyposis is highly suggestive of Cronkhite-Canada syndrome.

Suggested Readings
Kilcheski T, Kressel HY, Laufer I, et al: The radiographic appearance of the stomach in Cronkhite-Canada syndrome. *Radiology* 141: 57-60, 1981.

Kumar A, Quick CRG, Carr-Locke DL: Prolapsing gastric polyp, an unusual cause of gastric outlet obstruction: A review of the pathology and management of gastric polyps. *Endoscopy* 28:452-455, 1996.

WHAT THE REFERRING PHYSICIAN NEEDS TO KNOW
- In patients with familial adenomatous polyposis syndrome (FAPS), malignant potential of polyps and the risk of developing gastric and duodenal carcinoma make detection important.
- Periodic surveillance of the upper gastrointestinal tract should be performed on all patients with FAPS.
- Other polyposis syndromes involving the stomach and duodenum include Peutz-Jeghers syndrome, Cronkhite-Canada syndrome, juvenile polyposis, and Cowden disease.

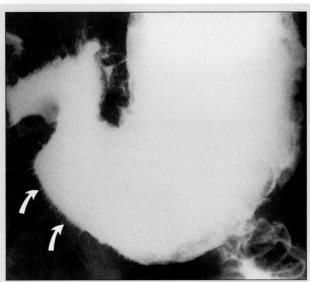

Figure 1. **Cronkhite-Canada syndrome involving the stomach.**
A single-contrast view shows whiskering *(arrows)* of the greater
curvature because of trapping of barium between tiny mucosal
excrescences. This finding is characteristic of gastric involvement by
Cronkhite-Canada syndrome.

Benign Gastrointestinal Stromal Tumors

DEFINITION: Benign mesenchymal tumors of the stomach and duodenum that test positive for CD117.

IMAGING

Radiography
Findings
- Typically appear on barium studies as discrete submucosal masses
- In profile: smooth surface etched in white on double contrast; borders form right angle or slightly obtuse angle with adjacent gastric or duodenal wall
- En face: intraluminal surface of tumors has abrupt, well-defined borders, normal overlying gastric mucosa.
- Gastric gastrointestinal stromal tumors (GISTs) vary in size from tiny lesions of several millimeters to enormous masses that encroach substantially on lumen.
- "Bull's-eye" or "target" lesion: central barium-filled crater within surrounding submucosal mass due to ulceration of GISTs larger than 2 cm in size
- Hanging droplet of barium from GIST on nondependent wall can mimic ulceration on single en face image.
- Spicule or dimple at apex of mass for intramural GISTs growing outward from bowel wall
- Benign GISTs in the stomach rarely may contain irregular streaks or clumps of mottled calcification.

Utility
- Barium study

CT
Findings
- Homogeneous or heterogeneous intramural mass
- Calcification of gastric GISTs occasionally seen

CLINICAL PRESENTATION

- Epigastric pain or upper gastrointestinal bleeding, manifested by hematemesis, melena, guaiac-positive stool, or iron-deficiency anemia
- Most patients with lesions smaller than 3 cm are asymptomatic.

DIAGNOSTIC PEARLS

- Discrete submucosal mass
- Bull's-eye or target lesions
- Central dimple or spicule at apex of mass

DIFFERENTIAL DIAGNOSIS

- Adenomatous polyps (stomach and duodenum)
- Other mesenchymal tumors (stomach and duodenum)

PATHOLOGY

- Believed to arise from interstitial cells of Cajal
- Identified using immunohistochemistry for expression of CD117, also known as c-kit protein (cell membrane receptor with tyrosine kinase activity)
- Histologic appearance: intersecting bundles of spindle-shaped cells in characteristic whorling pattern
- Gross appearance: endogastric, exogastric, or "dumbbell"-shaped lesions
- As these tumors enlarge, they often outgrow their blood supply, causing central necrosis and ulceration

INCIDENCE/PREVALENCE AND EPIDEMIOLOGY

- GISTs: 90% of mesenchymal tumors and 40% of all benign tumors in stomach and duodenum
- About 90% of gastric GISTs are found to be benign lesions.
- GISTs: most common benign submucosal tumors in stomach and duodenum
- Benign gastric and duodenal GISTs occur with about equal frequency in men and women.
- Affected individuals are usually older than 50 years of age.

WHAT THE REFERRING PHYSICIAN NEEDS TO KNOW

- It is often difficult to differentiate benign from malignant GISTs by histopathologic criteria.
- Ulceration and size larger than 2 cm should be considered indications for surgery.
- Ulcerated GIST in patient with contraindication for surgery may be treated medically.
- Radiologic criteria usually cannot differentiate GISTs from other discrete submucosal masses such as lipomas, neurofibromas, and hemangiomas.
- Small submucosal masses not causing symptoms should be followed up with repeat barium studies or endoscopy at yearly intervals.

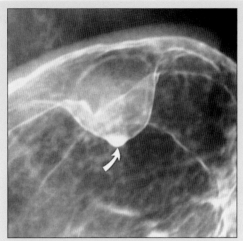

Figure 1. Benign GIST. A submucosal mass is seen in profile in the gastric fundus. The lesion has smooth borders that form slightly obtuse angles with the adjacent gastric wall. This view was taken with the patient upright, and a barium stalactite *(arrow)* is seen hanging down from the inferior surface of the lesion. *(From Laufer I, Levine MS [eds]: Double Contrast Gastrointestinal Radiology, 2nd ed. Philadelphia, WB Saunders, 1992.)*

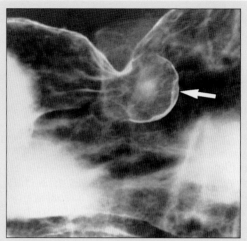

Figure 2. Benign GIST. In this patient, a small GIST is seen en face *(arrow)* in the gastric body. This lesion also has typical features of a submucosal mass with smooth, well-defined borders. A hanging droplet of barium or stalactite is visible on the surface of this anterior wall lesion. *(From Laufer I, Levine MS [eds]: Double Contrast Gastrointestinal Radiology, 2nd ed. Philadelphia, WB Saunders, 1992.)*

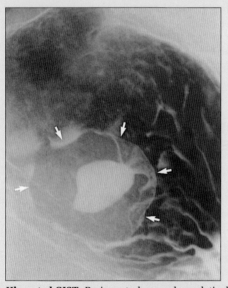

Figure 3. Ulcerated GIST. Barium study reveals a relatively large benign GIST *(arrows)* in the fundus with a central area of ulceration, producing a "bull's-eye" lesion. *(From O'Riordan D, Levine MS, Yeager BA: Complete healing of ulceration within a gastric leiomyoma. Gastrointest Radiol 10:47-49, 1985. With kind permission from Springer Science and Business Media.)*

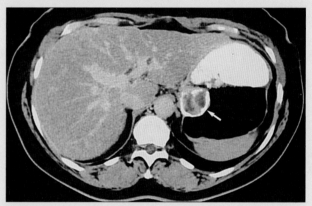

Figure 4. Benign GIST with gastric calcification. In this patient, a peripherally calcified benign GIST *(arrow)* is shown on a CT scan. *(Courtesy of Alec J. Megibow, MD, New York, NY.)*

Suggested Readings

Morrissey K, Cho ES, Gray GF, et al: Muscular tumors of the stomach: Clinical and pathological study of 113 cases. *Ann Surg* 178: 148-155, 1973.

O'Riordan D, Levine MS, Yeager BA: Complete healing of ulceration within a gastric leiomyoma. *Gastrointest Radiol* 10:47-49, 1985.

Sanders L, Silverman M, Rossi R, et al: Gastric smooth muscle tumors: Diagnostic dilemmas and factors affecting outcome. *World J Surg* 20:992-995, 1996.

Suster S: Gastrointestinal stromal tumors. *Semin Diagn Pathol* 13: 297-313, 1996.

Other Mesenchymal Tumors

DEFINITION: Tumors in the stomach and duodenum that arise from mesenchymal cells.

IMAGING

Radiography
Findings
- Large lipomas containing sufficient amount of fat may occasionally appear as radiolucent shadows on abdominal radiographs.
- Lipomas, hemangiomas, lymphangiomas, glomus tumors: smooth submucosal mass or centrally ulcerated bull's-eye lesions indistinguishable from benign gastrointestinal stromal tumors (GISTs).
- Presence of phleboliths within the lesion should be virtually pathognomonic of hemangioma.
- Glomus tumor may contain tiny flecks of calcification.
- Glomus tumor, lipoma, and lymphangioma may have a soft consistency, changing in shape with peristalsis or compression.

Utility
- Abdominal radiographs
- Barium studies

CT
Findings
- Lipomas typically appear as well-circumscribed lesions of uniform fatty density with attenuation of 70-120 Hounsfield units.
- CT may reveal linear strands of soft-tissue density or ulceration within tumor.

Utility
- Lipomas can be definitively diagnosed by CT; thus, endoscopy or surgery is unnecessary.

CLINICAL PRESENTATION

- Small lipomas cause no symptoms, but larger lesions may undergo ulceration, causing abdominal pain or upper gastrointestinal bleeding.
- Pedunculated antral lipomas may prolapse through the pylorus, causing intermittent gastric outlet obstruction with recurrent nausea and vomiting.
- Hemangiomas may produce massive upper gastrointestinal bleeding.

DIAGNOSTIC PEARLS

- Lipomas, hemangiomas, lymphangiomas, and glomus tumors: smooth submucosal masses or centrally ulcerated bull's-eye lesions that are indistinguishable from benign GISTs are seen.
- Presence of phleboliths within the lesion should be virtually pathognomonic of hemangioma.
- Glomus tumors, lipomas, and lymphangiomas have a soft consistency and change in shape with peristalsis or compression.
- Lipomas typically appear as well-circumscribed lesions of uniform fatty density with attenuation of 70-120 Hounsfield units.

- Lymphangiomas, when large enough, may cause obstruction or intussusception.
- Glomus tumors may contain ulceration, causing upper gastrointestinal bleeding.

DIFFERENTIAL DIAGNOSIS

- Benign gastrointestinal stromal tumors
- Malignant gastrointestinal stromal tumors

PATHOLOGY

- Lipomas are composed of mature fat cells surrounded by fibrous capsule; they occur as solitary lesions, most frequently in the gastric antrum.
- Hemangiomas appear on endoscopy as bluish-black submucosal lesions.
- Lymphangiomas consist histologically of irregularly dilated lymphatic channels lined by benign-appearing endothelial cells.
- Lymphangiomas may be developmental malformations arising from sequestered lymphatic tissue; the cystic appearance results from accumulation of fluid.

WHAT THE REFERRING PHYSICIAN NEEDS TO KNOW

- Larger lesions that cause symptoms should be resected.
- Gastric or duodenal lipomas can be definitively diagnosed by CT, avoiding the need for endoscopy or surgery.
- The presence of additional telangiectasias on the skin should suggest a diagnosis of hemangioma in patients with a submucosal mass in the stomach on barium study.
- Glomus tumor: Local excision is curative; high cellularity can mimic malignancy on frozen sections; thus, an unnecessarily extensive resection is sometimes performed.

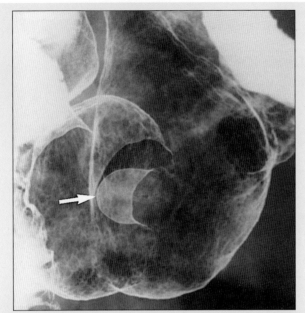

Figure 1. Gastric lipoma. Double-contrast view shows a smooth submucosal mass *(arrow)* in the antrum. *(From Laufer I, Levine MS [eds]: Double Contrast Gastrointestinal Radiology, 2nd ed. Philadelphia, WB Saunders, 1992.)*

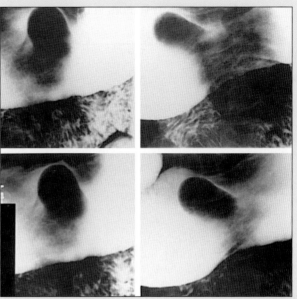

Figure 2. Gastric lipoma. Prone single-contrast views from same examination as in Figure 1 show how the lesion changes in size and shape with varying degrees of compression. This changing appearance should be highly suggestive of a lipoma. *(From Laufer I, Levine MS [eds]: Double Contrast Gastrointestinal Radiology, 2nd ed. Philadelphia, WB Saunders, 1992.)*

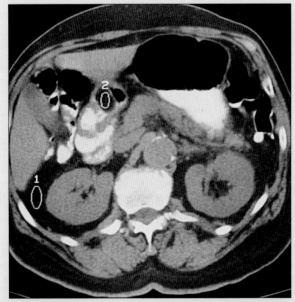

Figure 3. Gastric lipoma. CT scan from the same patient shown in Figures 1 and 2 shows how the lesion in the antrum *(cursor 2)* has the same density as perirenal fat *(cursor 1)*, confirming the presence of a lipoma. *(From Laufer I, Levine MS [eds]: Double Contrast Gastrointestinal Radiology, 2nd ed. Philadelphia, WB Saunders, 1992.)*

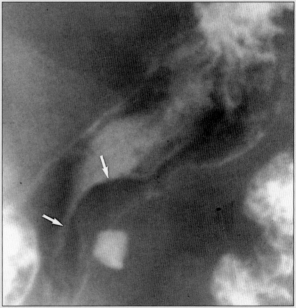

Figure 4. Glomus tumor. An ulcerated submucosal mass (bull's-eye lesion) *(arrows)* is seen on the greater curvature of the antrum. This lesion cannot be distinguished from other, more common mesenchymal tumors in the stomach. *(Courtesy of Bruce Knox, MD, Norfolk, VA.)*

- Glomus tumors are highly cellular, usually occurring as solitary lesions in the antrum ranging from 1-4 cm in size.

INCIDENCE/PREVALENCE AND EPIDEMIOLOGY

- Gastric lipomas are rare, constituting only approximately 5% of all gastrointestinal tract lipomas and less than 1% of all gastric neoplasms.
- Hemangiomas constitute less than 2% of all benign tumors in the stomach.
- Hemangiomas are even rarer in the duodenum.
- Lymphangiomas are rare benign tumors of the stomach and duodenum.
- Gastrointestinal hemangiomas may be associated with telangiectasias on the skin (Osler-Weber-Rendu syndrome).

Suggested Readings

Davis M, Fenoglio-Preiser C, Haque AK: Cavernous lymphangioma of the duodenum. *Gastrointest Radiol* 12:10-12, 1987.

Harig BM, Rosen Y, Dallemand S, et al: Glomus tumor of the stomach. *Am J Gastroenterol* 63:423-428, 1975.

Heiken JP, Forde KA, Gold RP: Computed tomography as a definitive method for diagnosing gastrointestinal lipomas. *Radiology* 142:409-414, 1982.

Kerekes ES: Gastric hemangioma. *Radiology* 82:468-469, 1964.

Maderal F, Hunter F, Fuselier G, et al: Gastric lipomas: An update of clinical presentation, diagnosis, and treatment. *Am J Gastroenterol* 79:964-967, 1984.

Megibow AJ, Redmond PE, Bosniak MA, et al: Diagnosis of gastrointestinal lipomas by CT. *AJR Am J Roentgenol* 133:743-745, 1979.

Simms SM: Gastric hemangioma associated with phleboliths. *Gastrointest Radiol* 10:51-53, 1985.

Taylor AJ, Stewart ET, Dodds WJ: Gastrointestinal lipomas: A radiologic and pathologic review. *Am J Gastroenterol* 155:1205-1210, 1990.

Ectopic Pancreatic Rests

DEFINITION: Ectopic pancreatic rests are pancreatic elements arranged haphazardly in organs other than normal pancreatic tissue.

ANATOMIC FINDINGS

Stomach
- Tend to be located on greater curvature of the distal antrum within 1-6 cm from pylorus

IMAGING

Radiography
Findings
- Pancreatic rests are smooth, broad-based submucosal masses, closely resembling benign gastrointestinal stromal tumors (GISTs) or other mesenchymal tumors but are almost always located on the greater curvature of the distal antrum within 1-6 cm from the pylorus.
- Lesions are solitary, ranging from 1-3 cm in size.
- Lesions may have a central umbilication, 1-5 mm in diameter, 5-10 mm in depth, mimicking a bull's-eye appearance of ulcerated GISTs or other mesenchymal tumors.
- Barium rarely may reflux into rudimentary ductal structures terminating in tiny club-shaped pouches; this finding is virtually pathognomonic of ectopic pancreatic rests.
- Occasionally found in proximal duodenum

Utility
- Barium studies

CLINICAL PRESENTATION

- Asymptomatic
- Epigastric pain or upper gastrointestinal bleeding

DIAGNOSTIC PEARLS

- Solitary lesions, ranging from 1-3 cm in size
- Smooth, broad-based submucosal masses
- Central umbilication
- Location on greater curvature of distal antrum

DIFFERENTIAL DIAGNOSIS

- GISTs (stomach and duodenum)
- Other mesenchymal tumors (stomach and duodenum)
- Metastases (stomach and duodenum)
- Lymphoma (stomach and duodenum)

PATHOLOGY

- Histologically consists of all pancreatic elements, including acini, ducts, and islet cells.
- Results from abnormal embryologic development with fragments of ventral or dorsal pancreatic anlage implanted in intestinal wall
- Primitive epithelial buds undergo differentiation toward mature glandular tissue.

Suggested Readings

Clark RE, Teplick SK: Ectopic pancreas causing massive gastrointestinal hemorrhage: Report of a case diagnosed angiographically. *Gastroenterology* 69:1331-1333, 1975.

Kilman WJ, Berk RN: The spectrum of radiographic features of aberrant pancreatic rests involving the stomach. *Radiology* 123:291-296, 1977.

Thoeni RF, Gedgaudas RK: Ectopic pancreas: Usual and unusual features. *Gastrointest Radiol* 5:37-42, 1980.

WHAT THE REFERRING PHYSICIAN NEEDS TO KNOW

- Ectopic pancreatic rests should be resected only if the patient is symptomatic or if significant neoplasm cannot be excluded nonoperatively.

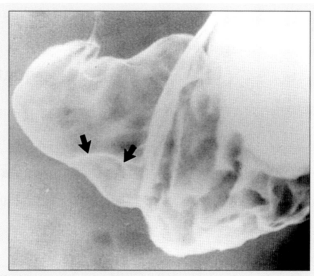

Figure 1. Ectopic pancreatic rest. The leison appears as a discrete submucosal mass *(arrows)* on the greater curvature of the distal antrum. This is a characteristic location for ectopic pancreatic rests. (*From Laufer 1. Levine MS [eds]:* Double Contrast Gastrointestinal Radiology, *2nd ed. Philadelphia, WB Saunders, 1992.*)

Brunner's Gland Hyperplasia (Duodenum)

DEFINITION: Diffuse enlargement of Brunner's glands throughout the proximal duodenum or massive enlargement of a single gland.

ANATOMIC FINDINGS

Duodenal Bulb
- Site of more abundant hyperplastic nodules

IMAGING

Radiography
Findings
- Hyperplasia: multiple small, rounded nodules in the proximal duodenum, producing *cobblestone* or *Swiss cheese* appearance, most abundant in duodenal bulb
- Central flecks of barium may be identified in the nodules.
- Brunner's gland hamartomas are submucosal or sessile lesions, ranging from several millimeters to several centimeters in size.
- Giant Brunner's gland hamartomas are large polypoid defects in the duodenum.
- Concomitant duodenitis: markedly thickened, irregular folds in the proximal duodenum
Utility
- Barium studies

CLINICAL PRESENTATION

- Diffuse form of Brunner's gland hyperplasia has no clinical significance except for its association with duodenal ulcers and gastric hypersecretory states.
- Brunner's gland hamartomas may cause obstructive symptoms, epigastric pain, or upper gastrointestinal bleeding because of ulceration of overlying mucosa.
- Rarely, large intramural masses cause mechanical obstruction of the duodenum or duodenojejunal intussusception.

DIAGNOSTIC PEARLS

- *Cobblestone* or *Swiss cheese* appearance
- Abundant nodules in the duodenal bulb
- Submucosal or sessile lesions

DIFFERENTIAL DIAGNOSIS

- Adenomatous or hyperplastic polyps (duodenum)
- Lymphoid hyperplasia
- Heterotopic gastric mucosa
- Ectopic pancreatic rest
- Carcinoid

PATHOLOGY

- Diffuse enlargement of Brunner's glands throughout the proximal duodenum or massive enlargement of a single gland
- Intimate admixture of ducts, acini, smooth muscle, and adipose tissue without evidence of cellular atypia; classified as hamartomas rather than true neoplasms

Suggested Readings

Dodd GD, Fishler JS, Park OK: Hyperplasia of Brunner's glands: Report of two cases with review of the literature. *Radiology* 60:814-823, 1953.

Franzin G, Musola R, Ghidini O, et al: Nodular hyperplasia of Brunner's glands. *Gastrointest Endosc* 31:374-378, 1985.

Kaplan EL, Dyson WL, Fitts WT: The relationship of gastric hyperacidity to hyperplasia of Brunner's glands. *Arch Surg* 98:636-639, 1969.

Nielson OF, Whitaker EG, Roberts FM: Adenoma of Brunner's glands. *Am J Surg* 110:977-980, 1965.

Osborne R, Toffler R, Lowman RM: Brunner's gland adenoma of the duodenum. *Am J Dig Dis* 18:689-694, 1973.

Strutynsky N, Posniak R, Mori K: Obstructing hamartoma of Brunner's glands of the duodenum. *Dig Dis Sci* 27:279-282, 1982.

WHAT THE REFERRING PHYSICIAN NEEDS TO KNOW

- Diffuse form of Brunner's hyperplasia requires no specific treatment.
- Solitary lesions should be resected if they cause symptoms or if the pathologic diagnosis is in doubt.
- Endoscopic polypectomy may be feasible if the lesion is small or pedunculated, but surgery may be required for larger lesions.

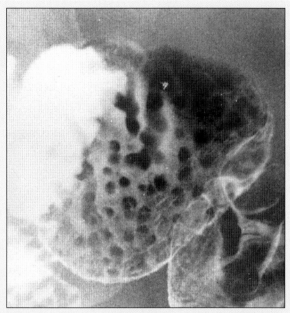

Figure 1. **Brunner's gland hyperplasia: spectrum of findings.** Multiple tiny, rounded nodules are present in the duodenal bulb in a patient with diffuse Brunner's gland hyperplasia. (*From Laufer I, Levine MS [eds]:* Double Contrast Gastrointestinal Radiology, *2nd ed. Philadelphia, WB Saunders, 1992.*)

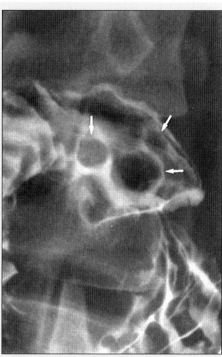

Figure 2. **Brunner's gland hyperplasia: spectrum of findings.** This patient has several Brunner's gland hamartomas in the duodenum, characterized by submucosal masses (*arrows*) in the bulb.

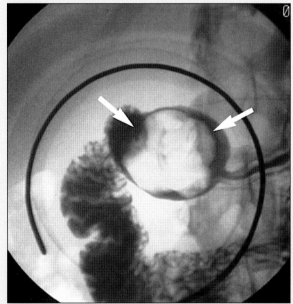

Figure 3. **Brunner's gland hyperplasia: spectrum of findings.** A large polypoid defect (*arrows*) is seen in the duodenal bulb in a patient with a giant Brunner's gland hamartoma. (*Courtesy of Jackie Brown, MD, Vancouver, Canada.*)

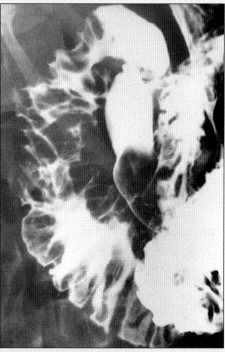

Figure 4. **Brunner's gland hyperplasia: spectrum of findings.** A patient with enlarged Brunner's glands has markedly thickened, disorganized folds in the descending duodenum because of concomitant duodenitis. (*Courtesy of Dean D. T. Maglinte, MD, Indianapolis, IN.*)

Part 18

CARCINOMA OF THE STOMACH AND DUODENUM

Gastric Carcinoma

DEFINITION: Gastric cancer is a group of primary gastric malignancies with papillary, tubular, mucinous, or signet-ring cell histology.

IMAGING

Radiography
Findings
- Early type I: small, sessile or pedunculated polyps
- Early type II: superficial lesions with elevated (IIa), flat (IIb), or depressed (IIc) components
- Early type III: shallow, irregular ulcer craters with nodularity of adjacent mucosa, and clubbing, fusion, or amputation of radiating folds
- Advanced carcinomas: lobulated or fungating masses that protrude into the lumen
- Scirrhous carcinomas: narrowed, tubular configuration of the gas-filled stomach (linitis plastica or *leather bottle* appearance)
- Mucin-producing scirrhous carcinomas: calcification that has a stippled, punctate, or sand-like appearance
- Ulcerated carcinomas: ulcer crater with scalloped, angular, or stellate borders, eccentrically located within the mass

Utility
- Barium studies
- Single-contrast examinations have an overall sensitivity of only 75% in diagnosing gastric carcinoma.
- Double-contrast examinations can detect 99% of these tumors.
- When the index of suspicion is low, a double-contrast barium study may be performed as a cost-effective test to confirm that the stomach is normal.

DIAGNOSTIC PEARLS
- Lobulated or fungating masses that protrude into the lumen
- Narrowed, tubular configuration of the gas-filled stomach produces a linitis plastica or *leather bottle* appearance.
- Ulcer craters have scalloped, angular, or stellate borders and are eccentrically placed within the mass.
- Calcification or low attenuation within the thickened gastric wall on CT suggests mucinous adenocarcinoma.
- Thickened muscularis propria on endoscopic ultrasonography is virtually pathognomonic of a malignant gastric tumor.

CT
Findings
- Polypoid, fungating, ulcerated, or infiltrating lesion
- After contrast: stratified enhancement with brightly enhancing mucosal and serosal layers and less enhancement of submucosal and muscular layers of gastric wall
- Calcification or low attenuation within the thickened gastric wall suggests mucinous adenocarcinoma.

Utility
- CT is a particularly sensitive technique for demonstrating calcification.

WHAT THE REFERRING PHYSICIAN NEEDS TO KNOW
- Gastric cancers have a relatively even distribution in the stomach (30% in the antrum, 30% in the body, 40% in the fundus or cardiac region).
- Gastric cardia and fundus must be carefully evaluated on barium studies or endoscopy to rule out carcinoma.
- Approximately 60% of patients have unresectable tumors; palliative resection or bypass procedure may be performed to prevent obstruction.
- Endoscopy and biopsy should be performed for all lesions with suspicious radiographic findings to avoid missing early cancers.
- When the index of suspicion is high, EUS is recommended to confirm the diagnosis.
- Radiographically demonstrated lesions at the cardia may occasionally be missed at endoscopy; barium study should be repeated in these patients to confirm presence of tumor.

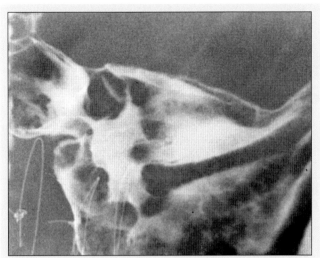

Figure 1. **Early gastric cancer.** A type III lesion is seen as a scalloped, irregular antral ulcer with nodular, clubbed folds surrounding the ulcer crater. (*From Levine MS, Creteur V, Kressel HY, et al: Benign gastric ulcers: Diagnosis and follow-up with double-contrast radiography.* Radiology *164:9-13, 1987.*)

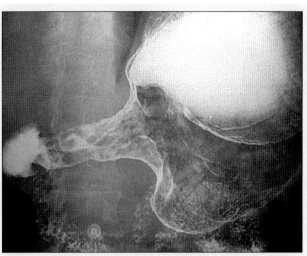

Figure 2. **Scirrhous carcinoma of the stomach.** Narrowing of the antrum is marked as a result of infiltration of the wall by tumor.

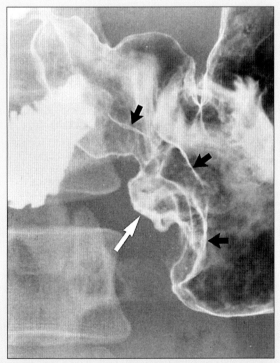

Figure 3. **Malignant gastric ulcer.** This patient has an ulcerated mass on the greater curvature of the antrum. Note how the ulcer (*white arrow*) has an intraluminal location. Also note how the mass itself is etched in white (*black arrows*).

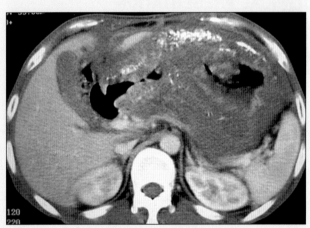

Figure 4. **Mucinous adenocarcinoma of the stomach.** CT image shows massive thickening of the gastric wall and marked luminal narrowing by an advanced, infiltrating carcinoma. Also note extensive calcification within the tumor. This type of calcification is characteristic of mucinous adenocarcinomas of the stomach.

- Multidetector CT is used to create high-quality images in all viewing planes.

Ultrasound
Findings
- Thickened muscularis propria is virtually pathognomonic of a malignant gastric tumor, most often gastric adenocarcinoma, and, less frequently, lymphoma.

Utility
- Endoscopic ultrasonography (EUS) has substantially improved accuracy for local staging of gastric carcinomas.
- EUS enables visualization of the gastric wall layers and perigastric lymph nodes and shows the relationship of the tumor to the surrounding tissues.
- EUS is best performed as a complementary test to cross-sectional imaging studies such as CT for local tumor staging.
- Overall diagnostic accuracy of EUS for determining nodal status (N classification) ranges from 70%-90%.
- Limitation of EUS is its inability to detect nonenlarged nodes more than 3 cm from the gastric wall.

CLINICAL PRESENTATION

- Epigastric pain, bloating, early satiety, nausea, vomiting, and dysphagia
- Anorexia and weight loss
- Signs or symptoms of upper gastrointestinal bleeding, such as hematemesis, melena, guaiac-positive stool, and iron-deficiency anemia
- Advanced gastric cancer: signs or symptoms of metastatic disease may be present.

DIFFERENTIAL DIAGNOSIS

- Adenocarcinoma of esophagus invading stomach
- Adult hypertrophic stenosis (stomach and duodenum)
- Antral gastritis
- Ménétrier disease (stomach)
- Ulcers (pyloric channel or distal gastric antrum) with marked surrounding edema

PATHOLOGY

- Gross features: polypoid carcinomas have a plaque-like, lobulated, or fungating appearance.
- Ulcerated carcinomas may contain deep, irregular and broad shallow areas of ulceration caused by necrosis and excavation of the tumor.
- *Scirrhous* tumors may produce a classic *linitis plastica* appearance as a result of submucosal thickening and fibrosis.
- Histology includes papillary, tubular, mucinous, and signet-ring cell types of tumor.

- As they infiltrate the gastric wall, signet-ring cell tumors often incite a marked desmoplastic response in the submucosa and muscularis propria, producing the classic pathologic features of primary scirrhous carcinoma.
- By definition, *advanced gastric cancers* have already invaded the muscularis propria.
- Early gastric cancers are defined histologically as cancers in which malignant invasion is limited to the mucosa or submucosa, regardless of the presence or absence of lymph node metastases.

INCIDENCE/PREVALENCE AND EPIDEMIOLOGY

- Gastric carcinoma is usually considered a disease of middle and late life, with a peak incidence between 50 and 70 years of age.
- Younger patients constitute 3%-5% of all patients with gastric carcinoma; they also tend to have more aggressive lesions.
- Gastric carcinoma is twice as common in men as in women.
- Carcinoma of the cardia has much greater predilection for men (7:1) than carcinomas elsewhere in stomach.
- Gastric carcinoma has striking geographic variations, with highest incidences reported in Japan, Chile, Finland, Poland, and Iceland.
- Dietary habits may be particularly important in explaining observed geographic differences in cancer risk.
- *Helicobacter pylori* infection, atrophic gastritis, pernicious anemia, gastric polyps, partial gastrectomy, and Ménétrier disease are risk factors for gastric carcinoma.

Suggested Readings

Correa P, Haenszel W, Cuello C, et al: Gastric precancerous process in a high risk population: Cross sectional studies. *Cancer Res* 50:4731-4736, 1990.
Forman D, Newell DG, Fullerton F, et al: Association between infection with *Helicobacter pylori* and risk of gastric cancer: Evidence from a prospective investigation. *BMJ* 302:1302-1305, 1991.
Levine MS, Kong V, Rubesin SE, et al: Scirrhous carcinoma of the stomach: Radiologic and endoscopic diagnosis. *Radiology* 175:151-154, 1990.
Low VHS, Levine MS, Rubesin SE, et al: Diagnosis of gastric carcinoma; sensitivity of double-contrast barium studies. *AJR Am J Roentgenol* 162:329-334, 1994.
Mirvish SS: Effects of vitamins C and E on N-nitroso compound formation, carcinogenesis, and cancer. *Cancer* 58:1842-1850, 1986.
Mirvish SS: The etiology of gastric cancer: Intragastric nitrosamide formation and other theories. *J Natl Cancer Inst* 71:629-647, 1983.
Neugut AI, Hayek M, Howe G: Epidemiology of gastric cancer. *Semin Oncol* 23:281-291, 1996.
Oiso T: Incidence of stomach cancer and its relation to dietary habits and nutrition in Japan between 1900 and 1975. *Cancer Res* 35:3254-3258, 1975.
Terry P, Lagergren J, Ye W, et al: Inverse association between intake of cereal fiber and risk of gastric cardia cancer. *Gastroenterology* 120:387-391, 2001.
White RM, Levine MS, Enterline HT, et al: Early gastric cancer: Recent experience. *Radiology* 155:25-27, 1985.

Duodenal Carcinoma

DEFINITION: Duodenal carcinoma is a malignant tumor of the duodenum.

ANATOMIC FINDINGS

Duodenum
- Almost all lesions are located at or distal to the ampulla of Vater.

IMAGING

Radiography
Findings
- Polypoid, ulcerated, or annular lesions are seen at or, more commonly, distal to the ampulla of Vater.
- Rarely, early duodenal cancers appear on double-contrast barium studies as small (less than 2 cm), sessile, polypoid, or ulcerated lesions.
- Infiltrating form of the tumor may produce marked narrowing, with a linitis plastica appearance.

Utility
- Barium studies

CT
Findings
- Localized area of wall thickening is seen, producing a soft-tissue mass.
- Infiltrating form of the tumor may produce a linitis plastica appearance.

Utility
- Features such as tumor necrosis and ulceration are readily identified.
- With duodenal mass containing central necrosis and ulceration, CT has a sensitivity of 100% and accuracy of 86% for detecting a malignant tumor.
- CT is useful for differentiating primary duodenal carcinoma from extrinsic tumors involving the duodenum.
- Three-dimensional multidetector CT is particularly helpful for localizing neoplasms and defining tumor extent.
- Hypotonic CT duodenography may be useful for differentiating pancreatic carcinoma from duodenal carcinoma.

CLINICAL PRESENTATION

- Clinical findings usually occur when the tumor is already at an advanced stage.
- Weight loss

DIAGNOSTIC PEARLS

- Polypoid, ulcerated, or annular lesions
- Ulcerated masses in the proximal descending duodenum or even the duodenal bulb
- Localized area of wall thickening
- Infiltrating forms of the tumor produce a linitis plastica appearance.

- Nausea, vomiting, and abdominal pain
- Signs or symptoms of upper gastrointestinal bleeding

DIFFERENTIAL DIAGNOSIS

- Lymphoma (duodenum)
- Ampullary carcinoma
- Pancreatic carcinoma
- Metastatic tumor

INCIDENCE/PREVALENCE AND EPIDEMIOLOGY

- Duodenal carcinoma accounts for less than 1% of all gastrointestinal neoplasms.
- Incidence is increased in patients with Gardner syndrome and celiac disease.
- Duodenal carcinoma has also been associated with Crohn disease and neurofibromatosis.

Suggested Readings

Bradford D, Levine MS, Hoang D, et al: Early duodenal cancer: Detection on double-contrast upper gastrointestinal radiography. *AJR Am J Roentgenol* 174:1564-1566, 2000.

Cortese AF, Cornell GN: Carcinoma of the duodenum. *Cancer* 29:1010-1015, 1972.

Itoh H, Iida M, Kuroiwa S, et al: Gardner's syndrome associated with carcinoma of the duodenal bulb: Report of a case. *Am J Gastroenterol* 80:248-250, 1985.

McGlinchey JJ, Santer GJ, Haggani MT: Primary adenocarcinoma of the duodenum associated with cutaneous neurofibromatosis. *Postgrad Med J* 58:115-116, 1982.

Meiselman MS, Ghahremani GG, Kaufman MW: Crohn's disease of the duodenum complicated by adenocarcinoma. *Gastrointest Radiol* 12:333-336, 1987.

WHAT THE REFERRING PHYSICIAN NEEDS TO KNOW

- Distinguishing ampullary and periampullary carcinomas from primary pancreatic carcinomas is important because ampullary tumors have a much better prognosis.
- The vast majority of duodenal ulcers are benign; endoscopy therefore should be considered only for lesions that have suspicious radiographic features.

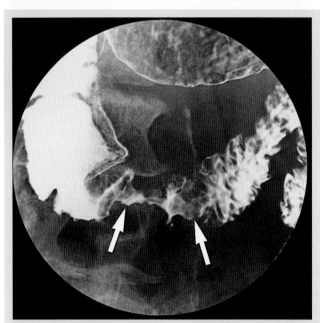

Figure 1. Duodenal carcinoma. An annular, ulcerated lesion *(arrows)* is seen in the third portion of the duodenum.

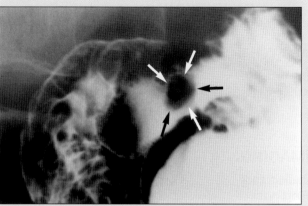

Figure 2. Early duodenal cancer. Double-contrast spot image of duodenum shows a sessile, slightly lobulated, 1.3-cm polypoid lesion *(arrows)* in the duodenal bulb. This cancer was an early cancer confined to the mucosa. (*Reprinted with permission from the American Journal of Roentgenology. From Bradford D, Levine MS, Hoang D, et al: Early duodenal cancer: Detection on double-contrast upper gastrointestinal radiography. AJR Am J Roentgenol 174:1564-1566, 2000.*)

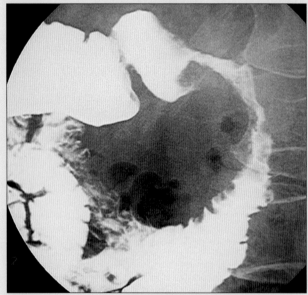

Figure 3. Duodenal carcinoma. Barium study shows an advanced infiltrating carcinoma of the descending duodenum, producing a linitis plastica appearance.

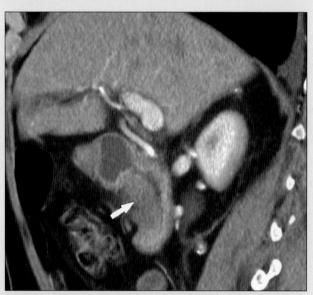

Figure 4. Duodenal carcinoma. Three-dimensional volume-rendered multidetector CT (MDCT) scan from same patient as in Figure 3 shows narrowing of the postbulbar duodenum by an eccentric soft-tissue mass arising in the wall *(arrow)*.

Metastases to the Stomach and Duodenum

DEFINITION: Metastases to the stomach and duodenum are blood- or lymph-borne deposits seeding from primary tumor.

IMAGING

Radiography

Findings

- Hematogenous metastases: one or, more commonly, multiple discrete submucosal masses
- Large masses with central necrosis and ulceration: classic "bull's-eye" or "target" lesion
- Superficial fissures may occasionally radiate toward central ulcer crater, producing characteristic spoke-wheel pattern.
- Cavitated metastases: amorphous collections of barium (usually 5-15 cm in size) that communicate with lumen
- Breast carcinoma metastases: linitis plastica appearance, with mucosal nodularity, spiculation, ulceration, and thickened, irregular folds on double-contrast studies, mimicking appearance of primary scirrhous carcinoma of stomach
- Retroperitoneal tumor involving duodenum may cause delayed gastric emptying with massive gastric dilatation out of proportion to duodenal dilation.
- Metastases to retroperitoneal lymph nodes near superior mesenteric root: extrinsic mass effect, nodular indentations, ulceration, and obstruction of distal duodenum

Utility

- Barium studies
- Larger, more lobulated masses can mimic malignant gastrointestinal stromal tumors (GISTs) or even polypoid carcinomas.

DIAGNOSTIC PEARLS

- Hematogenous metastases: one or, more commonly, multiple discrete submucosal masses
- Large masses with central necrosis and ulceration: classic "bull's-eye" or "target" lesions
- Retroperitoneal tumor involving duodenum may cause delayed gastric emptying with massive gastric dilation out of proportion to duodenal dilation.

CT

Findings

- Giant, cavitated lesions
- Breast carcinoma metastases: thickened gastric wall, producing linitis plastica appearance
- Some metastatic breast cancers may be manifested by focal wall thickening.
- Squamous cell metastases to lymph nodes in upper abdomen are seen as multiple low-attenuation masses relative to skeletal muscle.
- CT is extremely helpful for determining cause of widened duodenal sweep and for differentiating pancreatic mass from adjacent lymphadenopathy.

Utility

- CT is particularly well suited for demonstrating giant, cavitated metastases.
- Linitis plastica or "leather bottle" appearance of gastric metastases may be indistinguishable from that of primary scirrhous carcinoma of stomach

---

WHAT THE REFERRING PHYSICIAN NEEDS TO KNOW

- Possibility of metastatic disease should be considered in any patient with linitis plastica who has a history of breast carcinoma.
- Focal wall metastases reside deep within the gastric wall, making it difficult to obtain a definitive pathologic diagnosis by endoscopic biopsy.
- Carcinoma of the breast or kidney can metastasize to the stomach or duodenum many years after treatment of original tumor.
- Metastases that have a submucosal appearance can be mistaken for benign intramural lesions such as GISTs, lipomas, or ectopic pancreatic rests.
- Differential diagnosis for "bull's-eye" lesions includes lymphoma, Kaposi sarcoma, carcinoid tumors, and large varioliform erosions.
- Differential diagnosis for giant cavitated lesions includes lymphoma and malignant GISTs.
- Other considerations in differential diagnosis include multiple hyperplastic or adenomatous polyps and primary scirrhous carcinoma of stomach (linitis plastica).

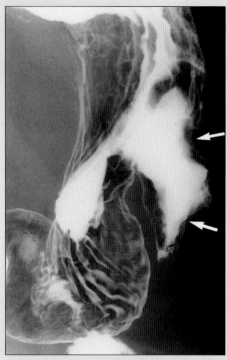

Figure 1. **Cavitated metastasis from malignant melanoma.** A giant, cavitated lesion *(arrows)* is seen on the greater curvature of the stomach. A malignant gastrointestinal stromal tumor or lymphoma could produce similar findings. *(From Laufer I, Levine MS [eds]:* Double Contrast Gastrointestinal Radiology, *2nd ed. Philadelphia, WB Saunders, 1992.)*

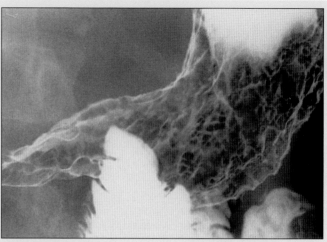

Figure 2. **Metastatic breast cancer involving the stomach with a linitis plastica appearance.** There is only mild loss of distensibility of the gastric antrum and body, but the mucosa has a nodular, irregular appearance because of infiltration by metastatic tumor. *(From Levine MS, Kong V, Rubesin SE, et al: Scirrhous carcinoma of the stomach: Radiologic and endoscopic diagnosis.* Radiology *175:151-154, 1990.)*

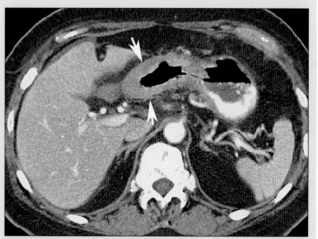

Figure 4. **Metastatic breast cancer to the stomach with a linitis plastica appearance on CT**. Multidetector CT (MDCT) image in an elderly woman with metastatic breast carcinoma and early satiety shows marked thickening of the wall of the gastric antrum *(arrows)*. The radiographic findings are indistinguishable from those of a primary scirrhous carcinoma of the stomach.

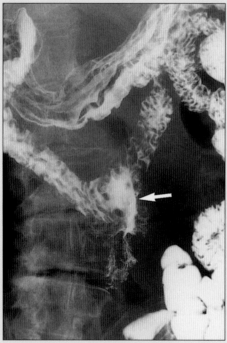

Figure 3. **Duodenal invasion by retroperitoneal adenopathy.** Barium study shows an ulcerated lesion *(arrow)* at the junction of the third and fourth portions of the duodenum.

PET
Findings
- Increased activity on fluorodeoxyglucose (FDG)-PET

CLINICAL PRESENTATION

- Most gastroduodenal metastases are discovered unexpectedly at surgery or autopsy.
- Some patients with ulcerated metastases may develop signs or symptoms of upper gastrointestinal bleeding, such as hematemesis, melena, and guaiac-positive stool.
- Others may present with epigastric pain, nausea, vomiting, early satiety, anorexia, or weight loss.
- Most patients with gastroduodenal metastases have known underlying malignancy.
- Occasionally, metastases to the stomach or duodenum may occur as the initial manifestation of an occult primary tumor.

DIFFERENTIAL DIAGNOSIS

- Lymphoma (stomach and duodenum)
- Kaposi sarcoma (stomach and duodenum)
- Carcinoid tumor (stomach and duodenum)
- GIST (stomach and duodenum)
- Primary scirrhous carcinoma (stomach)

PATHOLOGY

- Gastric metastases are most commonly from malignant melanoma or breast carcinoma, and, less frequently, other remote malignant tumors such as thyroid or testicular carcinoma.
- Esophageal squamous cell carcinoma metastases to stomach are caused by tumor emboli via submucosal esophageal lymphatics extending subdiaphragmatically.
- Duodenum is occasionally involved by peripancreatic lymphadenopathy from pancreatic carcinoma, lymphoma, or other malignant tumors.

- Linitis plastica appearance of metastatic breast carcinoma to stomach is caused by highly cellular infiltrates of metastatic tumor in gastric wall.

INCIDENCE/PREVALENCE AND EPIDEMIOLOGY

- Gastric metastases are found at autopsy in less than 2% of patients who die of carcinoma.
- Duodenal metastases are even rarer.
- Gastric metastases are found at autopsy in 2%-15% of patients who die of squamous cell carcinoma of the esophagus.
- In two studies, metastases to the stomach were detected on CT in 5%-27% of patients with breast carcinoma.
- Malignant melanoma has the highest percentage of hematogenous metastases to the gastrointestinal tract, followed by breast cancer.

Suggested Readings

Asch MJ, Wiedel PD, Habif DV: Gastrointestinal metastases from carcinoma of the breast: Autopsy study and 18 cases requiring operative intervention. *Arch Surg* 96:840-843, 1968.

Chang SF, Burrell MI, Brand MH, et al: The protean gastrointestinal manifestations of metastatic breast carcinoma. *Radiology* 126:611-617, 1978.

Das Gupta TK, Brasfield RD: Metastatic melanoma of the gastrointestinal tract. *Arch Surg* 88:969-973, 1964.

Hsu CC, Chen JJ, Changchien CS: Endoscopic features of metastatic tumors in the upper gastrointestinal tract. *Endoscopy* 28:249-253, 1996.

Khilnani MT, Wolf BS: Late involvement of the alimentary tract by carcinoma of the kidney. *Am J Dig Dis* 5:529-540, 1960.

Klein MS, Sherlock P: Gastric and colonic metastases from breast carcinoma. *Am J Dig Dis* 17:881-886, 1972.

Menuck LS, Amberg JR: Metastatic disease involving the stomach. *Am J Dig Dis* 20:903-913, 1975.

Meyers MA, McSweeney J: Secondary neoplasms of the bowel. *Radiology* 105:1-11, 1972.

Lymphoma

ANATOMIC FINDINGS

Esophagus
- "Volcano crater" on endoscopy
- Thickened, irregular folds, luminal narrowing, or polypoid mass in distal esophagus

Stomach
- Infiltrative gastric lymphomas: focal or diffuse rugal fold enlargement resulting from submucosal tumor spread; massively enlarged folds often have distorted, nodular contour.
- Non-Hodgkin lymphomas: linitis plastica with varying degrees of narrowing of gastric antrum, body, or fundus, and nodularity, ulceration, and thickened or effaced mucosal folds
- Ulcerative lymphomas: ulcerated lesions are occasionally surrounded by smooth mound of tumor or symmetric, radiating folds, mimicking benign gastric ulcers.
- Ulcers' irregular configuration is associated with surrounding nodular mucosa or thickened, irregular folds resulting from lymphomatous infiltration of gastric wall.
- Giant, cavitated lesions result from necrosis and excavation of tumor.
- Polypoid gastric lymphomas: one or more lobulated intraluminal masses

DIAGNOSTIC PEARLS
- Presence of lymphadenopathy beyond expected drainage pathways of primary gastric carcinoma should suggest diagnosis of gastric lymphoma.
- Infiltrative gastric lymphomas: focal or diffuse enlargement of rugal folds resulting from submucosal spread of tumor; massively enlarged folds often have distorted, nodular contour.
- Ulcerative lymphomas: ulcerated lesions occasionally are surrounded by smooth mound of tumor or symmetric, radiating folds, mimicking benign gastric ulcers.
- Polypoid gastric lymphomas: one or more lobulated intraluminal masses are seen in the stomach.
- Nodular form of gastric lymphoma: multiple submucosal nodules or masses, ranging from several millimeters to several centimeters, are seen in the stomach.

- Nodular form of gastric lymphoma: multiple submucosal nodules or masses, ranging from several millimeters to several centimeters in size
- Submucosal masses often ulcerate, producing typical bull's-eye or target lesions

WHAT THE REFERRING PHYSICIAN NEEDS TO KNOW
- Failure to obtain biopsy specimens from advanced lesion that is assumed to be inoperable gastric cancer may deprive the patient of the opportunity for cure or long-term palliation.
- Proper staging of the tumor is important so that a rational decision can be made about prognosis and treatment options such as surgery, radiation therapy, and chemotherapy.
- Endoscopic biopsy specimens should be obtained for definitive diagnosis when low-grade mucosa-associated lymphoid tissue (MALT) lymphomas are suspected on the basis of radiographic findings.
- Patients with advanced gastric lymphoma are sometimes treated exclusively with radiation therapy or chemotherapy.
- Follow-up barium studies or CT scans are useful in documenting treatment response, gastrointestinal bleeding, or other symptoms that develop after treatment.
- Endoscopic biopsy specimens are required for definitive diagnosis; superficial biopsy specimens may be nondiagnostic because lymphomas often infiltrate the gastric wall beneath an intact mucosa.
- Whenever possible, multiple brushings and biopsy specimens should be obtained from ulcerated or polypoid areas where tumor is more likely to be present.
- Deep biopsy specimens should be obtained when the overlying mucosa appears normal; with adequate cytologic and biopsy specimens, endoscopy has a reported sensitivity of 85%-95% in diagnosing gastric lymphoma.

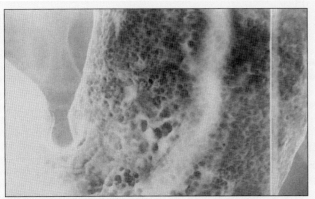

Figure 1. Low-grade mucosa-associated lymphoid tissue (MALT) lymphoma with regression after treatment. Initial double-contrast study shows confluent, varying-sized nodules in the gastric body resulting from a low-grade B-cell MALT lymphoma. (*From Yoo CC, Levine MS, Furth EE, et al: Gastric mucosa-associated lymphoid tissue lymphoma: Radiographic findings in six patients.* Radiology *208:239-243, 1998.*)

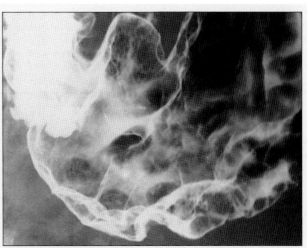

Figure 2. Forms of gastric lymphoma. Diffusely thickened, irregular folds are present in the stomach due to lymphomatous infiltration of the gastric wall. (*From Laufer I, Levine MS [eds]:* Double Contrast Gastrointestinal Radiology, *2nd ed. Philadelphia, WB Saunders, 1992.*)

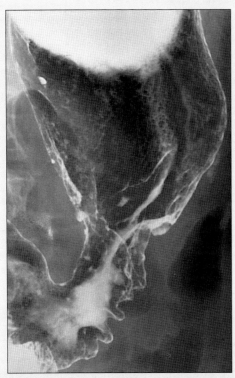

Figure 3. Forms of gastric lymphoma. This patient has linitis plastica, manifested by focal narrowing of the gastric body with nodularity and succulation of the adjacent greater curvature. (*From Levine MS, Pantongrag-Brown L, Aguilera NS, et al: Non-Hodgkin lymphoma of the stomach: A cause of linitis plastica.* Radiology *201:375-378, 1996.*)

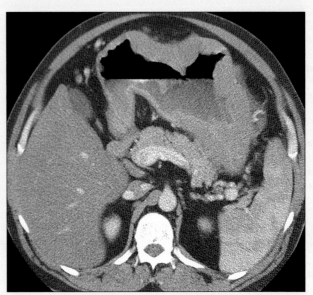

Figure 4. Gastric lymphoma on CT. CT scan shows marked thickening of the gastric wall with homogeneous enhancement due to the infiltrative form of gastric lymphoma. Small perigastric lymph nodes are present in the adjacent fat.

Duodenum

- Infiltrative, ulcerative, polypoid, and nodular forms
- Marked soft tissue thickening of duodenal wall, ulcerated mass, or exaggerated folds in duodenum

IMAGING

Fluoroscopy

Findings

- Low-grade gastric MALT lymphomas: variably sized, rounded, often confluent nodules involving focal or, less frequently, diffuse segment of stomach on double-contrast studies
- Small polypoid or ulcerated lesions; shallow, irregular ulcers with nodular surrounding mucosa; or focally or diffusely distorted, enlarged rugal folds
- Linitis plastica appearance with varying degrees of narrowing, nodularity, and ulceration

Utility

- Follow-up barium study is useful in documenting treatment response, gastrointestinal bleeding, or evaluation of other symptoms that develop after treatment.

CT

Findings

- Gastric lymphoma: polypoid, infiltrating, or hypertrophic lesions
- Most common finding is marked thickening of the gastric wall due to tumor infiltration.
- Gastric wall: more uniform enhancement pattern than in patients with gastric cancer (unless areas of ulceration or cavitation are present)
- Substantially thickened rugal folds, preserved gastric contour
- Transpyloric spread of lymphoma into duodenum
- Duodenal lymphoma: marked soft tissue thickening of duodenal wall, an ulcerated mass, or exaggerated folds in duodenum

Utility

- Primary imaging modality for pretreatment evaluation of abdominal lymphoma
- Less sensitive technique for detecting low-grade gastric MALT lymphomas
- Follow-up is useful in evaluating treatment response, gastrointestinal bleeding, or other symptoms that develop after treatment.
- When gastric lymphoma is suspected, histologic confirmation should be obtained before treatment.

Ultrasound

Findings

- Non-Hodgkin gastric lymphoma: hypoechoic mass that disrupts normal wall layer pattern, selective thickening of second and third echogenic layers, or diffuse thickening of all five wall layers
- Linitis plastica produces hypoechoic or inhomogeneous mural thickening of stomach.

Utility

- Endoscopic ultrasonography (EUS) has been shown to be a valuable technique for staging patients with non-Hodgkin gastric lymphoma.
- Overall accuracy is approximately 90%.
- Findings on EUS may be highly suggestive of lymphoma.
- EUS is also useful for documenting response to therapy in nonoperative patients.

PET

Findings

- PET has corresponding levels of uptake in lymphoma of the stomach, with a higher standard uptake value (SUV) associated with high-grade malignancy and a lower SUV associated with low-grade tumors.

Utility

- Fluorodeoxyglucose (FDG)-PET is useful in diagnosing, staging, restaging, and evaluating treatment response in lymphoma, including that of the small bowel.

CLINICAL PRESENTATION

- Patients with advanced lesions may present with abdominal pain, nausea, vomiting, anorexia, weight loss, palpable epigastric mass, or signs or symptoms of upper gastrointestinal bleeding.
- Presence of lymphadenopahthy beyond expected drainage pathways of primary gastric carcinoma should suggest diagnosis of gastric lymphoma.
- Occasional patients may develop acute abdomen because of spontaneous perforation of ulcerated gastric lymphoma.
- Patients with generalized lymphoma may present with fever or other signs of systemic disease.
- Patients with early gastric lymphoma (particularly low-grade B-cell MALT lymphoma) may present with epigastric pain, dyspepsia, bloating, nausea, or vomiting.
- Symptoms at presentation are indistinguishable from those of gastric or duodenal ulcers, gastritis, or duodenitis. Most patients have underlying *Helicobacter pylori* gastritis.

PATHOLOGY

- Majority of gastric lymphomas are non-Hodgkin lymphomas that arise from low-grade MALT lymphomas classified as marginal zone B-cell MALT lymphomas by International Lymphoma Study Group.
- National Cancer Institute recognizes three non-Hodgkin lymphomas prognostic categories: low grade, intermediate grade, and high grade (advanced lesion is high-grade lymphoma or large cell or immunoblastic type).

- Chronic *H. pylori* gastritis leads to lymphoid follicle acquisitions and lamina propria aggregations (i.e., MALT) and subsequent development of low-grade B-cell MALT lymphomas in the stomach, which normally contains no organized lymphoid tissue.
- Almost all patients with low-grade MALT lymphomas have particular strains of *H. pylori*-containing cytotoxin-associated antigen (*cagA*) that may have an important role in pathogenesis of gastric MALT lymphoma.
- Gastric MALT lymphomas are manifested pathologically by infiltration of the epithelium with small centrocyte-like cells, giving rise to lymphoepithelial lesions that are characteristic of these tumors.
- Most non-Hodgkin gastric lymphomas originate as low-grade gastric MALT lymphomas, which subsequently undergo transformation to intermediate-grade or high-grade lymphomas.
- Primary gastric lymphoma is usually confined to the stomach or regional lymph nodes at the time of diagnosis; it extends into the duodenum by continuous transpyloric spread.
- Ann Arbor staging system: Stage IE lesions, gastric wall; Stage IIE lesions, regional lymph nodes in abdomen; Stage III lesions, lymph nodes above and below diaphragm; and Stage IV lesions, widely disseminated lymphomas that involve extra-abdominal lymph nodes as well as omentum, mesentery, peritoneum, liver, spleen, lungs, or brain

INCIDENCE/PREVALENCE AND EPIDEMIOLOGY

- Lymphoma involves the stomach more frequently than any other portion of the gastrointestinal tract, accounting for 50% of all gastrointestinal lymphomas.
- Majority of gastric lymphomas are non-Hodgkin lymphomas; they rarely are Hodgkin's disease.
- Gastric lymphoma occurs more frequently in men than in women, and average age at time of diagnosis is 55 to 60 years.
- Gastric lymphoma has a much better prognosis than gastric carcinoma, with overall 5-year survival rates of 50% to 60%.
- Major factors affecting survival of patients with primary gastric lymphoma are invasion of gastric wall and the presence or absence of nodal disease.
- Long-term survival depends primarily on tumor stage at time of diagnosis; 5-year survival rates range from 62%-90% for stage IE lesions and 29%-50% for stage IIE lesions; substantially lower rates are reported for stage III and stage IV lesions.
- Patients with low-grade gastric MALT lymphomas have a much better prognosis than patients with high-grade lymphomas; low-grade lymphomas are associated with 5-year survival rates of 75%-91%, whereas high grade MALT lymphomas are associated with 5-year survival rates of less than 60%.

- In various serious, 30%-40% of patients with gastric lymphoma have associated duodenal involvement on barium studies; gastric carcinoma invades the duodenum in only 5%-25% of patients.

DIFFERENTIAL DIAGNOSIS

- MALT lymphomas: severe gastritis, lymphoid hyperplasia, or even polyposis syndrome involving stomach
- Advanced infiltrative gastric lymphomas may be difficult to distinguish radiographically from other causes of thickened gastric folds (*H. pylori* gastritis, hypertrophic gastritis, Ménétrier disease, and gastric carcinoma).
- Infiltrative lymphomas may produce a linitis plastica appearance indistinguishable from that of a primary scirrhous carcinoma.
- Ulcerated gastric lymphomas may be impossible to distinguish radiographically from ulcerated carcinomas.
- When lymphoma is characterized by multiple areas of ulceration, differential diagnosis includes various inflammatory or infectious conditions involving stomach (e.g., Zollinger-Ellison syndrome, Crohn disease, tuberculosis, syphilis, and cytomegalovirus).
- Polypoid gastric lymphomas may be indistinguishable from polypoid carcinomas.
- Lymphomas that appear as submucosal masses can be mistaken for malignant gastrointestinal stromal tumors (GISTs); giant, cavitated lymphomas may be impossible to differentiate from cavitated GISTs or cavitated metastases.
- Bull's-eye lesions in the stomach may be caused not only by lymphoma but also by Kaposi sarcoma, carcinoid tumors, or metastases (particularly those from malignant melanoma).

Suggested Readings
Brady LW: Malignant lymphoma of the gastrointestinal tract. *Radiology* 137:291-298, 1980.
Brands F, Monig SP, Raab M: Treatment and prognosis of gastric lymphoma. *Eur J Surg* 163:803-813, 1997.
Brooks JJ, Enterline HT: Primary gastric lymphoma: A clinicopathologic study of 58 cases with long-term follow-up and literature review. *Cancer* 51:701-711, 1983.
Dworkin B, Lightdale CJ, Weingrad DN, et al: Primary gastric lymphoma: A review of 50 cases. *Dig Dis Sci* 27:986-992, 1982.
Farinha P, Gascoyne RD: *Helicobacter pylori* and MALT lymphoma. *Gastroenterology* 128:1579-1605, 2005.
Harris NL: Extranodal lymphoid infiltrates and mucosa-associated lymphoid tissue (MALT): A unifying concept. *Am J Surg Pathol* 15:879-884, 1991.
Kitamura K, Yamaguchi T, Okamoto K, et al: Early gastric lymphoma. *Cancer* 77:850-857, 1996.
Orr RK, Lininger JR, Lawrence W: Gastric pseudolymphoma: A challenging clinical problem. *Ann Surg* 200:185-194, 1984.
Papadimitriou CS, Papacharalampous NX, Kittas C: Primary gastrointestinal lymphoma: A morphologic and immunohistochemical study. *Cancer* 55:870-879, 1985.
Yoo CC, Levine MS, Furth EE, et al: Gastric mucosa-associated lymphoid tissue lymphoma: Radiographic findings in six patients. *Radiology* 208:239-243, 1998.

Malignant Gastrointestinal Stromal Tumors

DEFINITION: Malignant gastrointestinal stromal tumors (GISTs) are tyrosine kinase growth factor receptor (KIT-CD117)-positive mesenchymal sarcomas.

ANATOMIC FINDINGS

Stomach
- Malignant GISTs most commonly arise in the stomach.
- Approximately 90% of cases involve the fundus and body; the remaining 10% involve the antrum.
- Patterns of growth may be endogastric or exogastric, but these tumors have a propensity for exogastric growth.

Duodenum
- Approximately 80% of malignant duodenal GISTs are located in the second or third portion of the duodenum.

Liver and Peritoneum
- Malignant GISTs of the stomach most commonly metastasize to the liver and peritoneal cavity.
- Metastatic lesions are usually large and heterogeneous.

IMAGING

Radiography
Findings
- Soft-tissue mass indenting gastric bubble may be seen on abdominal radiographs.
- One or more extraluminal gas collections may also be seen in the left upper quadrant as result of necrosis and cavitation.
- Rarely, abdominal radiographs may reveal mottled areas of calcification.
- Intramural lesions typically appear as large, lobulated submucosal masses in the gastric fundus or body with large areas of ulceration.

DIAGNOSTIC PEARLS
- Peripheral enhancement corresponds to areas of viable tumor, whereas central areas of low attenuation correspond to areas of hemorrhage or necrosis.
- Exogastric lesions may be characterized by giant soft-tissue masses that cause extrinsic compression of the adjacent gastric wall with a central dimple or spicule at the site of the attachment or pedicle of the mass.
- Intramural lesions typically appear as large, lobulated submucosal masses in the gastric fundus or body with large ulceration.

- Malignant GISTs may contain one or more ulcers or, not infrequently, large areas of cavitation.
- Exogastric lesions are characterized by giant soft-tissue masses causing extrinsic compression of the adjacent gastric wall with a central dimple or spicule.
- Rarely, endogastric tumors may appear as polypoid intraluminal masses indistinguishable from primary gastric carcinomas.

Utility
- Abdominal radiographs generally have limited value for diagnosing malignant GISTs involving the stomach.
- Despite their large size, they rarely cause duodenal obstruction.
- Exoenteric mass growth pattern may be indistinguishable from that of pancreatic neoplasms, pancreatic pseudocysts, and other extrinsic mass lesions involving the duodenum.

WHAT THE REFERRING PHYSICIAN NEEDS TO KNOW
- Size has been shown to be the single most accurate predictive feature of malignancy.
- The physician must be aware of the limitations of endoscopy in diagnosing malignant GISTs because positive endoscopic biopsy specimens may not be obtained unless the overlying mucosa is ulcerated.
- Surgery is the only curative form of therapy.
- Because some malignant GISTs may be as small as 2 cm, distinguishing benign from malignant stromal tumors by radiographic criteria is not always possible.
- Major considerations in the differential diagnosis include lymphoma and other benign or malignant tumors of mesenchymal origin.
- Other considerations include mass lesions arising in the liver, pancreas, kidney, or mesentery, as well as exophytic adenocarcinomas and duplication cysts.
- Malignant GISTs of the stomach most commonly metastasize to the liver and peritoneal cavity.

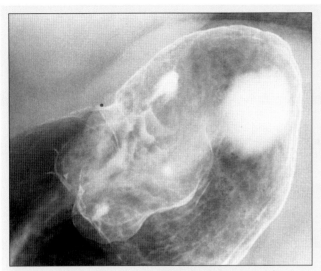

Figure 1. **Malignant gastrointestinal stromal tumor.** A large, lobulated submucosal mass is seen in the gastric fundus.

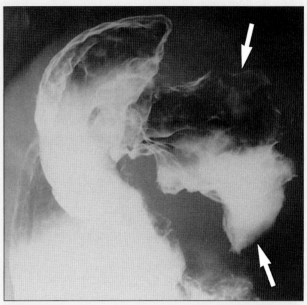

Figure 2. **Malignant gastrointestinal stromal tumor with cavitation.** A cavitated lesion is recognized by a giant extraluminal collection of barium *(arrows)*.

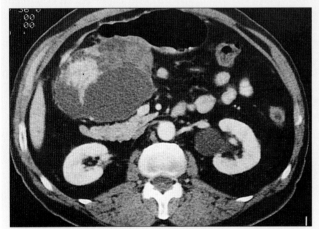

Figure 3. **Malignant gastrointestinal stromal tumor on CT.** In this patient, a heterogeneous exogastric mass is seen insinuating between the stomach and the pancreas.

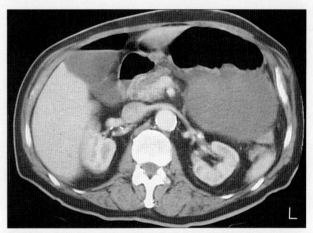

Figure 4. **Malignant gastrointestinal stromal tumor on CT.** In this patient, a gas- and fluid-filled mass projects posteriorly from the stomach. Although uncommon, this degree of necrosis can occur with malignant GISTs.

CT and Angiography

Findings

- Large and exophytic, heterogeneously enhancing mass containing gas, fluid, or contrast material caused by a variable degree of necrosis and ulceration.
- Peripheral enhancement corresponds to areas of viable tumor, whereas central areas of low attenuation correspond to hemorrhage or necrosis.
- Rarely, malignant GISTs may be so necrotic that they appear as water-density lesions.
- Lesions are seen on angiography as relatively well-circumscribed, hypervascular masses with huge feeding arteries, draining veins, and intense tumor staining.
- Peritoneal involvement by the tumor is similar to other intraperitoneal-seeded metastases.

Utility

- CT determines relationship of suspicious lesions to gastric wall.
- CT-guided needle aspiration biopsies of endoscopically inaccessible lesions may be performed.
- Extent of mass and invasion of adjacent structures is demonstrated
- Differentiating benign from malignant stromal tumors is not possible by angiographic criteria.
- Angiography cannot distinguish malignant GISTs from other hypervascular lesions (carcinoids, neurogenic tumors, or vascular metastases).

PET

Finding

- Similar to primary lesions, metastases may be multilocular lesions containing fluid levels and are usually positive on PET.

CLINICAL PRESENTATION

- Because malignant GISTs frequently ulcerate, patients may show signs of upper gastrointestinal bleeding, including hematemesis, melena, guaiac-positive stool, and iron-deficiency anemia.
- Other findings include nausea, vomiting, abdominal pain, weight loss, and palpable abdominal mass.
- Average duration of symptoms at the time of diagnosis is 4-6 months.
- Some patients with exogastric tumors may remain asymptomatic until lesions have reached enormous sizes.
- Duodenal GISTs may produce signs or symptoms of upper gastrointestinal bleeding, weight loss, abdominal pain, palpable mass, or obstructive jaundice.

DIFFERENTIAL DIAGNOSIS

- Lymphoma (stomach and duodenum)
- Other mesenchymal tumors (stomach and duodenum)
- Duplication cysts (stomach and duodenum)
- Exophytic adenocarcinomas (stomach and duodenum)

PATHOLOGY

- Tumors show a positive immunoreactivity for KIT-CD117 and tyrosine kinase growth factor receptor, allowing differentiation from true leiomyomas or leiomyosarcomas.
- GISTs usually consist histologically of interlacing whorls of spindle-shaped cells with eosinophilic cytoplasm and elongated nuclei.
- Occasionally, these tumors contain distinctive epithelioid cells with eccentric nuclei and perinuclear vacuolization.
- These tumors are mesenchymal lesions, usually originating from outer layer of muscularis propria.
- Malignant GISTs rarely metastasize to regional lymph nodes.
- GISTs larger than 10 cm and with more than five mitoses per 50 high-power fields are considered malignant.
- GISTs with more than 50 mitoses per 50 high-power fields are considered high-grade malignancies with an extremely aggressive malignant behavior.

INCIDENCE/PREVALENCE AND EPIDEMIOLOGY

- Malignant GISTs are uncommon tumors that constitute only 1%-3% of all malignant neoplasms in the stomach.
- GISTs are the most common mesenchymal tumors in the gastrointestinal tract.
- Malignant GISTs of the stomach are more common in men.
- Patients are usually older than 50 years of age.
- Malignant GISTs constitute only 10% of all malignant tumors in the duodenum, with sex distribution approximately equal.

Suggested Readings

Appelman HD, Helwig EB: Gastric epithelioid leiomyoma and leiomyosarcoma (leiomyoblastoma). *Cancer* 38:708-728, 1976.

Burkill GJC, Badran M, Al-Muderis O, et al: Malignant gastrointestinal stromal tumor: Distribution, imaging features, and pattern of metastatic spread. *Radiology* 226:527-532, 2003.

Franquemont DW: Differentiation and risk assessment of gastrointestinal stromal tumors. *Am J Clin Pathol* 103:41-47, 1995.

Levy AD, Remotti HE, Thompson WM, et al: Gastrointestinal stromal tumors: Radiologic features with pathologic correlation. *RadioGraphics* 23:283-304, 2003.

Ludwig DJ, Traverso LW: Gut stromal tumors and their clinical behavior. *Am J Surg* 173:390-394, 1997.

Miettinen M, Sarlomo-Rikala M, Lasota J: Gastrointestinal stromal tumors: Recent advances in understanding of their biology. *Hum Pathol* 30:1213-1220, 1999.

Sarlomo-Rikala M, Kovatich AJ, Barusevicius A, et al: CD117: A sensitive marker for gastrointestinal stromal tumors that is more specific than CD34. *Mod Pathol* 11:728-734, 1998.

Suster S: Gastrointestinal stromal tumors. *Semin Diagn Pathol* 13:297-313, 1996.

Kaposi Sarcoma

DEFINITION: Malignant tumor of the stomach and duodenum associated with slow-growing violaceous or hemorrhagic lesions on the lower extremities sometimes seen in patients with AIDS.

IMAGING

Radiography
Findings
- Submucosal defects ranging from 0.5-3.0 cm in size on barium studies
- Bull's-eye or target lesions
- Thickened, nodular folds or polypoid masses in the stomach or duodenum
- Linitis plastica appearance

Utility
- Barium studies
- Endoscopy is a more sensitive technique for detecting the earliest gastrointestinal lesions of Kaposi sarcoma.
- If suspicious lesions are found in the stomach and duodenum, small-bowel follow-through should be performed to search for additional lesions in the small bowel.

CT
Findings
- Tumor nodules or ulcers in the stomach or duodenum

Utility
- Used to determine whether retroperitoneal adenopathy, splenomegaly, or other evidence of Kaposi sarcoma is present in the abdomen.

CLINICAL PRESENTATION

- Gastrointestinal involvement by Kaposi sarcoma is almost always associated with cutaneous disease.
- Some patients complain of abdominal pain or upper gastrointestinal bleeding, but others are asymptomatic despite multiple lesions.
- Gastrointestinal symptoms more likely to result from recurrent opportunistic infections than from Kaposi sarcoma in patients with AIDS.
- AIDS patients with Kaposi sarcoma have worse prognosis than other patients with AIDS and are more likely to develop severe opportunistic infections.

DIAGNOSTIC PEARLS

- Bull's-eye or target lesions are often seen.
- Gastrointestinal symptoms usually result from recurrent opportunistic infection in patients with AIDS.
- Slow-growing violaceous or hemorrhagic lesions are seen on the lower extremities.

DIFFERENTIAL DIAGNOSIS

- Metastases (stomach and duodenum)
- Lymphoma (stomach and duodenum)
- Cytomegalovirus infection (stomach and duodenum)
- Leukemic infiltrates
- Multiple polyps
- Tuberculosis (stomach and duodenum)

PATHOLOGY

- Slow-growing violaceous or hemorrhagic lesions on the lower extremities
- Consist histologically of whorled bundles of spindle-shaped cells in vascular cleft matrix containing red blood cells and hemosiderin
- Endoscopic findings: flat, hemorrhagic patches or macular discolorations; raised, reddish-purple nodules; coalescent plaques or masses

INCIDENCE/PREVALENCE AND EPIDEMIOLOGY

- Approximately 35% of patients with AIDS have Kaposi sarcoma, and approximately 50% with Kaposi sarcoma have gastrointestinal involvement.
- Stomach, duodenum, and small bowel are the most common sites of involvement; the colon is affected less frequently; the esophagus is involved in rare instances.

WHAT THE REFERRING PHYSICIAN NEEDS TO KNOW

- Gastrointestinal involvement requires treatment if the patient is symptomatic.
- Radiation therapy or chemotherapy is occasionally used to treat gastrointestinal Kaposi sarcoma, but such therapy poses substantial risks in patients who are already immunocompromised.
- Patients with AIDS may develop an extremely aggressive form of Kaposi sarcoma characterized by widespread visceral lesions, particularly in the gastrointestinal tract.

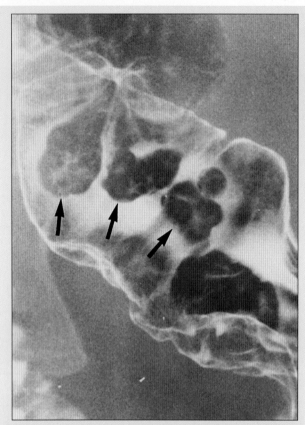

Figure 1. Kaposi sarcoma with bull's-eye lesions in a patient with AIDS. Multiple bull's-eye lesions or centrally ulcerated submucosal masses *(arrows)* are present in the gastric antrum.

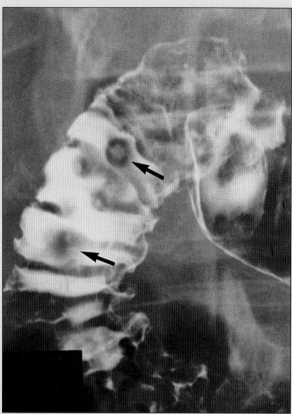

Figure 2. Kaposi sarcoma with bull's-eye lesions in a patient with AIDS. In this patient, several bull's-eye lesions *(arrows)* are seen in the descending duodenum. *(Courtesy of Robert Goren, MD, Philadelphia, PA.)*

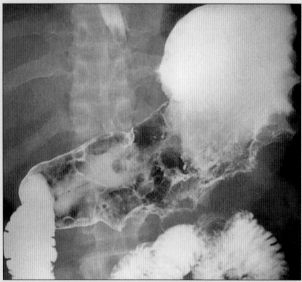

Figure 3. Kaposi sarcoma with a linitis plastica appearance in a patient with AIDS. The stomach has a markedly narrowed, irregular appearance caused by the infiltrating form of Kaposi sarcoma.

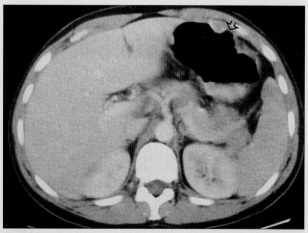

Figure 4. Kaposi sarcoma with bull's-eye lesion in a patient with AIDS. In this patient, CT scan shows an ulcerated submucosal mass on the anterior wall of the stomach. Gas outlines the ulcer *(arrow)*.

Suggested Readings

Balthazar EJ, Richman A: Kaposi's sarcoma of the stomach. *Am J Gastroenterol* 67:375-379, 1977.

Dunnick NR, Harell GS, Parker BR: Multiple "bull's-eye" lesions in gastric lymphoma. *AJR Am J Roentgenol* 126:965-969, 1976.

Ell C, Matek W, Gramatzki M, et al: Endoscopic findings in a case of Kaposi's sarcoma with involvement of the large and small bowel. *Endoscopy* 17:161-164, 1985.

Falcone S, Murphy BJ, Weinfeld A: Gastric manifestations of AIDS: Radiographic findings on upper gastrointestinal examination. *Gastrointest Radiol* 16:95-98, 1991.

Frager DH, Frager JD, Brandt LJ, et al: Gastrointestinal complications of AIDS: Radiologic features. *Radiology* 158:597-603, 1986.

Friedman SL: Gastrointestinal and hepatobiliary neoplasms in AIDS. *Gastroenterol Clin North Am* 17:465-486, 1988.

Friedman SL, Wright TL, Altman DF: Gastroenterology: Kaposi's sarcoma with acquired immunodeficiency syndrome. *Gastroenterology* 89:102-108, 1985.

Hadjiyane C, Lee YH, Stein L, et al: Kaposi's sarcoma presenting as linitis plastica. *Am J Gastroenterol* 86:1823-1825, 1991.

Henderson RG, Rahmatulla TD: An epidemic tumour. *Br J Radiol* 60:511-512, 1987.

Herts BR, Megibow AJ, Birnbaum BA, et al: High attenuation lymphadenopathy in AIDS patients: Significance of findings on CT. *Radiology* 185:777-781, 1992.

Hill CA, Harle TS, Mansell PWA: The prodrome, Kaposi sarcoma, and infections associated with acquired immunodeficiency syndrome: Radiologic findings in 39 patients. *Radiology* 149:393-399, 1983.

Jaffe HW, Bregman DJ, Selik RM: Acquired immune deficiency syndrome in the United States: The first 1,000 cases. *J Infect Dis* 148:339-345, 1983.

Jeffrey RB Jr, Goodman PC, Olsen WL, et al: Radiologic imaging of AIDS. *Curr Probl Diagn Radiol* 17:73-117, 1988.

Jeffrey RB, Nyberg DA, Bottles K, et al: Abdominal CT in acquired immunodeficiency syndrome. *AJR Am J Roentgenol* 146:7-13, 1986.

Leibman AJ, Gold BM: Gastric manifestations of autoimmune deficiency syndrome-related Kaposi's sarcoma on computed tomography. *J Comput Tomogr* 10:85-88, 1986.

Lustbader I, Sherman A: Primary gastrointestinal Kaposi's sarcoma in a patient with acquired immune deficiency syndrome. *Am J Gastroenterol* 82:894-895, 1987.

Rose HS, Balthazar EJ, Megibow AJ, et al: Alimentary tract involvement in Kaposi sarcoma: Radiographic and endoscopic findings in 25 homosexual men. *AJR Am J Roentgenol* 139:661-666, 1982.

Saltz RK, Kurtz RC, Lightdale CJ, et al: Kaposi's sarcoma: Gastrointestinal involvement correlation with skin findings and immunologic function. *Dig Dis Sci* 29:817-823, 1984.

Wall SD, Friedman SL, Margulis AR: Gastrointestinal Kaposi's sarcoma in AIDS: Radiographic manifestations. *J Clin Gastroenterol* 6:165-171, 1984.

Carcinoid Tumors

DEFINITION: Endocrine tumors that are capable of producing a variety of vasoactive substances.

IMAGING

Radiography
Findings
- Gastric carcinoid tumors: multiple small polyps in gastric fundus or body
- Sporadic carcinoids: one or more submucosal masses in stomach
- Masses may ulcerate, producing typical "bull's-eye" lesions
- Sessile or pedunculated lesions indistinguishable from hyperplastic or adenomatous polyps
- Large polypoid masses
- Duodenal carcinoids: discrete submucosal masses or intraluminal polyps

Utility
- Barium studies
- When gastric or duodenal carcinoids are detected radiographically, endoscopic biopsy specimens are required for a definitive diagnosis.

CT
Findings
- Enhancing polypoid or ulcerated lesions in stomach and duodenum

CLINICAL PRESENTATION

- Many patients are asymptomatic.
- Some may present with abdominal pain, nausea, vomiting, weight loss, anorexia, or signs and symptoms of upper gastrointestinal bleeding.
- Larger lesions are more likely to bleed, but massive bleeding of ulcerated carcinoids as small as 1 cm in size can occur.
- Patients with gastric or duodenal carcinoids almost never exhibit symptoms of carcinoid syndrome.

DIAGNOSTIC PEARLS

- Masses may ulcerate, producing typical "bull's-eye" lesions.
- Gastric carcinoids are associated with hypergastrinemia in patients with Zollinger-Ellison syndrome and with chronic atrophic gastritis.
- Gastric carcinoid tumors originate from enterochromaffin-like cells (Kulchitsky cells).

- Duodenal carcinoids may be associated with Zollinger-Ellison syndrome or neurofibromatosis type 1.

DIFFERENTIAL DIAGNOSIS

- Metastases (stomach and duodenum)
- Lymphoma (stomach and duodenum)
- Kaposi sarcoma (stomach and duodenum)

PATHOLOGY

- Low-grade, slow-growing malignant tumors that can eventually metastasize to liver or other structures
- Gastric carcinoids associated with primary hypergastrinemia in patients with Zollinger-Ellison syndrome and with secondary hypergastrinemia in patients with chronic atrophic gastritis
- Gastric carcinoid tumors originate from enterochromaffin-like cells (Kulchitsky cells), whereas duodenal carcinoids rarely arise from enterochromaffin cells
- Argyrophilic but argentaffin-negative tumors; lack enzyme required for synthesis of 5-hydroxytryptamine (serotonin); rarely show evidence of endocrine function

---

WHAT THE REFERRING PHYSICIAN NEEDS TO KNOW
- Carcinoids associated with hypergastrinemia have an excellent prognosis.
- Sporadic gastric carcinoids are more likely to exhibit invasive growth and to metastasize to distant sites.
- When gastric or duodenal carcinoids are detected radiographically, endoscopic biopsy specimens are required for a definitive diagnosis.
- Duodenal carcinoids may be associated with Zollinger-Ellison syndrome or neurofibromatosis type 1.

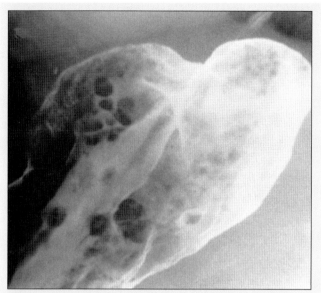

Figure 1. Gastric carcinoid tumors. This patient has multiple small nodules in the gastric fundus indistinguishable from hyperplastic polyps.

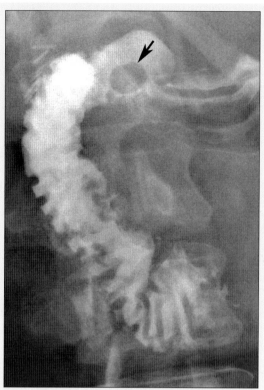

Figure 2. Duodenal carcinoid tumor. Barium study shows a smooth, round submucosal mass *(arrow)* in the duodenal bulb. At surgery, this patient was found to have a malignant duodenal carcinoid tumor involving periduodenal lymph nodes.

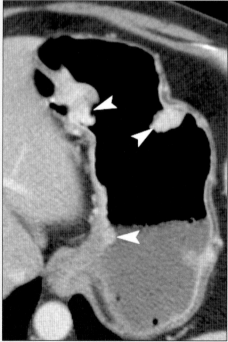

Figure 3. Gastric carcinoid tumors on CT. CT scan shows multiple carcinoid tumors as enhancing polypoid masses *(arrowheads)* in the proximal stomach.

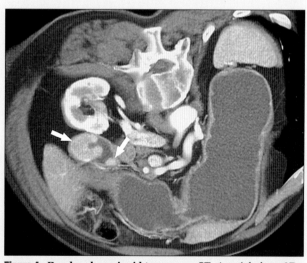

Figure 4. Duodenal carcinoid tumors on CT. Arterial phase 3D volume-rendered MDCT image shows two hyperdense masses *(arrows)* in the duodenal bulb. The larger mass contains a central area of ulceration. Endoscopic biopsy specimens revealed duodenal carcinoid tumors.

- Sporadic gastric carcinoids occur as solitary lesions more likely to exhibit invasive growth and to metastasize to distant sites.

INCIDENCE/PREVALENCE AND EPIDEMIOLOGY

- Only 2%-3% of all gastrointestinal carcinoids are located in the stomach or duodenum.
- Equal sex predilection for gastric carcinoids; usually occur in patients older than 40 years of age
- Metastases are found in 20%-30% of patients with gastric carcinoids at time of diagnosis.
- Long-term survival has been reported even when metastases are present.

Suggested Readings

Abrams JS: Multiple malignant carcinoids of the stomach. *Arch Surg* 115:1219-1221, 1980.

Balthazar EJ, Megibow A, Bryk D: Gastric carcinoid tumors: Radiographic features in eight cases. *AJR Am J Roentgenol* 139:1123-1127, 1982.

Berger MW, Stephens DH: Gastric carcinoid tumors associated with chronic hypergastrinemia in a patient with Zollinger-Ellison syndrome. *Radiology* 201:371-373, 1996.

Clements JL, Roche RR: Carcinoid of the duodenum: A report of six cases. *Gastrointest Radiol* 9:17-21, 1984.

Eschelman DJ, Duva-Frissora AD, Martin LC, et al: Metastatic carcinoid presenting as a duodenal mass. *AJR Am J Roentgenol* 156:1301-1302, 1991.

Levy AD, Taylor LD, Abbott RM, et al: Duodenal carcinoids: Imaging features with clinical-pathologic comparison. *Radiology* 237:967-972, 2005.

Modlin IM, Sandor A, Tang LH, et al: A 40-year analysis of 265 gastric carcinoids. *Am J Gastroenterol* 92:633-638, 1997.

Modlin IM, Tang LH: The gastric enterochromaffin-like cell: An enigmatic cellular link. *Gastroenterology* 111:783-810, 1996.

Rindi G, Luinetti O, Cornaggia M, et al: Three subtypes of gastric argyrophil carcinoid and the gastric neuroendocrine carcinoma: A clinicopathologic study. *Gastroenterology* 104:994-1006, 1993.

Sculco D, Bilgrami S: Pernicious anemia and gastric carcinoid tumor: Case report and review. *Am J Gastroenterol* 92:1378-1380, 1997.

Seymour EQ, Griffin CN, Kurtz SM: Carcinoid tumors of the duodenal cap presenting as multiple polypoid defects. *Gastrointest Radiol* 7:19-21, 1982.

Wengrower D, Fich A: Primary duodenal carcinoid. *Am J Gastroenterol* 82:1069-1070, 1987.

Part 20 MISCELLANEOUS ABNORMALITIES OF THE STOMACH AND DUODENUM

Varices

DEFINITION: Increased portal and splenic venous pressures lead to reversal of blood flow through the gastric veins into the venous plexus, producing varices.

IMAGING

Radiography
Findings
- Lobulated soft-tissue densities in the gas-filled fundus
- Splenomegaly, ascites, and pancreatic calcification

Utility
- Chest or abdominal radiographs
- Abdominal radiographs

Fluoroscopy
Findings
- Discrete, round submucosal filling defects in the gastric fundus (*bunch-of-grapes* appearance)
- Large polyploid mass secondary to a conglomerate mass of gastric varices (*tumorous* gastric varices)
- Thickened, tortuous folds in the body of the stomach
- Thickened, serpiginous folds in the proximal duodenum (duodenal varices)

Utility
- Barium studies

CT
Findings
- Enhancing, well-defined, round or tubular densities on the posterior or posteromedial wall of the gastric fundus

Utility
- More sensitive than conventional radiologic examinations in detecting varices

Interventional Radiology
Findings
- Absent visualization of the portal and splenic veins on angiography

DIAGNOSTIC PEARLS

- *Bunch of grapes* appearance
- Thickened, serpiginous folds in proximal duodenum (duodenal varices)
- Enhancing, well-defined, round or tubular densities on the posterior or posteromedial wall of the gastric fundus on CT

Utility
- Portal hypertension can be differentiated from splenic vein obstruction by angiography.

CLINICAL PRESENTATION

- Gastrointestinal bleeding
- Abdominal pain and weight loss
- Splenomegaly

DIFFERENTIAL DIAGNOSIS

- Hypertrophic gastritis
- Ménétrier's disease (stomach and duodenum)
- Lymphoma (stomach and duodenum)
- Portal hypertensive gastropathy

PATHOLOGY

- Increased portal and splenic venous pressures lead to reversal of blood flow through the gastric veins into the venous plexus, producing varices.

WHAT THE REFERRING PHYSICIAN NEEDS TO KNOW

- Varices are more likely to form in the esophagus than in the stomach, despite comparable elevations in pressure.
- Gastric varices are less likely to bleed than esophageal varices because of their subserosal location and the greater thickness of gastric tissue.
- Presence of combined esophageal and gastric varices almost always indicates portal hypertension as the underlying cause.
- Presence of isolated gastric varices should raise the possibility of splenic vein obstruction with a patent portal vein.
- Patients with splenic vein obstruction are almost always cured by a simple splenectomy because portal venous pressure is normal in these individuals.

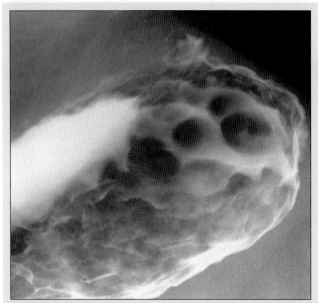

Figure 1. Gastric varices. Tortuous folds and submucosal filling defects are seen in the gastric fundus, resembling the appearance of a bunch of grapes. (*From Levine MS, Kieu K, Rubesin SE, et al: Isolated gastric varices: Splenic vein obstruction or portal hypertension?* Gastrointest Radiol *15:188-192, 1990. With kind permission from Springer Science and Business Media.*)

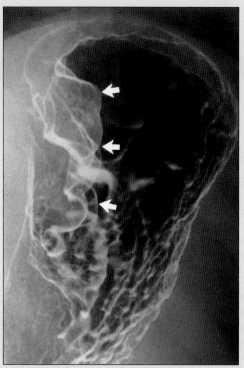

Figure 2. Conglomerate mass of gastric varices (also known as tumorous varices). Barium study shows a large, lobulated submucosal mass *(arrows)* on the medial aspect of the gastric fundus. Although this lesion can be mistaken for a malignant gastrointestinal stromal tumor or even a polypoid carcinoma, note its smooth, undulating contour.

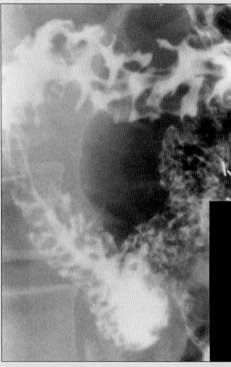

Figure 3. Duodenal varices. Thickened, serpiginous folds are seen in the proximal descending duodenum.

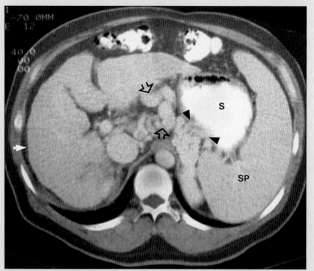

Figure 4. Gastric varices on CT. Enhancing collaterals are seen in the gastric wall *(arrowheads)*, gastrohepatic ligament *(open arrows)*, and left retroperitoneal space. This patient also has cirrhosis with splenomegaly and minimal ascites *(solid arrow)* caused by portal hypertension. (*S*, Stomach; *SP*, spleen.) (*Courtesy of Richard M. Gore, MD, Evanston, IL.*)

- Increased splenic vein pressure beyond the obstruction leads to reversal of flow through the short gastric veins to the fundal plexus of the veins.
- Portal hypertension results in gastric varices with associated esophageal varices.
- Splenic vein obstruction results in isolated varices in the gastric fundus without varices in the esophagus.
- Splenic vein obstruction results from intrinsic thrombosis or from extrinsic compression of the splenic vein.

INCIDENCE/PREVALENCE AND EPIDEMIOLOGY

- Gastric varices develop in 20% of patients with portal hypertension.
- Duodenal varices are almost always associated with esophageal varices.

Suggested Readings

Cho KJ, Martel W: Recognition of splenic vein occlusion. *AJR Am J Roentgenol* 131:439-443, 1978.

Goldstein GB: Splenic vein thrombosis causing gastric varices and bleeding. *Am J Gastroenterol* 58:319-325, 1972.

Hershfield NB, Morrow I: Gastric bleeding due to splenic vein thrombosis. *Can Med Assoc J* 98:649-652, 1968.

Itzchak Y, Glickman MG: Splenic vein thrombosis in patients with a normal size spleen. *Invest Radiol* 12:158-163, 1977.

Lavender S, Lloyd-Davies RW, Thomas ML: Retroperitoneal fibrosis causing localized portal hypertension. *BMJ* 3:627-628, 1970.

Levine MS, Kieu K, Rubesin SE, et al: Isolated gastric varices: Splenic vein obstruction or portal hypertension? *Gastrointest Radiol* 15:188-192, 1990.

Muhletaler C, Gerlock J, Goncharenko V, et al: Gastric varices secondary to splenic vein occlusion: Radiographic diagnosis and clinical significance. *Radiology* 132:593-598, 1979.

Okuda K, Yasumoto M, Goto A, et al: Endoscopic observations of gastric varices. *Am J Gastroenterol* 60:357-365, 1973.

Sutton JP, Yarborough DY, Richards JT: Isolated splenic vein occlusion. *Arch Surg* 100:623-626, 1970.

Portal Hypertensive Gastropathy

DEFINITION: Portal hypertensive gastropathy is a distinct pathologic entity caused by chronic portal hypertension.

IMAGING

Radiography
Findings
- Thickened, nodular gastric folds with undulating contours and indistinct borders
- In contrast, gastric varices may appear as thickened folds with a serpentine configuration, associated with discrete submucosal masses.

Utility
- Barium studies

CLINICAL PRESENTATION

- Acute and chronic upper gastrointestinal bleeding

DIFFERENTIAL DIAGNOSIS

- *Helicobacter pylori* gastritis
- Lymphoma (stomach)
- Ménétrier disease (stomach)

PATHOLOGY

- Chronic venous congestion in the stomach causes mucosal hyperemia and increased submucosal arteriovenous communications with dilated arterioles, capillaries, and veins in the gastric wall.
- Gastric fundus is predominantly involved.

DIAGNOSTIC PEARLS

- Thickened, nodular gastric folds with undulating contours and indistinct borders
- Gastric varices may appear as thickened folds with a serpentine configuration and are associated with discrete submucosal masses.
- Varices resemble a bunch of grapes.

INCIDENCE/PREVALENCE AND EPIDEMIOLOGY

- Condition occurs more frequently in patients with cirrhosis than in other patients with portal hypertension.

Suggested Readings

Balan KK, Grime JS, Sutton R, et al: Do alterations in the rate of gastric emptying after injection sclerotherapy for esophageal varices play any role in the development of portal hypertensive gastropathy? *HPB Surg* 11:141-148, 1999.

Chang D, Levine MS, Ginsberg GG, et al: Portal hypertensive gastropathy: Radiographic findings in eight patients. *AJR Am J Roentgenol* 175:1609-1612, 2000.

Panes J, Bordas JM, Pique JM, et al: Increased gastric mucosal perfusion in cirrhotic patients with portal hypertensive gastropathy. *Gastroenterology* 103:1875-1882, 1992.

Smart HL, Triger DR: Clinical features, pathophysiology, and relevance of portal hypertensive gastropathy. *Endoscopy* 23: 224-228, 1991.

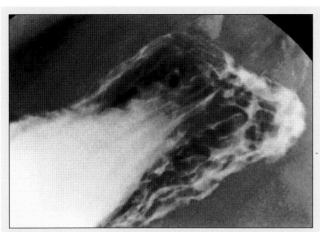

Figure 1. Portal hypertensive gastropathy. Thickened, nodular folds are seen in the gastric fundus. Note how the folds have an undulating contour and indistinct borders. Although gastric varices can produce a similar appearance, they tend to have a more serpentine configuration and are often associated with discrete submucosal masses. (*From Chang D, Levine MS, Ginsberg GG, et al: Portal hypertensive gastropathy: Radiographic findings in eight patients. AJR Am J Roentgenol 175:1609-1612, 2000, © by American Roentgen Ray Society.*)

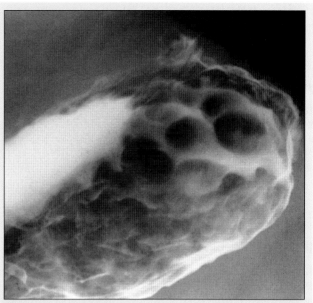

Figure 2. Gastric varices. Tortuous folds and submucosal filling defects are seen in the gastric fundus, resembling the appearance of a bunch of grapes. (*From Levine MS, Kieu K, Rubesin SE, et al: Isolated gastric varices: Splenic vein obstruction or portal hypertension. Gastrointest Radiol 15:188-192, 1990. With kind permission from Springer Science and Business Media.*)

Diverticula

DEFINITION: Diverticula are acquired lesions consisting of a sac of mucosal and submucosal layers herniating through a muscular defect.

ANATOMIC FINDINGS

Duodenum
- Most duodenal diverticula are located on the medial border of the descending duodenum in the periampullary region.
- Duodenal diverticula are also seen on the third or fourth portion of the duodenum and the lateral border of the descending duodenum.

IMAGING

Radiography
Findings
- True gastric diverticula almost always arise from the posterior wall of the gastric fundus; barium in the diverticulum can mimic an ulcer.
- Tiny collection of barium extending outside the contour of the adjacent gastric wall (partial gastric diverticulum) is usually located on the greater curvature of the distal antrum.
- Smooth, round outpouching arises from the medial border of the descending duodenum (duodenal diverticulum).
- *Halo sign* (intraluminal duodenal diverticulum) is rare.
- Localized retroperitoneal gas adjacent to the duodenum and upper pole of the right kidney when duodenal diverticula perforate.

Utility
- Barium studies
- Lack of inflammatory reaction differentiates duodenal diverticulum from a postbulbar duodenal ulcer.
- Abdominal radiographs

CT
Findings
- Fluid-filled cystic lesion or presence of intradiverticular gas

Utility
- Helpful for differentiating duodenal diverticulum from cystic lesion in adjacent pancreas

Nuclear Medicine
Utility
- Required to localize the site of upper gastrointestinal bleeding

DIAGNOSTIC PEARLS
- Smooth, round outpouching arising from the medial border of the descending duodenum (duodenal diverticulum)
- *Halo sign* (intraluminal duodenal diverticulum)
- Tiny collection of barium extending outside the contour of the adjacent gastric wall (partial gastric diverticulum)

CLINICAL PRESENTATION
- Ninety percent of patients with duodenal diverticula are asymptomatic.
- Patients with duodenal diverticula may occasionally exhibit duodenal diverticulitis, upper gastrointestinal bleeding, gastric outlet obstruction, or pancreaticobiliary disease.
- Patients with intraluminal duodenal diverticula can develop nausea and vomiting from associated duodenal obstruction.

DIFFERENTIAL DIAGNOSIS
- Acute cholecystitis
- Chronic cholecystitis
- Peptic ulcer disease
- Acute pancreatitis
- Chronic pancreatitis
- Duodenal ulcers

PATHOLOGY
- Diverticula are acquired lesions consisting of sacs of mucosal and submucosal layers herniating through a muscular defect.
- Diverticula often fill and empty by gravity as result of pressure generated by duodenal peristalsis.
- Intraluminal duodenal diverticulum forms from a congenital duodenal web that elongates intraluminally over time.
- Pseudodiverticula are exaggerated outpouchings or sacculations of inferior and superior recesses of the duodenal bulb related to acute or chronic duodenal ulcer disease.

WHAT THE REFERRING PHYSICIAN NEEDS TO KNOW
- Perforation can occur without clinical signs of peritonitis or radiographic signs of free intraperitoneal air.

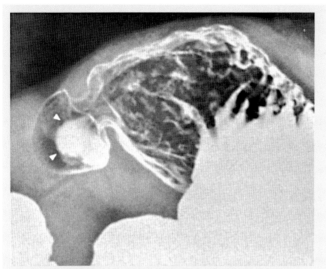

Figure 1. Gastric diverticulum. A large diverticulum is seen arising from the posterior wall of the fundus. Pooling of barium (*arrowheads*) in the diverticulum can be mistaken for an area of ulceration. (*From Eisenberg RL:* Gastrointestinal Radiology: A Pattern Approach, *3rd ed. Philadelphia, JB Lippincott, 1996.*)

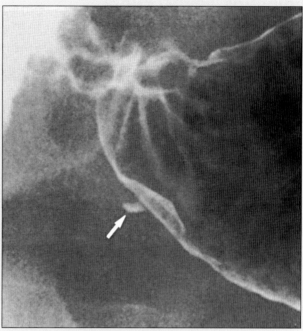

Figure 2. Intramural or partial gastric diverticulum. A tiny, barium-filled outpouching *(arrow)* is seen on the greater curvature of the distal antrum. A heaped-up area is seen overlying the diverticulum that can be mistaken for an ectopic pancreatic rest.

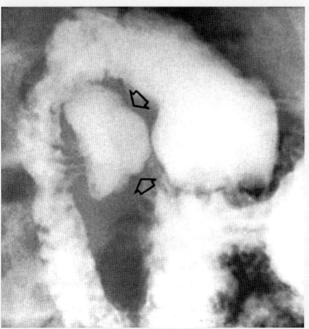

Figure 3. Duodenal diverticulum. A typical diverticulum *(arrows)* is seen arising from the medial border of the descending duodenum. (*From Eisenberg RL:* Gastrointestinal Radiology: A Pattern Approach, *3rd ed. Philadelphia, JB Lippincott, 1996.*)

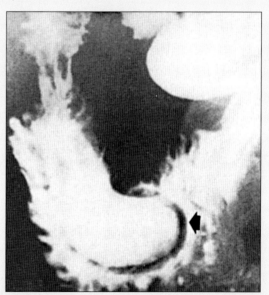

Figure 4. Intraluminal duodenal diverticulum. In this patient, the intraluminal finger-like sac is separated from barium in the adjacent duodenal lumen by a radiolucent band *(arrow)* representing the wall of the diverticulum. (*From Laudan JCH, Norton GI: Intraluminal duodenal diverticulum.* AJR Am J Roentgenol *90:756-760, 1963, © by American Roentgen Ray Society.*)

INCIDENCE/PREVALENCE AND EPIDEMIOLOGY

- Gastric diverticula almost always arise from posterior wall of the fundus.
- Intramural or partial gastric diverticulum is characterized by focal invagination of the mucosa into the muscular layer of the gastric wall; it is almost always located on the greater curvature of the distal antrum.
- Duodenal diverticula are detected as incidental findings on barium studies of upper gastrointestinal tract in up to 15% of patients.
- Most duodenal diverticula are located on the medial border of the descending duodenum in the periampullary region.
- Duodenal diverticula are less commonly found in the third or fourth portion of the duodenum and even the lateral border of the descending duodenum.

Suggested Readings

Afridi SA, Fichtenbaum CJ, Taubin H: Review of duodenal diverticula. *Am J Gastroenterol* 86:935-938, 1991.

Gore RM, Ghahremani GG, Kirsch MD, et al: Diverticulitis of the duodenum: Clinical and radiological manifestations of seven cases. *Am J Gastroenterol* 86:981-985, 1991.

Macari M, Lazarus D, Israel G, et al: Duodenal diverticula mimicking cystic neoplasms of the pancreas: CT and MR imaging findings in seven patients. *AJR Am J Roentgenol* 180:195-199, 2003.

Millard JR, Ziter FMH, Slover WP: Giant duodenal diverticula. *Am J Roentgenol Radium Ther Nucl Med* 121:334-337, 1974.

Nelson JA, Burhenne HJ: Anomalous biliary and pancreatic duct insertion into duodenal diverticula. *Radiology* 120:49-52, 1976.

Pugash RA, O'Brien SE, Stevenson GW: Perforating duodenal diverticulitis. *Gastrointest Radiol* 15:156-158, 1990.

Rioux L, Des Groseilliers S, Fortin M, et al: Massive upper gastrointestinal bleeding originating from a fourth-stage duodenal diverticulum. *Can J Surg* 39:510-512, 1996.

Treichel J, Gerstenberg E, Palme G, et al: Diagnosis of partial gastric diverticula. *Radiology* 119:13-18, 1976.

Wolfe RD, Pearl MJ: Acute perforation of duodenal diverticulum with roentgenographic demonstration of localized retroperitoneal emphysema. *Radiology* 104:301-302, 1972.

Webs and Diaphragms

DEFINITION: Antral webs and diaphragms are thin, membranous septa that are usually located within 3 cm of the pyloric canal and are oriented perpendicular to the long axis of the stomach.

IMAGING

Radiography
Findings
- Antral mucosal diaphragm or web: persistent, sharply defined, 2- to 3-cm-wide band-like defect in the barium column
- Gastric emptying is greatly delayed.
- Barium passes in a thin stream (jet phenomenon) through the center of the orifice.
- Duodenal web or diaphragm: thin, radiolucent line extending across the lumen associated with proximal duodenal dilation (congenital duodenal web).

Utility
- Barium studies
- Antrum distal to web or diaphragm can be mistaken radiographically for duodenal bulb.

CLINICAL PRESENTATION

- Epigastric pain, fullness, and vomiting, especially after heavy meals

DIFFERENTIAL DIAGNOSIS

- Prominent transverse antral fold
- Scarring from peptic ulcer disease
- Antral tumor
- Antral spasm

PATHOLOGY

- Antral webs and diaphragms are thin, membranous septa located 3 cm from the pyloric canal.

DIAGNOSTIC PEARLS

- Persistent, sharply defined, 2- to 3-cm-wide band-like defects in the barium column
- Barium passes in a thin stream (jet phenomenon) through the center of the orifice.
- Thin, radiolucent line extending across the lumen associated with proximal duodenal dilation (congenital duodenal web)

- Duodenal webs and diaphragms are web-like projections in the duodenal lumen that cause varying degrees of obstruction.
- Reported cases involve the second portion of the duodenum near the ampulla of Vater (duodenal webs and diaphragms).

INCIDENCE/PREVALENCE AND EPIDEMIOLOGY

- Vast majority of duodenal webs and diaphragms are thought to be congenital.

Suggested Readings

Bjorgvinsson E, Rudzki C, Lewicki AM: Antral web. *Am J Gastroenterol* 79:663-665, 1984.

Clements JL, Jinkins JR, Torres WE, et al: Antral mucosal diaphragms in adults. *AJR Am J Roentgenol* 133:1105-1111, 1979.

Pratt AD: Current concepts of the obstructing duodenal diaphragm. *Radiology* 100:637-643, 1971.

Rha SE, Lee JH, Lee SY, et al: Duodenal diaphragm associated with long-term use of nonsteroidal antiinflammatory drugs: A rare cause of duodenal obstruction in an adult. *AJR Am J Roentgenol* 175:920-921, 2000.

WHAT THE REFERRING PHYSICIAN NEEDS TO KNOW
- Symptoms of obstruction do not occur if the diameter of the aperture is greater than 1 cm.

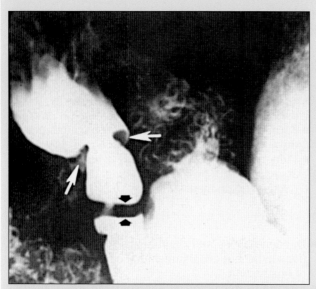

Figure 1. Antral mucosal diaphragm. A band-like defect *(black arrows)* is seen arising at right angles to the gastric wall. The web is approximately 5 mm in thickness. The pyloric channel is denoted by white arrows. *(From Bjorgvinsson E, Rudzki C, Lewicki AM: Antral web.* Am J Gastroenterol *79:663-665, 1984, © by The American College of Gastroenterology.)*

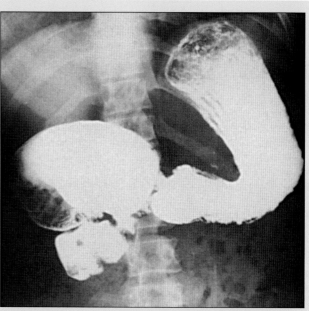

Figure 2. Duodenal web. High-grade stenosis of the second portion of the duodenum is seen. The presence of gas in the bowel distal to the web indicates that the obstruction is incomplete. *(From Eisenberg RL:* Gastrointestinal Radiology: A Pattern Approach, *3rd ed. Philadelphia, JB Lippincott, 1996.)*

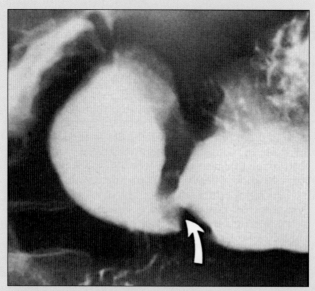

Figure 3. Antral mucosal diaphragm. The lumen is so narrowed by the diaphragm *(arrow)* that the antrum distal to the diaphragm can be mistaken for the duodenal bulb. *(From Eisenberg RL:* Gastrointestinal Radiology: A Pattern Approach, *3rd ed. Philadelphia, JB Lippincott, 1996.)*

Adult Hypertrophic Pyloric Stenosis

DEFINITION: Adult hypertrophic pyloric stenosis is typically characterized by elongation and narrowing of the pyloric canal.

IMAGING

Radiography
Findings
- Elongation and narrowing of pyloric canal
- Concave indentation on base of duodenal bulb

Utility
- Barium studies
- Pylorus can measure 2-4 cm in length (normal length is less than 1 cm in adults).

CLINICAL PRESENTATION

- Nausea and vomiting, epigastric pain, weight loss, or anorexia
- Associated with gastric ulcers

DIFFERENTIAL DIAGNOSIS

- Gastric carcinoma
- Scarring from peptic ulcer disease
- Antral spasm

DIAGNOSTIC PEARLS

- Elongation and narrowing of the pyloric canal
- Concave indentation on the base of the duodenal bulb

PATHOLOGY

- Ulcers probably develop as a result of delayed gastric emptying with increased gastrin production and hyperacidity.
- Pylorus is narrowed as result of hypertrophy of musculature.

INCIDENCE/PREVALENCE AND EPIDEMIOLOGY

- Approximately 50% of patients with adult hypertrophic pyloric stenosis have associated gastric ulcers.

Suggested Readings

Balthazar EJ: Hypertrophic pyloric stenosis in adults: Radiographic features. *Am J Gastroenterol* 78:449-453, 1983.

WHAT THE REFERRING PHYSICIAN NEEDS TO KNOW

- Histologic, anatomic, and radiographic abnormalities in adult hypertrophic pyloric stenosis are indistinguishable from the infantile form.
- Disease in adults represents a milder form of the same entity observed in infants and children.

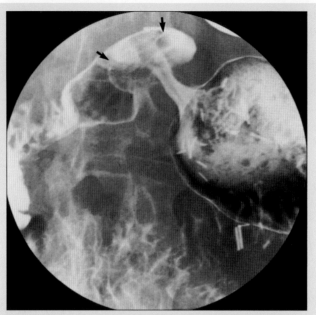

Figure 1. Adult hypertrophic pyloric stenosis. The pyloric canal is narrowed and elongated with a characteristic concave indentation *(arrows)* on the base of the duodenal bulb due to bulging of the pyloric muscle mass into the duodenum.

Gastric Outlet Obstruction

DEFINITION: Gastric outlet obstruction is usually secondary to peptic ulcer disease or a mass in the pylorus or distal antrum.

IMAGING

Radiography
Findings
- Dilated, gas-filled stomach

Utility
- Abdominal radiographs

Fluoroscopy
Findings
- Narrowing of gastric antrum if secondary to scarring
- Mottled density of nonopaque debris in the stomach
- Dilution of barium by retained fluid in the stomach
- Marked delay in gastric emptying of contrast (up to 24 hours or more)
- Narrowing and tapering of the antrum
- Dilated stomach
- Intraluminal filling defect at the base of the duodenal bulb

Utility
- Barium studies
- Persistent barium collection within duodenal bulb, pyloric channel, or prepyloric gastric antrum should suggest peptic ulcer disease as the cause of the obstruction.
- Presence of discrete mass, nodularity, or irregularity in adjacent antrum should suggest a malignant tumor.

CLINICAL PRESENTATION

- Acute or chronic vomiting
- Abdominal pain and weight loss

DIFFERENTIAL DIAGNOSIS

- Peptic ulcer disease
- Gastric carcinoma
- Crohn disease (gastrointestinal)
- Sarcoidosis
- Congenital syphilis
- Primary tuberculosis

DIAGNOSTIC PEARLS

- Dilated, gas-filled stomach
- Marked delay in gastric emptying of contrast (24 hours or more)
- Narrowing and tapering of antrum

- Acute pancreatitis
- Chronic pancreatitis

PATHOLOGY

- Ulcers are usually located in the duodenal bulb; they are also located in the pyloric channel or gastric antrum or body.
- Luminal narrowing in peptic ulcer disease can result from spasm, acute inflammation, edema, muscular hypertrophy, fibrosis, and scarring.
- Obstruction of gastric outlet can also be caused by annular carcinoma of the distal antrum or pylorus.

INCIDENCE/PREVALENCE AND EPIDEMIOLOGY

- Peptic ulcer disease is the most common cause of gastric outlet obstruction in adults, accounting for two thirds of cases.
- Annular carcinoma of the distal antrum or pylorus is the second most common cause of gastric outlet obstruction.

Suggested Readings

Aranha GV, Prinz RA, Greenlee HB, et al: Gastric outlet and duodenal obstruction from inflammatory pancreatic disease. *Arch Surg* 119:833-835, 1984.

Balthazar EJ, Rosenberg H, Davidian MM: Scirrhous carcinoma of the pyloric channel and distal antrum. *AJR Am J Roentgenol* 134:669-674, 1980.

WHAT THE REFERRING PHYSICIAN NEEDS TO KNOW

- Gastric carcinoma should be suspected when gastric outlet obstruction develops in previously asymptomatic patients.
- Radiologist must always attempt to differentiate benign lesion from malignant lesion as the cause of the obstruction on barium studies.
- When gastric carcinoma cannot be excluded, endoscopy or surgical exploration may be required for a definitive diagnosis.

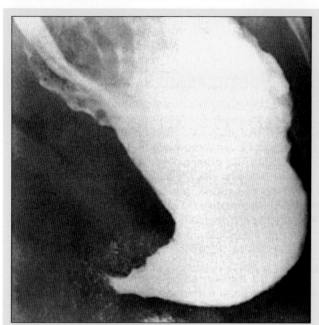

Figure 1. Gastric outlet obstruction caused by Crohn disease. Tapered narrowing of the distal antrum is caused by Crohn disease involving the stomach. (*From Eisenberg RL: Gastrointestinal Radiology: A Pattern Approach, 3rd ed. Philadelphia, JB Lippincott, 1996.*)

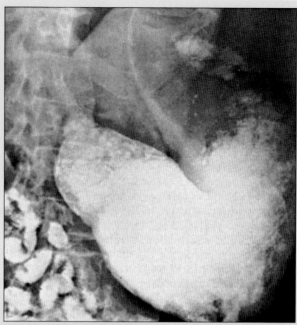

Figure 2. Gastric outlet obstruction caused by peptic ulcer disease. Note gastric distention and dilution of the barium by retained fluid in the stomach. (*From Eisenberg RL: Gastrointestinal Radiology: A Pattern Approach, 3rd ed. Philadelphia, JB Lippincott, 1996.*)

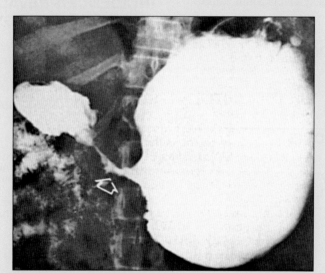

Figure 3. Gastric outlet obstruction caused by an annular carcinoma of the antrum. Note the irregular narrowing of the distal antrum (*arrow*) with proximal dilatation of the stomach. (*From Eisenberg RL: Gastrointestinal Radiology: A Pattern Approach, 3rd ed. Philadelphia, JB Lippincott, 1996.*)

Gastric Dilation Without Gastric Outlet Obstruction

DEFINITION: Acute or chronic dilation of the stomach with prolonged retention of food and barium can occur without any organic gastric outlet obstruction.

IMAGING

Radiography

Findings

- Large quantities of air and fluid fill the massively enlarged stomach extending to or above pelvic floor.
- Marked amount of particulate material is seen in the dilated stomach.

Utility

- Nonobstructive gastric dilation is indistinguishable from organic gastric outlet obstruction on abdominal radiographs.

Fluoroscopy

Findings

- Dilated stomach with retained fluid or debris. (A true bezoar sometimes develops.)
- Peristalsis that is irregular, sluggish, and ineffectual

Utility

- Can differentiate gastroparesis from mechanical gastric outlet obstruction as cause of gastric dilation

CLINICAL PRESENTATION

- Signs include vomiting, dehydration, and peripheral vascular collapse
- Aspiration, fluid and electrolyte disturbances, perforation, peritonitis, and shock also occur.
- Pain is seldom severe until the patient has marked gastric dilation.
- Patient may experience chronic nausea, vomiting, and postprandial abdominal fullness (chronic gastric dilation and gastroparesis).

PATHOLOGY

- Acute gastric dilation is characterized by sudden and severe distention of stomach by gas and fluid.
- Within minutes to hours, the normal stomach can expand into a hyperemic, cyanotic, atonic sac that fills the abdomen.
- Gastric retention with vomiting of food eaten more than 6 hours earlier

DIAGNOSTIC PEARLS

- Large quantities of air and fluid fill the massively enlarged stomach extending to or above pelvic floor.
- Marked amount of particulate material is seen in the dilated stomach.
- Peristalsis is irregular, sluggish, and ineffectual.

- Acute gastric dilation can occur as a complication of medical or surgical conditions, including abdominal trauma and peritoneal inflammatory processes.
- Most common causes of chronic gastric dilation and gastroparesis are diabetes and narcotics.
- Marked gastric dilation may develop in patients with scleroderma, polymyositis, dermatomyositis, and myotonic muscular dystrophy.

INCIDENCE/PREVALENCE AND EPIDEMIOLOGY

- Most cases of acute gastric dilation occur during the first several days after abdominal surgery.
- Most common causes of chronic gastric dilation and gastroparesis are diabetes and narcotics.
- Forty percent of patients with diabetes have dilated stomach with decreased or absent gastric peristalsis and delayed gastric emptying.
- Narcotic medications may also cause marked gastroparesis that gradually resolves after withdrawal of the offending agents.

Suggested Readings

Gramm HF, Reuter K, Costello P: The radiologic manifestations of diabetic gastric neuropathy and its differential diagnosis. *Gastrointest Radiol* 3:151-155, 1978.

Horowitz M, Fraser RJ: Gastroparesis. Diagnosis and management. *Scand J Gastroenterol Suppl* 213:7-16, 1995.

Parkman HP, Hasler WL, Fisher RS: American Gastroenterological Association medical position statement: Diagnosis and treatment of gastroparesis. *Gastroenterology* 127:1589-1591, 2004.

Rimer DG: Gastric retention without mechanical obstruction. *Arch Intern Med* 117:287-299, 1966.

WHAT THE REFERRING PHYSICIAN NEEDS TO KNOW

- Gastric retention may cause vomiting of food eaten more than 6 hours earlier.
- Gastric retention is not synonymous with gastric outlet obstruction, and *corrective* surgery is not always indicated.
- Appropriate therapy usually produces rapid clinical response, but, if untreated, acute gastric dilation may be life threatening.

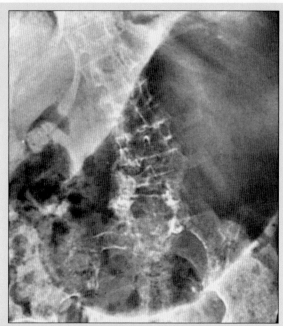

Figure 1. Massive gastric dilation. Abdominal radiograph shows an enormous amount of gas filling a markedly dilated stomach that extends inferiorly into the pelvis. (*From Eisenberg RL: Gastrointestinal Radiology: A Pattern Approach, 3rd ed. Philadelphia, JB Lippincott, 1996.*)

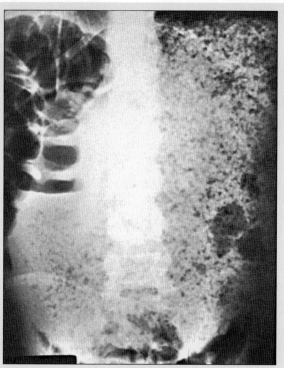

Figure 2. Chronic gastric dilation caused by severe electrolyte and acid-base imbalance. Abdominal radiograph shows a marked amount of particulate material in a massively dilated stomach.

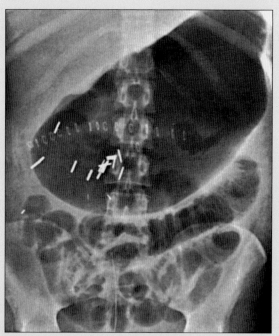

Figure 3. Acute gastric dilation resulting from recent abdominal surgery. (*From Eisenberg RL: Gastrointestinal Radiology: A Pattern Approach, 3rd ed. Philadelphia, JB Lippincott, 1996.*)

Superior Mesenteric Root Syndrome

DEFINITION: Superior mesenteric root syndrome is a type of duodenal obstruction that occurs when some degree of compression of the transverse portion of the duodenum exists.

IMAGING

Radiography

Findings
- Mild, variable dilation of the proximal duodenum
- Extrinsic, vertically oriented, band-like defect on the third portion of the duodenum by the superior mesenteric root
- Variably delayed emptying of barium into the fourth portion of the duodenum and the proximal small bowel with proximal dilatation of the duodenum

Utility
- Barium studies

CLINICAL PRESENTATION

- Nausea and vomiting if obstruction is present

PATHOLOGY

- Any process that closes the aorticomesenteric angle results in some degree of compression of the transverse portion of duodenum.
- Prolonged bed rest causes the mesenteric root to compress the anterior aspect of the transverse duodenum, resulting in duodenal obstruction.
- Superior mesenteric root syndrome occurs in patients with scleroderma and a dilated, atonic duodenum proximal to the level of the superior mesenteric root.
- Space-occupying processes within the aorticomesenteric angle can also compress the transverse duodenum.

DIAGNOSTIC PEARLS

- Mild, inconstant dilation of proximal duodenum
- Transient delay of barium where the transverse duodenum crosses spine
- Extrinsic, vertically oriented, band-like defect on the third portion of the duodenum by the superior mesenteric root

INCIDENCE/PREVALENCE AND EPIDEMIOLOGY

- Superior mesenteric root syndrome is most likely to occur in asthenic persons, particularly those who rapidly lose weight because of a debilitating illness.

Suggested Readings

Berk RN, Coulson DB: The body cast syndrome. *Radiology* 94:303-305, 1970.

Shammash JB, Rubesin SE, Levine MS: Massive gastric distention due to duodenal involvement by retroperitoneal tumors. *Gastrointest Radiol* 17:214-216, 1992.

Simon M, Lerner MA: Duodenal compression by the mesenteric root in acute pancreatitis and in inflammatory conditions of the bowel. *Radiology* 79:75-81, 1962.

Wallace RG, Howard WB: Acute superior mesenteric artery syndrome in the severely burned patient. *Radiology* 94:307-310, 1970.

WHAT THE REFERRING PHYSICIAN NEEDS TO KNOW

- Extrinsic, vertically oriented band-like defect on the third portion of the duodenum is characteristic of indentation by superior mesenteric root.
- This finding is often encountered as an incidental observation in thin patients who are asymptomatic.
- If the indentation by the superior mesenteric root is associated with radiographic signs of obstruction in patients with nausea and vomiting, then the patient has the superior mesenteric root syndrome as the cause of this obstruction.

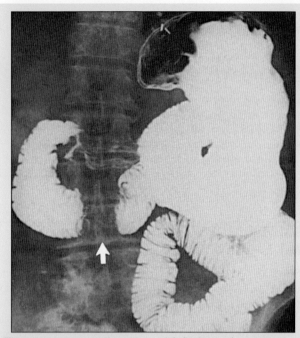

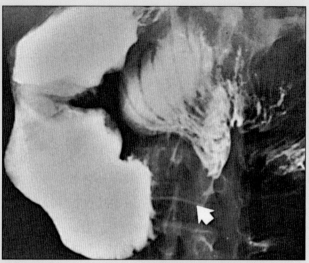

Figure 2. Superior mesenteric root syndrome caused by scleroderma. The duodenum is markedly dilated and atonic proximal to an extrinsic, vertically oriented, band-like defect *(arrow)* at the aorticomesenteric angle. This patient had nausea and vomiting due to duodenal obstruction by superior mesenteric root. (*From Eisenberg RL:* Gastrointestinal Radiology: A Pattern Approach, *3rd ed. Philadelphia, JB Lippincott, 1996.*)

Figure 1. Asymptomatic patient with findings of superior mesenteric root syndrome. Frontal view shows an extrinsic, vertically oriented, band-like defect *(arrow)* without significant obstruction of the third portion of the duodenum by the superior mesenteric root.

Extrinsic Masses

DEFINITION: Extrinsic impressions on the stomach and duodenum may be caused by prominence or pathologic enlargement of adjacent organs.

IMAGING

Radiography
Findings
- Large tubular defect in duodenal bulb with oblique orientation characteristic of extrinsic impression by dilated common bile duct
- Displacement of the duodenum
- Extrinsic impressions on the anterior aspect of the stomach

Utility
- Barium study

CT
Utility
- CT can aid in differentiating extrinsic defects from true intragastric lesions.

PATHOLOGY

- Impressions on the stomach are caused by a prominent left hepatic lobe, an aberrant spleen or kidney, or pathologic enlargement of adjacent structures.
- Common bile duct may produce a linear or small, rounded impression on the duodenal bulb.
- Hepatomegaly or anomalous lobes of liver cause leftward displacement of the duodenal bulb and sweep.
- Carcinoma of right side of the colon, especially hepatic flexure, results in extrinsic impression on the outer border of the descending duodenum.

DIAGNOSTIC PEARLS

- Large tubular defect in the duodenal bulb with oblique orientation is characteristic of extrinsic impression by dilated common bile duct.
- Extrinsic impressions on the stomach and duodenum caused by a variety of adjacent mass lesions

INCIDENCE/PREVALENCE AND EPIDEMIOLOGY

- Approximately 3% of patients exhibit a close positional relationship between the duodenum and the transverse colon, resulting in a mutual indentation.

Suggested Readings

Bluth I, Vitale P: Right renal enlargement causing alterations in the descending duodenum: A radiographic demonstration. *Radiology* 76:777-784, 1961.

Chon H, Arger PH, Miller WT: Displacement of duodenum by an enlarged liver. *Am J Roentgenol Radium Ther Nucl Med* 119:85-88, 1973.

Poppel MH: Duodenocolic apposition. *Am J Roentgenol Radium Ther Nucl Med* 83:851-856, 1960.

Shimkin PM, Pearson KD: Unusual arterial impressions upon the duodenum. *Radiology* 103:295-297, 1972.

Treitel H, Meyers MA, Maza V: Changes in the duodenal loop secondary to carcinoma of the hepatic flexure of the colon. *Br J Radiol* 43:209-213, 1970.

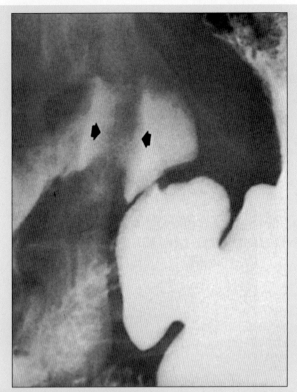

Figure 1. Duodenal impression by a dilated common bile duct.
The dilated duct produces a characteristic tubular impression
(arrows) on the duodenum near the apex of the bulb. (*From
Eisenberg RL:* Gastrointestinal Radiology: A Pattern Approach,
3rd ed. Philadelphia, JB Lippincott, 1996.)

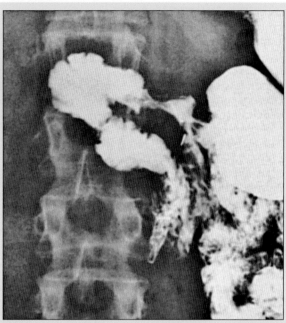

Figure 2. Duodenal impression by a polycystic right kidney.
The duodenum is displaced to the left of the spine by a polycystic
kidney. (*From Eisenberg RL:* Gastrointestinal Radiology: A Pattern
Approach, *3rd ed. Philadelphia, JB Lippincott, 1996.*)

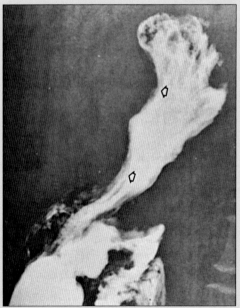

Figure 3. Gastric impressions by a polycystic liver. Two large
extrinsic impressions *(arrows)* on the anterior aspect of the stomach
can be mistaken for intramural lesions. (*From Eisenberg RL:*
Gastrointestinal Radiology: A Pattern Approach, *3rd ed. Philadelphia,
JB Lippincott, 1996.*)

Widening of the Duodenal Sweep

DEFINITION: True widening of the duodenal sweep may be caused by pancreatic neoplasms or by benign pancreatic disease.

IMAGING

Radiography
Findings
- Double contour on the medial border of the duodenum with associated widening of the duodenal sweep

Utility
- Barium studies

CT
Findings
- Mass in head of pancreas

Utility
- CT should be obtained for a more definitive diagnosis of pancreatic abnormalities.

CLINICAL PRESENTATION

- Signs and symptoms of underlying pancreatic disease

DIFFERENTIAL DIAGNOSIS

- Enlarged head of pancreas
- Peripancreatic lymphadenopathy

DIAGNOSTIC PEARLS

- Double contour on the medial border of duodenum

- Other retroperitoneal masses
- Choledochal cyst

PATHOLOGY

- Widening of the duodenal sweep is most commonly caused by an enlarged head of the pancreas secondary to pancreatic neoplasms, pancreatitis, or pancreatic pseudocysts.
- Lymphoma, metastases, and inflammation involving the pancreaticoduodenal and subpyloric lymph nodes may cause peripancreatic node enlargement and widening of the duodenal sweep.
- Retroperitoneal masses can widen the duodenal sweep.
- Choledochal cyst near the ampulla of Vater can result in generalized widening of the duodenal sweep.

Suggested Readings
Zeman RK, Schiebler M, Clark LR, et al: The clinical and imaging spectrum of pancreaticoduodenal lymph node enlargement. *AJR Am J Roentgenol* 144:1223-1227, 1985.

WHAT THE REFERRING PHYSICIAN NEEDS TO KNOW

- Great variation can be found in the configuration of the duodenal sweep, and slight widening is difficult to recognize with confidence on barium studies.

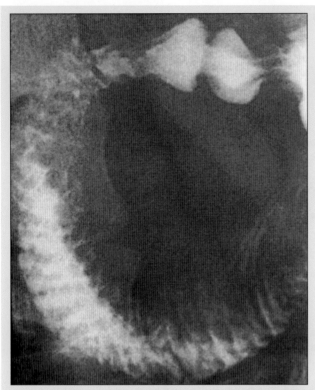

Figure 1. Widening of the duodenal sweep by peripancreatic lymphoma. Enlarged peripancreatic lymph nodes have produced a double contour on the medial border of the duodenum with associated spiculation. Pancreatitis or pancreatic carcinoma can produce similar findings. (*From Eisenberg RL:* Gastrointestinal Radiology: A Pattern Approach, *3rd ed. Philadelphia, JB Lippincott, 1996.*)

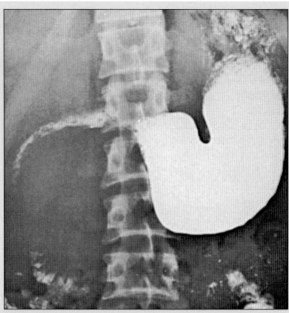

Figure 2. Widening of the duodenal sweep caused by acute pancreatitis. (*From Eisenberg RL:* Gastrointestinal Radiology: A Pattern Approach, *3rd ed. Philadelphia, JB Lippincott, 1996.*)

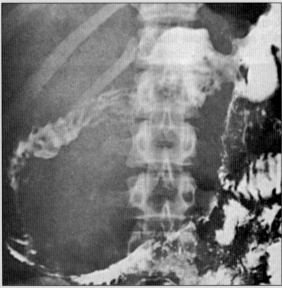

Figure 3. Widening of the duodenal sweep by a pancreatic pseudocyst. Pancreatitis or pancreatic carcinoma can produce similar findings. (*From Eisenberg RL:* Gastrointestinal Radiology: A Pattern Approach, *3rd ed. Philadelphia, JB Lippincott, 1996.*)

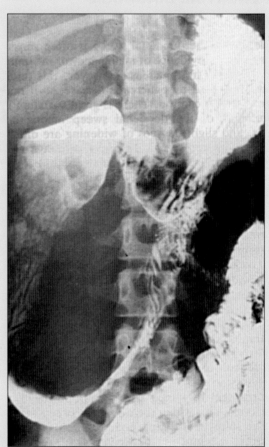

Figure 4. *Widening of the duodenal sweep by a choledochal cyst.* (*From Eisenberg RL:* Gastrointestinal Radiology: A Pattern Approach, *3rd ed. Philadelphia, JB Lippincott, 1996.*)

Pancreatic Diseases Affecting the Stomach and Duodenum

DEFINITION: The pancreas is an organ adjacent to both the stomach and the duodenum and can cause displacement or indentation of either organ in the setting of pancreatic enlargement.

IMAGING

Radiography
Findings
- Double-contour effect
- *Inverted-3 sign* of Frostberg
- Fine or coarse sharpening and elongation of barium-filled crevices between the duodenal folds
- *Antral pad sign*
- Irregular gastric contour with spiculated, tethered mucosal folds on the greater curvature
- Extrinsic compression, flattening, or spiculation of the posterior wall of the gastric fundus or body

Utility
- Results from differential filling of duodenum
- Nonspecific
- May be caused by mucosal edema or irritation

CT
Findings
- Compression or displacement of stomach

CLINICAL PRESENTATION

- Signs and symptoms of underlying pancreatic disease

DIAGNOSTIC PEARLS

- Double contour effect
- *Inverted-3 sign* of Frostberg
- *Antral pad sign*

DIFFERENTIAL DIAGNOSIS

- Peripancreatic lymphadenopathy
- Aortic aneurysm
- Other retroperitoneal masses

PATHOLOGY

- Duodenal involvement by pancreatitis, pancreatic pseudocysts, or pancreatic carcinoma may be manifested by development of ulcers, cavities, and pancreaticoduodenal fistulas.
- Pancreatic enlargement may cause displacement or indentation of either the stomach or the duodenum.

Suggested Readings
Asrani AV: The antral pad sign. *Radiology* 229:421-422, 2003.

WHAT THE REFERRING PHYSICIAN NEEDS TO KNOW
- CT, MR, or ultrasonography should be performed for a more definitive diagnosis.

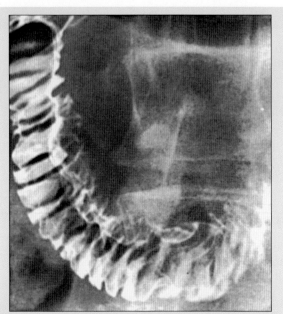

Figure 1. Duodenal involvement by pancreatic carcinoma. An enlarged pancreatic head produces a double contour on the medial border of the duodenum. Also note spiculated folds in this region. (*From Eisenberg RL: Gastrointestinal Radiology: A Pattern Approach, 3rd ed. Philadelphia, JB Lippincott, 1996.*)

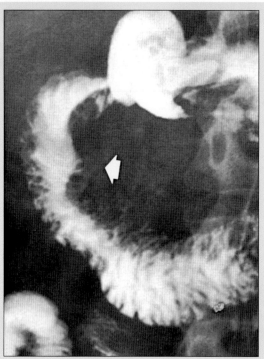

Figure 2. The inverted-3 sign of Frostberg. Note the widened duodenal sweep with fixation of the duodenal wall at the papilla *(arrow)*, producing the inverted-3 sign. This patient had acute pancreatitis; thus, the inverted-3 sign is not specific for pancreatic carcinoma.

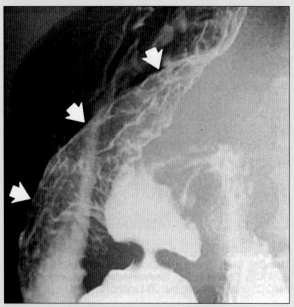

Figure 3. Gastric involvement by a pancreatic pseudocyst. Lateral view of a stomach shows a retrogastric mass *(arrows)* in profile. (*From Laufer I, Levine MS [eds]: Double-Contrast Gastrointestinal Radiology, 2nd ed. Philadelphia, WB Saunders, 1992.*)

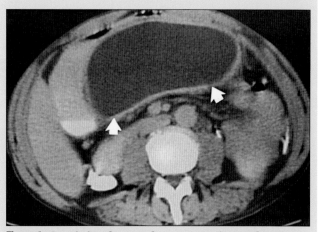

Figure 4. Gastric involvement by a pancreatic pseudocyst (same patient as in Figure 3). CT scan reveals a large pancreatic pseudocyst *(arrows)* compressing and displacing the stomach. (*From Laufer I, Levine MS [eds]: Double-Contrast Gastrointestinal Radiology, 2nd ed. Philadelphia, WB Saunders, 1992.*)

Gastric Bezoars

DEFINITION: A bezoar is an intragastric mass consisting of accumulated ingested material.

IMAGING

Radiography

Findings

- Soft-tissue mass is seen floating in the stomach at the air-fluid interface.
- Mottled appearance is caused by barium trapped in interstices of the bezoar.
- Bezoar may be unusually smooth, simulating an enormous gas bubble.

Utility

- With changes in patient position, most bezoars are freely movable within the gastric lumen.

CT

Findings

- Inhomogeneous intraluminal mass with mottled gas pattern in the lesion

CLINICAL PRESENTATION

- Signs include crampy epigastric pain and a sense of fullness or heaviness in the upper abdomen.
- Prevalence of associated peptic ulcers is high, especially with abrasive phytobezoars.
- Large bezoars may cause symptoms of gastric outlet obstruction.

PATHOLOGY

- Accumulated, matted mass of hair may enlarge to occupy the entire lumen of the stomach, assuming the shape of the stomach.

DIAGNOSTIC PEARLS

- Soft-tissue mass floating in the stomach at the air-fluid interface
- Mottled appearance caused by barium trapped in the interstices of the bezoar
- Inhomogeneous intraluminal mass with a mottled gas pattern on CT

- Bezoar may form in gastric remnant after a partial gastrectomy, particularly when strictures develop at the gastroduodenal or gastrojejunal anastomosis.

INCIDENCE/PREVALENCE AND EPIDEMIOLOGY

- Trichobezoars (composed of hair) occur predominantly in women, especially those with schizophrenia or other mental illnesses.
- Small percentage of bezoars are composed of both hair and vegetable matter (called trichophytobezoars).

Suggested Readings

Ripolles T, Garcia-Aguayo G, Martinez MJ, et al: Gastrointestinal bezoars: Sonographic and CT characteristics. *AJR Am J Roentgenol* 177:65-69, 2001.

WHAT THE REFERRING PHYSICIAN NEEDS TO KNOW

- Phytobezoars (composed of undigested vegetable matter) are associated with the eating of unripe persimmons.

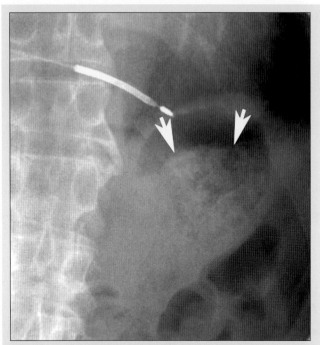

Figure 1. Gastric bezoar. Supine abdominal radiograph shows a gastric bezoar as a mottled soft-tissue mass *(arrows)* floating in the stomach at the air-fluid interface.

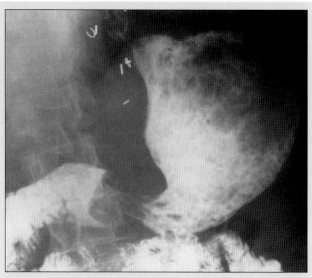

Figure 2. Gastric bezoar. The bezoar is characterized by a conglomerate mass of debris with barium trapped in its interstices, producing a characteristic mottled appearance.

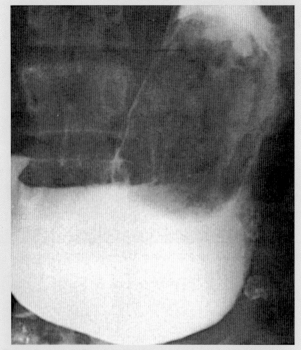

Figure 3. Gastric bezoar. The bezoar appears as a smooth filling defect in the stomach that can be mistaken for an enormous gas bubble. This patient was a model airplane builder who had been ingesting glue. (*From Eisenberg RL:* Gastrointestinal Radiology: A Pattern Approach, *3rd ed. Philadelphia, JB Lippincott, 1996.*)

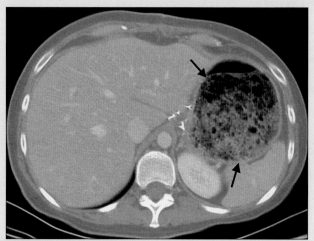

Figure 4. Gastric bezoar on CT. The bezoar is characterized on CT by an inhomogeneous intraluminal mass with a mottled gas pattern *(arrows)*. This patient had undergone a partial gastrectomy with a bezoar in the gastric remnant because of a stricture at the gastrojejunal anastomosis (not visualized on this image). (*From Woodfield CA, Levine MS: The postoperative stomach.* Eur J Radiol *53:341-352, 2005.*)

Gastric Volvulus

DEFINITION: Gastric volvulus is an uncommon acquired twist of the stomach on itself that can lead to obstruction or strangulation, with potentially life-threatening gastric infarction.

IMAGING

Radiography
Findings
- Intrathoracic stomach with double air-fluid level

Utility
- Upright chest radiograph

Fluoroscopy
Findings
- Upside-down intrathoracic stomach

Utility
- Barium studies are useful for showing gastric outlet obstruction.

CT
Findings
- Enlarged, twisted stomach in thorax with identification of one or more sites of torsion

Utility
- CT is useful for showing signs of ischemia.

CLINICAL PRESENTATION

- Patients with gastric volvulus may be asymptomatic if no gastric outlet obstruction or vascular compromise exists.
- There is a triad of retching with little vomitus, constant severe epigastric pain, and inability to advance nasogastric tube beyond distal esophagus.
- Postprandial pain or vomiting occurs if the patient has gastric outlet obstruction.
- Vascular occlusion causes gastric necrosis, perforation, and shock.

DIFFERENTIAL DIAGNOSIS

- Paraesophageal hernia
- Giant hiatal hernia with floppy fundus

DIAGNOSTIC PEARLS

- Intrathoracic stomach with double air-fluid level on abdominal radiographs
- Upside-down intrathoracic stomach on barium studies
- Enlarged, twisted stomach in the thorax with identification of one or more sites of torsion on CT

PATHOLOGY

- Acquired twist of stomach on itself, leading to obstruction or strangulation with potentially life-threatening gastric infarction
- Torsion of stomach may occur with significant degrees of gastric herniation.
- With small herniations, the proximal portion of stomach enters the hernial sac first.
- Organoaxial volvulus refers to rotation of stomach upward around its long axis.
- In mesenteroaxial volvulus, stomach rotates from right to left or left to right along the long axis of the gastrohepatic omentum.

Suggested Readings

Allen MS, Trastek VF, Deschamps C, et al: Intrathoracic stomach: Presentation and results of operation. *J Thorac Cardiovasc Surg* 105:253-258, 1993.
Chiechi MV, Hamrick-Turner J, Abbitt PL: Gastric herniation and volvulus: CT and MR appearance. *Gastrointest Radiol* 17:99-101, 1992.
Gerson DE, Lewicki AM: Intrathoracic stomach: When does it obstruct? *Radiology* 119:257-264, 1976.
Scott RL, Felker R, Winer-Muram H, et al: The differential retrocardiac air-fluid level: A sign of intrathoracic gastric volvulus. *J Can Assoc Radiol* 37:119-121, 1986.

WHAT THE REFERRING PHYSICIAN NEEDS TO KNOW

- Gastric volvulus may be associated with eventration or paralysis of the diaphragm without a true hernia.
- Acute gastric volvulus may be a surgical emergency if the vascular supply to the stomach is compromised.

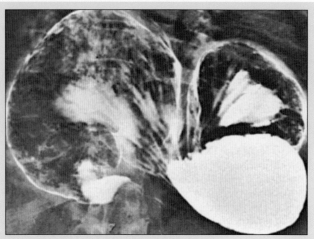

Figure 1. Gastric volvulus. This patient has an organoaxial volvulus of the stomach causing gastric outlet obstruction. The stomach is located above the diaphragm with inversion of the greater curvature above the lesser curvature and downward pointing of the pylorus. (*From Eisenberg RL:* Gastrointestinal Radiology: A Pattern Approach, *3rd ed. Philadelphia, JB Lippincott, 1996.*)

Gastroduodenal and Duodenojejunal Intussusception

DEFINITION: Gastroduodenal and duodenojejunal intussusceptions are associated with gastric or duodenal tumors that serve as the lead point for the intussusception.

IMAGING

Radiography

Findings

- Foreshortening and narrowing of the gastric antrum with telescoping mucosal folds in the antrum or duodenum (gastroduodenal intussusception)
- Converging or telescoping mucosal folds in the antrum or duodenum
- Prepyloric collar-shaped outpouchings
- Widening of the pyloric channel (gastroduodenal intussusception)
- Coil-spring appearance (gastroduodenal and duodenojejunal intussusception)
- Tumor serving as lead point may be identified as a mass.

CT

Findings

- CT may reveal target sign of intussusception with fat drawn into lumen.
- CT may also show tumor serving as lead point as a mass in the lumen or wall of bowel.

CLINICAL PRESENTATION

- Acute onset of vomiting
- Variable abdominal pain

DIAGNOSTIC PEARLS

- Telescoping mucosal folds in the antrum or duodenum (gastroduodenal intussusception)
- Prepyloric collar-shaped outpouchings and widening of the pyloric channel (gastroduodenal intussusception)
- Coil-spring appearance

PATHOLOGY

- Associated with gastric or duodenal tumors that serve as lead point

Suggested Readings

Choi SH, Han JK, Kim SH, et al: Intussusception in adults: From stomach to rectum. *AJR Am J Roentgenol* 183:691-698, 2004.

Meyers MA: Gastroduodenal intussusception. *Am J Med Sci* 254: 347-355, 1967.

Van Beers B, Trigau JP, Pringot J: Duodenojejunal intussusception secondary to duodenal tumors. *Gastrointest Radiol* 13:24-26, 1988.

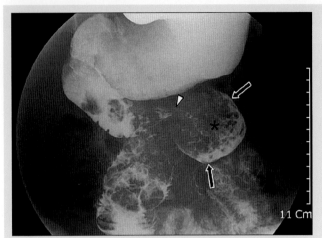

Figure 1. Duodenal intussusception. Small-bowel follow-through shows an elongation of the duodenum *(arrowhead)* and duodenojejunal intussusception *(arrows)* with a large, lobulate, cauliflower-surfaced polypoid intramural mass arising from the duodenum *(asterisk)* as the lead point for the intussusception. Note multiple polypoid masses throughout the stomach and small bowel. (*From Jeon SJ, Yoon SE, Lee YH, et al: Acute pancreatitis secondary to duodenojejunal intussusception in Peutz-Jegher syndrome. Clin Radiol 62:88-91, 2007.*)

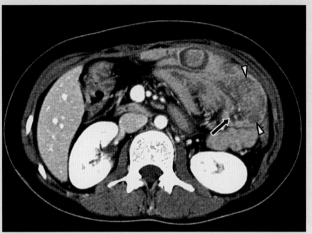

Figure 2. Duodenal intussusception. CT image shows duodenojejunal intussusception with surrounding fat and vessels invaginated into the proximal jejunum *(arrow)*. Note a large, lobulated, intramural mass as a lead point *(arrowheads)*. (*From Jeon SJ, Yoon SE, Lee YH, et al: Acute pancreatitis secondary to duodenojejunal intussusception in Peutz-Jegher syndrome. Clin Radiol 62:88-91, 2007.*)

Fistulas

DEFINITION: Fistulous communications between the stomach and duodenum and other abdominal organs may occur as a complication of benign or malignant disease.

IMAGING

Radiography
Findings
- Barium may enters fistulous tracts.
- Fistula may exert mass effect on the adjacent structure.
- Malignant tumors causing gastrocolic or duodenocolic fistulas are usually bulky, infiltrating lesions associated with marked inflammatory reaction.

Utility
- Malignant gastrocolic fistulas are frequently demonstrated on barium enema but are rarely detected on upper gastrointestinal series.
- Increased intraluminal pressure in the colon during a barium enema overcomes resistance of the rigid fistula, allowing passage of barium into the stomach.

CLINICAL PRESENTATION

- Diarrhea, weight loss, pain, vomiting, and bleeding occur in one third to one half of gastrocolic fistulas.
- Aortoduodenal fistula is characterized by abdominal pain, gastrointestinal bleeding, and a palpable, pulsatile mass.

PATHOLOGY

- Benign greater curvature ulcers caused by nonsteroidal anti-inflammatory drugs (NSAIDs) may penetrate inferiorly via the gastrocolic ligament into the superior border of the transverse colon.
- Malignant tumors causing gastrocolic or duodenocolic fistulas usually appear as bulky, infiltrating lesions that are associated with marked inflammatory reaction.
- Acute cholecystitis commonly results in development of cholecystoduodenal fistula.
- Aortoduodenal fistulas can occur as a complication of abdominal aortic aneurysms or prosthetic vascular grafts.
- Pressure necrosis of the third portion of the duodenum leads to aortic wall digestion by enteric secretions with the development of aortoduodenal fistulas.

DIAGNOSTIC PEARLS

- Barium fills the cholecystoduodenal fistula.
- Compression or displacement of the third portion of the duodenum by an extrinsic mass (aortoduodenal fistula)

- Fistulas between the duodenum and the right kidney occasionally develop as a complication of pyelonephritis.
- Duodenorenal fistulas can result from rupture of a perirenal abscess into the duodenum.

INCIDENCE/PREVALENCE AND EPIDEMIOLOGY

- Gastrocolic fistulas are most commonly caused by NSAIDs and, less frequently, by primary carcinoma of the stomach or colon, tuberculosis, radiation, and Crohn disease.
- Gastrocolic fistulas are associated with a high mortality rate, especially if the diagnosis of the fistula is delayed.
- Fistulas between the gallbladder and the duodenum may be caused by acute cholecystitis (90%) or severe peptic ulcer disease (less than 10%).

Suggested Readings

Haff RC, Wise L, Ballinger WF: Biliary-enteric fistulas. *Surg Gynecol Obstet* 133:84-88, 1971.

Levine MS, Kelly MR, Laufer I, et al: Gastrocolic fistulas: The increasing role of aspirin. *Radiology* 187:359-361, 1993.

Martinez LO, Manheimer LH, Casal GL, et al: Malignant fistulae of the gastrointestinal tract. *AJR Am J Roentgenol* 131:215-218, 1978.

Smith DL, Dockerty MD, Black BM: Gastrocolic fistulas of malignant origin. *Surg Gynecol Obstet* 134:829-832, 1972.

Swartz MJ, Paustian FF, Chleborad WJ: Recurrent gastric ulcer with spontaneous gastrojejunal and gastrocolic fistulas. *Gastroenterology* 44:527-531, 1963.

Wyatt GM, Rauchway MI, Spitz HB: Roentgen findings in aortoenteric fistulae. *AJR Am J Roentgenol* 126:714-722, 1976.

WHAT THE REFERRING PHYSICIAN NEEDS TO KNOW

- Gastrojejunocolic and gastrocolic fistulas represent serious complications of marginal ulceration after gastric surgery for peptic ulcer disease.
- In patients with severe peptic ulcer disease, penetrating gastric or duodenal ulcers can perforate into the transverse colon, gallbladder, or bile duct.

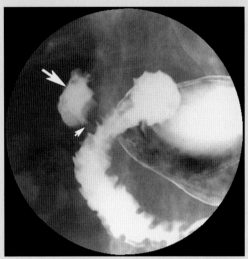

Figure 1. Cholecystoduodenal fistula. Barium study shows barium filling the gallbladder *(large arrow)* via a fistula *(small arrow)* from the descending duodenum. Also note thickened folds and decreased distensibility of the duodenum in this patient with a long-standing history of ulcer disease. The fistula presumably developed as a complication of a penetrating postbulbar duodenal ulcer.

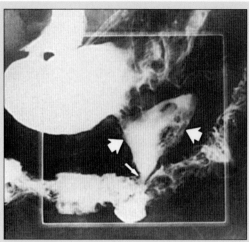

Figure 2. Gastrocolic fistula caused by a benign greater curvature ulcer. Upper gastrointestinal study shows a giant ulcer *(large arrows)* on the greater curvature of the stomach with barium entering a fistula *(small arrow)* that communicates with the superior border of the transverse colon. *(From Levine MS, Kelly MR, Laufer I, et al: Gastrocolic fistulas: The increasing role of aspirin.* Radiology *187:359-361, 1993.)*

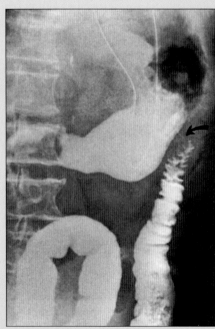

Figure 3. Gastrocolic fistula caused by carcinoma of the splenic flexure. Barium enema shows an annular carcinoma of the splenic flexure with barium entering the stomach via a gastrocolic fistula *(arrow)*. *(From Eisenberg RL: Gastrointestinal Radiology: A Pattern Approach, 3rd ed. Philadelphia, JB Lippincott, 1996.)*

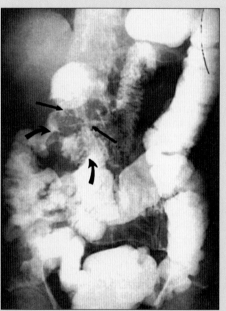

Figure 4. Duodenocolic fistula caused by carcinoma of the proximal transverse colon. Barium enema shows an annular carcinoma *(curved arrows)* of the proximal transverse colon, with barium entering the duodenum via a duodenocolic fistula *(straight arrows)*. *(From Vieta JO, Blanco R, Valentini GR: Malignant duodenocolic fistula: Report of two cases, each with one or more synchronous gastrointestinal cancers.* Dis Colon Rectum *19:542-552, 1976, © by American Society of Colon and Rectal Surgeons, Inc.)*

Perforation

DEFINITION: Perforation of the stomach or duodenum secondary to peptic ulcer disease is the most common cause of pneumoperitoneum.

IMAGING

Radiography
Findings
- Absence of gas within the stomach and the presence of gas in the small and large bowels
- Free intraperitoneal air

Utility
- The above findings suggest gastric perforation as cause of pneumoperitoneum.
- No evidence of free intraperitoneal air was seen on abdominal radiographs in 30% of patients with perforated duodenal ulcers.

Fluoroscopy
Findings
- Extravasation of contrast agent from the stomach or duodenum

Utility
- Diagnosis of site of perforation requires study with a water-soluble contrast agent.

CT
Findings
- Extraluminal gas or extravasated contrast material in the right anterior pararenal space

Utility
- Helpful in differentiating duodenal perforation from hematoma without perforation
- Particularly helpful for showing contained perforation

CLINICAL PRESENTATION

- Peritoneal signs and symptoms are classic.
- Perforation can occur without clinical signs of peritonitis in some patients with perforated duodenal ulcers.

DIAGNOSTIC PEARLS

- Absence of gas within the stomach and the presence of gas in the small and large bowels
- Free extravasation of the contrast agent from the stomach or duodenum
- Extraluminal gas or extravasated contrast material in the right anterior pararenal space

PATHOLOGY

- Perforated duodenal ulcer is the most common cause of pneumoperitoneum.

INCIDENCE/PREVALENCE AND EPIDEMIOLOGY

- Most frequent cause of pneumoperitoneum in patients with peritonitis is a perforated duodenal ulcer.
- Mortality rate of perforation approximately 30%

Suggested Readings

Kunin JR, Korobkin M, Ellis JH, et al: Duodenal injuries caused by blunt abdominal trauma: Value of CT in differentiating perforation from hematoma. *AJR Am J Roentgenol* 160:221-223, 1993.

Miller RE: The radiological evaluation of intraperitoneal gas (pneumoperitoneum). *CRC Crit Rev Clin Radiol Nucl Med* 4:61-85, 1973.

Wolfe RD, Pearl MJ: Acute perforation of duodenal diverticulum with roentgenographic demonstration of localized retroperitoneal emphysema. *Radiology* 104:301-302, 1972.

WHAT THE REFERRING PHYSICIAN NEEDS TO KNOW

- Failure to demonstrate pneumoperitoneum is of little value in excluding the possibility of a perforated ulcer.
- Absence of colonic gas and presence of gastric air-fluid level and small bowel distention make colonic perforation more likely.

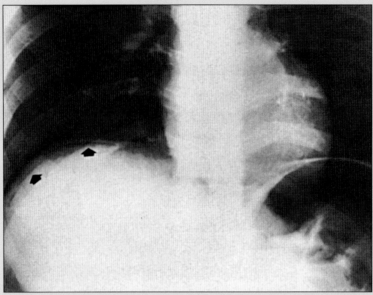

Figure 1. Pneumoperitoneum caused by a perforated duodenal ulcer. Free intraperitoneal air is seen beneath the right hemidiaphragm *(arrows).* (*From Eisenberg RL:* Gastrointestinal Radiology: A Pattern Approach, *3rd ed. Philadelphia, JB Lippincott, 1996.*)

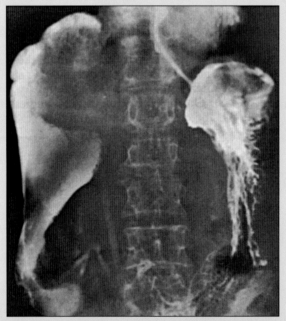

Figure 2. Pneumoperitoneum caused by a perforated duodenal ulcer. Study using a water-soluble contrast agent shows free extravasation of the contrast agent from the duodenum into the right side of the peritoneal cavity. (*From Eisenberg RL:* Gastrointestinal Radiology: A Pattern Approach, *3rd ed. Philadelphia, JB Lippincott, 1996.*)

Other Miscellaneous Abnormalities of the Stomach and Duodenum

DEFINITION: Miscellaneous abnormalities of the stomach and duodenum include benign gastric emphysema and changes caused by amyloidosis and cystic fibrosis.

IMAGING

Radiography

Findings

- Benign gastric emphysema: linear collections of gas within the gastric wall
- Amyloidosis: marked narrowing and rigidity of the gastric wall (especially the antrum), producing linitis plastica appearance
- Amyloidosis: thickened, nodular folds in the stomach
- Cystic fibrosis: thickened, coarse fold pattern, with nodular indentations in the duodenum
- Cystic fibrosis: associated findings include nodular indentations; poor definition of mucosal fold pattern; and redundancy, distortion, and kinking of the duodenum
- Cystic fibrosis changes are usually confined to the first and second portions of the duodenum but occasionally extend into the proximal jejunum.

Utility

- Barium studies

DIFFERENTIAL DIAGNOSIS

- Other causes of thickened gastric folds, including gastritis, lymphoma, and Ménétrier's disease
- Other causes of thickened duodenal folds, including duodenitis and Crohn disease

DIAGNOSTIC PEARLS

- Linear collections of gas within the gastric wall (benign gastric emphysema)
- Thickened, nodular folds in the stomach (amyloidosis)
- Nodular indentations on the duodenal wall (cystic fibrosis)

PATHOLOGY

- Benign gastric emphysema has no known underlying cause.
- Deposition of an amorphous, eosinophilic, extracellular protein-polysaccharide complex of amyloid in the stomach causes gastric abnormalities in amyloidosis.
- Lack of secretion of pancreatic bicarbonate results in inadequate buffering of gastric acid in cystic fibrosis.

Suggested Readings

Agrons GA, Corse WR, Markowitz RI, et al: Gastrointestinal manifestations of cystic fibrosis: Radiologic-pathologic correlation. *Radiographics* 16:871-893, 1996.

Carlson HC, Breen JF: Amyloidosis and plasma cell dyscrasias: Gastrointestinal involvement. *Semin Roentgenol* 21:128-138, 1986.

Lee S, Rutledge JN: Gastric emphysema. *Am J Gastroenterol* 79: 899-904, 1984.

Phelan MS, Fine DR, Zentler-Munro L, et al: Radiographic abnormalities of the duodenum in cystic fibrosis. *Clin Radiol* 34:573-577, 1983.

WHAT THE REFERRING PHYSICIAN NEEDS TO KNOW

- Benign gastric emphysema can be differentiated from gastric infarction by absence of acute symptoms of bowel ischemia and infarction.

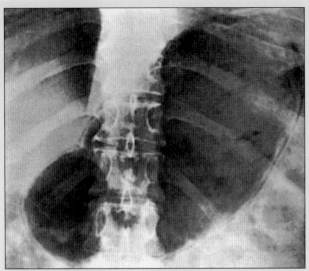

Figure 1. Benign gastric emphysema. Linear collections of gas are seen in the gastric wall as a complication of endoscopy. (*From Eisenberg RL:* Gastrointestinal Radiology: A Pattern Approach, *3rd ed. Philadelphia, JB Lippincott, 1996.*)

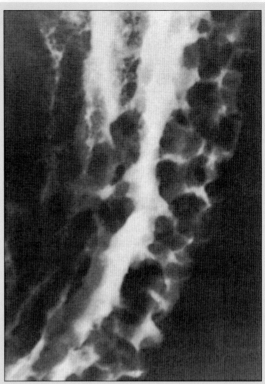

Figure 2. Gastric involvement by amyloidosis. Thickened, nodular folds in the stomach are caused by infiltration of the gastric wall by amyloidosis. (*From Eisenberg RL:* Gastrointestinal Radiology: A Pattern Approach, *3rd ed. Philadelphia, JB Lippincott, 1996.*)

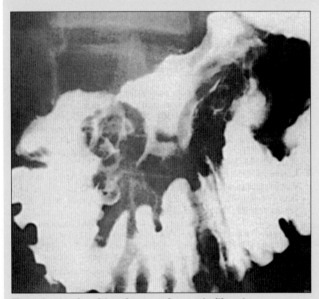

Figure 3. Duodenal involvement by cystic fibrosis. A thickened, coarse fold pattern is seen in the duodenum. (*From Eisenberg RL:* Gastrointestinal Radiology: A Pattern Approach, *3rd ed. Philadelphia, JB Lippincott, 1996.*)

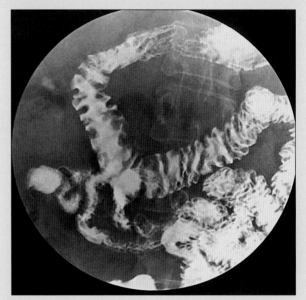

Figure 4. Duodenal involvement by cystic fibrosis. A thickened, coarse fold pattern is seen in the duodenum.

Small Bowel

Part 21

CROHN DISEASE OF THE SMALL BOWEL

Crohn Disease

DEFINITION: Crohn disease is an idiopathic inflammatory disease that can affect any part of the gastrointestinal tract from the mouth to the anus.

ANATOMIC FINDINGS

Bowel
- Small bowel is involved in 80% of patients, with the terminal ileum by far the most common location.
- Ileocecal and enteroenteric fistulas are common and are often multiple.
- Crohn-related fistulas between the transverse colon and the duodenum are not unusual.
- Neoterminal ileum is involved in recurrent disease.

Abdominal Lymph Nodes
- Prominent perienteric lymph nodes (located in sub-peritoneal space of small bowel mesentery) are seen in the active inflammatory phase.

IMAGING

Radiography and Fluoroscopy
Findings
- Smooth, symmetric fold thickening progressing to partial or complete fold obliteration in active inflammatory disease
- Shallow mucosal erosions progressing to stellate or linear ulcers to deep clefts and fissures, with cobblestone appearance in active inflammatory disease
- Thickening and retraction of the adjacent mesentery while the unaffected antimesenteric border becomes pleated, disappearing later on with the spread of involvement

DIAGNOSTIC PEARLS
- Cobblestone mucosa
- *Comb sign* consists of short, parallel, linear structures that are perpendicular to the intestinal long axis of the bowel, best seen on contrast-enhanced T1-weighted images.
- Mural thickening, with or without submucosal edema, is seen.
- Prominent mesenteric lymph nodes are noted.

- Nodular-pattern bowel segment containing many inflammatory polyps separated by curving lines of barium occupying crevices between elevations
- Changes associated with linear mesenteric ulceration advance in caudad direction as the disease progresses.
- Strictures: *string sign*; possibly associated with aneurysmal dilation in the proximal segment
- Fistulizing or perforating disease: barium possibly entering the abscess cavity, collection of tracts, or multiple small spaces within the inflammatory mass
- High-grade or low-grade partial small bowel obstruction
- Presence of prestenotic dilation
Utility
- Has traditionally been used to radiographically establish the diagnosis, detect complications, and follow disease course

---

WHAT THE REFERRING PHYSICIAN NEEDS TO KNOW
- Ileocolonoscopy allows an accurate diagnosis of Crohn disease of the colon and terminal ileum.
- Endoscopy provides assessment of disease activity and consequences of inflammation, including strictures, mass lesions, bleeding, and the development of dysplasia or malignancy.
- Comb sign and enhancing the mesenteric nodes may be useful in differentiating lymphoma and metastases, which are usually hypovascular lesions.
- Fibrofatty proliferation is a hallmark of Crohn disease, which can aid in the distinction between ulcerative colitis and Crohn disease.
- Differentiation between fibrotic and edematous stenosis based on magnetic resonance properties helps in selecting patients for medical versus surgical treatment.
- Video capsule endoscopy is a sensitive means of diagnosing nonstricturing Crohn disease; a stricture is a contraindication to the procedure.
- Increased prevalence of small bowel carcinoma has been reported in patients with Crohn disease involving the small bowel.

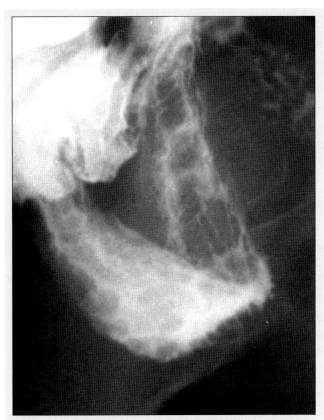

Figure 1. Active inflammatory Crohn disease: cobblestone mucosa. Multiple transverse and longitudinal ulcerations of the terminal ileum are identified on conventional small bowel examination performed in this patient with Crohn disease.

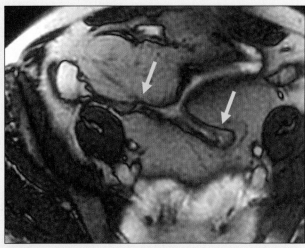

Figure 2. Fistulizing or perforating Crohn disease: MRI finding. Axial true FISP image shows multiple ileoileal fistulas that contain high-signal-intensity fluid *(arrows)*.

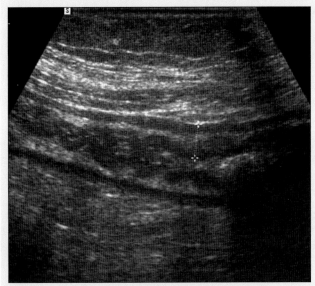

Figure 3. Crohn disease: sonographic features. Mural thickening is the sonographic hallmark of Crohn disease. *(Courtesy of Dr. Pierre-Jean Valette, Lyons, France.)*

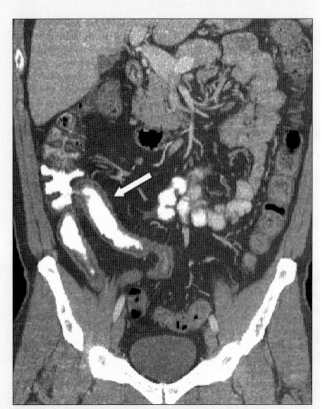

Figure 4. Mural thickening in Crohn disease: CT and pathologic findings. Coronal reformatted image also shows abnormal mural thickening and submucosal edema *(arrow)*.

MRI

Findings

- Blunting, flattening, thickening, distortion of small bowel folds, mucosal nodularity, and aphthous-type ulcers in early disease
- Ulcers: thin lines of high signal intensity within the thickened bowel wall; cobblestoning
- Mucosal hyperemia, submucosal edema: inner ring of mucosal enhancement highlighted against a low-intensity ring in gadolinium-enhanced fat-saturated T1-weighted sequences
- Bowel wall thickening, usually ranging from 1-2 cm, is the most consistent feature of Crohn disease on MRI.
- Target pattern that is often observed on gadolinium-enhanced T1-weighted images in patients with acute Crohn disease
- Sinus tracts, fistulas, abscess; fibrofatty proliferation (*creeping fat*) of the mesentery that causes bowel loop separation
- *Comb sign*: short, parallel, linear structures perpendicular to the intestinal long axis of the bowel best seen on contrast-enhanced T1-weighted images

Utility

- MRI helps confirm the diagnosis; localize lesions; assess the severity, extent, and inflammatory activity; and identify extraintestinal complications that may require surgical intervention.
- Adequate distention of the bowel lumen is very important because collapsed bowel loops can hide the lesions or mimic an abnormality.
- T2-weighted half-Fourier rapid acquisition with relaxation enhancement (RARE), half-Fourier acquisition single-shot turbo spin-echo, T1-weighted gadolinium-enhanced spoiled gradient-echo are important in the evaluation of Crohn disease.
- True fast imaging with steady-state precision (FISP) sequence is particularly good for obtaining information about mural and extraintestinal complications.
- MR enteroclysis is an emerging diagnostic tool that combines the advantages of conventional enteroclysis and MRI.
- MR fluoroscopic images can be reviewed in a cine-loop format to obtain functional information concerning bowel obstruction.

Ultrasound

Findings

- Mural thickening with stratification in acute disease, which is lost in the chronic stage
- Creeping fat of the mesentery manifesting as a uniform echogenic halo around the mesenteric border of encased gut, separating the bowel loops
- Prominent lymph nodes: spherical hypoechoic masses without the normal echogenic streak from nodal hilum in patients with active inflammatory disease
- Crohn disease strictures showing mural thickening with luminal surfaces of the involved segments in apposition
- Fistula appearing as linear bands of varying echogenicity extending from the gut to the bladder, another segment of the bowel, or bladder

- Empty or partially closed tract appearing as hypoechoic segment of the bowel, or bladder
- Abscesses on ultrasound look like a fluid-filled or complex mass that may contain gas.

Utility

- Ultrasound is inferior to CT and MRI in the depiction of serosal and mesenteric complications of Crohn disease.

Doppler Ultrasound

Findings

- Increased superior and inferior mesenteric artery blood flow, an increased pulsatility index, a decreased resistive index, increased portal vein velocity
- Increased systolic and diastolic flow through the superior mesenteric artery also possibly seen, attesting to disease activity
- Color Doppler imaging typically shows hyperemia.

Utility

- This technique has been used in assessing disease activity.

CT

Findings

- Mural hyperenhancement and increased mural thickness are the most sensitive CT findings of active Crohn disease.
- Cobblestone mucosa can be appreciated as deep longitudinal and transverse ulcers with thickened, edematous mucosa interposed.
- Target sign of active inflammation is inner mucosal and outer muscularis propria and serosa enhancement; intermediate low-density ring reflects submucosal edema.
- Patients with active Crohn disease also show engorgement of the vasa rectae (*comb sign*).
- Creeping fat of the mesentery is also well depicted on multidetector CT (MDCT).
- Fistula formation, perforation, and abscesses are seen.
- Fibrostenotic phase manifests as fixed narrowing of the bowel with uniformly enhanced mural thickening.

Utility

- CT enterography employs MDCT with narrow-section thickness and reconstruction intervals, intravenous contrast material, and neutral contrast agent to distend the lumen.
- MDCT has become the primary means of diagnosing and treating Crohn disease–related abscesses.

CLINICAL PRESENTATION

- Crohn disease is a chronic relapsing disease, usually characterized by periods of symptom exacerbation alternating with periods of clinical remission.
- Abdominal pain, mild diarrhea, weight loss, and pyrexia are common clinical findings.
- Other patients may have a right lower quadrant mass, representing a diseased ileum or cecum.
- Combination of decreased food absorption and intermittent obstruction may lead to significant weight loss in these patients.

- Crohn disease in the small bowel has a slightly better prognosis than colonic disease.
- Complications such as abscesses, fistulas, and obstruction are more likely than with colon disease.

DIFFERENTIAL DIAGNOSIS

- Metastases to the small bowel
- Lymphoma (gastrointestinal)
- Bacterial infections
- Gastric outlet obstruction (stomach and duodenum)
- Lipomas (and fatty infiltration of the ileocecal valve) (colon)
- Parasitic infections
- Peritoneal carcinomatosis

PATHOLOGY

- Crohn disease is an idiopathic inflammatory disease that can affect any part of gastrointestinal tract from the mouth to the anus.
- Types include active inflammatory, fibrostenotic, fistulizing or perforating, and reparative or regenerative.
- Different phases of the disease may be present within different segments of the small bowel in the same patient.
- Earliest histologic changes consist of hyperplasia of lymphoid tissue and obstructive lymphedema in the submucosa.
- Strictures of small-bowel Crohn disease are caused by collagen deposition, predominantly in the submucosa.

- Fistulas occur as result of the transmural extension of the disease.
- Cobblestoning reflects severe edema between the longitudinal and the transverse ulcerations.

INCIDENCE/PREVALENCE AND EPIDEMIOLOGY

- With the exception of malignant neoplasms, Crohn disease can be the most devastating disease to involve the gastrointestinal tract.
- Crohn disease has worldwide distribution but is most common in northern Europe, North America, and Japan.
- Prevalence has increased, mostly in younger age groups, with peak age between 15 and 25 years.
- Both sexes are equally affected.
- Familial tendency has frequently been described.

Suggested Readings

Hara AK, Leighton JA, Heigh RI, et al: Crohn disease of the small bowel: Preliminary comparison among CT enterography, capsule endoscopy, small-bowel follow-through, and ileoscopy. *Radiology* 238:128-134, 2006.

Maglinte DDT, Gourtsoyiannis N, Rex D, et al: Classification of small bowel Crohn's subtypes based on multimodality imaging. *Radiol Clin North Am* 41:285-303, 2003.

Munkholm P, Binder V: Clinical features and natural history of Crohn's disease. In Sartor RB, Sandborn WJ (eds): *Kirsner's Inflammatory Bowel Diseases*, 6th ed. Edinburgh, Saunders, 2004, pp 289-300.

Part 22

INFLAMMATORY DISORDERS OF THE SMALL BOWEL (OTHER THAN CROHN DISEASE)

Parasitic Infections

DEFINITION: Colonization of parasites (nematodes, cestodes, trematodes, protozoans) in the small bowel.

IMAGING

Radiography
Findings
- Ascariasis: long tubular filling defects in the intestinal lumen and thickened small bowel folds
- Ancylostomiasis: jejunal fold thickening
- Strongyloidiasis: small bowel folds thickened, effaced, or obliterated. (The jejunum has narrowed, tubular configuration, sometimes associated with fold thickening.)
- Anisakiasis: focal, irregular small bowel fold thickening
- Giardiasis: thickened folds and irritability in the duodenum and jejunum
- Trypanosomiasis: dilation of the small bowel with delayed transit

Utility
- Barium studies
- Enteroclysis

CT
Findings
- Ascariasis: long tubular filling defects in the intestinal lumen
- Anisakiasis: mesenteric mass or abscess

CLINICAL PRESENTATION

- Ascariasis: small-bowel obstruction, malabsorption, and abdominal pain
- Strongyloidiasis: abdominal pain, diarrhea, malabsorption, and weight loss
- Ancylostomiasis: iron-deficiency anemia, peripheral eosinophilia, and acute gastrointestinal bleeding

DIAGNOSTIC PEARLS

- Ascariasis: long tubular filling defects in the intestinal lumen and enlarged bowel folds
- Giardiasis: thickened folds and irritability in the duodenum and jejunum
- Ancylostomiasis, strongyloidiasis: jejunal fold thickening
- Trypanosomiasis: dilation of the small bowel with delayed transit
- Strongyloidiasis: small bowel folds effaced or obliterated. (The jejunum has a narrowed, tubular configuration.)

- *Diphyllobothrium latum* may cause vitamin B_{12} deficiency and macrocytic anemia.
- Trypanosomiasis may cause secondary achalasia, megaduodenum, and megacolon.

DIFFERENTIAL DIAGNOSIS

- Crohn disease (small bowel)
- Bacterial infections (small bowel)
- Viral infections (small bowel)

PATHOLOGY

- *Ascaris* larvae penetrate the mucosa, enter the bowel wall vessels, reaching the portal venous system, then migrate to the liver, heart, and lungs.
- Ancylostomiasis results from filarial invasion of the feet (in people who walk barefoot) or hands.

WHAT THE REFERRING PHYSICIAN NEEDS TO KNOW
- Radiographic diagnosis can be confirmed by detection of ova in stool specimens.
- Hookworms have not been demonstrated on barium studies.
- Strongyloidiasis autoinfection may occur; infections may be life threatening in immunocompromised hosts.
- Mild infestation by strongyloidiasis cannot be detected on imaging studies.
- Tapeworm infection usually causes no symptoms.
- Colonic infection by schistosomiasis is more common than small-bowel infection.

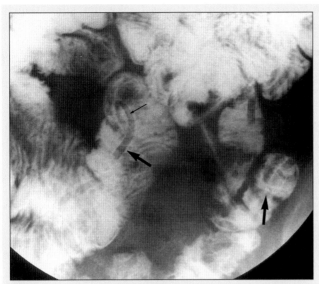

Figure 1. Ascariasis. A young man complained of crampy abdominal pain and mild diarrhea 1 month after returning from a vacation in Central America. Spot image of the ileum from a small bowel follow-through shows numerous smooth, tubular filling defects in the barium column (representative ascarids identified by *thick arrows*). Barium faintly stains the body cavity of one worm *(thin arrow)*. *(From Forbes A, Misiewicz JJ, Compton CC, et al: Atlas of Clinical Gastroenterology, 3rd ed. Edinburgh, Elsevier-Mosby, 2005.)*

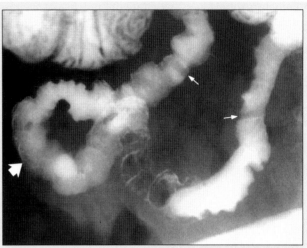

Figure 2. Strongyloidiasis. Coned-down view of overhead radiograph from a small bowel follow-through shows markedly thickened folds *(thin arrows)* in several loops of jejunum. In some areas, the inflammatory process is so severe that the folds are effaced or lost *(thick arrow)*. *(Courtesy of Jack Farman, MD, New York; from the teaching file of Hans Herlinger, MD.)*

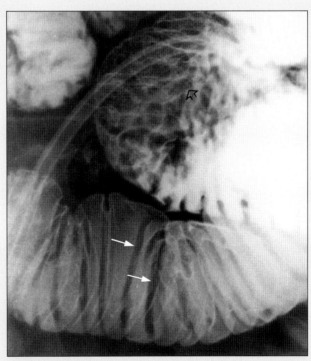

Figure 3. Giardiasis. Spot image of the jejunum from an enteroclysis examination shows mildly thickened folds *(arrows)*. Tiny mucosal nodules *(open arrow)* reflect enlargement of villi. *(From the teaching file of Hans Herlinger, MD.)*

- Female *Strongyloides* penetrate the mucosa of the duodenum and proximal jejunum and live in the superficial layers of the proximal small bowel.
- Edema and inflammation develop at the site of attempted *Anisakis* larval penetration.
- After the cestode-infected flesh is ingested, the cysticercus breaks down, releasing the scolex, which attaches to the upper jejunum.
- *Giardia* trophozoites remain in the intestinal lumen or penetrate the mucous gel layer of the proximal intestine, attaching to the glycocalyx of enterocytes.
- *Trypanosoma cruzi* produces a neurotoxin that attacks autonomic ganglion cells throughout the body.

INCIDENCE/PREVALENCE AND EPIDEMIOLOGY

- Worms and protozoa infect more than one fourth of the world's population.
- *Ascaris lumbricoides* infects one fourth of the world's population, frequently people living in the tropics and subtropics.
- Hookworms infect almost 1 billion people worldwide.
- *Ancylostoma duodenale* is found in southern Europe, the Mediterranean, the western coast of South America, India, and Southeast Asia.

- *Necator americanus* causes hookworm infestation in the southern United States, Caribbean, South America, India, and Southeast Asia.
- *Strongyloides stercoralis* is found in the tropics and subtropics.
- *Schistosoma* infects more than 150 million people worldwide.

Suggested Readings

Blumenthal DS, Schultz MG: Incidence of intestinal obstruction in children infected with *Ascaris lumbricoides*. *Am J Trop Med Hyg* 24:801-804, 1975.

Dallemand S, Waxman M, Farman J: Radiological manifestations of *Strongyloides stercoralis*. *Gastrointest Radiol* 8:45-51, 1983.

Drasin GF, Moss JPO, Cheng SH: *Strongyloides stercoralis* colitis: Findings in four cases. *Radiology* 126:619-621, 1978.

Herlinger H: Parasitic and bacterial inflammatory diseases. In Herlinger H, Maglinte DDT, Birnbaum BA (eds): *Clinical Imaging of the Small Intestine*, 2nd ed. New York, Springer, 1999, pp 291-309.

Hommeyer SC, Hamill GS, Johnson JA: CT diagnosis of intestinal ascariasis. *Abdom Imaging* 20:315-316, 1995.

Markell EK, Voge M: *Medical Parasitology*, 4th ed. Philadelphia, WB Saunders, 1976.

Muraoka A, Suehiro I, Fuigii M, et al: Acute gastric anisakiasis: 28 cases during the last 10 years. *Dig Dis Sci* 41:2362-2365, 1996.

Pawloski ZS: Ascariasis. Host-pathogen biology. *Rev Infect Dis* 4:806-814, 1982.

Wynne JM, Ellman BAH: Bolus obstruction by *Ascaris lumbricoides*. *S Afr Med J* 63:644-646, 1983.

Bacterial Infections

DEFINITION: Bacterial infections involving the small bowel may cause pathologic changes that can be confused with Crohn disease.

ANATOMIC FINDINGS

Ileum
- Intestinal tuberculosis occurs primarily in the ileocecal region.
- Yersiniosis occurs in the terminal ileum, where aphthoid ulcers overlie hyperplastic lymphoid follicles.
- Salmonellosis occurs in the distal ileum, where ulcers are found overlying Peyer patches.
- Campylobacteriosis occurs in the distal and terminal ileum as well as the ileocecal valve.

IMAGING

Fluoroscopy
Findings
- Tuberculosis: 3- to 6-mm perpendicular, stellate, or longitudinal ulcers with heaped-up margins, strictures, and nodular mucosa
- Yersiniosis: aphthoid ulcers and thickened folds in the early stage; thickened, undulating folds that persist while ulcers disappear in the late stage
- Yersiniosis versus Crohn disease: absence of luminal narrowing, fissures, and fistulas makes yersiniosis more likely
- Salmonellosis: longitudinally oriented ulcers, prominent lymphoid follicles, vascular thrombosis, and fold thickening
- Campylobacteriosis: multiple superficial ulcers, thickened folds, and aphthoid ulcers

Utility
- Barium studies
- Radiographic findings in campylobacteriosis, early yersiniosis, and early Crohn disease may be indistinguishable.

DIAGNOSTIC PEARLS
- Tuberculosis: 3- to 6-mm perpendicular, stellate, or longitudinal ulcers with heaped-up margins, strictures, and nodular mucosa
- Yersiniosis: aphthoid ulcers and thickened folds in the early stage; thickened, undulating folds persisting while ulcers disappear in the late stage
- Salmonellosis: longitudinally oriented ulcers, prominent lymphoid hyperplasia, vascular thrombosis, and fold thickening
- Campylobacteriosis: multiple superficial ulcers, thickened folds, and aphthoid ulcers

CT
Findings
- Tuberculosis: thickening of the ileocecal valve and pericecal lymphadenopathy
- Salmonellosis: circumferential thickening of the terminal ileum

CLINICAL PRESENTATION
- *Yersinia*: ileitis, colitis, mesenteric adenitis, periappendicitis, and hemolytic-uremic syndrome; the inflammatory process usually resolves in 4-6 weeks.
- Salmonellosis (typhoid fever): brief diarrhea, followed by febrile illness lasting for 3 weeks, with headaches, malaise, abdominal discomfort, and arthralgias
- Typhoid ileitis: gastrointestinal bleeding, perforation, peritonitis, adynamic ileus, right lower quadrant pain, hepatosplenomegaly, and fever

---

WHAT THE REFERRING PHYSICIAN NEEDS TO KNOW
- Intestinal tuberculosis frequently occurs without radiographic evidence of pulmonary disease; endoscopic biopsy specimens and tissue cultures are frequently negative.
- Tuberculosis versus Crohn disease: clinical history and patient demographics should help suggest the correct diagnosis.
- The diagnosis of tuberculosis is often made only by pathologic examination of resected surgical specimens.
- Cross-reactivity of *Campylobacter jejuni* and neural antigens may result in Guillain-Barré syndrome.
- Bacterial multiplication of *Yersinia* in lymph nodes can result in chronic hepatitis, ankylosing spondylitis, and lung or kidney infections.
- Bacteremia in salmonellosis can lead to other infections, including meningitis, pericarditis, orchitis, and splenic or liver abscesses.

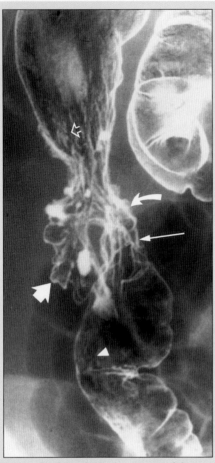

Figure 1. Ileocecal tuberculosis. Spot image of the ascending colon from a double-contrast barium enema shows disproportionately severe disease in the cecum versus the terminal ileum. The cecum is contracted and sacculated *(large arrow)*. Granular and nodular mucosa *(open arrow)* is present in the cecum and ascending colon. The ileocecal valve is gaping *(curved arrow)*. Only the distal 2 cm of the terminal ileum is narrowed *(thin arrow)*. The remainder of the terminal ileum has a finely nodular mucosa *(arrowhead)*. (From Rubesin SE, Bartram CI, Laufer I: Inflammatory bowel disease. In Levine MS, Rubesin SE, Laufer I [eds]: Double Contrast Gastrointestinal Radiology, *3rd ed. Philadelphia, WB Saunders, 2000, pp 417-470.)*

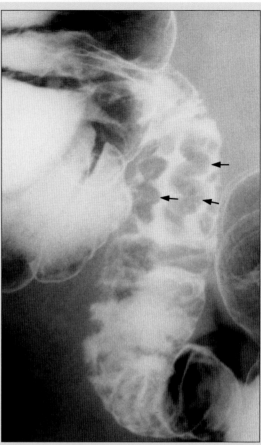

Figure 2. *Yersinia* ileitis. Spot image of the terminal ileum from a double-contrast barium enema shows thickened, undulating folds *(arrows)* in the terminal ileum. No ileal narrowing is seen.

- Campylobacteriosis: acute enteritis or colitis; fulminant colitis with gastrointestinal bleeding, toxic megacolon, and systemic manifestations, including arthritis, endocarditis, genital infections, and urinary tract infections

DIFFERENTIAL DIAGNOSIS

- Crohn disease (small bowel)
- Parasitic infections (small bowel)

PATHOLOGY

- Gastrointestinal tuberculosis includes ulcerative, hypertrophic, and ulcerohypertrophic forms.

- Sloughing of mucosa overlying submucosal tubercles results in ulceration, whereas inflammation and fibrosis of the bowel wall result in a hypertrophic form associated with extensive mesenteric lymphadenopathy and adhesions.
- Tubercle bacilli are found primarily in necrotic mesenteric lymph nodes rather than the intestinal wall.
- *Yersinia* invades epithelial cells, enters Peyer patches in the lamina propria or submucosa, spreads to mesenteric lymph nodes, and causes massive lymphadenopathy, vasculitis, and ischemia.
- *Salmonella* enters and multiplies in M cells and enterocytes, then disseminates to lymphoid tissue, macrophages in the submucosa, and mesenteric lymph nodes.

INCIDENCE/PREVALENCE AND EPIDEMIOLOGY

- Tuberculosis is endemic in Asia; incidence is uncommon, but is rising, in Western countries.
- Gastrointestinal tuberculosis occurs in the homeless, alcoholics, inmates, farmers, immigrants, and people with human immunodeficiency virus.
- *Yersinia enterocolitica* is more frequently encountered than *Y. pseudotuberculosis* in the United States.
- Food-borne *Salmonella* outbreaks are more common than fecal-oral spread from human reservoirs.

Suggested Readings

Ahmed FB: Tuberculous enteritis: A serious possibility in some patients. Grand Rounds-Hammersmith Hospital. *BMJ* 31:215-217, 1996.

Fantry GT, Fantry LE, James SP: Chronic infections of the small intestine. In Yamada T, Alpers DH, Kaplowitz N, et al (eds): *Textbook of Gastroenterology*, 4th ed. Philadelphia, Lippincott Williams & Wilkins, 2003, pp 1561-1579.

Fenoglio-Preiser CM, Noffsinger AE, Stemmermann GN, et al: Non-neoplastic lesions of the small intestine. In *Gastrointestinal Pathology: An Atlas and Text*. Philadelphia, Lippincott-Raven, 1999, pp 309-358.

Greenberg HB, Matsui SM, Holodniy M: Small intestine: Infections with common bacterial and viral pathogens. In *Textbook of Gastroenterology*, 4th ed. Philadelphia, Lippincott Williams & Wilkins, 2003, pp 1530-1560.

Herlinger H: Parasitic and bacterial inflammatory diseases. In Herlinger H, Maglinte DDT, Birnbaum BA (eds): *Clinical Imaging of the Small Intestine*, 2nd ed. New York, Springer, 1999, pp 291-308.

Nakano H, Jaramillo E, Watanabe M, et al: Intestinal tuberculosis: Findings on double-contrast barium enema. *Gastrointest Radiol* 17:108-114, 1992.

Saebo A, Lasser J: *Yersinia enterocolitica*, an inducer of chronic inflammations. *Int J Tissue React* 16:51-57, 1994.

Histoplasmosis and Other Infections

DEFINITION: Infections of the small bowel caused by *Histoplasma* fungi and viruses.

IMAGING

Radiography
Findings
- Histoplasmosis of ileocecal region: ulceration, mucosal nodularity, strictures, and lymphadenopathy
- Intestinal perforation and peritonitis
Utility
- Contrast study

CT
Findings
- Thickening of bowel wall

CLINICAL PRESENTATION

- Viral infection of the small intestine results in acute diarrhea.
- Histoplasmosis of the small intestine causes minimal symptoms.

DIFFERENTIAL DIAGNOSIS

- Crohn disease (small bowel)
- Bacterial infections (small bowel)
- Parasitic infections (small bowel)

PATHOLOGY

- *Histoplasma capsulatum* fungus occurs in mycelial form at ambient temperature and in yeast form at body temperature.
- Various viruses infect the small intestine.

DIAGNOSTIC PEARLS

- Histoplasmosis of the ileocecal region produces ulceration, mucosal nodularity, strictures, and lymphadenopathy.
- Diagnosis of acute diarrhea caused by viral infection can be made by viral cultures or by enzyme-linked immunosorbent assay or electron microscopy of stool specimens.

INCIDENCE/PREVALENCE AND EPIDEMIOLOGY

- Fungus usually infects elderly patients or immuno-compromised hosts.
- Small bowel infection is common in patients with disseminated disease.
- *H. capsulatum* is a dimorphic fungus commonly found in the Mississippi and Ohio River valleys.

Suggested Readings

Alterman DD, Cho KC: Histoplasmosis involving the omentum in an AIDS patient: CT demonstration. *J Comput Assist Tomogr* 12: 664-665, 1988.

Fantry GT, Fantry LE, James SP: Chronic infections of the small intestine. In Yamada T, Alpers DH, Kaplowitz N, et al (eds): *Textbook of Gastroenterology*, 4th ed. Philadelphia, Lippincott Williams & Wilkins, 2003, pp 1561-1579.

Greenberg HB, Matsui SM, Holodniy M: Small intestine: Infections with common bacterial and viral pathogens. In Yamada T, Alpers DH, Kaplowitz N, et al (eds): *Textbook of Gastroenterology*, 4th ed. Philadelphia, Lippincott Williams & Wilkins, 2003, pp 1530-1560.

Heneghan SJ, Li J, Petrossian E, Bizer LS: Intestinal perforation from gastrointestinal histoplasmosis in acquired immunodeficiency syndrome: Case report and review of the literature. *Arch Surg* 128:464-466, 1993.

WHAT THE REFERRING PHYSICIAN NEEDS TO KNOW

- Radiologic studies are rarely performed in patients with acute diarrhea secondary to viral infection.
- Diagnosis can be made by viral cultures or by enzyme-linked immunosorbent assay or electron microscopy of stool specimens.
- Histoplasmosis may cause intestinal perforation and peritonitis.

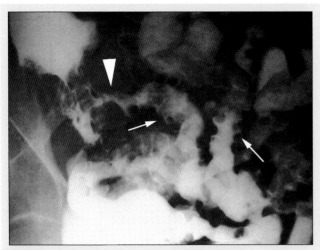

Figure 1. Histoplasmosis. Small bowel fluoroscopic image reveals multiple small bowel loops with thickened, nodular folds and slight separation of bowel loops *(arrows)*. Terminal ileum is narrowed *(arrowhead)*, especially near the ileocecal valve. This appearance resembles Stierlin's sign, which is more often seen in tuberculosis.

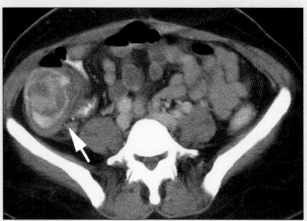

Figure 2. Histoplasmosis colitis. Axial CT image reveals marked thickening of ascending colonic wall *(arrow)*. *(From Mazzie JP, Wilson SR, Sadler MA, et al: Imaging of gastrointestinal tract infection. Semin Roentgenol 42:102-116, 2007.)*

Drug-Induced Disorders

DEFINITION: Drugs may cause a variety of abnormalities in the small intestine, usually characterized by ulcers and diarrhea.

ANATOMIC FINDINGS

Ileum
- Nonsteroidal anti-inflammatory drug (NSAID)-related injury is found primarily in the ileum.
- Fluorinated antipyrimidines may cause marked wall thickening of the distal ileum.

Duodenum
- Ulcers and inflammation secondary to fluorinated pyrimidine chemotherapy

IMAGING

Radiography
Findings
- NSAIDs may cause ulcers, strictures, and webs.
- Ulcers are punctate, linear, or circumferential.
- Thin webs may be difficult to differentiate from prominent small bowel folds.
- Thick webs are seen as 2- to 5-mm-thick rings encircling the bowel, with a tapered contour.
- 5-Fluorouracil (5-FU) and 5-floxuridine (5-FUDR) may cause thickened or effaced ileal folds.

Utility
- Barium studies
- Enteroclysis

CT
Findings
- 5-FU and 5-FUDR: marked wall thickening within distal ileum

Utility
- Enteritis related to chemotherapy can sometimes be detected on CT scans.

CLINICAL PRESENTATION
- NSAIDs may cause gastrointestinal bleeding or perforation.
- Enteritis related to chemotherapy may cause abdominal pain and diarrhea.
- 5-FU and 5-FUDR may cause nausea, vomiting, and diarrhea.

DIAGNOSTIC PEARLS
- 2- to 5-mm thick rings encircling the bowel associated with a tapered contour
- Marked wall thickening within the distal ileum
- Small bowel strictures
- NSAIDs: ulcers, strictures, and webs

DIFFERENTIAL DIAGNOSIS
- Crohn disease (small bowel)
- Ischemia (small bowel)
- Cytomegalovirus enteritis
- Chronic graft-versus-host disease (small bowel)
- Chronic ulcerative jejunoileitis

PATHOLOGY
- NSAIDs cause bowel injury by unknown mechanisms.
- Chronic inflammation and scarring lead to formation of characteristic web-like diaphragms and ring-like areas of narrowing.
- Mucosal diaphragms vary from slightly enlarged valvulae conniventes to thick, rigid, ring-like areas of narrowing.
- Thick layers of hyalinized collagen are found to interdigitate with the muscularis mucosae.
- Enteritis may be caused by chemotherapeutic agents such as dactinomycin, bleomycin, cytarabine, doxorubicin, methotrexate, 5-FU, and vincristine.

INCIDENCE/PREVALENCE AND EPIDEMIOLOGY
- NSAID-related lesions are being detected with increased frequency by capsule endoscopy, enteroscopy, and enteroclysis.
- Small bowel ulcers are found at autopsy in approximately 8% of people who take NSAIDs.

WHAT THE REFERRING PHYSICIAN NEEDS TO KNOW

- Ischemia results from systemic hypotension, hypovolemia, mesenteric arterial vasoconstriction, and slow mesenteric flow with venous thrombosis.
- Consider the age, travel history, medical history, and immune status of the patient before suggesting the diagnosis.
- Diagnosis of chemotherapy-induced enteritis is confirmed by resolution of symptoms after cessation of chemotherapy with regression of radiologic abnormalities on follow-up studies.

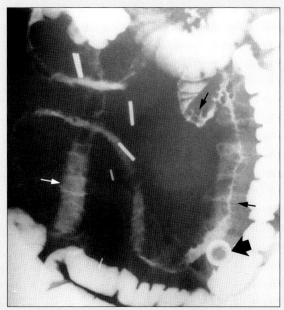

Figure 1. 5-FUDR chemotoxicity. Spot image of the right lower quadrant shows three loops of neoterminal ileum with markedly thickened, relatively smooth folds *(thin arrows)* perpendicular to the longitudinal axis of the bowel. A portion of the infusion pump is identified *(thick arrow)*. The ascending colon and cecum are surgically absent after a right hemicolectomy for colonic cancer.

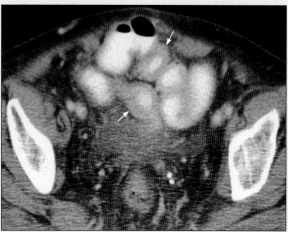

Figure 2. 5-FUDR chemotoxicity. CT through the upper pelvis shows thickening of the wall of several ileal loops *(arrows)*.

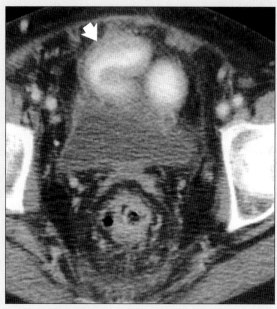

Figure 3. 5-FUDR chemotoxicity. CT at the level of the acetabula shows wall thickening of an ileal loop in profile *(arrow)*.

Suggested Readings

Allison MC, Howatson AG, Torrance CJ, et al: Gastrointestinal damage associated with the use of nonsteroidal antiinflammatory drugs. *N Engl J Med* 327:749-754, 1992.

Bjarnason I, Price AB, Zanelli G, et al: Clinicopathological features of nonsteroidal antiinflammatory drug-induced small intestinal strictures. *Gastroenterology* 94:1070-1074, 1988.

Carucci LR, Rubesin SE, Pretorius ES, et al: Toxic effects of fluorouracil on the small bowel. RSNA Gastrointestinal cases of the day. *RSNA*:[serial online]. RSNA Link Web, 2002.

Hiehle JF, Levine MS: Gastrointestinal toxicity of 5-FU and 5-FUDR: Radiographic findings. *Can Assoc Radiol J* 42:109-112, 1991.

Lang J, Price AB, Levi AJ, et al: Diaphragm disease: Pathology of disease of the small intestine induced by non-steroidal anti-inflammatory drugs. *J Clin Pathol* 41:516-526, 1988.

Levi S, deLacey G, Price AB, et al: "Diaphragm-like" strictures of the small bowel in patients treated with non-steroidal antiinflammatory drugs. *Br J Radiol* 63:186-189, 1990.

Levin MS: Miscellaneous diseases of the small intestine. In Yamada T, Alpers DH, Kaplowitz N, et al (eds): *Textbook of Gastroenterology*, 4th ed. Philadelphia, Lippincott Williams & Wilkins, 2003, pp 1663-1684.

Morris AJ, Madhok R, Sturrock RD, et al: Enteroscopic diagnosis of small bowel ulceration in patients receiving non-steroidal antiinflammatory drugs. *Lancet* 337:520, 1991.

Wilson IH, Cooley NV, Luibel FJ: Nonspecific stenosing small bowel ulcers. *Am J Gastroenterol* 50:449-455, 1968.

Graft-Versus-Host Disease

DEFINITION: In graft-versus-host disease (GVHD), the CD4+ T lymphocytes from the graft recognize the host histocompatibility antigens as foreign, leading to a T cell–mediated attack on the host tissue.

IMAGING

Radiography
Findings
- Thickened or effaced folds and nodular mucosa
- Tubular (*ribbon-like* or *toothpaste*) bowel
- Barium may adhere to the necrotic bowel surface; detected on radiographs or CT performed after the initial barium study.

Utility
- Barium studies may confirm diagnosis of acute or chronic GVHD and show extent of disease.

CT
Findings
- Thickened small bowel wall
- Extensive submucosal edema
- Pneumatosis
- Engorged mesentery
- Ascites

CLINICAL PRESENTATION

- Diarrhea, anorexia, vomiting, abdominal pain, gastrointestinal bleeding, protein loss, and secondary infections may occur.
- Maculopapular rash may be present on the palms, soles, and trunk.
- Acute GVHD develops 3-11 weeks after marrow transplantation.
- Chronic GVHD develops 3-13 months after transplantation without prior acute disease.

DIFFERENTIAL DIAGNOSIS

- Cytomegalovirus infection (small bowel)

DIAGNOSTIC PEARLS

- Thickened folds and nodular mucosa
- Tubular (*ribbon-like* or *toothpaste*) bowel
- Diffusely thickened small bowel wall

PATHOLOGY

- CD4+ T lymphocytes from the graft recognize host histocompatibility antigens as foreign, leading to a T cell–mediated attack on the host tissue.
- Acute GVHD biopsy findings vary from crypt cell death to total necrosis of epithelium; submucosal edema is present.
- Chronic GVHD is characterized by patchy fibrosis of the lamina propria and submucosa with bacterial overgrowth.

INCIDENCE/PREVALENCE AND EPIDEMIOLOGY

- Acute GVHD develops in 30%-50% of patients.
- Chronic GVHD develops in 25% of patients.

Suggested Readings

Fisk JD, Shulman HM, Greening RR, et al: Gastrointestinal radiographic features of human graft-versus-host-disease. *AJR Am J Roentgenol* 136:329-336, 1981.

McDonald GB, Sullivan KM, Plumley TF: Radiographic features of esophageal involvement in chronic graft-versus-host disease in humans. *AJR Am J Roentgenol* 142:501-506, 1984.

Rosenberg HK, Serota FT, Koch, et al: Radiographic features of gastrointestinal graft-versus-host disease. *Radiology* 38:371-374, 1981.

Shanahan F: Gastrointestinal manifestations of immunologic disorders. In Yamada T, Alpers DH, Kaplowitz N, et al (eds): *Textbook of Gastroenterology*, 4th ed. Philadelphia, Lippincott Williams & Wilkins, 2003, pp 2705-2722.

WHAT THE REFERRING PHYSICIAN NEEDS TO KNOW

- Tissue damage is clinically evident in the skin, liver, mucous membranes, eyes, and gastrointestinal tract.
- Acute GVHD is often complicated by cytomegalovirus, astrovirus, adenovirus, and *Clostridium difficile* infections.

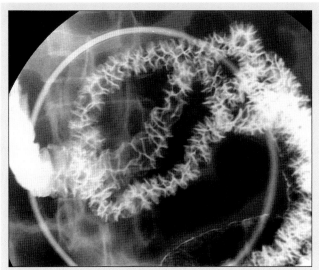

Figure 1. Graft-versus-host disease. Spot image from small bowel follow-through shows diffuse fold thickening in the jejunum.

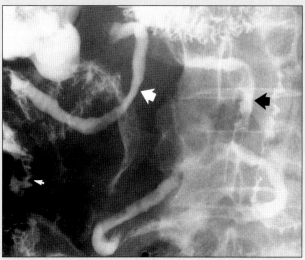

Figure 2. Graft-versus-host disease. Spot image from small bowel follow-through shows that the jejunum and upper ileum have a diffusely narrowed, tubular appearance. In some loops, the folds are markedly thickened *(small arrow),* whereas in other loops the folds are completely effaced *(large arrows).*

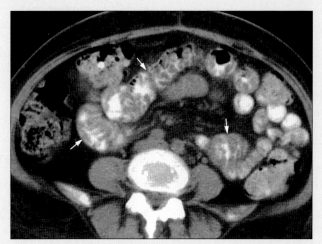

Figure 3. Graft-versus-host disease. CT through the top of the iliac crest shows extensive fold thickening *(arrows)* in mid small bowel loops.

Opportunistic Infections in Acquired Immunodeficiency Syndrome

DEFINITION: Opportunistic infections in patients with AIDS are caused by viruses, bacteria, and fungi that affect immunocompromised individuals and usually cause lymphadenopathy and diarrhea.

ANATOMIC FINDINGS

Duodenum
- Cryptosporidiosis
- Isosporiasis

Jejunum
- Cryptosporidiosis
- Isosporiasis
- *Mycobacterium avium-intracellulare* complex (MAC) in jejunum or ileum, or both

Ileum
- Cytomegalovirus (CMV) infection: ulceration usually involves the distal small bowel and terminal ileum.
- Gastrointestinal actinomycosis most frequently involves the terminal ileum and appendix.
- MAC infection typically occurs in the jejunum or ileum, or both.

IMAGING

Radiography
Findings
- CMV infection: discrete erosions and penetrating ulcers separated by normal mucosa, and lymphoid hyperplasia
- Cryptosporidiosis: variable degree of fold thickening in the duodenum and mesenteric small bowel.
- MAC: thickened small bowel folds and fine mucosal nodularity. (Aphthoid ulcers have also been described.)
- Isosporiasis: thickened small bowel folds, primarily in the duodenum and proximal small bowel
- Actinomycosis: transmural infection mimicking Crohn disease. (Fistulas are often present.)
- Candidiasis: ulceration, perforation, thickened small bowel fold

Utility
- Barium studies

DIAGNOSTIC PEARLS

- Ulceration in the distal small bowel, terminal ileum, cecum, and ascending colon (CMV infection)
- Extrinsic mass impressions on the mesenteric border of mid-jejunal loops (MAC)
- Mucosal nodularity and irregular fold thickening in the terminal ileum (actinomycosis)
- Variable degree of fold thickening in the duodenum and mesenteric small bowel (cryptosporidiosis)
- Ulceration, perforation, and thickened small bowel folds (candidiasis)

CT
Findings
- CMV: ulceration
- MAC: mesenteric lymphadenopathy with normal or low attenuation
- Gastrointestinal tuberculosis: similar to tuberculosis in immunocompetent patients
- Tuberculous peritonitis: high-attenuation ascites, peritoneal and omental nodules, and low-attenuation lymphadenopathy

CLINICAL PRESENTATION

- Regardless of the causative organism, the most common manifestation of infectious enteritis is diarrhea.
- Malabsorption may occur.
- Ulceration and perforation (candidiasis, CMV infection) may occur.
- MAC produces chronic diarrhea, abdominal pain, malabsorption, and weight loss; hepatomegaly, splenomegaly, and ascites occur with disseminated infection.
- Gastrointestinal tuberculosis may lead to peritonitis.

WHAT THE REFERRING PHYSICIAN NEEDS TO KNOW

- Wide variety of viruses, bacteria, protozoa, and fungi can infect the small bowel of patients with AIDS.
- *M. avium-intracellulare* infection is unique to AIDS.
- Imaging studies show the presence of small bowel disease and can aid in the differential diagnosis of these conditions.
- Small intestine is the most severely infected portion of gastrointestinal tract in MAC infection.
- Fungal spores of *Candida* may be found as a result of noninvasive colonization of blind loops or necrotic tissue.

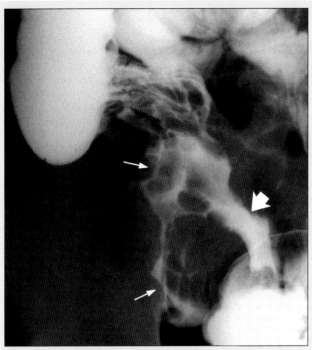

Figure 1. Cytomegalovirus infection in a patient with AIDS. Spot image of the terminal ileum from a small bowel follow-through shows large, lobulated folds *(thin arrows)* and barium-filled grooves caused by ulceration. Localized perforation is manifested by a barium-filled track *(thick arrow)* extending into the mesentery. *(Courtesy of Emil J. Balthazar, MD, New York; from the teaching files of Hans Herlinger, MD.)*

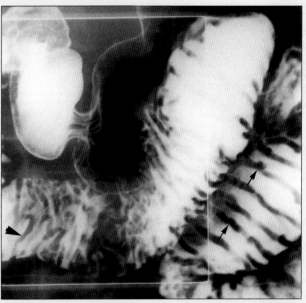

Figure 2. Proximal small bowel fold thickening in a patient with AIDS. Spot image from a small bowel follow-through shows mildly thickened undulating folds *(thin arrows)* in a proximal loop of jejunum. Compare these jejunal folds with folds in the third portion of the duodenum *(thick arrow)*. Normal duodenal folds should be slightly thicker than jejunal folds. Enteroscopic biopsy specimens revealed cryptosporidiosis.

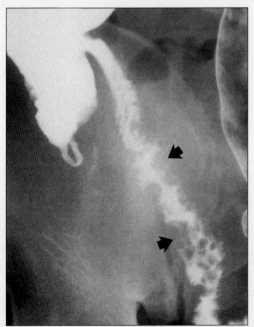

Figure 3. Actinomycosis in a patient with AIDS. Spot image from a double-contrast barium enema shows mucosal nodularity *(arrows)* and irregular fold thickening in the terminal ileum.

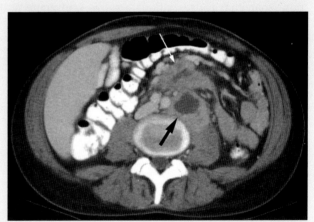

Figure 4. Mesenteric and retroperitoneal lymphadenopathy in a patient with *Mycobacterium avium-intracellulare* **complex enteritis.** CT through the tip of the liver shows a large left para-aortic nodal mass with a low-attenuation center *(black arrow)*. Mass-like infiltration of the small bowel mesentery *(white arrow)* is also present.

DIFFERENTIAL DIAGNOSIS

- Whipple disease (small bowel)
- Intestinal lymphangiectasia (small bowel)
- Mastocytosis (small bowel)
- Amyloidosis (small bowel)
- Abetalipoproteinemia (small bowel)
- Crohn disease (small bowel)

PATHOLOGY

- Human immunodeficiency virus (HIV) enteritis: HIV infection causes villous atrophy, crypt hyperplasia, edema, and chronic inflammation.
- CMV (double-stranded DNA virus) accumulates in various cells of the gastrointestinal tract, resulting in inflammation and necrosis; endothelial cell damage causes submucosal ischemia, with secondary epithelial ulceration.
- *Cryptosporidium parvum* is a protozoan found in villous epithelial cells; findings range from a normal histologic appearance to villous atrophy with severe inflammation.
- *Isospora belli* is an obligate intracellular protozoan; microscopically, villous atrophy and inflammation occur, often associated with extensive eosinophilic infiltration of the small bowel wall.
- *Cyclospora cayetanensis* is an obligate intracellular protozoan that causes villous atrophy and acute and chronic inflammation in normal or immunocompromised people.
- Microsporidia are spore-forming, obligate intracellular protozoans that infect the small intestine or disseminate to other organs.
- MAC (*M. avium* and *M. avium-intracellulare*) form a complex; infiltration of the lamina propria and submucosa by macrophages packed with acid-fast organisms occurs.

INCIDENCE/PREVALENCE AND EPIDEMIOLOGY

- One-half of patients infected with HIV have chronic diarrhea related to enteropathy, infectious enteritis, or colitis.
- *Enterocytozoon bieneusi* infects 10% to 34% of patients with HIV infection and CD4+ counts of less than 50 cells/mm^3.

Suggested Readings

Dworkin B, Wormser GP, Rosenthal WS, et al: Gastrointestinal manifestations of the acquired immunodeficiency syndrome: A review of 22 cases. *Am J Gastroenterol* 80:774-778, 1985.

Poles M, Fuerst M, McGowan I, et al: HIV-related diarrhea is multifactorial and fat malabsorption is commonly present, independent of HAART. *Am J Gastroenterol* 96:1831-1837, 2001.

Smith PD, Janoff EN: Gastrointestinal complications of the acquired immunodeficiency syndrome. In Yamada T, Alpers DH, Kaplowitz N, et al (eds): *Textbook of Gastroenterology*, 4th ed. Philadelphia, Lippincott Williams & Wilkins, 2003, pp 2567-2589.

Malabsorption (Small Bowel)

DEFINITION: Malabsorption is the inability or marked inefficiency of the intestines in absorbing nutrients as a result of various abnormalities affecting the digestive tract.

ANATOMIC FINDINGS

Jejunum
- Decreased number of folds
- Moderately thickened, nodular folds

Duodenum
- Moderately thickened, nodular folds

Ileum
- Moderately thickened, nodular folds

IMAGING

Fluoroscopy
Findings
- Celiac disease: decreased number of folds in the proximal jejunum.
- Abetalipoproteinemia: moderately thickened, nodular folds in the duodenum and proximal jejunum
- Eosinophilic gastroenteritis: smooth or nodular, thickened folds perpendicular to the longitudinal axis of the small bowel
- *Hidebound bowel* of scleroderma: patchy fibrosis of circular muscle layer leads to bunching of small bowel folds.
- Tropical sprue: thickened folds are seen in the jejunum and ileum.
- Whipple disease: fine mucosal nodularity
- Giardiasis: rapid transit of barium and spasm in the proximal small bowel

Utility
- Enteroclysis

DIAGNOSTIC PEARLS

- Moderately thickened, nodular folds in the duodenum and proximal jejunum (abetalipoproteinemia)
- *Hidebound bowel:* patchy, predominant fibrosis of circular muscle layer leads to bunching of small bowel folds (scleroderma).
- Numerous low-attenuation lymph nodes within the root of the small bowel mesentery and in the retroperitoneum (celiac disease)

CT
Findings
- Celiac disease: numerous low-attenuation lymph nodes within the root of the small bowel mesentery and in the retroperitoneum
- Whipple disease: enlarged, low-attenuation lymph nodes in the mesentery and retroperitoneum

CLINICAL PRESENTATION

- Children may have diarrhea, abdominal distention, weight loss, and failure to thrive (celiac disease).
- Mild steatorrhea (eosinophilic gastroenteritis) may occur.
- Megaloblastic anemia (tropical sprue) may occur.
- Cardiac involvement is characterized by pericarditis, valvular defects, and congestive heart failure (Whipple disease).

WHAT THE REFERRING PHYSICIAN NEEDS TO KNOW

- Removal of wheat products from the diet reverses mucosal damage in celiac disease.
- Eosinophilic enteritis can mimic radiographic findings of other diseases causing submucosal bleeding in small bowel.
- Transient intussusceptions and pneumatosis intestinalis may occur in scleroderma with or without pneumoperitoneum.
- Combined folate and vitamin B_{12} deficiency in tropical sprue can lead to megaloblastic anemia.
- Other causes of low-attenuation mesenteric and retroperitoneal lymphadenopathy include *Mycobacterium avium-intracellulare* infection in acquired immunodeficiency syndrome and metastatic testicular carcinoma.

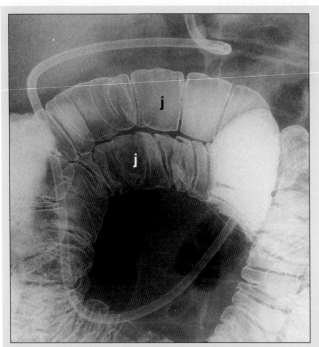

Figure 1. Celiac disease. Spot radiograph from enteroclysis shows a paucity of folds (two to three folds per inch) in two loops of jejunum (j). However, the folds are of normal thickness.

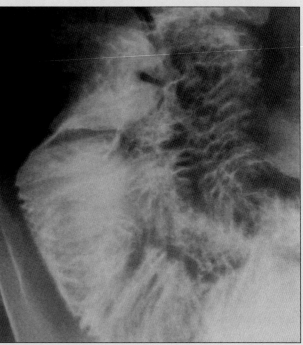

Figure 2. Abetalipoproteinemia. Spot radiograph of the small bowel shows mildly thickened, irregular folds, possibly because of intestinal secretions that prevent barium from adequately coating the mucosal surface, given that the microscopic pathology does not explain the apparent fold thickening in this condition. (*From the teaching files of Hans Herlinger, MD.*)

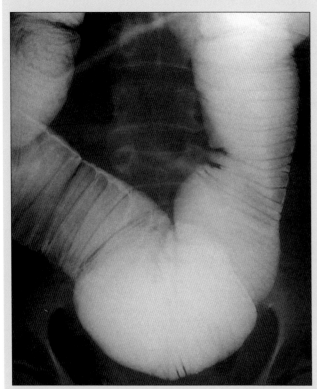

Figure 3. Scleroderma. Spot radiograph from enteroclysis shows massively dilated small bowel. (Compare the diameter of the lumen with the size of a lumbar vertebral body.) In addition, an increased number of folds per inch is seen, producing the hidebound sign.

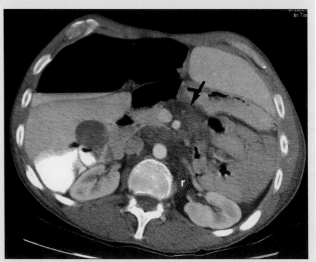

Figure 4. Lymphadenopathy in celiac disease. CT shows numerous low-attenuation lymph nodes *(arrow)* in the root of the small bowel mesentery and in the retroperitoneum (r).

PATHOLOGY

- Celiac disease is a chronic disease in which the gliadin fraction of wheat gluten causes damage to the small bowel mucosa.
- Malabsorption is sometimes linked to a defect in the microsomal triglyceride transport protein in abetalipoproteinemia.
- Circular muscle layer degenerates and is replaced by collagen in scleroderma.
- Researchers have postulated that colonization of the small intestine by toxigenic strains of coliform bacteria causes tropical sprue.
- Villous blunting in Whipple disease is caused by lamina propria expansion by lacteals distended with fat and macrophages.
- *Giardia lamblia* attaches to the mucosal surface of intestine, causing little damage to underlying small bowel.

INCIDENCE/PREVALENCE AND EPIDEMIOLOGY

- Increased incidence of squamous cell carcinoma of the pharynx and esophagus as well as adenocarcinoma and lymphoma of the small bowel in patients with celiac disease

- Abetalipoproteinemia is rare.
- Eosinophilic enteritis usually develops during the third to sixth decades of life.
- Tropical sprue is endemic in tropical and subtropical areas such as the Caribbean, Southeast Asia, and India.
- Whipple disease has a male-female predominance of 6:1.
- *G. lamblia* is a frequent cause of endemic and epidemic diarrhea worldwide.

Suggested Readings

Ganapathy V, Ganapathy ME, Leibach FH: Protein digestion and assimilation. In *Textbook of Gastroenterology*, 4th ed. Philadelphia, Lippincott Williams & Wilkins, 2003, pp 438-449.

Powel DW: Approach to the patient with diarrhea. In *Textbook of Gastroenterology*, 4th ed. Philadelphia, Lippincott Williams & Wilkins, 2003, pp 844-894.

Rubesin SE: Diseases of small bowel causing malabsorption. In *Radiology: Diagnosis-Imaging-Intervention*. Philadelphia, JB Lippincott, 1993, pp 1-17.

Traber P: Carbohydrate assimilation. In *Textbook of Gastroenterology*, 4th ed. Philadelphia, Lippincott Williams & Wilkins, 2003, pp 389-413.

Jejunal Diverticulosis (Small Bowel)

DEFINITION: Jejunal diverticula are acquired protrusions of the mucosa and submucosa on the mesenteric border of the small bowel where the vasa recta pierce the muscularis propria.

IMAGING

Radiography
Findings
- Barium-filled 1- to 7-cm round sacs on mesenteric border of small bowel may be seen.
- The underlying small bowel may be obscured by numerous diverticular sacs.
- Mouths of diverticula are broad based, and the necks are variable in length.
- Decreased peristalsis, increased intraluminal fluid and gas, luminal dilation, and prolonged transit time may occur.
- Air-fluid levels may be present on upright views.

Utility
- Barium studies
- Best visualized on enteroclysis

CLINICAL PRESENTATION

- Most people with jejunal diverticulosis are asymptomatic.
- Small bowel dysmotility may cause pseudo-obstruction and malabsorption.
- Complications of jejunal diverticula, including gastrointestinal obstruction, bleeding, or perforation, may cause abdominal symptoms.

DIFFERENTIAL DIAGNOSIS

- Scleroderma with sacculations (small bowel)

PATHOLOGY

- Small-bowel diverticula are acquired protrusions of the mucosa and submucosa on the mesenteric border of the small bowel, where the vasa recta pierce the muscularis propria.

DIAGNOSTIC PEARLS

- Barium-filled 1- to 7-cm round sacs on mesenteric border of small bowel
- Air-fluid levels within diverticula

- Jejunal diverticula develop in a heterogeneous group of disorders associated with abnormalities of smooth muscle or myenteric plexus.
- In patients with numerous diverticula, stasis with bacterial overgrowth and malabsorption may occur.
- Mechanical obstruction may result from volvulus, enterolith impaction, or diverticulitis.

INCIDENCE/PREVALENCE AND EPIDEMIOLOGY

- Jejunal diverticulosis occurs in approximately 2% of the population.

Suggested Readings

Ganapathy V, Ganapathy ME, Leibach FH: Protein digestion and assimilation. In *Textbook of Gastroenterology*, 4th ed. Philadelphia, Lippincott Williams & Wilkins, 2003, pp 438-449.

Powel DW: Approach to the patient with diarrhea. In *Textbook of Gastroenterology*, 4th ed. Philadelphia, Lippincott Williams & Wilkins, 2003, pp 844-894.

Rubesin SE: Diseases of small bowel causing malabsorption. In *Radiology: Diagnosis-Imaging-Intervention*. Philadelphia, JB Lippincott, 1993, pp 1-17.

Rubesin SE, Rubin RA, Herlinger H: Small bowel malabsorption: Clinical perspectives. *Radiology* 184:297-305, 1992.

Traber P: Carbohydrate assimilation. In *Textbook of Gastroenterology*, 4th ed. Philadelphia, Lippincott Williams & Wilkins, 2003, pp 389-413.

WHAT THE REFERRING PHYSICIAN NEEDS TO KNOW

- Complications of jejunal diverticula include obstruction, perforation, and gastrointestinal bleeding.
- Jejunal diverticulosis may be complicated by pneumatosis cystoides intestinalis caused by the perforation.
- Mechanical obstruction may result from volvulus, enterolith impaction, or diverticulitis.
- Heterotopic tissue or neoplasms are rare complications.

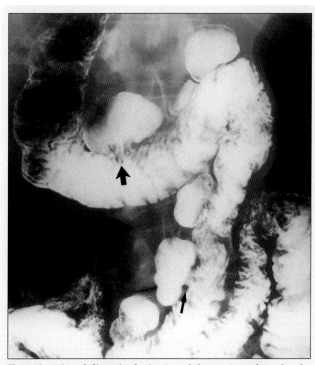

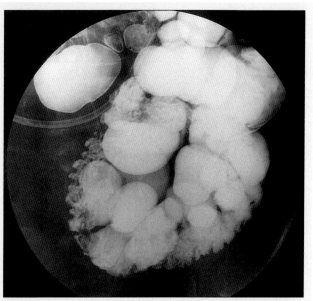

Figure 2. Jejunoileal diverticulosis causing malabsorption.
Spot image from enteroclysis shows innumerable barium-filled
diverticula obscuring the underlying small bowel loops from
which they arise.

Figure 1. Jejunal diverticulosis. Coned-down view of overhead
radiograph from small bowel follow-through shows multiple
large diverticula on the mesenteric border of the distal duodenum
and proximal jejunum. The sacs are smooth, but many have a
lobulated contour. The mouth *(small arrow)* of one diverticulum
is visualized in profile. Folds are seen radiating *(large arrow)*
into another diverticulum. This degree of diverticulosis does not
usually cause malabsorption.

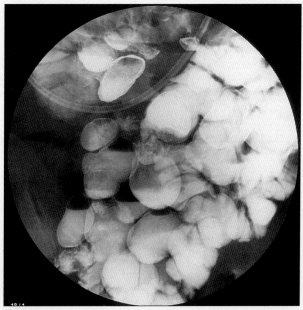

Figure 3. Jejunoileal diverticulosis causing malabsorption. Upright spot image shows multiple air-fluid levels and air-barium levels in
the diverticula.

Scleroderma (Small Bowel)

DEFINITION: Scleroderma is a disease in which the smooth muscle, especially that of the circular muscle layer in the small bowel wall, degenerates and is replaced by collagen.

IMAGING

Fluoroscopy
Findings
- Duodenal and jejunal dilation
- Hypomotility with prolonged small bowel transit time
- Hidebound bowel: patchy, predominant fibrosis of the circular muscle layer leads to bunching and crowding of small bowel folds (*hidebound sign*) with an increased number of folds, a finding that is virtually pathognomonic of scleroderma.
- Wide-mouthed sacculations, frequently on the mesenteric border of the small bowel and colon

Utility
- Small bowel follow-through
- Enteroclysis
- Double-contrast barium enema

CLINICAL PRESENTATION

- Malabsorption (diarrhea, steatorrhea, excessive gas, abdominal pain, and weight loss)

PATHOLOGY

- Circular muscle layer of bowel wall degenerates and is replaced by collagen.
- Asymmetric scarring leads to wide-mouthed sacculations.

DIAGNOSTIC PEARLS

- Hidebound bowel
- Duodenal and jejunal dilatation
- Wide-mouthed sacculations

INCIDENCE/PREVALENCE AND EPIDEMIOLOGY

- Small intestine is involved in approximately 40% of patients with progressive systemic sclerosis.

Suggested Readings

Ganapathy V, Ganapathy ME, Leibach FH: Protein digestion and assimilation. In *Textbook of Gastroenterology*, 4th ed. Philadelphia, Lippincott Williams & Wilkins, 2003, pp 438-449.

Powel DW: Approach to the patient with diarrhea. In *Textbook of Gastroenterology*, 4th ed. Philadelphia, Lippincott Williams & Wilkins, 2003, pp 844-894.

Rubesin SE: Diseases of small bowel causing malabsorption. In *Radiology: Diagnosis-Imaging-Intervention*. Philadelphia, JB Lippincott, 1993, pp 1-17.

Rubesin SE, Rubin RA, Herlinger H: Small bowel malabsorption: Clinical perspectives. *Radiology* 184:297-305, 1992.

Traber P: Carbohydrate assimilation. In *Textbook of Gastroenterology*, 4th ed. Philadelphia, Lippincott Williams & Wilkins, 2003, pp 389-413.

WHAT THE REFERRING PHYSICIAN NEEDS TO KNOW

- Transient intussusceptions and a benign form of pneumatosis intestinalis may occur with or without a benign asymptomatic pneumoperitoneum.

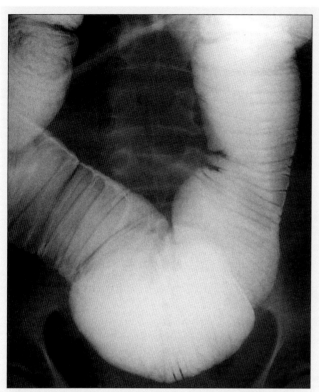

Figure 1. Scleroderma. Spot radiograph from enteroclysis shows a massively dilated small bowel. (Compare the diameter of the lumen with the size of a lumbar vertebral body.) Also seen is an increased number of folds per inch, producing the *hidebound sign.*

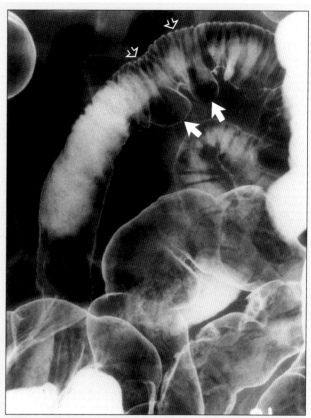

Figure 2. Scleroderma. Spot image from double-contrast barium enema shows sacculation of the mesenteric border *(closed arrows)* of the terminal ileum, with bunching of folds *(open arrows)* on the antimesenteric border caused by asymmetric fibrosis in the muscular layers of the bowel wall.

Celiac Disease (Small Bowel)

DEFINITION: Celiac disease is a chronic disease in which the gliadin fraction of wheat gluten causes damage to the small bowel mucosa.

IMAGING

Radiography
Findings
- Decreased number of folds in the proximal jejunum is virtually pathognomic of celiac disease.
- Finely reticular mucosal surface with polygonal radiolucent islands of mucosa surrounded by barium-filled grooves
- Ileal folds may be increased in number and thicker than normal (*jejunization* of the ileum).
- Superimposed small-bowel lymphoma may be manifested by short, annular lesion with central ulceration in jejunum or by thickened, nodular folds in longer segments of jejunum.

Utility
- Enteroclysis
- Barium studies

CT
Findings
- Lymphadenopathy in celiac disease may be characterized by numerous low-attenuation lymph nodes in the root of the small bowel mesentery and retroperitoneum.
- Superimposed cavitary mesenteric lymph node syndrome may be characterized by mesenteric or retroperitoneal masses of low attenuation with or without fat-fluid levels.

CLINICAL PRESENTATION

- Children may have diarrhea, abdominal distention, weight loss, or failure to thrive.
- Young adults may have diarrhea, steatorrhea, or infertility.
- Older adults may have steatorrhea, anemia, or weight loss.

DIAGNOSTIC PEARLS

- Decreased number of folds in proximal jejunum
- *Jejunization* of ileum
- Finely reticular mucosal surface with polygonal radiolucent islands of mucosa surrounded by barium-filled grooves

- Aphthous stomatitis
- Cheilosis
- Glossitis

PATHOLOGY

- Celiac disease (gluten-sensitive enteropathy or celiac sprue) is a chronic disease in which the gliadin fraction of wheat gluten causes damage to the small bowel mucosa.
- Suspension of normal immune tolerance to foreign food antigens stimulates an immune response, leading to mucosal inflammation and destruction.
- Loss of intestinal villi is associated with crypt hyperplasia and infiltration of the lamina propria by plasma cells and lymphocytes on histologic specimens.
- Lymphocytic infiltration may also occur in the stomach (lymphocytic gastritis) or colon.
- Immunoglobulin (Ig)A and IgG antibodies to gliadin are elevated in 75% to 85% of patients with celiac disease.

INCIDENCE/PREVALENCE AND EPIDEMIOLOGY

- Celiac disease is uncommon.
- Approximately 1 in 200 whites contract the disease.
- Disease is most frequently encountered in whites, particularly northern Europeans and people from Ireland.

WHAT THE REFERRING PHYSICIAN NEEDS TO KNOW

- Removal of wheat products from diet reverses mucosal damage.
- In adults, symptoms of celiac disease may be precipitated by pregnancy, respiratory therapy, or gastric surgery.
- Celiac disease can be associated with other skin diseases such as psoriasis, eczema, cutaneous amyloid, and mycosis fungoides.
- Endoscopic or capsular biopsy is required for a definitive diagnosis.
- Complications of celiac disease include malabsorption, hyposplenism, neuropathy, intestinal ulceration, lymphadenopathy, cavitary mesenteric lymph node syndrome, and malignancy.

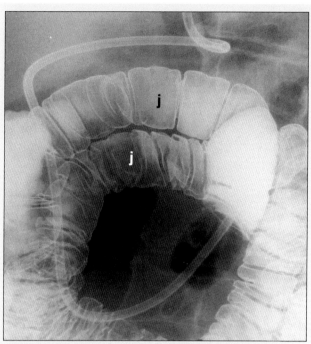

Figure 1. Celiac disease. Spot radiograph from enteroclysis shows a paucity of folds (two to three folds per inch) in two loops of jejunum (j). However, the folds are of normal thickness.

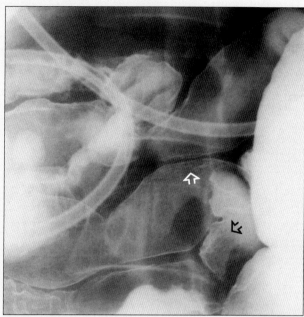

Figure 2. Mosaic pattern in celiac disease. Spot radiograph of the jejunum from enteroclysis shows a tubular configuration with nearly complete absence of folds. A subtle, finely nodular surface pattern is seen in some regions (*arrows*), reflecting the mosaic pattern of atrophic mucosa. (*From Rubesin SE, Herlinger H, Saul SH, et al: Adult celiac disease and its complications. RadioGraphics 9:1045-1066, 1989.*)

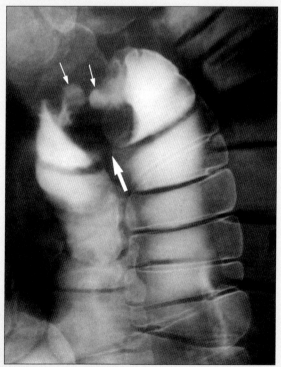

Figure 3. T-cell lymphoma complicating celiac disease. Spot radiograph from enteroclysis shows a short, annular lesion *(large arrow)* with central ulceration *(small arrows)* in the jejunum. Note the decreased number of jejunal folds proximal to the lesion caused by underlying celiac disease.

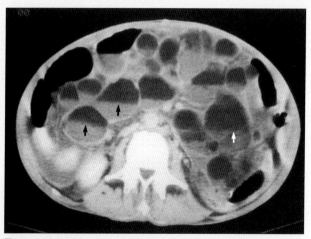

Figure 4. Cavitary mesenteric lymph node syndrome. CT shows numerous ovoid masses in the abdomen. The masses have fat or debris levels *(arrows)*. These represent enlarged, cavitary lymph nodes that can be mistaken for loops of small bowel with air-fluid levels. However, fat and fluid attenuation of the nodes and the lack of opacification by positive oral contrast should suggest the correct diagnosis. (*From Rubesin SE, Herlinger H, Saul SH, et al: Adult celiac disease and its complications. RadioGraphics 9:1045-1066, 1989.*)

- Transient intussusceptions occur in 25% of patients with celiac disease.
- Increased incidence of squamous cell carcinoma of the pharynx and esophagus and of adenocarcinoma and lymphoma of the small bowel occurs in patients with celiac disease.

Suggested Readings

Ganapathy V, Ganapathy ME, Leibach FH: Protein digestion and assimilation. In *Textbook of Gastroenterology*, 4th ed. Philadelphia, Lippincott Williams & Wilkins, 2003, pp 438-449.

Powel DW: Approach to the patient with diarrhea. In *Textbook of Gastroenterology*, 4th ed. Philadelphia, Lippincott Williams & Wilkins, 2003, pp 844-894.

Rubesin SE: Diseases of small bowel causing malabsorption. In *Radiology: Diagnosis-Imaging-Intervention*. Philadelphia, JB Lippincott, 1993, pp 1-17.

Rubesin SE, Rubin RA, Herlinger H: Small bowel malabsorption: Clinical perspectives. *Radiology* 184:297-305, 1992.

Traber P: Carbohydrate assimilation. In *Textbook of Gastroenterology*, 4th ed. Philadelphia, Lippincott Williams & Wilkins, 2003, pp 389-413.

Tropical Sprue (Small Bowel)

DEFINITION: Tropical sprue is a malabsorptive disease that is endemic in tropical or subtropical areas, possibly caused by toxigenic coliform bacteria.

IMAGING

Radiography
Findings
- Thickened folds in the jejunum and ileum
Utility
- Barium studies

CLINICAL PRESENTATION

- Patients initially suffer watery diarrheal illness that may remit or progress to chronic malabsorption.
- Megaloblastic anemia may occur.

DIFFERENTIAL DIAGNOSIS

- Whipple disease (small bowel)
- Intestinal lymphangiectasia (small bowel)
- Mastocytosis (small bowel)
- Amyloidosis (small bowel)
- Abetalipoproteinemia (small bowel)
- Opportunistic infections in AIDS (small bowel)

PATHOLOGY

- Researchers have postulated that colonization of the small intestine by toxigenic strains of coliform bacteria causes tropical sprue.
- In contrast to celiac disease, villous atrophy is partial, and crypt hyperplasia is not severe.

DIAGNOSTIC PEARLS

- Thickened jejunal and ileal folds
- Tropical sprue occurs in endemic tropical or subtropical areas.

INCIDENCE/PREVALENCE AND EPIDEMIOLOGY

- Tropical sprue is endemic in tropical or subtropical areas such as the Caribbean, Southeast Asia, and India.
- Visitors are affected only after a prolonged stay.
- Tropical sprue is uncommon in children.

Suggested Readings

Ganapathy V, Ganapathy ME, Leibach FH: Protein digestion and assimilation. In *Textbook of Gastroenterology,* 4th ed. Philadelphia, Lippincott Williams & Wilkins, 2003, pp 438-449.

Powel DW: Approach to the patient with diarrhea. In *Textbook of Gastroenterology,* 4th ed. Philadelphia, Lippincott Williams & Wilkins, 2003, pp 844-894.

Rubesin SE: Diseases of small bowel causing malabsorption. In *Radiology: Diagnosis-Imaging-Intervention.* Philadelphia, JB Lippincott, 1993, pp 1-17.

Rubesin SE, Rubin RA, Herlinger H: Small bowel malabsorption: Clinical perspectives. *Radiology* 184:297-305, 1992.

Traber P: Carbohydrate assimilation. In *Textbook of Gastroenterology,* 4th ed. Philadelphia, Lippincott Williams & Wilkins, 2003, pp 389-413.

WHAT THE REFERRING PHYSICIAN NEEDS TO KNOW

- Combined folate and vitamin-B_{12} deficiency in tropical sprue can lead to megaloblastic anemia.
- Tropical sprue responds to antibiotic and folate therapy.

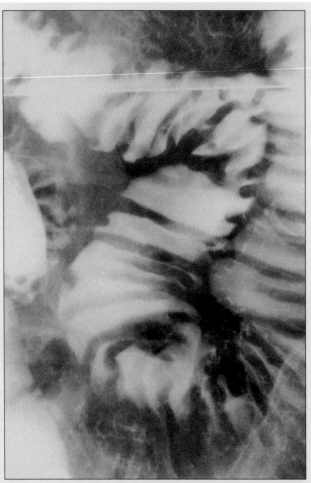

Figure 1. Tropical sprue. Spot radiograph from small bowel follow-through shows moderately thickened, slightly undulating folds in the jejunum. Unlike in celiac disease, the number of folds per inch in the jejunum is normal.

Giardiasis (Small Bowel)

DEFINITION: Malabsorption caused by small intestinal colonization of the protozoan *Giardia lamblia.*

IMAGING

Radiography
Findings
- Thickened folds in the distal duodenum and proximal jejunum
- Rapid transit of barium and spasm in the proximal small bowel

Utility
- Enteroclysis
- Barium small bowel follow-through

CLINICAL PRESENTATION

- Patient may complain of diarrhea.
- Rarely, giardiasis is heralded by malabsorptive symptoms.

DIFFERENTIAL DIAGNOSIS

- Opportunistic infections in AIDS (small bowel)

PATHOLOGY

- *G. lamblia* attaches to mucosal surface of intestine, causing little damage to the underlying small bowel.

DIAGNOSTIC PEARLS

- Thickened folds in the distal duodenum and proximal jejunum
- Rapid transit of barium and spasm in the proximal small bowel

INCIDENCE/PREVALENCE AND EPIDEMIOLOGY

- *G. lamblia* is frequent cause of endemic and epidemic diarrhea worldwide.
- Outbreaks of diarrhea caused by *G. lamblia* are less frequent in the United States.
- Giardiasis is a rare cause of malabsorption.

Suggested Readings

Ganapathy V, Ganapathy ME, Leibach FH: Protein digestion and assimilation. In *Textbook of Gastroenterology*, 4th ed. Philadelphia, Lippincott Williams & Wilkins, 2003, pp 438-449.

Powel DW: Approach to the patient with diarrhea. In *Textbook of Gastroenterology*, 4th ed. Philadelphia, Lippincott Williams & Wilkins, 2003, pp 844-894.

Rubesin SE: Diseases of small bowel causing malabsorption. In *Radiology: Diagnosis-Imaging-Intervention*. Philadelphia, JB Lippincott, 1993, pp 1-17.

Rubesin SE, Rubin RA, Herlinger H: Small bowel malabsorption: Clinical perspectives. *Radiology* 184:297-305, 1992.

Traber P: Carbohydrate assimilation. In *Textbook of Gastroenterology*, 4th ed. Philadelphia, Lippincott Williams & Wilkins, 2003, pp 389-413.

WHAT THE REFERRING PHYSICIAN NEEDS TO KNOW

- Barium studies in patients with giardiasis usually show no abnormalities.
- Other causes of malabsorption associated with intestinal hypermotility include Zollinger-Ellison syndrome and diabetes.

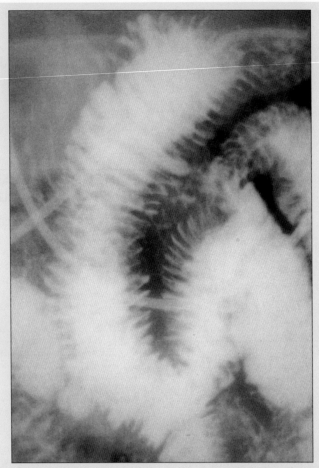

Figure 1. Giardiasis. Spot radiograph from enteroclysis shows mildly thickened, straight folds in the proximal jejunum. (*From Rubesin SE: Diseases of small bowel causing malabsorption. In Taveras JM, Ferrucci JT [eds]:* Radiology: Diagnosis-Imaging-Intervention. *Philadelphia, JB Lippincott, 1993, pp 1-17.*)

Whipple Disease (Small Bowel)

DEFINITION: Whipple disease is caused by small bowel colonization by *Tropheryma whippelii*.

IMAGING

Radiography
Findings
- Thickened, nodular folds, primarily in the distal duodenum and jejunum
- Fine mucosal nodularity

Utility
- Small bowel follow-through
- Enteroclysis

CT
Findings
- Enlarged, low-attenuation lymph nodes in the mesentery and retroperitoneum

CLINICAL PRESENTATION

- Gastrointestinal symptoms include bloating, weight loss, and steatorrhea.
- Extraintestinal manifestations include arthritis, arthralgias, cardiac disease, fever, and multiple central nervous findings (e.g., dementia, myoclonus).
- Arthritis is typically migratory, involving large and small joints.
- Cardiac involvement is characterized by pericarditis, valvular defects, and congestive heart failure.
- Peripheral lymphadenopathy is not uncommon.

DIFFERENTIAL DIAGNOSIS

- Intestinal lymphangiectasia (small bowel)
- Mastocytosis (small bowel)
- Amyloidosis (small bowel)
- Abetalipoproteinemia (small bowel)
- Opportunistic infections in AIDS (small bowel)

PATHOLOGY

- *T. whippelii* is a gram-positive bacillus with a thick wall and trilaminar membrane.

DIAGNOSTIC PEARLS

- Thickened, nodular folds, primarily in the distal duodenum and jejunum
- Fine mucosal nodularity
- Enlarged, low-attenuation lymph nodes in the mesentery and retroperitoneum

- Villous blunting is caused by expansion of the lamina propria by lacteals distended with fat and innumerable macrophages containing digested bacilli.
- Fat accumulation in obstructed lymph nodes accounts for low-attenuation lymphadenopathy.
- Diagnosis is confirmed on biopsy specimens showing lamina propria packed with periodic acid-Schiff–positive macrophages and gram-positive, acid-fast negative bacilli.

INCIDENCE/PREVALENCE AND EPIDEMIOLOGY

- Rare bacterial disease typically seen in middle-aged white men
- Male-female predominance is 6:1.

Suggested Readings

Ganapathy V, Ganapathy ME, Leibach FH: Protein digestion and assimilation. In *Textbook of Gastroenterology*, 4th ed. Philadelphia, Lippincott Williams & Wilkins, 2003, pp 438-449.

Powel DW: Approach to the patient with diarrhea. In *Textbook of Gastroenterology*, 4th ed. Philadelphia, Lippincott Williams & Wilkins, 2003, pp 844-894.

Rubesin SE: Diseases of small bowel causing malabsorption. In *Radiology: Diagnosis-Imaging-Intervention*. Philadelphia, JB Lippincott, 1993, pp 1-17.

Rubesin SE, Rubin RA, Herlinger H: Small bowel malabsorption: Clinical perspectives. *Radiology* 184:297-305, 1992.

Traber P: Carbohydrate assimilation. In *Textbook of Gastroenterology*, 4th ed. Philadelphia, Lippincott Williams & Wilkins, 2003, pp 389-413.

WHAT THE REFERRING PHYSICIAN NEEDS TO KNOW

- Diagnosis may be confirmed on small bowel biopsies.
- Other causes of low-attenuation mesenteric or retroperitoneal lymphadenopathy include *Mycobacterium avium-intracellulare* infection in patients with acquired immunodeficiency syndrome as well as celiac disease and metastatic testicular carcinoma.

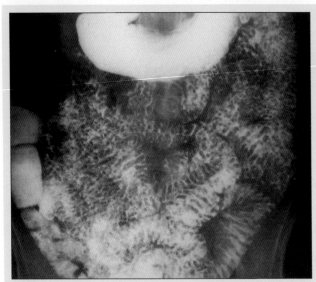

Figure 1. **Whipple disease.** Overhead radiograph from small bowel follow-through shows thickened, nodular folds in the proximal and mid small bowel.

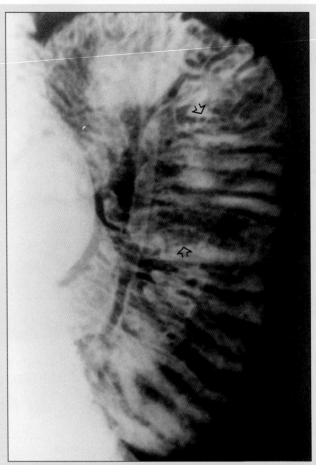

Figure 2. **Whipple disease.** Spot radiograph from enteroclysis shows mildly thickened folds in the proximal jejunum. Also note nodularity of the mucosa *(arrows)* caused by villous enlargement. (*From Rubesin SE: Diseases of small bowel causing malabsorption. In Taveras JM, Ferrucci JT [eds]:* Radiology: Diagnosis-Imaging-Intervention. *Philadelphia, JB Lippincott, 1993, pp 1-17.*)

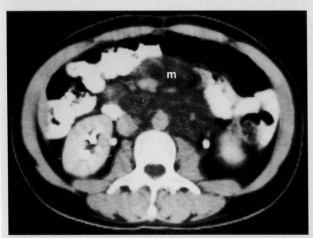

Figure 3. **Whipple disease.** CT shows expansion of the root of the small bowel mesentery (m), as well as the aortocaval and left para-aortic regions, with separation of vessels, lateral displacement of small bowel loops, and focally decreased attenuation of expanded mesenteric fat. At surgery, marked lymphadenopathy was seen, caused by lymphatic infiltration by Whipple disease rather than abnormal mesenteric fat. (*From Rubesin SE, Rubin RA, Herlinger H:* Small bowel malabsorption: clinical perspectives, *Radiology 184:297-305, 1992.*)

Eosinophilic Gastroenteritis (Small Bowel)

DEFINITION: Eosinophilic enteritis is a rare heterogeneous group of disorders characterized by eosinophilic infiltration of various organs and various layers of the gastrointestinal tract.

IMAGING

Radiography
Findings
- Smooth or thickened, nodular folds perpendicular to the longitudinal axis of the small bowel
- Gastric disease: antral polyps, thickened, nodular antral folds
- Spasm

Utility
- Barium studies
- Eosinophilic enteritis can mimic radiographic findings of other diseases causing submucosal bleeding (e.g., ischemia) in small bowel.

CLINICAL PRESENTATION

- Patient may have small bowel mucosal and submucosal involvement with mild steatorrhea, protein loss, weight loss, and iron deficiency anemia.
- Muscularis propria involvement causes gastric outlet obstruction or small bowel obstruction.
- Serosal involvement causes eosinophilic ascites.
- Approximately 50% of patients have peripheral eosinophilia or an allergic history (including asthma, hay fever, drug sensitivity, or urticaria).

DIFFERENTIAL DIAGNOSIS

- Ischemia (small bowel)
- Vasculitis (small bowel)
- Radiation (small bowel)
- Hemorrhage (small bowel)

PATHOLOGY

- Eosinophilic gastroenteritis is a heterogeneous group of disorders characterized by eosinophilic infiltration of various organs and various layers of the gastrointestinal tract.

DIAGNOSTIC PEARLS

- Smooth or nodular, thickened folds perpendicular to the longitudinal axis of the small bowel
- Antral polyps
- Thickened, nodular antral folds

- Eosinophilic infiltration of the small bowel can involve the jejunum or the entire small bowel, is typically patchy, and can be unifocal or multifocal.

INCIDENCE/PREVALENCE AND EPIDEMIOLOGY

- Eosinophilic gastroenteritis is rare.
- It usually develops during the third to sixth decades of life.
- Eosinophilic infiltration, primarily of small bowel serosa, is rare.

Suggested Readings

Ganapathy V, Ganapathy ME, Leibach FH: Protein digestion and assimilation. In *Textbook of Gastroenterology,* 4th ed. Philadelphia, Lippincott Williams & Wilkins, 2003, pp 438-449.

Powel DW: Approach to the patient with diarrhea. In *Textbook of Gastroenterology,* 4th ed. Philadelphia, Lippincott Williams & Wilkins, 2003, pp 844-894.

Rubesin SE: Diseases of small bowel causing malabsorption. In *Radiology: Diagnosis-Imaging-Intervention.* Philadelphia, JB Lippincott, 1993, pp 1-17.

Rubesin SE, Rubin RA, Herlinger H: Small bowel malabsorption: Clinical perspectives. *Radiology* 184:297-305, 1992.

Traber P: Carbohydrate assimilation. In *Textbook of Gastroenterology* 4th ed. Philadelphia, Lippincott Williams & Wilkins, 2003, pp 389-413.

WHAT THE REFERRING PHYSICIAN NEEDS TO KNOW

- Eosinophilic enteritis can mimic radiographic findings of other diseases causing submucosal bleeding in the small bowel.
- Diagnosis requires biopsy confirmation of eosinophilic infiltration of the small bowel wall in the absence of extraintestinal disease or parasitic infection.
- Clues to the diagnosis include simultaneous involvement of the gastric antrum and small bowel, peripheral eosinophilia, and a history of allergic diseases.

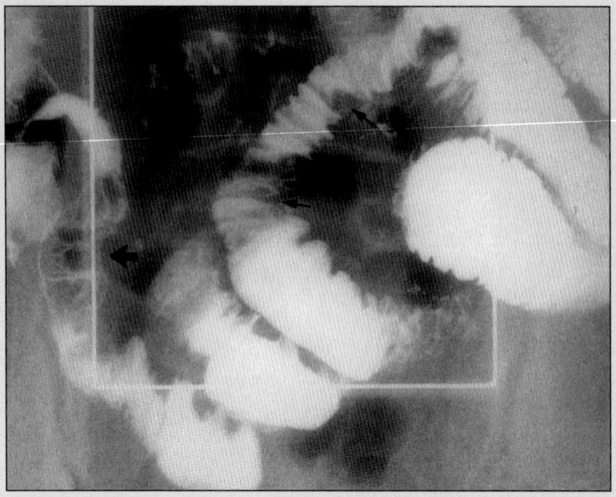

Figure 1. **Eosinophilic enteritis.** Spot radiograph from small bowel follow-through shows thickened, straight folds *(small arrows)* in several loops of the distal small bowel and an abnormal surface pattern *(large arrow)* in the terminal ileum.

Short-Gut Syndrome (Small Bowel)

DEFINITION: Extensive small bowel resection causes an acute diarrheal illness, and long-term malabsorptive state.

IMAGING

Radiography
Findings
- Increased height, thickness, and number of folds in the small bowel

Utility
- Barium studies can document the amount of remaining small intestine, the presence of residual or recurrent disease, and postsurgical complications such as adhesions and anastomotic strictures.

CLINICAL PRESENTATION

- Malabsorption (diarrhea, steatorrhea, excessive gas, abdominal pain, and weight loss)

PATHOLOGY

- Resection of large lengths of the small intestine results in acute diarrheal illness and a long-term malabsorptive state.
- In some patients, the remaining small intestine compensates by increasing thickness and number of folds to increase absorptive capability.

DIAGNOSTIC PEARLS

- Extensively shortened small bowel
- Increased thickening and number of small bowel folds

INCIDENCE/PREVALENCE AND EPIDEMIOLOGY

- Diseases leading to extensive resections include volvulus, superior mesenteric vessel obstruction, strangulated hernia, Crohn disease, radiation enteropathy, and abdominal trauma.

Suggested Readings

Ganapathy V, Ganapathy ME, Leibach FH: Protein digestion and assimilation. In *Textbook of Gastroenterology*, 4th ed. Philadelphia, Lippincott Williams & Wilkins, 2003, pp 438-449.

Powel DW: Approach to the patient with diarrhea. In *Textbook of Gastroenterology*, 4th ed. Philadelphia, Lippincott Williams & Wilkins, 2003, pp 844-894.

Rubesin SE: Diseases of small bowel causing malabsorption. In *Radiology: Diagnosis-Imaging-Intervention*. Philadelphia, JB Lippincott, 1993, pp 1-17.

Rubesin SE, Rubin RA, Herlinger H: Small bowel malabsorption: Clinical perspectives. *Radiology* 184:297-305, 1992.

Traber P: Carbohydrate assimilation. In *Textbook of Gastroenterology*, 4th ed. Philadelphia, Lippincott Williams & Wilkins, 2003, pp 389-413.

WHAT THE REFERRING PHYSICIAN NEEDS TO KNOW

- Barium studies are of value for documenting the amount of remaining small intestine.
- Ileal resection can lead to cholelithiasis.
- Other complications include gastric hypersecretion with ulcer formation and hyperoxaluria (after ileal resection) with renal calculi.

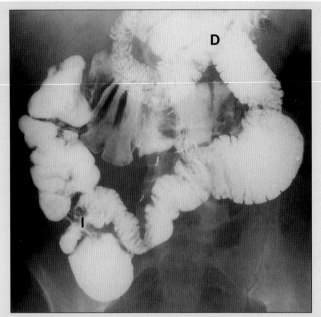

Figure 1. Short-gut syndrome. Overhead radiograph shows a total of only three loops of small bowel from the duodenojejunal junction (D) to the ileocecal valve (I). The small bowel is dilated but not obstructed.

Abetalipoproteinemia (Small Bowel)

DEFINITION: Abetalipoproteinemia is a rare, autosomally transmitted disorder that is heterogeneous at the molecular level.

IMAGING

Radiography
Findings
- Moderately thickened, nodular folds in the duodenum and proximal jejunum

Utility
- Small bowel follow-through
- Enteroclysis

CLINICAL PRESENTATION

- Vitamin E deficiency results in spinocerebellar degeneration and acanthocytosis.
- Vitamin A deficiency results in retinitis pigmentosa, which typically develops during the second decade of life.
- Mental retardation may also be present.

DIFFERENTIAL DIAGNOSIS

- Whipple disease (small bowel)
- Intestinal lymphangiectasia (small bowel)
- Mastocytosis (small bowel)
- Amyloidosis (small bowel)
- Opportunistic infections in AIDS (small bowel)

PATHOLOGY

- Abetalipoproteinemia is an autosomally transmitted disorder that is heterogeneous at the molecular level.
- Condition is linked to a defect in the microsomal triglyceride transfer protein (MTTP).

DIAGNOSTIC PEARLS

- Moderately thickened, nodular folds in the duodenum and proximal jejunum
- Resulting vitamin A and vitamin E deficiency

- Without functioning MTTP, apo-B cannot form the protein capable of transporting fats from the basal membrane of enterocytes.
- Result is an accumulation of absorbed fats and fat-soluble vitamins within enterocytes.
- Triglycerides also accumulate in hepatocytes.

INCIDENCE/PREVALENCE AND EPIDEMIOLOGY

- Symptoms and age of onset vary.
- Condition is a rare, autosomally transmitted disorder.

Suggested Readings

Ganapathy V, Ganapathy ME, Leibach FH: Protein digestion and assimilation. In *Textbook of Gastroenterology*, 4th ed. Philadelphia, Lippincott Williams & Wilkins, 2003, pp 438–449.
Powel DW: Approach to the patient with diarrhea. In *Textbook of Gastroenterology*, 4th ed. Philadelphia, Lippincott Williams & Wilkins, 2003, pp 844-894.
Rubesin SE: Diseases of small bowel causing malabsorption. In *Radiology: Diagnosis-Imaging-Intervention*. Philadelphia, JB Lippincott, 1993, pp 1-17.
Rubesin SE, Rubin RA, Herlinger H: Small bowel malabsorption: Clinical perspectives. *Radiology* 184:297-305, 1992.
Traber P: Carbohydrate assimilation. In *Textbook of Gastroenterology*, 4th ed. Philadelphia, Lippincott Williams & Wilkins, 2003, pp 389-413.

WHAT THE REFERRING PHYSICIAN NEEDS TO KNOW

- Although rare, abetalipoproteinemia should be considered in patients with thickened small bowel folds on barium studies who develop vitamin A deficiency or vitamin E deficiency, or both.

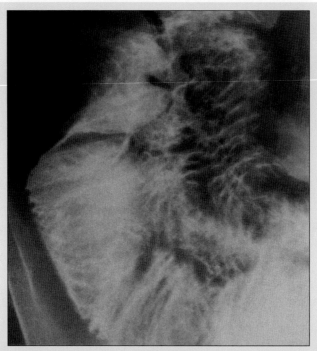

Figure 1. Abetalipoproteinemia of small bowel. Spot radiograph of small bowel shows mildly thickened, irregular folds, possibly because of intestinal secretions that prevent barium from adequately coating the mucosal surface, because the microscopic pathology does not explain the apparent fold thickening in this condition. (*From the teaching files of Hans Herlinger, MD.*)

Intestinal Lymphangiectasia (Small Bowel)

DEFINITION: Intestinal lymphangiectasia results from a congenital abnormality of lymphatic development or from lymphatic obstruction in the small bowel wall and mesentery.

IMAGING

Radiography
Findings
- Thickened, straight or undulating folds in the jejunum and ileum
- Villous distention: sharply defined 1-mm nodular radiolucencies within the small bowel

Utility
Barium studies

CT
Findings
- Thickened small bowel wall
- Lymphadenopathy of normal or low attenuation

CLINICAL PRESENTATION

- Diarrhea is present in 80% of patients.
- Steatorrhea is less common, occurring in 20% of patients.
- Edema of extremities and chylous pleural effusions are common.
- Chylous ascites may be present.

DIFFERENTIAL DIAGNOSIS

- Whipple disease (small bowel)
- Mastocytosis (small bowel)
- Amyloidosis (small bowel)
- Abetalipoproteinemia (small bowel)
- Opportunistic infections in AIDS (small bowel)

PATHOLOGY

- Intestinal lymphangiectasia results from a congenital abnormality of lymphatic development or from lymphatic obstruction in the small bowel wall and mesentery.
- Secondary lymphangiectasia is caused by cardiac failure, retroperitoneal fibrosis, radiation therapy, and mesenteric lymph node involvement by various diseases.

DIAGNOSTIC PEARLS

- Fold changes evenly distributed throughout the small bowel
- Thickened, straight or undulating folds in the jejunum and ileum
- Sharply defined 1-mm nodular radiolucencies within the small bowel

- Lymphatic obstruction results in abnormal absorption of chylomicrons and fat-soluble vitamins, excessive leakage of lymph into the lumen, and impaired circulation of enteric lymphocytes.
- Chylous ascites results from serosal and mesenteric lymphatic obstruction.
- Blockage of the thoracic duct causes chylous pleural effusions.
- Dilated lymphatic lacteals cause villous distention and blunting.
- Some patients develop hypogammaglobulinemia, lymphocytopenia (particularly of T lymphocytes), and hypoproteinemia.

INCIDENCE/PREVALENCE AND EPIDEMIOLOGY

- In primary lymphangiectasia, symptoms usually develop in older children and young adults.

Suggested Readings

Ganapathy V, Ganapathy ME, Leibach FH: Protein digestion and assimilation. In *Textbook of Gastroenterology*, 4th ed. Philadelphia, Lippincott Williams & Wilkins, 2003, pp 438-449.

Powel DW: Approach to the patient with diarrhea. In *Textbook of Gastroenterology*, 4th ed. Philadelphia, Lippincott Williams & Wilkins, 2003, pp 844-894.

Rubesin SE: Diseases of small bowel causing malabsorption. In *Radiology: Diagnosis-Imaging-Intervention*. Philadelphia, JB Lippincott, 1993, pp 1-17.

Rubesin SE, Rubin RA, Herlinger H: Small bowel malabsorption: Clinical perspectives. *Radiology* 184:297-305, 1992.

Traber P: Carbohydrate assimilation. In *Textbook of Gastroenterology*, 4th ed. Philadelphia, Lippincott Williams & Wilkins, 2003, pp 389-413.

WHAT THE REFERRING PHYSICIAN NEEDS TO KNOW

- Patients may develop hypogammaglobulinemia, lymphocytopenia (particularly of T lymphocytes), and hypoproteinemia.

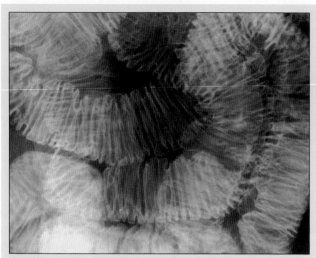

Figure 1. Intestinal lymphangiectasia. Spot radiograph of the jejunum from enteroclysis shows smooth, mildly thickened, slightly undulating folds.

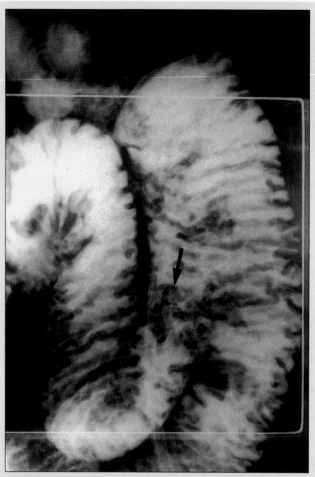

Figure 2. Intestinal lymphangiectasia. Spot radiograph from enteroclysis shows mildly thickened, irregular folds. Tiny mucosal nodules *(arrow)* are seen in one region as a result of enlarged, bulbous villi.

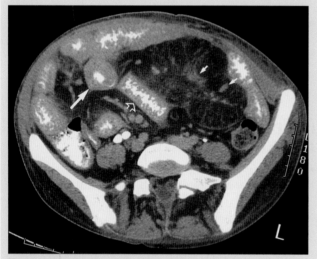

Figure 3. Intestinal lymphangiectasia. CT through upper pelvis shows diffuse thickening of the small bowel wall both in profile *(open arrow)* and en face *(large arrow)*. Stranding of the small bowel mesentery reflects dilated lymphatics and mild mesenteric lymph node enlargement *(small arrows)*.

Mastocytosis (Small Bowel)

DEFINITION: Mastocytosis causes thickened, nodular folds in the small bowel.

IMAGING

Radiography
Findings
- Multifocal thickened, nodular small bowel folds

Utility
- Barium studies

CLINICAL PRESENTATION

- Flushing
- Tachycardia
- Headaches
- Urticaria pigmentosa
- Malabsorption (with diarrhea, steatorrhea, excessive gas, abdominal pain, and weight loss) (rare)

DIFFERENTIAL DIAGNOSIS

- Whipple disease (small bowel)
- Intestinal lymphangiectasia (small bowel)
- Amyloidosis (small bowel)
- Abetalipoproteinemia (small bowel)
- Opportunistic infections in AIDS (small bowel)

PATHOLOGY

- Mastocytosis is a multisystem disorder in which there is accumulation of mast cells in multiple organs, including the skin, small bowel, liver, spleen, and bones.

DIAGNOSTIC PEARLS

- Thickened, nodular folds in small bowel
- Sclerotic foci in bones

- Because mast cells mediate the secretion of histamine, affected individuals may present with episodic flushing, tachycardia, and headaches.

Suggested Readings

Ganapathy V, Ganapathy ME, Leibach FH: Protein digestion and assimilation. In *Textbook of Gastroenterology*, 4th ed. Philadelphia, Lippincott Williams & Wilkins, 2003, pp 438-449.

Powel DW: Approach to the patient with diarrhea. In *Textbook of Gastroenterology*, 4th ed. Philadelphia, Lippincott Williams & Wilkins, 2003, pp 844-894.

Rubesin SE: Diseases of small bowel causing malabsorption. In *Radiology: Diagnosis-Imaging-Intervention*. Philadelphia, JB Lippincott, 1993, pp 1-17.

Rubesin SE, Rubin RA, Herlinger H: Small bowel malabsorption: Clinical perspectives. *Radiology* 184:297-305, 1992.

Traber P: Carbohydrate assimilation. In *Textbook of Gastroenterology*, 4th ed. Philadelphia, Lippincott Williams & Wilkins, 2003, pp 389-413.

WHAT THE REFERRING PHYSICIAN NEEDS TO KNOW

- Differential diagnosis includes Whipple disease, amyloidosis, eosinophilic enteritis, intestinal lymphangiectasia, and abetalipoproteinemia.

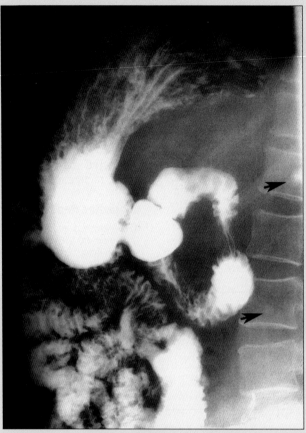

Figure 1. **Lateral overhead radiograph from small bowel follow-through shows thickened, irregular folds in the jejunum caused by accumulation of mastocytes in the lamina propria and submucosa in this patient with mastocytosis.** Also note sclerotic foci *(arrows)* in vertebral bodies caused by associated osseous involvement.

Part 24

BENIGN TUMORS OF THE SMALL BOWEL

Benign Tumors

DEFINITION: Nonmalignant tumors of the small intestine primarily include adenomas, leiomyomas, lipomas, and hemangiomas.

ANATOMIC FINDINGS

Jejunum
- Neurofibromas in neurofibromatosis type 1 are most common in the jejunum.
- Villous adenomas are sessile, lobulated polyps that are larger than most adenomatous polyps and have a strong predilection for the duodenum.

Ileum
- Inflammatory fibroid polyps (also called *inflammatory pseudotumors*) are found almost exclusively in the ileum.
- Lipomas usually occur in the ileum.

IMAGING

Radiography
Findings
- Adenoma: small (1-2 cm), smooth or slightly lobulated lesion seen as sessile or pedunculated intraluminal polyps or as small mural nodules.
- Adenoma: usually a solitary lesion, occasionally multiple in patients with polyposis syndromes.
- Gastrointestinal stromal tumor (GIST): smooth, round or semilunar mural defect demarcated by sharp angles with wall
- Lipoma: sharply demarcated, often pedunculated tumor that conforms to the contour of small bowel lumen; usually in distal ileum
- Hemangioma: nodular defect; usually on distal ileum, may contain calcified phleboliths
- Neurofibroma: solitary or multifocal intraluminal or intramural masses with scalloping of intestinal wall
- Inflammatory fibroid polyp: solitary, smooth, rounded mass in distal ileum

DIAGNOSTIC PEARLS
- Adenomas: small (1- to 2-cm), smooth or slightly lobulated lesions, sessile or pedunculated intraluminal polyps or small mural nodules
- GISTs: smooth, round or semilunar mural defects that are demarcated by sharp angles with the adjacent wall
- Lipoma: homogeneous mass between -80 and -120 Hounsfield units

Utility
- Barium-based enteroclysis is a reliable technique for the demonstration of small bowel tumors and for the evaluation of occult gastrointestinal bleeding and intestinal obstruction.
- Enteroclysis allows more accurate differentiation of benign small bowel tumors than small bowel follow-through studies.
- Enteroclysis allows an accurate preoperative diagnosis of GISTs in 83%-100% of cases.
- Lipoma: configuration may change at fluoroscopy with manual palpation or peristalsis of the small bowel as a result of the soft consistency of the lesion.

Interventional Radiology
Findings
- Hemangioma: intestinal vascular abnormality
Utility
- Mesenteric angiography

CT
Findings
- GIST: sharply defined spherical mass that displays homogeneous soft-tissue density and uniform contrast enhancement

WHAT THE REFERRING PHYSICIAN NEEDS TO KNOW
- Diagnosis may be difficult, but useful diagnostic observations can be made based on the number, location, and radiologic features of the tumors.
- In patients with vascular cutaneous lesions (tuberous sclerosis, Turner syndrome, or Osler-Weber-Rendu disease), suspicion for intestinal hemangiomas should be raised.
- Malignant GISTs are larger than benign GISTs, are less uniform in shape, and produce a more heterogeneous tissue attenuation.

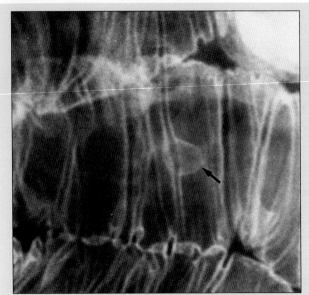

Figure 1. Adenoma. Enteroclysis shows a small (8-mm) jejunal adenoma as a smooth, sessile mucosal nodule *(arrow)*.

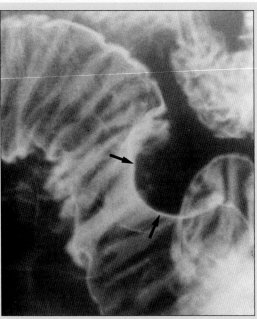

Figure 2. Benign gastrointestinal stromal tumor. The submucosal nature of the tumor is recognized on barium study by an area of semicircular mass effect within the lumen *(arrows)*. The smooth surface results from stretching of the overlying normal mucosa.

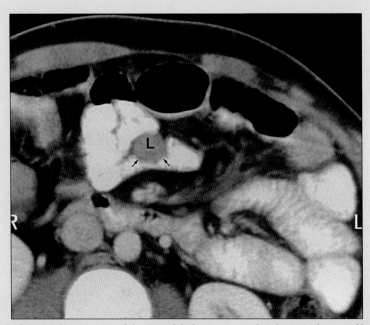

Figure 3. Benign gastrointestinal stromal tumor. CT of the GIST (L) shows a smooth submucosal mass of homogeneous soft-tissue (muscle) attenuation compressing the lumen *(arrows)*.

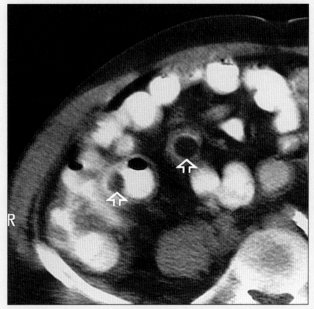

Figure 4. Lipoma. CT shows two lipomas protruding into the bowel lumen *(arrows)*. A well-circumscribed, intraluminal homogeneous mass with negative attenuation consistent with fat is characteristic of an enteric lipoma on CT.

- Lipoma: homogeneous mass between − 80 and − 120 Hounsfield units; soft-tissue stranding caused by fibrovascular changes associated with ulceration
- Neurofibromas: diffusely elongated tumor, sometimes characterized by mural thickening

Utility
- Cross-sectional imaging studies are ideal for showing extraluminal component of lesions.
- CT findings can differentiate benign and malignant small bowel tumors.
- CT allows for specific diagnosis of tumors such as lipomas and GISTs.
- CT enteroclysis combines techniques of small bowel infusion enteroclysis with imaging advantages inherent in cross-sectional imaging.
- CT is particularly useful in depicting nature and extent of small bowel GISTs.
- CT enteroclysis is an accurate method for diagnosis of small bowel neoplasms.

MRI
Utility
- MR enteroclysis is emerging as an improved imaging technique for investigation of small bowel neoplasms.

CLINICAL PRESENTATION
- Patients are mostly asymptomatic.
- Symptomatic patients may exhibit abdominal pain and other clinical features of partial or intermittent small bowel obstruction.
- Small bowel obstruction caused by intussusception may occur.

- Hemangiomas are more likely to cause gastrointestinal bleeding than other benign tumors.

DIFFERENTIAL DIAGNOSIS
- Metastasis (small bowel)
- Lymphoma (small bowel)
- Carcinoid (small bowel)
- Duplication cyst (small bowel)

PATHOLOGY
- Approximately 90% of benign small bowel neoplasms are adenomas, GISTs, lipomas, or hemangiomas.
- Adenomas: most are villous; others are tubular or tubulovillous; they may exhibit cellular atypia, a villous component, and larger sizes increase the risk for malignancy.
- Lipomas are well-circumscribed, solitary, relatively avascular submucosal proliferations of fat of variable size (1-6 cm) that usually grow intraluminally.
- Hemangiomas are most likely congenital submucosal hamartomatous vascular growths; microscopically, vascular sinuses are enlarged and lined by endothelium and are surrounded by minimal stromal tissue.
- Neurogenic tumors arise from the intramural neural plexus; neurofibromas are composed of Schwann cells and fibroblasts.
- Ganglioneuromas arise from the sympathetic ganglia and produce focal polypoid lesions, multifocal polyps (ganglioneuromatous polyposis), or diffusely infiltrating lesions (ganglioneuromatosis).

- Inflammatory fibroid polyps are composed of a vascular fibrous stroma with a diffuse inflammatory infiltrate.

INCIDENCE/PREVALENCE AND EPIDEMIOLOGY

- Benign neoplasms of small bowel constitute 1%-5% of all gastrointestinal neoplasms.
- Nearly 75% of small bowel tumors found at autopsy are benign.
- Benign neoplasms occur with equal frequency in men and women between 50 and 80 years of age.
- Approximately 90% of benign neoplasms are adenomas, GISTs, lipomas, or hemangiomas.
- Lipomas of the small bowel account for 20%-25% of all gastrointestinal lipomas.
- Although rare in the general population, neural tumors of the small bowel are reported in 10%-25% of patients with neurofibromatosis.

- Heterotopic gastric mucosa: associated with malformations such as a Meckel diverticulum or enteric duplication

Suggested Readings

Ciresi DL, Scholten DJ: The continuing dilemma of primary tumors of the small intestine. *Am Surg* 61:698-702, 1995.

Gill SS, Heuman DM, Mihas AA: Small intestinal neoplasms. *J Clin Gastroenterol* 33:267-282, 2001.

Gourtsoyiannis NC, Bays D, Papaioannou N, et al: Benign tumors of the small intestine: Preoperation evaluation with a barium infusion technique. *Eur J Radiol* 16:115-125, 1993.

Minardi AJ Jr, Zibari GB, Aultman DF, et al: Small-bowel tumors. *J Am Coll Surg* 186:664-668, 1998.

O'Riordan BG, Vilor M, Herrera L: Small bowel tumors: An overview. *Dig Dis Sci* 14:245-257, 1996.

Rangiah DS, Cox M, Richardson M, et al: Small bowel tumours: A 10-year experience in four Sydney teaching hospitals. *Aust NZ J Surg* 74:788-792, 2004.

Polyposis Syndromes

DEFINITION: Polyposis syndromes include familial adenomatous polyp syndrome (FAPS), Peutz-Jeghers syndrome (PJS), Cowden disease, and Cronkhite-Canada syndrome, which are characterized by multiple polyps in the gastrointestinal tract.

IMAGING

Radiography
Findings
- Peutz-Jeghers syndrome (PJS) produces luminal polyps of variable size; 2- to 3-cm polyps have a lobulated contour; normal loops may alternate with involved loops.
- Cowden disease is characterized by multiple polyps producing nodular mucosal surface pattern.
- Cronkhite-Canada syndrome is characterized by sparse to diffuse involvement of bowel with a few to innumerable polyps of various sizes, thickened folds, and increased secretions.

Utility
- Barium studies
- Enteroclysis is a reliable technique for demonstration of small bowel tumors.

CT
Findings
- PJS polyps: soft-tissue masses within the contrast-filled small bowel loops

Utility
- CT enteroclysis helps differentiate benign and malignant small bowel tumors.
- Accurate method for diagnosis of small bowel neoplasms.
- Ideal imaging test for detection of desmoids because it can show extent of tumor invasion.

CLINICAL PRESENTATION

- Abdominal pain and other clinical features of partial or intermittent small bowel obstruction
- Anemia, occult bleeding, or intermittent gastrointestinal hemorrhage
- PJS: pigmented macules on lips, mouth, hands, and feet. (Gastrointestinal polyps may cause gastrointestinal bleeding or abdominal pain as a result of intermittent intussusceptions.)
- Cowden disease: facial trichilemmomas, lipomas, and mucocutaneous keratoses

DIAGNOSTIC PEARLS

- PJS produces luminal polyps of variable size; 2- to 3-cm polyps have a lobulated contour; normal loops may alternate with involved loops.
- Cowden disease is characterized by multiple polyps producing a nodular mucosal surface pattern.
- Cronkhite-Canada syndrome is characterized by diffuse to sparse involvement of bowel with a few to innumerable small polyps (or scattered polyps of various sizes), thickened folds, and increased secretions.

- Cronkhite-Canada syndrome: gradual disease onset with abdominal pain, diarrhea, and anorexia that precede or occur together with alopecia, hyperpigmentation, and nail dystrophy

DIFFERENTIAL DIAGNOSIS

- Lymphoma (small bowel)
- Multifocal carcinoids (small bowel)

PATHOLOGY

- FAPS is a hereditary disorder caused by mutation of the adenomatous polyposis coli gene; the colon is typically involved, but the small bowel may also be involved.
- PJS is an autosomal dominant disorder, but 50% are new mutations; polyps are benign hamartomas containing a smooth muscle core and lined by intestinal epithelium.
- Cowden disease (multiple hamartoma syndrome) is an inherited condition characterized by hamartomas and other abnormalities of the skin, breast, thyroid gland, and gastrointestinal tract.
- Cronkhite-Canada syndrome is a nonfamilial condition characterized by diffuse gastrointestinal polyposis and ectodermal changes; polyps are inflammatory, consisting of dilated cystic interstitial glands.

WHAT THE REFERRING PHYSICIAN NEEDS TO KNOW

- FAPS: enteroclysis and capsule endoscopy may have an important role for diagnosis and surveillance in patients with duodenal polyps.
- PJS produces an increased risk of gastrointestinal and extraintestinal malignancies, including esophageal, gastric, small bowel, colorectal, breast, ovarian, and pancreatic cancers.
- Cowden disease is associated with a high risk of breast and thyroid cancers.

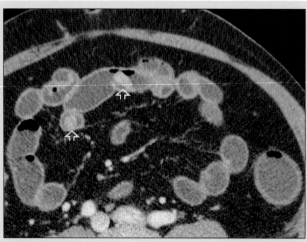

Figure 1. Peutz-Jeghers syndrome. CT enteroclysis performed with enteral water infusion and intravenous contrast enhancement shows multiple intraluminal polyps *(arrows)* within the jejunum. The fluid density of the neutral enteral contrast medium is juxtaposed to the enhancing bowel wall, increasing the conspicuity of the polyps.

INCIDENCE/PREVALENCE AND EPIDEMIOLOGY

- Polyposis syndromes occur with equal frequency in men and women, usually between 50 and 80 years of age.
- FAPS: 75% of patients with duodenal adenomas have adenomas in proximal jejunum on endoscopy.
- JPS: gastrointestinal polyposis is reported in 30%-60% of patients.
- Cronkhite-Canada syndrome: small bowel involvement is reported in more than 50% of patients.

Suggested Readings

Bronner MP: Gastrointestinal inherited polyposis syndromes. *Mod Pathol* 16:359-365, 2003.

Casillas J, Sais GJ, Greve JL, et al: Imaging of intra- and extraabdominal desmoid tumors. *RadioGraphics* 11:959-968, 1991.

Chen YM, Ott DJ, Wu WC, et al: Cowden's disease: A case report and literature review. *Gastrointest Radiol* 12:325-329, 1987.

Cho GJ, Bergquist K, Schwartz AM: Peutz-Jeghers syndrome and the hamartomatous polyposis syndromes: Radiologic-pathologic correlation. *RadioGraphics* 17:785-791, 1997.

Dachman AH, Buck JL, Burke AP, et al: Cronkhite-Canada syndrome: Radiologic features. *Gastrointest Radiol* 14:285-290, 1989.

Einstein DM, Tagliabue JR, Desai RK: Abdominal desmoids: CT findings in 25 patients. *AJR Am J Roentgenol* 157:275-279, 1991.

Knudsen AL, Bulow S: Desmoid tumour in familial adenomatous polyposis: A review of literature. *Fam Cancer* 1:111-119, 2001.

Schulmann K, Hollerbach S, Kraus K, et al: Feasibility and diagnostic utility of video capsule endoscopy for the detection of small bowel polyps in patients with hereditary polyposis syndromes. *Am J Gastroenterol* 100:27-37, 2005.

Wu JS, McGannon EA, Church JM: Incidence of neoplastic polyps in the ileal pouch of patients with familial adenomatous polyposis after restorative proctocolectomy. *Dis Colon Rectum* 41:552-556, 1998.

Small Bowel Carcinoma

DEFINITION: Primary malignant tumor of the small bowel.

IMAGING

Radiography
Findings
- The tumor may be manifested by a polypoid, ulcerated, or annular lesion, usually in the proximal jejunum.

CT
Findings
- Associated signs of small bowel obstruction may be present in patients with annular lesions.
- Focal wall thickening or soft-tissue mass in affected loop

Utility
- CT useful for showing extraintestinal spread of tumor in abdomen.

CLINICAL PRESENTATION

- Many patients have advanced tumors at the time of surgery because of delayed diagnosis.

DIFFERENTIAL DIAGNOSIS

- Metastases (small bowel)
- Lymphoma (small bowel)
- Carcinoid tumors (small bowel)
- Gastrointestinal stromal tumors (small bowel)

PATHOLOGY

- Similar features with colorectal carcinoma include development via an adenoma-carcinoma sequence and mutations in the *ki-RAS* and *TP53* genes.
- Gene mutations may explain the high incidence of associated extraintestinal malignant tumors in patients with small bowel cancer.

DIAGNOSTIC PEARLS

- Adenocarcinoma is more common in the jejunum than in the ileum, occurring predominantly in its first 30 cm.
- Tumors are usually well differentiated, even when metastases are present.
- Mucin-producing columnar epithelium is frequently identified.

- Adenocarcinoma is more common in the jejunum than in the ileum, occurring predominantly in its first 30 cm.
- These tumors are usually well differentiated, even when metastases are present.
- Mucin-producing columnar epithelium is frequently identified.

INCIDENCE/PREVALENCE AND EPIDEMIOLOGY

- Primary malignant tumors of small bowel constitute less than 2% of all gastrointestinal neoplasms.
- Adenocarcinomas constitute 45% of small bowel primary malignancies.
- Incidence of small bowel cancer is 50 times less than that of colorectal cancer.

Suggested Readings

Maglinte DD, O'Connor K, Bessette J, et al: The role of the physician in the late diagnosis of primary malignant tumors of the small intestine. *Am J Gastroenterol* 86:304-308, 1991.
Neugut AI, Marvin MR, Rella VA, Chabot JA: An overview of adenocarcinoma of the small intestine. *Oncology (Williston Park)* 11:529-536, 1997.

WHAT THE REFERRING PHYSICIAN NEEDS TO KNOW
- Low prevalence and nonspecific clinical symptoms underscore the need for imaging methods with high sensitivity and negative predictive value.

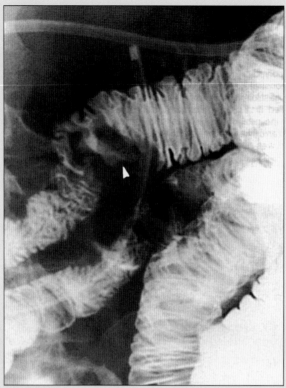

Figure 1. Atypical jejunal adenocarcinoma in a 63-year-old man with abdominal pain. Enteroclysis shows an eccentric, ulcerated mass *(arrowhead)* in the proximal jejunum. The radiographic findings are more suggestive of lymphoma, but the location is typical of adenocarcinoma, which was found at surgery.

Carcinoid Tumors

DEFINITION: Carcinoid tumors originate from the ectodermal cells of the neural crest and represent a heterogeneous group of tumors with different forms of biologic behavior.

ANATOMIC FINDINGS

Small Bowel
- Small bowel is the most common site of malignant carcinoid tumors.
- Distal 50 cm of the ileum is most common site of small bowel involvement.

IMAGING

Radiography
Findings
- Multiple smooth, rounded nodules or submucosal masses

Utility
- Barium studies

CT
Findings
- Primary tumor-enhancing polypoid mass in the wall of the bowel
- Tumor growth into the mesentery is characterized by spiculated mesenteric mass with curvilinear stranding and in-drawing of adjacent bowel loops.
- Smaller metastases are usually hypervascular.
- Larger lesions are often heterogeneous with peripheral hyperdensity.
- Calcification of mesenteric lesions is common.

Utility
- Multislice CT is performed with neutral oral and intravenous contrast media.
- In most cases, CT fails to reveal the primary tumor.
- Isotropic imaging with maximal-intensity projections and multiplanar reformats may help in planning surgery for carcinoid tumors.

DIAGNOSTIC PEARLS
- Enhancing polypoid mass is seen in the wall of the bowel.
- Tumor growth into the mesentery is characterized by a spiculated mesenteric mass with curvilinear stranding and in-drawing of adjacent bowel loops.
- Distal 50 cm of ileum is common site of small bowel involvement.

MRI
Findings
- Primary tumors: T1 hypointensity, T2 hyperintensity with postgadolinium intense enhancement

Nuclear Medicine
Utility
- Iodine-123 (^{123}I)-labeled metaiodobenzylguanidine (MIBG) has low sensitivity (55%-70%).
- Indium-111 or iodine-123 (^{111}In or ^{123}I)-labeled DTPA octreotide has a sensitivity of 80%-100% in diagnosing carcinoid tumors.

Single Photon Emission Computed Tomography (SPECT)
Utility
- Improves anatomic localization

PET
Utility
- Somatostatin receptor scanning has been claimed to be more cost effective than conventional imaging for detecting these tumors.

WHAT THE REFERRING PHYSICIAN NEEDS TO KNOW

- Invasiveness is a function of time, anatomic location, and size.
- Malignant nature of these tumors can be confirmed only if local invasion or distant metastases are observed.
- All small-bowel carcinoids are potentially malignant and should be resected with clear margin together with radical resection of regional lymph nodes.
- Radiation therapy can be used for palliation of pain from bone metastases.
- Optimal CT technique is achieved with oral and intravenous contrast media, isotropic imaging, and nonaxial reformats.
- Ninety-five percent of carcinoid tumors larger than 2 cm metastasize versus only 50% of tumors smaller than 1 cm.
- Survival rate is less than 20% in patients with metastatic disease at time of presentation.

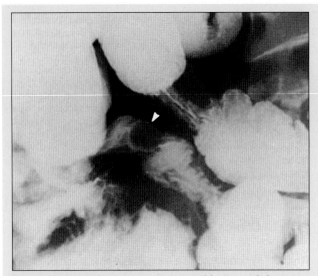

Figure 1. Carcinoid tumor in a 69-year-old man with lower gastrointestinal bleeding. Enteroclysis shows a small, rounded submucosal defect *(arrowhead)* in the terminal ileum. This was a proven ileal carcinoid. Adjacent lymph nodes were negative for metastases. Prior radionuclide scintigraphy, angiography, and CT (not shown) failed to reveal the lesion.

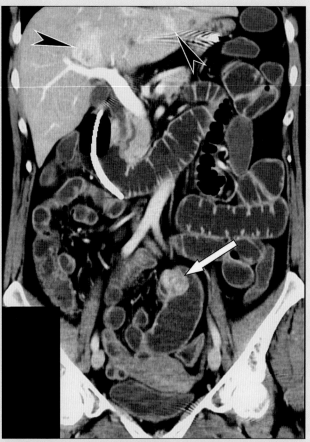

Figure 2. Metastatic carcinoid tumor in a 59-year-old woman with diarrhea and wheezing. Coronal reformat from isotropic resolution CT enteroclysis performed with neutral enteral contrast media shows a 3-cm hypervascular mass *(arrow)* in the distal ileum. Also seen are multiple hypervascular liver metastases *(arrowheads)*.

CLINICAL PRESENTATION

- Ileal carcinoids may cause no symptoms or nonspecific symptoms.
- Carcinoid syndrome produces periodic cutaneous flushing, diarrhea, and, less frequently, bronchospasm.
- Carcinoid syndrome may occur in the absence of hepatic disease.

DIFFERENTIAL DIAGNOSIS

- Lymphoma (small bowel)
- Metastases to the small bowel
- Gastrointestinal stromal tumors (small bowel)

PATHOLOGY

- Tumors originate from ectodermal cells of the neural crest.

- Condition is a heterogeneous group of tumors with different forms of biologic behavior.
- Tumors are classified as foregut, midgut, and hindgut lesions based on their embryonic origin.
- Tumor invasion of the muscle layer of the bowel causes mesenteric fibrosis.
- Occlusion of mesenteric vessels may cause bowel ischemia.
- Mesenteric metastases often exceed the primary tumor in size and endocrine activity.
- Advanced ileal carcinoid tumors can metastasize widely to the omentum, peritoneal surfaces, lymph nodes, liver, and lungs.

INCIDENCE/PREVALENCE AND EPIDEMIOLOGY

- Extension beyond the bowel wall is found in 30%-67% of ileal lesions at the time of diagnosis.
- Carcinoid syndrome occurs in approximately 10% of patients with ileal carcinoids.

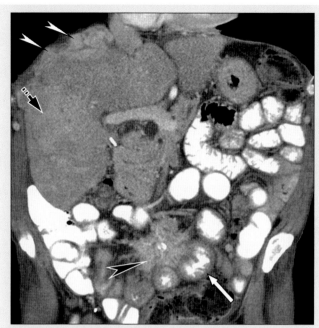

Figure 3. Carcinoid syndrome in a 69-year-old man. Coronal CT reformat shows a spiculated mass *(black arrowhead)* in the mesentery with calcification. The superior mesenteric artery is encased by this mass. Associated wall thickening *(white arrow)* of an adjacent small bowel loop caused by proven ischemia is seen. Also note liver parenchymal *(dashed arrow)* and surface *(white arrowheads)* metastases.

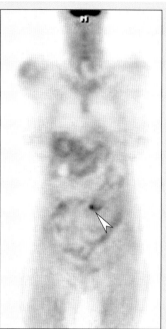

Figure 4. Carcinoid syndrome in a 59-year-old woman. CT and octreotide scans *(not shown)* failed to reveal the primary tumor or evidence of metastases. Fluoro-18-deoxyglucose PET scan shows intense uptake *(arrowhead)* in the mid small bowel corresponding to the primary carcinoid tumor. This patient presumably had the carcinoid syndrome because the venous drainage of the tumor communicated with the systemic circulation via retroperitoneal veins.

■ Extensive hepatic metastases are present in 95% of patients with carcinoid syndrome.

Suggested Readings

Bader TR, Semelka RC, Chiu VC, et al: MRI of carcinoid tumors: Spectrum of appearances in the gastrointestinal tract and liver. *J Magn Reson Imaging* 14:261-269, 2001.

Gore RM, Berlin JW, Mehta UK, et al: GI carcinoid tumours: Appearance of the primary and detecting metastases. *Best Pract Res Clin Endocrinol Metab* 19:245-263, 2005.

Horton KM, Kamel I, Hofmann L, Fishman EK: Carcinoid tumors of the small bowel: A multitechnique imaging approach. *AJR Am J Roentgenol* 182:559-567, 2004.

Oberg K, Eriksson B: Nuclear medicine in the detection, staging and treatment of gastrointestinal carcinoid tumours. *Best Pract Res Clin Endocrinol Metab* 19:265-276, 2005.

Orlefors H, Sundin A, Garske U, et al: Whole-body (11)C-5-hydroxy-tryptophan positron emission tomography as a universal imaging technique for neuroendocrine tumors: Comparison with somatostatin receptor scintigraphy and computed tomography. *J Clin Endocrinol Metab* 90:3392-3400, 2005.

Sugimoto E, Lorelius LE, Eriksson B, Oberg K: Midgut carcinoid tumours: CT appearance. *Acta Radiol* 36:337-367, 1995.

Gastrointestinal Stromal Tumors

DEFINITION: Gastrointestinal stromal tumors (GISTs) are characterized by expression of the tyrosine kinase growth factor receptor.

IMAGING

CT
Findings
- Large tumors (>5 cm in size) are seen as heterogeneously enhancing exophytic masses.
- Homogeneous, intense enhancement may sometimes be seen with tumors less than 5 cm in size.
- Marked expansion of lumen or aneurysmal dilation of the affected bowel is seen.
- Calcification is uncommon at presentation but may be detected in metastatic lesions after chemotherapy.

Utility
- CT is better at detecting mesenteric metastases than MRI.
- Small liver metastases are usually hypervascular on CT before chemotherapy.
- Cystic changes on CT are predictive of successful tumor response.

MRI
Findings
- Mesenteric masses: smooth surfaced without spiculation or in-drawing of the mesentery
- Metastases: low or intermediate signal intensity on precontrast T1-weighted image and marginally bright signal intensity on T2-weighted image
- Mucosal ulceration

Utility
- MRI is superior to single-phase CT in assessing viability of metastases.
- Changes in T2-weighted signal intensity on MRI are predictive of successful tumor response.
- Tumor size measurements are less accurate in charting tumor response.
- One of first signs of relapse may be new enhancing focus within stable cystic metastasis.

DIAGNOSTIC PEARLS
- Heterogeneously or homogeneously enhancing exophytic mass
- Aneurysmal dilatation of affected bowel
- Expression of tyrosine kinase growth factor receptor (also called KIT receptor or CD117)

PET
Utility
- Uptake of ^{18}F-FDG (fluorodeoxyglucose) by metastatic GISTs is variable.
- PET is not as sensitive as CT in detecting metastases.
- PET may determine response of metastatic GISTs to imatinib earlier than CT.

CLINICAL PRESENTATION
- Clinical presentation is often nonspecific.
- Abdominal pain or distention may occur.
- Gastrointestinal bleeding and unexplained anemia may occur.
- Intestinal obstruction is rare.

DIFFERENTIAL DIAGNOSIS
- Lymphoma (small bowel)
- Metastases (small bowel)
- Carcinoma (small bowel)

PATHOLOGY
- GISTs are characterized by expression of tyrosine kinase growth factor receptor, also called KIT receptor or CD117.

WHAT THE REFERRING PHYSICIAN NEEDS TO KNOW

- GISTs will eventually become malignant.
- In absence of metastatic disease, complete surgical excision of GISTs should be undertaken.
- Imatinib mesylate is effective as chemotherapy for 80% of patients with metastatic or large (>10 cm in size) GISTs.
- Tumor relapse after initial response is sometimes seen after the first year of therapy.
- Small-bowel GISTs have worse prognosis than gastric GISTs.
- CT and MRI help determine tumor response to therapy.
- Features indicating worse prognosis include distal small bowel location, large tumor size, and high mitotic activity.

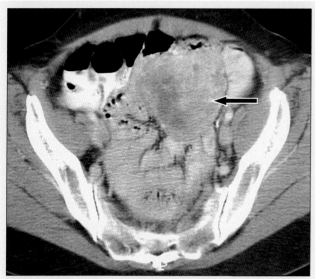

Figure 1. Gastrointestinal stromal tumor in a 50-year-old woman with chronic abdominal pain. CT of the pelvis shows a heterogeneously enhancing exophytic mass *(arrow)* adherent to small bowel loops. This mass was a proven GIST.

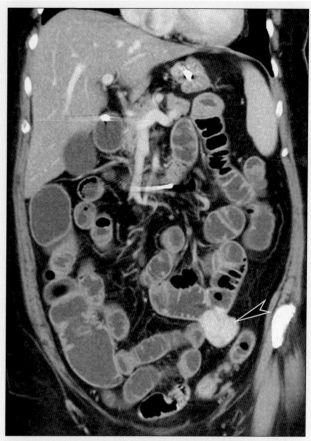

Figure 2. Gastrointestinal stromal tumor in a 63-year-old woman with unexplained gastrointestinal bleeding. CT enteroclysis shows a 3-cm hypervascular submucosal mass *(arrowhead)* arising from the mid–small bowel. This mass was a proven GIST at surgery. Prior capsule endoscopy showed jejunal angioectasia (not shown) but not the small bowel tumor.

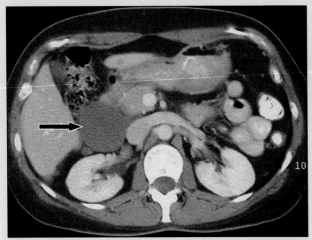

Figure 3. **A 49-year-old woman with a history of a leiomyosarcoma and recurrent abdominal pain.** Previous CT showed a solid mesenteric metastasis. After 3 months of imatinib therapy a repeat CT shows that the mass *(arrow)* has decreased in size; a substantial decrease in the density of the lesion (which now resembles a benign cyst) has also occurred.

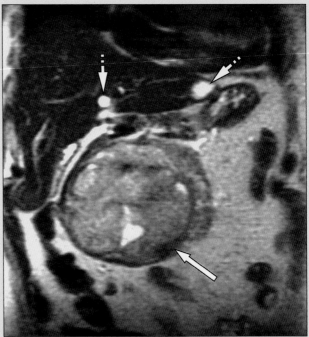

Figure 4. **A 75-year-old woman receiving treatment with imatinib for a known gastrointestinal stromal tumor.** T2-weighted coronal fast spin-echo MRI sequence shows a 10-cm mildly hyperintense abdominal mass *(solid arrow)* caused by mesenteric metastases from her known GIST. Note how the mass has a smooth surface. Hyperintense liver metastases *(dashed arrows)* are also seen.

- Histologic classification is based on predominant cell type, either spindle cell or epithelioid.
- Most GISTs occur as a result of single gain-of-function mutation of KIT gene.
- GISTs originate from stem cells that normally express CD117.
- Exophytic growth pattern is often seen.
- Damage in myenteric plexus causes luminal dilation.

INCIDENCE/PREVALENCE AND EPIDEMIOLOGY

- GISTs are found to be malignant at the time of presentation in 20%-30% of cases.
- Tumors smaller than 2 cm usually do not metastasize, whereas those greater than 5 cm are usually malignant.
- Hepatic or mesenteric recurrences occur in 40%-90% of patients after surgery.

Suggested Readings

Choi H, Charnsangavej C, de Castro FS, et al: CT evaluation of the response of gastrointestinal stromal tumors after imatinib mesylate treatment: A quantitative analysis correlated with FDG PET findings. *AJR Am J Roentgenol* 183:619-628, 2004.

Gayed I, Vu T, Iyer R, et al: The role of 18F-FDG PET in staging and early prediction of response to therapy of recurrent gastrointestinal stromal tumors. *J Nucl Med* 45:17-21, 2004.

Goerres GW, Stupp R, Barghouth G, et al: The value of PET, CT and in-line PET/CT in patients with gastrointestinal stromal tumours: Long-term outcome of treatment with imatinib mesylate. *Eur J Nucl Med Mol Imaging* 32:153-162, 2005.

Sandrasegaran K, Rajesh A, Rushing DA, et al: Gastrointestinal stromal tumors: CT and MRI findings. *Eur Radiol* 15:1407-1414, 2005.

Sandrasegaran K, Rajesh A, Rydberg J, et al: Gastrointestinal stromal tumors: Clinical, radiologic, and pathologic features. *AJR Am J Roentgenol* 184:803-811, 2005.

Non-Hodgkin Lymphoma

DEFINITION: Lymphocytic cell neoplasm of the small bowel.

IMAGING

Radiography
Findings
- Nodular form: multiple small (0.5- to 2.0-cm) submucosal nodules, often containing central areas of umbilication or ulceration (bull's-eye lesions)
- Mesenteric nodal lymphoma: displacement and compression of loops by adjacent mesenteric masses
- Transmural infiltration: localized perforation, resulting in a sealed-off mesenteric cavity

Utility
- Barium studies

CT
Findings
- Mesenteric nodal lymphoma: lobulated mesenteric masses encase adjacent small bowel loops, producing classic *sandwich* appearance.
- One or more segments of circumferential bowel wall thickening, with mild or moderate homogeneous enhancement
- Aneurysmal bowel dilation: focally ballooned segments of the bowel, showing reduced peristalsis and no proximal obstruction

Utility
- CT with intravenous contrast media

MRI
Findings
- Homogeneous low-signal and heterogeneous high-signal intensity on T1- and T2-weighted images

Utility
- MRI has not gained widespread acceptance in the diagnosis or staging of non-Hodgkin lymphoma.

PET
Utility
- Positive FDG (fluorodeoxyglucose) PET scan after completion of chemotherapy is a strong predictor of relapse.
- FDG-PET has higher accuracy than CT in detecting residual disease after therapy.

DIAGNOSTIC PEARLS

- Multiple, small (0.5- to 2.0-cm), submucosal nodules in the small bowel in nodular form
- One or more segments of circumferential wall thickening with mild or moderate homogeneous enhancement on CT
- Mesenteric nodal lymphoma: lobulated mesenteric masses that encase adjacent small bowel loops, producing a classic *sandwich* appearance on CT

CLINICAL PRESENTATION

- Patient may complain of abdominal pain, often associated with nausea or vomiting, anemia, weight loss, and pyrexia.
- Palpable abdominal mass or small bowel obstruction may occur.
- Malabsorption and diarrhea are rare features in the Western form of lymphoma.
- Overall prognosis of primary small bowel lymphoma is only fair, with 5-year survival rates of 25%-30%.

DIFFERENTIAL DIAGNOSIS

- Carcinoid tumors (small bowel)
- Metastases (small bowel)
- Kaposi sarcoma (small bowel)

PATHOLOGY

- Stage IE: disease confined to a single extranodal site (i.e., the small bowel)
- Stage IIE1: associated involvement of a group of regional lymph nodes
- Stage IIE2: more extensive subdiaphragmatic nodal involvement
- Stage IIIE: small bowel lymphoma with lymphadenopathy on both sides of the diaphragm.

WHAT THE REFERRING PHYSICIAN NEEDS TO KNOW

- Secondary gastrointestinal lymphoma usually affects multiple sites.
- Immunohistochemical methods are used in combination with the histologic findings to classify tumors.
- Staging of non-Hodgkin lymphoma is more relevant for selecting treatment options than the histologic classification of tumor.
- Patients with stage IE and IIE should have complete resection of the tumor before chemotherapy is instituted.
- Cavitary form of lymphoma requires extensive bowel resection.
- Poor prognosis seen in stages greater than IIE2, tumor size greater than 10 cm, immunoblastic histology, and T-cell type

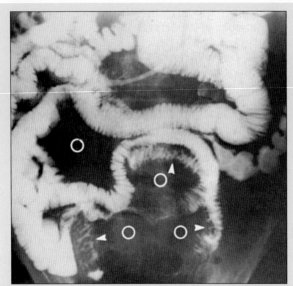

Figure 1.   **Mesenteric nodal form of non-Hodgkin lymphoma in a 71-year-old man.** Multiple loops of small bowel are displaced by mesenteric masses *(open circles)*. Involved folds are thickened and nodular *(arrowheads)*. No evidence of obstruction is seen.

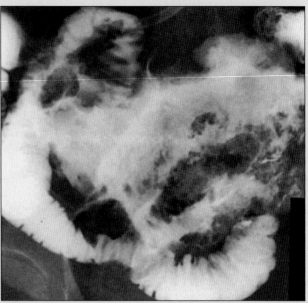

Figure 2.   **Cavitary non-Hodgkin lymphoma in an elderly woman with abdominal pain and weight loss for 5 months.** Spot image from enteroclysis examination shows a large barium-, air-, and debris-filled cavity occupying the mesenteric border of several small bowel loops. *(From Fishman EK, Kuhlman JE, Jones RC: CT of lymphoma: Spectrum of disease.* RadioGraphics *11:647-669, 1991.)*

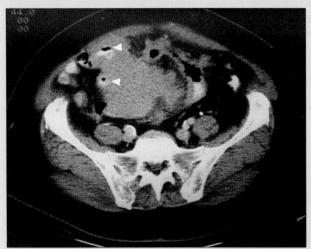

Figure 3.   **Mesenteric nodal form of non-Hodgkin lymphoma in a 71-year-old man.** CT shows a large mesenteric mass displacing and compressing loops of ileum. Two segments of small bowel *(arrowheads)* are surrounded by the nodal mass, producing a typical *sandwich* appearance.

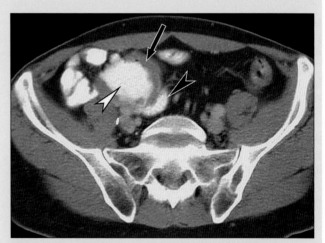

Figure 4.   **Non-Hodgkin lymphoma causing aneurysmal dilation in a 64-year-old man with night sweats and weight loss.** CT shows a small bowel mass *(arrow)* with a markedly dilated lumen *(white arrowhead)*. The bowel serosa or lymphomatous mass itself surrounds the distended lumen, differentiating this from the cavitary form of lymphoma. Note nondilated small bowel *(black arrowhead)* more proximally.

- Stage IV: widespread organ dissemination
- Gastrointestinal lymphomas are classified as infiltrating, cavitary, aneurysmal (saccular), nodular, and mesenteric nodal forms.

INCIDENCE/PREVALENCE AND EPIDEMIOLOGY

- Primary gastrointestinal lymphoma involves the stomach (40%-75%), small intestine (20%-40%), ileocecal region (10%-20%), colon (10%-15%), and esophagus (less than 1%).
- Small bowel lesion may be primary or secondary.
- Gross or microscopic evidence of gastrointestinal involvement has been found at autopsy in approximately 50% of cases of disseminated lymphoma.

- Infiltrating form is most frequent, followed by cavitary form.

Suggested Readings

Chou CK, Chen LT, Sheu RS, et al: MRI manifestations of gastrointestinal lymphoma. *Abdom Imaging* 19:495-500, 1994.

Fishman EK, Kuhlman JE, Jones RJ: CT of lymphoma: Spectrum of disease. *RadioGraphics* 11:647-669, 1991.

Goerg C, Schwerk WB, Goerg K: Gastrointestinal lymphoma: Sonographic findings in 54 patients. *AJR Am J Roentgenol* 155: 795-798, 1990.

Kumar R, Xiu Y, Potenta S, et al: F-FDG PET for evaluation of the treatment response in patients with gastrointestinal tract lymphomas. *J Nucl Med* 45:1796-1803, 2004.

Rubesin SE, Gilchrist AM, Bronner M, et al: Non-Hodgkin lymphoma of the small intestine. *RadioGraphics* 10:985-998, 1990.

Metastases to the Small Bowel

DEFINITION: Secondary lesion from hematogenous, intraperitoneal, or direct spread of a primary malignancy.

ANATOMIC FINDINGS

Small Bowel
- Hematogenous metastases are usually on the antimesenteric border of the bowel.
- Lymph node metastases from left-sided colon carcinoma can invade the proximal jejunum near the ligament of Treitz.
- Residual tumor after resection of a cecal carcinoma or gynecologic malignancy can involve the distal ileum.

Mesentery of the Small Intestine
- Intraperitoneal metastases usually involve the small bowel mesentery near the ileocecal valve.

IMAGING

Radiography
Findings
- Smoothly rounded polypoid lesions of different sizes are seen on the antimesenteric border (centrally located submucosal masses) of the bowel.
- *Target* or *bull's-eye* lesions are seen.
- Spokewheel pattern of fissuring is seen extending from the edge of the central ulcer to the periphery of the mass.
- Large melanoma deposits may grow through the small bowel wall and cavitate, simulating aneurysmal dilation.
- Desmoplasia with bowel obstruction is more often seen with metastases from lung cancer.

Utility
- Intestinal obstruction is rare unless an associated intussusception is present.
- Barium studies are not sensitive for identifying the number and location of metastases from metastatic melanoma to the small bowel.
- Nodules with central ulcers (bull's-eye lesions) occur less often in the mesenteric small intestine than in the stomach.

CT
Findings
- Rounded, nodular defects or focal enhancement of the bowel wall are characteristic of metastases.

DIAGNOSTIC PEARLS
- Rounded, nodular defects or focal enhancement of the bowel wall
- Bull's-eye on CT and spokewheel pattern on barium studies
- Smoothly rounded polypoid lesions of different sizes on the antimesenteric border of the bowel

- Smoothly rounded polypoid lesions of different sizes are seen on the antimesenteric border of the bowel.
- Large melanoma deposits may grow through the small bowel wall and cavitate, simulating aneurysmal dilation.
- Desmoplasia with bowel obstruction is more often seen with metastases from lung cancer.

Utility
- CT is the most common technique for detecting intraperitoneally seeded metastases.
- Sensitivity is improved by optimizing distention of the bowel lumen (CT enteroclysis).
- Irregular wall thickening of pelvic small bowel loops with normal thickness of abdominal bowel loops is likely radiation enteropathy.
- Sharp zone of transition (often adjacent to the anterior parietal peritoneum) indicates adhesions.
- CT is not sensitive in identifying the number and location of metastases from metastatic melanoma to the small bowel.

CLINICAL PRESENTATION
- Patients with hematogenous metastases usually exhibit gastrointestinal bleeding and generalized deterioration rather than intestinal obstruction.
- Clinical features of primary tumor usually overshadow symptoms caused by metastases.

DIFFERENTIAL DIAGNOSIS
- Lymphoma (small bowel)
- Kaposi sarcoma (small bowel)
- Carcinoid (small bowel)

WHAT THE REFERRING PHYSICIAN NEEDS TO KNOW
- Metastases from breast cancer or melanoma may be detected many years after diagnosis and treatment of the original tumor.
- No lag time exists with carcinoma of the lung.
- Optimal CT technique includes the use of neutral oral and intravenous contrast media and isotropic imaging with high-quality nonaxial reformats.
- Imaging is required to assess tumor extent and response to therapy.

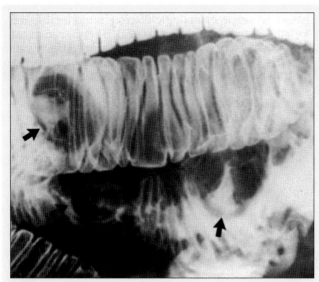

Figure 1. **A 65-year-old man with a history of malignant melanoma.** At least two bull's-eye lesions *(arrows)* are present in the jejunum. Note the large size of the ulcers. *(From Herlinger H, Maglinte D [eds]:* Clinical Radiology of the Small Intestine. *Philadelphia, WB Saunders, 1989.)*

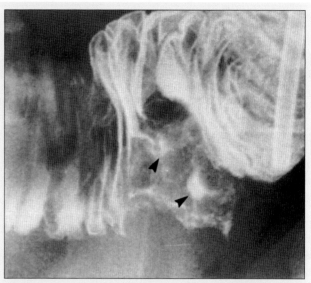

Figure 2. **A 65-year-old man with a history of malignant melanoma.** A larger polypoid metastasis with radiating linear ulcerations *(arrowheads)* produces the typical spokewheel pattern of metastases from malignant melanoma. Note how no evidence of small-bowel obstruction is seen. *(From Herlinger H, Maglinte D [eds]:* Clinical Radiology of the Small Intestine. *Philadelphia, WB Saunders, 1989.)*

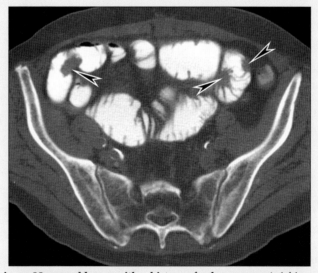

Figure 3. **Small-bowel obstruction in an 80-year-old man with a history of colon cancer.** Axial image from positive-contrast CT enteroclysis shows multiple masses *(arrowheads)* in the small bowel wall compatible with serosal metastases as the cause of this patient's small-bowel obstruction.

PATHOLOGY

- Pathways of spread include intraperitoneal seeding, hematogenous dissemination, and extension from an adjacent tumor.
- Etiology of small bowel obstruction after therapy for abdominal malignancy includes adhesions, metastases, and radiation enteropathy.
- Hematogenous metastases to the small bowel are most commonly from malignant melanoma, breast cancer, and lung cancer.

Suggested Readings

Bender GN, Maglinte DD, McLarney JH, et al: Malignant melanoma: Patterns of metastasis to the small bowel, reliability of imaging studies, and clinical relevance. *Am J Gastroenterol* 96:2392-2400, 2001.

Oliphant M, Berne AS, Meyers MA: Imaging the direct bidirectional spread of disease between the abdomen and the female pelvis via the subperitoneal space. *Gastrointest Radiol* 3:285-298, 1988.

Part 26

VASCULAR DISORDERS OF THE SMALL INTESTINE

Vasculitis

DEFINITION: Inflammation and necrosis of blood vessels.

IMAGING

Radiography
Findings
- Thickened, straight folds in segmental distribution

CT
Findings
- Polyarteritis nodosa: mural thickening of superior mesenteric artery
- Systemic lupus erythematosus: small bowel ischemia with bowel wall thickening, edema, intramural hemorrhage, pneumatosis, and mesenteric venous gas
- Henoch-Schönlein syndrome: wall thickening, luminal narrowing, fold thickening, target sign, and ulceration

Utility
- CT angiography
- CT directly visualizes mural changes.
- Three-dimensional imaging of mesenteric vessels may also be useful for detection of thrombus in mesenteric vessels.

Angiography
Findings
- Wall of superior mesenteric artery (SMA) appears thickened, similar in appearance to atherosclerotic disease.
- Significant stenosis of SMA can occur along with poststenotic dilation, aneurysm, and, in severe cases, occlusion with collateral vessel formation.
- Demonstration of aneurysm

CLINICAL PRESENTATION

- Takayasu arteritis: abdominal pain, gastrointestinal bleeding, and obstructive symptoms
- Polyarteritis nodosa: abdominal pain caused by ischemia
- Henoch-Schönlein purpura: petechial rash with purpura, often on the lower extremities

DIAGNOSTIC PEARLS

- Mural thickening or stenosis of SMA on angiography
- Small bowel fold thickening on barium studies
- Small bowel wall thickening on CT

DIFFERENTIAL DIAGNOSIS

- Ischemia (small bowel)
- Radiation enteritis (small bowel)
- Hemorrhage (small bowel)
- Eosinophilic enteritis (small bowel)

PATHOLOGY

- Vasculitis is a general term used for a group of diseases that result in inflammation and necrosis of blood vessels.
- Vasculitis is classified according to size of affected blood vessels.
- Large-vessel vasculitis affects the aorta and its major branches; includes giant cell arteritis and Takayasu arteritis.
- Medium-vessel vasculitis involves the visceral arteries and their branches; includes polyarteritis nodosa and Kawasaki disease.
- Small-vessel vasculitis affects the arterioles, venules, and capillaries; includes Wegener granulomatosis, Henoch-Schönlein purpura, systemic lupus erythematosus, and Behçet disease.

INCIDENCE/PREVALENCE AND EPIDEMIOLOGY

- Women are affected 10 times more often than men by Takayasu arteritis.
- Small bowel and mesenteric vessels are involved in more than 50% of patients with polyarteritis nodosa.

WHAT THE REFERRING PHYSICIAN NEEDS TO KNOW

- Intestinal Behçet disease can mimic Crohn disease on barium studies and CT, with inflammatory changes most pronounced in the ileum.
- Polypoid lesions are more common in patients without complications, whereas bowel wall thickening is more common in patients with complications.
- Severe mesenteric infiltration is more common in patients with complications such as peritonitis or perforation.

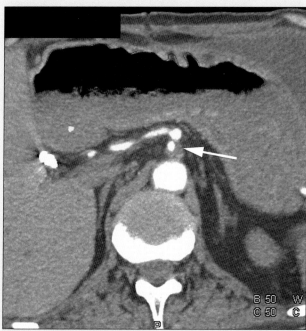

Figure 1. Patient with abdominal pain and polyarteritis nodosa. Axial contrast-enhanced CT demonstrates mural thickening of the SMA *(arrow)* in a patient with polyarteritis nodosa.

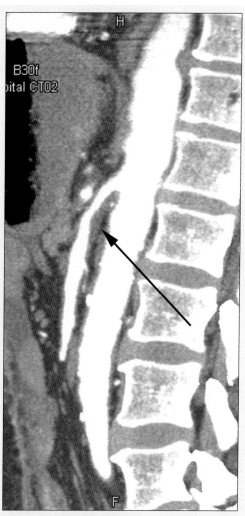

Figure 2. Patient with abdominal pain and polyarteritis nodosa. Sagittal multiplanar reconstruction image demonstrates mural thickening *(arrow)* of the proximal portion of the SMA, a classic finding in polyarteritis nodosa.

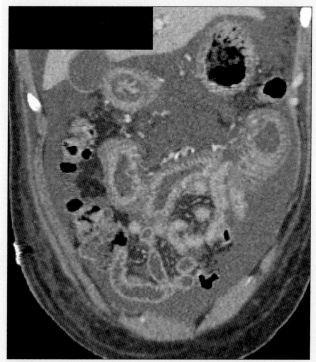

Figure 3. A 32-year-old woman with systemic lupus erythematosus, abdominal pain, and elevated lactic acid level. Coronal contrast-enhanced multiplanar CT reconstruction image shows moderate ascites. The small bowel in the mid abdomen and left upper quadrant is thickened. Mucosal hyperemia is seen, and low density is seen in the submucosa.

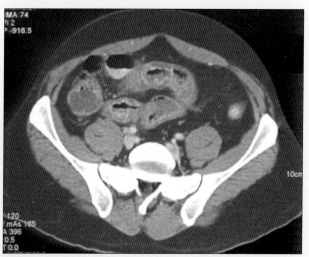

Figure 4. Henoch-Schönlein purpura. Contrast-enhanced CT demonstrates moderate small bowel thickening with submucosal edema, producing a target appearance. This patient had pathologically proven Henoch-Schönlein purpura.

- Henoch-Schönlein purpura is a small-vessel vasculitis most commonly affecting children; involvement of gastrointestinal tract occurs in up to 60% of adults.
- Patients with lupus have antiphospholipid syndrome and are at risk for development of mesenteric arterial or venous thrombosis in 27%-42% of cases.
- Behçet disease usually affects boys and men between 10 and 30 years of age.

Suggested Readings

Andrews P, Frampton G, Cameron J: Antiphospholipid syndrome and systemic lupus erythematosus. *Lancet* 342:988-989, 1993.

Bassel K, Harford W: Gastrointestinal manifestation of collagen vascular disease. *Semin Gastrointest Dis* 6:228-240, 1995.

Espinosa G, Cervera R, Font J, Shoenfeld Y: Antiphospholipid syndrome: Pathogenic mechanisms. *Autoimmune Rev* 2:677-696, 2003.

Ha H, Lee S, Rha S, et al: Radiologic features of vasculitis involving the gastrointestinal tract. *RadioGraphics* 20:779-794, 2000.

Ha H, Lee H, Yang S, et al: Intestinal Behçet syndrome: CT features of patients with and without complications. *Radiology* 209:449-454, 1998.

Jeong Y, Ha H, Yoon C, et al: Gastrointestinal involvement in Henoch-Schönlein syndrome: CT findings. *AJR Am J Roentgenol* 168:965-968, 1997.

Kato T, Fujii K, Ishii E, et al: A case of polyarteritis nodosa with lesions of the superior mesenteric artery illustrating the diagnostic usefulness of three-dimensional computed tomographic angiography. *Clin Rheumatol* 24:628-631, 2005.

Lalani T, Kanne J, Hatfield G, Chen P: Imaging findings in systemic lupus erythematosus. *RadioGraphics* 24:1069-1086, 2004.

Levine S, Hellman D, Stone J: Gastrointestinal involvement in polyarteritis nodosa (1986–2000): Presentation and outcomes in 24 patients. *Am J Med* 112:386-391, 2002.

Mills J, Michel B, Bloch D, et al: The American College of Rheumatology 1990 criteria for the classification of Henoch-Schönlein purpura. *Arth Rheum* 33:1114-1121, 1990.

Siskind B, Burrell M, Pun H, et al: CT demonstration of gastrointestinal involvement in Henoch-Schönlein syndrome. *Gastrointest Radiol* 10:352-354, 1985.

Trauma

DEFINITION: Bowel and mesenteric injury after significant blunt abdominal trauma.

ANATOMIC FINDINGS

Small Intestine
- Wall thickening with adjacent foci of free intraperitoneal air

IMAGING

Radiography
Findings
- Any fluid or increased density in the mesentery must be viewed with suspicion even in the absence of pneumoperitoneum.
- Small bowel wall thickening with adjacent foci of free intraperitoneal air

PATHOLOGY

- Some patient's have small bowel and mesenteric injury after significant blunt-force abdominal trauma.
- Mesenteric border of small bowel is more vulnerable to vascular tears and mesenteric hematomas.

DIAGNOSTIC PEARLS

- Fluid or increased density in the mesentery
- Antimesenteric border of small bowel is more likely to perforate.
- Mesenteric border of small bowel is more likely to develop hematomas.

- Antimesenteric border of small bowel is more likely to perforate.
- Mesenteric injuries are notoriously difficult to detect.

INCIDENCE/PREVALENCE AND EPIDEMIOLOGY

- Mesenteric injuries are found in 5% of patients undergoing laparotomy after significant blunt abdominal trauma.

Suggested Readings

Corbetti F, Vigo M, Bulzacchi A, et al: CT diagnosis of spontaneous dissection of the superior mesenteric artery. *J Comput Assist Tomogr* 13:965-967, 1989.
Nghiem H, Jeffrey R, Mindelzun R: CT of blunt trauma to the bowel and mesentery. *AJR Am J Roentgenol* 160:53-58, 1993.

WHAT THE REFERRING PHYSICIAN NEEDS TO KNOW
- Mesenteric injuries are difficult to detect.
- Any fluid or increased density in the mesentery must be viewed with suspicion even in the absence of pneumoperitoneum.

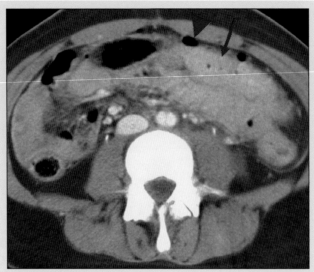

Figure 1. Small bowel wall thickening with adjacent gas. A 16-year-old girl was evaluated after a high-speed motor-vehicle collision and partial ejection from vehicle. CT scan shows small bowel wall thickening *(arrow)* with adjacent foci of free intraperitoneal air *(arrowhead)*. A transmural jejunal injury 30 cm distal to the ligament of Treitz was found at laparotomy.

Radiation Enteritis

DEFINITION: Inflammation, immobility, and adhesions of the intestine secondary to radiation therapy.

IMAGING

Radiography
Findings
- Thickening of small bowel folds as well as mucosal ulceration
- Intramural hemorrhage or edema
- Stenosis, adhesions, or fistulas
- *Ribbon* or *toothpaste* bowel

Utility
- Barium studies
- Enteroclysis
- Helps confirm the diagnosis and determine the severity and extent of small bowel involvement

CT
Findings
- Thickening of small bowel folds and wall, as well as mucosal ulceration
- Intramural hemorrhage or edema
- Stenosis, adhesions, or fistulas
- *Ribbon* or *toothpaste* bowel

Utility
- Helps confirm the diagnosis and determine the severity and extent of small bowel involvement

CLINICAL PRESENTATION

- Pain, diarrhea, and bleeding during or shortly after radiation therapy
- Chronic radiation injury: abdominal pain, small bowel obstruction, and malabsorption, which can develop as long as 25 years after therapy

DIFFERENTIAL DIAGNOSIS

- Ischemia (small bowel)
- Vasculitis (small bowel)

DIAGNOSTIC PEARLS

- Thickening of small bowel fold and wall as well as mucosal ulceration
- *Ribbon* or *toothpaste* bowel
- Stenosis, adhesions, or fistulas

- Hemorrhage (small bowel)
- Eosinophilic enteritis (small bowel)

PATHOLOGY

- Patients with previous intra-abdominal surgery or peritonitis are more susceptible because of immobility of the small intestine caused by adhesions.
- Patients with diabetes or atherosclerotic disease are at increased risk for radiation enteropathy, given that radiation causes endarteritis and, ultimately, fibrosis.

INCIDENCE/PREVALENCE AND EPIDEMIOLOGY

- Small intestine is the most common site of injury in patients receiving high doses of radiation over a relatively short period.
- Patients with diabetes or atherosclerotic disease are at increased risk for radiation enteropathy.

Suggested Readings

Fujimoto T, Fukuda T, Uetani M, et al: Helical CT signs in the diagnosis of intestinal ischemia in small bowel obstruction. *AJR Am J Roentgenol* 176:1167-1171, 2000.

Horton K, Corl F, Fishman E: CT of nonneoplastic diseases of the small bowel: Spectrum of disease. *J Comput Assist Tomogr* 23: 417-428, 1999.

Okino Y, Kiyosue H, Mori H, et al: Root of the small-bowel mesentery: Correlative anatomy and CT features of pathologic conditions. *RadioGraphics* 21:1475-1490, 2001.

WHAT THE REFERRING PHYSICIAN NEEDS TO KNOW

- Diagnosis is usually made clinically.
- Small bowel follow-through, enteroclysis, and CT can help confirm the diagnosis and determine the severity and extent of small bowel involvement.

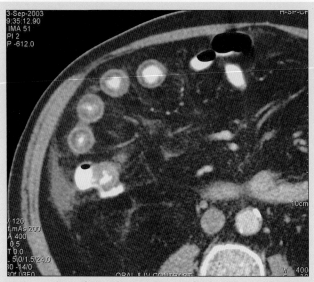

Figure 1. **Axial contrast-enhanced CT in a patient after radiation therapy for lymphoma shows moderate thickening of several small bowel loops in the right abdomen, compatible with radiation enteritis.** Minimal mesenteric stranding and ascites are seen.

Splanchnic Artery Aneurysm

DEFINITION: Aneurysmal dilation of the splanchnic arteries.

IMAGING

CT
Findings
- Aneurysm

Utility
- Contrast-enhanced CT is the most sensitive means of establishing the diagnosis.

MRI
Findings
- Aneurysm

Utility
- Contrast-enhanced MRI is more accurate than ultrasound in showing the full extent of these aneurysms.

Ultrasound
Findings
- Aneurysm

Utility
- Because of bowel gas and fat, ultrasound may not show the full extent of these aneurysms.

CLINICAL PRESENTATION

- Most patients with splanchnic artery aneurysms are asymptomatic, and the diagnosis is usually made incidentally.
- These aneurysms can rupture, causing abdominal pain and bleeding.
- Seventy-five percent of patients with celiac artery aneurysms will have symptoms, typically pain.

PATHOLOGY

- Splanchnic artery aneurysms are rare.
- Splenic artery is the most commonly involved, as well as the hepatic artery, superior mesenteric artery (SMA), celiac artery, pancreatic arteries, and gastroduodenal artery.

DIAGNOSTIC PEARLS

- Aneurysmal dilation of the celiac axis is seen.
- Dilation begins approximately 1.5 cm distal to the origin of the celiac axis.

- Most common location for SMA aneurysm is within first 5 cm of its origin.
- SMA aneurysm: Most common causes are endocarditis, atherosclerosis, and pancreatitis.
- Complications include thrombosis, ischemia, and rupture and carry high mortality rates.
- Celiac artery aneurysms: Most common cause is atherosclerosis, and most aneurysms develop at or near the vessel origin.

INCIDENCE/PREVALENCE AND EPIDEMIOLOGY

- Routine autopsy shows a 0.01%-0.25% incidence.
- Celiac artery aneurysms occur more often in men, and 75% will have symptoms.
- Risk of rupture is 13%, with a 100% mortality rate when rupture occurs.

Suggested Readings

Messina L, Shanley C: Visceral artery aneurysms. *Surg Clin North Am* 77:425-442, 1997.

Pilleul F, Beuf O: Diagnosis of splanchnic artery aneurysms and pseudoaneurysms, with special reference to contrast enhanced 3D magnetic angiography: A review. *Acta Radiol* 45:702-708, 2004.

Rokke O, Sondenaa K, Amundsen S, et al: The diagnosis and management of splanchnic artery aneurysms. *Scand J Gastroenterol* 1:737-743, 1996.

Shanley C, Shah N: Uncommon splanchnic artery aneurysms: Splenic, hepatic and celiac. *Ann Vasc Surg* 10:506-515, 1996.

Stanley J, Thompson N, Fry W: Splanchnic artery aneurysms. *Arch Surg* 101:689-697, 1970.

WHAT THE REFERRING PHYSICIAN NEEDS TO KNOW

- Patients are usually asymptomatic, and the diagnosis is usually made incidentally.

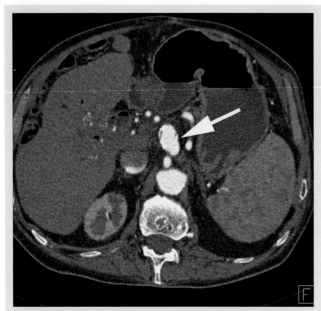

Figure 1. Celiac axis aneurysm. Axial contrast-enhanced CT in the arterial phase shows an aneurysm *(arrow)* of the celiac axis.

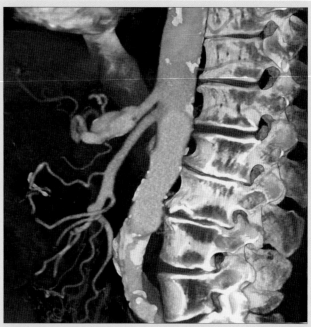

Figure 2. Celiac axis aneurysm. Volume-rendered CT angiogram nicely demonstrates the complex shape of the celiac axis aneurysm, which begins approximately 1.5 cm distal to the origin.

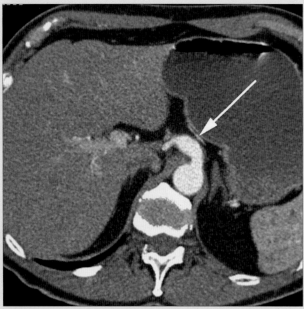

Figure 3. Celiac artery aneurysm. Aneurysmal dilation of the celiac axis *(arrow)* is identified on the axial axis image.

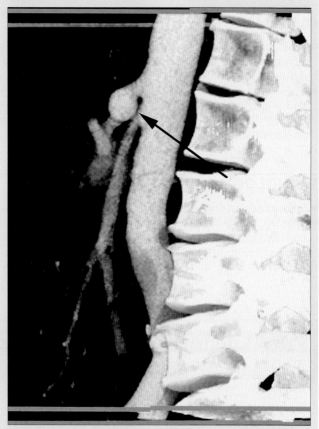

Figure 4. Celiac artery aneurysm. Aneurysmal dilation of the celiac axis *(arrow)* is identified on the sagittal axis image.

Median Arcuate Ligament Syndrome

DEFINITION: Low insertion of the ligament across the origin of the celiac axis that causes gastrointestinal symptoms.

IMAGING

CT Angiography
Findings
- *Hooked* appearance is seen; low insertion of the median arcuate ligament results in a characteristic impression on the proximal celiac axis.
- Poststenotic dilation and collateral flow from the superior mesenteric artery through the gastroduodenal and peripancreatic arteries is seen when compression is hemodynamically significant.

Utility
- The most sensitive means of establishing the diagnosis

Ultrasound
Findings
- Doppler ultrasound will show the stenosis and provide velocity of flow in the region of poststenotic dilation.

Utility
- Doppler can assess the degree of celiac artery stenosis.

MR Angiography
Findings
- *Hooked* appearance is seen; low insertion of the median arcuate ligament results in a characteristic impression on the proximal celiac axis.
- Poststenotic dilation and collateral flow from the superior mesenteric artery through the gastroduodenal and peripancreatic arteries is seen when compression is hemodynamically significant.

CLINICAL PRESENTATION

- Patient exhibits symptoms similar to those of chronic mesenteric ischemia and abdominal pain associated with meals and weight loss.
- Pain is a result of compromised blood flow or celiac plexus compression.

DIFFERENTIAL DIAGNOSIS

- Celiac artery embolism
- Celiac artery thrombus

DIAGNOSTIC PEARLS

- Impression on the proximal celiac axis, *hooked* appearance
- Low insertion across the origin of the celiac axis
- Collateral flow to the celiac artery from the superior mesenteric artery

PATHOLOGY

- Ligament has low insertion across the origin of the celiac axis.
- Compression can be hemodynamically significant, resulting in collateral flow to the celiac artery from the superior mesenteric artery.

INCIDENCE/PREVALENCE AND EPIDEMIOLOGY

- In 10%-24% of people, the ligament has a low insertion across the origin of the celiac axis.

Suggested Readings

Cognet F, Salem D, Dranssart M, et al: Chronic mesenteric ischemia: Imaging and percutaneous treatment. *RadioGraphics* 22:863-879, 2002.

Horton K, Talamini M, Fishman E: Median arcuate ligament syndrome: Evaluation with CT angiography. *RadioGraphics* 25:1177-1182, 2005.

Linder H, Kemprud E: A clinicoanatomic study of the arcuate ligament of the diaphragm. *Arch Surg* 103:600-605, 1971.

Matsumoto A, Tegtmeyer C, Fitzcharles E, et al: Percutaneous transluminal angioplasty of visceral arterial stenosis: Results and long term clinical follow-up. *J Vasc Interv Radiol* 6:165-174, 1995.

Nyman O, Ivancey K, Lindle M, Uher P: Endovascular treatment of chronic mesenteric ischemia: Report of five cases. *Cardiovasc Intervent Radiol* 31:305-313, 1998.

Roayaie S, Jossart G, Gitlitz D, et al: Laparoscopic release of celiac artery compression syndrome facilitated by laparoscopic ultrasound scanning to confirm restoration of blood flow. *J Vasc Surg* 32:814-817, 2000.

WHAT THE REFERRING PHYSICIAN NEEDS TO KNOW

- Diagnosis is typically made with catheter angiography but has also been reported with MRI, ultrasonography, and CT.
- Percutaneous transluminal angioplasty or stent placement may be required to relieve pain.

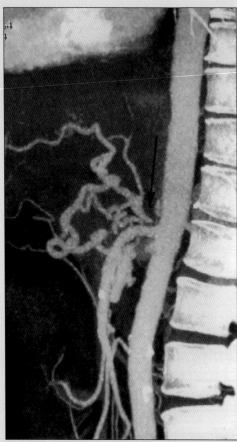

Figure 1. **Median arcuate ligament syndrome.** Sagittal contrast-enhanced multiplanar reconstruction image shows the *hooked* appearance *(arrow)* of the proximal celiac axis, which is narrowed.

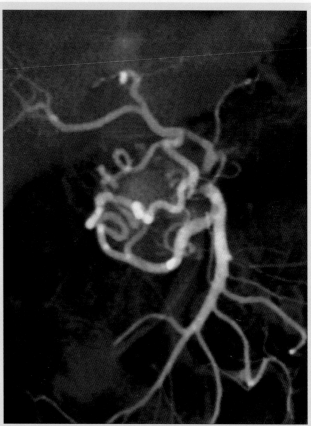

Figure 2. **Median arcuate ligament syndrome.** Coronal three-dimensional CT angiogram shows enlarged and dilated collateral supplying the celiac artery from the superior mesenteric artery.

Enterectomy and Anastomosis

DEFINITION: Resection of the small bowel and reattachment to a distant segment.

INDICATIONS

- Performed for a variety of conditions, including neoplasms of small intestine
- Extensive resection of small bowel performed in adults with infarction, strangulated internal hernias, volvulus, Crohn disease, or intestinal trauma
- Extensive resection of small bowel performed in children with necrotizing enterocolitis, intestinal atresia, or gastroschisis

ANATOMY AND APPROACH

- When minimal disparity exists in the luminal size between the proximal and distal loops, end-to-end anastomosis is the preferred technique for reestablishing continuity of small bowel.
- Side-to-side anastomosis in close proximity to the closed ends is another technique for producing functional end-to-end anastomosis.
- End-to-side anastomosis is used to compensate for disproportionate proximal and distal luminal sizes.
- Side-to-side anastomosis is also used to bypass intestinal obstruction (e.g., extensive neoplastic disease of small bowel).

TECHNIQUE

- When end-to-side anastomosis is performed, the end of the proximal intestinal lumen is anastomosed to the side of the distal lumen.

OUTCOMES

- Intestinal perforation from anastomotic dehiscence may be recognized by the presence of free intraperitoneal air on abdominal radiographs.
- Water-soluble contrast studies or CT may be performed to demonstrate anastomotic leaks.

- Extraintestinal fluid collections are suggestive of anastomotic disruption on CT; extravasation of enteric contrast is diagnostic of this complication.
- Blind pouch is suggested by a fluid-filled soft-tissue mass or gas-filled structure of variable size and shape.
- Small bowel contrast studies, particularly enteroclysis and CT enteroclysis, should demonstrate the pouch and its anastomotic relationships.
- Blind intestinal pouch may be recognized on CT as a distinct saccular enteric structure with surgical clips abutting this structure.

COMPLICATIONS

- Intestinal obstruction related to the development of strictures or kinking at anastomotic site is uncommon.
- Dehiscence of small bowel anastomoses may lead to anastomotic leaks.
- Blind intestinal pouch dilation of blind-ending segments usually develops 5-15 years after surgery.
- Postoperative blind pouch may cause inflammation, ulceration, gastrointestinal bleeding, and blind pouch syndrome with stasis, bacterial overgrowth, and diarrhea.
- Short-bowel syndrome may occur.
- Localized perianastomotic inflammatory process or phlegmon may develop, causing partial small bowel obstruction.

Suggested Readings

Lappas JC, Maglinte DDT: Radiological approach to investigation of the small intestine. In Gourtsoyiannis N (ed): *Medical Radiology: Diagnostic Imaging and Radiological Imaging of the Small Intestine*. New York, Springer-Verlag, 2002, pp 447-463.

Lui KIM, Walker FW: Surgical procedures on the small intestine. In Zuidema GD (ed): *Surgery of the Alimentary Tract*, 4th ed. Philadelphia, WB Saunders, 1996, pp 267-288.

Maglinte DDT, Bender GN, Heitkamp DE, et al: Multidetector-row helical CT enteroclysis. *Radiol Clin North Am* 41:249-262, 2003.

Maglinte DDT, Lappas JC, Heitkamp DE, et al: Technical refinements in enteroclysis. *Radiol Clin North Am* 41:213-229, 2003.

WHAT THE REFERRING PHYSICIAN NEEDS TO KNOW

- When disparity in luminal size between loops is minimal, end-to-end anastomosis is the preferred technique for reestablishing continuity of the small bowel.

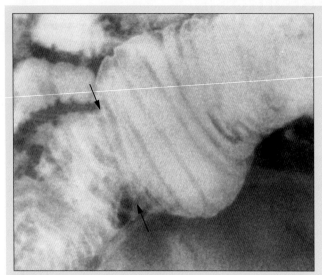

Figure 1. Jejunal end-to-end anastomosis. Luminal distention achieved by enteroclysis infusion facilitates accurate delineation of a normal anastomosis *(arrows)*.

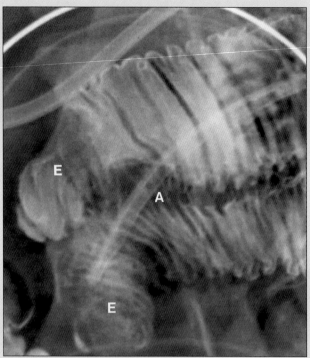

Figure 2. Intestinal anastomoses. Functional end-to-end jejunal anastomosis (created by an anatomic side-to-side technique) is shown on enteroclysis with short oversewn ends (E) in close proximity to a broad anastomotic lumen (A) traversed by the catheter. (*From Lappas JC, Maglinte DDT: Imaging of the postsurgical small bowel.* Radiol Clin North Am *41:305-326, 2003.*)

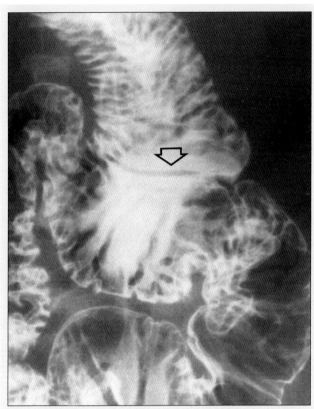

Figure 3. Intestinal anastomoses. End-to-side anastomosis *(arrow)*. (*From Lappas JC, Maglinte DDT: Imaging of the postsurgical small bowel.* Radiol Clin North Am *41:305-326, 2003.*)

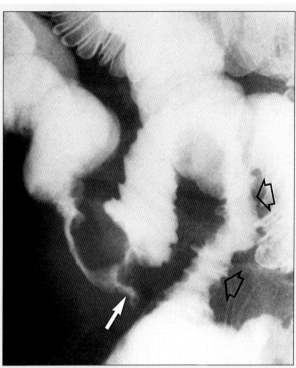

Figure 4. Perianastomotic phlegmon with intestinal narrowing. Symptoms of obstruction developed in this patient shortly after a segmental ileal resection with an end-to-end anastomosis had been performed for benign disease. Enteroclysis shows a short segment of luminal narrowing with a tiny leak *(closed arrow)* and thickened folds *(open arrows)* in the adjacent ileal loop. At surgery, ischemic dehiscence of the anastomosis was associated with a localized inflammatory reaction and mural edema of the proximal small bowel segment.

Enterostomy (Jejunostomy and Ileostomy)

DEFINITION: Enterostomy refers to an intestinal opening that is surgically designed to communicate with the skin.

INDICATIONS

- Surgical feeding jejunostomies are placed in malnourished patients with a lengthy anticipated postoperative course.
- Indications include patients with upper gastrointestinal conditions—gastroparesis, malignant tumors, fistulas, or anastomotic leaks proximal to potential jejunostomy site.
- Indications include patients who are not candidates for endoscopic, fluoroscopic, or laparoscopic insertion of feeding jejunostomies or patients who have failed these approaches.
- Ileostomy is primarily used for the evacuation of intestinal contents in patients with diseases that necessitate total colectomy.
- Ileostomy is usually restricted to elderly adults or to patients with extensive Crohn proctocolitis, anal sphincter dysfunction, or reservoir failure.
- Loop (double-barrel) ileostomy is sometimes performed for temporary intestinal diversion in patients with acute intestinal obstruction or Crohn disease.
- Double-barrel ileostomy is also performed as an adjunct to complex operations requiring protection of a distal enteric anastomosis to promote healing.

ANATOMY AND APPROACH

- Enterostomy is made in segments that are sufficiently mobile to be brought in contact with the anterior abdominal wall.
- Direct intubated jejunostomies satisfy temporary nutritional requirements.
- Long-term jejunal feeding is best accomplished by a Roux-en-Y–type jejunostomy.
- Conventional ileostomy or double-barrel ileostomy may be performed, depending on indications.

TECHNIQUE

- The jejunostomy should be placed at least 70 cm distal to the duodenojejunal junction.

- Some surgeons prefer to have the jejunostomy catheter routinely injected with water-soluble contrast medium before initiating enteric feeding.
- Creation of conventional Brooke or everting end-ileostomy involves transection of the ileum.
- Mobilization of a 5-cm ileal segment through the abdominal wall defect is performed.
- Specific suturing techniques are used to allow for ileostomy maturation.

OUTCOMES

- Jejunostomy is used to provide a route for administering nutritional support.
- Conventional (end) ileostomy with total proctocolectomy provides a relatively simple and often curative surgical approach.
- Loss of fecal continence and its attendant physical and psychological problems are seen in patients with end ileostomies.

COMPLICATIONS

- Jejunostomy: complications related to catheter placement include enterogastric reflux of alimentation fluid, malpositioning of catheter and dislodgement with intra-abdominal leakage.
- Small bowel obstruction may occur at or near the jejunostomy site.
- Malfunction of the ileostomy may result from adhesions, prestomal narrowing of ileal lumen, paraileostomy hernias, and recurrent disease.
- Fascial scarring with narrowing of the prestomal segment of the ileum may cause intestinal obstruction and resulting ileostomy dysfunction.
- Parastomal hernias are relatively common.

POSTPROCEDURAL AND FOLLOW-UP CARE

- Evaluation of patients with an ileostomy and ileostomy complications can be safely performed by retrograde ileostomy examinations.

KEY POINTS

- Jejunostomy is indicated as a means of creating a route for nutritional support in patients with upper gastrointestinal abnormalities.
- Ileostomy creates a means for evacuation of the bowel in patients with colonic or anal abnormalities.

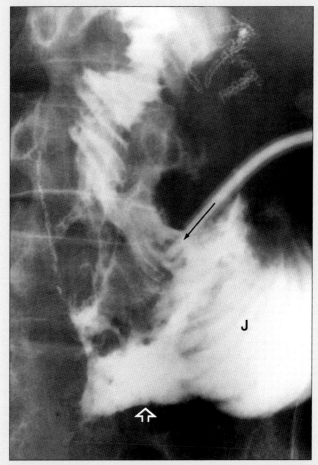

Figure 1. Jejunostomy catheter malpositioning. Injection of water-soluble contrast medium *(closed arrow)* shows incomplete purchase of the catheter within the jejunal lumen (J), resulting in tracking of contrast medium into a focal extraluminal collection *(open arrow)*. Proper positioning of the catheter may be achieved by manipulating the catheter under fluoroscopic guidance.

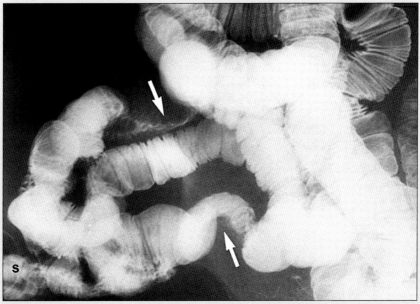

Figure 2. Parastomal ileostomy hernia. Lateral view during enteroclysis shows small bowel loops herniating through the anterior abdominal wall, with mild luminal compression *(arrows)* at the site of the abdominal wall defect. Antegrade infusion more accurately depicts the functional degree of obstruction in patients with an ileostomy. (*S*, Ileostomy stoma.)

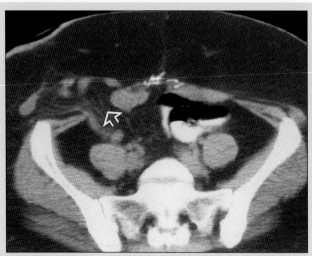

Figure 3. CT of parastomal ileostomy hernia. CT shows a large anterior abdominal wall defect *(arrow)* with herniation of small bowel loops and adjacent mesentery. This diagnosis requires careful review of several scan slices, because the herniated loops and ileostomy stoma are often in different axial scan planes.

■ In cases of partial small bowel obstruction, antegrade enteroclysis may accurately demonstrate the presence of functionally significant adhesions.

■ CT can accurately detect parastomal ileostomy hernias; a retrograde ileostomy examination may also be helpful in patients with unexplained stoma-related abdominal symptoms.

Suggested Readings

Lappas JC, Maglinte DDT: Radiological approach to investigation of the small intestine. In Gourtsoyiannis N (ed): *Medical Radiology: Diagnostic Imaging and Radiological Imaging of the Small Intestine.* New York, Springer-Verlag, 2002, pp 447–463.

Lui KIM, Walker FW: Surgical procedures on the small intestine. In Zuidema GD (ed): *Surgery of the Alimentary Tract*, 4th ed. Philadelphia, WB Saunders, 1996, pp 267–288.

Maglinte DDT, Bender GN, Heitkamp DE, et al: Multidetector-row helical CT enteroclysis. *Radiol Clin North Am* 41:249-262, 2003.

Maglinte DDT, Lappas JC, Heitkamp DE, et al: Technical refinements in enteroclysis. *Radiol Clin North Am* 41:213-229, 2003.

Ileal Reservoirs

DEFINITION: Continence-preserving surgical procedures that offer patients the advantage of improved body image and active lifestyle.

INDICATIONS

- Koch pouch construction: prior colectomy and conventional ileostomy or failed or contraindicated ileoanal pouch surgery
- Ileoanal pouches: primary colonic mucosal disease, including chronic ulcerative colitis and familial adenomatous polyposis syndrome

CONTRAINDICATIONS

- Crohn disease

ANATOMY AND APPROACH

- Koch pouch: construction of continent ileostomy reservoir
- Ileoanal pouch: creation of ileal reservoir with ileoanal anastomosis after colectomy and rectal mucosectomy
- J-pouch configuration of ileoanal pouch preferred because of simplicity of construction, adequate reservoir capacity, ease of emptying, and no potentially obstructing efferent limb

TECHNIQUE

- Koch pouch: distal 45 cm of ileum is used to construct pouch; most proximal ileal segment is fashioned into a spherical reservoir by suturing techniques.
- Suturing of pouch to anterior abdominal wall provides stability and prevents volvulus of pouch and peripouch herniation.
- Ileoanal J-pouch is constructed from distal 25 cm of ileum fashioned into a J shape.
- J-pouch is secured by side-to-side anastomosis of two adjacent loops.
- Anorectal mucosectomy and rectal transection preserves the integrity of the anal sphincter.
- Constructed ileal pouch is anastomosed to dentate line of the rectal cuff.
- Proximal diverting ileostomy is often performed.
- Extensive anastomoses in the ileoanal pouch are allowed to heal for a period of 8-12 weeks before closure of the protective diverting ileostomy.

OUTCOMES

- Ileal reservoirs are continence-preserving procedures.
- Successful construction of the Koch pouch eliminates the need for an external ileostomy appliance; the contents of the reservoir are evacuated by stomal intubation.
- Barium studies of the normal reservoir show typical small bowel fold patterns interrupted by a linear mucosal ridge representing the suture line.
- Ileoanal pouch after proctocolectomy removes the potential disease-bearing mucosa while preserving anal continence and a normal defecatory pathway.
- Normal J-pouch is depicted on contrast studies as an ovoid structure with distinctive vertical raphes corresponding to the lines of anastomosis.
- CT may reveal a thin, surgically stapled pouch wall with normal adjacent fat.

COMPLICATIONS

- Koch pouch complications include valve dysfunction, pouch ileitis, and fistulas, usually occurring months after surgery.
- Ileoanal pouch complications include pouchitis, small bowel obstruction, anastomotic dehiscence or strictures, fistulas, and pelvic abscesses.
- Ileoanal pouch failure occurs in approximately 10% of patients.
- Adhesions, volvulus, and anastomotic strictures may develop as a result of extensive surgical resection and bowel manipulations.

POSTPROCEDURAL AND FOLLOW-UP CARE

- Retrograde barium examination after cleansing irrigation of the reservoir is the recommended technique for evaluation of the Koch pouch.
- Radiography with the patient in oblique or lateral positions is required to visualize the efferent ileal segment and the ileostomy stoma adequately.
- If clinical suspicion exists of suture dehiscence postoperatively or pouch perforation after intubation, the pouch should be evaluated with a water-soluble contrast agent.

KEY POINTS

- Ileal reservoirs are indicated in patients who need to undergo a total colectomy, except for those with Crohn disease.

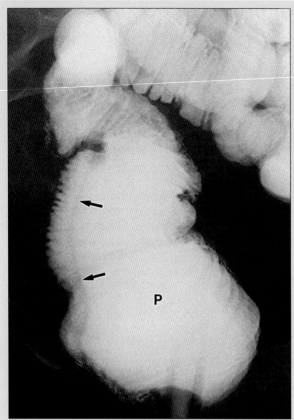

Figure 1. Ileoanal J-pouch. Normal pouchogram shows characteristic vertical raphe *(arrows)* created by the anastomotic line. (P, pouch.) *(From Lappas JC, Maglinte DDT: Imaging of the postsurgical small bowel. Radiol Clin North Am 41:305-326, 2003.)*

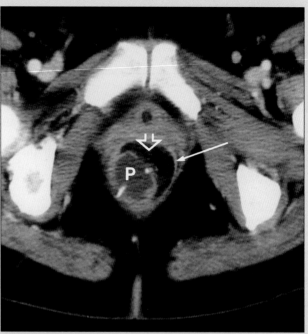

Figure 2. Ileoanal J-pouch. CT of normal pouch (P) with surrounding ileal mesentery *(open arrow)* and thin muscular anorectal wall *(closed arrow)*. *(From Lappas JC, Maglinte DDT: Imaging of the postsurgical small bowel. Radiol Clin North Am 41:305-326, 2003.)*

- Although the Koch pouch achieves reasonable functional results with long-term continence, surgical revision of the continent ileostomy is often required.
- Surveillance of the reservoir is required in patients who underwent surgery for any of the polyposis syndromes.
- Radiologic evaluation of the ileoanal reservoir is required to assess its function and to exclude anastomotic leaks or other postoperative complications.
- Water-soluble contrast agents are used for early postoperative examinations, whereas barium is used for routine evaluation of the pouch.

Suggested Readings

Lappas JC, Maglinte DDT: Radiological approach to investigation of the small intestine. In Gourtsoyiannis N (ed): *Medical Radiology: Diagnostic Imaging and Radiological Imaging of the Small Intestine.* New York, Springer-Verlag, 2002, pp 447–463.

Lui KIM, Walker FW: Surgical procedures on the small intestine. In Zuidema GD (ed): *Surgery of the Alimentary Tract,* 4th ed. Philadelphia, WB Saunders, 1996, pp 267–288.

Maglinte DDT, Bender GN, Heitkamp DE, et al: Multidetector-row helical CT enteroclysis. *Radiol Clin North Am* 41:249-262, 2003.

Maglinte DDT, Lappas JC, Heitkamp DE, et al: Technical refinements in enteroclysis. *Radiol Clin North Am* 41:213-229, 2003.

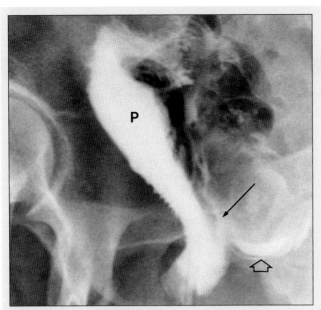

Figure 3. Peri-pouch abscess. J-pouch ileogram shows breakdown *(closed arrow)* of the ileoanal anastomosis with extravasation of water-soluble contrast medium *(open arrow)* into the pelvis. Adjacent pelvic inflammation results in narrowing and irregularity of the pouch (P). (*From Lappas JC, Maglinte DDT: Imaging of the postsurgical small bowel.* Radiol Clin North Am *41:305-326, 2003.*)

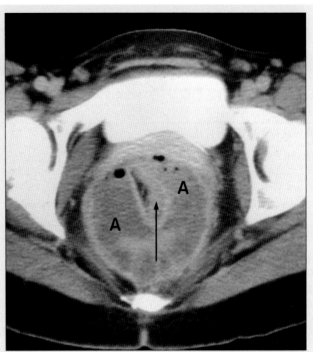

Figure 4. Peri-pouch abscess. CT shows a large multilocular abscess (A) encircling the collapsed pouch and its fat-density mesentery *(arrow)*. Note how the inflammatory process causes rectal wall thickening and stranding of the perirectal fat. (*From Lappas JC, Maglinte DDT: Imaging of the postsurgical small bowel.* Radiol Clin North Am *41:305-326, 2003.*)

Part 28

MISCELLANEOUS ABNORMALITIES OF THE SMALL BOWEL

Meckel Diverticulum

DEFINITION: Persistence of the omphalomesenteric duct at its attachment to the ileum.

ANATOMIC FINDINGS

Ileum
- Meckel diverticulum arises from the antimesenteric border of the ileum within 100 cm of the ileocecal valve.

IMAGING

Radiography and Fluoroscopy
Findings
- Abdominal radiographs occasionally may reveal radiopaque enteroliths or dilated, gas-filled diverticulum in right lower quadrant.
- Blind-ending tubular or cystic sac communicating with antimesenteric border of distal ileum is seen on barium studies.
- Triradiate fold pattern is seen at the junction of the sac with the intestinal lumen.
- Surface of diverticulum may be abnormal, containing granular mucosa, focal ulceration, or focal mound of ectopic gastric mucosa.
- Inverted Meckel diverticulum may be seen as a polypoid intraluminal mass; it may act as the lead point for a small bowel intussusception.

Utility
- Enteroclysis is the best radiologic test for detecting Meckel diverticulum in adults without gastrointestinal bleeding.

Nuclear Medicine
Findings
- Presence of ectopic gastric mucosa in patients with acute or chronic gastrointestinal bleeding

Utility
- Technetium pertechnetate scintigraphy has a sensitivity of 85% for detecting Meckel diverticulum in patients with gastrointestinal bleeding.

DIAGNOSTIC PEARLS

- Blind-ending tubular or cystic sac communicating with antimesenteric border of distal ileum
- Triradiate fold pattern at junction of sac with intestinal lumen on enteroclysis
- Presence of ectopic gastric mucosa in patients who have acute or chronic gastrointestinal bleeding on technetium pertechnetate scintigraphy

- Scintigraphy has a poor sensitivity in patients without gastrointestinal bleeding.

CT
Findings
- Cystic or tubular structure attached to small bowel in right lower quadrant

Utility
- Poor sensitivity

Ultrasound
Findings
- Cystic or tubular structure attached to small bowel in right lower quadrant

Utility
- Poor sensitivity

CLINICAL PRESENTATION

- Affected individuals may present with gastrointestinal bleeding or signs and symptoms of small bowel obstruction or perforation.
- Majority of people with this congenital anomaly never develop symptoms.

WHAT THE REFERRING PHYSICIAN NEEDS TO KNOW

- Except enteroclysis, all imaging modalities have poor sensitivity for the detection of Meckel diverticulum.
- Inverted Meckel diverticulum sometimes acts as the lead point for small bowel intussusception.
- Diverticulitis results from ulceration and focal perforation of the diverticulum caused by ectopic gastric mucosa, enterolith, or foreign-body impaction.
- Obstruction may result from intussusception, volvulus around a persistent fibrous or adhesive band, or ileal narrowing related to ulceration.
- Diverticulum may become incarcerated in an inguinal, femoral, or umbilical hernia.
- Tumors may arise in Meckel diverticulum, including carcinoid tumors, adenocarcinomas, and benign or malignant mesenchymal tumors.

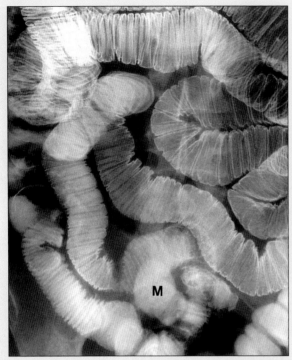

Figure 1. Meckel diverticulum. Overhead radiograph from enteroclysis shows a saccular structure (M) in a pelvic loop of ileum. Note how this portion of the bowel is blind-ending and does not contain normal folds.

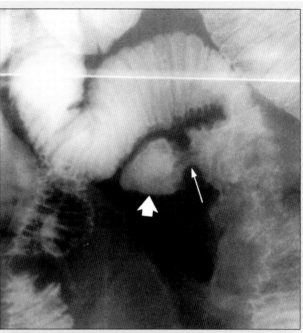

Figure 2. Meckel diverticulum. (Same patient as in Figure 1.) A spot image when the diverticulum was incompletely distended shows a triangular sac *(thick arrow)* arising from the distal ileum. Smooth folds *(thin arrow)* radiate to the origin of the diverticulum. Note how this Meckel diverticulum appears to arise from the concave border of the bowel. This image demonstrates how the concave border of a small bowel loop is not always its true mesenteric border, given that the Meckel diverticulum arises from the antimesenteric border of the ileum.

DIFFERENTIAL DIAGNOSIS

- Diverticulum (small bowel)
- Sacculation (small bowel)

PATHOLOGY

- Meckel diverticulum results from persistence of the omphalomesenteric duct at its attachment to the ileum.
- Meckel diverticulum contains all layers of the intestinal wall.
- Diverticulum usually varies from 2-15 cm in length and is approximately 2 cm in width.
- Diverticulum is lined by small bowel epithelium and often contains heterotopic gastric or pancreatic tissue or Brunner glands.
- Diverticulum may be connected to the umbilicus by a fibrous band or to other intestinal loops by congenital bands or adhesions.

INCIDENCE/PREVALENCE AND EPIDEMIOLOGY

- Meckel diverticulum is the most common congenital abnormality of the gastrointestinal tract.
- Prevalence at autopsy is 1%-4%.

Suggested Readings

Levy A, Hobbs CM: Meckel diverticulum: Radiologic features with pathologic correlation. *RadioGraphics* 24:565-587, 2004.
Mackey WC, Dineen P: A fifty-year experience with Meckel's diverticulum. *Surg Gynecol Obstet* 156:56-64, 1983.
Perlman JA, Hoover HC, Safer PK: Femoral hernia with strangulated Meckel's diverticulum (Littre's hernia). *Am J Surg* 139:286-289, 1980.
Sfakianakis GN, Conway JJ: Detection of ectopic gastric mucosa in Meckel's diverticulum and in other aberrations by scintigraphy: Indications and methods—a 10-year experience. *J Nucl Med* 22 (part I):647-654, (part II): 732-738:1981.

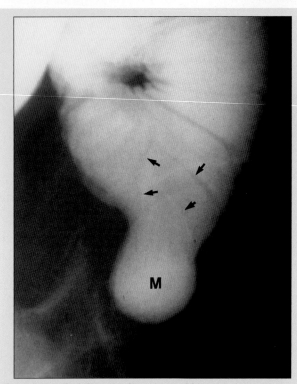

Figure 3. **Meckel diverticulum.** Steep oblique spot image shows a blind-ending saccular structure (M) arising from the antimesenteric border of the ileum. Note how folds *(arrows)* radiate to the edges of the diverticulum and its opening. *(From Herlinger H, Jones B, Jacobs JE: Miscellaneous abnormalities of the small bowel. In Gore RM, Levine MS [eds]: Textbook of Gastrointestinal Radiology. Philadelphia, WB Saunders, 2000, pp 865-883.)*

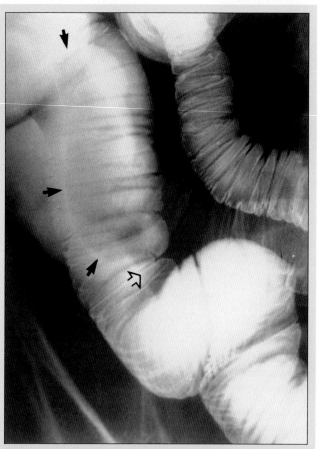

Figure 4. **Inverted Meckel diverticulum.** Enteroclysis shows a long, smooth-surfaced, polypoid intraluminal filling defect *(closed arrows)* in the distal ileum. A tubular radiolucent filling defect *(open arrow)* resembles a stalk. This inverted Meckel diverticulum can be mistaken for a pedunculated ileal polyp such as a lipoma or inflammatory fibroid polyp. *(Reprinted with permission from Rubesin SE, Herlinger H, DeGaeta L: Interlude: Test your skills. Inverted Meckel's diverticulum. Radiology 176:636 and 644, 1990.)*

Segmental Dilation

DEFINITION: Focally dilated and aperistaltic small intestinal segment.

ANATOMIC FINDINGS

Ileum
- The isolated atonic loop is usually in the distal ileum.

IMAGING

Fluoroscopy
Findings
- Focally dilated, spherical or tubular segment of distal ileum in direct contiguity with adjacent inflow and outflow loops of ileum
- Effacement or obliteration of folds in dilated loop
- Ulcerated mucosa may be present in some patients.

Utility
- Barium studies

CLINICAL PRESENTATION

- Partial small bowel obstruction (functional obstruction caused by atonic ileal segment)

DIFFERENTIAL DIAGNOSIS

- Meckel's diverticulum (small bowel)
- Lymphoma with aneurysmal dilation (small bowel)
- Crohn disease with dilated segment between two strictures (small bowel)

PATHOLOGY

- Ileal dysgenesis may be the result of congenital neuromuscular dysfunction.
- Ectopic mucosa (especially gastric mucosa) may be found in the dilated segment and may cause ulceration.

DIAGNOSTIC PEARLS

- Focally dilated, spherical or tubular segment of distal ileum in direct contiguity with the adjacent inflow and outflow loops of ileum
- Isolated atonic loop of distal ileum in most cases
- Ectopic gastric mucosa may be present with ulceration.

- Aperistaltic segment functions as a barrier to intestinal flow, resulting in partial small bowel obstruction.

INCIDENCE/PREVALENCE AND EPIDEMIOLOGY

- In children, ileal dysgenesis is associated with Meckel diverticulum and omphalocele.

Suggested Readings

Bell BR, Ternberg JL, Bower RJ: Ileal dysgenesis in infants and children. *J Pediatr Surg* 17:395-399, 1982.

Musselman JA, Ghahremai GG, Bordin GM, et al: Idiopathic localized dilatation of the ileum in adults. *Gastrointest Radiol* 6:267-268, 1981.

Ratcliffe J, Tait J, Lisle D, et al: Segmental dilatation of the small bowel: Report of three cases and literature review. *Radiology* 171:827-830, 1989.

WHAT THE REFERRING PHYSICIAN NEEDS TO KNOW

- Ulcerated mucosa may be present (rare).
- Segmental dilation is distinguished from Meckel diverticulum by direct continuity with adjacent ileal loops.
- Ileal dysgenesis is distinguished from primary small bowel lymphoma with aneurysmal dilation by the normal mucosal surface of the atonic segment.

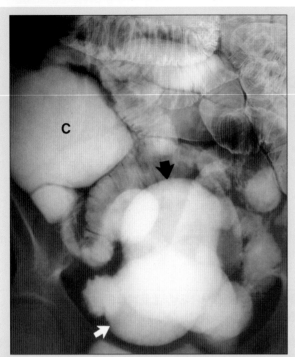

Figure 1. **Ileal dysgenesis.** Overhead radiograph from enteroclysis shows several round, focal, markedly dilated segments of pelvic ileum *(arrows)*. The cecum (C) is identified. Normal-sized ileal loops were seen entering and exiting the dilated ileum at fluoroscopy.

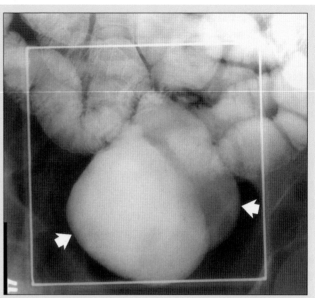

Figure 2. **Ileal dysgenesis.** Enteroclysis shows a large bilobed ileal segment *(arrows)*. Normal entry and exit loops of pelvic ileum were seen on other views.

Intestinal Malrotation

DEFINITION: Intestinal malrotation results in variations in small bowel location based on the degree of rotation of the midgut when it returns to the coelomic cavity.

ANATOMIC FINDINGS

Small Bowel
- Malrotation: The small bowel lies in the right or mid-abdomen; the duodenojejunal junction lies inferior to the duodenal bulb and to the right of the spine.
- Nonrotation: The third and fourth portions of the duodenum and duodenojejunal flexure are absent; the jejunum directly connects to the second portion of the duodenum.
- Nonrotation: The jejunum and ileum lie in the right side of the abdomen, with the terminal ileum entering the cecum from its right side.

Superior Mesenteric Vein and Artery
- In malrotation, the superior mesenteric vein lies anterior and to the left of the superior mesenteric artery.

IMAGING

Radiography
Findings
- Twisting and obstruction of the proximal small bowel manifested by duodenal dilation and slow transit on barium studies
- Malrotation: *corkscrew sign* of midgut volvulus in infants

Utility
- Barium studies

CT
Findings
- In malrotation, the superior mesenteric vein lies anterior and to the left of the superior mesenteric artery.

DIAGNOSTIC PEARLS
- Malrotation: The small bowel lies in the right or mid-abdomen; the duodenojejunal junction lies inferior to the duodenal bulb and to the right of the spine.
- Nonrotation: The third and fourth portions of the duodenum and duodenojejunal flexure are absent; the jejunum directly connects to the second portion of the duodenum.
- In malrotation, the superior mesenteric vein lies anterior to and to the left of the artery on CT.

MRI
Findings
- In malrotation, the superior mesenteric vein lies anterior to and to the left of the superior mesenteric artery.

Ultrasound
Findings
- In malrotation, the superior mesenteric vein lies anterior to and to the left of the superior mesenteric artery.

CLINICAL PRESENTATION
- Symptomatic patients are usually infants or children with high-grade obstruction caused by midgut volvulus or Ladd bands.
- Adult patients are usually asymptomatic or have vague abdominal complaints.
- Adults may occasionally complain of vomiting or abdominal pain.

WHAT THE REFERRING PHYSICIAN NEEDS TO KNOW
- Symptomatic patients with intestinal malrotation are usually infants or children with high-grade obstruction caused by midgut volvulus or Ladd's bands.
- Adults with intestinal malrotation are usually asymptomatic or have vague abdominal complaints.
- Location of the duodenojejunal junction should be ascertained in any adult who experiences vomiting or abdominal pain.
- An abnormally positioned duodenojejunal junction is important because it may cause twisting and obstruction of the proximal small bowel.

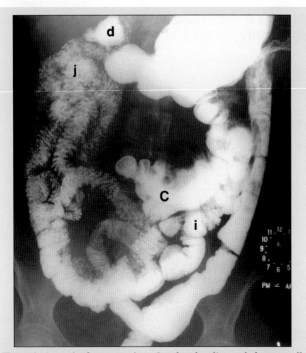

Figure 1. Intestinal nonrotation. Overhead radiograph from small bowel follow-through shows the duodenal bulb (d) in a normal location with absence of the third and fourth portions of the duodenum and absence of a duodenojejunal junction to the left of the spine. The jejunum (j) is in the right upper quadrant, and most of the ileum is also in the right abdomen, with the distal ileum (i) crossing to the left to join a midline cecum (C). The colon lies in the left abdomen.

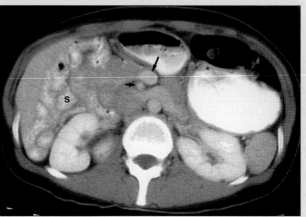

Figure 2. Intestinal malrotation. Axial CT through the tip of the liver shows that the superior mesenteric vein (*long arrow*) lies anterior and to the left of the superior mesenteric artery (*short arrow*). The jejunum (s) lies in the right upper quadrant.

DIFFERENTIAL DIAGNOSIS

■ Paraduodenal hernia
■ Floppy mesentery

PATHOLOGY

■ Intestinal malrotation encompasses different variations based on the degree of rotation of the midgut when it returns to the coelomic cavity.
■ Intestinal malrotation: The midgut fails to complete its 180-degree counterclockwise rotation.
■ Intestinal hyper-rotation: The small intestine has rotated more than the usual 180 degrees.
■ Nonrotation: Small bowel rotation has stopped at 90 degrees of counterclockwise rotation.
■ Reversed rotation: The bowel enters the abdomen via clockwise rotation.

Suggested Readings

Balthazar EJ: Intestinal malrotation in adults: Roentgenographic assessment with emphasis on isolated complete and partial nonrotations. *AJR Am J Roentgenol* 126:358-367, 1976.

Kern IB, Curie BG: The presentation of malrotation of the intestine in adults. *Ann R Coll Surg Engl* 72:239-242, 1990.

Houston CS, Wittenborg MH: Roentgen evaluation of anomalies of rotation and fixation of the bowel in children. *Radiology* 84:1-17, 1965.

Paraduodenal Hernia

DEFINITION: Paraduodenal hernias are hernias into the mesenteries of the ascending or descending colon.

ANATOMIC FINDINGS

Mesentery of the Descending Colon
- Left paraduodenal hernia is a hernia into the mesentery of the descending colon with an opening at the fossa of Landzert.
- Landzert fossa is present when the inferior mesenteric vein and ascending left colonic artery are incompletely fixed to the retroperitoneum.
- Landzert fossa is lateral to the fourth portion of the duodenum.

Mesentery of the Ascending Colon
- Right paraduodenal hernia is a hernia into the mesentery of the ascending colon through the mesentericoparietal fossa (Waldeyer fossa).
- Waldeyer fossa lies in the upper portion of the jejunal mesentery behind the superior mesenteric artery and inferior to the third portion of the duodenum.
- Waldeyer fossa orifice is bounded superiorly by the superior mesenteric artery and vein leading beneath the mesenteries of the transverse and ascending colon.

IMAGING

Radiography
Findings
- Left paraduodenal hernia: jejunal loops are clumped together in the left upper quadrant lateral to the fourth portion of the duodenum.
- Right paraduodenal hernia: jejunal loops are clumped together in the right abdomen inferior to the third portion of the duodenum.
- Focal narrowing of the inlet and outlet loops are seen at the orifice of the hernia.
- Herniated loops may be dilated with delayed emptying of barium from these loops.

Utility
- Barium studies

CT
Findings
- Left paraduodenal hernia: clustered small bowel loops are lateral to the duodenum between the adrenal gland and the transverse or descending colon.
- Right paraduodenal hernia: jejunal loops are clustered in the right side of the abdomen inferior to the duodenum.
- Right paraduodenal hernia: branches of the superior mesenteric artery and vein are whirled posteriorly and to the right behind these vessels.

MRI
Findings
- Right paraduodenal hernia: jejunal loops are clustered in the right side of the abdomen inferior to the duodenum.

DIAGNOSTIC PEARLS
- Left duodenal hernia: jejunal loops are clustered together in the left upper quadrant lateral to the fourth portion of the duodenum.
- Right duodenal hernia: jejunal loops are clustered together in the right abdomen inferior to the third portion of the duodenum.
- Focal narrowing of the inlet and outlet loops at the hernia orifice is seen.
- Herniated loops may be dilated with delayed emptying of barium.

- Right paraduodenal hernia: branches of the superior mesenteric artery and vein are whirled posteriorly and to the right behind these vessels.

CLINICAL PRESENTATION
- Small bowel obstruction

DIFFERENTIAL DIAGNOSIS
- Floppy mesentery
- Displacement of small bowel by abdominal mass
- Closed-loop small bowel obstruction secondary to adhesions or other causes
- Intestinal malrotation

PATHOLOGY
- Abnormalities of small bowel development

INCIDENCE/PREVALENCE AND EPIDEMIOLOGY
- Paraduodenal hernias are the most common internal abdominal hernias, accounting for approximately 50% of all such hernias.
- Fossa of Landzert is found in approximately 2% of patients at autopsy.
- Waldeyer fossa is found in approximately 1% of patients at autopsy.

Suggested Readings
Meyers MA: Internal abdominal hernias. In Meyers MA (ed): *Dynamic Radiology of the Abdomen*, 5th ed. New York, Springer, 2000, pp 712-728.

Olazabal A, Guasch I, Casas D: Case report: CT diagnosis of nonobstructive left paraduodenal hernia. *Clin Radiol* 46:288-289, 1992.

Parsons PB: Paradudodenal hernia. *AJR Am J Roentgenol 69*:563-589, 1953.

Suchato C, Pekanan P, Panjapiyakul C: CT findings in symptomatic left paraduodenal hernia. *Abdom Imaging* 21:148-149, 1996.

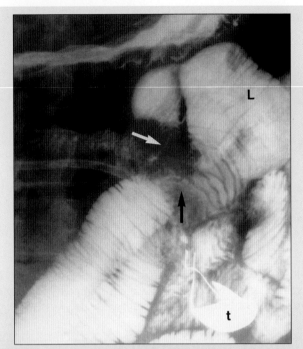

Figure 1. Left paraduodenal hernia. Coned-down image from an overhead radiograph on enteroclysis performed via a Kantor tube (t) shows a cluster of jejunal loops (L) in the left upper quadrant. These loops are extrinsically compressed *(arrows)* at the entry site to the fossa of Landzert. *(From the teaching files of Hans Herlinger, MD.)*

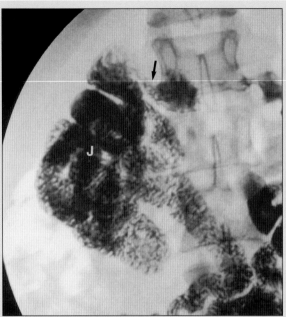

Figure 2. Right paraduodenal hernia. Low-power spot image from a small bowel follow-through shows a large cluster of jejunal loops (J) clumped together in the right upper quadrant. Note compression of one loop *(arrow)* at the inlet to the fossa of Waldeyer.

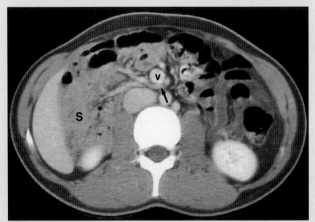

Figure 3. Right paraduodenal hernia. Axial CT through the tip of the liver shows collapsed small bowel (S) in the right upper quadrant. A tributary *(arrow)* of the superior mesenteric vein is looping behind this vein (V). *(Reprinted with permission from Herlinger H, Jones B, Jacobs JE: Miscellaneous abnormalities of the small bowel. In Gore RM, Levine MS [eds]:* Textbook of Gastrointestinal Radiology. *Philadelphia, WB Saunders, 2000, pp 865-883.)*

Endometriosis

DEFINITION: Endometrial tissue found outside the uterus.

IMAGING

Radiography
Findings
- Focal or multifocal areas of extrinsic mass effect are seen on ileal loops.
- Endometriosis is associated with spiculation of small bowel contour and tethering of mucosal folds.
- Circumferential narrowing may be present, but the mucosal folds are preserved.
- Findings can mimic those of carcinoid tumors or intraperitoneal-seeded metastases to the bowel.

Utility
- Barium studies

CT
Findings
- Findings can mimic those of carcinoid tumors or intraperitoneal-seeded metastases to the bowel.

CLINICAL PRESENTATION

- Crampy abdominal or pelvic pain
- Symptoms of intestinal obstruction
- Cyclic pain associated with menses in a minority of patients

DIFFERENTIAL DIAGNOSIS

- Carcinoid tumors (small bowel)
- Metastases (small bowel)

PATHOLOGY

- Ectopic endometrial tissue usually has a serosal or subserosal location.

DIAGNOSTIC PEARLS

- Focal or multifocal areas of extrinsic mass effect on ileal loops
- Endometriosis is associated with spiculation of small bowel contour and tethering of mucosal folds.
- Circumferential narrowing may be present, but mucosal folds are preserved.

- Ectopic endometrial tissue may burrow into the muscularis propria, submucosa, or even the mucosa.
- Ectopic endometrial tissue goes through proliferative and secretory phases of menstrual cycle, with sloughing, bleeding, and subsequent regeneration of endometrial tissue and fibrosis.

INCIDENCE/PREVALENCE AND EPIDEMIOLOGY

- Colonic involvement is found in 15%-37% of women who undergo surgery for endometriosis.
- Ileal involvement is much less frequent, found in only 1%-7% of surgical cases.
- Cyclic pain associated with menses is found in a minority of patients (14%-40%).

Suggested Readings

Aronchick CA, Brooks FP, Dyson WL, et al: Ileocecal endometriosis presenting with abdominal pain and gastrointestinal bleeding. *Dig Dis Sci* 28:566-572, 1983.

Brosens JA: Endometriosis. Current issues in diagnosis and medical management. *J Reprod Med* 43:281-286, 1998.

LiVolsi VA, Perzin KH: Endometriosis of the small intestine producing intestinal obstruction or simulating neoplasm. *Am J Dig Dis* 19:100-107, 1974.

Martinbeau PW, Pratt JH, Gaffy TA: Small bowel obstruction secondary to endometriosis. *Mayo Clin Proc* 50:239-243, 1975.

WHAT THE REFERRING PHYSICIAN NEEDS TO KNOW

- Endometriosis implants in the small bowel can mimic the findings of carcinoid tumors or intraperitoneal-seeded metastases to the bowel on barium studies and CT.
- Rarely, a solitary deposit of ileal endometriosis can mimic a primary carcinoid tumor or appendicitis.

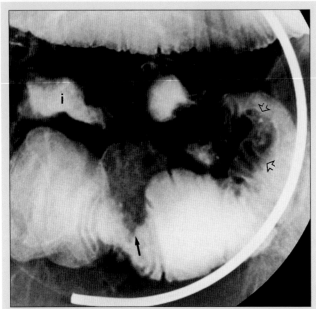

Figure 1. **Ileal endometriosis.** Spot image obtained during enteroclysis shows a focal, smooth, extrinsic mass impression *(open arrows)* on the mesenteric border of a pelvic loop of ileum. A second site reveals another focal extrinsic mass impression *(arrow)* and tethering of folds toward the mesenteric border. The ileal mucosa is preserved. The distal ileum (i) is collapsed. These endometriosis implants in the ileum are indistinguishable from intraperitoneal metastases to the small bowel.

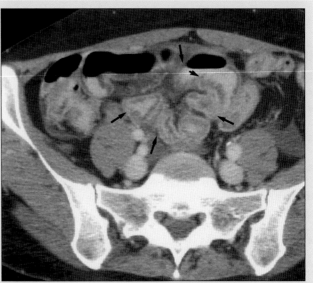

Figure 2. **Ileal endometriosis.** Axial CT through the pelvis shows ileal loops *(long arrows)* pulled toward the mesentery with associated tethering of folds *(small arrow)*. The submucosa has slightly low attenuation.

Pneumatosis Intestinalis

DEFINITION: Pneumatosis intestinalis is a condition in which gas is present in the bowel wall.

ANATOMIC FINDINGS

Bowel
- Multiple gas-filled cysts in wall of bowel

IMAGING

Radiography
Findings
- Round, ovoid, or linear collections of gas are seen along the margins of the bowel wall.
- Gas in the portomesenteric venous system is indicative of nonviable bowel.

Utility
- Abdominal radiographs

CT
Findings
- Linear or cystic collections in various layers of bowel wall
- Portomesenteric venous gas

Utility
- CT is a more sensitive technique for detecting pneumatosis.
- Parameters for ischemia include bowel wall thickness, postcontrast bowel wall enhancement, vascular engorgement or fluid in adjacent mesentery, and portomesenteric venous gas.

CLINICAL PRESENTATION

- Pneumatosis intestinalis is a secondary finding in patients with a wide variety of conditions.

PATHOLOGY

- Multiple gas-filled cysts are present in the submucosa and subserosa but rarely in the muscularis propria.
- Cysts contain the disorganized lining of flat cells and giant cells, often associated with mild surrounding inflammatory infiltrate.

DIAGNOSTIC PEARLS

- Round, ovoid, or linear collections of gas are seen along margins of bowel wall.
- Gas in portomesenteric venous system is indicative of nonviable bowel.
- Cysts do not communicate macroscopically with the bowel wall and are found to contain gas but not fluid.

- Cysts do not communicate macroscopically with bowel wall and are found to contain gas but not fluid.
- Gas in cyst does not have same composition as intestinal air.
- Pneumatosis intestinalis may be related to increased intraluminal pressure or bacterial invasion.

INCIDENCE/PREVALENCE AND EPIDEMIOLOGY

- Associated diseases include small bowel obstruction, diarrhea, barotrauma, Crohn disease, ischemic bowel disease, asthma, cystic fibrosis, and scleroderma.

Suggested Readings

Feczko PJ, Mezwa DG, Farah MC, et al: Clinical significance of pneumatosis of the bowel wall. *RadioGraphics* 12:1069-1078, 1992.

Heng Y, Schuffler MD, Haggitt RC, et al: Pneumatosis intestinalis: A review. *Am J Gastroenterol* 90:1747-1758, 1995.

Kelvin FM, Korobkin M, Rauch RF, et al: Computed tomography of pneumatosis intestinalis. *J Comput Assist Tomogr* 8:276-280, 1984.

Scheidler J, Stabler A, Kleber G, et al: Computed tomography in pneumatosis intestinalis: Differential diagnosis and therapeutic consequences. *Abdom Imaging* 20:523-528, 1995.

WHAT THE REFERRING PHYSICIAN NEEDS TO KNOW

- Bowel nonviability indicated by portomesenteric venous gas on abdominal radiograph or CT in patient with pneumatosis intestinalis.
- Presence of parameters for ischemia

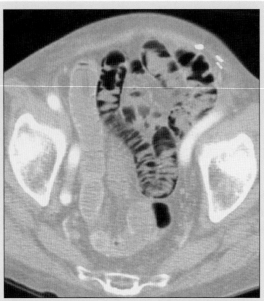

Figure 1. **Small bowel infarction with small bowel pneumatosis intestinalis and portal venous gas.** CT scan of the pelvis shows intramural gas in several ileal segments.

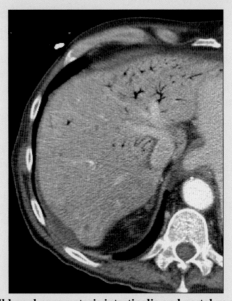

Figure 2. **Small bowel infarction with small bowel pneumatosis intestinalis and portal venous gas.** CT scan of the liver in same patient as in Figure 1 shows branching portal venous gas.

Intestinal Edema

DEFINITION: Increased interstitial fluid and dilation of mucosal and submucosal lymphatics in the small bowel wall.

ANATOMIC FINDINGS

Small Bowel Wall
- Dilation of mucosal and submucosal lymphatics and increased interstitial fluid

IMAGING

Radiography
Findings
- Smooth, straight or slightly undulating, mildly thickened folds that are diffusely distributed
- Luminal diameter of jejunum is slightly increased.

Utility
- Barium studies
- Generally best visualized in the jejunum

CT
Findings
- Edema of small bowel wall

CLINICAL PRESENTATION

- Signs and symptoms of hypoalbuminemia

DIFFERENTIAL DIAGNOSIS

- Ischemia (small bowel)
- Vasculitis (small bowel)
- Radiation (small bowel)
- Eosinophilic enteritis (small bowel)

PATHOLOGY

- Dilation of the mucosal and submucosal lymphatics and increased interstitial fluid
- Increased size and number of capillaries and venules in the lamina propria and submucosa of the jejunum in patients with cirrhosis

DIAGNOSTIC PEARLS

- Smooth, straight or slightly undulating, mildly thickened folds that are diffusely distributed
- Luminal diameter of the jejunum is slightly increased.
- CT shows edema of small bowel wall.

INCIDENCE/PREVALENCE AND EPIDEMIOLOGY

- Isolated edema of small bowel wall usually results from diseases that cause hypoalbuminemia.
- Two most common causes are cirrhosis and nephrotic syndrome.
- CT can show edema of the small bowel mesentery in 86% of patients.
- Omental and retroperitoneal edema is seen in 56% of patients.

Suggested Readings

Balthazar EJ, Gade MF: Gastrointestinal edema in cirrhotics: Radiographic manifestations with emphasis on colonic involvement. *Gastrointest Radiol* 1:215-223, 1976.

Chopra S, Dodd GD, Chintapalli KN, et al: Mesenteric, omental and retroperitoneal edema in cirrhosis: Frequency and spectrum of CT findings. *Radiology* 211:737-742, 1999.

Farthing MJG, Madewell JE, Bartram CI, et al: Radiologic features of the jejunum in hypoalbuminemia. *AJR Am J Roentgenol* 136: 883-886, 1981.

Marshak RH, Khilnani M, Eliasoph J, Wolf BS: Intestinal edema. *AJR* 101:379-387, 1967.

WHAT THE REFERRING PHYSICIAN NEEDS TO KNOW

- Intestinal edema usually results from diseases that cause hypoalbuminemia.
- The two most common causes of small-bowel edema are cirrhosis and nephrotic syndrome.
- In cirrhosis, congestive changes in jejunum are similar to portal hypertensive gastropathy in stomach.

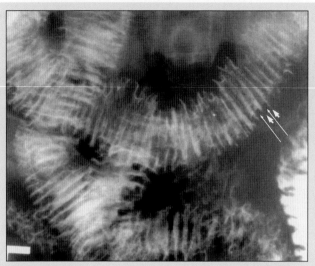

Figure 1. Small bowel edema in a patient with cirrhosis and hypoalbuminemia. Spot image from a small bowel follow-through shows diffusely thickened, smooth, straight folds *(long arrows)* that are perpendicular to the longitudinal axis of the bowel. Barium trapped between the folds forms the so-called interspace spikes *(short arrows)*.

Enteroliths and Bezoars

DEFINITION: Bezoars are composed of indigestible organic substances such as hair or fruit found inside the intestine.

ANATOMIC FINDINGS

Ileum
- Typical site of bezoar location

IMAGING

Radiography
Findings
- Masses containing air, soft tissue, or calcium

CT
Findings
- Intraluminal masses of mixed density or attenuation are seen.
- Peripheral or laminated calcification may be present.
- No air is identified in the biliary tree.

Utility
- Bezoars can be confused with ectopic gallstones in the small bowel associated with gallstone ileus.

DIFFERENTIAL DIAGNOSIS

- Intraluminal gallstones

PATHOLOGY

- Small intestinal bezoars are composed of indigestible materials, including hair, undigested food, and medications such as nonabsorbable antacids.

DIAGNOSTIC PEARLS

- Intraluminal masses of mixed density or attenuation are seen.
- Peripheral or laminated calcification may be present.
- Mass is differentiated from a gallstone by the lack of air in the biliary tree.

- Bezoars form in areas of stasis such as diverticula and small bowel proximal to strictures or in the terminal ileum.

INCIDENCE/PREVALENCE AND EPIDEMIOLOGY

- Bezoars and enteroliths are uncommon in the small bowel.
- In areas where persimmons are eaten, most phytobezoars are related to ingestion of unripe persimmons.

Suggested Readings

Javors BR, Bryk D: Enterolithiasis: Report of four cases. *Gastrointest Radiol* 8:359-362, 1983.

Kaplan O, Klausner JM, Lelcuk S, et al: Persimmon bezoars as a cause of intestinal obstruction: Pitfalls in their surgical management. *Br J Surg* 72:242-243, 1985.

Verstandig AG, Klin B, Bloom RA, et al: Small bowel phytobezoars: Detection with radiography. *Radiology* 172:705-707, 1989.

WHAT THE REFERRING PHYSICIAN NEEDS TO KNOW

- Small intestinal bezoars are typically found in the distal ileum or just proximal to pathologic areas of narrowing, such as strictures, anastomoses, or tumors.
- Bezoars can be confused with ectopic gallstones in the small bowel associated with gallstone ileus.

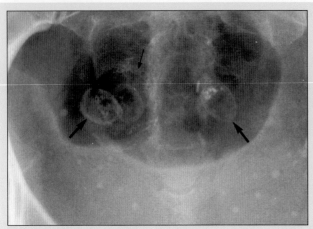

Figure 1. Calcified enteroliths. Coned-down view from abdominal radiograph shows three peripherally calcified ovoid structures *(large arrows)* near an anastomotic staple line *(small arrow)*. These structures are calcified enteroliths.

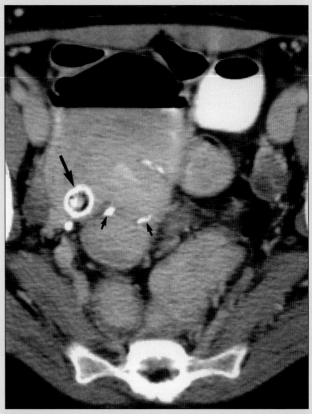

Figure 2. Calcified enteroliths. Axial CT image through the pelvis in the same patient as in Figure 1 shows one of the enteroliths as a peripherally calcified structure *(large arrow)* containing central bubbles of air and soft-tissue attenuation. Part of the staple line *(small arrows)* is identified.

Colon

Diverticulosis

DEFINITION: Small outpouchings of the colon, representing mucosal herniation.

ANATOMIC FINDINGS

Colon
- Mucosal and submucosal herniation through the muscularis
- Immature intramural diverticula that measure 1-2 mm high
- Mature diverticula that measure 0.5-1.0 cm
- Seen on either side of the taenia mesocolica and the mesenteric side of the antimesenteric taenia
- Commonly associated with myochosis

IMAGING

Radiography
Findings
- *Bubbly* appearance of the sigmoid colon on abdominal radiographs
- Thick circular muscle and *concertina* or zigzag appearance, representing myochosis
- Immature diverticula, conical or triangular when seen in profile
- Flask-like outward protrusions that are joined to the wall by a fairly long, large neck
- En face, possibly appearing as a ring shadow and a well-marginated barium collection or *bowler hat sign*
- Possibly inverting into the lumen to simulate polyp

Utility
- Barium studies are used.
- Immature diverticula en face may simulate aphthae; two views are needed to confirm.

CT
Findings
- Outpouchings that contain air, stool, or contrast agent
- Mural thickening of the colon in myochosis

Utility
- CT primarily is used to detect complications of diverticulosis, such as diverticulitis.

CLINICAL PRESENTATION

- Incidental finding in most patients
- Possible symptoms of irritable bowel syndrome such as chronic or intermittent postprandial lower abdominal pain relieved by defecation

DIAGNOSTIC PEARLS

- Small flask-like outward protrusions of the colon wall
- Found along taenia mesocolica and mesenteric side of other taenia
- Evidence of wall thickening with *concertina* haustra

DIFFERENTIAL DIAGNOSIS

- Collar-button ulcers in inflammatory bowel disease
- Deep ulcerations in ischemic infectious colitis

PATHOLOGY

- Multiple small outpouchings of the colon are seen, representing mucosal herniation.
- Low-residue diet results in tenacious stool, requiring increased propulsive effort.
- Pressure gradient between the lumen and serosa and the areas of relative bowel wall weakness contributes to diverticula formation.
- Most colonic diverticula are false diverticula, or pseudodiverticula, because they contain mucosa and submucosa but not the muscularis propria.
- Usually 0.5-1.0 cm, outpouchings penetrate the clefts between the bundles of circular muscle fibers at points where nutrient arteries pass through the submucosa.
- In an uninflamed state, diverticula are elastic and compressible, have tendency to empty poorly, and fill with inspissated stool.
- Sigmoid diverticula have myochosis, which is a disorder with thickening of the circular muscle layer, shortening of the taeniae, and narrowing of the lumen.

INCIDENCE/PREVALENCE AND EPIDEMIOLOGY

- Diverticulosis is the most common colonic disease in the Western world but is much less prevalent in underdeveloped areas of Asia and Africa.
- It occurs in 5% of the population by 40 years of age, 33%-50% after 50 years, and greater than 50% after 80 years.

DIVERTICULA OF THE COLON

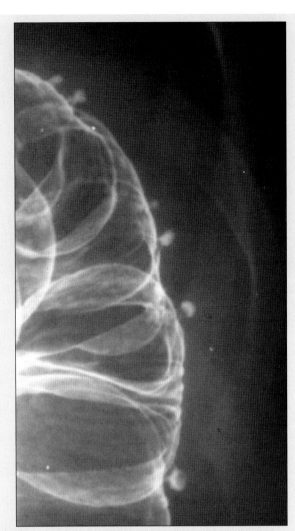

Figure 1. Colonic diverticulosis: double-contrast barium enema features. Multiple barium-filled outpouchings are identified along the lateral aspect of the proximal descending colon.

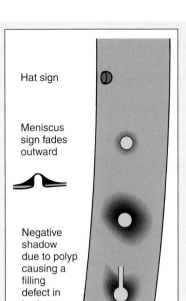

Hat sign

Meniscus sign fades outward

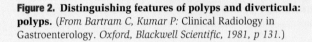

Negative shadow due to polyp causing a filling defect in barium

Figure 2. Distinguishing features of polyps and diverticula: polyps. (*From Bartram C, Kumar P:* Clinical Radiology in Gastroenterology. *Oxford, Blackwell Scientific, 1981, p 131.*)

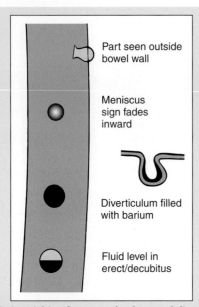

Figure 3. Distinguishing features of polyps and diverticula: diverticula. (*From Bartram C, Kumar P:* Clinical Radiology in Gastroenterology. *Oxford, Blackwell Scientific, 1981, p 131.*)

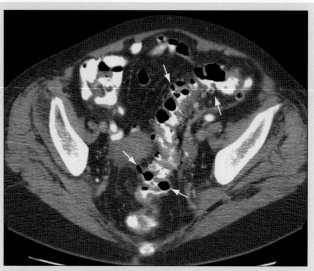

Figure 4. Diverticulosis: CT findings. CT scan at the level of the sigmoid colon shows multiple air- and contrast-filled diverticula (*arrows*).

- In individuals from low-prevalence areas who migrate to Western communities, the frequency of diverticula increases within 10 years.
- Sigmoid colon is involved in up to 95% of patients; the cecum is involved in 5% of patients.
- In Japan, patients with right-sided diverticulosis outnumber those with left-sided disease by a ratio of 5:1.
- Four to five percent of all patients harbor diverticula; 20% of those whose disease is clinically recognized will develop some complication.

Suggested Readings

Keller CE, Halpert RD, Feczko PJ, et al: Radiologic recognition of colonic diverticula simulating polyps. *AJR Am J Roentgenol* 143:93-97, 1984.

Miller WT, Levine MS, Rubesin SE, et al: Bowler-hat sign: A simple principle for differentiating polyps from diverticula. *Radiology* 173:615-617, 1989.

Papaconstantinou HT, Simmang CL: Diverticular disease. In Weinstein WM, Hawkey CJ, Bosch J (eds): *Clinical Gastroenterology and Hepatology.* New York, Elsevier, 2005, pp 463–472.

Simmang CL, Shires GT: Diverticular disease of the colon. In Feldman M, Friedman LS, Sleisenger MH (eds): *Gastrointestinal and Liver Disease.* Philadelphia, WB Saunders, 2002, pp 2100–2112.

Diverticulitis

DEFINITION: Diverticular perforation with subsequent surrounding inflammation.

ANATOMIC FINDINGS

Colon
- Diverticular perforation
- Intramural abscess if the intramural diverticulum ruptures intramurally
- Adjacent pericolic inflammatory changes
- Possible development of abscess, sinus tract, or fistula

IMAGING

Radiography
Findings
- Free intraperitoneal air or sealed-off perforations and pelvic extraluminal air
- Ill-defined, left-sided pelvic mass, localized ileus, and fluid in the pelvis
- Extravasation of contrast material from the diverticulum into the abscess, sinus tract, fistula, or peritoneal cavity
- Distortion of individual diverticula, which is an indirect sign
- Smooth, well-defined, contour defect associated with adjacent diverticula representing an intramural inflammatory mass.
- Longitudinal intramural fistulous tracts

Utility
- Radiography is diagnostic only in most severe forms of diverticulitis.
- Radiography is unremarkable in most patients and does not contribute to the diagnosis.
- Barium studies cannot evaluate pericolic inflammatory process directly.
- Radiography may show features suggestive of carcinoma.

Ultrasound
Findings
- Hypoechoic segments of gut wall thickening are seen.
- Abscesses appear as loculated, thick-walled fluid collections that may contain gas.
- Inflamed diverticula are brightly echogenic reflectors with acoustic shadowing or a ring-down artifact.
- Inflammatory changes are seen as poorly defined, hypoechoic zones without obvious gas or fluid.

DIAGNOSTIC PEARLS
- Central diverticulum with surrounding inflammation
- Extravasation of intraluminal colonic contrast
- Colonic wall thickening without lymphadenopathy

- Intramural sinus tracts appear as high-amplitude linear echoes that often have a ring-down artifact.

Utility
- First study often ordered for nondescript abdominal pain
- This technique is less sensitive than CT in the depiction of diverticulitis.

CT
Findings
- Hallmark on CT are inflammatory changes in the pericolic fat with or without central hyperdense diverticulum.
- Mild cases have a slight increase in pericolic fat attenuation with an engorged vasa recta.
- Abscesses are seen as pericolic or intramural loculated fluid collections with the *caterpillar sign*.
- Severe pericolic heterogeneous soft-tissue densities represent phlegmon.
- Linear or branching fluid-filled tracts and fistulas are located intramurally or pericolic.
- Partial colonic obstruction with sigmoid narrowing, gradual zone of transition, preservation of mucosal folds, and associated diverticula is seen.

Utility
- Multidetector CT (MDCT) is the primary cross-sectional imaging study.
- Differentiation from carcinoma may be difficult.
- CT may be used to guide percutaneous abscess drainage.
- CT helps differentiate the condition from primary epiploic appendagitis.
- CT helps identify the normal appendix to rule out appendicitis in right-sided disease.
- Sensitivity: 90%-100%
- Specificity: 90%-100%
- Accuracy: 97%

WHAT THE REFERRING PHYSICIAN NEEDS TO KNOW
- Close clinical and radiologic evaluation is crucial to guiding treatment.
- Stage of diverticulitis is best evaluated by CT.
- Complications include fistulas, free perforation, bowel obstruction, and pyelophlebitis with liver abscess.

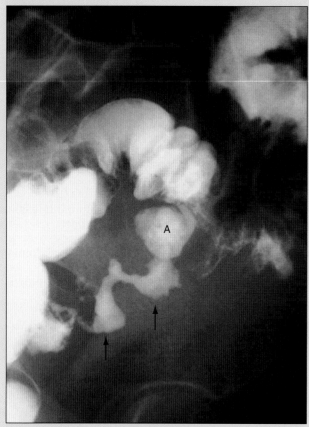

Figure 1. Diverticulitis with pericolonic abscess: barium enema features. Spot image from a barium enema shows filling of an abscess (A) and a sinus tract *(arrows)* along the inferior aspect of the sigmoid colon.

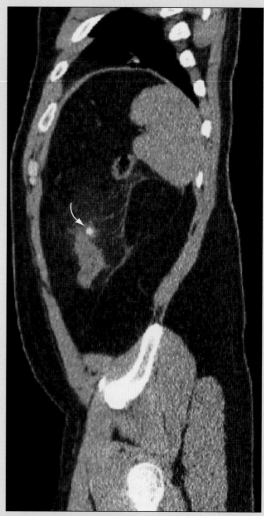

Figure 2. Diverticulitis: MDCT findings on non–contrast-enhanced scans. Sagittal image shows the hyperdense offending diverticulum *(curved arrow)* at the center of the pericolonic inflammation. Note the thickening of the anterior and lateroconal interfascial planes.

MRI

Findings

- Mural thickening of the colon and diverticular abscesses are seen.
- Sinus tracts, fistulas, and abscess walls are enhanced in the background of suppressed fat.

Utility

- MRI has little role in the primary evaluation of patients.

CLINICAL PRESENTATION

- Patients experience abdominal pain, tenderness, fever, and leukocytosis.
- Certain patients produce only minimal or unremarkable clinical symptoms.
- Patients younger than 40 years often develop severe forms.

DIFFERENTIAL DIAGNOSIS

- Crohn disease (gastrointestinal)
- Ulcerative colitis
- Drug-induced colitis
- Infectious enterocolitides
- *Clostridium difficile* colitis
- Epiploic appendagitis
- Abdominal aortic disease
- Bowel obstruction
- Colon carcinoma
- Foreign-body perforation of the colon
- Ischemic colitis
- Nonspecific colitis

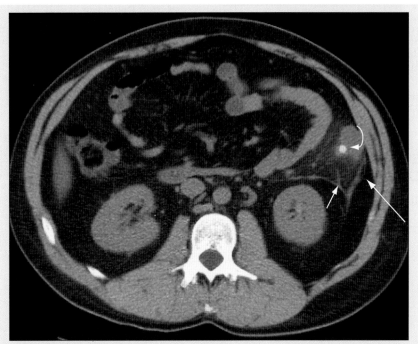

Figure 3. Diverticulitis: MDCT findings on non–contrast-enhanced scans. Axial image shows the hyperdense offending diverticulum *(curved arrow)* at the center of the pericolonic inflammation. Note the thickening of the anterior *(small straight arrow)* and lateroconal *(large straight arrow)* interfascial planes.

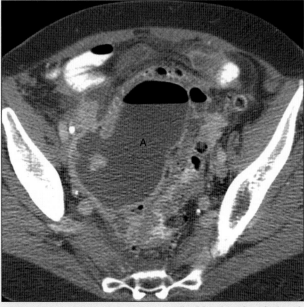

Figure 4. MDCT of diverticulitis: abscess. A large abscess (A) with an air-fluid level is identified in the pelvis.

PATHOLOGY

- Stagnation of nonsterile, inspissated fecal material within the diverticulum
- Inflammatory erosion of the mucosal lining with eventual perforation
- Subsequent fibrinous exudate, abscess formation, local adhesions, or peritonitis

INCIDENCE/PREVALENCE AND EPIDEMIOLOGY

- Diverticular perforation is the most common complication of diverticulosis.
- It occurs in 10%-20% of patients with known diverticulosis.

Suggested Readings

Ambrosetti P, Becker C, Terrier F: Colonic diverticulitis: Impact of imaging on surgical management—a prospective study of 542 patients. *Eur Radiol* 12:1145-1149, 2002.

Buckley O, Geoghegan T, McAuley G, et al: Pictorial review: Magnetic resonance imaging of colonic diverticulitis. *Eur Radiol* 17:221-227, 2007.

Kaiser AM, Jiang JK, Lake JP, et al: The management of complicated diverticulitis and the role of computed tomography. *Am J Gastroenterol* 100:910-917, 2005.

Vijayaraghavan SB: High-resolution sonographic spectrum of diverticulosis, diverticulitis, and their complications. *J Ultrasound Med* 25:75-85, 2006.

Zaidi E, Daly B: CT and clinical features of acute diverticulitis in an urban U.S. population: Rising frequency in young, obese adults. *AJR Am J Roentgenol* 187:689-694, 2006.

Diverticular Hemorrhage

DEFINITION: Bleeding from a colonic diverticulum.

IMAGING

Catheter Angiography
Findings
- Only specific criterion for diverticular hemorrhage is extravasation into the offending diverticulum.

Utility
- Angiography can locate the bleeding site.
- Effects transcatheter control to obviate surgery or stabilize the patient before surgery

CT Angiography
Findings
- Extravasation of contrast medium

Utility
- Multidetector CT is being used with greater frequency to detect diverticular bleeds.

CLINICAL PRESENTATION

- Patient experiences a sudden onset of mild abdominal cramps and the urge to defecate.
- Large volume of bright-red blood or clots (or both) are seen; dark-red, maroon, or black stool is passed rectally.
- Bleeding may spontaneously resolve or intermittently recur.
- Patients typically exhibit acute, painless, bright-red blood or clots (or both) and dark-red, maroon, or black stool passed rectally (hematochezia).

DIFFERENTIAL DIAGNOSIS

- Inflammatory bowel disease
- Hemorrhoids
- Colon cancer
- Ischemic colitis
- Infectious colitis

DIAGNOSTIC PEARLS

- Patient experiences a sudden onset of mild abdominal cramps and the urge to defecate.
- Bleeding may spontaneously resolve or intermittently recur.
- Severe hemorrhage originates from the right colon in two thirds of patients.

PATHOLOGY

- Severe hemorrhage originates from the right colon (related to wider necks) and the domes of the right-sided diverticula, permitting arterial exposure to injury.
- Hemorrhage results when the vas rectum of the colonic artery ruptures into the dome of the diverticulum from pressure erosion.
- Source is typically a single diverticulum.
- Diverticulum develops through the cleft for the vas rectum.
- Diverticular enlargement results in the vas rectum position adjacent to the lumen.
- Intraluminal injurious factor causes eccentric intimal thickening of vas rectum.
- Subsequent weakening and rupture of vas rectum may occur.

INCIDENCE/PREVALENCE AND EPIDEMIOLOGY

- Diverticular hemorrhage occurs in 30% of patients with diverticulosis.
- Forty-three percent of elderly patients experience major rectal bleeding.
- Thirty-five percent of elderly patients experience minor rectal bleeding.

WHAT THE REFERRING PHYSICIAN NEEDS TO KNOW

- Twenty-five percent of patients rebleed; occurrence of rebleed increases the chance of further rebleeding.
- Selective catheterization and infusion of intra-arterial vasopressin work to control hemorrhage in most patients.
- In older patients, emergency surgery is necessary to remove the portion of the colon containing the bleeding site.
- Embolization is considered as a temporizing measure to stop bleeding while the patient is prepared for surgery or if the condition poses surgical high risk.
- Intra-arterial vasopressin therapy is most effective in patients who have diverticular bleeding.

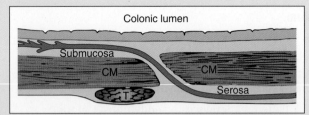

Figure 1. Diverticulum formation and vascular relationships.
The vas rectum penetrates the colon wall from the serosa to the submucosa through an obliquely oriented connective tissue septum in the circular muscle (CM). This penetration occurs near the mesenteric side of the taenia (T).

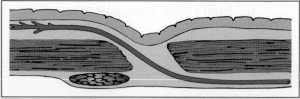

Figure 2. Diverticulum formation and vascular relationships.
The diverticulum develops through and widens this connective tissue cleft. The mucosal protrusion begins to elevate the artery.

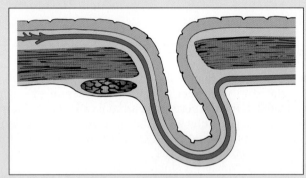

Figure 3. Diverticulum formation and vascular relationships.
As the diverticulum extends transmurally, the vas rectum is placed over its dome, penetrating to the submucosa on the antimesenteric border of its neck and orifice. (*From Meyers MA, Volberg F, Katzen B, et al: Angioarchitecture of colonic diverticula: Significance in bleeding diverticulosis.* Radiology *108:249-261, 1973.*)

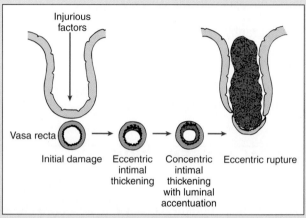

Figure 4. Pathogenesis of colonic diverticular hemorrhage.
Progressive eccentric changes weaken the wall of the vas rectum, which eventually ruptures into the lumen of the diverticulum.
(*From Meyers MA, Alonso DR, Gray GF, et al: Pathogenesis of bleeding colonic diverticulosis.* Gastroenterology *71:577-583, 1976.*)

- Significant diverticular bleeding occurs in only 3% of patients with diverticulosis.
- Diverticular hemorrhage is the most common cause of major gastrointestinal hemorrhage in the Western world.

Suggested Readings

Kaiser AM, Jiang JK, Lake JP, et al: The management of complicated diverticulitis and the role of computed tomography. *Am J Gastroenterol* 100:910-917, 2005.

Salzman H, Lillie D: Diverticular disease: Diagnosis and treatment. *Am Fam Physician* 72:1229-1234, 2005.

West BA: The pathology of diverticulosis: Classical concepts and mucosal changes in diverticula. *J Clin Gastroenterol* 40(7 Suppl 3): S126-S131, 2006.

Giant Sigmoid Diverticulum

DEFINITION: Cystic enlargement of a sigmoid diverticulum.

IMAGING

Radiography
Findings
- Large gas-filled structure is seen in the lower to middle pelvis with possible air-fluid level.
- Structure may change in size on interval studies.
- Colonic barium may fill the cyst.
- Connection between the cyst and the gut lumen may be demonstrated.
- Presence of colonic diverticula is seen.

Utility
- Barium enema will fill diverticulum only if its mouth is patent.

CT
Findings
- Large gas-filled structures adjacent to the sigmoid colon

Utility
- Best means of establishing the diagnosis
- May be difficult to differentiate from large diverticular abscess

CLINICAL PRESENTATION

- History of chronic, vague, abdominal discomfort or acute symptoms suggesting diverticulitis
- Palpable mass, which is hyper-resonant on percussion
- Lower abdominal pain
- Diverticulitis
- Hemorrhage
- Peritonitis

DIFFERENTIAL DIAGNOSIS

- Meckel diverticulum (small bowel)
- Diverticula (small bowel)
- Fistulas

DIAGNOSTIC PEARLS

- Cystic structure of more than 6 cm
- Anatomic connection between the cyst and the gut lumen
- Large gas-filled structure in the lower to middle pelvis, with possible air-fluid level

PATHOLOGY

- Cystic enlargement of the colonic diverticulum rarely results from diverticulitis.
- It may result from subserosal perforation and inflammation of the diverticulum with subsequent air trapping and cyst formation resulting from the ball-valve mechanism.
- Inflammatory and granulation tissue replaces the mucosal lining of the cyst wall.
- Trapped air in the cyst increases during defecation and is vented irregularly.
- Cysts range in size between 6 and 27 cm, with a mean diameter of 13 cm.

INCIDENCE/PREVALENCE AND EPIDEMIOLOGY

- Disease of elderly adults
- Less common than colonic diverticulosis

Suggested Readings

Abou-Nukta F, Bakhos C, Ikekpeazu N, et al: Ruptured giant colonic diverticulum. *Am Surg* 71:1073-1074, 2005.
Chaiyasate K, Yavuzer R, Mittal V: Giant sigmoid diverticulum. *Surgery* 139:276-277, 2006.
Muhletaler CA, Berger JL, Robinette CL: Pathogenesis of giant colonic diverticula. *Gastrointest Radiol* 6:217-222, 1981.

WHAT THE REFERRING PHYSICIAN NEEDS TO KNOW

- Giant colonic diverticula have been reported to perforate, causing volvulus and infarction and small-bowel obstruction, and may contain a carcinoma.
- Accepted therapy is surgical excision.

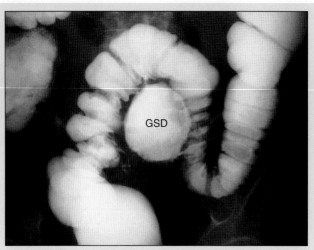

Figure 1. Giant sigmoid colon diverticulum (GSD) is demonstrated in a barium enema study.

Appendicitis

ANATOMIC FINDINGS

Appendix
- Acute appendicitis with or without presence of appendicolith and periappendiceal fat inflammation
- Fluid-filled distended tubular structure
- Circumferential and symmetrical appendiceal wall thickening
- Appendiceal abscess
- Appendiceal phlegmon
- Perforated acute appendicitis
- Ileus with minimal small bowel obstruction

IMAGING

Conventional Radiography
Findings
- Appendicolith is the most specific sign; it is usually solitary, but two or three adjacent small calcifications are not unusual.
- Appendiceal abscess: extraluminal bubbles of air associated with an ill-defined soft tissue mass indicate an abscess.
- Severe localized ileus with ileal and cecal dilation and air-fluid levels due to severe inflammatory process may mimic mechanical distal small bowel obstruction.

Utility
- Inadequate for diagnosis of appendicitis but has become an important adjunct to clinical evaluation
- Can sometimes determine alternate conditions as cause of patient's pain when appendix is normal

Fluoroscopy
Findings
- Complete filling of appendix to its bulbous tip effectively excludes diagnosis of acute appendicitis.

DIAGNOSTIC PEARLS

- Classic presentations are poorly localized periumbilical pain, followed by nausea and vomiting, then pain migration to right lower quadrant, which occurs in only one half to two thirds of all patients.
- Abnormal appendix appears as thick-walled, fluid-filled, distended tubular structure, associated with or without calcified appendicolith and periappendiceal or pericecal inflammation.
- Continued tissue ischemia results in appendiceal infarction and perforation, which can cause localized or generalized peritonitis.

- Extravasation of barium in patient with sealed-off, perforative appendicitis
- Appendiceal abscess shows compression of cecal caput and obstruction of base of appendix.

Utility
- Barium enema was the primary radiologic test used in diagnosis of appendicitis before the 1990s.
- Performed quickly and safely with single-column technique
- Diagnostic accuracy of barium enema in patient with acute appendicitis is reportedly as high as 91.5%.

CT
Findings
- Abnormal appendix may appear as a fluid-filled, minimally distended tubular structure greater than 5-6 mm in diameter with no periappendiceal inflammation, with calcified appendicolith and pericecal inflammation.
- Circumferentially, symmetrically thickened appendiceal wall; mural enhancement may be homogenous or exhibit target sign appearance after contrast administration.

WHAT THE REFERRING PHYSICIAN NEEDS TO KNOW

- Serial white blood cell (WBC) count may help; WBC count increases 4-8 hours after admission unless the appendix is perforated (in which case WBC count typically decreases).
- Normal WBC count, however, does not exclude the diagnosis of appendicitis.
- Elevated C-reactive protein (CRP) >0.8 mg/dL is more common when symptoms are present for more than 12 hours.
- Urinalysis is positive, which includes bacteriuria, mild pyuria, and hematuria; it is more commonly observed in women versus men.
- Differential diagnosis includes cecal or ileal diverticulitis, Crohn disease, mesenteric adenitis, epiploic appendagitis, inflamed Meckel diverticulum, infection or ischemic ileitis, typhlitis, perforated cecal carcinoma, and pelvic inflammatory disease.

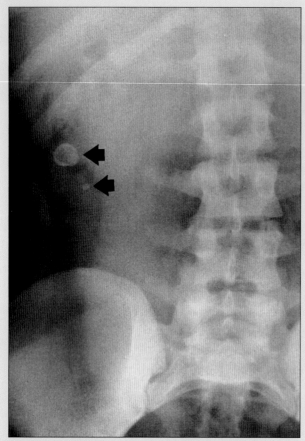

Figure 1. **Appendicoliths.** Two appendicoliths (*arrows*) are present in the right upper quadrant. The patient had a long retrocolic subhepatic appendix with acute appendicitis.

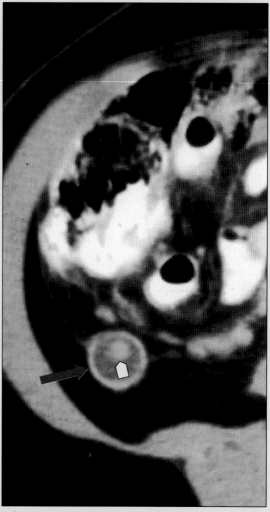

Figure 2. **Acute appendicitis on enhanced CT.** The distended appendix (*red arrow*) is seen in cross-section and demonstrates abnormal mural thickening and enhancement. In addition, an intraluminal appendicolith (*yellow arrowhead*) is present.

- Cecal arrowhead sign: triangular "arrowhead" configuration of oral contrast funneling into focally thickened, spastic cecum and pointing toward appendiceal orifice.
- Cecal bar sign: linear inflammatory soft tissue at base of appendix that separates contrast-filled cecum from appendix.
- Perforated appendicitis, extraluminal air, marked ileocecal wall thickening, localized lymphadenopathy, pericecal phlegmon, or abscess, peritonitis, and/or small bowel obstruction may be present.
- Appendicitis can be confined to distal or tip of appendix, referred to as "distal" or "tip" appendicitis.

Utility
- Use of CT has significantly diminished negative appendectomy rate.
- Highly effective and accurate means of diagnosing acute appendicitis, abscess, and phlegmon; staging complications; and suggesting other alternative diagnosis.
- Reported sensitivities of 90%, specificities of 91%-99%, accuracies of 94%-98%, positive predictive values of 92%-98%, negative predictive values of 95%-100%
- Performance of thin-section scans with coronal and sagittal reformations improves sensitivity of identifying abnormal appendix.
- Contrast non-usage: immediate scan of symptomatic patient eliminates potential risk of contrast reaction, with reduced costs, but has potential for misinterpretation.
- Contrast usage: able to rapidly achieve identification and increase sensitivity in diagnosing acute appendicitis but causes patient discomfort; contrast reaction is a potential risk and it is costly.

Ultrasonography
Findings
- Abnormal appendix appears as blind-ending, noncompressible, thick-walled tubular structure larger than 6 mm in diameter with laminated wall. It is fluid-filled and distended.

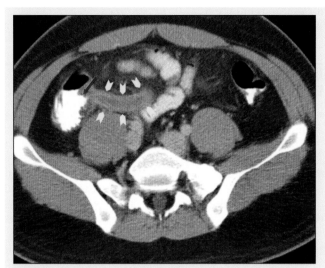

Figure 3. Acute appendicitis on enhanced CT. The appendix (*yellow arrowheads*) is distended, with enhancement of the thickened appendiceal wall and periappendiceal soft tissue stranding. Note the funneling of enteric contrast in the thickened cecum toward the appendiceal orifice, the "arrowhead" sign (*red arrows*).

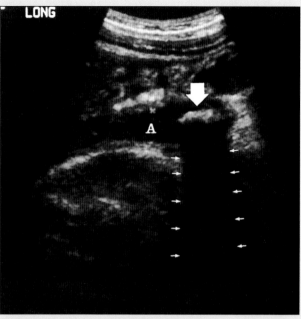

Figure 4. Sonogram of an inflamed appendix containing an appendicolith. Longitudinal image shows a thick-walled, fluid-filled appendix (*A*). The layers of the appendiceal wall are not well defined. An appendicolith (*large arrow*) is identified as an echogenic focus with acoustic shadowing (*small arrows*).

- Presence of appendicolith appears as a rounded, echogenic foci with clean distal acoustic shadowing; it is strongly associated with appendicitis.
- Periappendiceal fat inflammation appears as an echogenic region that may cause mass effect and separate inflamed bowel segment from surrounding structure.
- Periappendiceal phlegmon appears as a hypoechoic, poorly marginated area within fat adjacent to appendix.
- Periappendiceal abscess is recognized as focal collections of fluid that may or may not contain gas.

Utility
- Use of ultrasonography has diminished negative appendectomy rate.
- Widely available, relatively inexpensive, noninvasive; more importantly, poses no ionizing radiation risk (significant in pediatrics and pregnant patients)
- Diagnostic accuracy varies; meta-analysis showed an overall sensitivity of 85% and specificity of 92%.
- Limitations are operator dependent. It is difficult to perform in patients with severe abdominal pain, with a large amount of bowel gas, and in obese patients.
- US diagnostic sensitivity for perforated appendicitis is lower than for nonperforated appendicitis.
- Best used as initial imaging modality in children, adolescents, thin adults, women of reproductive age.

MRI
Findings
- Appendiceal wall thickening with high intensity; dilated lumen filled with high intensity material; increased intensity of periappendiceal tissues

Utility
- Use of T2-weighted fast spin-echo and fat-suppressed spectral presaturation inversion recovery images
- Has proven to be accurate for diagnosing acute appendicitis
- Benefits are its multiplanar image acquisition capabilities, its high intrinsic soft tissue contrast, no need for contrast material, and lack of ionizing radiation
- Indicated in pregnant patients when results of nonionizing diagnostic tests are inconclusive or inadequate and used for important treatment decisions concerning fetus or mother

CLINICAL PRESENTATION

- Poorly localized periumbilical pain, followed by nausea and vomiting, then migration of pain to right lower quadrant, which occurs in only one half to two thirds of all patients
- Visceral epigastric or periumbilical pain is perceived during initial distention and increased intraluminal pressure in obstructed appendix.
- Somatic pain with classic shift of pain to right lower quadrant is perceived when inflamed appendix comes in contact with parietal peritoneum.
- Abdominal tenderness typically localized at or near McBurney's point is the most common physical finding, occurring in more than 85% of patients.

- *Rovsing's sign* is pain referred to an area of maximal tenderness during palpation or percussion of left lower quadrant.
- *Psoas sign* is right lower quadrant pain with hip extension, whereas *obturator sign* is right lower quadrant pain with flexion and internal right hip rotation.
- Voluntary muscle guarding in right lower quadrant is common and typically precedes localized rebound tenderness.
- Nausea, vomiting, and anorexia occur in varying degrees, but they are usually present in more than one half of all cases.
- Diagnostic sensitivity is improved by 97%-100% when elevated CRP (>0.8 mg/dL), elevated WBC (>10,000/mL), and neutrophilia (>75%) coexist.

PATHOLOGY

- Initiating event in acute appendicitis is luminal obstruction, which may be caused by fecaliths or appendicoliths (most common), lymphoid hyperplasia, primary and metastatic tumor, parasites, foreign bodies, Crohn disease, or adhesions.
- Appendicolith forms around a nidus (e.g., vegetable matter); inspissated feces and calcium salts may adhere to nidus, eventually reaching a size that occludes appendiceal lumen.
- Continued mucus secretion into appendix after luminal obstruction results in distention and concurrent luminal pressure elevation.
- When luminal pressure exceeds capillary perfusion pressure, lymphatic and venous drainage are impaired and arterial compromise and tissue ischemia result.
- Breakdown of epithelial mucosal barrier occurs, luminal bacteria multiply, and lumen fills with purulent exudates and invades the appendiceal wall, causing periappendiceal, transmural inflammation and gangrenous changes.
- Continued tissue ischemia results in appendiceal infarction and perforation, which can cause localized or generalized peritonitis.
- Appendiceal calculi (hard, noncrushable calcified stones) are less common but are more commonly associated with appendiceal perforation and periappendiceal abscess formation.

DIFFERENTIAL DIAGNOSIS

- Mesenteric adenitis
- Infectious enterocolitis
- Crohn disease
- Epiploic appendagitis
- Omental infarction
- Right-sided ileal diverticulitis
- Meckel diverticulitis
- Neutropenic colitis (typhlitis)
- Ischemia
- Cecal carcinoma
- Pelvic inflammatory disease

INCIDENCE/PREVALENCE AND EPIDEMIOLOGY

- Appendicitis is the most frequent cause of acute abdominal pain requiring surgical intervention; its incidence has been declining steadily since the late 1940s.
- Acute appendicitis is the most common abdominal surgical emergency, affecting approximately 250,000 people annually in the United States.
- Currently, lifetime appendicitis risk is 8.6% for males and 6.7% for females.
- In teenagers and young adults, there is a 3:2 male gender predilection; continuous slight male predominance with a rate of 1.4:1 occurs in adults.
- Acute appendicitis is the most common nonobstetric surgical emergency in pregnant patients, occurring in approximately 1 in 766 pregnancies.
- Mortality and morbidity rates for acute appendicitis are 0.24% and 6.1%, respectively, but increase to 1.7 and 19% for perforated appendicitis.
- Complications occur in 1%-5% of all patients with appendicitis, and wound infections account for nearly one third of all morbidity, which increases to 20%-40% with perforated appendicitis; gangrene increases morbidity 5-fold and perforation 10-fold.
- Appendiceal perforation occurs in 16%-39% of patients, with a median of 20%; it is inversely proportional to patient's age, and markedly higher for children younger than 5 years.
- Appendicoliths are found in only 10% of patients with acute appendicitis, and, when present, incidence of perforation is nearly 50%.

Suggested Readings

Addiss DG, Shaffer N, Fowler BS, et al: The epidemiology of appendicitis and appendectomy in the United States. *Am J Epidemiol* 132:910-925, 1990.

Birnbaum BA, Wilson SR: Appendicitis at the millennium. *Radiology* 215:337-348, 2000.

Dueholm S, Bagi P, Bud M: Laboratory aid in the diagnosis of acute appendicitis. *Dis Colon Rectum* 32:855-859, 1989.

Flum DR, Koepsell T: The clinical and economic correlates of misdiagnosed appendicitis. *Arch Surg* 137:799-804, 2002.

Gough IR: A study of diagnostic accuracy in acute appendicitis. *Aust N Z J Surg* 58:555-560, 1988.

Noudeh YJ, Sadigh N, Ahmadnia AY: Epidemiologic features of acute appendicitis. *Int J Surg* 5:95-98, 2007.

Rothrock SG, Pagane J: Acute appendicitis in children: Emergency department diagnosis and management. *Ann Emerg Med* 6:39-51, 2000.

Shelton T, McKinlay R, Schwartz RW: Acute appendicitis: Current diagnosis and treatment. *Curr Surg* 60:502-505, 2003.

Walker ARP, Segal I: What causes appendicitis [editorial]? *J Clin Gastroenterol* 12:127-129, 1990.

Wilcox RT, Traverso LW: Have the evaluation and treatment of acute appendicitis changed with a new technology? *Surg Clin North Am* 77:1355-1370, 1970.

Appendiceal Mucocele

DEFINITION: Cystic dilation of the appendiceal lumen by mucinous secretions.

ANATOMIC FINDINGS

Appendix
- Obstructing lesion
- Thin-walled cystic structure measuring 3-6 cm
- Possible calcification of the wall or lumen
- Myxoglobulosis variant results in numerous small globules.

Cecum
- Obstructing lesion may arise from the cecum.

IMAGING

Radiography
Findings
- Well-defined right lower quadrant mass
- Rim-like calcifications may be present.
- Myxoglobulosis is manifested by multiple mobile 1- to 10-mm round to oval calcifications.
- Appendix fails to fill on barium enema, and cecum is indented by a smooth-walled mass.

Utility
- Abdominal radiographs are normal in most patients.
- 15%-20% of normal appendices do not routinely fill on barium enema.

Ultrasound
Findings
- Fluid-filled anechoic masses with increased through-transmission
- Possible septations and gravity-dependent echoes

Utility
- Sagittal, transverse, and oblique imaging of the abdomen and pelvis is performed.
- Transvaginal examination in women may be helpful if transabdominal images are equivocal.
- Ultrasound is operator dependent; use is limited in certain patient populations and clinical situations.

DIAGNOSTIC PEARLS
- Water or soft-tissue density masses on CT
- Fluid-filled anechoic masses with increased through-transmission on ultrasound
- Thin, curvilinear wall calcification

CT
Findings
- Water or soft-tissue density masses are seen.
- Calcification may be detected within the wall or lumen.

Utility
- CT uses both enteric and intravenous contrast material.

MRI
Findings
- If predominantly fluid-filled, the mass has a low T1- and a high T2-weighted intensity.
- If predominantly mucin-filled, the mass appears intense on both T1- and T2-weighted images.

CLINICAL PRESENTATION
- Chronic right lower quadrant pain
- Possible abdominal swelling, anemia, or mucous fistula
- Right lower quadrant tenderness or palpable mass on physical examination

DIFFERENTIAL DIAGNOSIS
- Appendiceal cystadenoma–cystadenocarcinoma
- Ovarian serous cystadenomas and mucinous cystadenomas
- Primary neoplasms of the mesentery
- Omental and mesenteric cysts
- Duplication cyst
- Mesenteric hematoma
- Mesenteric tumor

WHAT THE REFERRING PHYSICIAN NEEDS TO KNOW
- Complications include rupture with pseudomyxoma peritonei, torsion with gangrene and hemorrhage, and intussusception.
- Cystic dilation of the appendix may be indistinguishable from cystadenocarcinoma clinically, radiographically, and on gross inspection.

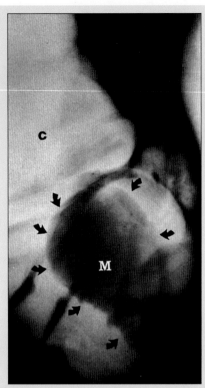

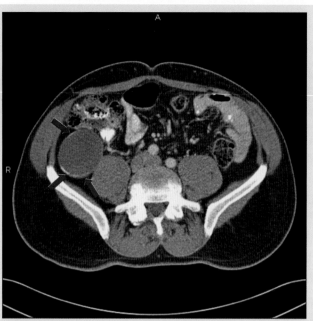

Figure 2. **Mucocele of the appendix on CT.** This ovoid-shaped, fluid-filled appendiceal mucocele contains mural calcifications *(arrows).*

Figure 1. **Mucocele of the appendix.** Barium enema study shows a sharply contoured, large intraluminal cecal defect (M). Note how the intussuscepting mucocele *(arrows)* arises from the tip of the cecum (c) and the appendix is not filled.

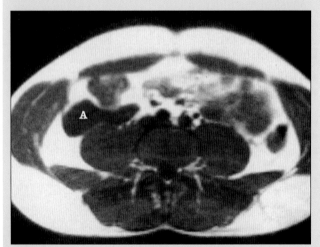

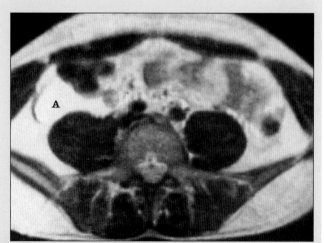

Figure 3. **Mucocele of the appendix visualized by MRI.** T1-weighted MR image (250/15) shows a distended appendix (A) of low signal intensity. *(Courtesy of Charles A. Whelan, MD, Montclair, NJ.)*

Figure 4. **Mucocele of the appendix visualized by MRI in same patient as in Figure 3.** T2-weighted MR image (2000/60) shows a bright structure of high signal intensity, representing the distended, fluid-filled appendix (A). *(Courtesy of Charles A. Whelan, MD, Montclair, NJ.)*

PATHOLOGY

- Cystic dilation of the appendiceal lumen secondary to mucinous secretions
- Slow accumulation of mucin in the obstructed lumen; most commonly secondary scarring from appendicitis
- Appendix becomes a thin-walled, cystic structure.
- Histologically classified into three groups: focal or diffuse hyperplasia, mucinous cystadenoma, and mucinous cystadenocarcinoma

INCIDENCE/PREVALENCE AND EPIDEMIOLOGY

- Uncommon; found in 0.3% of appendectomy specimens
- Female-to-male ratio of 4:1
- Mean age of 55 years at presentation

Suggested Readings

Higa E, Rosai J, Pizzimbono CA, et al: Mucosal hyperplasia, mucinous cystadenoma and mucinous cystadenocarcinoma of the appendix: A re-evaluation of appendiceal mucocele. *Cancer* 32:1525-1541, 1973.

Isaacs KL, Warshauer DM: Mucocele of the appendix: Computed tomographic, endoscopic, and pathologic correlation. *Am J Gastroenterol* 87:787-789, 1992.

Kim SH, Lim HK, Lee WJ, et al: Mucocele of the appendix: Ultrasonographic and CT findings. *Abdom Imaging* 23:292-296, 1998.

Madwell D, Mindelzun R, Jeffrey RB: Mucocele of the appendix: Imaging findings. *AJR Am J Roentgenol* 159:69-72, 1992.

Skaane P: Radiological features of mucocele of the appendix. *Rofo* 149:624-628, 1988.

Appendiceal Cystadenoma— Cystadenocarcinoma

DEFINITION: Cystic adenoma or adenocarcinoma of the appendix.

ANATOMIC FINDINGS

Appendix
- Mass may be confined to mucosa only.
- Mass may have associated mucocele.

IMAGING

CT
Findings
- Heterogeneous mass with nodular areas of soft tissue or a cystic mass with soft-tissue components.
- Calcification may be seen within the wall or lumen.
- Soft-tissue stranding of the periappendiceal fat.

Utility
- Both enteric and intravenous contrast material are used.
- Differentiation of lesions from mucocele by imaging alone is difficult; histopathologic correlation therefore is necessary.

CLINICAL PRESENTATION

- Patients with appendiceal cystadenomas may present with clinical signs and symptoms of appendicitis.

DIFFERENTIAL DIAGNOSIS

- Appendiceal mucocele
- Other appendiceal neoplasms

DIAGNOSTIC PEARLS

- Heterogeneous mass with nodular soft-tissue areas
- Cystic mass with soft-tissue components
- Periappendiceal mesenteric stranding

INCIDENCE/PREVALENCE AND EPIDEMIOLOGY

- Patients with mucoceles, including cystadenomas and cystadenocarcinomas, have a mean age of 55 years at presentation.

Suggested Readings

Gustafson KD, Karnaze GC, Hattery RR, et al: Pseudomyxoma peritonei associated with mucinous adenocarcinoma of the pancreas: CT findings and CT-guided biopsy. *J Comput Assist Tomogr* 8:335-338, 1984.

Higa E, Rosai J, Pizzimbono CA, et al: Mucosal hyperplasia, mucinous cystadenoma and mucinous cystadenocarcinoma of the appendix: A re-evaluation of appendiceal mucocele. *Cancer* 32:1525-1541, 1973.

McGinnis HD, Chew FS: Mucin-producing adenoma of the appendix. *AJR Am J Roentgenol* 160:1046, 1993.

Wackym PA, Gray GF: Tumors of the appendix: I. Neoplastic and nonneoplastic mucoceles. *South Med J* 77:283-287, 1984.

WHAT THE REFERRING PHYSICIAN NEEDS TO KNOW

- Complications include rupture, appendicitis, and pseudomyxoma peritonei.
- Appendiceal cystadenoma may be indistinguishable from a mucocele clinically, radiographically, and on gross inspection.

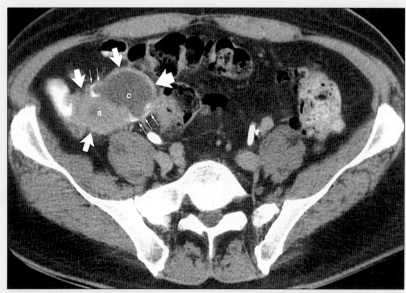

Figure 1. Mucinous cystadenocarcinoma of the appendix. CT shows a mass with solid (s) and cystic (c) components in the right pelvis inferior and medial to the cecum *(large arrows)*. Peripheral calcifications are seen in the cystic component *(small arrows)*.

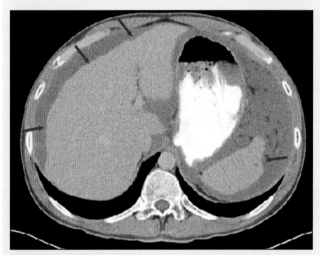

Figure 2. Pseudomyxoma peritonei is seen in the upper abdomen. Note ascites with a scalloped contour to the liver and spleen *(arrows)*.

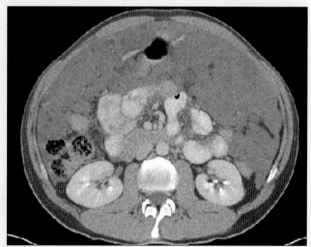

Figure 3. Pseudomyxoma peritonei. Massive ascites is seen in the mid-abdomen with heterogeneous attenuated fluid and septations causing mass effect on adjacent bowel loops.

Appendiceal Carcinoid

DEFINITION: Carcinoid tumor of the appendix.

ANATOMIC FINDINGS

Appendix
- Tumor is usually less than 2 cm.
- Most common site (70%) is the appendiceal tip.
- Other sites are the appendiceal body (22%) and base (7%).

IMAGING

CT
Findings
- Homogeneous soft-tissue mass is seen.
- Mass may infiltrate into the cecum and mesentery.

Utility
- Both enteric and intravenous contrast material are used.

CLINICAL PRESENTATION

- Most patients are asymptomatic, but symptoms of appendicitis can occur when the lumen is obstructed.
- Tendency exists to exhibit coexistent tumors.
- Tumors are typically found incidentally during surgery.
- Low metastatic potential exists.

DIFFERENTIAL DIAGNOSIS

- Other appendiceal masses
- Appendicitis

DIAGNOSTIC PEARLS

- Homogeneous soft-tissue mass
- Usually less than 2 cm
- Possible infiltration into the cecum and mesentery

INCIDENCE/PREVALENCE AND EPIDEMIOLOGY

- Carcinoid tumor is the most common neoplasm of the appendix.
- Incidence is 0.32% in appendectomy specimens.
- Incidence is 0.054% at autopsy.
- Carcinoid tumors of the appendix comprise 18.9% of all gastrointestinal carcinoid tumors.
- Average age at presentation is 42 years.
- Female predominance is found.

Suggested Readings

Chiou YY, Pitman MB, Hahn PF, et al: Rare benign and malignant appendiceal lesions: Spectrum of computed tomography findings with pathologic correlation. *J Comput Assist Tomogr* 27:297-306, 2003.

Modlin IM, Sandor A: An analysis of 8305 cases of carcinoid tumors. *Cancer* 79:813-829, 1997.

Pelage JP, Soyer P, Boudiaf M, et al: Carcinoid tumors of the abdomen: CT features. *Abdom Imaging* 24:240-245, 1999.

Sandor A, Modlin IM: A retrospective analysis of 1570 appendiceal carcinoids. *Am J Gastroenterol* 93:422-428, 1998.

WHAT THE REFERRING PHYSICIAN NEEDS TO KNOW

- Tumor size is important for management.
- Carcinoids smaller than 2 cm are treated with appendectomy.
- Carcinoids greater than 2 cm or those accompanied by evidence of mesoappendiceal invasion necessitate a right hemicolectomy.

Ulcerative Colitis

DEFINITION: A contiguous, confluent, circumferential, symmetric, and diffuse inflammatory disease of unknown origin that begins in the rectum and extends proximally.

ANATOMIC FINDINGS

Colon
- Ulceration of the mucosa

IMAGING

Radiography
Findings
- Distal extent of formed fecal residue gives a good indication, although not absolute, of the proximal extent of the colitis.
- With progressive edema and hyperemia, the mucosa develops a granular pattern.
- Crypt abscesses: ulcers deepen, and barium flecks become adherent to them, producing mucosal stippling.
- Mucosal defect is small relative to the degree of undermining and produces a flask-like, *collar-button* ulcer.
- Polyps, pseudopolyps, widened presacral space, and strictures are seen.
- Chronic pancolitis is associated with a patulous and fixed ileocecal valve that easily refluxes with persistent dilation of the terminal ileum.
- Backwash ileitis, haustral folds are edematous, thickened or blunted, and completely lost.

DIAGNOSTIC PEARLS
- Mucosal defect that is small relative to the degree of undermining and produces a flask-like, *collar-button* ulcer
- Backwash ileitis usually occurs in patients with pancolitis.
- Mural changes that produce a *target* or *halo* appearance when axially imaged on CT or MR

Utility
- Barium enema confirms the clinical diagnosis and assesses the extent and severity of the disease.
- It can also differentiate ulcerative colitis from Crohn disease and other colitides; can follow the course of the disease; and can detect complications.

CT
Findings
- Inflammatory pseudopolyps are seen.
- Mural thickening and luminal narrowing are seen, as well as subacute and chronic ulcerative colitis.
- Mural changes produce a *target* or *halo* appearance when axially imaged.
- Rectal narrowing and widening of the presacral space are radiologic hallmarks of chronic ulcerative colitis.

WHAT THE REFERRING PHYSICIAN NEEDS TO KNOW

- Diagnosis is based on clinical symptoms and the presence of inflamed mucosa on colonoscopy and is confirmed by mucosal biopsy.
- Treatment depends on the severity, extent, and distribution of the disease.
- 5-ASA-based medications are effective in the treatment of acute ulcerative colitis and in reducing both the frequency and the severity of recurrent attacks.
- Corticosteroids are effective in patients with moderate to severe ulcerative colitis; topical hydrocortisone is the mainstay of therapy for distal proctocolitis.
- Azathioprine, 6-mercaptopurine, chloroquine, hydroxychloroquine sulfate (Plaquenil), methotrexate, infliximamib, and cyclosporine are alternative therapies in patients with refractory disease.
- Indications for surgery include massive or unremitting hemorrhage, toxic megacolon with perforation, fulminant colitis that is unresponsive to medical therapy, obstruction, and suspicion or demonstration of cancer.
- Proctocolectomy is always curative for ulcerative colitis.

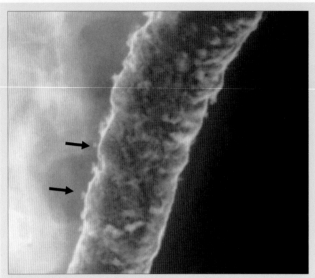

Figure 1. Ulcerative colitis: *collar-button* **ulcers.** Spot film of the splenic flexure shows multiple flask-like ulcers *(arrows)* with a flat base. The ulceration is limited to the layers superficial to the muscularis propria.

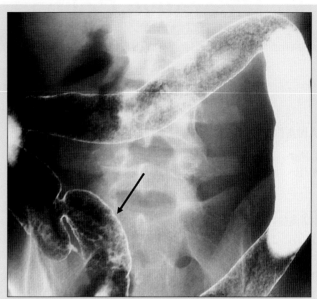

Figure 2. Ulcerative colitis: backwash ileitis. Backwash ileitis *(arrow)* is demonstrated in this patient with chronic ulcerative pancolitis.

Utility
- CT is helpful in determining the urgency of surgery in patients with stable abdominal radiographs yet with a deteriorating clinical course.

Ultrasound
Findings
- Thickening of the colon wall and preservation of wall stratification are seen.
- On transverse section, alternate hyperechoic and hypoechoic layers give rise to a *target* appearance.
- With progressive disease, haustral septations are lost.
Utility
- This technique is very operator-dependent and can be limited by large body habitus.

MRI
Findings
- Thickening and abnormal hypointensity of the mucosal and submucosal layers on T1-weighted and T2-weighted images
Utility
- MRI is capable of identifying the mural stratification present in ulcerative colitis.

Nuclear Medicine
Findings
- Increased leukocyte tracer uptake
Utility
- Scintigraphic techniques are useful when a danger of bowel perforation exists; they are also used for the assessment of disease extent and activity.

- PET scans and indium-111 (^{111}In)-labeled leukocyte scans are useful in patients with inflammatory bowel disease.

PET
Findings
- Tracer uptake is increased in areas of active inflammation resulting from hyperemia and increased metabolic activity.
Utility
- PET scanning using ^{18}F-fluorodeoxyglucose is used to assess disease activity and can monitor responses to therapy.

CLINICAL PRESENTATION
- Ulcerative colitis is highly variable in clinical course, severity, and prognosis; disease activity waxes and wanes.
- Acute exacerbations of bloody diarrhea are seen that resolve either spontaneously or after therapy.
- Diarrhea, abdominal pain, rectal bleeding, weight loss, and tenesmus may be seen; vomiting, fever, constipation, and arthralgias occur less commonly.
- Physical examination discloses fever, prostration, dehydration, and postural hypotension in the most severe cases.
- Protuberant abdomen may be seen because of colonic atony and distention.
- Abdominal tenderness over colon and absent bowel sounds are ominous signs suggesting toxic megacolon or early perforation.

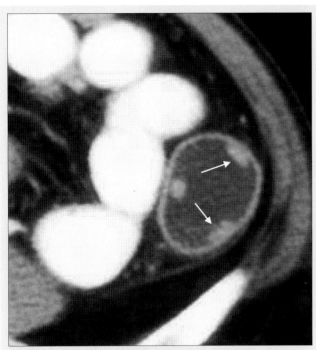

Figure 3. Mucosal disease in acute ulcerative colitis: CT features. Magnified CT image of the distal descending colon shows residual islands of inflamed mucosa protruding above the denuded colonic surface—so-called inflammatory pseudopolyps *(arrows)*. *(From Gore RM, Balthazar E, Ghahremani GG, et al: CT features of ulcerative colitis and Crohn's disease. AJR Am J Roentgenol 167:3-15, 1996. Reprinted with permission from the American Journal of Roentgenology.)*

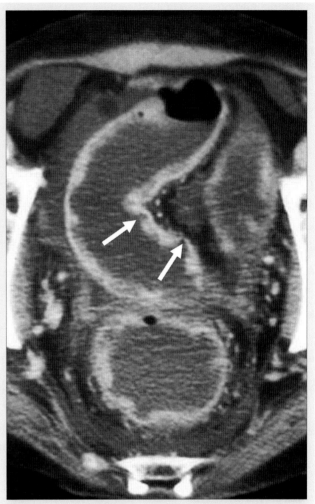

Figure 4. Mucosal disease in acute ulcerative colitis: CT features. Pelvic CT reveals diffuse mucosal thickening of the fluid-filled rectum and sigmoid. Deep ulcerations *(arrows)* are visualized. Note the normal lumen caliber and ascites. *(From Gore RM, Balthazar E, Ghahremani GG, et al: CT features of ulcerative colitis and Crohn's disease. AJR Am J Roentgenol 167:3-15, 1996. Reprinted with permission from the American Journal of Roentgenology.)*

- Patients with milder involvement exhibit pallor, low-grade fever, weight loss, and mild abdominal tenderness.

DIFFERENTIAL DIAGNOSIS

- Noninfectious colitis
- Crohn disease
- *Clostridium difficile* colitis
- Infectious colitis
- Ischemic colitis
- Radiation-induced colitis

PATHOLOGY

- Ulcerative colitis is a diffuse inflammatory disease of unknown origin involving primarily the colorectal mucosa but later extending to other layers of the bowel wall.
- Human leukocyte antigen (HLA) phenotypes B5, Bw52, and DR2 also have a significant association with ulcerative colitis.
- Ulcerative colitis is associated with autoimmune disorders, sacroiliitis, ankylosing spondylitis, enteropathic oligoarthritis, and anterior uveitis, which are associated with the HLA-B27 antigen.
- Signs include abnormal mucin production and intraluminal bacterial products, and toxins that attack the mucosa.

- Enteric nervous system and nerves containing substance P and vasoactive intestinal polypeptide become straight, thick, and highly immunoreactive.
- Alteration of the relative representation of macrophages and T-cell and B-cell populations is seen, as well as an increase in the numbers of immunoglobulin G–bearing cells.
- Also seen is activation of the arachidonic cascade with increased release of chemical mediators, superoxide radicals, prostaglandins, leukotrienes, and thromboxane.

INCIDENCE/PREVALENCE AND EPIDEMIOLOGY

- Annual incidence of 2-10 cases per 100,000 population has been documented; worldwide prevalence ranges from 35-100 cases per 100,000 population.
- Ulcerative colitis is most prevalent in the developed countries of northern Europe, Scandinavia, the British Isles, the United States, and Israel.
- Twofold to fourfold increase occurs among Jews; the incidence is lower in Sephardic than in Ashkenazi Jews in Israel.
- Peak age at onset is between 15 and 25 years, with a smaller peak at ages 55-65 years.
- Ulcerative colitis is more common than Crohn disease in children younger than 10 years and is more common in urban than rural populations.
- Incidence among first-degree relatives is 30-100 times greater than in the general population; 10%-20% of patients have a similarly affected first-degree relative.

- Mortality rate is 1 per 100,000 ages 20-29 years and 3-4 per 100,000 for ages 50-59 years.

Suggested Readings

Aburano T, Saito Y, Shuke N, et al: Tc-99m leukocyte imaging for evaluating disease severity and monitoring treatment response in ulcerative colitis: Comparison with colonoscopy. *Clin Nucl Med* 23:509-513, 1998.
Bartram CI: Radiology in the current assessment of ulcerative colitis. *Gastrointest Radiol* 1:383-392, 1977.
Caprilli R, Vernia P, Latella G, et al: Early recognition of toxic megacolon. *J Clin Gastroenterol* 9:160-164, 1987.
Gabrielsson N, Grandvist S, Sundelin P, et al: Extent of inflammatory lesions in ulcerative colitis assessed by radiology, colonoscopy, and endoscopic biopsies. *Gastrointest Radiol* 4:395-400, 1979.
Gore RM: Characteristic morphologic changes in chronic ulcerative colitis. *Abdom Imaging* 20:275-278, 1995.
Gore RM, Marn CS, Kirby DF, et al: CT findings in ulcerative, granulomatous, and indeterminate colitis. *AJR Am J Roentgenol* 143:279-284, 1984.
Laufer I: The radiologic demonstration of early changes in ulcerative colitis by double contrast techniques. *Can Assoc Radiol J* 26:116-121, 1975.
Laufer I, Mullens JE, Hamilton J: Correlation of endoscopy and double-contrast radiography in the early stages of ulcerative and granulomatous colitis. *Radiology* 118:15, 1988.
McConnell F, Hanelin J, Robbins LL: Plain film diagnosis of fulminating ulcerative colitis. *Radiology* 71:674-682, 1958.
Prantera C, Lorenzetti R, Cerro P, et al: The plain abdominal film accurately estimates extent of active ulcerative colitis. *J Clin Gastroenterol* 13:231-234, 1991.
Rice RP: Plain abdominal film roentgenographic diagnosis of ulcerative disease of the colon. *Radiology* 104:544-550, 1968.
Simpson SA, Lewis JR: Plain roentgenography in diagnosis of chronic ulcerative colitis and terminal ileitis. *Radiology* 84:306-315, 1960.
Suekane H, Iida M, Matsui T, et al: Radiographic demonstration of longitudinal ulcers in patients with ulcerative colitis. *Gastrointest Radiol* 4:103-112, 1980.

Part 32

OTHER INFLAMMATORY CONDITIONS OF THE COLON

Bacterial Infections

DEFINITION: Infection of the colon caused by bacterial organisms.

IMAGING

Radiography
Findings
- *Salmonella typhi* or *S. paratyphi* produces narrowing, loss of haustrations in the cecum, and aphthoid ulcers in the ascending colon.
- *Shigella* spp. produce predominantly left-sided colitis with deep ulcers that have a collar-button appearance; aphthoid ulcers may also be seen.
- *Campylobacter* spp. produce pancolitis with diffuse granularity, loss of haustration (simulating ulcerative colitis), and aphthous ulcers resembling Crohn disease.
- *Yersinia enterocolitica* produces aphthous ulcers located predominantly in the right side of the colon.
- *Escherichia coli* (O157:H7) produces effects similar to those of ischemic colitis, with thumbprinting, narrowing, and spasm of involved tissue.
- Tuberculosis mimics Crohn disease: loss of ileum-colon anatomic demarcation (Stierlin's sign) and right-angle intersection between the ileum and the cecum (Fleischner's sign).
- *Actinomyces israelii* produces extrinsic masses, reactive changes, distortion, and strictures with or without fistula formation.

Utility
- Single- and double-contrast studies may be performed if stool cultures yield negative results.
- This technique has largely been replaced by colonoscopy.

CT
Findings
- *E. coli* (O157:H7) causes low-density thickening of the wall as a result of edema.
- Tuberculosis causes markedly enlarged low-density lymph nodes, ascites, narrowing, deep ulceration, and mucosal granulation with nodularity and inflammatory polyps.
- *A. israelii* causes large inflammatory masses.

DIAGNOSTIC PEARLS
- Ulceration, signs of inflammation, and loss of haustration may occur.
- Lymphadenopathy and ischemic bowel signs may occur.
- Diagnosis is readily established with routine stool cultures.
- Typical presentation of acute onset of dysenteric symptoms is seen, consisting of fever, crampy abdominal pain and tenderness (with or without vomiting), tenesmus, and small-volume diarrhea (frequently bloody).

Utility
- CT is now the most common noninvasive imaging test in evaluating patients with known or suspected enterocolitis.

CLINICAL PRESENTATION
- Patient exhibits acute onset of dysenteric symptoms.
- Fever and crampy abdominal pain and tenderness, with or without vomiting, tenesmus, and diarrhea (usually bloody) are noted.
- In campylobacteriosis, the patient may have a 24-hour prodrome consisting of headaches, nausea and vomiting, and arthralgias.
- With *Yersinia* enterocolitis, the patient may have rashes such as erythema nodosum or erythema multiforme.
- In colitis caused by *E. coli,* symptoms may progress over several days to hemorrhagic colitis.
- Chronic symptoms such as weight loss may be seen in tuberculosis.
- Palpable mass may develop in actinomycosis.

WHAT THE REFERRING PHYSICIAN NEEDS TO KNOW
- Imaging studies are not usually performed for patients with bacterial colitis because the diagnosis is readily established with routine stool cultures.
- Routine cultures occasionally yield false-negative results; therefore specialized cultures are required; in this setting, imaging may be of use.
- In patients with toxic megacolon, antispasmodics are contraindicated because they may aggravate the patient's condition.

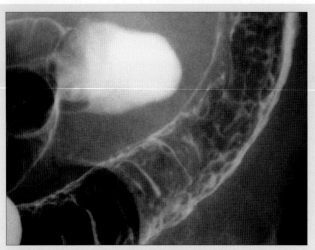

Figure 1. *Shigella* **colitis.** Ulcerations of the sigmoid colon are present on double-contrast barium enema.

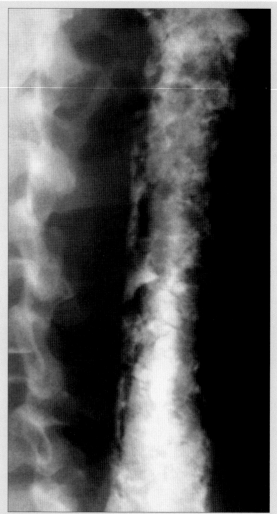

Figure 2. **Colitis caused by** *E. coli* **O157:H7.** Deep ulcerations are identified in the descending colon.

DIFFERENTIAL DIAGNOSIS

- Crohn disease
- Ulcerative colitis
- Ischemic colitis
- Radiation colitis
- Collagenous colitis
- Drug-induced colitis
- Behçet disease
- Tuberculous colitis

PATHOLOGY

- Causative organisms include *Salmonella* serotypes, *Campylobacter fetus* ssp. *jejuni*, *Y. enterocolitica*, *E. coli* subtype O157:H7, tuberculosis, and *A. israelii.*

- Actinomycosis: Contact with tissues not normally exposed (through trauma, intrauterine devices) to the organism results in an infection.
- *E. coli*: Changes are caused predominantly by ischemia; histologic specimens may resemble pseudomembranous colitis.

INCIDENCE/PREVALENCE AND EPIDEMIOLOGY

- Hemorrhage and perforation occur in 1%-3% of salmonellosis cases.
- Mortality rate is 10%-20% in immunocompromised patients or in patients with bacteremia caused by shigellosis.

- Campylobacteriosis is the most common cause of bacterial colitis.
- *E. coli* O157:H7 colitis mortality rate is as high as 33%.
- Most reported cases involve the transverse colon.

Suggested Readings

Grundy A, Gilks CF: Typhoid: An unusual cause of gastrointestinal bleeding. *Br J Radiol* 57:344-346, 1984.
Nakamura S, Iida M, Tominaga M, et al: *Salmonella* colitis: Assessment with double-contrast barium enema examination in seven patients. *Radiology* 184:537-540, 1992.
Saffouri B, Bartolomeo RS, Fuchs B: Colonic involvement in salmonellosis. *Dig Dis Sci* 24:203-208, 1979.
Speelman P, Kabir I, Islam M: Distribution and spread of colonic lesions in shigellosis: A colonoscopic study. *J Infect* 150:899-903, 1984.
Tedesco FJ, Hardin RD, Harper RN, et al: Infectious colitis endoscopically simulating inflammatory bowel disease: A prospective evaluation. *Gastrointest Endosc* 29:195-197, 1983.
Vender RJ, Marignani P: *Salmonella* colitis presenting as a segmental colitis resembling Crohn's disease. *Dig Dis Sci* 28:848-851, 1983.

Parasitic Infections

DEFINITION: Parasitic infections of the colon include amebiasis, anisakiasis, schistosomiasis, strongyloidiasis, and trichuriasis.

IMAGING

Radiography
Findings
- Anisakiasis: segmental thumbprinting; actual larvae appearing as thin, linear filling defects 12-20 mm long and 0.7 mm wide
- Amebiasis: skip lesions, ameboma, deep ulcers, bowel wall edema, discrete ulcers appearing as marginal defects, and granularity with barium flecks
- Ascariasis: numerous smooth, tubular filling defects in the barium column
- Schistosomiasis: inflammatory polyps, narrowing, loss of haustration, and ulceration
- Strongyloidiasis: diffuse ulcerative colitis, aphthous ulcers, fistulas, and sinus tracts; also markedly thickened folds in several loops of the jejunum
- Trichuriasis: clumping, granularity; worms identified as wavy, linear lucencies 3-5 cm in length, terminating in the ring with central barium collection

Utility
- Colonoscopy has replaced barium studies in the evaluation of parasitic infections of the colon.

CT
Findings
- Calcification of the bowel wall or liver, which is most often associated with *Schistosoma haematobium* but also with *Schistosoma japonicum*

Utility
- CT is particularly sensitive to changes in bowels caused by schistosomiasis involvement.

CLINICAL PRESENTATION

- Abdominal pain, fever, nausea and vomiting, diarrhea, and bleeding
- Schistosomiasis: usually bloody diarrhea but also possibly chronic abdominal pain, intermittent diarrhea, and palpable abdominal mass

DIAGNOSTIC PEARLS

- Diagnosis of anisakiasis can be suggested when double-contrast barium enemas show the actual larvae as thin, linear filling defects.
- Diagnosis of amebiasis is usually established by the presence of trophozoites in the stool or on a rectal smear.
- Hallmark of schistosomiasis is the presence of inflammatory polyps as a result of granulation reaction to the deposition of eggs in the bowel wall.
- Diagnosis of strongyloidiasis requires the identification of the cysts, larvae, or both, in the stool.
- *Trichuris trichiura* are identified as wavy, linear lucencies 3-5 cm in length, sometimes terminating in a ring shape with central barium collection.

- Trichuriasis: bleeding, anemia, diarrhea, malaise, cramps; also commonly intussusception and rectal prolapse

DIFFERENTIAL DIAGNOSIS

- Ulcerative colitis
- Crohn disease
- Ischemic colitis
- Behçet disease
- Pyogenic infectious colitis

PATHOLOGY

- *T. trichiura* invades the bowel mucosa, then causes intussusception and rectal prolapse.
- *Strongyloides stercoralis* penetrates the skin, spreads to the lungs, and is subsequently ingested, which

---

WHAT THE REFERRING PHYSICIAN NEEDS TO KNOW

- Imaging studies have a role in assessing severity, in monitoring the course of the disease, and in determining the presence of complications.
- Anisakiasis: Serologic studies may be performed to confirm the diagnosis.
- Diagnosis of amebiasis is usually established by the presence of trophozoites in the stool or on rectal smear.
- Serologic studies for amebae are also quite sensitive.
- When amebiasis is suspected, trial therapy may be warranted even if the diagnosis is not confirmed.
- Schistosomiasis: The diagnosis can be established by demonstrating the eggs in biopsy specimens or in the stool.
- Strongyloidiasis: Diagnosis requires identification of cysts, larvae, or both, in the stool.

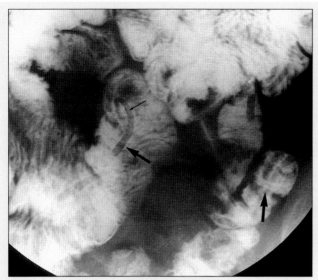

Figure 1. **Ascariasis: a young man with crampy abdominal pain and mild diarrhea 1 month after returning from a vacation in Central America.** Spot image of the ileum from a small bowel follow-through shows numerous smooth, tubular filling defects in the barium column (representative ascarids identified by thick arrows). Barium faintly opacifies the body cavity of one worm *(thin arrow)*. *(From Forbes A, Misiewicz JJ, Comptom CC, et al: Atlas of Clinical Gastroenterology, 3rd ed. Edinburgh, Elsevier-Mosby, 2005.)*

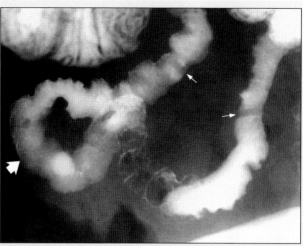

Figure 2. **Strongyloidiasis.** Coned-down view of overhead radiograph from a small bowel follow-through shows markedly thickened folds *(thin arrows)* in several loops of jejunum. In some areas, the inflammatory process is so severe that the folds are effaced or lost *(thick arrow)*. *(Courtesy of Jack Farman, MD, New York; from the teaching files of Hans Herlinger, MD.)*

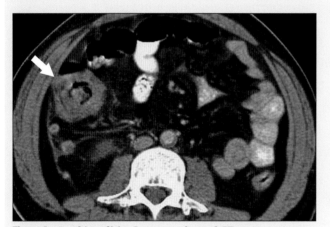

Figure 3. **Amebic colitis.** Contrast-enhanced CT scan illustrates concentric wall thickening involving the right colon *(arrow)*. *(From Restrepo CS, Raut AA, Riascos R, et al: Imaging manifestations of tropical parasitic infections. Semin Roentgenol 42:37-48, 2007.)*

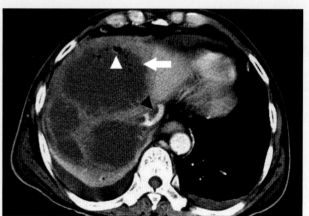

Figure 4. **Multiple amebic liver abscesses.** Contrast-enhanced CT scan demonstrates multiple hepatic abscesses *(white arrow)* with associated nonocclusive thrombosis involving the inferior vena cava *(black arrowhead)*. Presence of gas *(white arrowhead)* within the fluid collection is pathognomic of an abscess. *(From Restrepo CS, Raut AA, Riascos R, et al: Imaging manifestations of tropical parasitic infections. Semin Roentgenol 42:37-48, 2007.)*

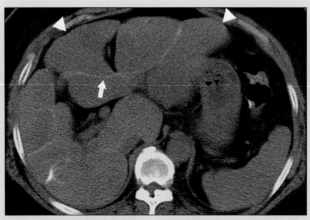

Figure 5. Hepatic schistosomiasis. Noncontrast CT scan shows the characteristic *tortoise-shell* appearance of the liver *(arrowheads)* and septal calcifications *(arrow)*. (*From Restrepo CS, Raut AA, Riascos R, et al: Imaging manifestations of tropical parasitic infections.* Semin Roentgenol *42:37-48, 2007.*)

involves the stomach, duodenum, and proximal small bowel, and a host-parasite relationship ensues.

- Amebiasis: The cyst is ingested then becomes an invasive trophozoite, causing ameboma and ulcers in the colon.
- Schistosomiasis: The larva penetrates the skin, matures in the liver, and migrates to the colon, causing granulation reaction to the eggs in the bowel wall.

INCIDENCE/PREVALENCE AND EPIDEMIOLOGY

- 20% of world's population harbors amebae.
- *Schistosoma mansoni* is found in the United States, Puerto Rico, and in the tropics.
- *S. haematobium* is found in Africa and southern Asia.

- *T. trichiura* involves predominantly children in tropical areas.
- In underdeveloped countries, parasitic infestation is the frequent form of colonic infection.

Suggested Readings

Cevallos AM, Farthing MJG: Parasitic infections of the gastrointestinal tract. *Curr Opin Gastroenterol* 9:96-102, 1993.

Dallemand S, Waxman M, Farman J: Radiological manifestations of *Strongyloides stercoralis. Gastrointest Radiol* 8:45-51, 1983.

Kolawole TM, Lewis EA: Radiologic observations on intestinal amebiasis. *AJR Am J Roentgenol* 122:257-265, 1974.

Matsui T, Iida M, Murakami M, et al: Intestinal anisakiasis: Clinical and radiologic features. *Radiology* 157:299-302, 1985.

Medina JT, Seaman WB, Guzman-Acosta C, et al: The roentgen appearance of *Schistosoma mansoni* involving the colon. *Radiology* 85:682-688, 1965.

Viral Infections

DEFINITION: Colon inflammation caused by a virus, usually cytomegalovirus (CMV), in patients with AIDS.

ANATOMIC FINDINGS

Colon
- Inflammation often involves the cecum and proximal colon.

IMAGING

Radiography
Findings
- Multifocal ulcerations appearing as shallow, well-defined ulcers scattered on otherwise normal background mucosa
- Deeper ulcers and marked thickening of the colonic wall
- Pancolitis with diffuse, contiguous involvement of the bowel

Utility
- Colonoscopy has replaced barium studies in the evaluation of the colonic mucosa in patients with known or suspected viral infection.

CT
Findings
- Deeper ulcers and marked thickening of the colonic wall
- Enhancement of the mucosa and serosa with hypodense thickening of the intervening bowel wall caused by edema
- In severe disease, possible increased attenuation, reflecting a hemorrhagic component

Utility
- CT is used to detect complications, associated adenopathy, and abdominal masses

CLINICAL PRESENTATION

- Hemorrhage
- Diarrhea
- Abdominal pain
- Weight loss, fatigue, malaise, myalgias, and rigors

DIAGNOSTIC PEARLS

- Patient exhibits multifocal ulcerations appearing as shallow, well-defined ulcers scattered on otherwise normal background mucosa.
- Also seen is enhancement of the mucosa and serosa, with hypodense thickening of the intervening bowel wall caused by edema.
- CMV colitis usually involves the cecum, proximal colon, and distal ileum.
- Diagnosis can be confirmed by the presence of characteristic viral inclusion bodies on endoscopic brushings or biopsy specimens.

DIFFERENTIAL DIAGNOSIS

- Ulcerative colitis
- Crohn disease
- Bacterial infectious colitis
- Ischemic colitis
- Parasitic colitis
- Tuberculous colitis
- Behçet disease

PATHOLOGY

- CMV-induced ischemic vasculitis causes gastrointestinal abnormalities such as colitis.

INCIDENCE/PREVALENCE AND EPIDEMIOLOGY

- CMV infection is a frequent complication of AIDS.

Suggested Readings

Balthazar EJ, Megibow AJ, Fazzini E: Cytomegalovirus colitis in AIDS: Radiographic findings in 11 patients. *Radiology* 155:585-589, 1985.
Thoeni RF, Cello JP: CT imaging of colitis. *Radiology* 240:623-638, 2006.

WHAT THE REFERRING PHYSICIAN NEEDS TO KNOW

- Increased attenuation in CT scan reflects hemorrhage, which can be fatal in patients with AIDS.
- Diagnosis can be confirmed by the presence of characteristic intranuclear inclusions (viral inclusion bodies) on endoscopic brushings or biopsy specimens.

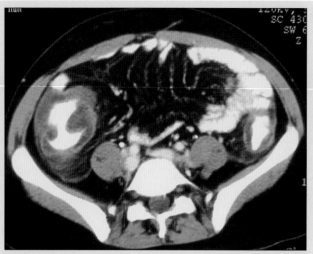

Figure 1. Cytomegalovirus (CMV) colitis. Enhanced CT scan of the pelvis demonstrates marked mural thickening of the ascending colon in this patient with AIDS and CMV colitis. Note the edematous low-density wall with enhancement of the mucosa and serosa.

Noninfectious Colitis

DEFINITION: Inflammation of colon from noninfectious causes, including nonspecific colonic ulcer, microscopic colitis, eosinophilic colitis, graft-versus-host disease (GVHD), retractile mesenteritis, and reactive inflammation.

ANATOMIC FINDINGS

Colon
- Nonspecific ulcer: the majority of ulcers are on the right colon near the ileocecal valve on the antimesenteric border; 20% are multiple.
- Retractile mesenteritis: the sigmoid colon and transverse colon are most likely to be involved because of the intimate relationship to the mesentery.

Cecum
- Typhlitis (neutropenic colitis confined to the cecum): diffuse hyperemia, edema, and superficial ulceration

IMAGING

Radiography
Findings
- Nonspecific ulcer: barium enema finding of a focal mass, with or without ulceration, and, occasionally, a short stricture (segmental colitis)
- Nonspecific ulcer: inflammatory surface abnormalities predominantly in the rectosigmoid region
- Eosinophilic colitis: primary findings on barium study revealing thumbprinting, spasm, and narrowing
- GVHD: mural fold thickening, loss of mucosal features (*ribbon bowel*), nonspecific colitis, and a granular surface pattern
- Retractile mesenteritis: long segments of narrowing, thumbprinting, strictures, and extrinsic masses with reactive changes on the contiguous bowel margin
- Reactive inflammation: area involved depending on primary diseased organ; extrinsic mass effect, reactive spiculation, and concentric narrowing

DIAGNOSTIC PEARLS
- Nonspecific ulcer occurs in the antimesenteric border and is suspected if biopsy results are negative for other causes.
- Neutropenic colitis is confined to the right side of the colon, specifically the cecum, and develops in immunocompromised patients.
- Microscopic collagenous colitis occurs in elderly women with a history of intermittent or chronic watery diarrhea, usually with normal diagnostic and laboratory studies.
- Eosinophilic colitis involves the stomach or small bowel, the right side of the colon with thumbprinting, and spasm and narrowing on barium study.
- GVHD produces a ribbon-like appearance of the bowel and nonspecific colitis.
- Retractile mesenteritis usually involves the mesenteric fat of the small intestine seen as long-segment narrowing, thumbprinting, strictures, or extrinsic masses on barium study.
- Site of reactive inflammation in the colon correlates with the site of primary inflammatory processes from other organs and with variable appearance.

Utility
- Microscopic colitis: barium enema is generally considered incapable of detecting changes of microscopic colitis.
- Colonoscopy has replaced barium studies in the evaluation of patients with known or suspected noninfectious colitis.

WHAT THE REFERRING PHYSICIAN NEEDS TO KNOW
- Colonoscopic findings of neutropenic enterocolitis are difficult to distinguish from idiopathic ulcerative colitis and infectious colitis, except for the location.
- Prompt diagnosis of neutropenic enterocolitis, supportive therapy with broad-spectrum (including antifungal) antibiotics, and supplemental nutrition are necessary to prevent necrosis and perforation.
- Nonspecific ulcer is rarely diagnosed preoperatively, but it may be suspected when the ulcer is seen at colonoscopy and biopsy results are negative for other causes.
- GVHD or viral infection (or both conditions combined) is indistinguishable on colonoscopy and imaging.
- In retractile mesenteritis, surgery is often performed to relieve obstructive symptoms, but corticosteroid therapy may also be beneficial.
- In microscopic (collagenous) colitis, laboratory studies and diagnostic procedures, including endoscopy, are usually normal.

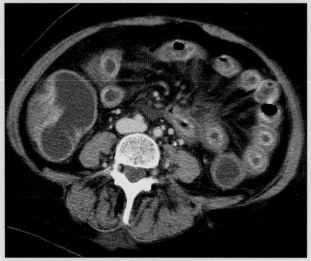

Figure 1. Graft-versus-host disease. Axial contrast-enhanced scan shows edema in the mesentery, small- and large-bowel wall thickening, and mucosal and serosal enhancement.

CT

Findings
- Nonspecific ulcer: colonic mass with mesenteric stranding
- GVHD: edema in the mesentery, bowel wall thickening, and mucosal and serosal enhancement
- Retractile mesenteritis: markedly increased density in the mesentery with or without discrete and fibrotic soft-tissue masses
- Mural thickening with or without loss of mural stratification

Utility
- CT can depict the mural changes and extramural complications of these colitides.
- CT scan combined with appropriate laboratory studies may allow an accurate diagnosis.

Ultrasound

Findings
- Mural thickening of the involved colon with or without loss of mural stratification

Utility
- CT more reliably depicts the mural changes of these colitides than does ultrasound.

CLINICAL PRESENTATION

- Nonspecific ulcer produces a clinical presentation that can mimic that of appendicitis or even carcinoma.
- Typhlitis produces fever, right lower quadrant pain, and diarrhea.
- Microscopic (collagenous) colitis is characterized by a history of variable (but usually long) duration, intermittent, or chronic watery diarrhea.
- Retractile mesenteritis symptoms include abdominal pain, diarrhea, and weight loss.

DIFFERENTIAL DIAGNOSIS

- Ulcerative colitis
- *Clostridium difficile* colitis
- Viral infections
- Crohn disease
- Infectious colitis
- Ischemic colitis
- Radiation colitis
- Behçet disease

PATHOLOGY

- Reactive inflammation may occur in the colon as a result of the extension of primary inflammatory processes from other organs or from adjacent abscesses.
- In retractile mesenteritis, autoimmune factors cause inflammatory and fibrotic pathologic changes in the mesenteric fat, which can extend to the intestinal wall.
- In GVHD, donor immune cells may recognize host tissue as foreign cells, and thus attack it.
- Infection has an important role in neutropenic colitis (typhlitis).
- Microscopic (collagenous) colitis causes increased lymphocytes in the surface epithelium; in variant collagenous colitis, the width of the subepithelial collagen band increases.
- In eosinophilic gastroenteritis, ascites is common, and peripheral eosinophilia is usually present.

INCIDENCE/PREVALENCE AND EPIDEMIOLOGY

- Microscopic colitis occurs predominantly in middle-aged and elderly women.

■ Retractile mesenteritis: the patient's age may range from the second to the eighth decade of life, with slight male predominance.

■ Neutropenic colitis develops in profoundly immunocompromised patients, especially patients with leukemia, acquired immunodeficiency syndrome, profound neutropenia caused by chemotherapy, and transplantation.

Suggested Readings

Abramson SJ, Berdon WE, Baker DH: Childhood typhlitis: Its increasing association with acute myelogenous leukemia. *Radiology* 146:61-64, 1983.

Brodey PA, Hill RP, Baron S: Benign ulceration of the cecum. *Radiology* 122:323-327, 1977.

Feczko PJ, Mezwa DG: Nonspecific radiographic abnormalities in collagenous colitis. *Gastrointest Radiol* 16:128-132, 1991.

Frick MP, Maile CW, Crass JR, et al: Computed tomography of neutropenic colitis. *AJR Am J Roentgenol* 143:763-765, 1984.

Gardiner GA, Bird CR: Nonspecific ulcers of the colon resembling annular carcinoma. *Radiology* 137:331-334, 1980.

Glick SN, Teplick SK, Amenta PS: Microscopic (collagenous) colitis. *AJR Am J Roentgenol* 153:995-996, 1989.

Han SY, Koehler RE, Keller FS, et al: Retractile mesenteritis involving the colon: Pathologic and radiologic correlation. *AJR Am J Roentgenol* 147:268-270, 1986.

Kalantari BN, Mortele KJ, Cantisani V, et al: CT features with pathologic correlation of acute gastrointestinal graft-versus-host disease after bone marrow transplantation in adults. *AJR Am J Roentgenol* 181:1621-1625, 2003.

MacCarty RL, Talley NJ: Barium studies in diffuse eosinophilic gastroenteritis. *Gastrointest Radiol* 15:183-187, 1990.

Periz-Fontan FJ, Soler R, Sanchez J, et al: Retractile mesenteritis involving the colon: Barium enema, sonographic, and CT findings. *AJR Am J Roentgenol* 147:937-940, 1986.

Thompson GT, Fitzgerald EF, Somers SS: Retractile mesenteritis of the sigmoid colon. *Br J Radiol* 58:266-267, 1985.

Clostridium difficile Colitis

DEFINITION: Exposure to and colonization by *Clostridium difficile*, causing colonic damage.

ANATOMIC FINDINGS

Colon
- Inflammatory changes in the superficial epithelium
- Necrosis of full thickness of the mucosa with formation of the pseudomembrane
- Ulcers

IMAGING

CT
Findings
- Marked low-density mural thickening with swollen haustra projecting into the lumen between the thin streaks of contrast medium

Utility
- Images may be obtained as an initial diagnostic test to rule out abscess.

Radiography
Findings
- In severe cases, plain-film radiography shows massive thumbprinting throughout the colon, sometimes associated with a shaggy margin.
- Megacolon can be rarely seen.
- Double-contrast studies reveal small, subtly elevated, round nodules or a small, irregular, plaque-like filling.
- Single-contrast studies reveal coarse polypoid defects or shaggy marginal irregularities in advanced cases.

Utility
- Contrast enema is contraindicated in patients with megacolon or severe colitis.
- Has been replaced primarily by colonoscopy

CLINICAL PRESENTATION

- Watery diarrhea, fever, abdominal tenderness, and leukocytosis are seen.
- Onset usually occurs within 2 days to 2 weeks after the start of antibiotic therapy.
- Some symptoms may develop 8 weeks after the discontinuation of antibiotic therapy.

DIAGNOSTIC PEARLS

- Marked low-density mural thickening with swollen haustra projecting into the lumen between the thin streaks of the contrast medium is seen.
- In severe cases, plain-film radiography shows massive thumbprinting throughout the colon, sometimes associated with a shaggy margin.
- Double-contrast studies reveal small, subtly elevated, round nodules or a small, irregular plaque-like filling.
- Megacolon can rarely be seen.

DIFFERENTIAL DIAGNOSIS

- Noninfectious colitis
- Ulcerative colitis
- Crohn disease
- Other infectious colitides
- Ischemic colitis
- Collagenous colitis
- Behçet disease

PATHOLOGY

- Antibiotics disturb normal colonic microflora.
- Normal colonic microflora disturbance leads to *C. difficile* colonization, the production of toxin and toxin-mediated inflammation and injury, and colonic damage.
- Colitis is pancolonic in the majority of patients, but some may have the disease confined to the right colon or, less commonly, the left side of the colon.

INCIDENCE/PREVALENCE AND EPIDEMIOLOGY

- *C. difficile* colitis may occur in immunosuppressed patients.

WHAT THE REFERRING PHYSICIAN NEEDS TO KNOW

- Discontinuation of the causative drug is often sufficient treatment.
- Vancomycin is the treatment of choice for patients with more severe disease.

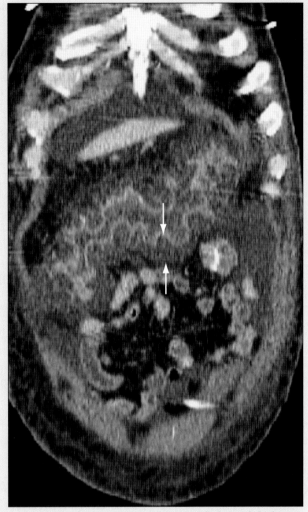

Figure 1. *C. difficile* **colitis: CT features.** Coronal reformatted image shows marked mural thickening *(arrows)* of the transverse colon with enhancing mucosa and submucosal edema. A small amount of intraperitoneal fluid is also present.

- As many as 20% of asymptomatic hospitalized patients are found to have *C. difficile.*
- Many patients are hospitalized and have had recent surgery.
- In approximately 40% of cases, the rectum is normal or harbors nonspecific changes on proctosigmoidoscopy.
- Relapses have been reported in 10%-39% of treated patients.

Suggested Readings

Ash L, Baker ME, O'Malley CM Jr, et al: Colonic abnormalities on CT in adult hospitalized patients with *Clostridium difficile* colitis: Prevalence and significance of findings. *AJR Am J Roentgenol* 186:1393-1400, 2006.

Cho KJ, Ting YM, Chuang VP, et al: Roentgenographic features in antibiotic-associated pseudomembranous colitis. *Australas Radiol* 20:38-41, 1976.

Fishman EK, Kavuru M, Jones B, et al: Pseudomembranous colitis: CT evaluation of 26 cases. *Radiology* 180:57-60, 1991.

Gerding DN, Olson MM, Peterson LR, et al: *Clostridium difficile*–associated diarrhea and colitis in adults. *Arch Intern Med* 146:95-100, 1986.

Kirkpatrick ID, Greenberg HM: Gastrointestinal complications in the neutropenic patient: Characterization and differentiation with abdominal CT. *Radiology* 226:668-674, 2003.

Stanley RJ, Melson GL, Tedesco FJ: The spectrum of radiographic findings in antibiotic-related pseudomembranous colitis. *Radiology* 111:519-524, 1974.

Strada M, Meregaglia D, Donzelli R: Double-contrast enema in antibiotic-related pseudomembranous colitis. *Gastrointest Radiol* 8:67-69, 1983.

Drug-Induced Colitis

DEFINITION: Inflammation of the colon caused by pharmaceutical agents.

ANATOMIC FINDINGS

Colon
- Diffuse or segmental colitis is seen.
- Any segment of the colon can be involved but more commonly the cecum.

IMAGING

CT
Findings
- Mural thickening of the colon
- Submucosal edema
- Inflammatory changes in adjacent fat
- Intraperitoneal fluid

Utility
- CT is useful in diagnosing complications of the colitis, such as perforation, pneumatosis, or obstruction.

Radiography
Findings
- Diffuse or segmental colitis to scattered discrete ulcers involving any segment of the colon, particularly the cecum

Utility
- Barium studies have been replaced by colonoscopy to directly inspect the colonic mucosa.

CLINICAL PRESENTATION

- Diarrhea
- Hematochezia
- Abdominal pain
- Sepsis

DIFFERENTIAL DIAGNOSIS

- Ulcerative colitis
- Crohn disease
- Ischemic colitis
- Radiation colitis
- Collagenous colitis
- Infectious colitis
- Behçet disease

DIAGNOSTIC PEARLS

- Diffuse or segmental colitis produces scattered ulcers involving any segment of colon, particularly the cecum.
- Vasoconstrictive drugs, antihypertensive medications, and oral contraceptives may cause ischemia-related inflammation.
- Penicillin, ampicillin, amoxicillin, and erythromycin cause right-sided hemorrhagic colitis that subsides spontaneously when these antibiotics are withdrawn.

PATHOLOGY

- Cancer chemotherapeutic agents cause an inhibitory effect on mucosal epithelial cells, resulting in ulceration and inflammation.
- Drug-induced neutropenia may result in typhlitis.
- Vasoconstrictive drugs, antihypertensive medications, and oral contraceptives may cause ischemia-related inflammation.
- Hypersensitivity reaction may occur.
- Right-sided hemorrhagic colitis subsides spontaneously when antibiotics such as penicillin, ampicillin, amoxicillin, and erythromycin are withdrawn.
- Inhibition of prostaglandin synthesis by nonsteroidal anti-inflammatory drugs causes colonic injury.

INCIDENCE/PREVALENCE AND EPIDEMIOLOGY

- Drug-induced colitis is seen in patients undergoing chemotherapy and those taking vasoconstrictive drugs, antihypertensive medications and oral contraceptives, antibiotics, and nonsteroidal anti-inflammatory drugs.

Suggested Readings

Fortson WC, Tedesco FJ: Drug-induced colitis: A review. *Am J Gastroenterol* 79:878-883, 1984.

Gerding DN, Olson MM, Peterson LR, et al: *Clostridium difficile*–associated diarrhea and colitis in adults. *Arch Intern Med* 146: 95-100, 1986.

Gibson GR, Whitacre EB, Ricotti CA: Colitis induced by nonsteroidal anti-inflammatory drugs. *Arch Intern Med* 152:625-632, 1992.

WHAT THE REFERRING PHYSICIAN NEEDS TO KNOW

- Imaging findings combined with the patient's history, symptoms, and laboratory and pathologic findings help narrow the diagnostic possibilities.
- Imaging studies may have a role in assessing the severity, in monitoring the course of disease, and in determining complications.

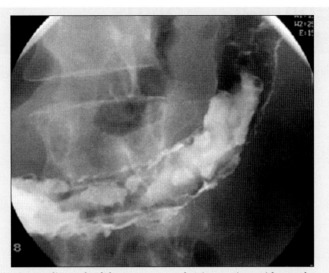

Figure 1. Pseudomembranous colitis. Spot radiograph of the transverse colon in a patient with pseudomembranous colitis caused by overgrowth of *C. difficile* secondary to antibiotics administered for a sinus infection 10 days before this barium enema examination.

Benign Epithelial Polyps

DEFINITION: Polyp refers to a focal, protruded lesion within the bowel, which may be neoplastic or non-neoplastic.

ANATOMIC FINDINGS

Colon
- Polypoid masses

Rectum
- Polypoid masses

IMAGING

Radiography
Findings
- Radiolucent filling defect
- Contour defect
- Ring shadow
- *Bowler hat sign* and *Mexican hat sign*
- Reticular or granular mucosal surface seen with villous adenomas
- Large villous adenoma: large, bulky polypoid mass with barium caught between frond-like protrusions, producing a lacy surface pattern
- Carpet lesion: a flat, lobulated lesion characterized primarily by an alteration in the bowel surface texture

Utility
- Barium enema

CT
Findings
- Sessile soft-tissue masses that protrude into bowel lumen
- Large polypoid mass representing the combined polyp and stalk
- Villous adenomas: homogeneous water density occupying more than one half of lesion, with eccentric location on luminal side of mass

Utility
- CT colonography is increasingly used as a means of diagnosing colorectal polyps and cancers.
- CT can also be used as the initial noninvasive means of staging colorectal cancer.

DIAGNOSTIC PEARLS
- Large villous adenomas are large, bulky, polypoid masses with barium caught between the frond-like protrusions, producing a lacy surface pattern.
- *Bowler hat sign* and *Mexican hat sign* are sometimes seen.
- Villous adenomas are characterized on CT by homogeneous water density occupying more than one half of the lesion, with eccentric location on the luminal side of the mass.
- Sessile soft-tissue masses that protrude into the bowel lumen

MRI
Findings
- Low-intensity structures on T1-weighted images

Utility
- T1-weighted spin-echo sequences are obtained.
- Intensity increases as the mucin content increases.

Ultrasound
Findings
- Ultrasound demonstrates the depth of invasion by a sessile mass.

Utility
- Transrectal ultrasound (TRUS) is performed for assessing the depth of mural involvement of sessile rectal polyps.
- TRUS is the easiest imaging technique for showing the various layers of the colonic wall.
- TRUS can suggest adenopathy in normal-sized nodes.

CLINICAL PRESENTATION
- Polyps usually do not cause symptoms.
- Some patients may present with signs of acute or chronic gastrointestinal bleeding.

WHAT THE REFERRING PHYSICIAN NEEDS TO KNOW
- Risk of carcinoma is related to the amount of villous change in the adenoma and its size.
- Multidetector CT (MDCT) is the gold standard for staging colon cancer.
- TRUS is used to assess the depth of polyp invasion and the presence of adenopathy.

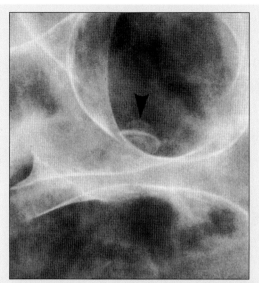

Figure 1. Colonic polyp with a bowler hat sign on a double-contrast barium enema. Note how the head of the polyp or dome of the hat (*arrowhead*) points toward the lumen in this patient with a sessile polyp viewed obliquely on a double-contrast radiograph. (*From Laufer I, Levine MS [eds]: Double-Contrast Gastrointestinal Radiology, 3rd ed. Philadelphia, WB Saunders, 2000.*)

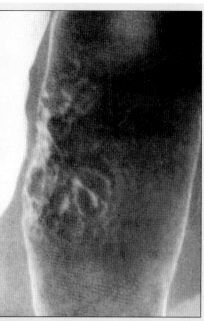

Figure 2. Villous adenoma. A flat tumor in the descending colon with an irregular surface suggestive of a villous adenoma. This was a villous polyp. (*From Laufer I, Levine MS [eds]: Double-Contrast Gastrointestinal Radiology, 3rd ed. Philadelphia, WB Saunders, 2000.*)

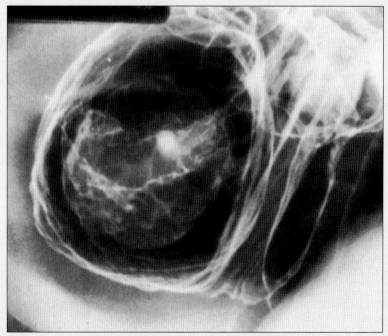

Figure 3. Villous adenoma. Typical villous tumor in the sigmoid colon. This tumor exhibits the typical, irregular, frond-like surface of a villous tumor. It was a malignant villous adenoma. (*From Laufer I, Levine MS [eds]: Double Contrast Gastrointestinal Radiology, 3rd ed. Philadelphia, WB Saunders, 2000.*)

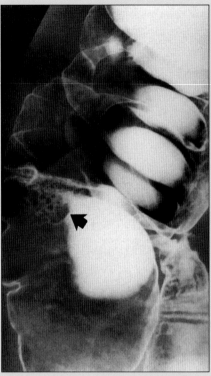

Figure 4. Carpet lesion. Typical carpet lesion *(arrow)* in the cecum manifested by confluent nodularity of the mucosa without a discrete mass. Carpet lesions are almost always villous adenocarcinomas. *(From Laufer I, Levine MS [eds]: Double Contrast Gastrointestinal Radiology, 3rd ed. Philadelphia, WB Saunders, 2000.)*

DIFFERENTIAL DIAGNOSIS

■ Carcinoma (colon)

PATHOLOGY

■ Most non-neoplastic polyps are either inflammatory or hyperplastic, which are generally small and occur most frequently in the distal colon.
■ Of the neoplastic lesions, adenomas are most important because they serve as precursors to colorectal carcinoma.
■ Most colonic adenomas are tubular adenomas.
■ Tubular adenomas have various degrees of villous change; as the polyp becomes larger, the degree of villous change increases, and the risk of developing a cancer increases as well.
■ Other non-neoplastic polyps include juvenile polyps, the hamartomatous polyps of Peutz-Jeghers syndrome, and the inflammatory polyps of Cronkhite-Canada syndrome.

INCIDENCE/PREVALENCE AND EPIDEMIOLOGY

■ Incidence rises dramatically with increasing age.
■ Polyps are found in 10%-12.5% of patients studied with double-contrast techniques.

Suggested Readings

Smith TR: Pedunculated malignant colonic polyps with superficial invasion of the stalk. *Radiology* 115:593-596, 1975.
Winawer SJ, Zauber AG, O'Brien MJ, et al: The national polyp study: Design, methods, and characteristics of patients with newly diagnosed polyps. *Cancer* 70:1236-1245, 1992.
Yuan Y, Han HJ, Zheng S, et al: Germline mutations of *hMLH1* and *hMSH2* genes in patients with suspected hereditary nonpolyposis colorectal cancer and sporadic early-onset colorectal cancer. *Dis Colon Rectum* 41:434-440, 1998.

Adenocarcinoma

DEFINITION: Early carcinoma of the colon is typically a flat, sessile lesion, whereas advanced tumors are generally polypoid or annular lesions.

IMAGING

Radiography
Findings
- Typical early colon cancer is a flat, sessile lesion that may produce a contour defect.
- Long, thin stalk is generally a sign of a benign polyp; conversely, a short, thick stalk is often associated with carcinoma.
- Advanced cancers are generally manifested by polypoid or annular lesions.
- Plaque-like lesions can produce abnormal lines on double-contrast barium studies.
- Annular or semiannular lesions have higher rates of serosal invasion and lymph node metastases.
- Linitis plastica–type of carcinoma has radiologic appearance suggestive of an inflammatory stricture.
- Perforation of the colon may lead to a fistula to adjacent organs.

Utility
- Single- or double-contrast barium enema

CT
Findings
- CT may visualize a discrete mass or focal wall thickening that may be circumferential, without or with extension beyond the bowel wall.
- Asymmetric mural thickening with or without an irregular surface contour is suggestive of a neoplastic process.
- Tumor invasion beyond the bowel is suggested by a mass with nodular or spiculated borders.
- Desmoplastic reaction to tumor leads to overstaging as a result of difficulty distinguishing between fibrosis alone and fibrosis that contains tumor cells.

DIAGNOSTIC PEARLS

- Carcinoma is virtually nonexistent in polyps smaller than 5 mm.
- If definite evidence can be found of polyp growth on serial examinations, malignancy should be suspected.
- CT frequently understages patients with microinvasion of pericolonic or perirectal fat or small tumor foci in normal-sized nodes.

- Extracolonic tumor spread is suggested by loss of tissue fat planes between the large bowel and surrounding muscles; this type of tumor invades the uterus.
- Liver metastases usually appear hypodense; foci of calcification can often be seen within metastatic mucinous adenocarcinomas.
- Metastases show early rim enhancement, become partially hyperdense, go through an isodense phase, and then become low-density lesions again.

Utility
- CT is better suited for evaluation of tumor stage.
- CT cannot detect microscopic invasion of fat surrounding the colon or rectum and tends to understage patients.

MRI
Findings
- When T1-weighted spin-echo images are used, rectosigmoid tumors may be manifested by wall thickening, with a signal intensity similar to or slightly higher than that of skeletal muscle.
- Accurately staged tumor, extension of tumor beyond the rectal wall, and lymph node and liver metastases are seen.

WHAT THE REFERRING PHYSICIAN NEEDS TO KNOW

- If definite evidence exists of polyp growth on serial examinations, malignancy should be suspected.
- Presence of a long, thin stalk is generally a sign of a benign polyp; conversely, a short, thick stalk is often associated with carcinoma.
- Carcinomas are particularly difficult to detect in patients with extensive diverticular disease of the sigmoid colon.
- If the tumor is contained within the wall of the colon or rectum, CT cannot reliably assess the depth of mural penetration.
- Desmoplastic reaction to tumor frequently leads to overstaging by MRI.
- CT frequently understages patients with microinvasion of pericolonic or perirectal fat or those with small tumor foci in normal-sized nodes.
- Most polyps detected radiographically should be removed if they are more than 5 mm in diameter.

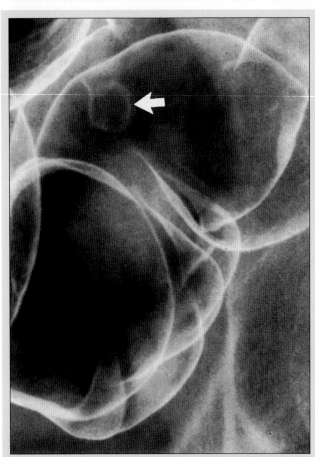

Figure 1. Pedunculated early cancer on double-contrast barium enema. Early carcinoma *(arrow)* with a short, thick stalk. *(From Laufer I, Levine MS [eds]:* Double-Contrast Gastrointestinal Radiology, *3rd ed. Philadelphia, WB Saunders, 2000.)*

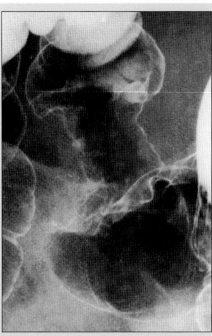

Figure 2. Advanced colon cancer. Double-contrast barium enema shows an annular, *apple core* lesion with circumferential narrowing, obliteration of mucosal folds, and abrupt, shelf-like margins. *(From Laufer I, Levine MS [eds]:* Double-Contrast Gastrointestinal Radiology, *3rd ed. Philadelphia, WB Saunders, 2000.)*

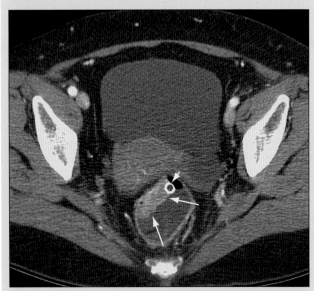

Figure 3. Rectal carcinoma confined to the bowel wall (T2N0M0 (Dukes' stage B1). Axial thin-section (2.5 mm) MDCT scan of the rectum in the arterial phase and with rectal administration of water demonstrates focal thickening of the anterior and right lateral rectal wall *(arrows)*. The outer margin of the rectum is smooth and well preserved. The rectal tube also is seen *(arrowhead)*. No abnormal lymph nodes are identified (CT stage II).

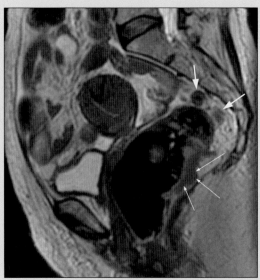

Figure 4. MR image of rectal adenocarcinoma with extension beyond the bowel wall (T3N1M0 or Dukes' stage C2). Sagittal T2-weighted fast spin-echo image shows enlarged lymph nodes *(large arrows)* in the presacral space. Nodular outer margin of the rectal mass *(thin arrows)* is well demonstrated on sagittal view, suggesting invasive tumor (T3).

- When T2-weighted spin-echo images are used, the signal intensity of the tumor increases relative to that of the muscle.
- MRI can distinguish between tumors localized to the mucosa and submucosa.
- Edema, granulation tissue, and fibrosis can lead to overstaging in patients who undergo MRI after neoadjuvant chemotherapy and irradiation.

Utility
- MRI is used to detect and stage rectosigmoid tumors more accurately.
- Rectal air insufflation (with prone positioning and an antispasmodic agent) may be helpful in better depicting the extent of tumor.
- MRI is superior to CT in demonstrating levator ani invasion.
- Endoluminal MRI and endoluminal ultrasound are the two most accurate methods for staging early or superficial rectal cancer.

Ultrasound

Findings
- Ultrasound depicts the various layers of the colon wall.
- Ultrasound also can be used to determine the depth of mural tumor penetration; perirectal fat invasion is visualized by disruption of the outermost hyperechoic ring.
- Colorectal tumors are characterized by a hypoechoic mass.
- Elements of the rectal wall appear as rings of different echogenicities.

Utility
- Transrectal ultrasound (TRUS)
- Ultrasonographic staging system is based on the TNM (tumor, lymph node, metastasis) classification.

PET

Findings
- Increased fluorodeoxyglucose uptake

Utility
- PET is used for the detection of primary and recurrent tumors as well as metastases.
- PET is also used to identify distant metastatic foci and occasionally unexpected primary malignant tumors in patients with other colorectal neoplasms.
- PET is excellent for the depiction of distant nodal or extranodal metastases.

CLINICAL PRESENTATION

- Approximately 5% of patients with colon carcinoma have additional, synchronous carcinomas elsewhere in the colon.
- Most symptomatic patients with colorectal carcinoma have advanced lesions.
- Major complications of colorectal cancer include bleeding, bowel obstruction, and perforation.

DIFFERENTIAL DIAGNOSIS

- Benign epithelial polyps (colon)
- Lymphoma (colon)

PATHOLOGY

- Carcinoma is virtually nonexistent in polyps smaller than 5 mm.
- Typical early colon cancers are flat, sessile lesions that produce a contour defect.
- Malignant polyps tend to grow more quickly than benign polyps.
- The presence of a long, thin stalk is generally a sign of a benign polyp; conversely, a short, thick stalk is often associated with carcinoma.
- Advanced cancers are generally polypoid or annular lesions; polypoid carcinomas have a higher rate of serosal invasion and lymph node metastases than polypoid carcinomas.
- Advanced cancers are often associated with *sentinel* polyps or additional polyps elsewhere in the colon.
- Linitis plastica–type of carcinoma is characterized by submucosal infiltration and fibrous reaction and is more likely to develop in patients with ulcerative colitis.

INCIDENCE/PREVALENCE AND EPIDEMIOLOGY

- Colon cancer is the most common significant cancer in the United States and is the second most common cause of cancer mortality.
- Colon cancer ranks third to lung and prostate cancer in men and third to lung and breast cancer in women.
- Colon cancer is more common in North America, Europe, and New Zealand; the incidence is low in South America, Africa, and Asia.
- Overall colorectal tumor incidence increases with age, and race and sex can independently predict the location of the cancer.
- Risk factors include a diet high in saturated fat but low in fiber, excess alcohol, sedentary lifestyle, obesity, and inflammatory bowel disease.
- Cancer incidence is nonexistent in polyps less than 5 mm, but increases to approximately 1% in polyps in the 5- to 10-mm range.
- Cancer incidence is 10% in polyps between 1 and 2 cm and greater than 25% in polyps larger than 2 cm.

Suggested Readings

Chen CD, Yen MF, Wang WM, et al: A case-cohort study for the disease natural history of adenoma-carcinoma and de novo carcinoma and surveillance of colon and rectum after polypectomy: Implication for efficacy of colonoscopy. *Br J Cancer* 88:1866-1873, 2003.

Ribeiro MB, Greenstein AJ, Sachar DB, et al: Colorectal adenocarcinoma in Crohn's disease. *Ann Surg* 223:186-193, 1996.

Lymphoma

ANATOMIC FINDINGS

Colon
- Bulky polypoid or cavitary mass shows smooth-surfaced lesions, frequently located near the ileocecal valve.
- Annular, infiltrating form involves the long segment of the colon, appearing as a concentric area of narrowing or as a cavitary mass.
- Annular, infiltrating form has an irregular contour; the mucosal surface is smooth, suggesting submucosal infiltration rather than mucosal ulceration.
- Diffuse, multinodular form appears as nonuniform, smooth, sessile nodules—varying from 2-25 mm—that carpet the colonic surface.
- Multinodular lymphomas involve the long segment of the colon or the entire colon.

IMAGING

Fluoroscopy
Findings
- Bulky polypoid masses appear as smooth-surfaced, broad-based, sessile lesions with or without ulcerations that vary from 4-20 cm.
- Annular, infiltrating colonic lymphoma appears as a concentric area of narrowing that involves the long segment of the colon or as a cavitary mass.
- Annular, infiltrating colonic lymphoma has an irregular, lobulated contour; overlying mucosal surface is smooth, suggesting submucosal infiltration.

DIAGNOSTIC PEARLS

- Primary form of colonic lymphoma involves the ileocecal valve, cecum, or rectum; primary localized form may be manifested by a polypoid or cavitary mass or circumferential mural lesion on radiographs.
- Bulky polypoid masses represent the most common form of primary colonic lymphoma.
- The most frequent finding is palpable abdominal mass; abdominal pain, weight loss, and altered bowel habits occur in 60%-90% of patients; rectal bleeding or diarrhea occurs in 25%.

- More than 100 nonuniform, smooth, sessile nodules varying from 2-25 mm carpet the colonic surface in diffuse, multinodular form.
- Extension of cecal lymphoma into terminal ileum

CT
Findings
- Large soft tissue mass, lobular wall thickening of colon
- This mural thickening is homogeneous.

Ultrasound
Utility
- Appearances of gastrointestinal lymphoma have been described.
- Ultrasound has not gained widespread acceptance in diagnosis or staging of non-Hodgkin lymphoma.

WHAT THE REFERRING PHYSICIAN NEEDS TO KNOW

- Primary gastrointestinal lymphoma: (1) lymphadenopathy is confined to the area of bowel abnormality; (2) peripheral white blood cell counts and bone marrow spirates are normal; (3) there is no evidence of disease in liver or spleen.
- Secondary gastrointestinal lymphoma usually affects multiple sites.
- Patients with disseminated lymphoma involving the colon are usually asymptomatic and do not undergo barium studies.
- Differential diagnosis of annular, infiltrating lymphoma includes submucosal hemorrhage and edema (caused by ischemia or bleeding diathesis) and unusual colonic carcinoma.
- Differential diagnosis of cavitary lymphoma includes perforated colonic carcinoma and mesenchymal tumor (e.g., gastrointestinal stromal tumor).
- Diffuse, multinodular colonic lymphoma (lymphomatous polyposis) is associated with disseminated disease from nodal primary lymphoma or occurs as true primary gastrointestinal lymphoma.
- Multinodular form of colonic lymphoma may be confused radiographically with familial polyposis, lymphoid hyperplasia, inflammatory bowel disease, or infectious diseases (pseudomembranous colitis or schistosomiasis).

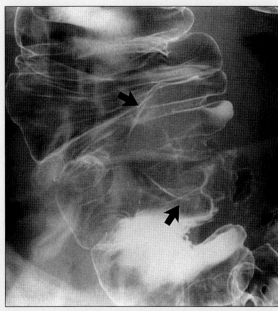

Figure 1. Lymphoma of the ileocecal valve. Spot image from a double-contrast barium enema shows a smooth-surfaced mass (*arrows*) replacing the ileocecal valve.

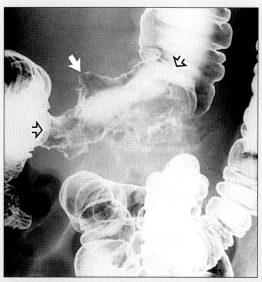

Figure 2. Lymphoma of the transverse colon. Spot image from a double-contrast barium enema shows a long (limits denoted by *open arrows*), concentric lesion in the transverse colon with an irregular contour. Note protrusion of the contour superiorly outside the expected lumen of the bowel (*white arrow*); this finding indicates cavitation of the mass.

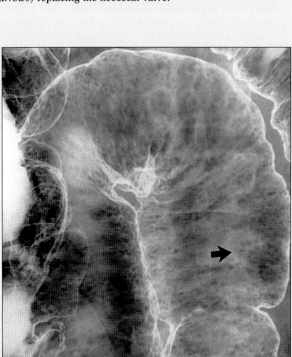

Figure 3. Disseminated lymphoma of the colon. Spot image from a double-contrast barium enema shows innumerable small (1-3 mm), nonuniform nodules (representative area shown by *arrow*) carpeting the surface of the sigmoid colon. This is an unusual appearance for disseminated lymphoma involving the colon because the nodules tend to be larger.

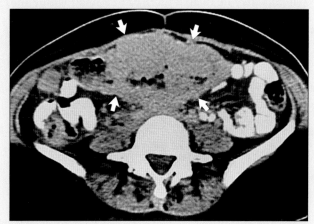

Figure 4. Lymphoma of the transverse colon. CT shows a large soft tissue mass (*arrows*) with lobular thickening of the walls of the transverse colon.

MRI

Findings
- Generally, homogeneous low-signal and heterogeneous high-signal intensity on T1- and T2-weighted MRI sequences, respectively

Utility
- Appearances of gastrointestinal lymphoma have been described.
- MRI has not gained widespread acceptance in diagnosis or staging of non-Hodgkin lymphoma.

PET

Utility
- PET has higher accuracy than CT in detection of residual disease after therapy.

CLINICAL PRESENTATION

- Abdominal pain, weight loss, and altered bowel habits occur in 60%-90% of patients; rectal bleeding or diarrhea occurs in 25%.
- Most frequent physical finding is palpable abdominal mass.
- Long-standing inflammatory bowel disease appears to be a predisposing condition, but lymphoma in these patients may be related more to treatment with immunosuppressive agent than to disease itself.
- Extranodal presentation of post-transplant lymphoproliferative disorders is typical, and B-cell lymphomas may arise in the colon after solid organ transplantation.
- Patients with disseminated lymphoma involving the colon are usually asymptomatic and do not undergo barium studies.
- Colonic lumen in annular, infiltrating form of colonic lymphoma may be narrowed, but obstruction is uncommon.
- Associated mesenteric lymph nodes are usually enlarged in multinodular colonic lymphoma; conglomerate cecal mass is seen in almost 50% of cases.

PATHOLOGY

- Bulky polypoid masses usually appear as smooth-surfaced, broad-based, sessile lesions with or without central depressions or ulcerations; they vary from 4-20 cm.
- Annular, infiltrating form of colonic lymphoma is usually characterized by a discrete lesion with thickened, irregular haustral folds and nodular surface pattern.
- Large infiltrating tumors may extend into mesentery or exhibit central cavitation, which results in a bulky, cavitary mass lesion.
- Histologically, diffuse multinodular colonic lymphoma (lymphomatous polyposis) is usually mantle cell lymphoma derived from mantle zone cell subpopulations.
- Lymphomatous polyposis disseminates rapidly to liver, spleen, peripheral lymph nodes, and bone marrow.

- Multinodular colonic lymphoma has more than 100 nonuniform, smooth, sessile nodules varying from 2-25 mm that carpet the colonic surface.
- Nodules are occasionally elongated, pedunculated, umbilicated, or filiform.

INCIDENCE/PREVALENCE AND EPIDEMIOLOGY

- In primary gastrointestinal lymphoma, the colon is the third most commonly involved (6%-12%), after stomach and small bowel.
- Primary lymphoma of the colon is rare, comprising less than 1% of all primary malignant tumors of the colon.
- Bulky polypoid masses represent the most common form of primary colonic lymphoma.
- Colonic involvement by systemic lymphoma is relatively common, with microscopic evidence of tumor in up to 44% of cases at autopsy.
- Non-Hodgkin lymphoma accounts for almost all colonic lymphomas; Hodgkin disease is extremely rare.
- Large cell lymphoma is most common primary non-Hodgkin lymphoma subtype.
- Rarely, diffuse colonic lymphoma may be associated with acute toxic dilation or pneumatosis coli.
- Primary non-Hodgkin lymphoma in the colon is usually seen in middle-aged or elderly persons.
- Males are more frequently affected than females by a ratio of 2:1.

DIFFERENTIAL DIAGNOSIS

- Familial polyposis
- Lymphoid hyperplasia
- Inflammatory bowel disease
- Infectious disease (pseudomembranous colitis, schistosomiasis)
- Submucosal hemorrhage and edema (caused by ischemia or bleeding diathesis)
- Colonic carcinoma
- Gastrointestinal stromal tumor in colon
- Large stromal tumors

Suggested Readings

Dragosics B, Bauer P, Radaszkiewicz T: Primary gastrointestinal non-Hodgkin lymphomas: A retrospective clinicopathologic study of 150 cases. *Cancer* 55:1060-1073, 1985.
Herrman R, Panahon AM, Barcos MP, et al: Gastrointestinal involvement in non-Hodgkin's lymphoma. *Cancer* 46:215-222, 1980.
Lewin KJ, Ranchod M, Dorfman RF: Lymphomas of the gastrointestinal tract: A study of 117 cases presenting with gastrointestinal disease. *Cancer* 2:693-707, 1987.
Messinger NH, Bobroff LM, Beneventano TC: Lymphosarcoma of the colon. *AJR Am J Roentgenol* 117:281-286, 1973.
Weinsrad D, DeCosse JJ, Sherlock P, et al: Primary gastrointestinal lymphoma. *Cancer* 49:1258-1265, 1982.
Wychulis AR, Beahrs OH, Woolner LB: Malignant lymphoma of the colon. *Arch Surg* 93:215-225, 1966.

Vascular Lesions

DEFINITION: Vascular abnormalities in the colon that cause rectal bleeding.

IMAGING

Radiography
Findings
- Hemangiomas may be manifested by multiple phleboliths along the course of the bowel.
- Circumferential lesions have scalloped contours and a nodular mucosal surface pattern.
- Polypoid form of hemangiomas: smooth, sessile, broad-based submucosal masses
- Lymphangiomas: solitary, 2-4 cm, often pedunculated polypoid lesions or smooth, submucosal masses
- Angiodysplasia: tangle of small vessels at the end of the cecal or right colonic artery
- Kaposi sarcoma: flat or plaque-like lesions, small polypoid nodules, or polypoid submucosal-appearing masses with or without central umbilication

Utility
- Abdominal radiographs for detection of phleboliths
- Barium enema

CT
Findings
- Usually vascular, sometimes containing multiple phleboliths
- Occasionally hypovascular or avascular
- Lymphangioma: cystic or multicystic mass or a smooth, unilocular or multilocular submucosal mass of water attenuation

Utility
- CT better delineates the true dimensions of the mass and involvement of adjacent structures.
- Angiography to assess vascular supply and vascularity

Ultrasound
Findings
- Cystic or multicystic mass

Utility
- Endoscopic ultrasonography

CLINICAL PRESENTATION

- Colonic hemangiomas occur at a young age with acute, recurrent, or chronic rectal bleeding.

DIAGNOSTIC PEARLS

- Abdominal radiographs show multiple phleboliths along the course of the bowel in 50% of cases.
- CT better delineates the true dimensions of the mass and involvement of adjacent structures such as the urinary bladder.
- Barium enema examinations usually reveal a circumferential lesion with scalloped contours and a nodular mucosal surface pattern.

- Colonic hemangiomas: some patients may have severe, life-threatening rectal bleeding.
- Patients with anorectal lesions may complain of tenesmus or constipation.
- Colonic lymphangiomas may cause abdominal pain, rectal bleeding, watery diarrhea, or altered bowel habits.
- Angiodysplasia is a common cause of chronic, low-grade or acute massive lower gastrointestinal bleeding.

DIFFERENTIAL DIAGNOSIS

- Lymphoma (colon)
- Ischemia (colon)
- Pneumatosis coli (colon)

PATHOLOGY

- Cavernous hemangiomas (most common form): unencapsulated lesions arising in submucosa with large, multiloculated, thin-walled vessels separated by loose connective tissue
- Capillary hemangiomas: solitary, sharply circumscribed, submucosal masses in asymptomatic patients; small vessels lined by well-differentiated endothelial cells
- Colonic hemangiomas: no propensity for malignant transformation; should be distinguished from their true neoplastic counterpart, angiosarcomas
- Lymphangiomas: cluster of lymphatic spaces lined by endothelial cells and separated by connective tissue septa

---

WHAT THE REFERRING PHYSICIAN NEEDS TO KNOW

- Hemangiomas may be misdiagnosed at endoscopy and have a high mortality rate related to severe gastrointestinal bleeding.
- Hemangiomas may be suspected if abdominal radiographs demonstrate phleboliths along the expected course of the bowel in young patients with gastrointestinal bleeding.

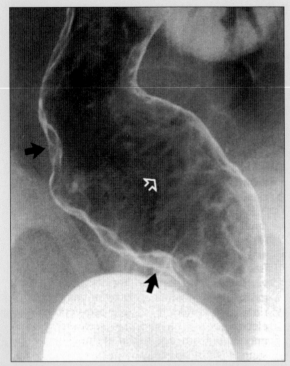

Figure 1. Hemangioma of the colon. Prone, angled view of the rectosigmoid junction shows a subtle circumferential lesion with a lobulated contour *(solid arrows)* and a finely lobulated mucosal surface *(open arrow).* (*From Margulis AR: Case: Cavernous hemangioma of the rectum.* Gastrointest Radiol *16:363-364, 1981.*)

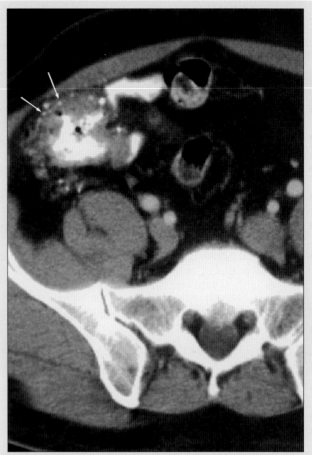

Figure 2. Hemangioma of the colon. CT shows lobulated thickening of the circumference of the wall of the cecum with numerous calcified phleboliths *(arrows)* in the subserosa.

- Angiodysplasia: clusters of dilated, tortuous, thin-walled veins, venules, and capillaries localized in the colonic mucosa and submucosa
- Kaposi sarcoma involving the colon: usually occurs in patients with AIDS

INCIDENCE/PREVALENCE AND EPIDEMIOLOGY

- Colonic lymphangiomas usually occur in the fourth to sixth decades of life.
- Angiodysplasia occurs in elderly patients.
- Kaposi sarcoma involving the colon usually occurs in patients with AIDS.

Suggested Readings

Agha FP, Francis IR, Simms SM: Cystic lymphangioma of the colon. *AJR Am J Roentgenol* 141:709-710, 1983.

Allred HW Jr, Spencer RJ: Hemangiomas of the colon, rectum, and anus. *Mayo Clin Proc* 49:739-741, 1974.

Camilleri M, Satti MB, Wood CB: Cystic lymphangioma of the colon. *Dis Colon Rectum* 25:813-816, 1982.

Dachman AH, Ros PR, Shekitka KM, et al: Colorectal hemangioma: Radiologic findings. *Radiology* 167:31-34, 1988.

Gandolfi L, Rossi A, Stasi G, Tonti R: The Klippel-Trenaunay syndrome. *Gastrointest Endosc* 33:442-445, 1987.

Goboes K: Rare and secondary (metastatic) tumors. In Whitehead R (ed): *Gastrointestinal and Oesphageal Pathology.* Edinburgh, Churchill Livingstone, 1995, pp 910-924.

Kawamoto K, Ueyama T, Iwashita I, et al: Colonic submucosal tumors: Comparison of endoscopic US and target air-enema CT with barium enema study and colonoscopy. *Radiology* 192:697-702, 1994.

Lyon DT, Mantea AG: Large-bowel hemangiomas. *Dis Colon Rectum* 27:404-414, 1984.

Margulis AR: Selected cases from the film interpretation session of the Society of Gastrointestinal Radiologists. Case 1: Hemangioma of the rectum. *Gastrointest Radiol* 6:363-364, 1981.

Perez C, Andreu J, Llauger J, et al: Hemangioma of the rectum: CT appearance. *Gastrointest Radiol* 12:347-349, 1987.

Puy-Montbrun T, Pigot F, Vuong PN, et al: Kaposi's sarcoma of the colon in a young HIV-negative woman with Crohn's disease. *Dig Dis Sci* 36:528-531, 1991.

Reinhart WH, Staubli M, Mordasini C, et al: Abnormalities of the gut vessels in Turner's syndrome. *Postgrad Med J* 59:122-124, 1983.

Thompson GB, Pemberton JH, Morris S, et al: Kaposi's sarcoma of the colon in a young HIV-negative man with chronic ulcerative colitis. *Dis Colon Rectum* 32:73-76, 1989.

Young T-H, Ho A-S, Tang HS, et al: Cystic lymphangioma of the transverse colon: Report of a case and review of the literature. *Abdom Imaging* 21:415-417, 1996.

Carcinoid Tumors

DEFINITION: Neuroendocrine cells that give rise to gastrointestinal tumors.

IMAGING

Radiography

Findings

- Neuroendocrine tumors of colon may appear as large (> 5 cm), fungating, intraluminal masses or as irregular annular lesions.
- Neuroendocrine tumors of colon may also appear as smooth, polypoid submucosal masses in some patients.
- Neuroendocrine tumors of rectum may be seen as smooth submucosal polypoid lesions less than 2 cm in diameter.
- Large rectal carcinoids are occasionally seen as irregular, ulcerated masses.

Utility

- Barium enemas

CLINICAL PRESENTATION

- Symptoms include abdominal pain, distention, and a palpable abdominal mass.
- Rectal bleeding and diarrhea are seen in approximately one third of patients.

DIFFERENTIAL DIAGNOSIS

- Polypoid or annular carcinoma (colon)
- Lipoma (colon)
- Metastatic disease (colon)

PATHOLOGY

- Endocrine cells synthesize and secrete a variety of peptide hormones and biogenic amines, which are then scattered throughout the gastrointestinal tract.

DIAGNOSTIC PEARLS

- Smooth submucosal polypoid lesions less than 2 cm in diameter (rectal)
- Large (> 5 cm), fungating, intraluminal masses or irregular annular lesions (colon excluding rectum)

- Midgut neuroendocrine tumors involve the cecum and ascending or transverse colon; they synthesize, store, and secrete serotonin.
- Hindgut neuroendocrine tumors involve the descending colon, sigmoid colon, and rectum; they synthesize and store gastrin, somatostatin, glucagon, and vasoactive intestinal polypeptides.
- Rectal neuroendocrine tumors appear as small, smooth, submucosal polypoid lesions less than 2 cm in diameter in the lower two thirds of the rectum, usually detected as incidental findings.
- Neuroendocrine tumors in the colon are large, aggressive lesions associated with a poor prognosis, located in the cecum or ascending colon.

INCIDENCE/PREVALENCE AND EPIDEMIOLOGY

- Most common sites of carcinoids include the appendix (35%), ileum (16%), lung (14%), and rectum (13%).
- Neuroendocrine tumors arising in the remainder of the colon constitute only 2%-3% of all carcinoid tumors.
- Patients with rectal carcinoids have an overall 5-year survival rate of approximately 85%.
- Fifty to sixty percent of patients with large neuroendocrine tumors have metastases to the liver, lymph nodes, mesentery, or peritoneum at the time of diagnosis.
- Overall 5-year survival rates of approximately 50% have been reported.

WHAT THE REFERRING PHYSICIAN NEEDS TO KNOW

- Most cases are discovered incidentally during a screening barium enema examination or endoscopy or during a workup for rectal pain or bleeding.
- Small rectal carcinoids have a low malignant potential and are cured by simple, complete excision (*low-grade* neuroendocrine tumors).
- Larger tumors have a greater chance of metastases at the time of diagnosis; large rectal carcinoids appear as irregular, ulcerated masses.
- Neuroendocrine tumors in the colon (exclusive of the rectum) are associated with a poor prognosis.
- Diagnosis usually occurs in the sixth decade of life.

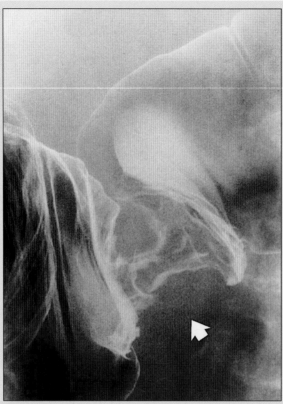

Figure 1. Neuroendocrine carcinoma of the colon. Spot image from a double-contrast barium enema shows a short, annular lesion *(arrow)* with shelf-like margins in the hepatic flexure of the colon. These radiographic findings are similar to those of an annular carcinoma of the colon, but the mucosa is smoother than that usually found with an annular carcinoma. (*Courtesy of Seth N. Glick, MD, Philadelphia, PA.*)

Suggested Readings

Balthazar EJ: Carcinoid tumors of the alimentary tract. *Gastrointest Radiol* 3:47-56, 1978.

Berardi RS: Carcinoid tumors of the colon (exclusive of the rectum): Review of the literature. *Dis Colon Rectum* 15:383-391, 1972.

Crittenden JJ, Byllesby J, Dodds W: Carcinoid tumor presenting as an annular lesion in the ascending colon. *Radiology* 97:85-86, 1970.

Fioca R, Capella C, Bufta R, et al: Glucagon-like, glicentin-like and pancreatic polypeptide-like immunoreactivities in rectal carcinoids and related colorectal cells. *Am J Pathol* 100:81-92, 1980.

Jetmore AB, Ray JE, Gathright JB, et al: Rectal carcinoids: The most frequent rectal tumor. *Dis Colon Rectum* 35:717-725, 1992.

Martensson H, Nobin A, Sundler F: Carcinoid tumours in the gastrointestinal tract—an analysis of 156 cases. *Acta Chir Scand* 149:607-616, 1983.

Sato T, Sakai Y, Sonoyama A, et al: Radiologic spectrum of rectal carcinoid tumors. *Gastrointest Radiol* 9:23-26, 1984.

Shulman H, Giustra P: Invasive carcinoids of the colon. *Radiology* 98:139-143, 1971.

Lipomas and Fatty Infiltration of the Ileocecal Valve

DEFINITION: Fatty infiltration of the ileocecal valve results from localized, massive accumulation of submucosal fat. Colonic lipomas are encapsulated, and these masses of mature adipose tissue are usually confined to the submucosa.

IMAGING

Radiography
Findings
- Smooth, sessile submucosal masses or smooth polypoid lesions on a broad-based pedicle
- Lipomas: round, ovoid, or pear-shaped, sharply demarcated masses that form obtuse angles with the adjacent colonic wall
- Fatty infiltration of ileocecal valve: large ileocecal valve with smooth or lobulated contours and a smooth mucosal surface without a discrete polypoid mass

Utility
- Barium enemas

CT
Findings
- Lipomas characterized by masses of uniform fat density (–60 to –120 HU) without septa or other large areas of nonfatty tissue
- Intussuscepting lipoma may be seen as a soft-tissue mass with a small focus of fat attenuation (may be confused with an intussuscepting carcinoma).

Utility
- CT provides a definitive diagnosis of a colonic lipoma.
- CT can obviate the need for surgery in patients without symptoms or complications or in those who represent poor operative risks.
- Imaging should be tailored with thin sections through the lesion to minimize the partial volume effect of surrounding contrast material or air.

Ultrasound
Findings
- Lipomas are seen as smooth, broad-based hemispheric masses of increased or intermediate echogenicity.

CLINICAL PRESENTATION

- Most patients are asymptomatic.
- When patients are symptomatic, abdominal pain and discomfort may occur.

DIAGNOSTIC PEARLS

- Mass of uniform fat density (–60 to –120 HU) without septa or other large areas of nonfatty tissue characteristic of lipoma on CT
- Variably enlarged ileocecal valve (> 4 cm), with a smooth or slightly lobulated contour, and a smooth mucosal surface may be seen in patients with fatty infiltration of the ileocecal valve.

DIFFERENTIAL DIAGNOSIS

- Metastatic disease (colon)
- Adenoma (colon)
- Carcinoid (colon)

PATHOLOGY

- Colonic lipomas are usually less than 3 cm in diameter, but those that cause symptoms tend to be larger lesions.
- Colonic lipomas are encapsulated masses of mature adipose tissue, usually confined to the submucosa.
- Two thirds of these tumors are pedunculated, with a broad-based pedicle covered by normal colonic mucosa.
- Local trauma and mechanical irritation can lead to focal ulceration and fat necrosis; continuing inflammation causes fibrosis and calcification.
- Tumors change shape on barium enema with palpation and patient position; colonic distention and elongation occur during colonic spasm or after colonic evacuation.
- Fatty infiltration of the ileocecal valve is not associated with a true capsule.

INCIDENCE/PREVALENCE AND EPIDEMIOLOGY

- Colonic lipomas are uncommon lesions, occurring at autopsy in less than 1% of cases.

WHAT THE REFERRING PHYSICIAN NEEDS TO KNOW

- Lack of a capsule in fatty infiltration of the ileocecal valve differentiates this finding from a true lipoma.

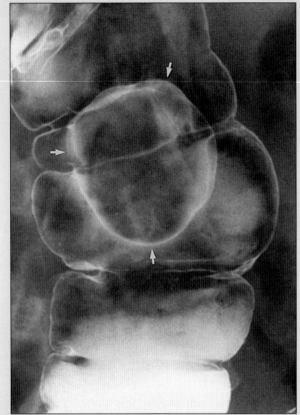

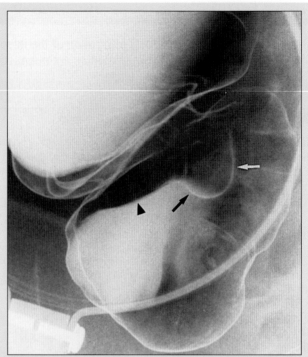

Figure 2. Lipoma of the ileocecal valve. A small, smooth-surfaced submucosal lesion *(arrows)* is seen arising from the inferior lip of the ileocecal valve *(arrowhead).*

Figure 1. Lipoma of the descending colon. Spot image from a double-contrast barium enema shows a 3-cm smooth-surfaced submucosal mass *(arrows)* with a slightly lobulated contour.

- Most colonic lipomas are found in the right colon: 90% originate in the submucosa, and the remaining 10% arise in the appendices epiploicae.
- Multiple lipomas are found in up to 25% of patients.

Suggested Readings

Berk RN, Werner LG: The radiology corner: Lipoma of the colon. *Am J Gastroenterol* 61:145-150, 1974.

Buetow PC, Buck JL, Carr NJ, et al: Intussuscepted colonic lipomas: Loss of fat attenuation on CT with pathologic correlation in 10 cases. *Abdom Imaging* 21:153-156, 1996.

Castro DB, Stearns MW: Lipomas of the large intestine. *Dis Colon Rectum* 15:441-444, 1972.

Deeths TM, Dodds WJ: Lipoma of the colon. *Am J Gastroenterol* 58:326-331, 1972.

Heiken JP, Forde KA, Gold RP: Computed tomography as a definitive method for diagnosing gastrointestinal lipomas. *Radiology* 142:409-414, 1982.

Hurwitz MH, Redleaf PD, Williams HJ, et al: Lipomas of the gastrointestinal tract. *AJR Am J Roentgenol* 99:84-89, 1967.

Kabaalioglu A, Gelen T, Aktan S, et al: Acute colonic obstruction caused by intussusception and extrusion of a sigmoid lipoma through the anus after barium enema. *Abdom Imaging* 22:389-391, 1997.

Liessi G, Pavanello M, Cesari S, et al: Large lipomas of the colon: CT and MR findings in three symptomatic cases. *Abdom Imaging* 21:150-152, 1996.

Margulis AR, Jovanovich A: The roentgen diagnosis of submucous lipomas of the colon. *AJR Am J Roentgenol* 84:1114-1120, 1960.

Megibow AJ, Redmond PE, Bosniak MA, et al: Diagnosis of gastrointestinal lipomas by CT. *AJR Am J Roentgenol* 133:743-745, 1979.

Wulff C, Jespersen N: Colo-colic intussusception caused by lipoma: Case report. *Acta Radiol* 36:478-480, 1995.

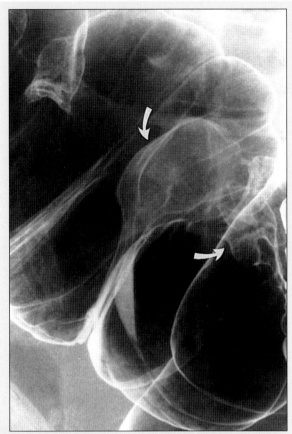

Figure 3. Fatty infiltration of the ileocecal valve. Close-up view from a right-side-down decubitus overhead radiograph of the colon shows smooth, slightly lobulated enlargement of the ileocecal valve *(arrows)*. Fatty infiltration was confirmed at colonoscopy performed for other reasons.

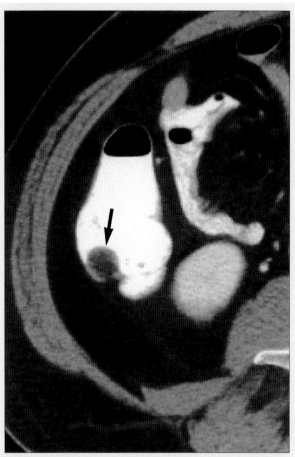

Figure 4. Lipoma of the cecum. CT shows a 1.5-cm smooth-surfaced ovoid mass *(arrow)* in the cecum with the same attenuation value as nearby mesenteric fat.

Gastrointestinal Stromal Tumors

DEFINITION: Undifferentiated stromal neoplasms originating from the interstitial cells of Cajal.

ANATOMIC FINDINGS

Colon
- Small polypoid lesions may be sessile or pedunculated.

IMAGING

Radiography
Findings
- Small rectal lesions may be seen as sessile or pedunculated polyps with a smooth or slightly irregular surface.
- Large gastrointestinal stromal tumors (GISTs) may appear as annular lesions or cavitating masses with a prominent extraluminal component or as submucosal masses with or without central ulceration.
- Cavitation may lead to superimposed infection or to perforation with abscess formation.

Utility
- Barium enemas

CT
Findings
- Large GISTs: annular lesions and cavitating masses with a prominent extraluminal component or submucosal masses with or without central ulceration

CLINICAL PRESENTATION

- Some patients with small polypoid rectal lesions complain of rectal discomfort, pain, and bleeding; other patients are asymptomatic.
- Large colonic GISTs may produce pain, gastrointestinal bleeding, and altered bowel habits but rarely cause obstruction.

DIFFERENTIAL DIAGNOSIS

- Lymphoma (colon)
- Carcinoma (colon)
- Metastatic disease (colon)

PATHOLOGY

- Spindle and epithelioid cell tumors of gastrointestinal tract are undifferentiated stromal neoplasms, termed GISTs.

DIAGNOSTIC PEARLS

- Large GISTs may appear on barium enemas or CT as annular lesions or cavitating masses with a prominent extraluminal component or as submucosal masses with or without central ulceration.
- These lesions may be confused radiographically with colonic lymphomas or perforated colonic carcinomas.
- Small rectal lesions appear on barium enema as sessile or pedunculated polyps with a smooth or slightly irregular surface.

- GISTs originate from the interstitial cells of Cajal, express CD34, and their development depends on the proto-oncogenic receptor tyrosine kinase (KIT).
- Two macroscopic types of colonic stromal tumors: small polypoid lesions and large, bulky masses
- Small polypoid lesions are sessile or pedunculated, arise from the muscularis mucosae, are histologically benign, do not recur after excision, and have no malignant potential.
- Small polypoid lesions are *true* leiomyomas of the colon; they demonstrate smooth-muscle differentiation by their desmin positivity and ultrastructural characteristics.
- Large lesions arise from the muscularis propria, have a high rate of local recurrence (60%), are associated with a poor prognosis, and are found mainly in the rectum.

INCIDENCE/PREVALENCE AND EPIDEMIOLOGY

- Colonic GISTs are usually located in the rectum.
- Only 1% of all gastrointestinal tumors are of stromal origin; these lesions are least commonly found in the colon.

Suggested Readings

Hirtoa S, Isozaki K, Moriyama Y, et al: Gain-of-function mutations of c-kit in human gastrointestinal stromal tumors. *Science* 279:577-580, 1998.

WHAT THE REFERRING PHYSICIAN NEEDS TO KNOW

- GISTs may be confused radiographically with colonic lymphomas or perforated colonic carcinomas.
- GISTs typically metastasize to peritoneal surfaces as well as to the lungs and liver.

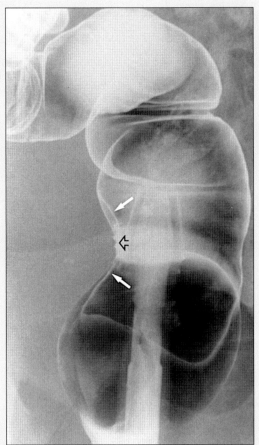

Figure 1. Gastrointestinal stromal tumor of the rectum. Steep oblique view of the rectum from a double-contrast barium enema shows a relatively broad-based mass *(solid arrows)* with focal spiculation of the contour *(open arrow)*.

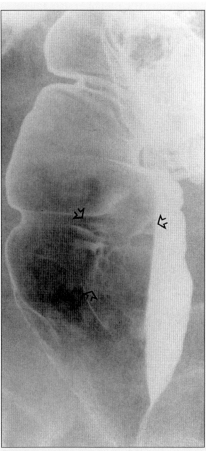

Figure 2. Gastrointestinal stromal tumor of the rectum. Close-up view from a left-side-down decubitus overhead radiograph in the same patient as in Figure 1 shows focal nodularity of the mucosa *(arrows)* corresponding to the area of spiculation on the earlier view.

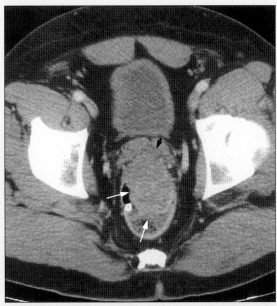

Figure 3. Malignant gastrointestinal stromal tumor of the rectum. CT scan shows a large soft tissue mass *(white arrows)* arising from the left anterolateral wall of the rectum. The mass enhances to the same degree as the adjacent muscle. Infiltration of the fat plane between the rectum and the seminal vesicles *(black arrow)* is present. (*Reproduced with permission from Forbes A, Rubesin SE, et al: Colon II. In* Atlas of Clinical Gastroenterology, *3rd ed. Edinburgh, Elsevier Mosby, 2005, p 183.*)

Kempson RL, Henrickson WR: Gastrointestinal stromal (smooth muscle) tumors. In Whitehead R (ed): *Gastrointestinal and Oesophageal Pathology*. Edinburgh, Churchill Livingstone, 1995, pp 727-739.

Ma CK, De Peralta MN, Amin MB, et al: Small intestinal stromal tumors: A clinicopathologic study of 20 cases with immunohistochemical assessment of cell differentiation and the prognostic role of proliferation antigens. *Am J Clin Pathol* 108:641-651, 1997.

Saul SH, Rast ML, Brooks JJ: The immunohistochemistry of gastrointestinal stromal tumors: Evidence supporting an origin from smooth muscle. *Am J Surg Pathol* 11:464-473, 1987.

Sugimura H, Tamura S, Yamada H, et al: Benign nerve sheath tumor of the sigmoid colon. *Clin Imaging* 17:64-66, 1993.

Cloacogenic Carcinoma

DEFINITION: Cloacogenic carcinomas are malignant epithelial tumors arising at the junction of the anal canal and rectum.

IMAGING

Radiography
Findings
- Submucosal masses with a smooth or ulcerated surface
- Broad-based, sessile polypoid masses or infiltrative lesions

Utility
- Barium enema

CLINICAL PRESENTATION

- Patients usually complain of rectal bleeding or pain or altered bowel habits.

DIFFERENTIAL DIAGNOSIS

- Adenocarcinoma (rectum)
- Squamous cell carcinoma (anorectal junction)
- Carcinoid (rectum)
- Metastatic disease (rectum)

PATHOLOGY

- Transitional zone is the area in which metaplasia and reserve cell hyperplasia occurs.
- Tumors arise in this region in areas of chronic inflammation or squamous metaplasia or reserve cell hyperplasia, resulting in dysplasia and subsequent carcinoma.
- Tumors appear as flat, infiltrative, annular, or ulcerative lesions with rolled borders.
- Hematogenous metastases may result from spread of tumor via the portal venous system and inferior vena cava.

DIAGNOSTIC PEARLS

- Junction of the anal canal and rectum
- Submucosal masses with a smooth or ulcerated surface
- Broad-based, sessile polypoid masses or infiltrative lesions

INCIDENCE/PREVALENCE AND EPIDEMIOLOGY

- Metastases to sacral, internal iliac, and common iliac lymph nodes are found in approximately 50% of patients.
- Patients with basaloid carcinoma have 5-year survival rates of approximately 50%.

Suggested Readings
Fenger C: The anal canal epithelium: A review. *Scand J Gastroenterol* 14(Suppl):114-117, 1979.

Gillespie JJ, MacKay B: Histogenesis of cloacogenic carcinoma: Fine structure of anal transitional epithelium and cloacogenic carcinoma. *Hum Pathol* 9:579-587, 1978.

Glickman MG, Margulis AR: Cloacogenic carcinoma. *AJR Am J Roentgenol* 107:175-180, 1969.

Kyaw MM, Gallagher T, Haines JO: Cloacogenic carcinoma. *AJR Am J Roentgenal* 115:384-391, 1972.

WHAT THE REFERRING PHYSICIAN NEEDS TO KNOW

- Transitional zone (the junction of the anal canal and rectum) has both urothelium and squamous epithelium compatible with a cloacogenic origin.
- Primary tumors at the anorectal junction are classified according to architectural and cellular differentiation.
- The most common malignant tumor of the anal canal is not of cloacogenic origin but is adenocarcinoma.

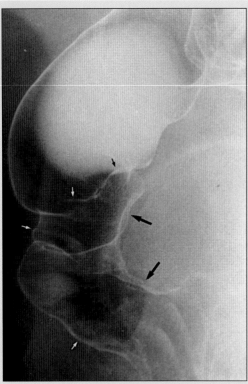

Figure 1. Cloacogenic carcinoma. Lateral view of the rectum shows a large submucosal mass *(large arrows)* indenting the anterior wall of the mid-rectum. Diffuse infiltration by tumor is characterized by smooth narrowing of the distal rectum *(small arrows)*.

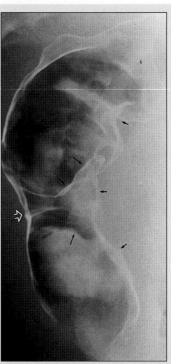

Figure 2. Cloacogenic carcinoma. Lateral view of the rectum shows the infiltrative pattern of cloacogenic carcinoma. The anterior wall of the rectum is moderately flattened and lobulated *(short arrows)*, with thickened, nodular folds traversing the rectum *(long arrows)*. The rectal mucosa is relatively smooth. Focal circumferential extension of the tumor around the rectum is seen as flattening of the posterior rectal wall *(open arrow)*.

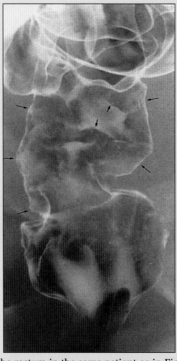

Figure 3. Cloacogenic carcinoma. Prone view of the rectum in the same patient as in Figure 2 shows mild in-bowing and irregularity of the contour of the lateral walls of the rectum *(long arrows)* and thickened, nodular folds en face *(short arrows)*.

Metastases to the Colon

DEFINITION: Spread of malignant tumor to the colon.

ANATOMIC FINDINGS

Colon
- Mass effect, mucosal pleating, and a tethered or spiculated contour

IMAGING

Radiography
Findings
- Extrinsic mass effect, mucosal pleating, tethering en face, and a spiculated contour in profile are seen in patients with intraperitoneal-seeded metastases to the colon.
- Advanced prostatic carcinoma: the rectum is circumferentially narrowed, with a widened presacral space, and a spiculated contour.
- Direct invasion by ovarian carcinoma may be characterized by sigmoid loop angulation, contour spiculation, mucosal fold tethering, and angulation.
- Spread of gastric carcinoma is characterized by mass effect, fixation, and fold spiculation along the superior border of the transverse colon, with sacculation of the uninvolved inferior border.
- Pancreatic carcinoma may spread to the inferior border of the transverse colon.
- Omental tumor invading the transverse colon may also be manifested by extrinsic mass effect, spiculation, and tethering, predominantly on its superior border.
- Metastatic melanoma is characterized by umbilicated or ulcerated submucosal masses or by bulky, polypoid intraluminal masses.
- Metastatic carcinoma of the breast is characterized by mural nodules, eccentric strictures, or irregular areas of circumferential narrowing, producing a linitis plastica appearance.

Utility
- Barium enemas

CT
Fingings
- Large prostatic mass displacing and invading the rectum
- Enlargement and increased attenuation of greater omentum caused by omental cakes

DIAGNOSTIC PEARLS
- Extrinsic mass effect, mucosal pleating, and tethering are seen en face, and a spiculated contour is seen in profile.
- The rectum is circumferentially narrowed, with a widened presacral space and spiculated contour in patients with prostatic carcinoma invading the rectum.
- Mural nodules, eccentric strictures, or irregular areas of circumferential narrowing may produce a linitis plastica appearance.

CLINICAL PRESENTATION
- Prostatic carcinoma: affected individuals may exhibit obstructive symptoms, constipation, or rectal bleeding.
- Patients with embolic metastases to the colon may exhibit rectal bleeding or incomplete obstruction.

DIFFERENTIAL DIAGNOSIS
- Diverticulitis
- Primary linitis plastica of the colon

PATHOLOGY
- Colonic metastases may result from direct invasion by a contiguous primary tumor or noncontiguous primary tumor; intraperitoneal seeding and embolic metastases are also seen.
- Tumors that directly invade the colon include carcinoma of the ovary, kidney, uterus, cervix, prostate, and gallbladder.
- Malignancies may spread into the subperitoneal space or by lymphatic permeation.
- Tumors that seed the peritoneal cavity include ovarian carcinoma in women and gastric, pancreatic, and colonic carcinomas in men.
- Primary tumors resulting in embolic metastases to the colon include malignant melanoma and carcinoma of the breast and lung.

WHAT THE REFERRING PHYSICIAN NEEDS TO KNOW
- Endoscopic biopsy specimens with stains for prostate-specific antigen or prostatic acid phosphatase may be obtained to confirm the radiologic diagnosis of prostatic carcinoma in patients with suspected recto-sigmoid invasion.

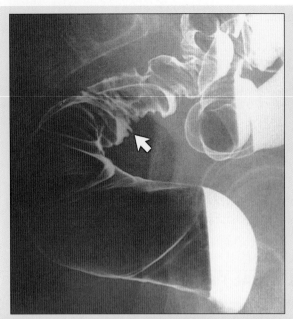

Figure 1. Ovarian carcinoma with intraperitoneal metastases to the rectosigmoid junction. Prone cross-table lateral view of the rectosigmoid junction shows spiculation *(arrow)* and tethering of folds along the anterior wall of the rectosigmoid junction. Pleating of the mucosa is seen en face.

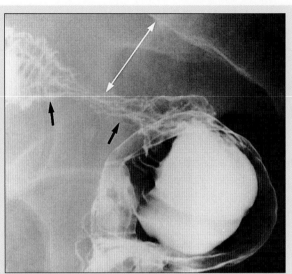

Figure 2. Direct invasion of the rectosigmoid colon by prostatic carcinoma. Lateral view of the rectum shows circumferential mass effect, especially on the anterior wall of the distal sigmoid colon *(arrows)*. Note the spiculated colonic contour and widening of the presacral space *(double-ended arrow)*.

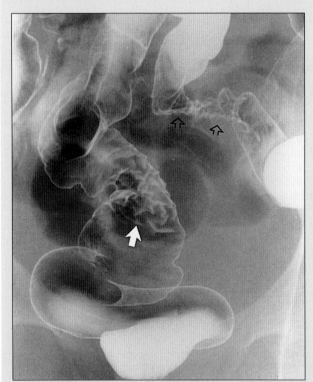

Figure 3. Direct colonic invasion by left ovarian carcinoma. Close-up view of an overhead radiograph from a double-contrast barium enema shows spiculation and mass effect along the inferior border of the sigmoid colon *(open arrows)* and pleating of the mucosa of the rectosigmoid junction en face *(solid arrow)*.

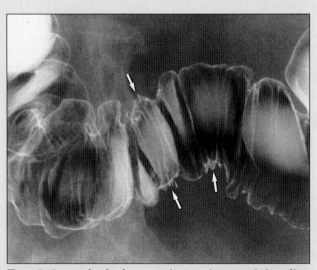

Figure 4. Omental cake from ovarian carcinomatosis invading the transverse colon. Spot image from a double-contrast barium enema shows spiculation of the colonic contour *(arrows)* and thin transverse stripes traversing the colon as a result of pleating of the mucosa en face.

INCIDENCE/PREVALENCE AND EPIDEMIOLOGY

- Rectal involvement by prostatic carcinoma occurs in 0.5%-11.5% of patients.
- The pouch of Douglas or rectovesical space is the most common site for intraperitoneal metastases, occurring in 56% of cases.

Suggested Readings

Aigen AB, Schapira HE: Metastatic carcinoma of prostate and bladder causing intestinal obstruction. *Urology* 21:464-466, 1983.

Bachman AL: Roentgen appearance of gastric invasion from carcinoma of the colon. *Radiology* 63:814-822, 1954.

Becker JA: Prostatic carcinoma involving the rectum and sigmoid colon. *AJR Am J Roentgenol* 94:421-428, 1965.

Fry DE, Amin M, Harbrecht PJ: Rectal obstruction secondary to carcinoma of the prostate. *Ann Surg* 189:488-492, 1979.

Gedgaudas RK, Kelvin FM, Thompson WM, et al: The value of preoperative barium enema in the assessment of pelvic masses. *Radiology* 146:609-613, 1983.

Gengler L, Baer J, Finby N: Rectal and sigmoid involvement secondary to carcinoma of the prostate. *AJR Am J Roentgenol* 125:910-917, 1975.

Goodman P, Balachandran S: Direct invasion of the transverse colon by a cecal tumor. *Abdom Imaging* 18:20-22, 1993.

Honda H, Lu CH, Barloon TT, et al: Sigmoid colon fistula complicating ovarian cystadenocarcinoma—a rare finding. *Gastrointest Radiol* 15:78-81, 1990.

Huang TY, Yam LT, Li CY: Unusual radiologic features of metastatic prostatic carcinoma confirmed by immunohistochemical study. *Urology* 23:218-223, 1984.

Khilnani MT, Wolf BS: Late involvement of the alimentary tract by carcinoma of the kidney. *Am J Dig Dis* 5:529-540, 1960.

Li CY, Lam WKW, Yam LT: Immunohistochemical diagnosis of prostatic cancer with metastasis. *Cancer* 46:706-712, 1980.

Meyers MA: Distribution of intra-abdominal malignant seeding: Dependency on dynamics of flow of ascitic fluid. *AJR Am J Roentgenol* 119:198-206, 1973.

Meyers MA: *Dynamic Radiology of the Abdomen: Normal and Pathologic Anatomy*, 3rd ed. New York, Springer, 1988.

Meyers MA: Intraperitoneal spread of malignancies and its effect on the bowel. *Clin Radiol* 32:129-146, 1981.

Meyers MA, McSweeney J: Secondary neoplasms of the bowel. *Radiology* 105:1-11, 1972.

Rubesin SE, Levine MS: Omental cakes: Colonic involvement by omental metastases. *Radiology* 154:593-596, 1985.

Rubesin SE, Levine MS, Bezzi M, et al: Rectal involvement by prostatic carcinoma: Radiographic findings. *AJR Am J Roentgenol* 152:53-57, 1989.

Wigh R: Tapley NduV. Metastatic lesions to the large intestine. *Radiology* 70:222-228, 1958.

Winter CC: The problem of rectal involvement by prostatic cancer. *Surg Gynecol Obstet* 105:136-140, 1957.

Familial Adenomatous Polyposis Syndrome

DEFINITION: Autosomal-dominant polyposis syndrome associated with the development of adenomas and specific clinical syndromes.

ANATOMIC FINDINGS

Colon
- Innumerable adenomatous polyps may be seen as small or moderate-sized filling defects carpeting the entire colon but are sometimes widely scattered.
- Patients are at high risk for the development of colonic carcinoma via an adenoma-carcinoma sequence.

Stomach
- Most common gastric manifestation is fundic gland polyps, which are almost always confined to the fundus and body of the stomach.
- Invariably multiple, appearing as small, sessile lesions ranging from 1-5 mm in diameter
- Also, tubular and villous gastric adenomas, usually in the distal stomach
- Gastric adenomas are typically sessile polyps, 5-10 mm in diameter, and multiple in greater than 50% of reported cases.

Duodenum
- Polyps are usually found in the second portion of the duodenum, clustered around the papilla.
- Villous adenomas are also commonly found and tend to be located in the periampullary region of the duodenum and jejunum.
- Small adenomas may be scattered throughout the duodenum.

Ileum
- Small adenomas may be scattered throughout ileum.
- Ileal lymphoid hyperplasia occurs more frequently.

Bile Duct
- Biliary polyps are commonly found.

DIAGNOSTIC PEARLS
- Innumerable small or moderate-sized filling defects carpeting the entire colon
- Polyps and adenomas involving the stomach, small bowel, and sometimes the bile ducts
- Association with sebaceous cysts, osteomas, fibrous proliferation, and tumors of the central nervous system, thyroid, liver, and pancreas

IMAGING

Radiography
Findings
- Innumerable small or moderate-sized filling defects may carpet the entire colon but are sometimes widely scattered.

Utility
- Barium studies

CLINICAL PRESENTATION
- Many patients are asymptomatic.
- Most common signs encountered are rectal bleeding and diarrhea; abdominal pain, anemia, and mucus discharge occur less frequently.
- Familial adenomatous polyposis syndrome may be associated with specific extraintestinal manifestations, producing various clinical syndromes.

DIFFERENTIAL DIAGNOSIS
- Cronkhite-Canada syndrome (gastrointestinal)
- Peutz-Jeghers syndrome (gastrointestinal)

WHAT THE REFERRING PHYSICIAN NEEDS TO KNOW
- Barium enemas markedly underestimate the number of polyps, especially in young patients whose polyps are often less than 3 mm in diameter.
- Surgical intervention is necessary once the condition is diagnosed, with continuous surveillance afterward because of the extremely high risk of malignant degeneration of adenomatous polyps and the development of carcinoma.
- DNA testing or serial colonic examinations after 10 years of age are recommended for other family members at risk.

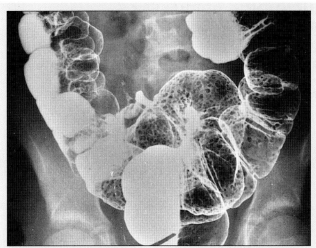

Figure 1. Various appearances of colonic involvement by familial adenomatous polyposis syndrome. In a 10-year-old boy, a double-contrast barium enema demonstrates innumerable small polyps in the colon, particularly carpeting the rectosigmoid region.

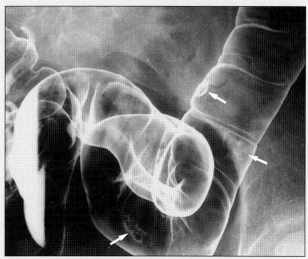

Figure 2. Various appearances of colonic involvement by familial adenomatous polyposis syndrome. In a 17-year-old girl, a double-contrast barium enema shows scattered, small to moderate-sized polyps *(arrows)* in the sigmoid colon.

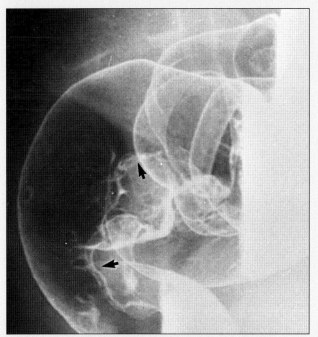

Figure 3. Colon carcinoma in a 32-year-old woman with familial adenomatous polyposis syndrome. A saddle carcinoma *(arrows)* is seen on the anterior wall of the rectum. Scattered small polyps are also present.

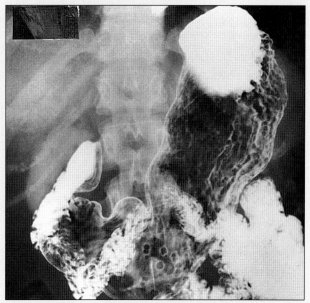

Figure 4. Fundic gland polyposis of the stomach in a 25-year-old woman with familial adenomatous polyposis syndrome. Double-contrast upper gastrointestinal study demonstrates multiple small filling defects in the fundus and body of the stomach. The antrum is not involved. The gallbladder is faintly opacified from a prior oral cholecystogram.

- Multiple hamartoma syndrome (Cowden disease) (gastrointestinal)
- Juvenile polyposis (gastrointestinal)

PATHOLOGY

- Most cases are caused by an abnormal tumor suppressor gene (*APC* gene) on the long arm of chromosome 5.
- Cases show an autosomal-dominant pattern of inheritance; however, up to 30% of patients have no family history of polyposis.
- Familial adenomatous polyposis syndrome may be associated with spontaneous mutations or different mutations.
- Autosomal-dominant polyposis syndrome is associated with the development of adenomas.
- Polyps may be tubular, tubulovillous, or villous adenomas, depending on the location.
- Most commonly affected site is the colon, followed, in order, by the stomach, duodenum, and small bowel.

INCIDENCE/PREVALENCE AND EPIDEMIOLOGY

- Men and women are equally affected.
- Condition is relatively rare but is the most common polyposis syndrome.
- Associations with sebaceous cysts, osteomas, fibrous proliferation, and tumors of central nervous system, thyroid, liver, and pancreas

Suggested Readings

Jagelman DG: Extracolonic manifestations of familial polyposis coli. *Cancer Genet Cytogenet* 27:319-325, 1987.

Lal G, Gallinger S: Familial adenomatous polyposis. *Semin Surg Oncol* 18:314-323, 2000.

Ushio K, Sasagawa M, Doi H, et al: Lesions associated with familial polyposis coli: Studies of lesions of the stomach, duodenum, bones, and teeth. *Gastrointest Radiol* 1:67-80, 1976.

Wallace MH, Phillips RKS: Upper gastrointestinal disease in patients with familial adenomatous polyposis. *Br J Surg* 85:742-750, 1998.

Watne AL: The syndromes of intestinal polyposis. *Curr Probl Surg* 24:269-340, 1987.

Peutz-Jeghers Syndrome

DEFINITION: Inherited condition characterized by gastrointestinal hamartomas, mucocutaneous pigmentation, extraintestinal neoplasms, and an increased risk for gastrointestinal carcinoma.

ANATOMIC FINDINGS

Gastrointestinal Tract
- In Peutz-Jeghers syndrome (PJS), hamartomas are found predominantly in the jejunum and ileum, followed by the duodenum, colon, and stomach.
- Pedunculated polyps are usually found in the small bowel or colon.
- Sessile polyps are more common in the stomach.

IMAGING

Radiography
Findings
- Individual polyps vary in size and may be pedunculated or sessile.
- Polyps tend to occur in clusters rather than as lesions that carpet the bowel.
- Intussusception is a frequent complication.

Utility
- Barium studies

CLINICAL PRESENTATION

- Majority of patients have recurrent episodes of abdominal pain related to intussusceptions caused by hamartomatous polyps.
- Mucocutaneous brown or bluish-black macules on lips and buccal mucosa are a characteristic feature.
- Less frequently, patients may have rectal bleeding or melena.

DIFFERENTIAL DIAGNOSIS

- Familial adenomatous polyposis syndrome (gastrointestinal)
- Cronkhite-Canada syndrome (gastrointestinal)
- Juvenile polyposis (gastrointestinal)
- Multiple hamartoma syndrome (Cowden disease) (gastrointestinal)

DIAGNOSTIC PEARLS

- Individual polyps vary in size and may be pedunculated or sessile.
- PJS hamartomas are found predominantly in the jejunum and ileum, followed by the duodenum, colon, and stomach.
- Mucocutaneous pigmentation, extraintestinal neoplasms, and an increased risk for gastrointestinal carcinoma may occur.

PATHOLOGY

- Autosomal-dominant pattern of inheritance has been noted.
- PJS is associated with the tumor-suppressor gene *STK11,* also known as the *LKB1* gene, located on chromosome 19.
- Characteristic histologic feature of PJS hamartoma is a smooth muscle core arising from the muscularis mucosae and extending into the polyp.
- Mucosa covering the polyp is similar to that normally found in the portion of the gut in which the polyp arises.

INCIDENCE/PREVALENCE AND EPIDEMIOLOGY

- PJS affects men and women equally.
- Studies suggest that at least 10% of patients with PJS develop gastrointestinal cancer.
- Women are more likely to develop gastrointestinal cancer.

Suggested Readings

Buck JL, Harned RK, Lichtenstein JE, et al: Peutz-Jeghers syndrome. *RadioGraphics* 12:365-378, 1992.
Flageole H, Stavros R, Trude JL, et al: Progression toward malignancy of hamartomas in a patient with Peutz-Jeghers syndrome: Case report and literature review. *Can J Surg* 37:231-236, 1994.
Parker MC, Michell MJ: Polyposis. The Peutz-Jeghers syndrome. *Br J Surg* 83:865-875, 1996.
Sener RN, Kumcuoglu Z, Elmasn N, et al: Peutz-Jeghers syndrome: CT and US demonstration of small bowel polyps. *Gastrointest Radiol* 16:21-23, 1991.

WHAT THE REFERRING PHYSICIAN NEEDS TO KNOW

- Patients with PJS have an increased risk for malignancies, most commonly gastrointestinal carcinoma or carcinoma of the pancreas, breast, and ovary.

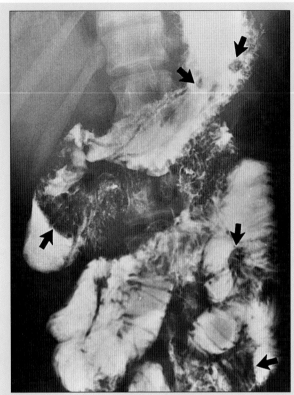

Figure 1. Peutz-Jeghers syndrome in a 22-year-old woman. Multiple hamartomas are present throughout the gastrointestinal tract. Upper gastrointestinal study shows hamartomatous polyps *(arrows)* in the stomach, duodenum, and jejunum.

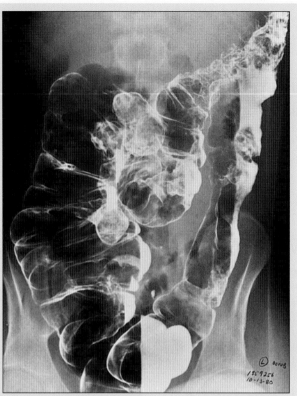

Figure 2. Peutz-Jeghers syndrome in a 22-year-old woman. Double-contrast barium enema shows large hamartomas in all segments of the colon.

Multiple Hamartoma Syndrome (Cowden Disease)

DEFINITION: Genodermatosis characterized by hamartomas and neoplasms of ectodermal, mesodermal, and endodermal origin, affecting multiple organs and organ systems.

ANATOMIC FINDINGS

Gastrointestinal Tract
- Most commonly involves rectosigmoid colon, followed, in decreasing order of frequency, by the stomach, duodenum, small bowel, and esophagus.

IMAGING

Radiography
Findings
- Multiple small, sessile lesions with a segmental or diffuse distribution
Utility
- Barium studies

CLINICAL PRESENTATION

- Mucocutaneous lesions are present in almost all patients and are considered to be a hallmark of the disease.
- Gastrointestinal polyps cause no symptoms and are usually found incidentally or during screening.
- Thyroid gland and central nervous system abnormalities (i.e., Lhermitte-Duclos disease) and breast carcinoma are consistent clinical features.
- Many patients have facial or skeletal abnormalities.

DIFFERENTIAL DIAGNOSIS

- Familial adenomatous polyposis syndrome (gastrointestinal)
- Cronkhite-Canada syndrome (gastrointestinal)
- Juvenile polyposis (gastrointestinal)
- Peutz-Jeghers syndrome (gastrointestinal)

DIAGNOSTIC PEARLS

- Multiple small, sessile lesions with a segmental or diffuse distribution, most commonly located in the rectosigmoid colon
- Thyroid gland and central nervous system abnormalities (i.e., Lhermitte-Duclos disease) and breast carcinoma are consistent clinical features.
- Mucocutaneous lesions are present in almost all patients and are considered to be a hallmark of the disease.

PATHOLOGY

- Autosomal-dominant pattern of inheritance has been established.
- Eighty percent of patients have a mutation in the tumor suppressor gene *PTEN* located on the long arm of chromosome 10.
- Multiple hamartoma syndrome (MHS) is classified as a genodermatosis.
- MHS is characterized by hamartomas and neoplasms of ectodermal, mesodermal, and endodermal origin, affecting multiple organs and organ systems.

INCIDENCE/PREVALENCE AND EPIDEMIOLOGY

- Prevalence of MHS is 1 per 200,000.
- MHS usually occurs in the patient's late teens or early 20s, with almost all cases occurring by the late 30s.

Suggested Readings

Brownstein MH, Mehregan AH, Bikowski JB: The dermatopathology of Cowden's disease: Analysis of fourteen new cases. *Br J Dermatol* 11:1127-1134, 1984.

WHAT THE REFERRING PHYSICIAN NEEDS TO KNOW

- Regular surveillance and possible screening mammography should be encouraged in young women with MHS.
- Lhermitte-Duclos disease (dysplastic gangliocytomas of cerebellar cortex), readily diagnosed by MRI, is considered to be a major criterion for the diagnosis of MHS.
- After MHS or Lhermitte-Duclos disease has been diagnosed, thorough evaluation of the patient for the other entity is crucial.

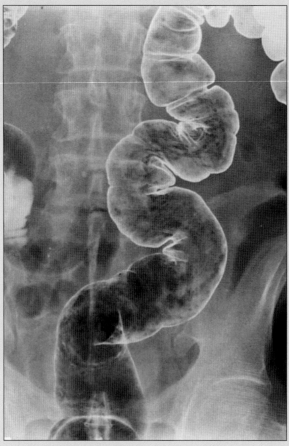

Figure 1. Multiple hamartoma syndrome in a 53-year-old man. Tiny sessile hamartomatous polyps are present in the rectosigmoid colon. Hamartomas were also present in the esophagus.

Carlson GJ, Nivatrongs S, Snover DC: Colorectal polyps in Cowden's disease/multiple hamartoma syndrome. *Am J Pathol* 8:703-707, 1984.

Hanssen AMN, Fryns JP: Cowden syndrome. *J Med Genet* 32:117-119, 1995.

Hizawa K, Iida M, Matsumoto T, et al: Gastrointestinal manifestations of Cowden's disease—report of four cases. *J Clin Gastroenterol* 18:13-18, 1994.

Lashner BA, Riddell RH, Winans CS: Ganglioneuromatosis of the colon and extensive glycogenic acanthosis in Cowden's disease. *Dig Dis Sci* 31:212-216, 1986.

Marra G, Armelao F, Vecchio FM, et al: Cowden's disease with extensive gastrointestinal polyposis. *J Clin Gastroenterol* 18:42-47, 1994.

Taylor AJ, Dodds WJ, Stewart ET: Alimentary tract lesions in Cowden's disease. *Br J Radiol* 62:890-892, 1989.

Thomas DW, Lewis MAO: Lhermitte-Duclos disease associated with Cowden's disease. *Int J Oral Maxillofac Surg* 24:369-371, 1995.

Juvenile Polyposis

DEFINITION: Juvenile polyposis (JP) is characterized by the presence of multiple polyps anywhere in the gastrointestinal tract from the stomach to the rectum, occurring before adulthood.

ANATOMIC FINDINGS

Gastrointestinal Tract
- In decreasing order of frequency, polyps occur in the colon, stomach, small bowel, and duodenum.
- Colonic polyps vary in size but tend to be large, with a diameter of 1 cm or greater.
- Gastric polyps are predominantly located in the gastric antrum.

IMAGING

Radiography
Findings
- Polyps can be sessile or pedunculated.
- Polyps may occur in clusters.

Utility
- Barium studies

CLINICAL PRESENTATION

- Affected individuals may exhibit bleeding, obstruction, and intussusception.
- Many patients are asymptomatic.
- Various congenital anomalies occur in 25% of non-familial cases.
- JP of infancy occurs in first 2 years of life with devastating mucoid or bloody diarrhea.
- Anemia, hypoproteinemia, and repeated episodes of bronchopulmonary infection and small bowel intussusception are seen.
- Ectodermal changes resembling adult Cronkhite-Canada syndrome and congenital anomalies have been reported.

DIFFERENTIAL DIAGNOSIS

- Familial adenomatous polyposis syndrome (gastrointestinal)
- Cronkhite-Canada syndrome (gastrointestinal)

DIAGNOSTIC PEARLS

- Polyps can be sessile or pedunculated, sometimes occurring in clusters.
- Diagnostic criteria include more than five juvenile polyps in the colon and rectum and juvenile polyps throughout the gastrointestinal tract in any number in patients with a family history.

- Multiple hamartoma syndrome (Cowden disease) (gastrointestinal)
- Peutz-Jeghers syndrome (gastrointestinal)

PATHOLOGY

- Polyps can be sessile or pedunculated.
- Diagnostic criteria include more than five juvenile polyps in the colon and rectum and juvenile polyps throughout gastrointestinal tract of any number in patients with a family history of JP.
- Genetics is not precisely defined, but JP appears to have an autosomal-dominant pattern of inheritance.
- Two genes have been implicated in development of JP: *MADH4* in chromosome 18 and *BMPR1A* in chromosome 10.

INCIDENCE/PREVALENCE AND EPIDEMIOLOGY

- JP is rare.
- Approximately 25% of newly diagnosed cases of JP are sporadic.
- Remaining 75% of patients have family history of JP.
- Age at onset is variable, but most cases occur during the second decade of life.

Suggested Readings

Coburn MC, Pricolo VE, Deluca FG, et al: Malignant potential in intestinal juvenile polyposis syndromes. *Ann Surg Oncol* 2:386-391, 1995.

WHAT THE REFERRING PHYSICIAN NEEDS TO KNOW

- Patients are at increased risk for developing malignant tumors of the colon, stomach, small intestine, and pancreas.
- Screening recommendations for patients with JP include colonoscopy every 1-2 years beginning at 15 years of age.
- Upper endoscopy also recommended, beginning at 25 years of age.
- Family members of patients may also be at risk for developing malignant tumors of the gastrointestinal tract.

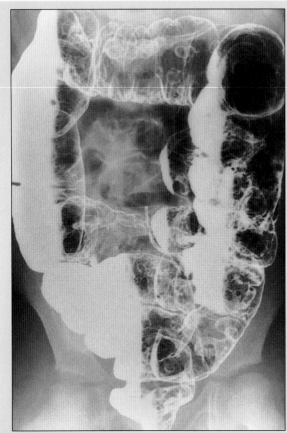

Figure 1. Juvenile polyposis in a 9-year-old girl. A double-contrast barium enema shows clusters of large juvenile polyps throughout the colon.

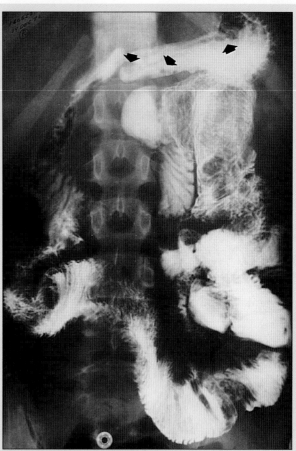

Figure 2. Juvenile polyposis of the gastrointestinal tract in a 21-year-old man with diarrhea and rectal bleeding for 5 years. Upper gastrointestinal study shows juvenile polyps in the stomach (*arrows*) and small bowel.

Desai DC, Neale KF, Talbot IC, et al: Juvenile polyposis. *Br J Surg* 82:14-17, 1995.

Hess KF, Schaffner D, Ricketts RR, et al: Malignant risk in juvenile polyposis coli: Increasing documentation in the pediatric age group. *J Pediatr Surg* 28:1188-1193, 1993.

Jarvinen H, Franssila KO: Familial juvenile polyposis coli: Increased risk of colorectal cancer. *Gut* 25:792-800, 1984.

Jass JR, Williams CB, Bussey HR, et al: Juvenile polyposis: A precancerous condition. *Histopathology* 13:619-630, 1988.

O'Riordain DS, O'Dwyer PJ, Cullen AF, et al: Familial juvenile polyposis coli and colorectal cancer. *Cancer* 68:889-892, 1991.

Radin DR: Hereditary generalized juvenile polyposis: Association with arteriovenous malformation and risk of malignancy. *Abdom Imaging* 19:140-142, 1994.

Vaiphei K, Thapa BR: Juvenile polyposis (coli)—high incidence of dysplastic epithelium. *J Pediatr Surg* 32:1287-1290, 1997.

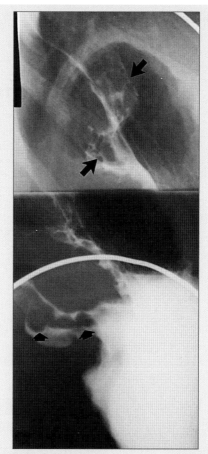

Figure 3. **Juvenile polyposis of the gastrointestinal tract in a 21-year-old man with diarrhea and rectal bleeding for 5 years.** Spot images of the stomach show large juvenile polyps in the fundus *(large arrows)* and smaller polyps in the antrum *(small arrows)*. Multiple juvenile polyps were also present in the colon.

Cronkhite-Canada Syndrome

DEFINITION: Nonfamilial polyposis syndrome characterized by multiple polyps from the stomach to the rectum.

IMAGING

Radiography
Findings
- Polyps are small, sessile, or, less commonly, pedunculated lesions.
- Distribution is throughout the stomach, small bowel, and colon.
- In the stomach, small to moderate-sized polyps carpet the mucosal surface, usually superimposed on thickened rugal folds.

Utility
- Barium studies

CLINICAL PRESENTATION

- Patients typically complain of abdominal pain, anorexia, severe protein-losing diarrhea, malabsorption, and weight loss.
- Severe diarrhea causes electrolyte disturbances, anemia, and hypoproteinemia.
- Ectodermal abnormalities of the skin, hair, and nails generally follow the onset of gastrointestinal symptoms.
- Hair loss involving scalp or body hair occurs abruptly.
- Brown macules develop on the palmar and plantar skin surfaces.
- Prognosis is usually poor, with mortality rate of greater than 50%.

DIFFERENTIAL DIAGNOSIS

- Familial adenomatous polyposis syndrome (gastrointestinal)
- Peutz-Jeghers syndrome (gastrointestinal)
- Multiple hamartoma syndrome (Cowden disease) (gastrointestinal)
- Juvenile polyposis (gastrointestinal)

PATHOLOGY

- Cronkhite-Canada syndrome (CCS) is a nonfamilial polyposis syndrome characterized by multiple polyps from the stomach to the rectum.

DIAGNOSTIC PEARLS

- Polyps are small, sessile, or, less commonly, pedunculated lesions.
- Distribution occurs throughout the stomach, small bowel, and colon.
- In stomach, small to moderate-sized polyps carpet the mucosal surface, usually superimposed on thickened rugal folds.
- Ectodermal abnormalities of the skin, hair, and nails develop.

- Lesions are believed to be inflammatory polyps, but adenomatous, hyperplastic, and hamartomatous polyps have also been reported in smaller numbers.
- Mental and physical stress has been suggested as an important factor in the development of this disorder.

INCIDENCE/PREVALENCE AND EPIDEMIOLOGY

- Average age at onset is 60 years, with an age distribution of 31-76 years.
- Colon cancer has been reported in approximately 12% of 387 documented cases of CCS to date.

Suggested Readings

Burke AP, Sobin LH: The pathology of Cronkhite-Canada syndrome polyps. *Am J Surg Pathol* 13:940-946, 1989.
Daniel ES, Ludwig SL, Lewin KL, et al: The Cronkhite-Canada syndrome: An analysis of clinical and pathological features and therapy in 55 patients. *Medicine (Baltimore)* 61:293-309, 1982.
Diner WC: The Cronkhite-Canada syndrome. *Radiology* 105:715-716, 1972.
Kilcheski T, Kressel HY, Laufer I, et al: The radiographic appearance of the stomach in the Cronkhite-Canada syndrome. *Radiology* 141:57-60, 1981.

WHAT THE REFERRING PHYSICIAN NEEDS TO KNOW

- Recent reports suggest a more favorable prognosis after intense therapy with steroids and nutritional support.

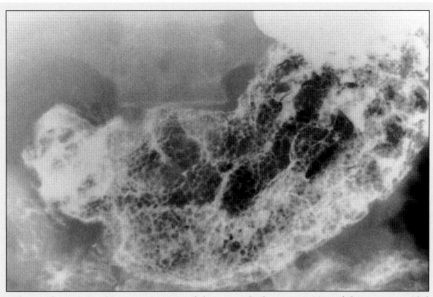

Figure 1. Cronkhite-Canada syndrome. Double-contrast view of the stomach shows carpeting of the mucosa with hamartomatous polyps superimposed on enlarged rugal folds.

Part 36

MISCELLANEOUS ABNORMALITIES OF THE COLON

Colonic Obstruction

DEFINITION: Colonic obstruction is usually caused by a neoplasm or another abnormality, including diverticulitis, volvulus, intussusception, adhesions, hernias, and strictures, among others.

IMAGING

Radiography
Findings
- Colon is dilated proximal to the obstruction.
- If the ileocecal valve is incompetent, the appearance may mimic small bowel obstruction.
- Progressive tapering of two limbs leading to a twist in volvulus is the *beak* seen on barium enema.
- Classic *coil spring* appearance of intussusception is seen on barium study; contrast is trapped between the intussusceptum and the intussuscipiens.
- On barium enema, adhesions appear as a circumferential narrowing with intact mucosa or as smooth, broad-based filling defect.

Utility
- Abdominal radiographs should be taken in supine and erect or the left lateral decubitus positions.
- Radiography may confirm the diagnosis and locate the site of the obstruction and may sometimes identify the nature of the obstruction.

CT
Findings
- Distended bowel loops are seen proximal to the collapsed loops.
- *Whirl* sign constitutes afferent and efferent limbs leading into the volvulus; twisted mesentery and the bowel comprise the central portion of the whirl.
- Intussusceptions are of three different patterns: the *target* sign, a sausage-shaped mass, and a reniform mass.

DIAGNOSTIC PEARLS
- Colon is dilated proximal to the obstruction.
- Progressive tapering of the two limbs leading to twist in volvulus is the *beak* seen on barium study.
- Classic *coil spring* appearance of intussusception is seen on barium study.

Utility
- CT is the primary imaging technique in all patients with suspected obstruction.

Ultrasound
Findings
- Target-like lesion in intussusception, a hypoechoic halo in intussuscipiens, and a hyperechoic center in intussusceptum

Utility
- Ultrasound is often the initial cross-sectional test ordered in infants with suspected bowel obstruction.

CLINICAL PRESENTATION
- Right colon lesions: Signs and symptoms are insidious because the lumen is large and the contents are semiliquid; they include pain, palpable mass, and anemia.
- Left-sided lesions cause progressive constipation, obstipation with abdominal distention, and pain.

WHAT THE REFERRING PHYSICIAN NEEDS TO KNOW
- After plain-film radiography, a water-soluble enema is the next step for large-bowel obstruction or if the level of the obstruction is unknown.
- Water-soluble enema can be therapeutic in patients with fecal impactions.
- Patients with suspected nonobstructing diverticulitis may benefit from a CT examination as the initial study.
- Anything that causes colon distention, including pseudo-obstruction, distal tumor, endoscopy, enemas, and postoperative ileus, may precipitate cecal volvulus.
- In infants and young children, hydrostatic or pneumatic intussusception reduction should be attempted and may be definitive therapy.
- In adult intussusception, the high incidence of organic lesions, often malignant, precludes hydrostatic or pneumatic reduction.
- Internal hernias, through the foramen of Winslow, can cause colon obstruction; diagnosis is made by radiography, barium enema, or CT.

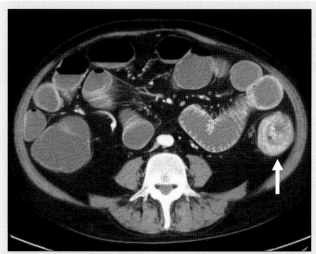

Figure 1. CT in the evaluation of large-bowel obstruction.
Axial image shows an enhancing, obstructing mass *(arrow)* at
the junction of the descending colon and sigmoid colon.

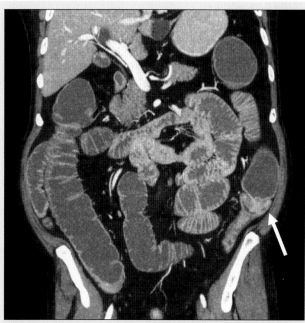

Figure 2. CT in the evaluation of large-bowel obstruction.
Coronal reformatted image demonstrates the obstructing cancer
(arrow) and dilated, fluid-filled colon and small bowel.

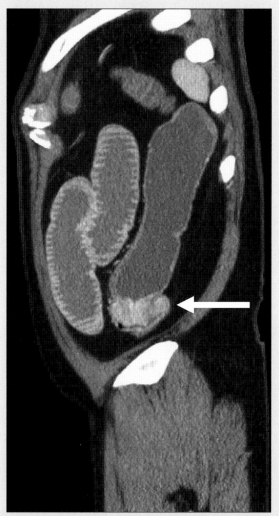

Figure 3. CT in the evaluation of large-bowel obstruction.
Sagittal depiction of the cancer *(arrow)* and dilated, fluid-filled
colon and small bowel.

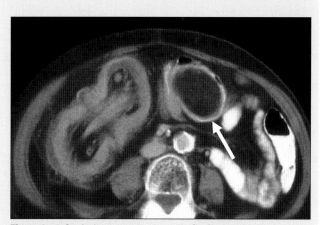

Figure 4. Colonic intussusception: CT findings. The lead
point of this colonic intussusception is a lipoma *(arrow)*. The
outer layer represents the intussuscipiens and the inner layer
represents the intussusceptum.

- If the ileocecal valve is incompetent, retrograde decompression produces a gradual onset of distention and, eventually, feculent vomiting.
- Lesions at the ileocecal valve or ileocolic intussusception cause more acute symptoms of small bowel obstruction: abdominal pain, distention, vomiting, and obstipation.
- In patients with volvulus, pain and distention occur rapidly; if a closed-loop obstruction and bowel ischemia are present, an abdominal mass and distention can be present.
- Bowel sounds are often hyperactive, particularly with a superimposed small bowel obstruction, marked tenderness, or rebound, which suggests perforation or strangulation.

DIFFERENTIAL DIAGNOSIS

- Toxic megacolon
- Colonic pseudo-obstruction
- Parkinson disease, electrolyte imbalance, antimotility medications, hormonal disorders

PATHOLOGY

- Swallowed air proximal to the obstruction causes dilation, but third spacing of the fluid in the gut lumen is not seen.
- Strangulation rarely occurs, except in occasional cases of volvulus.
- Colonic response to mechanical obstruction depends on the competency of the ileocecal valve; the small bowel decompresses the colon when the valve is incompetent.
- A closed-loop obstruction develops when the valve is competent because the colon cannot decompress.
- In the cecum, which has the largest diameter, the wall develops the highest tension, according to Laplace's law (wall tension = intraluminal pressure × radius).
- Dissection of the air into the wall results in pneumatosis and precedes frank perforation.
- Ischemia and bacterial overgrowth also play a role in cecal perforation and the systemic effects seen with strangulation obstruction.

INCIDENCE/PREVALENCE AND EPIDEMIOLOGY

- Large bowel obstruction is caused by intrinsic colon carcinoma in approximately 55% of cases.
- Nearly 20% of colon cancers have some obstruction; 5%-10% are complete obstructions that require emergent surgery.

- Large bowel volvulus accounts for approximately 10% of colon obstructions.
- Sigmoid colon is the most frequent site of colonic volvulus, especially in patients older than 60 years.
- In infants and children, intussusception represents 80%-90% of bowel obstructions, the second most common cause of acute abdominal emergency in children.
- Adult intussusception accounts for 1%-3% of mechanical intestinal obstructions, with demonstrable cause in 80% of cases.

Suggested Readings

Alessi V, Salerno G: The "hay-fork" sign in the ultrasonographic diagnosis of intussusception. *Gastrointest Radiol* 10:177-179, 1985.

Ballantyne GH, Brandner ML, Beart RW, et al: Volvulus of the colon: Incidence and mortality. *Ann Surg* 202:83-92, 1985.

Cohn I, Chappuis CW: Bowel obstruction. In Taylor MB (ed): *Gastrointestinal Emergencies*, 2nd ed. Baltimore, Williams & Wilkins, 1997, pp 515-536.

Cotlar AM, Cohn I: Intussusception in adults. *Am J Surg* 101:114-120, 1961.

Culp WC: Relief of severe rectal impactions with water-soluble contrast enemas. *Radiology* 115:9-12, 1975.

Del-Pozo G, Albillos JC, Tejedor D: Intussusception: US findings with pathologic correlation—the crescent-in-doughnut sign. *Radiology* 199:688-692, 1996.

Erkan N, Haciyanli M, Yildirim M, et al: Intussusception in adults: An unusual and challenging condition for surgeons. *Int J Colorectal Dis* 20:452-456, 2005.

Garcia-Valdecasas JC, Llovera JM, deLacy AM, et al: Obstructing colorectal carcinomas: A prospective study. *Dis Colon Rectum* 34:759-762, 1991.

Hirao K, Kikawada M, Hanyu H, et al: Sigmoid volvulus showing "a whirl sign" on CT. *Intern Med* 45:331-332, 2006.

Iko BO, Teal JS, Siram SM, et al: Computed tomography of adult colonic intussusception: Clinical and experimental studies. *AJR Am J Roentgenol* 143:769-772, 1984.

Jones DJ, Dharmeratnam R, Langstaff RJ: Large bowel obstruction due to pelvic lipomatosis. *Ann Surg* 71:309-311, 1985.

Lou CJ: Intussusception in adults: An analysis of 92 cases. *Clin Med J* 95:297-300, 1982.

McKay R: Ileocecal intussusception in an adult: The laparoscopic approach. *JSLS* 10:250-253, 2006.

Parienty RA, LePreux JF, Gruson B: Sonography and CT features of ileocolic intussusception. *AJR Am J Roentgenol* 136:608-610, 1981.

Phillips RKS, Hittinger R, Fry JS, et al: Malignant large bowel obstruction. *Br J Surg* 72:296-302, 1985.

Rao BK, Fleischer AC: Sonography of the gastrointestinal tract. *Curr Opin Radiol* 2:207-212, 1990.

Richards WO, Williams L Jr: Obstruction of the large and small intestine. *Surg Clin North Am* 68:355-376, 1988.

Russell JC, Welch JP: Pathophysiology of bowel obstruction. In Welch JP (ed): *Bowel Obstruction*. Philadelphia, WB Saunders, 1990, pp 28-58.

Sarr MG, Nagorney DM, McIlrath DC: Postoperative intussusception in the adult: A previously unrecognized entity. *Arch Surg* 116:144-148, 1981.

Turnage RH, Bergen PC: Intestinal obstruction and ileus. In Feldman M, Scharschmidt BF, Sleisenger MH (eds): *Gastrointestinal and Liver Disease*, 6th ed. Philadelphia, WB Saunders, 1998, pp 1799-1809.

Endometriosis Involving the Gastrointestinal Tract

DEFINITION: Endometriosis is the presence of ectopic tissue containing endometrial epithelial and stromal elements outside the uterine cavity.

IMAGING

Radiography
Findings
- Implants appear as an extrinsic serosal mass effect with mucosal preservation on double-contrast barium enema studies.
- Mass may appear as a polypoid mass extending into the lumen of the colon, a stricture, or a short annular lesion on barium enema.
- Serosal spiculation and fine crenulations of the mucosa are seen.

Utility
- Nonspecific and may be seen in drop metastases or abscess
- Possibly difficult to distinguish radiographically from carcinoma

Ultrasound
Findings
- Solid or complex cystic masses

Utility
- Not specific and may be indistinguishable from neoplasm or abscess

CT
Findings
- Solid or complex cystic masses

Utility
- Not specific and may be indistinguishable from neoplasm or abscess

MRI
Findings
- Detects hemorrhage within the masses

Utility
- More sensitive and specific for detection of hemorrhage within masses

CLINICAL PRESENTATION

- Endometriosis rarely causes acute obstruction, gastrointestinal bleeding, or perforation necessitating resection.
- Abdominal pain often coinciding with menstrual period

DIAGNOSTIC PEARLS

- Implants appear as an extrinsic serosal mass effect with mucosal preservation on double-contrast barium enema studies.
- MRI is more sensitive and specific for the detection of hemorrhage within masses.
- Solid or complex cystic masses on ultrasound and CT are difficult to differentiate from an abscess or carcinoma.

DIFFERENTIAL DIAGNOSIS

- Serosal tumor implant in patients with carcinomatosis due to cancer of the ovary, appendix, colon, stomach, small bowel, or pancreas
- Primary colon cancer
- Primary colon infection

PATHOLOGY

- Endometriosis is the presence of ectopic tissue containing endometrial epithelial and stromal elements outside the uterine cavity.
- Endometrial implants on the bowel are usually extrinsic or serosal but may be intramural or, rarely, intraluminal.

INCIDENCE/PREVALENCE AND EPIDEMIOLOGY

- Endometriosis affects 8%-18% of women during the active menstrual years, between 30 and 45 years of age.
- Gastrointestinal tract involvement in endometriosis has been reported in 5%-37% of patients.
- Rectosigmoid colon is the most frequently involved site, followed by the rectovaginal septum, small intestine, cecum, and appendix.
- Anterior wall of the rectosigmoid colon adjacent to the pouch of Douglas is the most frequent site of gastrointestinal tract involvement.

WHAT THE REFERRING PHYSICIAN NEEDS TO KNOW
- Endometriosis is common in women during their active menstrual years, between 30 and 45 years of age.

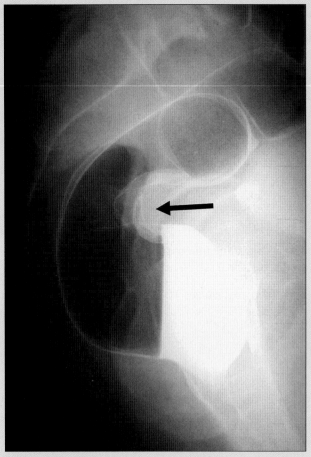

Figure 1. Endometrioma in the pouch of Douglas. Barium enema examination shows an extrinsic mass on the anterior serosal aspect of the rectum *(arrow)*.

Suggested Readings

Athey PA, Diment DD: The spectrum of sonographic findings in endometriomas. *J Ultrasound Med* 8:491-497, 1989.

Brown DL, Frates MC, Laing FC, et al: Ovarian masses: Can benign and malignant lesions be differentiated with color and pulsed Doppler US? *Radiology* 190:333-336, 1994.

Coronado C, Franklin RR, Lotze EC, et al: Surgical treatment of symptomatic colorectal endometriosis. *Fertil Steril* 53:411-416, 1990.

Fagan CJ: Endometriosis: Clinical and roentgenographic manifestations. *Radiol Clin North Am* 12:109-125, 1974.

Fishman EK, Scatarige JC, Saksouk FA, et al: Computed tomography of endometriosis. *J Comput Assist Tomogr* 7:257-264, 1983.

Goodman P, Raval B, Zimmerman G: Perforation of the colon due to endometriosis. *Gastrointest Radiol* 15:346-348, 1990.

Gordon RL, Evers K, Kressel HY, et al: Double-contrast enema in pelvic endometriosis. *AJR Am J Roentgenol* 138:549-552, 1982.

McCaffee CHG, Greer HLH: Intestinal endometriosis: A report of 29 cases and a survey of the literature. *J Obstet Gynecol* 67:539-555, 1960.

Nezhat F, Nezhat C, Pennington E, et al: Laparoscopic segmental resection for infiltrating endometriosis of the rectosigmoid colon: A preliminary report. *Surg Laparosc Endosc* 2:212-216, 1992.

Prystowsky JB, Stryker SJ, Ujiki GT, et al: Gastrointestinal endometriosis: Incidence and indications for resection. *Arch Surg* 123:855-858, 1988.

Sievert W, Sellin JH, Stringer CA: Pelvic endometriosis simulating colonic malignant neoplasm. *Arch Intern Med* 149:935-938, 1989.

Tate GT: Acute obstruction of the large bowel due to endometriosis. *Br J Surg* 50:771-773, 1963.

Togashi K, Nishimura K, Kimura I, et al: Endometrial cysts: Diagnosis with MR imaging. *Radiology* 180:73-78, 1991.

Zwas FR, Lyon DT: Endometriosis: An important condition in clinical gastroenterology. *Dig Dis Sci* 36:353-364, 1991.

Benign and Malignant Gynecologic Conditions Affecting the Colon

DEFINITION: Variety of gynecologic diseases may involve the gastrointestinal tract and may mimic a primary disease of the gastrointestinal tract.

IMAGING

Radiography

Findings
- Peritoneal implants in ovarian carcinoma appear as extrinsic masses with serosal spiculation and tethering on barium enema.
- Invasion of the colon by ovarian cancer can also show gross invasion and annular constriction to complete obstruction on barium enema.
- On barium enema, fibroids show extrinsic mass effect on the sigmoid colon, displacing and stretching the colon if the tumor is large.

Utility
- Implant in the cul-de-sac may be indistinguishable from an abscess or endometrioma.
- Barium enema provides important information for staging and planning surgical resection of pelvic malignancy.

CT

Findings
- Teratomas usually contain fat or calcification.

Utility
- CT can show mass effect on the colon and small bowel.

CLINICAL PRESENTATION

- Patients with ovarian carcinoma have vague abdominal symptoms, increasing abdominal girth, and a large palpable mass.
- Intestinal symptoms or colonic obstruction may be the first manifestation of ovarian cancer.
- Uterine leiomyomas or fibroids are mostly small and are asymptomatic.

DIFFERENTIAL DIAGNOSIS

- Carcinoma of the colon
- Stricture related to inflammatory bowel disease
- Peritoneal carcinomatosis from colonic, gastric, small bowel, pancreatic, or hepatobiliary malignancy

DIAGNOSTIC PEARLS

- Peritoneal implants in ovarian carcinoma appear as extrinsic masses with serosal spiculation and tethering on barium enema.
- On barium enema, fibroids show extrinsic mass effect on the sigmoid colon, displacing and stretching the colon if the tumor is large.
- Teratomas usually contain fat or calcification that can be seen on plain CT.

PATHOLOGY

- Subperitoneal space forms a pathway for the spread of ovarian carcinoma from the pelvis to the abdomen.
- Carcinoma of the endometrium, vagina, and fallopian tubes can spread by peritoneal seeding or lymphatic extension.
- Leiomyosarcoma of the uterus may spread by hematogenous metastasis to the gut.

INCIDENCE/PREVALENCE AND EPIDEMIOLOGY

- Ovarian carcinoma is the most common primary malignancy to invade the colon directly.
- Ovarian carcinoma is the fifth leading cause of cancer death in women.
- Prevalence of ovarian carcinoma increases with age and peaks around age 60 years.
- Cervical carcinoma is the sixth leading cause of cancer death in women in the United States.
- Invasive cervical carcinoma has a peak prevalence at age 54 years.
- Uterine leiomyomas or fibroids are present in 25% to 50% of women.
- Uterine leiomyomas are the most common pelvic tumor, with a peak incidence in the fifth decade of life.

WHAT THE REFERRING PHYSICIAN NEEDS TO KNOW

- A variety of gynecologic and other extracolonic diseases may secondarily involve the gastrointestinal tract.
- Involvement may mimic a primary disease of the gastrointestinal tract.
- Familiarity with the patterns of gastrointestinal tract involvement is important for the accurate interpretation of imaging studies.

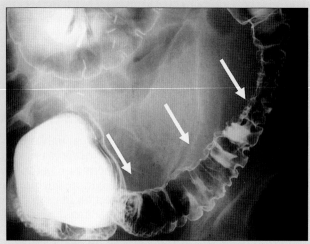

Figure 1. Ovarian carcinomatosis. Multiple serosal implants *(arrows)* are identified along the medial aspect of the sigmoid colon.

Suggested Readings

Ellis JH, Francis IR, Rhodes M, et al: CT findings in tuboovarian abscess. *J Comput Assist Tomogr* 15:589-592, 1991.

Feller E, Schiffman FJ: Colonic obstruction as the first manifestation of ovarian carcinoma. *Am J Gastroenterol* 82:25-28, 1987.

Gedgaudas K, Kelvin FM, Thompson WM, et al: The value of the preoperative barium-enema examination in the assessment of pelvic masses. *Radiology* 146:609-613, 1983.

Hawnaur JM: Staging of cervical and endometrial carcinoma. *Clin Radiol* 47:7-13, 1993.

Krestin GP, Beyer D, Lorenz R: Secondary involvement of the transverse colon by tumors of the pelvis: Spread of malignancies along the greater omentum. *Gastrointest Radiol* 10:283-288, 1985.

Landis SH, Murray T, Bolden S, et al: *Cancer Statistics CA* 48:6-29, 2006.

Levitt RG, Koehler RE, Sagel SS, et al: Metastatic disease of the mesentery and omentum. *Radiol Clin North Am* 20:501-510, 1982.

Meyers MA: Intraperitoneal spread of malignancies and its effect on the bowel. *Clin Radiol* 32:129-146, 1981.

Oliphant M, Berne AS, Meyers MA: Imaging the direct bidirectional spread of disease between the abdomen and the female pelvis via the subperitoneal space. *Gastrointest Radiol* 13:285-298, 1988.

Oliphant M, Berne AS, Meyers MA: Bidirectional spread of disease via the subperitoneal space: The lower abdomen and left pelvis. *Abdom Imaging* 18:117-125, 1993.

Rubesin SE, Levine MS: Omental cakes: Colonic involvement by omental metastases. *Radiology* 154:593-596, 1985.

Rubesin SE, Levine MS, Glick SN: Gastric involvement by omental cakes: Radiographic findings. *Gastrointest Radiol* 11:223-228, 1986.

Radiation Colitis

DEFINITION: Injuries to the colon caused by radiation exposure in patients receiving radiotherapy for pelvic, genitourinary, and gastrointestinal tumors.

ANATOMIC FINDINGS

Colon
- Diffuse or focal narrowing
- Distorted mucosal pattern

Presacral Space
- Widened

IMAGING

Radiography
Findings
- Diffuse or focal narrowing of the rectum and sigmoid colon is seen, usually with tapered margins.
- Mucosal pattern is usually preserved but may be distorted or disrupted because of edema or intramural hemorrhage.
- Rectal stricture is seen.
- Rectovaginal fistula is seen.

Utility
- Barium enema

CLINICAL PRESENTATION

- Rectal bleeding, pain, and diarrhea
- Proctitis

DIFFERENTIAL DIAGNOSIS

- Ischemic colitis
- Ulcerative colitis
- Crohn disease
- Infectious colitis
- Behçet disease

PATHOLOGY

- Radiation-injured cells by direct cytotoxic effect and by causing damage to the fine vasculature and connective tissue of the intestine.
- In decreasing order of radiation tolerance are the duodenum, jejunum, ileum, transverse colon, sigmoid colon, esophagus, and rectum.

DIAGNOSTIC PEARLS

- Radiation colitis occurs in patients receiving radiotherapy for pelvic genitourinary tumors.
- Diffuse or focal narrowing of rectum and sigmoid colon is seen, usually with tapered margins.
- Mucosal pattern is usually preserved but may be distorted or disrupted because of edema or intramural hemorrhage.

- Tolerance dose is 4500 cGy for the small bowel and colon and 5000 cGy for the rectum.
- Edema, hyperemia, and extensive inflammatory cell infiltration resulting from radiation-induced ischemic changes are seen.
- Pathologically, abnormal epithelial cell proliferation and maturation are associated with a decrease in crypt cell mitosis.

INCIDENCE/PREVALENCE AND EPIDEMIOLOGY

- Radiation colitis occurs in patients receiving radiation treatment for pelvic genitourinary tumors.
- It typically develops after a 2-year latent period.

Suggested Readings

Capps GW, Fulcher AS, Szucs RA, et al: Imaging features of radiation induced changes in the abdomen. *RadioGraphics* 17:1455-1473, 1997.

Carr ND, Pullen BR, Hasleton PS, et al: Microvascular studies in human radiation bowel disease. *Gut* 25:448-454, 1984.

Donner CS: Pathophysiology and therapy of chronic radiation-induced injury to the colon. *Dig Dis* 16:253-258, 1998.

Jeffrey RB, McGahan JP: Gastrointestinal tract and peritoneal cavity. In McGahan JP, Goldberg BB (eds): *Diagnostic Ultrasound: A Logical Approach*. Philadelphia, Lippincott-Raven, 1998, pp 511-560.

Schrock TR: Examination and diseases of the anorectum. In Feldman M, Scharschmidt BF, Sleisenger MH (eds): *Gastrointestinal and Liver Disease*, 6th ed. Philadelphia, WB Saunders, 1998, pp 1960-1976.

Wilson SR: The gastrointestinal tract. In Rumack CM, Wilson SR, Charboneau JW (eds): *Diagnostic Ultrasound*, 2nd ed. St. Louis, Mosby-Year Book, 1998, pp 279-328.

WHAT THE REFERRING PHYSICIAN NEEDS TO KNOW
- When symptoms such as obstruction or fistula become intolerable, surgical resection may be needed.
- Development of colon carcinoma has been suggested as a possible late sequela of pelvic irradiation.

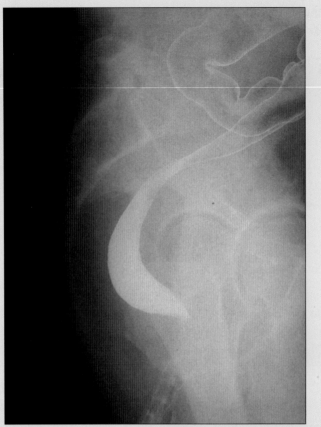

Figure 1. Radiation-induced rectosigmoid stricture. A long segment of narrowing occurs in the rectosigmoid demonstrated on this barium enema examination. The presacral space is widened as well.

Vascular Lesions of the Anorectum

DEFINITION: Disorders of different causes characterized by damage to the anorectal vasculature, leading to bleeding.

IMAGING

Radiography
Findings
- Internal hemorrhoids: lobulation; solitary or cluster of smooth polyps are seen in the anorectal folds less than 3 cm from the anorectal junction.
- Rectal varices appear as smooth, serpiginous folds coursing along the rectal mucosa or as small, smooth-surfaced submucosal nodules in profile.

Utility
- Double-contrast barium enema examination is a relatively accurate technique for diagnosing internal hemorrhoids.
- Purpose of the barium enema in patients with internal hemorrhoids is to investigate for serious causes of bleeding or pain.
- Internal hemorrhoids seen as solitary polyps cannot be distinguished from inflammatory, benign, or neoplastic rectal polyps.
- Internal hemorrhoids appearing as large, lobulated infiltrative folds are indistinguishable from proctitis or an infiltrating neoplasm.

CLINICAL PRESENTATION

- Hemorrhoids cause brisk rectal bleeding and painful swelling.
- Rectal varices cause lower gastrointestinal bleeding.

DIFFERENTIAL DIAGNOSIS

- Cloacogenic carcinoma (colon)
- Anal cancer
- Rectal cancer
- Ulcerative proctitis
- Crohn proctitis

PATHOLOGY

- Internal hemorrhoids appear as thick-walled submucosal veins with accompanying arteries and dilated capillaries and with abundant arteriovenous anastomoses.

DIAGNOSTIC PEARLS

- Internal hemorrhoids are associated with lobulation and a solitary or cluster of smooth polyps in the anorectal folds, less than 3 cm from the anorectal junction.
- Rectal varices appear as smooth serpiginous folds coursing along the rectal mucosa.
- Cloacogenic carcinoma may appear as a submucosal mass with a smooth or ulcerated surface, broad-based sessile polyps, or infiltrative lesions.
- Solitary rectal ulcer syndrome is associated with diffuse, finely nodular mucosa in the distal rectum and with focal, small ulcer or ulcers on the anterior or anterolateral wall.

INCIDENCE/PREVALENCE AND EPIDEMIOLOGY

- Rectal varices are a rare cause of lower gastrointestinal bleeding and are usually seen in patients with portal hypertension.

Suggested Readings

Feczko PJ, O'Connell DJ, Riddell RH, et al: Solitary rectal ulcer syndrome: Radiologic manifestations. *AJR Am J Roentgenol* 135:499-506, 1980.

Gillespie JJ, Mackay B: Histogenesis of cloacogenic carcinoma: Fine structure of anal transitional epithelium and cloacogenic carcinoma. *Hum Pathol* 9:579-587, 1978.

Glickman MG, Margulis AR: Cloacogenic carcinoma. *AJR Am J Roentgenol* 107:175-180, 1969.

Kelvin FM, Gardiner R (eds): *Clinical Imaging of the Colon and Rectum*. New York, Raven, 1987, pp 422-460.

Kyaw MM, Gallagher T, Haines JO: Cloacogenic carcinoma of the anorectal junction: Roentgenologic diagnosis. *AJR Am J Roentgenol* 115:384-391, 1972.

Levine MS, Piccolello ML, Sollenberger LC, et al: Solitary rectal ulcer syndrome: A radiologic diagnosis? *Gastrointest Radiol* 11:187-193, 1986.

Manzi D, Samanta AK: Adhesion-related colonic varices. *J Clin Gastroenterol* 7:71-75, 1985.

McCormack TT, Bailey HR, Simms JM, et al: Rectal varices are not piles. *Br J Surg* 71:163-168, 1984.

Millward SF, Bayjoo P, Dixon MF, et al: The barium enema appearances in solitary rectal ulcer syndrome. *Clin Radiol* 36:185-189, 1985.

Schrock TR: Examination and diseases of the anorectum. In Feldman M, Scharschmidt BF, Sleisenger MH (eds): *Gastrointestinal and Liver Disease*, 6th ed. Philadelphia, WB Saunders, 1998, pp 1960-1976.

Thoeni RF, Venbrux AC: The anal canal: Distinction of internal hemorrhoids from small cancers by double-contrast barium enema examination. *Radiology* 145:17-19, 1982.

Vaizey CJ, van den Bogaerde JB, Emmanuel AV, et al: Solitary rectal ulcer syndrome. *Br J Surg* 85:1617-1623, 1998.

WHAT THE REFERRING PHYSICIAN NEEDS TO KNOW

- With strangulation of hemorrhoids, mucosal infarction, necrosis, and superinfection may occur.
- Internal hemorrhoids may also be a complication of distal rectal carcinoma.

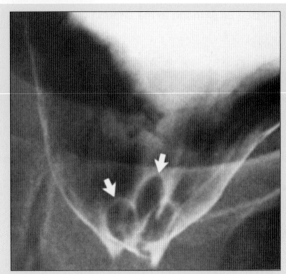

Figure 1. **Radiographic appearance of internal hemorrhoids.** *Bunch of grapes.* Three smooth-surfaced polyps *(arrows)* are clustered above the anorectal junction. This radiographic appearance is typical of internal hemorrhoids.

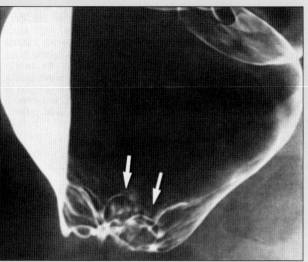

Figure 2. **Radiographic appearance of internal hemorrhoids.** Multiple polypoid folds. Large, polypoid folds *(arrows)* with a nodular surface pattern in the distal rectum. Although these radiographic findings are typically seen with internal hemorrhoids, they may also be caused by solitary rectal ulcer syndrome, various forms of proctitis, or an unusual infiltrating tumor.

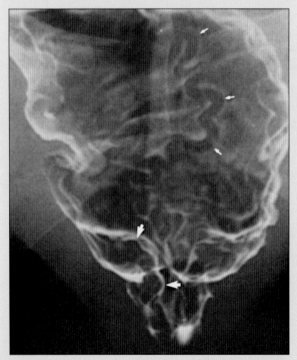

Figure 3. **Rectal varices.** Spot film of the distal rectum shows the en face appearance of rectal varices as serpentine folds etched in white *(small arrows).* In profile, smooth, lobulated folds disrupt the contour of the bowel, extending from the anorectal junction proximally *(large arrows).* *(From Rubesin SE, Saul SH, Laufer I, et al: Carpet lesions of the colon.* RadioGraphics *5:537-552, 1985.)*

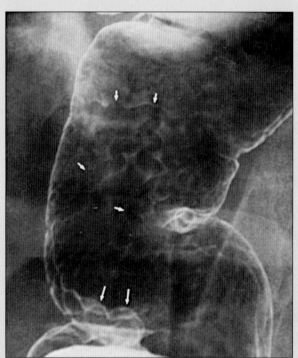

Figure 4. **Rectal varices.** In another patient, spot film of the proximal rectum shows serpentine folds etched in white *(short arrows).* In profile, a valve of Houston is expanded by a smooth, lobulated submucosal process compatible with a rectal varix *(long arrows).* *(From Rubesin SE, Saul SH, Laufer I, et al: Carpet lesions of the colon.* RadioGraphics *5:537-552, 1985.)*

Functional Disorders of the Colon

DEFINITION: Disorders largely caused by functional abnormalities rather than mechanical obstruction.

IMAGING

Fluoroscopy
Findings
- Irritable bowel syndrome (IBS) may be characterized by exaggerated haustral markings and scybalous (pellet-like) stool.
- Regions of hypertonicity and spasm, sigmoid myochosis, and diverticula have also been associated with IBS.
- Delayed transit time in chronic constipation is seen.
- Tremendously dilated, tortuous colon and rectum filled with large fecal residue are seen in nonobstructive megacolon.
- Smooth and wide diverticula, retaining barium on postevacuation films, are seen in scleroderma.
- Ileus, thumbprinting, pneumatosis intestinalis, and pseudo-obstruction are seen in systemic lupus erythematosus (SLE).
- Fecal impaction and obstruction may be observed in diabetics.

Utility
- Barium enema studies are used.
- Role of radiology in IBS is to exclude structural abnormalities such as inflammatory bowel disease, strictures, and cancer.

Radiography
Findings
- IBS may be associated with exaggerated haustral markings and scybalous stool.
- Delayed transit time in chronic constipation is seen.
- Tremendously dilated, tortuous colon and rectum filled with large fecal residue are seen in nonobstructive megacolon.
- Smooth and wide diverticula, retaining barium on postevacuation films, are seen in scleroderma.
- Ileus, thumbprinting, pneumatosis intestinalis, and pseudo-obstruction are seen in SLE.
- Fecal impaction and obstruction may be observed in diabetics.

Utility
- Double-contrast barium studies are being used less frequently in the evaluation of patients with functional colonic disorders.

DIAGNOSTIC PEARLS
- Tremendously dilated, tortuous colon and rectum filled with large fecal residue, are seen in nonobstructive megacolon.
- IBS may be associated with exaggerated haustral markings and scybalous stool.
- Smooth and wide diverticula, retaining barium on postevacuation films, are seen in scleroderma.

CLINICAL PRESENTATION
- IBS causes altered bowel habits, abdominal pain relieved by defecation, bloating, dyspepsia, nausea and vomiting, and heartburn.
- Nonobstructive megacolon causes vague rectal fullness, nonspecific abdominal discomfort, and overflow diarrhea as seen in fecal impaction.
- Systemic lupus erythematosus leads to peritoneal serositis, pancreatitis, ascites, and enteritis.
- Constipation is the most common gastrointestinal symptom of diabetic patients and is typically intermittent and alternates with diarrhea.
- Fecal impaction may be sufficiently severe to produce mechanical obstruction.

DIFFERENTIAL DIAGNOSIS
- Intestinal pseudo-obstruction
- Adhesions
- Parkinson disease
- Electrolyte and hormonal disorders
- Antimotility medication

PATHOLOGY
- These disorders are mostly caused by functional abnormalities rather than a mechanical obstruction.
- They may be caused by abnormal myoelectric and motor activities in the gut, neuropathy, or severe neurologic or psychological disorders.

WHAT THE REFERRING PHYSICIAN NEEDS TO KNOW
- In patients older than 50 years, the risk of colon cancer is such that evaluation by barium enema or colonoscopy is indicated.
- Role of radiology in IBS is to exclude structural abnormalities such as inflammatory bowel disease, strictures, and cancer.
- In IBS, metabolic and endocrine, drug-induced, and neurologic causes must be excluded by thorough history taking and physical and laboratory examinations.

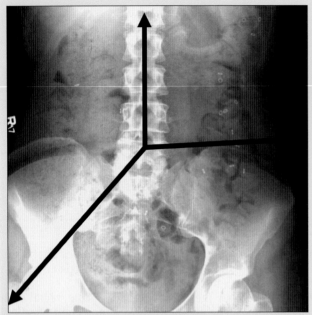

Figure 1. Colon transit study. Plain film demonstrates radiopaque markers *(arrows)*. For the purpose of counting, the colon is divided into three segments: left colon, right colon, and rectosigmoid.

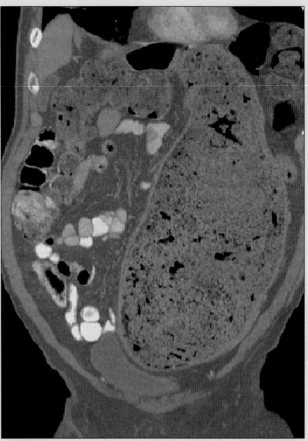

Figure 2. A large rectal fecal impaction with stool distending a dilated and elongated sigmoid colon in this patient with colonic inertia.

INCIDENCE/PREVALENCE AND EPIDEMIOLOGY

- Incidence of IBS is as high as 14% and accounts for one third to one half of outpatient referrals to gastroenterologists.
- IBS ranks close to the common cold as the leading cause of absenteeism from work because of illness.
- Symptoms of IBS begin before 35 years of age in one half of patients, and 40% of patients are 35 to 50 years of age.
- Female patients outnumber male patients 2:1 in IBS, and it is more common in white and Jewish populations.
- Colonic involvement in scleroderma occurs less frequently than in the esophagus and small bowel.

Suggested Readings

Chiao GZ, Rey D: Motor disorders of the colon. In DiMarino AJ, Benjamin SB (eds): *Gastrointestinal Disease: An Endoscopic Approach*. Malden, MA, Blackwell Scientific, 1997, pp 659-683.

Hasler WL, Owyang C: Irritable bowel syndrome. In Yamada T (ed): *Textbook of Gastroenterology*. Philadelphia, JB Lippincott, 1995, pp 1832-1855.

Karasick S, Ehrlich SM: Is constipation a disorder of defecation or impaired motility? Distinction based on defecography and colonic transit studies. *AJR Am J Roentgenol* 166:63-67, 1996.

Lennard-Jones JE, Feldman M, Scharschmidt BF, Sleisenger MH: Constipation. In *Gastrointestinal and Liver Disease*, 6th ed. Philadelphia, WB Saunders, 1998, pp 174-197.

Olden KW, Schuster MM: Irritable bowel syndrome. In Feldman M, Scharschmidt BF, Sleisenger MH (eds): *Gastrointestinal and Liver Disease*, 6th ed. Philadelphia, WB Saunders, 1998, pp 1536-1556.

Phillips SF: Motility disorders of the colon. In Yamada T, (ed): *Textbook of Gastroenterology*, 2nd ed. Philadelphia, JB Lippincott, 1995, pp 1856-1875.

Phillips SF, Pemberton JH: Megacolon: Congenital and acquired. In Feldman M, Scharschmidt BF, Sleisenger MH (eds): *Gastrointestinal and Liver Disease*, 6th ed. Philadelphia, WB Saunders, 1998, pp 1810-1819.

Rose S, Young MA, Reynolds JC: Gastrointestinal manifestations of scleroderma. *Gastroenterol Clin North Am* 27:563-594, 1998.

Sartor RB, Murphy ME, Rydzak E: Miscellaneous inflammatory and structural disorders of the colon. In Yamada T (ed): *Textbook of Gastroenterology*, 2nd ed. Philadelphia, JB Lippincott, 1995, pp 1806-1831.

Schrock TR: Examination and diseases of the anorectum. In Feldman M, Scharschmidt BF, Sleisenger MH (eds): *Gastrointestinal and Liver Disease*, 6th ed. Philadelphia, WB Saunders, 1998, pp 1960-1976.

General Radiologic Principles for Imaging and Intervention of the Solid Viscera

Complications of Percutaneous Abscess Drainage

DEFINITION: Complications of percutaneous abscess drainage include sepsis, drainage failure, catheter malposition, bowel injury, hemorrhage, pneumothorax, hemothorax, cardiorespiratory arrest, and peritonitis.

IMAGING

CT
Findings
- Normal course: fistula to the small bowel from the cavity
- Normal course: resolution of the abscess cavity and no enteric fistula
- Hemorrhage, drainage failure, pneumothorax, hemothorax

Utility
- CT scan can be obtained to confirm the resolution of the cavity.
- CT offers exquisite anatomic detail regarding the extent of the cavity, the relationship to the surrounding structures, and the presence of unfavorable factors for percutaneous abscess drainage.
- Disadvantage of using CT is that an occult fistula to the bowel cannot be detected.

Ultrasound
Findings
- Hemorrhage, drainage failure

Utility
- Ultrasound is less sensitive in the detection of these complications.

CLINICAL PRESENTATION

- Patients with sepsis may become symptomatic (e.g., sudden onset of rigor, fever, and hypotension) within 1-2 hours after the procedure.

DIAGNOSTIC PEARLS

- Abscess may be multilocular, poorly defined, or not mature and liquefied enough to be drained effectively.
- Patients are symptomatic (e.g., sudden onset of rigor, fever, or hypotension) within 1-2 hours after the procedure.
- Complications include sepsis, drainage failure, catheter malposition, bowel injury, hemorrhage, pneumothorax, hemothorax, cardiorespiratory arrest, and peritonitis.

PATHOLOGY

- Complications include sepsis, drainage failure, catheter malposition, bowel injury, hemorrhage, pneumothorax, hemothorax, cardiorespiratory arrest, and peritonitis.
- Drainage failure is usually related to characteristics of collection rather than the technique.
- The abscess may be multilocular, poorly defined, or not mature and liquefied enough to be drained effectively.
- Other causes include the presence of necrotic tumor, fungal contamination, and Crohn disease.

INCIDENCE/PREVALENCE AND EPIDEMIOLOGY

- Complications of percutaneous abscess drainage occur in 0.5%-8% of procedures.
- Hepatic or splenic interventions, especially those that transgress the pleural space, are associated with an increased incidence of complications.

WHAT THE REFERRING PHYSICIAN NEEDS TO KNOW

- Thorough preprocedure planning is the key to preventing many of these pitfalls.
- Once a catheter is placed, catheter manipulation should be minimal.
- Vigorous irrigation of the cavity or a high-volume abscessogram should also be avoided to prevent episodes of bacteremia during the procedure.
- Septic patients should be treated with aggressive fluid resuscitation, antibiotics, and vasopressors necessary to maintain an acceptable blood pressure.
- As always, the route of drainage should be carefully considered, and superficial vessels should be avoided.
- In subphrenic abscess drainage, the pleura should be avoided because of the risk of pneumothorax, hemothorax, or empyema.

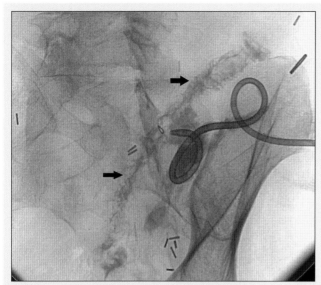

Figure 1. Typical course of catheter drainage. Interval abscessogram demonstrating a fistula to the small bowel from the cavity *(arrows)*.

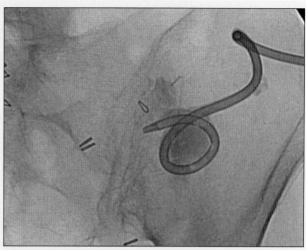

Figure 2. Typical course of catheter drainage. Final tube check demonstrates near complete resolution of the cavity and no enteric fistula. If the patient is clinically stable with minimal output from the drain, the catheter can be safely removed.

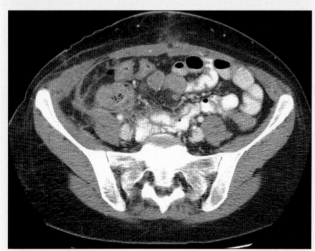

Figure 3. Appendiceal abscess drainage. Follow-up CT scan after catheter removal shows complete resolution of the abscess.

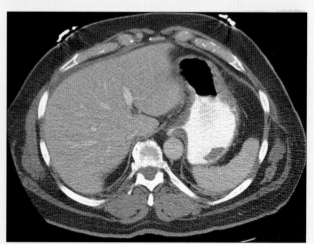

Figure 4. Liver abscess drainage. CT obtained several months after drain removal shows complete resolution of the abscess.

Imaging Findings in Abdominal Abscess

DEFINITION: Encapsulated liquid, septic focus in the abdomen.

IMAGING

CT

Findings

- A well-circumscribed fluid collection, spherical or ovoid in shape or conforming to the shape of compartment where located, is seen.
- Within peritoneum, abscesses displace the surrounding viscera.
- Gas is seen in the form of microbubbles or larger pockets of gas resulting in the air-fluid level.
- Because of the inflammation by the abscess, mesenteric fat shows increased attenuation, often associated with thickening of adjacent fascial planes.
- Density of the abscess typically ranges from 0 to +30 HU, depending on the degree of liquefaction and the presence of gas.
- Abscess contents do not typically enhance; the presence of such enhancement should raise concern for the presence of a necrotic tumor.
- Abscess walls are often enhanced.

Utility

- CT is the modality of choice for the diagnosis of intra-abdominal abscesses.
- Contrast-enhanced CT is performed to demonstrate the enhancing abscess wall if present.
- CT offers exquisite anatomic detail, extent of the cavity, and the relationship to the surrounding structures.
- Oral or rectal contrast is given to help distinguish the bowel from the extraluminal fluid collections.
- When in doubt, delayed scan or scanning in a different position demonstrates changes in appearance around a questionable structure.
- Sensitivity: 85%-100%
- Specificity: 90%-95%

Ultrasound

Findings

- Anechoic, cystic structure to complex, multiloculated, echogenic mass is seen.
- Abscesses assume the configuration of the compartment where they are located or displace the surrounding structures.
- Gas within the abscess produces a highly echogenic, ill-defined area with *dirty* posterior acoustic shadowing.

DIAGNOSTIC PEARLS

- Abdominal abscess is a well-circumscribed fluid collection that is spherical and ovoid in shape or conforms to the shape of the compartment where located.
- Gas is seen in form of microbubbles or larger pockets of gas resulting in air-fluid level.
- Density of abscess typically ranges from 0 to +30 HU, depending on degree of liquefaction and the presence of gas.

Utility

- Ultrasound is a readily available modality used to detect intra-abdominal abscesses.
- It enables the diagnosis of the abscess in intensive care unit patients because of its portability.
- Appearance of the abscess on ultrasound is not specific, resembling any intra-abdominal fluid collection.
- It can distinguish the abscess from the loop of the bowel based on the presence of peristalsis or definite visualization of the bowel wall itself.
- Ultrasound is highly operator dependent.
- Patient body habitus, overlying bowel gas, wounds, drains, and dressings can limit adequate visualization of abdominal structures.
- Sensitivity: 50%-60%
- Specificity: 80%-90%

MRI

Findings

- Inhomogeneous areas of low T1-weighted signal intensity
- Mural enhancement after intravenous contrast administration
- T2-weighted images displaying intermediate to high signal intensities

Utility

- MRI is used more frequently in intra-abdominal abscess diagnosis because of its multiplanar imaging capabilities and characterization of the nature of the suspected abscess.

WHAT THE REFERRING PHYSICIAN NEEDS TO KNOW

- CT offers exquisite anatomic detail and shows the extent of the cavity and the relationship to the surrounding structures.
- Oral contrast is given to help distinguish the bowel from the extraluminal fluid collections.
- Appearance of the abscess on ultrasound is not specific and resembles any intra-abdominal fluid collection.

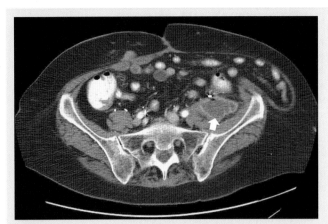

Figure 1. Typical course of catheter drainage. CT scan of the pelvis demonstrates a fluid collection in the left psoas muscle *(arrow)*.

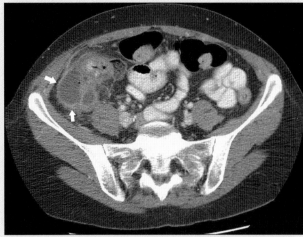

Figure 2. Appendiceal abscess drainage. A 19-year-old patient with fever and right lower quadrant pain. CT scan shows an appendiceal abscess *(arrows)*.

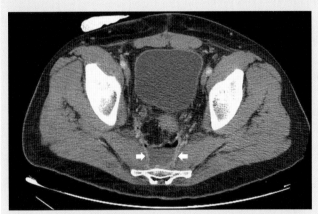

Figure 3. Transgluteal abscess drainage. CT scan demonstrates a small enhancing presacral cavity containing fluid and gas *(arrows)*.

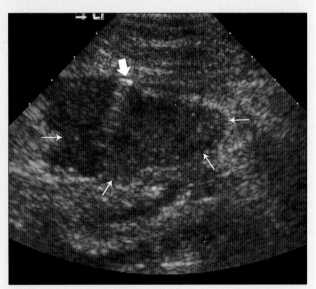

Figure 4. Diverticular abscess drainage. A 77-year-old patient with fever and abdominal pain. Ultrasound shows the cavity *(thin arrows)* with a hyperechoic focus *(large arrow)* exhibiting a ring-down artifact consistent with gas.

- Use of intravascular gadolinium provides information similar to CT while avoiding nephrotoxic effects or allergies to iodinated CT contrast.
- Sensitivity: 75%-90%
- Specificity: 85%-90%

Nuclear Medicine
Findings
- Accumulation of labeled white cells at the abscess site
Utility
- Nuclear scintigraphy is useful in septic patients without any localizing signs in whom CT, MRI, and ultrasound failed to identify the abscess.
- Gallium-67– and indium-111–labeled white cells are standard isotopes used in abscess detection.
- False-positive indium-labeled white cell scans can result in patients with bowel infarction or hemorrhage and after repeated enemas.
- Gallium scans are sensitive but less specific in detecting abscesses.
- False-positive gallium-labeled white cell scans occur with tumors, such as lymphoma, granulomatous lesions, wounds, and normal gut.
- Major disadvantage is relatively poor anatomic detail provided, but this may change with increasing use of image fusion technology.
- Sensitivity: 80%-85%
- Specificity: 60%-70%

Radiology
Findings
- Abnormal gas pattern, soft-tissue mass, and loss of the normal fat–soft tissue interface
Utility
- Radiography is an insensitive method for the detection of intra-abdominal abscesses.
- It has little role in the primary diagnosis of abscesses.
- Sensitivity: 5%
- Specificity: 25%

CLINICAL PRESENTATION

- Fever
- Elevated white cell count
- Sepsis

DIFFERENTIAL DIAGNOSIS

- Appendiceal mucocele
- Hematoma
- Adenopathy
- Unopacified bowel
- Neoplasm

PATHOLOGY

- Cause of intra-abdominal abscesses is multifactorial.
- Initially, existing intra-abdominal fluid collection becomes superinfected or the abscess cavity forms de novo from an infectious nidus.
- Mature cavity forms, which is encapsulated by a wall of fibrin, collagen, neovasculature, and leukocytes.
- As the contents of the abscess become more liquefied because of leukocyte action and enzymes, the cavity assumes a spherical or ovoid configuration.

Suggested Readings
Haaga JR, Weinstein AJ: CT-guided percutaneous aspiration and drainage of abscesses. *AJR Am J Roentgenol* 135:1187-1194, 1980.

Jaques P, Mauro M, Safrit H, et al: CT features of intraabdominal abscesses: Prediction of successful percutaneous drainage. *AJR Am J Roentgenol* 146:1041-1045, 1986.

Knochel JQ, Koehler PR, Lee TG, et al: Diagnosis of abdominal abscesses with computed tomography, ultrasound, and ^{111}In leukocyte scans. *Radiology* 137:425-432, 1980.

Levitt RG, Biello DR, Sagel SS, et al: Computed tomography and ^{67}Ga citrate radionuclide imaging for evaluating suspected abdominal abscess. *AJR Am J Roentgenol* 132:529-534, 1979.

Moir C, Robins RE: Role of ultrasonography, gallium scanning, and computed tomography in the diagnosis of intraabdominal abscess. *Am J Surg* 143:582-585, 1982.

Sheafor DH, Paulson EK, Simmons CM, et al: Abdominal percutaneous interventional procedures: Comparison of CT and US guidance. *Radiology* 207:705-710, 1998.

Gallbladder and Biliary Tract

Part 38

ENDOSCOPIC RETROGRADE CHOLANGIOPANCREATOGRAPHY

Biliary Tract Inflammation

DEFINITION: Inflammatory diseases of the biliary tract with various causes.

IMAGING

Interventional Radiology
Findings
- Stricture with or without upstream dilation is seen.
- Web-like narrowings with beading and a diverticular change in primary sclerosing cholangitis (PSC) is seen.
- Severe hepatic artery stenosis or occlusion shows diffuse intrahepatic biliary stricture or loss of duct integrity.
- Intraluminal filling defects are seen, consisting of sludge or stones (or both) in obstructive and recurrent pyogenic cholangitis.
- Long, smooth, gentle tapering of the intrapancreatic portion of common bile duct is seen in chronic pancreatitis.
- Hepatic abscesses are seen, resulting from ascending cholangitis, and subsequent duct disruption.
- Ducts appear splayed, angulated, or corkscrew-shaped secondary to cirrhosis.

Utility
- Endoscopic retrograde cholangiopancreatography (ERCP) can be used to dilate central strictures in an attempt to preserve hepatic function.
- ERCP can help confirm the disease, define the extent of the disease, and help in the relief of the obstruction.
- ERCP can define the stricture appearance, site, and narrowing in relationship to the hilum, according to the Bismuth classification.
- Sweeping the duct with a balloon can help clear central duct debris.

CLINICAL PRESENTATION

- Charcot triad of abdominal pain, fever, and jaundice is frequently present in ascending cholangitis.

DIAGNOSTIC PEARLS

- Ductal irregularity, strictures with or without upstream dilation
- Intraluminal filling defects
- Adjacent inflammatory processes

- PSC is characterized by an incidental elevation of alkaline phosphatase, nonspecific signs and symptoms, and the stigmata of portal hypertension.
- Recurrent pyogenic cholangitis will produce ascending cholangitis, abdominal pain without cholangitis, and, less frequently, pancreatitis.
- PSC is an indolent process of chronic cholestasis.

DIFFERENTIAL DIAGNOSIS

- Cholangiocarcinoma
- Metastases
- AIDS cholangiopathy

PATHOLOGY

- Ascending cholangitis is a biliary bacterial infection that develops above an obstruction caused by stone disease or an inflammatory stricture.
- Cirrhosis can distort the intrahepatic biliary tract.
- Radiation therapy and intra-arterial chemotherapy can cause biliary tract strictures.
- Biliary tract can also be involved in adjacent inflammatory processes.

WHAT THE REFERRING PHYSICIAN NEEDS TO KNOW

- Causes of *secondary* sclerosing cholangitis need to be ruled out before a diagnosis of primary sclerosing cholangitis can be made.
- Correlation with ERCP findings, cross-sectional imaging, and laboratory values may be needed to resolve the stricture's true cause.
- Right upper quadrant pain, fever, and a dilated bile duct are considered to be ascending cholangitis until proven otherwise.
- Biliary tract infections are the most common cause of pyogenic liver abscess.

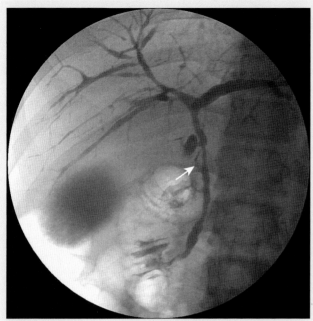

Figure 1. Primary sclerosing cholangitis. Mild changes of PSC with diffuse irregularity of both the intrahepatic and the extrahepatic biliary tree are present. Even with multiple strictures, no significant upstream dilation is seen. Note the aberrant low insertion of the right posterior segment *(arrow)*.

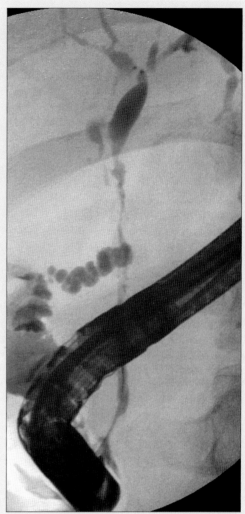

Figure 2. Primary sclerosing cholangitis (PSC). Endoscopic retrograde cholangiopancreatography (ERCP) in this patient shows more severe PSC changes. Marked stricture disease with some dilation of the proximal common hepatic duct is noted.

■ Autoimmune processes and ischemia also cause inflammatory cholangitis.

INCIDENCE/PREVALENCE AND EPIDEMIOLOGY

■ PSC is typically seen in young to middle-aged men.

Suggested Readings

Abdo AA, Bain VG, Kichian K, Lee SS: Evolution of autoimmune hepatitis to primary sclerosing cholangitis: A sequential syndrome. *Hepatology* 36:1393, 2002.

Altman C, Fabre M, Adrien C, et al: Cholangiographic features in fibrosis and cirrhosis of the liver. *Dig Dis Sci* 40:2128-2133, 1995.

Baron TH, Fleischer DE: Past, present, and future of endoscopic retrograde cholangiopancreatography: Perspectives on the National Institutes of Health consensus conference. *Mayo Clin Proc* 77:407-412, 2002.

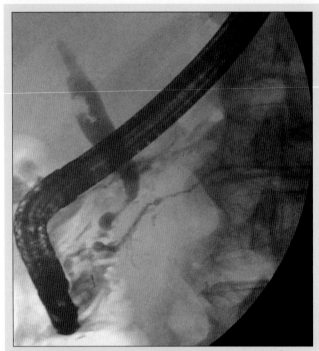

Figure 3. Autoimmune pancreatitis. The distal extrahepatic biliary tree is strictured along with the diffusely irregular and narrowed pancreatic duct.

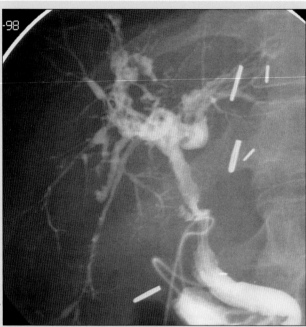

Figure 4. Ischemic cholangiopathy in hepatic transplantation. The T-tube cholangiogram in this patient, status post–orthotopic liver transplant with hepatic artery thrombosis, shows diffuse stricturing of the transplant biliary tract. Areas of ill-defined duct borders compatible with the beginning of loss of ductal integrity are seen.

Biliary Tract Neoplasia

DEFINITION: Benign and malignant primary, as well as metastatic, tumors involving the biliary tract.

IMAGING

Interventional Radiology
Findings
- Irregular ductal narrowing is seen in sclerosing cholangiocarcinoma and at the hilum in Klatskin tumor.
- Splayed intrahepatic biliary tree with occasional intraluminal component is seen in biliary cystadenoma.
- Filling defect is seen within the extrahepatic biliary tree, which may be solitary (adenoma) or multiple (papilloma).
- Periampullary tumor is seen as a nodular filling defect or stricture in the pancreatic or common bile duct.
- Lymphoma causes extra- or intrahepatic duct system narrowing or displacement.
- Gallbladder carcinoma invading biliary duct appears as medial splaying of the mid and proximal extrahepatic ducts.
- In a granular cell tumor, the bile duct is obstructed by a relatively short, smooth, annular-appearing stricture.

Utility
- Cholangiography is used.
- Cholangiographic malignant strictures usually produce a longer segment of irregular, asymmetric narrowing with a nodular or rounded shoulder.
- Benign strictures usually have a longer transition zone with smooth concentric narrowing.

CT
Findings
- Intrahepatic cholangiocarcinoma is seen as an intrahepatic mass on cross-sectional imaging studies.

MRI
Findings
- Intrahepatic cholangiocarcinoma is seen as an intrahepatic mass on cross-sectional imaging studies.

DIAGNOSTIC PEARLS

- Ductal narrowing or stricture, intraluminal filling defect, and irregularities are seen.
- Malignant strictures produce a longer segment of irregular, asymmetric narrowing with a nodular or rounded shoulder.
- Benign strictures have a longer transition zone with smooth concentric narrowing.

CLINICAL PRESENTATION

- Patients with hilar and common hepatic and common bile duct cancers present early with jaundice, pain, and weight loss.
- Patients with intrahepatic cholangiocarcinomas present late with weight loss, abdominal pain, and ultimately jaundice.
- Patients with gallbladder cancer typically present with signs and symptoms of gallstones: abdominal pain, cholangitis, and weight loss.
- Early gallbladder cancers may be found serendipitously at the time of cholelecystectomy for calculus disease.

DIFFERENTIAL DIAGNOSIS

- Sclerosing cholangitis
- Primary biliary cirrhosis
- Biliary tract stone or hemorrhage
- AIDS cholangitis
- Biliary metastasis
- Biliary parasite
- Autoimmune cholangitis

WHAT THE REFERRING PHYSICIAN NEEDS TO KNOW
- Cholangiographic appearance must be correlated with CT, MRI, and ultrasound, as well as the patient's clinical course.
- Benign appearance may have a malignant cause.
- Pancreatic neck lesions invade the mid extrahepatic biliary tract.
- Pancreatic body or tail lesions metastasize to peribiliary lymph nodes of the proximal extrahepatic biliary tree or hilum.
- Biliary tract is at risk for metastatic disease because of its location within the liver, the porta hepatis and hepatoduodenal ligament, and the pancreas.

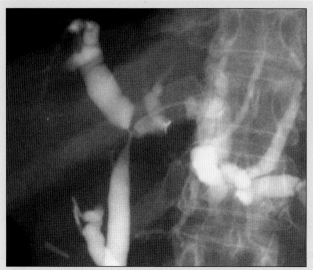

Figure 1. Cholangiocarcinoma. In this patient with a Klatskin tumor, the malignant stricture is unusual in its smooth appearance as it narrows the proximal CHD continuing proximally to involve both the right and left hepatic ducts.

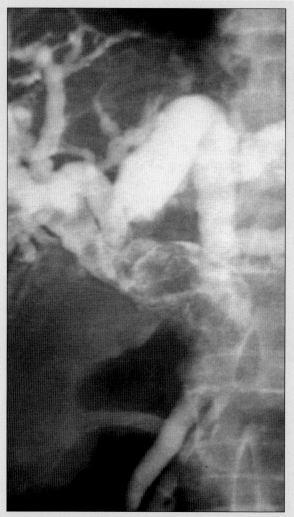

Figure 2. Papillomatosis. At cholangiography, multiple rounded filling defects are seen in the extrahepatic duct system. Malignant cells were retrieved at brushing.

PATHOLOGY

- Biliary tract may be involved in benign and malignant primary tumors and metastatic disease.
- Infections and inflammatory disease can lead to ductal narrowing.
- Biliary cystadenoma has a bile duct origin but usually has ovarian stromal tissue present.

INCIDENCE/PREVALENCE AND EPIDEMIOLOGY

- Biliary cystadenoma involves women almost exclusively in the fifth to sixth decades of life.
- Papilloma can appear in the sixth to seventh decades without gender predisposition.
- Granular cell tumors occur almost exclusively in young to middle-aged black women.

Suggested Readings

Baron TH, Fleischer DE: Past, present, and future of endoscopic retrograde cholangiopancreatography: Perspectives on the National Institutes of Health consensus conference. *Mayo Clin Proc* 77:407-412, 2002.

Brugge WR: Endoscopic techniques to diagnose and manage biliary tumors. *J Clin Oncol* 23:4561-4565, 2005.

Domagk D, Poremba C, Dietl KH, et al: Endoscopic transpapillary biopsies and intraductal ultrasonography in the diagnostics of bile duct strictures: A prospective study. *Gut* 51:240-244, 2005.

Rosch T, Meining A, Fruhmorgen S, et al: A prospective comparison of the diagnostic accuracy of ERCP, MRCP, CT, and EUS in biliary strictures. *Gastrointest Endosc* 55:870-876, 2002.

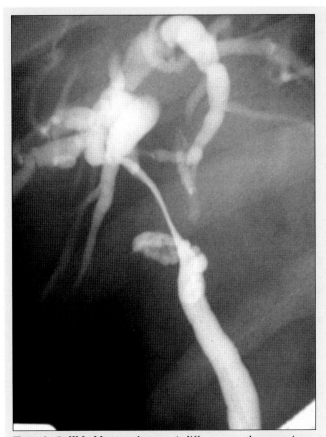

Figure 3. Gallbladder carcinoma. A diffuse, smooth narrowing of the CHD with mild bowing is present. Partial filling of the cystic duct is also seen.

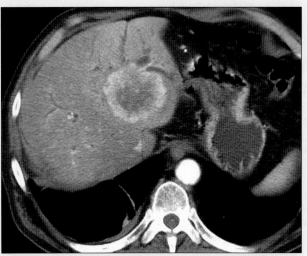

Figure 4. Intrahepatic cholangiocarcinoma. A late arterial phase CT shows the peripherally enhancing mass in the left lobe of the liver.

Pancreatic Inflammation

DEFINITION: Autoimmune pancreatitis refers to diffuse infiltration of the biliary tract and pancreatic ducts by a lymphoplasmacytic inflammatory process that can progress to a fibrotic infiltrate.

IMAGING

Radiography
Findings
- Calcified pancreatic concretions

Utility
- If not seen, endoscopic retrograde pancreatogram can be used.

Interventional Radiology
Findings
- Autoimmune pancreatitis: mild irregularity of the main duct in the early stage progressing to a diffuse irregularity in the advanced stage
- Ectasia: ostial narrowing and filling defects and cystic change in chronic pancreatitis
- Focal strictures with the ectatic duct *chain-of-lakes* appearance in the late stage of chronic pancreatitis

Utility
- Pancreatography is the presurgical road map in chronic pancreatitis.
- Side branches need to be filled adequately when diagnosing chronic pancreatitis, but overinjection will cause acinarization.

CLINICAL PRESENTATION
- Abdominal pain and pancreatic insufficiency

DIFFERENTIAL DIAGNOSIS
- Pancreatic neoplasia
- Pancreatic metastases
- Pancreatic hematoma
- Diverticulitis of duodenal diverticulum

PATHOLOGY
- Inflammation of the pancreas is divided into three major categories: acute, chronic, and acute relapsing pancreatitis.
- Inflammation is frequently seen with alcohol ingestion or gallstone disease.

DIAGNOSTIC PEARLS
- Ectasia, ostial narrowing, filling defects, and cystic change
- Calcified pancreatic concretions on plain films
- *Chain-of-lakes* appearance on endoscopic retrograde cholangiopancreatography
- Autoimmune pancreatitis: mild irregularity of the main duct in the early stage progressing to a diffuse irregularity in the advanced stage

- Acute relapsing pancreatitis refers to recurrent bouts of pancreatitis without an obvious cause.
- Chronic pancreatitis is permanent parenchymal or ductal damage as a result of pancreatic inflammation.
- Autoimmune pancreatitis shows a diffusely or focally lymphoplasmacytic infiltration that can progress to a fibrotic infiltrate.

INCIDENCE/PREVALENCE AND EPIDEMIOLOGY
- Seventy percent of cases are related to alcohol intake.
- Autoimmune pancreatitis affects elderly men and young women.

Suggested Readings

Axon ATR: Endoscopic retrograde cholangiopancreatography in chronic pancreatitis. Cambridge classification. *Radiol Clin North Am* 27:39, 1989.

Baron TH, Fleischer DE: Past, present, and future of endoscopic retrograde cholangiopancreatography: Perspectives on the National Institutes of Health consensus conference. *Mayo Clin Proc* 77:407-412, 2002.

Kasugai T, Kuno N, Kobayashi S, et al: Endoscopic pancreatocholangiography. *Gastroenterology* 63:217, 1972.

Lehman GA: Role of ERCP and other endoscopic modalities in chronic pancreatitis. *Gastrointest Endosc* 56:S237-S240, 2002.

WHAT THE REFERRING PHYSICIAN NEEDS TO KNOW
- Endoscopic retrograde cholangiopancreatography should be deferred in patients with acute pancreatitis.
- Common duct stone removal helps decrease the severity of acute pancreatitis.
- Autoimmune pancreatitis mimics pancreatic carcinoma.
- Pancreatic ductal changes can be seen in a minority of patients with primary sclerosing cholangitis.

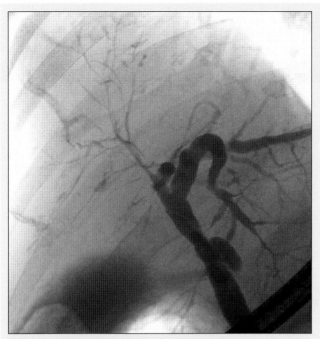

Figure 1. Autoimmune pancreatitis. This patient has severe intrahepatic biliary tree stricturing of the right intrahepatic duct system with mild irregularity of the extrahepatic biliary tree that can simulate primary sclerosing cholangitis.

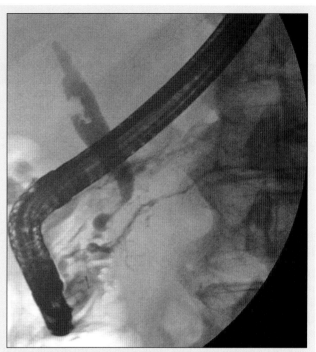

Figure 2. Autoimmune pancreatitis. The distal extrahepatic biliary tree is strictured along with the diffusely irregular and narrowed pancreatic duct.

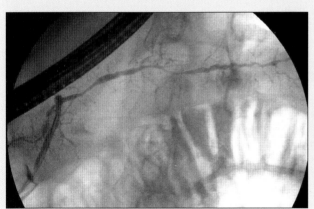

Figure 3. Chronic pancreatitis changes on endoscopic retrograde cholangiopancreatography. The irregular side branches with narrowings at the ductal origins, as well as a series of main pancreatic duct narrowings, leads to the diagnosis of chronic pancreatitis.

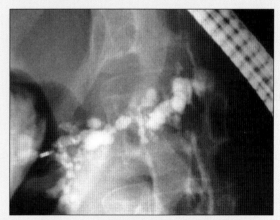

Figure 4. Chronic pancreatitis changes on endoscopic retrograde cholangiopancreatography. In this patient, severe chronic pancreatitis changes are seen with the so-called *chain-of-lakes* series of main duct strictures along with ectatic and truncated side branches.

Bile Duct Calculi

DEFINITION: Abnormal accumulations of bile salts in a bile duct.

Anatomic Findings

Gallbladder
- Well-defined, low signal intensity filling defect in high signal intensity bile

IMAGING

MRI
Findings
- Small, low signal intensity foci in the distal bile duct

Utility
- Sensitivity and specificity of MR cholangiopancreatography (MRCP) for detecting intrahepatic stones were 97% and 93%, respectively.
- Subsequent studies with state-of-the-art scanners and sequences demonstrated sensitivity and specificity of 90%-100%.
- It can detect stones as small as 2 mm even in normal-caliber ducts.
- Axial plane is helpful in detecting small stones and differentiating stones lying in the dependent portion of the duct from pneumobilia.

Ultrasound
Findings
- Echogenic filling defect often in dilated bile duct

Utility
- Sensitivity: 75%-90%
- Specificity: 90%-95%

CT
Findings
- Radiodense or radiolucent filling defect seen in a frequently dilated biliary tract.

Utility
- Sensitivity: 90%-100%
- Specificity: 90%-95%

DIAGNOSTIC PEARLS
- Well-defined, low signal intensity filling defect in high signal intensity bile

Endoscopic Retrograde Cholangiopancreatography (ERCP)
Findings
- Radiolucent filling defect often in a dilated biliary system

Utility
- Sensitivity: 90%-100%
- Specificity: 95%-100%

CLINICAL PRESENTATION
- Right upper quadrant pain, jaundice, sepsis, abnormal liver function tests, cholangitis

DIFFERENTIAL DIAGNOSIS
- Pneumobilia
- Blood clot
- Surgical clip
- Biliary parasite
- Cholangiocarcinoma
- Metastasis

PATHOLOGY
- Biliary duct calculi are often associated with biliary dilation.
- Biliary duct calculi are a leading cause of cholangitis.

WHAT THE REFERRING PHYSICIAN NEEDS TO KNOW
- MRCP provides images of the ducts similar to ERCP.
- MRCP depicts ducts proximal to the high-grade obstruction and ducts in patients with surgical alterations of the biliary and gastrointestinal tract.
- Major benefit of MRCP in the setting of suspected biliary calculi is reduction of unnecessary ERCPs.
- MRCP performs well in the detection of intrahepatic stones.
- Be aware of stone mimickers resulting in false-positive diagnoses such as pneumobilia and duct compression by an adjacent vessel.

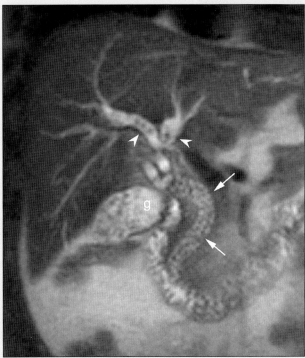

Figure 1. Multiple extrahepatic and intrahepatic bile duct calculi. Coronal HASTE MRCP provides a comprehensive image of the abdomen by showing multiple, low signal intensity calculi in the dilated extrahepatic bile duct *(arrows)*, central intrahepatic ducts *(arrowheads)*, and gallbladder (g). (*HASTE*, Half-Fourier acquisition single-shot turbo spin-echo.)

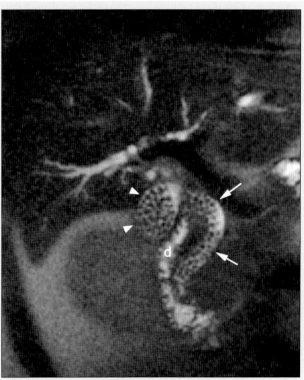

Figure 2. Multiple extrahepatic and intrahepatic bile duct calculi. Thin-slab MRCP focusing on the distal bile duct *(arrows)* shows multiple, intraductal calculi, as well as gallbladder calculi *(arrowheads)*. The fluid-filled duodenum (d) is noted.

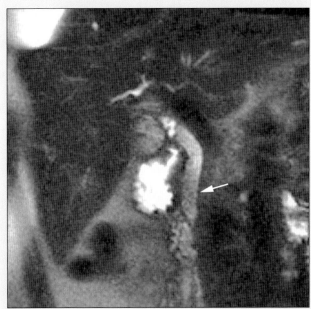

Figure 3. Small bile duct calculi: value of axial MRCP. Thin-slab MRCP reveals small, low signal intensity foci in the distal bile duct *(arrow)* later removed during therapeutic ERCP.

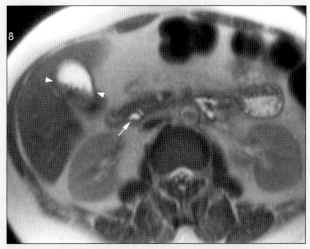

Figure 4. Small bile duct calculi: value of axial MRCP. Axial MRCP shows the small, low signal intensity stones layering in the dependent portion of the intrapancreatic bile duct *(arrow)* with high signal intensity bile seen anteriorly in the duct.
A similar stone-bile level *(arrowheads)* is present in the gallbladder.

- Passage of multiple small biliary tract calculi is a common cause of recurrent right upper quadrant pain and abnormal liver function tests.

INCIDENCE/PREVALENCE AND EPIDEMIOLOGY

- Occurs in 5%-13% of patients with symptomatic cholelithiasis
- Most biliary calculi in Western countries are cholesterol and secondary, arising in the gallbladder.
- Most biliary calculi in developing countries are primary pigment stones.

Suggested Readings

Becker CD, Grossholz M, Becker M, et al: Choledocholithiasis and bile duct stenosis: Diagnostic accuracy of MR cholangiopancreatography. *Radiology* 205:523-530, 1997.

Demartines N, Eisner L, Schnabel K, et al: Evaluation of magnetic resonance cholangiography in the management of bile duct stones. *Arch Surg* 135:148-152, 2000.

Reinhold C, Taourel P, Bret PM, et al: Choledocholithiasis: Evaluation of MR cholangiography for diagnosis. *Radiology* 209:435-442, 1998.

Soto JA, Barish MA, Alvarez O, et al: Detection of choledocholithiasis with MR cholangiography: Comparison of three-dimensional fast spin-echo and single- and multisection half-Fourier rapid acquisition with relaxation enhancement sequences. *Radiology* 215:737-745, 2000.

Cholangiocarcinoma

DEFINITION: Hilar cholangiocarcinoma causes a high-grade stricture of the confluence of the right and left hepatic ducts.

IMAGING

MRI
Findings
- Marked narrowing of the proximal extrahepatic bile duct with dilation proximal to the obstruction (hilar type)
- Strictures or intraductal, polypoid masses (distal type)

Utility
- MR cholangiopancreatography (MRCP) is an important tool in the evaluation of cholangiocarcinoma.
- MRI with MRCP offers the added advantage of demonstrating disease that has extended from the ducts into the liver and adjacent structures.
- It plays an important role in the noninvasive evaluation for hilar cholangiocarcinoma.
- It also facilitates planning of surgical, percutaneous, and radiation therapy procedures.

CT
Findings
- Homogeneous round or oval hypodense mass with irregular borders
- Early minimal rim enhancement with progressive concentric filling of contrast
- Clearing of contrast on delayed images
- Delayed enhancement (5-10 minutes) is typical.

Utility
- CT is often the first imaging test to suggest the diagnosis.

CLINICAL PRESENTATION

- Gradual onset of painless jaundice
- Cholangitis
- Weight loss and fatigue
- Epigastric pain
- Enlarged, tender liver

DIFFERENTIAL DIAGNOSIS

- Pancreatic carcinoma
- Primary sclerosing cholangitis
- Gallbladder carcinoma

DIAGNOSTIC PEARLS

- Marked narrowing of the proximal extrahepatic bile duct with dilation proximal to the obstruction
- Patients with intrahepatic cholangiocarcinomas that show delayed contrast enhancement tend to have poorer prognosis.

PATHOLOGY

- Hilar cholangiocarcinoma and high-grade stricture of the confluence of the right and left hepatic ducts
- Adenocarcinoma arising from the epithelium of a bile duct with prominent fibrosis and desmoplastic reaction; mucin and calcifications may be present.
- A well-differentiated sclerosing adenocarcinoma is found in two thirds of cases.
- In 11% of cases an anaplastic carcinoma is found.
- Ascending cholangitis
- One third of cases are intrahepatic in location.
- Two thirds of cases are extrahepatic in location.
- Tumor location for extrahepatic tumors: right/left hepatic duct—8%-13%; confluence of hepatic ducts—10%-26% (Klatskin tumor); common hepatic duct—14%-37%; proximal common bile duct—15%-30%; distal common bile duct—30%-50%

INCIDENCE/PREVALENCE AND EPIDEMIOLOGY

- Hilar cholangiocarcinoma is the most common manifestation of cholangiocarcinoma.
- Intrahepatic cholangiocarcinomas are the second most common primary hepatic neoplasm after hepatoma. These patients typically present in the sixth decade; it is more common in men.
- Extrahepatic cholangiocarcinomas present in the seventh decade and are more common in Asia.

WHAT THE REFERRING PHYSICIAN NEEDS TO KNOW

- MRCP is very useful in evaluating suspected malignancies of the pancreaticobiliary tract.
- When MRCP is supplemented by conventional MR and MR angiography, it permits the determination of resectability of neoplastic disease.
- MRCP depicts the entire biliary and pancreatic duct, even with high-grade strictures.
- Distal cholangiocarcinoma within the intrapancreatic bile duct is difficult to distinguish from pancreatic head carcinoma with MRCP or endoscopic retrograde cholangiopancreatography.

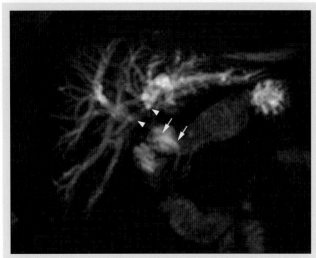

Figure 1. Hilar cholangiocarcinoma. Coronal thick-slab MRCP reveals high-grade, isolated obstructions of the central right and left hepatic ducts *(arrowheads)* caused by hilar cholangiocarcinoma. The extrahepatic bile duct distal to the obstruction *(arrows)* is seen adjacent to the fluid-filled duodenal bulb.

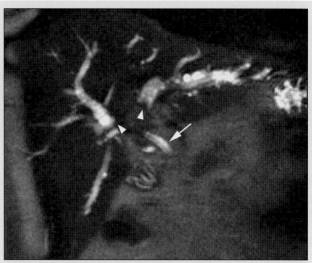

Figure 2. Hilar cholangiocarcinoma. Thin-slab MRCP reveals in greater detail the points of obstruction of the central right and left hepatic ducts *(arrowheads)* caused by cephalad extension of the hilar cholangiocarcinoma. The normal-caliber extrahepatic bile duct *(arrow)* located just distal to the tumor is noted.

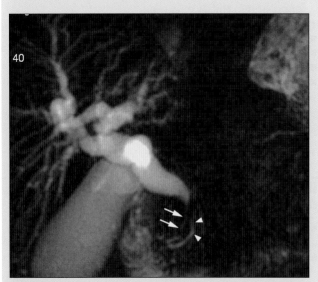

Figure 3. Distal duct cholangiocarcinoma. Coronal thick-slab MRCP shows a high-grade stricture of the intrapancreatic bile duct *(arrows)* resulting in proximal biliary ductal dilation. The pancreatic duct *(arrowheads)* is normal in caliber.

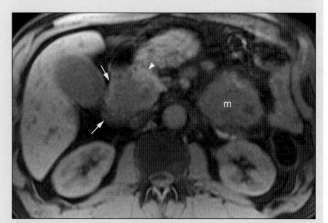

Figure 4. Distal duct cholangiocarcinoma. T1-weighted, fat-suppressed, unenhanced abdominal MRI shows a mass *(arrows)* involving the pancreatic head that is low in signal intensity relative to the adjacent normal pancreatic parenchyma *(arrowhead).* Pathologic analysis revealed cholangiocarcinoma. A large, mesenteric metastasis (m) was present at the time of diagnosis.

Suggested Readings

Fulcher AS, Turner MA: HASTE MR cholangiography in the evaluation of hilar cholangiocarcinoma. *AJR Am J Roentgenol* 169:1501-1505, 1997.

Lopera JE, Soto JA, Múnera F: Malignant hilar and perihilar biliary obstruction: Use of MR cholangiography to define the extent of biliary ductal involvement and plan percutaneous interventions. *Radiology* 220:90-96, 2001.

Park MS, Kim TK, Kim KW, et al: Differentiation of extrahepatic bile duct cholangiocarcinoma from benign stricture: Findings at MRCP versus ERCP. *Radiology* 233:234-240, 2004.

Intraductal Papillary Mucinous Neoplasms of the Pancreas

DEFINITION: Intraductal papillary mucinous neoplasms (IPMNs) are categorized as main duct type and branch duct type, depending on the duct of origin, and may be benign or malignant.

IMAGING

MRI
Findings
- Produces high signal intensity mucin within the ducts
- Main duct dilation
- Cystic dilation of the side branches
- Intraductal filling defects
- Lobulated cystic mass and nodular filling defects

Utility
- MR cholangiopancreatography is used.
- It can show communication between the tumor and the pancreatic duct.

CT
Findings
- Cystic dilation of side branches
- Dilation of main duct
- Intraluminal filling defects

Utility
- These lesions are most commonly found incidentally on CT.

CLINICAL PRESENTATION

- These lesions are usually found incidentally in asymptomatic patients.
- Malignant lesions may manifest with abdominal pain, weight loss, pancreatitis, and obstructive jaundice.

DIFFERENTIAL DIAGNOSIS

- Pancreatic carcinoma
- Pancreatic pseudocyst
- Serous cystadenoma
- Mucinous cystadenoma
- Mucinous cystadenocarcinoma

DIAGNOSTIC PEARLS

- Main duct dilation
- Intraductal filling defects
- Lobulated cystic mass

PATHOLOGY

- Main duct type and branch duct type, depending on duct of origin; may be benign or malignant
- Produces mucin
- Lesions that dilate the pancreatic duct are often malignant.
- Side-branch lesions are usually benign.

INCIDENCE/PREVALENCE AND EPIDEMIOLOGY

- Most commonly found in elderly male patients as an incidental finding.
- Second most common benign cystic tumor in elderly female patients after serous cystadenoma
- Male-to-female ratio of 3:1
- Most commonly found in the eighth and ninth decades of life

Suggested Readings

Irie H, Honda H, Aibe H, et al: MR cholangiopancreatographic differentiation of benign and malignant intraductal mucin-producing tumors of the pancreas. *AJR Am J Roentgenol* 174:1403-1408, 2000.

Koito K, Namieno T, Ichimura T, et al: Mucin-producing pancreatic tumors: Comparison of MR cholangiopancreatography with endoscopic retrograde cholangiopancreatography. *Radiology* 208:231-237, 1998.

Onaya H, Itai Y, Niitsu M, et al: Duct ectatic mucinous cystic neoplasms of the pancreas: Evaluation with MR cholangiopancreatography. *AJR Am J Roentgenol* 171:171-177, 1998.

WHAT THE REFERRING PHYSICIAN NEEDS TO KNOW

- Intraductal filling defects indicate malignancy.
- Diffuse main pancreatic duct dilation above 15 mm in main duct–type tumors indicates malignancy.
- In branch duct–type tumors, the absence of main pancreatic duct dilation suggests a benign tumor.

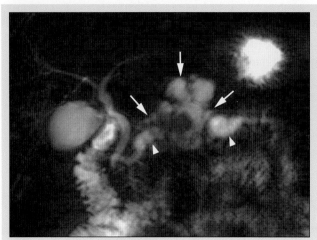

Figure 1. Malignant IPMN of the pancreas—main duct type.
Coronal thick-slab magnetic resonance cholangiopancreatography (MRCP) reveals a large cystic lesion *(arrows)* that contains nodular filling defects and that communicates with the main pancreatic duct in the pancreatic body *(arrowheads)*. Incidental note is made of pancreas divisum as evidenced by the horizontal orientation of the main pancreatic duct in the pancreatic head.

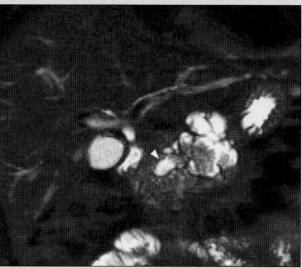

Figure 2. Malignant IPMN of the pancreas—main duct type.
Coronal-oblique thin-slab MRCP shows in detail the lobulated cystic mass and the nodular filling defects, as well as the dilated pancreatic duct *(arrowhead)* from which the mass arises.

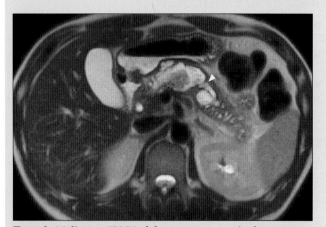

Figure 3. Malignant IPMN of the pancreas—main duct type.
Axial HASTE image shows in detail the lobulated cystic mass and the nodular filling defects, as well as the dilated pancreatic duct *(arrowhead)* from which the mass arises. *(HASTE,* Half-Fourier acquisition single-shot turbo spin-echo.)

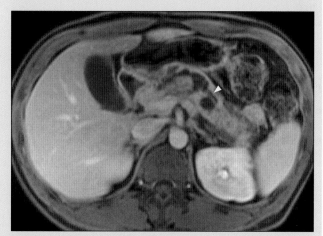

Figure 4. Malignant IPMN of the pancreas—main duct type.
Axial T1-weighted, fat-suppressed, contrast-enhanced abdominal MRI shows in detail the lobulated cystic mass and the nodular filling defects, as well as the dilated pancreatic duct *(arrowhead)* from which the mass arises.

Part 40

ANOMALIES AND ANATOMIC VARIANTS OF THE GALLBLADDER AND BILIARY TRACT

Abnormalities of Gallbladder Position

DEFINITION: Variations in gallbladder location are common.

IMAGING

CT

Findings
- Unusual location
- Herniated wandering gallbladder: cystic structure in the lesser sac
- Gallbladder torsion: gallbladder that is distended and may have an unusual location and mural thickening

Utility
- Sensitivity: 85%-95%
- Specificity: 95%-100%

Radiography

Findings
- Wandering gallbladder: gallbladder that may *disappear* into the pelvis on upright films and wander in front of spine and to the left of the abdomen
- Unusual angulation of the gallbladder when herniated into the foramen of Winslow

Utility
- Best seen using barium meal in conjunction with oral cholecystogram

MRI

Findings
- Herniated wandering gallbladder; a cystic structure in lesser sac
- Gallbladder torsion: gallbladder that is distended and may have an unusual location and mural thickening

Utility
- Sensitivity: 85%-95%
- Specificity: 95%-100%

Ultrasound

Findings
- Unusual location or gallbladder may not be visualized

DIAGNOSTIC PEARLS

- Wandering gallbladder: the gallbladder may *disappear* into the pelvis on upright films and wander in front of spine and to the left of the abdomen.
- In gallbladder torsion, the gallbladder is distended and may be in an unusual location; mural thickening may also be seen.
- In gallbladder torsion, the gallbladder is distended and may be in an unusual location and show mural thickening on CT.
- Anomalous positions of gallbladder include intrahepatic, left sided, transverse, retrodisplaced suprahepatic, retrohepatic, supradiaphragmatic, and retroperitoneal.

Utility
- Sensitivity: 30%-40%
- Specificity: 80%-85%

CLINICAL PRESENTATION

- Herniated wandering gallbladder that may cause intermittent abdominal pain
- Gallbladder torsion: leukocytosis, fever, and a right upper quadrant mass
- Ectopic gallbladder: often asymptomatic

DIFFERENTIAL DIAGNOSIS

- Hepatic cyst
- Renal cyst
- Omental cyst
- Mesenteric cyst

WHAT THE REFERRING PHYSICIAN NEEDS TO KNOW

- Wandering gallbladder can herniate through the foramen of Winslow into the lesser sac.
- Gallbladder torsion: Gangrene is common, particularly when pain has been present for more than 48 hours.
- Ectopic gallbladder may complicate the clinical diagnosis of acute cholecystitis as a result of the paucity of peritoneal signs because the gallbladder is far from the peritoneum.
- Ectopic gallbladder also makes cholecystectomy more difficult.

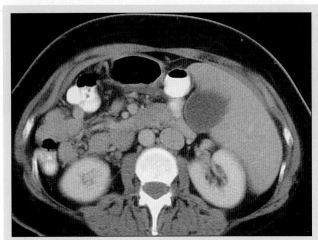

Figure 1. **Gallbladder ectopia.** Situs inversus with left-sided gallbladder.

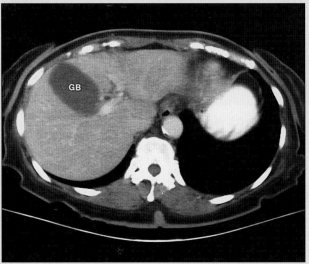

Figure 2. **Gallbladder ectopia.** Intrahepatic gallbladder (GB) demonstrated on CT scan.

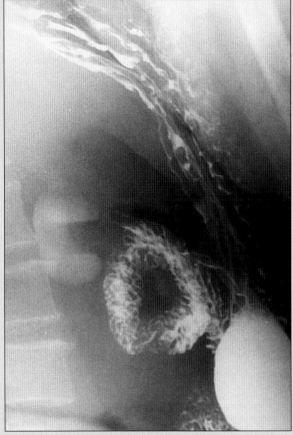

Figure 3. **Gallbladder ectopia.** Retrohepatic gallbladder shown on an oral cholecystogram.

PATHOLOGY

- Wandering gallbladder has an unusually long mesentery, permitting it to *wander* or *float*.
- Intrahepatic gallbladder is completely surrounded by hepatic parenchyma.
- In cirrhosis, small or absent right lobes, and chronic obstructive pulmonary disease, the gallbladder is often interposed between the liver and the diaphragm.
- Gallbladder torsion causes extreme mobility as a result of absent mesenteric or peritoneal investments, except for cystic duct and artery; long gallbladder mesentery may be noted.
- Presence of large stones in the gallbladder fundus causes lengthening and gallbladder mesenteric torsion.
- Kyphosis, vigorous gallbladder peristalsis, and atherosclerosis have also been implicated as other factors predisposing or contributing to torsion.

INCIDENCE/PREVALENCE AND EPIDEMIOLOGY

- Gallbladder torsion: the mesentery is sufficiently long to permit torsion in 4.5% of the population.
- Most cases of gallbladder torsion occur in women (female-male ratio of 3:1).

Suggested Readings

Blanton DE, Bream CA, Mandel SR: Gallbladder ectopia: A review of anomalies of position. *AJR Am J Roentgenol* 121:296-300, 1974.

Quinn SF, Fazzio F, Jones E: Torsion of the gallbladder: Findings on CT and sonography and role of percutaneous cholecystostomy. *AJR Am J Roentgenol* 148:881-882, 1987.

Senecail B, Texier F, Kergastel I, et al: Anatomic variability and congenital anomalies of the gallbladder: Ultrasonographic study of 1823 patients. *Morphologie* 84:35-39, 2000.

Choledochal Cysts

DEFINITION: Choledochal cyst is characterized by a cystic fusiform dilation of the majority of the extrahepatic bile duct.

IMAGING

MRI
Findings
- Fusiform dilation of the majority of the extrahepatic bile duct

Utility
- MR cholangiopancreatography (MRCP) has been proposed as the imaging modality of choice for choledochal cyst evaluation in adults.

Ultrasound
Findings
- Fusiform cyst beneath porta hepatis separate from gallbladder
- Communication with common hepatic and/or intrahepatic ducts present
- Abrupt change of caliber at junction of dilated segment and normal ducts

Utility
- Is typically the first imaging test employed when evaluating neonates, infants, and children with suspected hepatobiliary obstruction

CLINICAL PRESENTATION

- Intermittent obstructive jaundice
- Recurrent colicky right upper quadrant pain, back pain
- Intermittent palpable right upper quadrant abdominal pain
- Recurrent fever, chills, weight loss, and pruritus

PATHOLOGY/ANATOMIC FINDINGS

- The cyst wall is fibrous without an epithelial lining.
- Dilation, stenosis, or atresia of other portions of the biliary tract in 2% of patients
- Aplasia of or double gallbladder

DIAGNOSTIC PEARLS

- Fusiform dilation of the majority of the extrahepatic bile duct

- Failure of union of left and right hepatic ducts
- Pancreatic duct and accessory hepatic bile ducts may drain into cyst.

INCIDENCE/PREVALENCE AND EPIDEMIOLOGY

- Prevalence of 1 in 13,000 hospital admissions
- More prevalent in Japan
- Male-to-female ratio of 1:4
- 80% diagnosed during childhood
- 7% found during pregnancy

DIFFERENTIAL DIAGNOSIS

- Mesenteric, omental, renal, ovarian, adrenal, hepatic, or pancreatic cyst
- Gastrointestinal duplication
- Hydrops of gallbladder
- Hydronephrosis of right kidney

Suggested Readings

Irie H, Honda H, Jimi M, et al: Value of MR cholangiopancreatography in evaluating choledochal cysts. *AJR Am J Roentgenol* 171:1381-1385, 1998.

Lam WWM, Lam TPW, Saing H, et al: MR cholangiography and CT cholangiography of pediatric patients with choledochal cysts. *AJR Am J Roentgenol* 173:401-405, 1999.

Matos C, Nicaise N, Devière J, et al: Choledochal cysts: Comparison of findings at MR cholangiopancreatography and endoscopic retrograde cholangiopancreatography in eight patients. *Radiology* 209:443-448, 1998.

WHAT THE REFERRING PHYSICIAN NEEDS TO KNOW

- MRCP detects choledochal cysts in adults and children, providing diagnostic information equivalent to endoscopic retrograde cholangiopancreatography without complications.
- MRCP delineates the extent of cyst, detects anomalous pancreaticobiliary junctions, and defines critical factors in planning cyst excision and bile duct reconstruction.

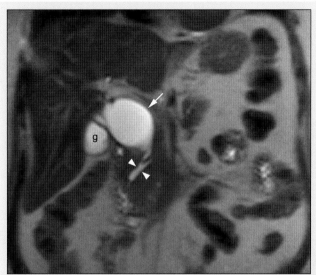

Figure 1. Type I choledochal or bile duct cyst. Coronal HASTE MRCP shows fusiform dilation of the majority of the extrahepatic bile duct *(arrow)* indicative of a type 1 choledochal or bile duct cyst. An anomalous pancreaticobiliary junction *(arrowheads)* is present. The gallbladder (g) lies lateral to the choledochal cyst. *(HASTE,* Half-Fourier acquisition single-shot turbo spin-echo.)

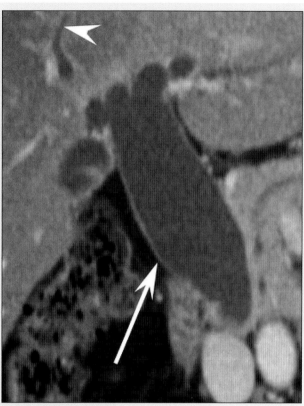

Figure 2. Type I choledochal cysts. Coronal oblique multiplanar reformatted image shows fusiform dilatation of the common bile duct *(arrow)*. Note also dilatation of the intrahepatic biliary tract *(arrowhead)*.

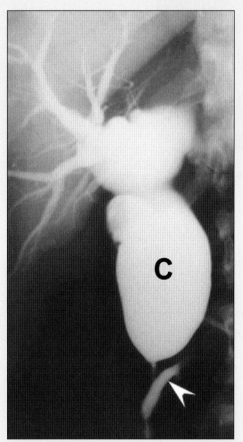

Figure 3. Type I choledochal cysts. Percutaneous transhepatic cholangiogram shows a large choledochal cyst (C) at the level of the extrahepatic bile duct. Note the aberrant entry of the common bile duct at the side of the pancreatic duct *(arrowhead)*.

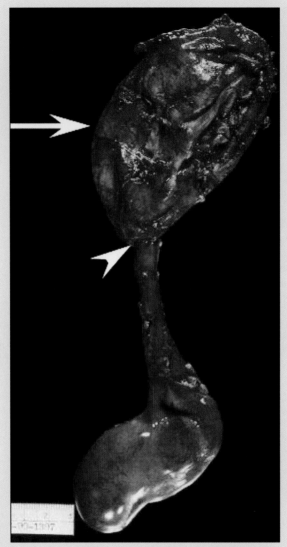

Figure 4. Type I choledochal cyst. Photograph shows an excised type I choledochal cyst of the common bile duct (*arrow*) in continuity with the cystic duct and the gallbladder (*arrowhead*). Scale is in centimeters. (*From Brancatelli G, Federle MP, Vilagrain V, et al: Fibropolycystic liver disease: CT and MR imaging findings. RadioGraphics 25:659-670, 2005.*)

Choledochocele

DEFINITION: Protrusion of a dilated common bile duct, intramural segment, into the duodenum, analogous to a ureterocele.

IMAGING

Fluoroscopy
Findings
- Smooth, well-defined intraluminal duodenal filling defect of the papilla that changes in shape with compression and peristalsis
- Should not be filled with barium

Utility
- Barium studies usually show secondary signs of this disorder.

Interventional Radiology
Findings
- Smooth club-like or sac-like dilation of the intramural segment of the common bile duct

Utility
- Cholangiography is the most diagnostic examination for this disorder.

MRI
Findings
- High signal intensity *cobra-head* appearance bulging into the duodenum on MR cholangiopancreatography (MRCP)

Utility
- MRI is less sensitive than direct cholangiography for making the diagnosis

CLINICAL PRESENTATION

- Choledochocele occurs in adulthood, with long-standing nausea, vomiting, and episodic abdominal pain.
- Choledocholithiasis with right upper quadrant pain, jaundice, and cholangitis
- Pancreatitis
- Nausea and vomiting

DIFFERENTIAL DIAGNOSIS

- Pancreatitis
- Peptic ulcer disease

DIAGNOSTIC PEARLS

- Smooth, well-defined intraluminal duodenal filling defect of the papilla that changes in shape with compression and peristalsis
- Smooth club-like or sac-like dilation of the intramural segment of the common bile duct
- High signal intensity *cobra-head* appearance bulging into the duodenum on MRCP

- Cholangitis
- Choledocholithiasis

PATHOLOGY

- Protrusion of the dilated common bile duct, intramural segment, into the duodenum; of unknown cause; may be partly acquired

INCIDENCE/PREVALENCE AND EPIDEMIOLOGY

- Choledochocele is often seen on cholangiograms in patients who have undergone a cholecystectomy.
- Patients are usually adults.

Suggested Readings
Catalano O: Conventional x-ray and CT findings in a case of intraluminal choledochocele. *Rofo* 169:210-212, 1998.

Scholz FJ, Carrera GF, Larsen CR: The choledochocele: Correlation of radiological, clinical and pathological findings. *Radiology* 118:28, 1976.

WHAT THE REFERRING PHYSICIAN NEEDS TO KNOW

- Choledochoceles can be congenital, originating from a tiny diverticulum of the distal common bile duct.
- More often they are acquired after surgery or after passage of a stone, with subsequent stenosis and inflammation.

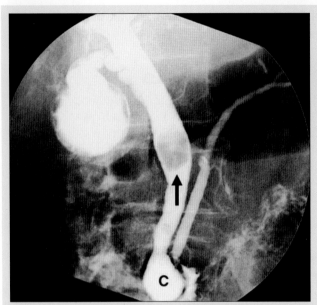

Figure 1. **Type III choledochocysts: choledochocele.** Endoscopic retrograde cholangiopancreatography shows saccular dilation of the distal common bile duct (C) and choledocholithiasis *(arrow)*.

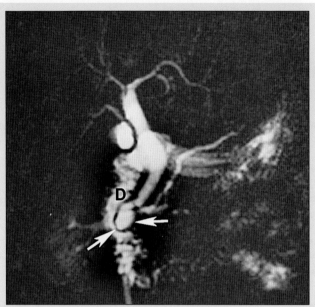

Figure 2. **Type III choledochocysts: choledochocele.** Coronal MRCP image demonstrates bulbous dilation of the intramural segment of the distal common bile duct *(arrows)*, which protrudes into the duodenum (D).

Part 41

CHOLELITHIASIS, CHOLECYSTITIS, CHOLEDOCHOLITHIASIS, AND HYPERPLASTIC CHOLECYSTOSES

Acute Acalculous Cholecystitis

DEFINITION: Gallbladder wall inflammation without stones.

IMAGING

Ultrasound
Findings
- Gallbladder wall thickening, distention, and sludge are seen.
- Gallstones are absent.

Utility
- Ultrasound is the reasonable first study for the diagnosis of acute acalculous cholecystitis.
- Reported sensitivity is 36%-92%.
- Unreliable sonographic Murphy sign is noted.

CT
Findings
- Pericholecystic inflammatory change and fluid
- Abnormalities of gallbladder wall or adjacent hepatic parenchyma
- Absence of gallstones
- CT findings that are similar to those of calculus cholecystitis

Utility
- CT provides a diagnostically more specific examination than sonography.
- It is helpful in patients who are stable enough to undergo imaging.

MRI and MR Cholangiopancreatography (MRCP)
Findings
- Pericholecystic inflammatory change and fluid
- Abnormalities of gallbladder wall or adjacent hepatic parenchyma
- Absence of gallstones
- MRI findings that are similar to those of calculus cholecystitis

DIAGNOSTIC PEARLS
- Gallbladder wall thickening, distention, and sludge are present on ultrasound.
- Gallstones are absent.

Utility
- MRCP has the advantage of depicting bile duct and occasionally cystic duct stones that are not seen on CT.

Nuclear Medicine
Findings
- Nonvisualization of the gallbladder

Utility
- Cholescintigraphy is used.
- False-positive rate of up to 40% was reported in patients with hepatocellular dysfunction, prolonged fasting, or severe illness.
- Specificity can be improved with the use of morphine.
- Combination of ultrasound and morphine scintigraphy may lead to greater diagnostic accuracy.

CLINICAL PRESENTATION
- Nonspecific findings of fever and leukocytosis
- Typically seen in critically ill patients in intensive care unit
- Possible demonstration of altered mental status in some patients
- Right upper quadrant pain
- Sepsis

WHAT THE REFERRING PHYSICIAN NEEDS TO KNOW
- Acute acalculous cholecystitis should be suspected in critically ill or injured patients who have fever with no apparent source.
- Negative cholescintigraphy is useful for excluding acalculous cholecystitis, but a positive study must be interpreted with caution.
- If no other source of sepsis is discovered in ill patients by CT or MRI, percutaneous cholecystostomy can be performed.

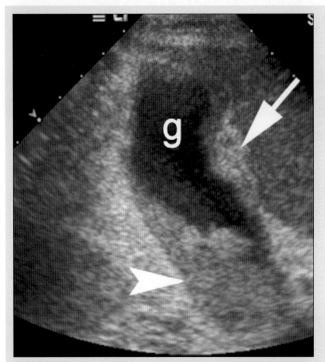

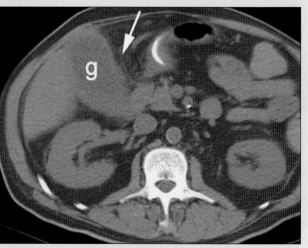

Figure 2. Acute acalculous cholecystitis: CT findings.
Noncontrast CT scan demonstrates gallbladder distention (g) with inflammatory changes in pericholecystic fat *(arrow)*, confirming presence of gallbladder inflammation.

Figure 1. Acute acalculous cholecystitis: ultrasound findings.
Gallbladder (g) is distended, with mural thickening *(arrow)*, and contains dependent echoes, indicating sludge *(arrowhead)*. These features are common ultrasound findings in acutely ill patients.

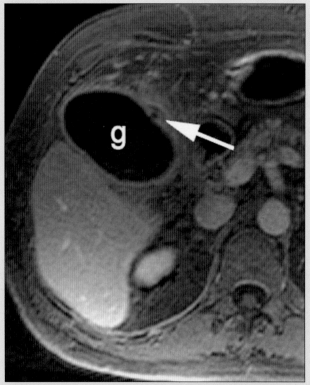

Figure 3. Acute acalculous cholecystitis: MR features. Axial T1-weighted fat-suppressed gradient-echo image with gadolinium enhancement demonstrates distended gallbladder (g), wall thickening, and pericholecystic inflammatory change. *Arrow* points to a small intramural abscess not suspected sonographically.

DIFFERENTIAL DIAGNOSIS

- Calculous cholecystitis
- Ascending cholangitis
- Hepatitis
- Gallbladder neoplasm
- Gallbladder metastases
- Pancreatitis
- Peptic ulcer disease

PATHOLOGY

- Bile stasis, gallbladder ischemia, cystic duct obstruction and systemic infection are important factors in the pathogenesis of acute acalculous cholecystitis.
- Histologic features include gallbladder wall inflammation and necrosis of blood vessels in the muscularis and serosa of the gallbladder.

INCIDENCE/PREVALENCE AND EPIDEMIOLOGY

- Reported incidence of acute acalculous cholecystitis ranges from approximately 5%-10%.
- Incidence is increased in critically ill patients or those with prolonged illness, such as patients with trauma or those in a prolonged stay in an intensive care unit.

Suggested Readings

Barie PS, Fischer E: Acute acalculous cholecystitis. *J Am Coll Surg* 180:232-244, 1995.

Boland GWL, Slater G, Lu DSK, et al: Prevalence and significance of gallbladder abnormalities seen on sonography in intensive care unit patients. *AJR Am J Roentgenol* 174:973-977, 2000.

Flancbaum L, Choban PS: Use of morphine cholescintigraphy in the diagnosis of acute cholecystitis in critically ill patients. *Intensive Care Med* 21:120-124, 1995.

Kalliafas S, Ziegler DW, Flancbaum L, et al: Acute acalculous cholecystitis: Incidence, risk factors, diagnosis, and outcome. *Am Surg* 64:471-475, 1998.

Mariat G, Mahul P, Prevot N, et al: Contribution of ultrasonography and cholescintigraphy to the diagnosis of acute acalculous cholecystitis in intensive care patients. *Intensive Care Med* 26:1658-1663, 2000.

Mirvis SE, Vainright JR, Nelson AW, et al: The diagnosis of acute acalculous cholecystitis: A comparison of sonography, scintigraphy and CT. *AJR Am J Roentgenol* 147:115-117, 1986.

Acute Cholecystitis

DEFINITION: Inflammation of the gallbladder mucosa caused by gallstones.

ANATOMIC FINDINGS

Gallbladder
- Obstruction of cystic duct or gallbladder neck with gallstones, resulting in gallbladder distention

IMAGING

Nuclear Medicine
Findings
- Prompt biliary excretion of tracer without demonstration of the gallbladder is the hallmark for acute cholecystitis.
Utility
- Cholescintigraphy is used.
- Recent studies showed accuracy of 91% for scintigraphy versus 77% for sonography.
- Longer time is needed to perform the procedure (up to 4 hours) compared with sonography.
- Cholescintigraphy cannot evaluate for nonbiliary conditions.
- Intravenous morphine is injected if the gallbladder is not visualized after 1 hour, with appearance of the biliary tree and duodenum.

Ultrasound
Findings
- Gallstones, gallbladder distention, wall thickening, and pericholecystic fluid
- Stone possibly impacted in the gallbladder neck or cystic duct
- Sonographic Murphy sign: maximal tenderness during compression with ultrasound transducer placed directly over the gallbladder
Utility
- Ultrasound can confirm the diagnosis of acute cholecystitis and distinguish from chronic cholecystitis with an accuracy of 95%-99%.
- It is readily available, can be rapidly performed without radiation, and allows for the detection of cholecystitis-related complications, as well as alternative diagnoses.
- Sonographic Murphy sign may be negative or impaired in patients with altered mental status and gangrenous cholecystitis.

DIAGNOSTIC PEARLS
- Gallstones, gallbladder distention, thickening of gallbladder wall, pericholecystic inflammation, and fluid are seen.
- Sonographic Murphy sign is maximal tenderness during compression with ultrasound transducer placed directly over the gallbladder.
- Greater than 80% contrast enhancement of gallbladder wall helps differentiate acute from chronic cholecystitis.

CT
Findings
- Gallstones, gallbladder distention, thickening of the gallbladder wall, pericholecystic inflammation, and fluid
- Ancillary finding of increased contrast enhancement in the liver parenchyma adjacent to the gallbladder
- Transient increase in hepatic enhancement around the gallbladder during the arterial phase of enhancement
Utility
- CT may be used as an initial study because it allows for a more comprehensive evaluation of the abdomen and pelvis.
- It identifies other acute inflammatory processes that may simulate acute cholecystitis.
- It is limited with respect to the detection of gallstones because up to only 75% are visualized.
- CT has an accuracy of 85% in the diagnosis of acute cholecystitis.

MRI
Findings
- Gallstones
- Gallbladder wall edema, which shows high signal intensity on T2-weighted images. (Greater than 80% contrast enhancement of the gallbladder wall helps differentiate acute from chronic cholecystitis.)
- Transient increase in hepatic enhancement around gallbladder during arterial phase of injection
Utility
- MRI is used when other imaging findings are equivocal or the clinical setting is ambiguous.
- It is superior to ultrasound for the detection of obstructing calculi in the gallbladder neck and the cystic duct.

WHAT THE REFERRING PHYSICIAN NEEDS TO KNOW
- Presence of acute cholecystitis is more likely if it can be demonstrated by ultrasound that the stone is impacted in the gallbladder neck or the cystic duct.
- Sonographic Murphy's sign may be blunted in patients receiving pain medications and those with altered mental status or in the presence of gangrenous cholecystitis.

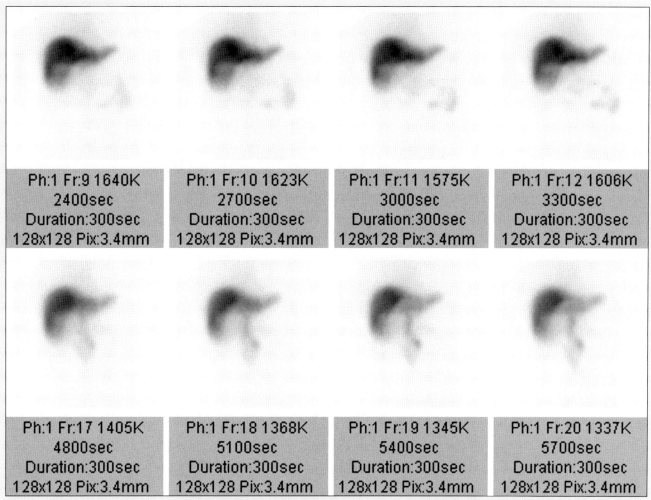

Figure 1. Cholescintigraphy. Positive hepatobiliary iminodiacetic acid scan. No filling of the gallbladder is seen, confirming obstruction of the cystic duct and the presence of acute cholecystitis. (*Courtesy of Dr. Elissa Kramer, Department of Nuclear Medicine, New York University Medical Center.*)

- It is helpful for identifying complications of acute cholecystitis.
- MRI has an accuracy of 87% in the diagnosis of acute cholecystitis.

CLINICAL PRESENTATION

- Fever, right upper quadrant pain, and elevated white blood cell count
- Clinically positive Murphy sign: focal tenderness over the gallbladder on inspiration

DIFFERENTIAL DIAGNOSIS

- Choledocholithiasis
- Cholelithiasis
- Omental infarction
- Diverticula (stomach and duodenum)
- Post-traumatic lesions of the gallbladder and biliary tract
- Gastric outlet obstruction (stomach and duodenum)
- Peptic ulcer disease
- Peritoneal carcinomatosis
- Acute pyelonephritis
- Appendicitis
- Right lower lobe pneumonia

PATHOLOGY

- Inflammation of gallbladder mucosa may result from chemical injury caused by bile salts or superimposed infection, or both.
- If untreated, inflammation eventually progresses to all layers of the gallbladder wall and may lead to necrosis, gangrene, and gallbladder perforation.

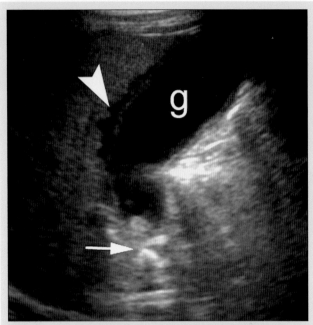

Figure 2. **Acute cholecystitis: ultrasound.** In the upright position, the gallbladder (g) is distended, and pericholecystic fluid is evident *(arrowhead)*. Stone *(arrow)* does not change location, confirming impaction in the gallbladder neck.

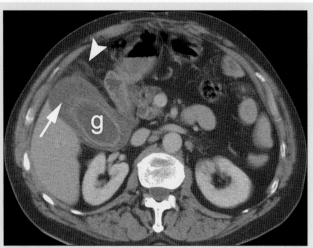

Figure 3. **Acute cholecystitis: CT features.** The gallbladder (g) is distended with marked mural thickening *(arrow)* and pericholecystic inflammatory changes *(arrowhead)*.

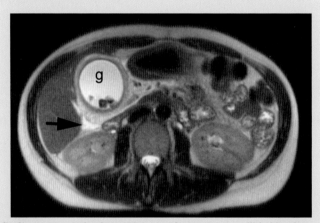

Figure 4. **Acute cholecystitis: MR findings.** T2-weighted HASTE image demonstrates gallbladder distention (g). Dependent low-signal gallstones are evident. Gallbladder wall is thickened, and pericholecystic fluid *(arrow)* can be seen. *(HASTE,* Half-Fourier acquisition single-shot turbo spin-echo.)

INCIDENCE/PREVALENCE AND EPIDEMIOLOGY

- Acute cholecystitis occurs in approximately one third of patients with gallstones.
- It is the most common cause of right upper quadrant pain.
- Approximately one third of patients show a clinically positive Murphy sign.
- Approximately one third of patients with presumptive diagnosis will not have acute cholecystitis on follow-up.

Suggested Readings

Laing FC: Ultrasonography of the acute abdomen. *Radiol Clin N Am* 30:389-404, 1992.

Laing FL, Federle MP, Jeffrey RB, et al: Ultrasonic evaluation of patients with acute right upper quadrant pain. *Radiology* 140:449-455, 1981.

Paulson EK: Acute cholecystitis: CT findings. *Semin Ultrasound CT MR* 21:56-63, 2000.

Ralls PW, Colletti PM, Halls JM, et al: Prospective evaluation of 99mTc-IDA cholescintigraphy and gray-scale ultrasound in the diagnosis of acute cholecystitis. *Radiology* 144:369-371, 1982.

Samuels BI, Freitas JE, Bree RL, et al: Comparison of radionuclide hepatobiliary imaging and real-time ultrasound for the detection of acute cholecystitis. *Radiology* 147:207-210, 1983.

Biliary Sludge

DEFINITION: Suspension of bile and particulate material in the gallbladder.

IMAGING

Ultrasound-Doppler
Findings
- Absence of vascularity intraluminally

Utility
- Ultrasound with or without Doppler is the primary means of establishing this diagnosis.
- Sensitivity: 90%-100%
- Specificity: 90%-100%

Ultrasound
Findings
- Low-level echoes are seen that layer dependently within the gallbladder lumen.
- *Hepatization* of gallbladder is seen when the lumen is entirely filled with sludge.
- Aggregate of intraluminal sludge can mimic a soft-tissue density mass (tumefactive sludge).

Utility
- Ultrasound with or without Doppler is the primary means of establishing this diagnosis.
- Sensitivity: 90%-100%
- Specificity: 85%-100%

MRI
Findings
- Nonenhancing gallbladder content

Utility
- Use of contrast and subtraction are helpful when findings are equivocal and when a suspicion of possible intraluminal mass exists.
- Sensitivity: 75%-90%
- Specificity: 90%-95%

CLINICAL PRESENTATION

- Biliary pain, cholecystitis, cholangitis, or pancreatitis

DIFFERENTIAL DIAGNOSIS

- Cholelithiasis
- Gallbladder mass

DIAGNOSTIC PEARLS

- Low-level echoes that layer dependently are seen within the gallbladder lumen on ultrasound.
- *Hepatization* of the gallbladder is seen when the lumen is entirely filled with sludge.
- Absence of vascularity on Doppler ultrasound confirms the diagnosis.

- Hemorrhage
- Parasites
- Vicarious excretion of contrast medium

PATHOLOGY

- Chemical composition consists of various proportions of calcium bilirubinate and cholesterol monohydrate crystals and gallbladder mucus.
- Combination of impaired gallbladder motility and alteration in nucleation factors leads to sludge formation.
- Precipitate aggregation results in gallstone formation.
- Fasting, pregnancy, total parenteral nutrition, and critical illness may lead to sludge formation.
- Sludge may resolve, have cyclical pattern of appearance and disappearance, or progress to stone formation.

INCIDENCE/PREVALENCE AND EPIDEMIOLOGY

- Sludge occurs in up to 80% of intensive care unit patients who are NPO.
- Sludge can be a precursor of gallstones and cholecystitis.
- There is an increased incidence of sludge formation in pregnant patients as well as those on hyperalimentation chemotherapy.

WHAT THE REFERRING PHYSICIAN NEEDS TO KNOW

- Aggregate of intraluminal sludge on ultrasound can mimic soft tissue density mass (tumefactive sludge).
- Use of color Doppler imaging is important to exclude other more significant abnormalities, such as intraluminal soft tissue masses.
- Doppler demonstration of vascularity within abnormality confirms the presence of a soft tissue mass.
- Absence of vascularity is less helpful; follow-up or assessment with precontrast and postcontrast CT or MRI is indicated.

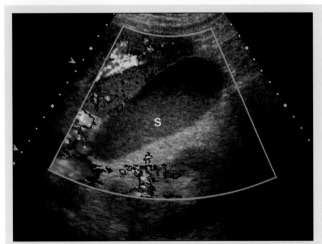

Figure 1. Sludge: sonographic findings. Color Doppler shows no vascularity in the sludge (s), helping to exclude a solid, intraluminal mass.

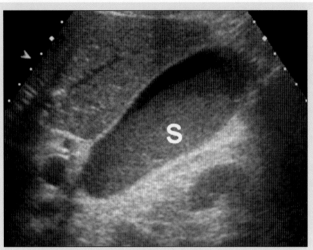

Figure 2. Sludge: sonographic findings. Ultrasound shows low-level, nonshadowing intraluminal echoes (s).

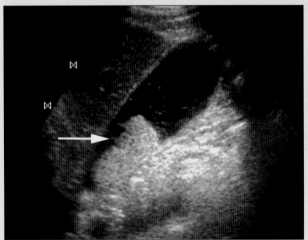

Figure 3. Aggregate of sludge on ultrasound. Sagittal ultrasound image of the gallbladder demonstrates an echogenic nonshadowing abnormality located dependently within the gallbladder lumen *(arrow)*.

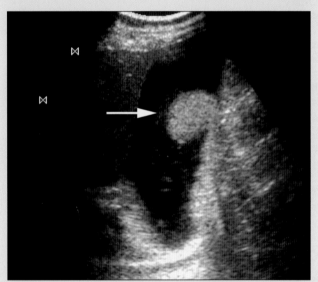

Figure 4. Aggregate of sludge on ultrasound. When the patient is imaged in the upright position, this abnormality changes location and configuration *(arrow)*, confirming aggregate of sludge rather than a soft tissue mass.

Suggested Readings

Jain R: Biliary sludge: When should it not be ignored? *Curr Treat Options Gastroenterol* 7:105-109, 2004.

Ko CW, Sekijima JH, Lee SP: Biliary sludge. *Ann Intern Med* 130:301-311, 1999.

Lee SP: Pathogenesis of biliary sludge. *Hepatology* 12:2005-2035, 1990.

Choledocholithiasis

DEFINITION: Presence of a gallstone in the bile duct.

IMAGING

Interventional Radiology
Utility
- Endoscopic retrograde cholangiopancreatography and percutaneous transhepatic cholangiography are used.
- Interventional radiology is highly accurate for the detection of choledocholithiasis and provides access for therapeutic intervention.
- It is an invasive procedure with risks of pancreatitis, hemorrhage, and sepsis.

Ultrasound
Findings
- Echogenic foci, which may or may not cause posterior acoustic shadowing, depending on the size and composition
Utility
- Ultrasound is the primary imaging modality for the evaluation of right upper quadrant pain.
- It is superior to CT in the initial imaging evaluation of biliary disease.
- Sensitivity of 22%-75% has been reported for common bile duct stones.
- Detection is improved by contrast enhancement and reduction of side-lobe artifacts by tissue-harmonic imaging.
- Scanning the patient in the erect right posterior oblique or right lateral decubitus position minimizes gas in the antrum and duodenum, improving detection.
- Limited sensitivity results from the inability to visualize the duct completely.
- Nonshadowing stones may be difficult to differentiate from aggregates of sludge or soft-tissue masses.

CT
Findings
- Stones may be calcified, have soft-tissue density, or have low density with respect to the bile.
- Calcified stones are most readily identified.
- *Target sign* refers to the central density, corresponding to the stone, surrounded by hypoattenuating bile or ampullary soft tissue.

DIAGNOSTIC PEARLS
- Echogenic foci, which may or may not cause posterior acoustic shadowing, depending on size and composition on ultrasound
- Target sign, rim sign, or crescent sign on CT
- Well-circumscribed low-signal-intensity filling defects in the biliary tract on MR cholangiopancreatography (MRCP)

- *Rim sign* refers to a faint rim of increased density along the margin of a low-density area.
- *Crescent sign* refers to calculus with increased density surrounded by crescent hypoattenuating bile.
- Indirect signs include abrupt termination of the dilated distal common bile duct without visible surrounding mass or biliary dilation.

Utility
- Unenhanced conventional CT has a sensitivity of 75% in the detection of choledocholithiasis.
- Multidetector CT has higher sensitivity, ranging from 65%-88%.
- Liver window settings improve visualization of non-calcified stones.
- CT cholangiography provides excellent visualization of biliary anatomy and filling defects, with 95% sensitivity for choledocholithiasis.

MRI
Findings
- Well-circumscribed low-signal-intensity filling defects in the biliary tract
Utility
- MRCP is used.
- MRCP is more sensitive than ultrasound and CT.
- It is highly accurate for the detection of common bile duct stones in patients with symptomatic gallstones.
- MRCP is also helpful but a noncalcified stone is difficult to differentiate from a soft-tissue mass.
- Diagnostic pitfalls include gas, blood, or other abnormality within the duct that can simulate stones.

WHAT THE REFERRING PHYSICIAN NEEDS TO KNOW
- Indirect signs on CT scan such as ductal dilation or abrupt termination of duct may be useful but are not conclusive.
- Unenhanced CT images are better for detection because most stones are slightly hyperdense.
- Reviewing coronal source and transverse T2-weighted images is important to prevent MRI diagnostic pitfalls.
- Stone that remains lodged in the common bile duct can lead to a potentially life-threatening emergency because of associated cholangitis.

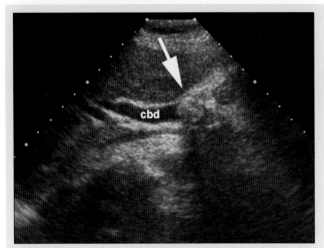

Figure 1. Choledocholithiasis: ultrasound features. Sagittal image demonstrates common bile duct (cbd) dilation. An intraductal echogenic shadowing focus can be seen *(arrow)*, consistent with a large stone.

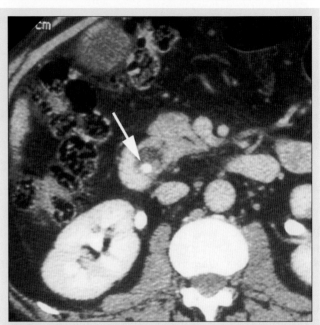

Figure 2. Choledocholithiasis: appearance at CT. Calcified stone *(arrow)* in the common bile duct.

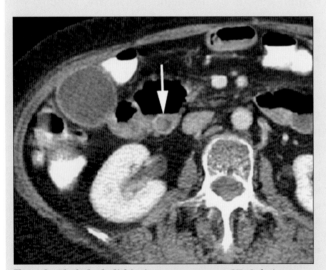

Figure 3. Choledocholithiasis: appearance at CT. Soft-tissue-density noncalcified stone *(arrow)* in the common bile duct with low-density crescent of bile.

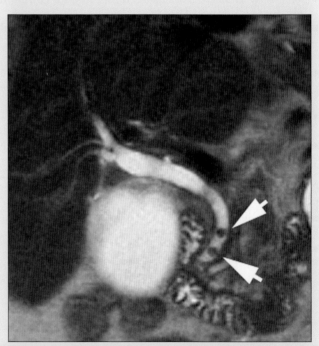

Figure 4. Choledocholithiasis: MR findings. T2-weighted coronal HASTE image shows low signal intensity common bile duct stones *(arrows)*. *(HASTE,* Half-Fourier acquisition single-shot turbo spin-echo.)

- Sensitivity: 90%-100%
- Specificity: 95%-100%
- Accuracy: 96%-98%

CLINICAL PRESENTATION

- Some patients may be asymptomatic, but others develop symptoms of biliary colic and acute pancreatitis.
- Jaundice, right upper quadrant pain, and abnormal liver function tests

DIFFERENTIAL DIAGNOSIS

- Pancreatic carcinoma
- Cholangiocarcinoma
- Ascending cholangitis
- Sclerosing cholangitis
- Biliary parasites
- Ampullary carcinoma
- Perivaterian duodenal diverticulum
- Oriental cholangiohepatitis

PATHOLOGY

- Primary stones are biliary stones that form within the biliary tract.
- Secondary stones are those that migrate from the gallbladder.
- Primary stones develop in the setting of bile stasis and the colonization of bile with enteric organisms.

- Obstruction of bile may be related to inflammatory or iatrogenic strictures, congenital strictures, or periampullary diverticula.
- Primary stones are associated with parasitic infections *(Ascaris lumbricoides),* which become nidi for stone and inflammatory stricture formation.

INCIDENCE/PREVALENCE AND EPIDEMIOLOGY

- Migration of gallstones among asymptomatic patients is estimated to occur in 3%-5% of patients per year.
- Around 1%-2% of patients per year develop symptoms, including biliary colic or acute pancreatitis.
- Between 7% and 20% of patients undergoing cholecystectomy are found to have stones in the common bile duct.
- In Western countries, most bile duct stones are secondary.
- In Asia, most bile duct stones are primary.

Suggested Readings

Lamont JT, Afdhal NH: Cholesterol gallstone disease: From pancreatitis to prevention. *Curr Opin Gastroenterol* 10:523-525, 1994.

Liu TH, Moody FG: Pathogenesis and presentation of common bile duct stones. *Semin Laparosc Surg* 7:224-231, 2000.

Lo SK, Chen J: The role of ERCP in choledocholithiasis. *Abdom Imaging* 21:120-132, 1996.

Makary MA, Duncan MD, Harmon JW, et al: The role of magnetic resonance cholangiography in the management of patients with gallstone pancreatitis. *Ann Surg* 241:119-124, 2005.

Raraty MG, Finch M, Neoptolemos JP: Acute cholangitis and pancreatitis secondary to common duct stones: Management update. *World J Surg* 22:115-116, 1998.

Cholelithiasis

DEFINITION: Stones in the gallbladder.

ANATOMIC FINDINGS

Gallbladder
- Stones may impact in the cystic duct.

IMAGING

Radiography
Findings
- Presence of calcified gallstones

Utility
- Radiography has a limited role in the detection of gallstones.
- Only 15%-20% of gallstones are calcified enough to be visualized on radiographs.

Ultrasound
Findings
- Highly reflective echo is seen that is generally mobile and is associated with posterior acoustic shadowing.
- Aggregate of sludge or sludge ball (tumefactive sludge) may be mobile but will not cast an acoustic shadow.
- Small stones produce a shadow only when imaged in the aggregate.
- If the gallbladder is contracted and the lumen is filled with shadowing stones, the wall-echo-shadow (WES) sign is seen.

Utility
- Ultrasound is the imaging tool of choice for the detection of gallstones, with reported accuracy of 96%.
- Performing studies at the patient's bedside is possible.
- It has no ionizing radiation.
- It also allows for the evaluation of other structures in right upper quadrant when alternative diagnoses are considered.
- Very small stones may not always cast a shadow.
- Use of tissue harmonic imaging has been shown to improve gallbladder calculi detection.
- It is important to evaluate the patient in more than one position.

CT
Findings
- Calcified stones are readily identified because they are denser than bile.

DIAGNOSTIC PEARLS
- Highly reflective echo is seen that is generally mobile and is associated with posterior acoustic shadowing.
- Presence of calcified gallstones is seen on radiographs.
- If the gallbladder is contracted and the lumen is filled with shadowing stones, the WES sign is seen.

- Stones with high concentration of cholesterol are less dense than bile.
- When stones degenerate, nitrogen gas may collect in the central fissures and create the *Mercedes-Benz sign.*
- Gas may also appear as a focal collection of gas located in the nondependent gallbladder lumen.

Utility
- Ability to detect stones on CT depends on differing densities of the stone and of bile.
- Reported sensitivity is 75%.

MRI and MR Cholangiopancreatography (MRCP)
Findings
- On T2-weighted MRI, gallstones show as the signal voids in high signal intensity bile.
- Cholesterol stones are isointense or hypointense on T1-weighted images.
- Pigment stones have high signal intensity on T1-weighted images.

Utility
- MRCP is useful in demonstrating common bile duct stone.

CLINICAL PRESENTATION
- Most common symptoms are biliary pain or colic.
- Gallstones are symptomatic in 20%-30% of patients.

DIFFERENTIAL DIAGNOSIS
- Biliary sludge
- Gallbladder cancer
- Biliary parasite

WHAT THE REFERRING PHYSICIAN NEEDS TO KNOW
- Both mobility and acoustic shadowing differentiate gallstones from other echogenic foci in the gallbladder lumen, such as sludge or solid masses.
- Solid mass will not be mobile, will not shadow, and may exhibit vascularity on color Doppler examination.
- Gallstones may not be detected sonographically if they are small in size or hidden behind the gallbladder fold or cystic duct.
- Evaluating the patient in more than one position is important.

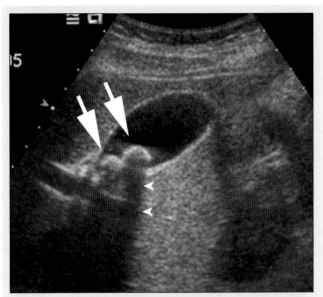

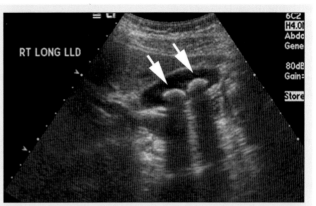

Figure 2. **Gallstones: sonography.** When the patient is imaged in the left lateral decubitus position, the gallstones *(arrows)* change location, indicating mobility.

Figure 1. **Gallstones: sonography.** Two highly reflective echoes *(arrows)* are located in the dependent portion of the gallbladder lumen with posterior acoustic shadowing *(arrowheads)*.

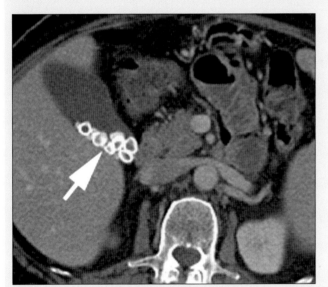

Figure 3. **CT appearance of gallstones.** Calcified stones are depicted as calcified dependent densities in gallbladder lumen *(arrow)*.

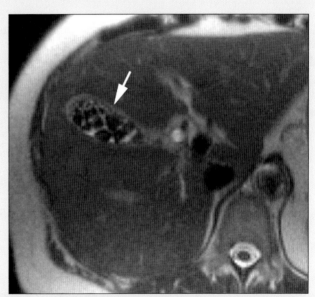

Figure 4. **MRI appearance of gallstones.** Axial T2-weighted HASTE image demonstrates multiple low signal intensity filling defects in gallbladder lumen *(arrow)*. *(HASTE,* Half-Fourier acquisition single-shot turbo-spin echo.)

- Gallbladder lumen pus
- Gallbladder lumen hemorrhage
- Gallbladder polyp

PATHOLOGY

- Gallstones are composed mainly of cholesterol, bilirubin, and calcium salts.
- Smaller amounts of protein and other materials, including bile acids, fatty acids, and inorganic salts, are also present.
- Stones form in the setting of supersaturation of various bile components.
- Black pigment stones consist of polymers of bilirubin with large amounts of mucin glycoproteins.
- Brown pigment stones are made up of calcium salts of unconjugated bilirubin with protein and cholesterol and are more commonly associated with bacterial infection.
- Lithogenic bile usually results from increased biliary cholesterol output, decreased bile acid synthesis, or a combination defect.
- Biliary dysmotility and prolonged intestinal transit may also be a factor.

INCIDENCE/PREVALENCE AND EPIDEMIOLOGY

- Gallstones are present in an estimated 10%-15% of men and 20%-40% of women over the age of 60 years.
- Risk for stones increases with a history of childbearing, estrogen replacement therapy, oral contraceptive use, and obesity.

- It is also associated with hypertriglyceridemia, Crohn disease, and parenteral hyperalimentation.
- In Western countries, cholesterol is the principal constituent of more than 75% of gallstones.
- Black pigment stones are more common in cirrhosis or chronic hemolytic anemias in which biliary excretion is increased.

Suggested Readings

Bortoff GA, Chen MYM, Ott DJ, et al: Gallbladder stones: Imaging and intervention. *RadioGraphics* 20:751-766, 2000.

Carroll BA: Gallstones: In vitro comparison of physical, radiographic and ultrasonic characteristics. *AJR Am J Roentgenol* 131:223, 1978.

Filly RA, Moss AA, Way LW: In vitro investigation of gallstone shadowing with ultrasound tomography. *J Clin Ultrasound* 7:255-262, 1979.

Grossman M: Cholelithiasis and acoustic shadowing. *J Clin Ultrasound* 6:182, 1978.

Johnston DE, Kaplan MM: Pathogenesis and treatment of gallstones. *N Engl J Med* 328:412-421, 1993.

Chronic Cholecystitis

DEFINITION: Chronic inflammation of the gallbladder.

ANATOMIC FINDINGS

Gallbladder
- Thickened and fibrotic gallbladder wall
- Gallbladder eventually becoming shrunken and distorted

IMAGING

Ultrasound
Findings
- Gallstones and a thickened gallbladder wall with contraction of the gallbladder that persists in the fasting state

Utility
- Findings are usually nonspecific.

CT
Findings
- Pericholecystic inflammatory change may be absent.

Utility
- Findings are usually nonspecific.

MRI
Findings
- Gallbladder wall thickening related to chronic inflammation demonstrates low signal intensity.

Utility
- Findings are usually nonspecific.

Nuclear Medicine Cholescintigraphy
Findings
- Delayed gallbladder visualization
- Visualization of bowel prior to gallbladder
- Noncontractility or decreased response after cholecystitis injection–decreased ejection fraction.

Utility
- Sensitivity: 45%
- Specificity: 90%

CLINICAL PRESENTATION

- Right upper quadrant pain
- Postprandial discomfort
- Weight loss

DIAGNOSTIC PEARLS

- Gallstones and thickened gallbladder wall with contraction of the gallbladder that persists in the fasting state
- Absent perihepatic contrast enhancement
- Gallbladder wall thickening related to chronic inflammation, demonstrating low signal intensity

DIFFERENTIAL DIAGNOSIS

- Biliary colic
- Hepatitis
- Choledocholithiasis
- Acute intermittent cholecystitis

PATHOLOGY

- Chronic inflammatory changes cause the gallbladder wall to become thickened and fibrotic.
- With increasing fibrosis, the gallbladder eventually becomes shrunken and distorted.
- If coexisting acute and chronic inflammatory changes are present, the term *chronic active cholecystitis* may be used.
- Chronic cholecystitis may occur after a single bout or multiple current episodes of acute cholecystitis.

INCIDENCE/PREVALENCE AND EPIDEMIOLOGY

- Chronic cholecystitis is associated with cholelithiasis in 95% of cases.

Suggested Readings

Grand D, Horton KM, Fishman E: CT of the gallbladder: Spectrum of disease. *AJR Am J Roentgenol* 183:163-170, 2004.
Pedrosa I, Rofsky NM: MR imaging in abdominal emergencies. *Magn Reson Imaging Clin North Am* 12:603-635, 2004.

WHAT THE REFERRING PHYSICIAN NEEDS TO KNOW

- Increased perihepatic contrast enhancement observed with acute cholecystitis can be helpful in differentiating acute from chronic inflammation.

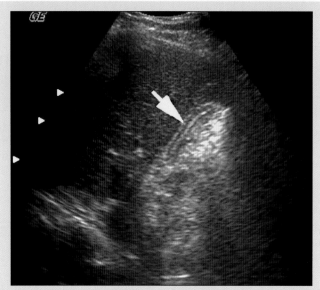

Figure 1. Chronic cholecystitis. Ultrasound demonstrates contracted gallbladder *(arrow)* in patient with repeated episodes of right upper quadrant pain. Patient was fasting at the time of the examination.

Gallbladder Hydrops

DEFINITION: Massive enlargement of the gallbladder.

ANATOMIC FINDINGS

Gallbladder
- Enlargement

IMAGING

Radiography
Findings
- Right upper quadrant mass indenting the lateral border of the duodenum

Utility
- Plain radiographs cannot establish a specific diagnosis.

Ultrasound
Findings
- Distended gallbladder (> 5 cm) with biconvex shape and normal wall thickness
- Possibly sludge and stones

Utility
- Sensitivity: 90%-100%
- Specificity: 90%-95%

CT
Findings
- Lumen distention with normal mural thickness

Utility
- Sensitivity: 90%-100%
- Specificity: 90%-95%

MRI
Findings
- Distended gallbladder lumen with high signal intensity on T1-weighted images
- Stones and sludge may be present.

Utility
- Sensitivity: 90%-100%
- Specificity: 90%-95%

CLINICAL PRESENTATION

- Patient usually has few symptoms but may have chronic right upper quadrant discomfort.
- Right upper quadrant mass may be palpable.

DIAGNOSTIC PEARLS

- Massive enlargement of the gallbladder proximal to an obstructing stone in the gallbladder neck or cystic duct.
- Right upper quadrant mass indents the lateral border of the duodenum.
- Lumen distention and normal mural thickness are seen.

DIFFERENTIAL DIAGNOSIS

- Acute cholecystitis
- Fasting
- Hyperalimentation
- Pregnancy

PATHOLOGY

- Massive enlargement of gallbladder is seen proximal to an obstructing stone in the gallbladder neck or cystic duct.
- Gallbladder lumen becomes progressively distended as a result of the accumulation of sterile mucus secreted by the epithelial cells.

Suggested Readings

Carroll BA: In vitro comparison of physical, radiographic and ultrasonic characteristics. *AJR Am J Roentgenol* 131:223, 1978.
Cooperberg P: Imaging of the gallbladder. *Radiology* 163:605, 1987.
McIntosh DM, Penney HF: Gray-scale ultrasonography as a screening procedure in the detection of gallbladder disease. *Radiology* 136:725-727, 1980.

WHAT THE REFERRING PHYSICIAN NEEDS TO KNOW
- Normal wall thickness is evident in gallbladder hydrops, as seen on ultrasound or CT.

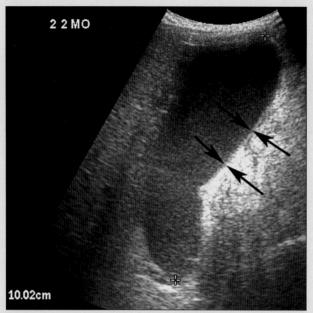

Figure 1. Gallbladder hydrops. The gallbladder is abnormally distended, measuring more than 10 cm long in this 22-month-old child after bone marrow transplantation. The gallbladder wall is thin *(arrows),* and echogenic sludge is noted within the lumen. The gallbladder was later drained with a cholecystostomy tube.

Hyperplastic Cholecystoses

DEFINITION: Noninflammatory pathologic processes resulting in benign proliferation of normal gallbladder tissue elements.

IMAGING

Radiography
Findings
- Cholesterolosis: numerous fixed filling defects in the lumen of the gallbladder
- Adenomyomatosis: radiopaque dots that parallel the gallbladder lumen; polyp-like appearance or circumferential narrowing of lumen

Utility
- Oral cholecystography is used.
- This technique is no longer widely performed.

Ultrasound
Findings
- Cholesterolosis: cholesterol polyps may appear as single or multiple nonshadowing foci adherent to the gallbladder wall and projecting into the gallbladder lumen
- Adenomyomatosis: diffuse or segmental thickening of the gallbladder wall; anechoic intramural diverticula
- Biliary sludge or gallstones within the diverticula, possibly appearing as echogenic foci
- V-shaped reverberation or comet-tail artifact possibly emanating from small cholesterol stones that are lodged in the Rokitansky-Aschoff sinus (RAS).
- Focal form of adenomyomatosis most commonly appearing as a sessile, polypoid mass in the region of the fundus protruding into the gallbladder lumen.

Utility
- Diffuse form of cholesterolosis cannot be diagnosed on imaging.
- Coexisting gallstones are a frequent finding, along with an increased incidence in the segmental form of adenomyomatosis.
- If a reverberation artifact is not observed, this focal mural thickening may be indistinguishable from gallbladder carcinoma.

DIAGNOSTIC PEARLS

- Cholesterolosis: cholesterol polyps possibly appearing as single or multiple nonshadowing foci adherent to the gallbladder wall and projecting into the gallbladder lumen
- Adenomyomatosis: diffuse or segmental thickening of the gallbladder wall and anechoic intramural diverticula
- Focal form of adenomyomatosis most commonly appearing as a sessile, polypoid mass in the region of the fundus protruding into the gallbladder lumen

CT
Findings
- Demonstration of gallbladder polyps on cholesterolosis
- Diffuse form of gallbladder adenomyomatosis exhibiting intramural diverticula
- Segmental and focal forms appearing as focal thickening of the gallbladder wall or a fundal intramural mass
- Small (< 1 cm) and multiple polypoid lesions are suggestive of benign cholesterol polyps.
- Single, sessile, and large polypoid lesions (> 10 mm), adenomas, and carcinomas should not be ruled out.
- CT is the least sensitive imaging test in the diagnosis of these disorders.

MRI
Findings
- High-signal-intensity foci in the gallbladder wall (*string-of-pearls sign*).

Utility
- MRI is a very helpful problem-solving tool in patients with gallbladder adenomyomatosis.

WHAT THE REFERRING PHYSICIAN NEEDS TO KNOW

- Polypoid lesions on ultrasound or CT should be followed up for 3-6 months and then 1-2 years to ensure stability.
- Segmental and focal forms of adenomyomatosis can be particularly difficult to differentiate from carcinoma.
- Findings of adenomyomatosis on CT may not be diagnostic, and follow-up with ultrasound may be necessary.
- If the findings of adenomyomatosis on ultrasound are equivocal, MR with MR cholangiopancreatography is the next best test.
- The incidence of gallbladder carcinoma is increased in patients with segmental adenomyomatosis; therefore these patients should be closely monitored.

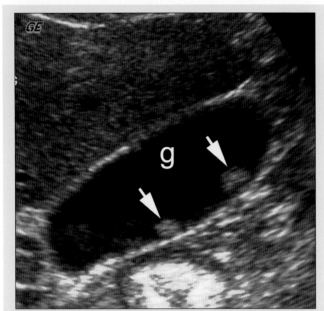

Figure 1. Cholesterol polyps: ultrasound and pathologic findings. Sagittal ultrasound image demonstrates two echogenic nonshadowing foci *(arrows)* adherent to the posterior wall of the gallbladder (g) consistent with cholesterol polyps.

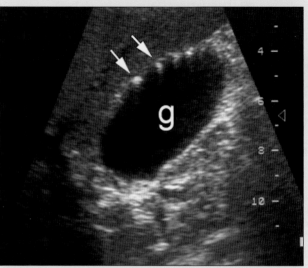

Figure 2. Adenomyomatosis: ultrasound and pathologic features. Ultrasound demonstrates multiple comet-tail artifacts *(arrows)* arising from the wall of the gallbladder (g).

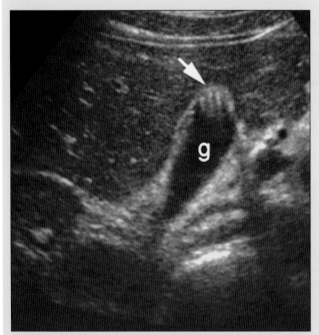

Figure 3. Focal fundal adenomyomatosis. Sagittal ultrasound image of the gallbladder (g) demonstrates focal fundal thickening *(arrow)* with multiple comet-tail artifacts.

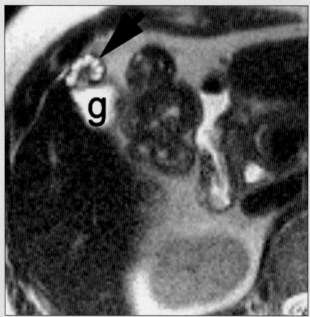

Figure 4. Focal fundal adenomyomatosis. Coronal T2-weighted HASTE MR image demonstrates multiple high signal intensity foci *(arrow)* in the region of the fundus of the gallbladder (g) corresponding to the dilated RAS. This sign has been called the *string-of-pearls sign. (HASTE,* Half-Fourier acquisition single-shot turbo-spin echo.)

- Using the half-Fourier RARE sequence was superior to helical CT and transabdominal ultrasound in detecting adenomyomatosis.
- It offers a more complete visualization of the gallbladder and more definitive identification of RAS.

CLINICAL PRESENTATION

- No specific clinical findings in cholesterolosis have been found; presentation is usually the result of complications such as cholelithiasis or cholecystitis.
- Adenomyomatosis may be asymptomatic or associated with symptoms of chronic cholecystitis.
- Many patients are asymptomatic and these disorders are often found incidentally on imaging or at autopsy.

DIFFERENTIAL DIAGNOSIS

- Gallbladder carcinoma
- Choleystitis
- Gallbladder metastases

PATHOLOGY

- In cholesterolosis, cholesterol is likely deposited initially in the epithelium and accumulates in the lamina propria and is subsequently taken up by macrophages.
- In cholesterolosis, hyperemia of the mucosa of the gallbladder results in a *strawberry gallbladder* appearance.
- Adenomyomatosis is characterized by excessive proliferation of the surface epithelium, with invaginations into the thickened, hypertrophied muscularis propria.
- Intramural diverticula are formed by epithelial invaginations into the muscularis, which are prominent features of adenomyomatosis.

- Pathogenesis related to mechanical obstruction of the gallbladder, chronic inflammation, and anomalous pancreaticobiliary ductal union.

INCIDENCE/PREVALENCE AND EPIDEMIOLOGY

- In cholesterolosis, the incidence of gallstones may be increased.
- Cholesterol polyps account for 60%-90% of gallbladder polyps and are not true neoplasms.
- Reported incidence of adenomyomatosis in cholecystectomy specimens is up to 8%.
- Over 90% of cases of adenomyomatosis are associated with gallstones, which may be responsible for the biliary symptoms.
- Adenocarcinoma of the gallbladder has been found in association with adenomyomatosis.

Suggested Readings

Berk RN, van der Vegt JH, Lichtenstein JE: The hyperplastic cholecystoses: Cholesterolosis and adenomyomatosis. *AJR Am J Roentgenol* 146:593-601, 1983.

Chattopadhyay D, Lochan R, Balupuri S, et al: Outcome of gallbladder polypoidal lesions detected by transabdominal ultrasound scanning: A nine year experience. *World J Gastroenterol* 11:2171-2173, 2005.

Gerard PS, Berman D, Zafaranloo S: CT and ultrasound of gallbladder adenomyomatosis mimicking carcinoma. *J Comput Assist Tomogr* 14:490-491, 1990.

Owen CC, Bilhartz LE: Gallbladder polyps, cholesterolosis, adenomyomatosis and acute acalculous cholecystitis. *Semin Gastrointest Dis* 14:178-188, 2003.

Yoshimitsu K, Honda H, Jimi M, et al: MR diagnosis of adenomyomatosis of the gallbladder and differentiation from gallbladder carcinoma: Importance of showing Rokitansky-Aschof sinuses. *AJR Am J Roentgenol* 172:1535-1540, 1999.

Milk of Calcium Bile

DEFINITION: Putty-like material in the gallbladder composed of calcium carbonate.

IMAGING

Radiography
Findings
- Visualized dense material

Utility
- Abdominal plain-film radiography

CT
Findings
- Hyperdense material in gallbladder lumen

Utility
- Most sensitive means of establishing the diagnosis

CLINICAL PRESENTATION

- Right upper quadrant pain
- Right upper quadrant mass

DIFFERENTIAL DIAGNOSIS

- Hemobilia
- Gallstones
- Sludge
- Parasites

PATHOLOGY

- Cystic duct obstructed by a gallstone
- Chronic gallbladder inflammation
- Putty-like material consisting of calcium carbonate in the gallbladder

DIAGNOSTIC PEARLS

- Visualized dense material on CT or radiograph

INCIDENCE/PREVALENCE AND EPIDEMIOLOGY

- Milk of calcium bile gallbladder is found in 0.32% of autopsy series.

Suggested Readings

Bortoff GA, Chen MYM, Ott DJ, et al: Gallbladder stones: Imaging and intervention. *RadioGraphics* 20:751-766, 2000.
Brakel K, Lameris JS, Nijs HG, et al: Predicting gallstone composition with CT: In vivo and in vitro analysis. *Radiology* 174:337-341, 1990.
Cooperberg P: Imaging of the gallbladder. *Radiology* 163:605, 1987.

WHAT THE REFERRING PHYSICIAN NEEDS TO KNOW
- Dense material in gallbladder can be visualized on both abdominal plain film and CT.

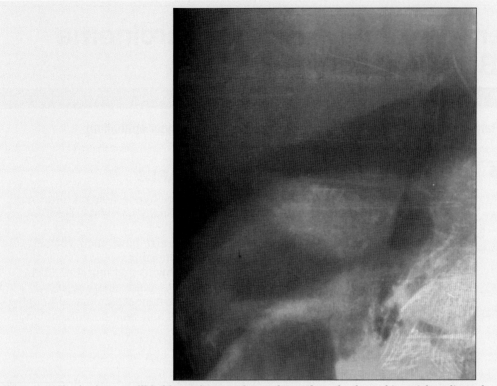

Figure 1. **Milk of calcium gallbladder.** Calcium carbonate layers dependently on this upright radiograph.

Part 42

NEOPLASMS OF THE GALLBLADDER AND BILIARY TRACT

Cystadenoma and Cystadenocarcinoma (Cystic Bile Duct Neoplasms)

DEFINITION: Rare cystic neoplasms lined by the mucin-secreting columnar epithelium.

ANATOMIC FINDINGS

Intrahepatic Bile Ducts
- Cystic mass

IMAGING

Ultrasound
Findings
- Hypoechoic intrahepatic masses
- Irregular, papillary growths and mural nodules along the internal septa and wall
- Papillary excrescences and solid portions, more commonly in cystadenocarcinoma
- Fine septal calcifications in cystadenoma
- Thick, coarse, mural and septal calcifications in cystadenocarcinoma

Utility
- Sonography is superior to CT in depicting internal morphologic features.

CT
Findings
- Irregular, papillary growths and mural nodules along the internal septa and wall
- Low-attenuation; uniloculated or multiloculated; cystic appearance

Utility
- CT is superior in demonstrating the size and extent of the tumors.
- Attenuation of the fluid component in biliary cystadenoma depends on the fluid content.

MRI
Findings
- Mostly nonenhancing mass with a thin enhancing septum.

Utility
- MRI is the best single noninvasive imaging test for evaluating these cystic neoplasms.

DIAGNOSTIC PEARLS

- Intrahepatic masses are hypoechoic on ultrasound.
- Cystadenomas occasionally have fine septal calcification.
- Cystadenocarcinomas may have thick, coarse, mural and septal calcifications.
- Irregular, papillary growths and mural nodules along the internal septa and wall are seen in cystadenoma and cystadenocarcinoma, although papillary excrescences and solid portions are more common in the latter.

CLINICAL PRESENTATION

- Abdominal pain
- Distention
- Jaundice

DIFFERENTIAL DIAGNOSIS

- Bacterial (pyogenic) hepatic abscesses
- Choledochal cysts
- Cystic metastases
- Cystic sarcoma
- Hematoma
- Hepatic cysts
- Hydatid cyst

PATHOLOGY

- Cystic neoplasms lined by a mucin-secreting columnar epithelium

INCIDENCE/PREVALENCE AND EPIDEMIOLOGY

- Rare cystic neoplasms
- Predominantly in middle-aged women

WHAT THE REFERRING PHYSICIAN NEEDS TO KNOW
- Cystadenomas can undergo malignant transformation to cystadenocarcinomas.

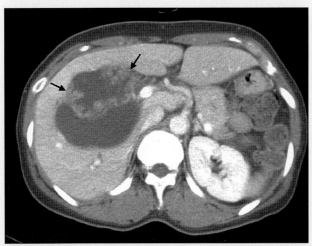

Figure 1. Biliary cystadenocarcinoma. CT scan shows a lobulated cystic mass with thick septation and enhancing mural nodules *(arrows)*.

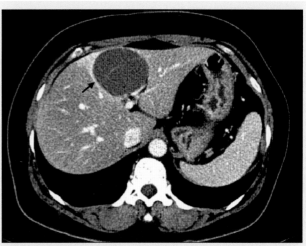

Figure 2. Biliary cystadenoma. CT scan shows a homogeneous, water-density mass *(arrow)* with thin septation in left lobe of liver.

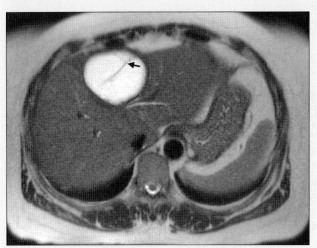

Figure 3. Biliary cystadenoma. Septations *(arrow)* in the cystadenoma are more easily seen on T2-weighted MR image than on CT scan.

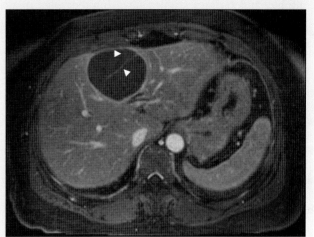

Figure 4. Biliary cystadenoma. Postcontrast T1-weighted MR image shows mostly nonenhancing mass with a thin enhancing septum *(arrowheads)* in left hepatic lobe.

Suggested Readings

American Joint Committee on Cancer, et al: Gallbladder and extrahepatic bile ducts. In Greene F, Page D, Fleming I (eds): *American Joint Committee on Cancer Staging Manual*, 6th ed. New York, Springer-Verlag, 2002, pp 139–150.

Berk RN, Ferrucci JT, Leopold GR: *Radiology of the Gallbladder and Bile Ducts*. Philadelphia, WB Saunders, 1983, p 54.

Simmons TC, Miller C, Pesigan AM, et al: Cystadenoma of the gallbladder. *Am J Gastroenterol* 84:1427-1430, 1989.

Gallbladder Carcinomas

DEFINITION: Carcinomas of the gallbladder are adenocarcinomas and anaplastic, squamous cell, or adenosquamous carcinomas that may produce an infiltrating, polypoid, or gallbladder fossa mass.

ANATOMIC FINDINGS

Gallbladder
- Fungating mass growing into the gallbladder lumen
- Diffuse gallbladder wall thickening

IMAGING

Radiography
Findings
- Calcified gallstones, porcelain gallbladder or, rarely, punctate calcifications from mucinous carcinomas
- Displacement or direct invasion of the duodenum or the anterior limb of the hepatic flexure

Utility
- Plain-film abdominal radiography, oral cholecystography, and barium studies have limited roles in the imaging of gallbladder carcinoma.
- Endoscopic retrograde cholangiopancreatography or percutaneous transhepatic cholangiography is helpful in planning the surgical procedure.

Ultrasound
Findings
- Focal or diffuse thickening of the gallbladder wall is seen.
- Marked mural thickening is seen, often with irregular and mixed echogenicity.
- Gallbladder may be contracted, normal size, or distended, and gallstones are usually present.
- Polypoid carcinomas usually have a homogeneous tissue texture and are fixed to the gallbladder wall, without an acoustic shadow.
- Polyp may be hyperechoic, hypoechoic, or isoechoic relative to the liver.
- It may be seen as a complex mass with regions of necrosis, pericholecystic fluid, stones within the mass, and invasion of the hepatic parenchyma.
- Biliary dilation is seen.

DIAGNOSTIC PEARLS

- Polypoid type shows homogeneous enhancement on CT and homogeneous texture without acoustic shadow on ultrasound.
- Pronounced wall thickening (> 1.0 cm) is demonstrated by ultrasonography, with associated mucosal irregularity or marked asymmetry.
- Large mass obscuring or replacing the gallbladder is the most common presentation of gallbladder carcinoma.
- Ill-defined early enhancement is seen on dynamic gadolinium-enhanced MRI and CT.

Utility
- Ultrasound has a diagnostic accuracy of 80%.
- It has limitations in tumor staging.
- Endoscopic ultrasound is useful in depicting the depth of tumor invasion and in characterizing polypoid lesions.

CT
Findings
- Marked mural thickening is seen, often with irregular and mixed echogenicity.
- Gallbladder may be thickened, contracted, normal size, or distended, and gallstones are usually present.
- Polypoid carcinomas are characterized by soft-tissue masses that are denser than the surrounding bile on CT scans.
- Polypoid carcinoma usually enhances homogeneously after the administration of contrast medium.
- Infiltrating carcinomas that replace the gallbladder often show irregular contrast enhancement, with scattered regions of internal necrosis.
- Other findings include invasion of the liver or hepatoduodenal ligament, satellite lesions, hepatic or nodal metastases, and bile duct dilation.

WHAT THE REFERRING PHYSICIAN NEEDS TO KNOW
- Fewer than 15% of all patients with gallbladder carcinoma are alive after 5 years.
- When the disease extends through the serosa, more radical procedures (e.g., extended cholecystectomy, pancreatoduodenectomy, major hepatic resection) can be performed.
- Survival is strongly influenced by the pathologic stage at presentation.
- Gallbladder carcinoma should be suspected in the setting of a focal mass, lymphadenopathy, hepatic metastases, and biliary obstruction at the level of the porta hepatis.
- Gallbladder carcinoma is staged surgically by the depth of the invasion, extension of the disease into adjacent structures, involvement of the lymph nodes, and the presence of metastases.

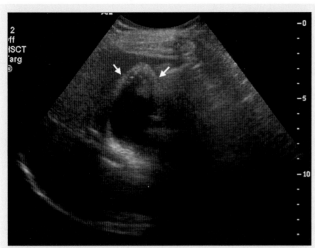

Figure 1. Gallbladder carcinoma: mural thickening. Subcostal sonogram shows a markedly thickened, inhomogeneous gallbladder wall *(arrows)*.

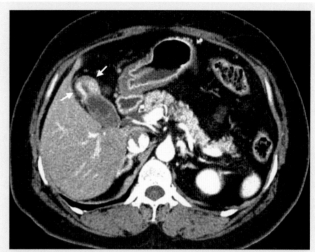

Figure 2. Gallbladder carcinoma: mural thickening. CT shows an enhancing, thick gallbladder wall *(white arrows)* with lumen narrowing.

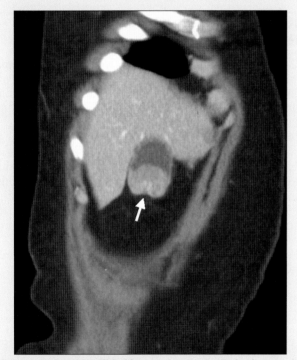

Figure 3. Polypoid gallbladder carcinoma. Sagittal reformatted image demonstrates a polypoid mass causing focal dimpling of the gallbladder wall *(arrow)*.

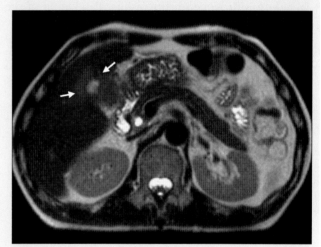

Figure 4. Gallbladder carcinoma: MRI features. T2-weighted MR image shows a thickened moderately hyperintense gallbladder wall *(arrows)*.

Utility
- CT is superior to ultrasound in assessing lymphadenopathy and the spread of the disease into the liver, porta hepatis, or adjacent structures.
- It is useful in predicting which patients will benefit from surgical therapy.
- CT is inferior to ultrasound for evaluating the gallbladder wall for mucosal irregularity, mural thickening, and cholelithiasis.

- CT is superior for evaluating the thickness of the portions of the gallbladder wall that are obscured by interposed gallstones or mural calcifications on ultrasound.
- Detection of hepatic invasion is improved by using narrow collimation and coronal or sagittal reformatting.
- Invasion of the hepatoduodenal ligament is often better demonstrated with coronal reformatted CT than with axial CT.

MRI
Findings
- Prolongation of T1 and T2 relaxation times is seen in gallbladder carcinoma.
- Lesions are heterogeneously hyperintense on T2-weighted images and hypointense on T1-weighted images compared with the liver parenchyma.
- Ill-defined early enhancement is the typical appearance of gallbladder carcinoma on dynamic gadolinium-enhanced MRI.
- Biliary dilation is seen.
Utility
- MRI is useful in assessing the cause of mural thickening and in helping to differentiate gallbladder cancer from adenomyomatosis and chronic cholecystitis.
- MR cholangiopancreatography (MRCP) provides more detailed information regarding biliary involvement of tumor than ultrasound or CT.
- MRI with MRCP offers the potential of evaluating parenchymal, vascular, biliary, and nodal involvement with a single noninvasive examination.
- Based on MRI alone, distinguishing carcinoma of the gallbladder from inflammatory and metastatic disease may be difficult.
- Invasion of the hepatoduodenal ligament is often better demonstrated with coronal reformatted CT or MRI than with axial CT.

CLINICAL PRESENTATION

- Right upper quadrant abdominal pain
- Weight loss
- Jaundice
- Abdominal mass
- Elevated serum α-fetoprotein and carcinoembryonic antigen

DIFFERENTIAL DIAGNOSIS

- Cirrhosis
- Hepatitis
- Renal failure
- Cholangiocarcinoma
- Pancreatic carcinoma
- Carcinoid tumor
- Hepatocellular carcinoma
- Hyperplastic cholecystoses
- Adenomyomatosis
- Complicated cholecystitis
- Gallbladder polyps
- Heart failure
- Hematoma
- Metastatic melanoma
- Mirizzi syndrome
- Xanthogranulomatous cholecystitis

PATHOLOGY

- Most carcinomas of the gallbladder are adenocarcinomas and can be papillary, tubular, mucinous, or signet-cell type.
- Carcinoma may produce mural thickening, a polypoid mass, or a gallbladder fossa mass.
- Invasion of the muscularis mucosae distinguishes T1 from T2 cancers.
- Gallbladder carcinoma spreads most commonly via direct invasion of the liver.
- Lymphatic metastases progress from the gallbladder fossa through the hepatoduodenal ligament to the nodal stations near the head of the pancreas.
- Approximately 60% of carcinomas originate in the fundus, 30% in the body, and 10% in the neck.

INCIDENCE/PREVALENCE AND EPIDEMIOLOGY

- Carcinoma of the gallbladder is the seventh most common malignancy of the gastrointestinal tract.
- It is two to three times more common in women than in men.
- Peak age at diagnosis is 70-75 years.
- Israelis, Native Americans, Spanish Americans in southwest United States, and Eskimos in Alaska have significantly higher risk of gallbladder carcinoma.
- Risk factors for developing gallbladder carcinoma include gallstones, porcelain gallbladder, the presence of gallbladder adenomas, anomalous pancreaticobiliary duct junction, and exposure to carcinogenic chemicals.
- Fewer than 15% of all patients with gallbladder carcinoma are alive after 5 years.

Suggested Readings

American Joint Committee on Cancer: Gallbladder and extrahepatic bile ducts. In Greene F, Page D, Fleming I, et al: *American Joint Committee on Cancer Staging Manual*, 6th ed. New York, Springer-Verlag, 2002, pp 139–150.

Berk RN, Ferrucci JT, Leopold GR: In *Radiology of the Gallbladder and Bile Ducts*. Philadelphia, WB Saunders, 1983, p 54.

Henson DE, Albores-Saavedra J, Corle D: Carcinoma of the gallbladder. Histologic types, stage of disease, grade and survival rates. *Cancer* 70:1493-1497, 1992.

Misra S, Chaturvedi A, Misra NC, Sharma ID: Carcinoma of the gallbladder. *Lancet Oncol* 4:167-176, 2003.

Wilbur AC, Sagireddy PB, Aizenstein RI: Carcinoma of the gallbladder: Color Doppler ultrasound and CT findings. *Abdom Imaging* 22:187-190, 1997.

Periampullary Carcinoma

DEFINITION: Tumors arising from or within 1 cm of the papilla of Vater.

ANATOMIC FINDINGS

Pancreatic Duct
- Dilated

Ampulla
- Mass

IMAGING

CT
Findings
- Abrupt termination of the dilated bile duct in the head of the pancreas
- Villous polypoid lesion in the distal common bile duct and duodenum
- Pancreatic duct dilation

Utility
- Masses tend to be small and may not be seen on CT.
- Sensitivity: 80%-95%
- Specificity: 90%-100%
- Accuracy: 90%

MRI
Findings
- Periampullary tumors appearing as a low signal intensity mass in the region of the ampulla on T1-weighted fat-suppressed images
- Areas of low signal intensity, reflecting a hypovascular character compared with the background pancreatic tissue on postgadolinium T1-weighted images
- On 2-minute postgadolinium fat-suppressed images, thin rim of enhancement commonly observed along the periphery of the tumor

Utility
- MR cholangiopancreatography (MRCP) and MRI can be useful in determining the origins of periampullary carcinomas.
- Superior to CT in the depiction of small masses

CLINICAL PRESENTATION

- Upper abdominal pain and weight loss
- Abnormal liver function tests and obstructive jaundice

DIAGNOSTIC PEARLS

- On T1-weighted, fat-suppressed images, periampullary tumors appear as a low-signal-intensity mass in the region of the ampulla.
- Biliary dilation to the level of the ampulla of Vater is seen in 75% of cases, and pancreatic ductal dilation is seen in 67%.
- Periampullary neoplasms tend to be polypoid and lower in grade than the more proximal biliary neoplasms.

DIFFERENTIAL DIAGNOSIS

- Lesser omental adenopathy
- Perivaterian duodenal diverticulum
- Annular pancreas

PATHOLOGY

- Periampullary carcinoma arises from or within 1 cm of the papilla of Vater and includes ampullary, pancreatic, bile duct, and duodenal cancers.
- Biliary dilation to level of the ampulla of Vater is seen in 75% of cases, and pancreatic ductal dilation is seen in 67%.

INCIDENCE/PREVALENCE AND EPIDEMIOLOGY

- Incidence is high in patients with familial adenomatous polyposis.
- Periampullary carcinomas tend to be polypoid and lower in grade.

Suggested Readings

Darweesh RMA, Thorsen MK, Dodds WJ, et al: Computed tomography examination of periampullary neoplasms. *J Comput Assist Tomogr* 12:36-41, 1988.

Heller SL, Lee VS: MR imaging of the gallbladder and biliary system. *Magn Reson Imaging Clin North Am* 13:295-311, 2005.

Pancreatic Section of the British Society of Gastroenterology: Guidelines for the management of patients with pancreatic cancer, periampullary and ampullary cancers. *Gut* 54(Suppl 5):v1-v16, 2005.

WHAT THE REFERRING PHYSICIAN NEEDS TO KNOW

- MRCP and sectional MRI can be useful in determining the origins of periampullary carcinomas.
- Incidence of tumors is high in patients with familial adenomatous polyposis, and cancer is often preceded by ampullary or duodenal adenomas.
- The patients typically have a better prognosis than most pancreatic and biliary tract neoplasms.

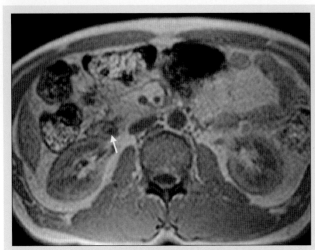

Figure 1. **Ampullary cancer.** T1-weighted MRI shows hypointense ampullary tumor *(arrow)*.

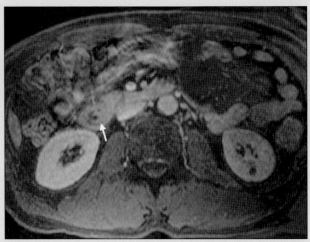

Figure 2. **Ampullary cancer.** Postgadolinium fat-suppressed MRI demonstrates a thin rim of enhancement along the periphery of the tumor.

Part 43 INFLAMMATORY DISORDERS OF THE BILIARY TRACT

Acquired Immunodeficiency Syndrome–Related Cholangitis

DEFINITION: Cholangitis caused by *Cryptosporidium* and cytomegalovirus, which is a common component of AIDS.

ANATOMIC FINDINGS

Bile Ducts
- Irregularities and strictures

Gallbladder
- Mural thickening

IMAGING

Radiography
Findings
- Irregularities and strictures of intrahepatic and extra-hepatic bile ducts with associated ductal dilation
- Papillary stenosis possibly seen as an isolated finding or associated with other findings.
- Polypoid intraluminal filling defects possibly seen as a result of granulation tissue

Utility
- Cholangiography

CT
Findings
- Gallbladder and bile duct mural thickening and abnormal mural enhancement

Utility
- MRI and MRCP are the preferred imaging tests.

Ultrasound
Findings
- Gallbladder and bile ducts show mural thickening.
- Hyperechoic nodule at the distal end of the common duct caused by inflammation and edema of the papilla of Vater

Utility
- MRI and MRCP are the preferred imaging tests.

DIAGNOSTIC PEARLS
- Cholangiograms show irregularities and strictures of the intrahepatic and extrahepatic bile ducts with associated ductal dilation.
- Papillary stenosis may be seen as an isolated finding or associated with other findings.
- Polypoid intraluminal filling defects may be seen as a result of granulation tissue.
- Mural thickening of gallbladder and bile ducts may be seen.

MRI and MR Cholangiopancreatography (MRCP)
Findings
- Ductal irregularities, strictures, and beading
- Mural thickening of the gallbladder and bile ducts
- Abnormal mural enhancement following intravenous gadolinium administration

CLINICAL PRESENTATION
- Biliary tract signs and symptoms
- Abdominal pain and diarrhea caused by cryptosporidial enteritis

DIFFERENTIAL DIAGNOSIS
- Bile duct injury and bile leak
- Bile duct strictures
- Sclerosing cholangitis
- Ascending cholangitis

WHAT THE REFERRING PHYSICIAN NEEDS TO KNOW
- AIDS-related cholangitis resembles primary sclerosing cholangitis.
- Usually related to CMV and *Cryptosporidium* infection

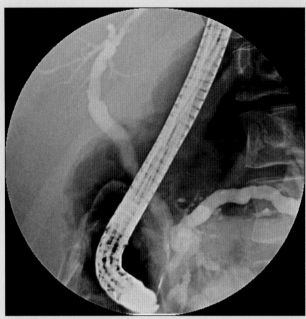

Figure 1. AIDS-related papillitis. Endoscopic retrograde cholangiopancreatography shows marked dilation of the common bile duct and pancreatic duct, a finding indicating low obstruction.

PATHOLOGY

- Inflammation of the bile ducts and gallbladder secondary to opportunistic infection by *Cryptosporidium*, cytomegalovirus, or both

INCIDENCE/PREVALENCE AND EPIDEMIOLOGY

- Common component of AIDS

Suggested Readings

Cockerill FR, Hurley DV, Malagelada JR, et al: Polymicrobial cholangitis and Kaposi's sarcoma in blood product transfusion-related acquired immune deficiency syndrome. *Am J Med* 80:1237-1241, 1986.

Collins CE, Forbes A, Harcourt-Webster JN, et al: Radiological and pathological features of AIDS-related polypoid cholangitis. *Clin Radiol* 48:307-310, 1993.

Da Silva F, Boudghene F, Lecomte I, et al: Sonography in AIDS-related cholangitis: Prevalence and cause of an echogenic nodule in the distal end of the common bile duct. *AJR Am J Roentgenol* 160:1205-1207, 1993.

Dolmatch BL, Laing FC, Federle MP, et al: AIDS-related cholangitis: Radiographic findings in nine patients. *Radiology* 163:313-316, 1987.

McCarty M, Choudhri AH, Helbert M, et al: Radiological features of AIDS-related cholangitis. *Clin Radiol* 40:582-585, 1989.

Obstructive Cholangitis

DEFINITION: Cholangitis is caused by a bacterial infection as a result of biliary stasis in the obstructed bile duct.

ANATOMIC FINDINGS

Biliary Tree
- Obstruction (choledocholith, surgical anastomotic stricture, papillary stenosis, or neoplasm)
- Ductal strictures in recurrent cases
- Purulent material

Liver
- Abscess
- Cirrhosis in recurrent cases

IMAGING

Ultrasound
Findings
- Obstruction
- Purulent bile identified as intraluminal echogenic material within the involved ducts
- Hepatic abscesses

CT
Findings
- Obstruction
- Purulent bile appearing as high-density intraductal material
- Hepatic abscesses

Interventional Radiology
Findings
- Obstruction
- Irregular tubular filling defects in the dilated ducts above the obstruction
- Hepatic abscesses in communication with the biliary tract

Utility
- Cholangiography is used.
- Injection of contrast medium under pressure above the obstruction may exacerbate the existing infection and can introduce infection into the sterile biliary tract.

DIAGNOSTIC PEARLS
- Obstruction
- Purulent bile identified as an intraluminal echogenic material within the involved ducts on ultrasound
- Irregular tubular filling defects in the dilated ducts above the obstruction

CLINICAL PRESENTATION
- Right upper quadrant abdominal pain, chills, fever, and jaundice

DIFFERENTIAL DIAGNOSIS
- Primary sclerosing cholangitis
- Recurrent pyogenic cholangitis (oriental cholangiohepatitis)
- Acquired immune deficiency syndrome–related cholangitis
- Bile duct injury and bile leak
- Bile duct strictures

PATHOLOGY
- Biliary obstruction (choledocholithiasis, surgical anastomotic stricture, papillary stenosis, or neoplasm) induces bile stasis and predisposes the patient to bacterial infection.
- *Escherichia coli* is the most common infecting organism, but most infections are polymicrobial.

INCIDENCE/PREVALENCE AND EPIDEMIOLOGY
- Obstructive cholangitis is associated with a congenital cystic disease, including Caroli disease.
- Obstructive cholangitis is the most common cause.

WHAT THE REFERRING PHYSICIAN NEEDS TO KNOW
- Nature and level of the obstruction must be ascertained.
- Injection of contrast medium under pressure above the obstruction may exacerbate existing infection or introduce an infection into the previously sterile biliary tree.
- Prompt biliary drainage and broad-spectrum antibiotic coverage are mandatory.

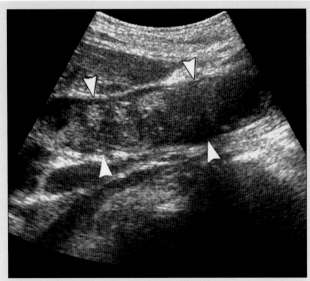

Figure 1. Ascending obstructive cholangitis. Sagittal sonogram shows a markedly dilated common bile duct *(arrowheads)* filled with sludge and stones. (*From Hanbidge AE, Buckler PM, O'Malley ME, et al: Imaging evaluation for acute pain in the upper abdomen. RadioGraphics 24:1117-1135, 2004.*)

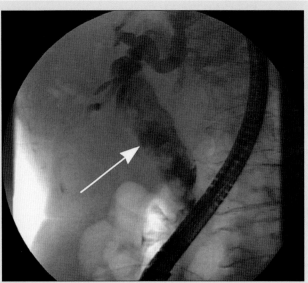

Figure 2. Ascending obstructive cholangitis. Endoscopic retrograde cholangiopancreatography shows a dilated intrahepatic and extrahepatic biliary system with multiple filling defects *(arrow)*. The patient recovered after urgent papillotomy and the administration of antibiotics and intravenous fluids. (*From Hanbidge AE, Buckler PM, O'Malley ME, et al: Imaging evaluation for acute pain in the upper abdomen. RadioGraphics 24:1117-1135, 2004.*)

Suggested Readings

Bass NM: Sclerosing cholangitis and recurrent pyogenic cholangitis. In Feldman M, Scharschmidt BF, Sleisenger MH (eds): *Sleisenger and Fordtran's Gastrointestinal and Liver Disease*, 6th ed. Philadelphia, WB Saunders, 1998, pp 1275-1283.

Carpenter HA: Bacterial and parasitic cholangitis. *Mayo Clin Proc* 73:473-478, 1998.

Dodd GD 3rd, Niedzwiecki GA, Campbell WL, Baron RL: Bile duct calculi in patients with primary sclerosing cholangitis. *Radiology* 203:443-447, 1997.

Pokorny CS, McCaughan GW, Gallagher ND, et al: Sclerosing cholangitis and biliary tract calculi: Primary or secondary. *Gut* 33:1376-1380, 1992.

Biliary Tract: Parasitic Infestations

DEFINITION: Infestation of the biliary tract by parasites, including *Ascaris, Clonorchis,* and *Echinococcus* species.

ANATOMIC FINDINGS

Bile Ducts
- *Ascaris:* longitudinal filling defects
- Liver flukes: filling defects within dilated intrahepatic bile ducts; extrahepatic duct sparing
- Echinococcosis: biliary tree compression, obstruction, and inflammation

IMAGING

Interventional Radiology
Findings
- *Ascaris:* longitudinal filling defects up to several inches in length on direct or intravenous cholangiograms
- Clonorchiasis: appearing as ellipsoid, leaf-like filling defects measuring 2-10 mm in length on cholangiograms
Utility
- Endoscopic retrograde cholangiopancreatography (ERCP) can be used to make the diagnosis and perform a sphincterotomy to assist parasite removal.

Ultrasound
Findings
- *Ascaris:* thin, long, or coiled echogenic intraluminal structures; *bull's-eye* appearance; central anechoic component representing the worm's digestive tract
- Liver flukes: small intrahepatic duct dilation, wall and periductal tissue thickening, fluke and fluke aggregates within the duct
Utility
- Real-time ultrasound confirms the diagnosis by demonstrating the *Ascaris* worm's motility.
- Ultrasound more easily identifies the fluke and fluke aggregates than CT.

CT
Findings
- Liver flukes: branching, low-density structures representing small intrahepatic duct dilation and periductal fibrosis on unenhanced scan
- With contrast enhancement periductal tissue component increasing in density and blending in with surrounding parenchyma

DIAGNOSTIC PEARLS
- *Ascaris:* longitudinal filling defects up to several inches in length on direct cholangiograms
- Clonorchiasis: appearing as ellipsoid, leaf-like filling defects measuring 2-10 mm in length on cholangiograms
- Liver flukes: small intrahepatic duct dilation, wall and periductal tissue thickening, and fluke and fluke aggregates within duct
- Stippled or powder-like areas of high attenuation in *Clonorchis*-associated cholangiocarcinoma

CLINICAL PRESENTATION
- Ascariasis: intestinal obstruction, acute appendicitis and pancreatitis, and biliary colic
- Clonorchiasis: anorexia, dyspepsia, abdominal fullness, and right upper quadrant discomfort in moderate infection; palpitations, weight loss, and diarrhea in severe disease

PATHOLOGY
- Ascariasis is acquired by the ingestion of ova; the larvae migrate through the liver and lungs, causing scarring, granuloma, or abscess formation.
- Clonorchiasis is acquired by the ingestion of infested raw fish, later causing periductal fibrosis, ductal epithelial hyperplasia, and cholangiocarcinoma.
- *Fasciola hepatica, Opisthorchis felineus,* and *Opisthorchis viverrini* infections share many features with *Camellia sinensis* infection, except the association with cholangiocarcinoma.
- *Echinococcus granulosus* and *Echinococcus multilocularis* are small tapeworms, the larvae of which may lodge in human livers.

WHAT THE REFERRING PHYSICIAN NEEDS TO KNOW
- Complications of clonorchiasis include intraductal calculus formation, suppurative cholangitis, cholangiohepatitis, and liver abscess.
- *Clonorchis*-associated carcinomas tend to occur peripherally where flukes are most concentrated; therefore jaundice is often absent.
- Ascariasis cholangitis is a life-threatening complication that may ensue and includes inflammation and thrombosis (pyelophlebitis) in the portal and hepatic veins and liver abscesses.

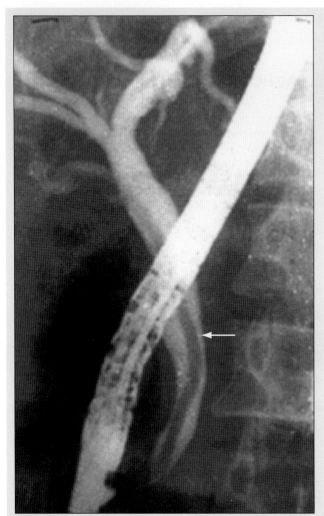

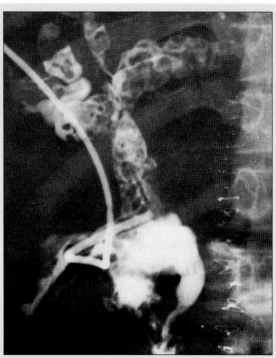

Figure 2. Clonorchiasis. T-tube cholangiogram shows innumerable 1- to 2-cm filling defects within the dilated bile ducts. The flukes can be identified by their typical comma-shaped or crescentic outlines; other filling defects may represent associated stones and biliary sludge. Short strictures and gross dilations of the ducts are present as a result of chronic obstruction and cholangitis. (*Courtesy of Joan Kendall, MD.*)

Figure 1. Ascariasis. Endoscopic retrograde cholangiopancreatography shows a linear filling defect (*arrow*) in the common bile duct, which is the *Ascaris* worm.

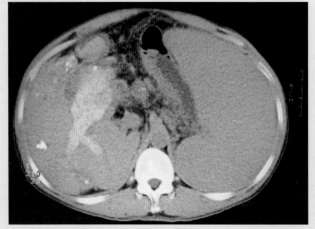

Figure 3. Clonorchiasis. Nonenhanced CT scan in the same patient as in Figure 2 shows hyperdense material within grossly distended major intrahepatic bile ducts, which on pathologic examination was proven to be a combination of pigmented biliary stones and sludge and *Clonorchis* flukes. Several calcified stones can be seen in peripheral ducts. The spleen is enlarged. (*Courtesy of Joan Kendall, MD.*)

INCIDENCE/PREVALENCE AND EPIDEMIOLOGY

- *Ascaris lumbricoides* is the most prevalent human helminth worldwide; it is more frequent and severe in children.
- Clonorchiasis is endemic in Asia but may be seen in Western countries as a result of travel and immigration.
- Clonorchiasis is associated with the development of cholangiocarcinoma.

Suggested Readings

Cerri GG, Leite GJ, Simoes JB, et al: Ultrasonic evaluation of *Ascaris* in the biliary tract. *Radiology* 146:753-754, 1983.

Choi BI, Kim HJ, Han MC, et al: CT findings of clonorchiasis. *AJR Am J Roentgenol* 152:281-284, 1989.

Choi BI, Park JH, Kim YI, et al: Peripheral cholangiocarcinoma and clonorchiasis: CT findings. *Radiology* 169:149-153, 1988.

Larrubia JR, Ladero JM, Mendoza JL, et al: The role of sonography in the early diagnosis of biliopancreatic *Ascaris* infestation. *J Clin Gastroenterol* 22:48-50, 1996.

Lim JH: Radiologic findings of clonorchiasis. *AJR Am J Roentgenol* 155:1001-1008, 1990.

Ooms HWA, Puylaert JBCM, van der Werf SDJ: Biliary fascioliasis: US and endoscopic retrograde cholangiopancreatography findings. *Eur Radiol* 2:1-4, 1994.

Primary Biliary Cirrhosis

DEFINITION: Chronic cholestatic syndrome of unknown cause characterized by the destruction of small bile ducts.

ANATOMIC FINDINGS

Intrahepatic Bile Ducts
- Tortuous and attenuated

Liver
- Hepatomegaly initially, then cirrhosis later as primary biliary cirrhosis (PBC) progresses

IMAGING

Radiography
Findings
- Intrahepatic bile ducts become tortuous and attenuated in response to the surrounding cirrhosis.
- In areas of parenchymal atrophy, the ducts become crowded and tortuous.
- In areas of compensatory hypertrophy or nodular regeneration, the ducts become splayed or displaced.
- Extrinsic compression of common bile duct caused by lymphadenopathy is seen within the porta hepatis.
- Bile duct deformities are less severe and are confined to the intrahepatic bile ducts, in contrast to primary sclerosing cholangitis (PSC).
Utility
- Cholangiograms are normal during the early stages of the disease.
- Cholangiography can be helpful in differentiating PSC from primary biliary cirrhosis.

CT
Findings
- Hepatomegaly is seen.
- Later, liver volume decreases with atrophy of the right hepatic lobe and relative hypertrophy of the caudate and left hepatic lobes.
- Lace-like pattern of thin or thick bands of low attenuation surround the regenerating nodules.
- Regenerating nodules are seen as small, rounded, hyperdense foci on unenhanced scans.
- Lymphadenopathy is seen within the porta hepatis and portacaval locations.
Utility
- CT is less sensitive than MRI and MR cholangiopancreatography (MRCP) in establishing the diagnosis.

DIAGNOSTIC PEARLS
- Intrahepatic bile ducts become tortuous and attenuated in response to the surrounding cirrhosis.
- Bile duct deformities are less severe and confined to the intrahepatic bile ducts, in contrast to PSC.
- Hepatomegaly is seen, later progressing to cirrhosis.

Ultrasound
Findings
- Hepatomegaly is seen.
- Later, liver volume decreases with atrophy of the right hepatic lobe and relative hypertrophy of the caudate and left hepatic lobes.
- Lace-like pattern of thin or thick bands surrounds the regenerating nodules.
- Sonographic findings are typically nonspecific in these patients.

MRI
Findings
- Hepatomegaly is seen.
- Later, liver volume decreases with atrophy of the right hepatic lobe and relative hypertrophy of the caudate and left hepatic lobes.
- Lace-like pattern of thin or thick bands surrounds the regenerating nodules.
- Lymphadenopathy is seen within the porta hepatis and portacaval locations.
- *Periportal halo sign* denotes a small (5-mm to 1-cm) rounded lesion of decreased T1 and T2 signal intensity surrounding the portal venous branch.
Utility
- MRI and MRCP are the most accurate means of noninvasively establishing the diagnosis.

CLINICAL PRESENTATION
- Insidious onset of diffuse pruritus is seen followed by cutaneous jaundice in 6 months to 2 years.
- In the later stages of the disease, osteomalacia, liver failure, and portal hypertension are seen.

WHAT THE REFERRING PHYSICIAN NEEDS TO KNOW
- Diagnosis is usually based on clinical features and laboratory evaluation.
- Cross-sectional imaging is used to stage the liver disease by demonstrating portal hypertension and cirrhosis.
- Imaging is useful to detect the development of hepatic malignancies.

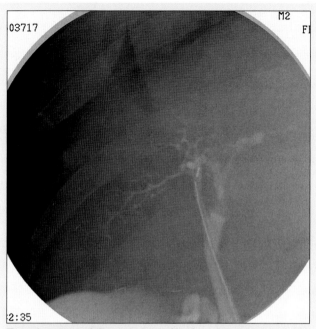

Figure 1. Primary biliary cirrhosis (PBC): endoscopic retrograde cholangiopancreatographic findings. The intrahepatic bile ducts are small and attenuated, giving the *pruned-tree* appearance. The extrahepatic ducts are normal. In PSC, the intrahepatic and extrahepatic ductal systems are usually involved together.

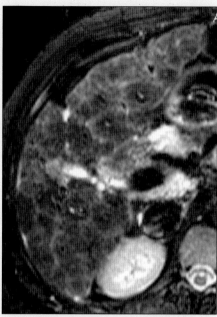

Figure 2. PBC: MRI features. Patients with PBC have a distinctive, conspicuous, low-signal-intensity abnormality centered around portal venous branches on T1- and T2-weighted MR images, the *periportal halo sign*. This abnormality consists of a rounded lesion centered on a portal venous branch, 5 mm to 1 cm in size. These lesions are numerous and involve all hepatic segments with low signal intensity on T1- and T2-weighted images and no mass effect. These criteria allow differentiation of this finding from regenerating nodules, which are usually of various sizes and signal intensities, may exert mass effect, and are not centered on portal venous branches. (*Case courtesy of Glenn Krinsky, MD.*)

- Serum alkaline phosphatase levels are elevated, and serum bilirubin values fluctuate and are seldom significantly elevated at presentation.
- Mean survival in symptomatic patients is 5.5-6.0 years, with range of 3-11 years.

DIFFERENTIAL DIAGNOSIS

- Primary sclerosing cholangitis
- Alcohol-related cirrhosis
- Viral-related cirrhosis

PATHOLOGY

- Cell-based immunity is altered.
- Antimitochondrial antibodies are frequently present in high titers.
- Sensitized T lymphocytes—and possibly B lymphocytes—may mediate duct injury.
- Small-duct destruction is accompanied by inflammatory cellular infiltrate (lymphocytes, plasma cells, histiocytes, and eosinophils) and granuloma formation.

INCIDENCE/PREVALENCE AND EPIDEMIOLOGY

- Ninety percent of patients with PBC are women.
- PSC is associated with autoimmune and collagen vascular diseases.

Suggested Readings

Blachar A, Federle MP, Brancatelli G: Primary biliary cirrhosis: Clinical, pathologic, and helical CT findings in 53 patients. *Radiology* 220:329-336, 2001.

Nakanuma Y: Distribution of B lymphocytes in nonsuppurative cholangitis in primary biliary cirrhosis. *Hepatology* 18:570-575, 1993.

Poupon R, Poupon RE: Primary biliary cirrhosis. In Zakim D, Boyer TD (eds): *Hepatology: A Textbook of Liver Disease*, 3rd ed. Philadelphia, WB Saunders, 1996, pp 1329–1365.

Summerfield JA, Elias E, Hungerford GD, et al: The biliary system in primary biliary cirrhosis: A study by endoscopic retrograde cholangiopancreatography. *Gastroenterology* 70:240-243, 1976.

Wenzel JS, Donohoe A, Ford KL, et al: Primary biliary cirrhosis: MR imaging findings and description of MR imaging periportal halo sign. *AJR Am J Roentgenol* 176:885-889, 2001.

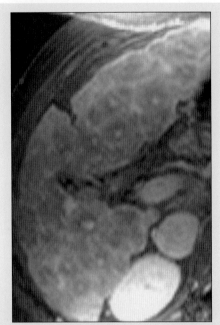

Figure 3. PBC: MRI features. Patients with PBC have a distinctive, conspicuous, low-signal-intensity abnormality centered around portal venous branches on T1- and T2-weighted MR images, the *periportal halo sign*. This abnormality consists of a rounded lesion centered on a portal venous branch, 5 mm to 1 cm in size. These lesions are numerous and involve all hepatic segments with low signal intensity on T1- and T2-weighted images and no mass effect. These criteria allow differentiation of this finding from regenerating nodules, which are usually of various sizes and signal intensities, may exert mass effect, and are not centered on portal venous branches. (*Case courtesy of Glenn Krinsky, MD.*)

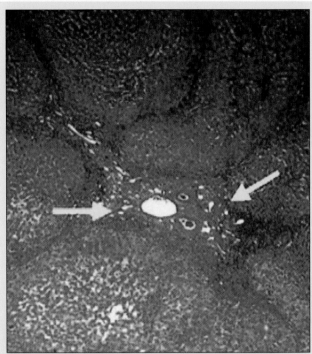

Figure 4. PBC: pathologic findings. Photomicrograph of liver tissue from a 41-year-old woman with primary biliary cirrhosis with a positive MR periportal halo sign. Stellate areas of hepatocellular parenchymal extinction *(arrows)* around the portal triads can be seen. Larger and more variably sized regenerating nodules encircle the fibrotic portal triads. (*From Wenzel JS, Donohue A, Ford KL, et al: Primary biliary cirrhosis: MR imaging findings and description of MR imaging periportal halo sign. AJR Am J Roentgenol 176: 885-889, 2001. Reprinted with permission from the American Journal of Roentgenology.*)

Primary Sclerosing Cholangitis

DEFINITION: Chronic cholestatic liver disease of unknown cause.

ANATOMIC FINDINGS

Bile Duct
- Segmental strictures
- Diverticular duct outpouchings
- Mural thickening and irregularities
- Intrahepatic and extrahepatic biliary calculi

IMAGING

Interventional Radiology
Findings
- Multiple segmental strictures involving both the intrahepatic and extrahepatic bile ducts
- Normal or less-involved duct segments that alternate with segmental strictures, producing the classic beaded appearance
- *Pruned tree* appearance when the peripheral ducts are obliterated
- Diverticular outpouchings
- Mural irregularity from a fine, brush-border appearance to a coarse, shaggy, or frankly nodular appearance
- Combined findings of short strictures, beading, pruning, diverticula, and mural irregularities are nearly pathognomonic for primary sclerosing cholangitis (PSC).
- Cholangiography is either by endoscopic retrograde cholangiopancreatography (ERCP) or percutaneous transhepatic cholangiography.
Utility
- Sensitivity: 80%-95%
- Specificity: 80%-100%
- Accuracy: 89%

Ultrasound
Findings
- Duct dilation and wall thickening of the common bile duct or the intrahepatic ducts in a smooth or irregular manner
- Thickened bile ducts that appear as two parallel echogenic lines with a central hypoechoic stripe
- Intrahepatic bile duct thickening is a subtle finding and not always readily apparent.
Utility
- Ultrasound is inexpensive and can effectively evaluate the biliary system.

DIAGNOSTIC PEARLS
- Combined findings of short strictures, beading, pruning, diverticula, and mural irregularities are nearly pathognomonic for PSC.
- Calculi
- Upper abdominal lymphadenopathy
- Macronodular cirrhosis

- Commonly, ultrasound is the initial imaging modality used in the evaluation of cholestatic liver disease.
- Sensitivity: 60%-85%
- Specificity: 75%-90%
- Accuracy: 83%

CT
Findings
- Segmental intrahepatic biliary duct dilation with focal constrictions
- Intrahepatic bile duct calculi appearing as foci of faint high attenuation or as coarse calcifications
- Upper abdominal lymphadenopathy
- Liver that is markedly deformed with severe contour lobulations, creating a rounded-appearing organ
Utility
- CT cholangiography allows for cross-sectional imaging of the biliary tract in patients with contraindications to MRI.
- Sensitivity: 75%-90%
- Specificity: 80%-90%
- Accuracy: 85%

MRI
Findings
- Multifocal segmental strictures alternating with normal or slightly dilated bile duct segments
- Obliterated peripheral bile ducts, resulting in the *pruned tree* appearance, with progressive fibrosis
- Extrahepatic bile duct wall thickening (1.5 mm or greater) and enhancement
- Increased signal intensity in a peripheral wedge-shaped or fine reticular pattern on T2-weighted images
- Macronodular cirrhosis with nodules greater than 3 cm within the central liver portion and isointense on T1- and hypointense on T2-weighted images.

WHAT THE REFERRING PHYSICIAN NEEDS TO KNOW
- Cross-sectional imaging allows for the detection of complications such as cirrhosis and malignancy.
- No known therapy, short of liver transplantation, has been proved effective.
- Biopsy specimens of the extrahepatic ducts should not be obtained unless cholangiocarcinoma must be ruled out.

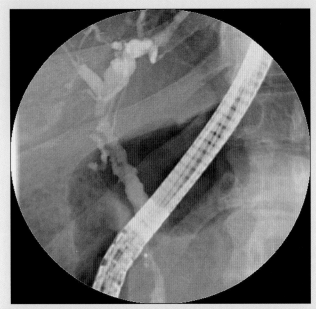

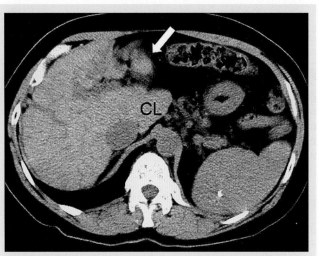

Figure 2. PSC: CT findings. Noncontrast scans demonstrate a nodular liver with marked atrophy of the lateral segment of the left lobe *(arrow)* and enlargement of the caudate lobe (CL).

Figure 1. PSC: ERCP findings. Multifocal, irregular strictures and dilations involving the intra- and extrahepatic bile ducts with a predilection for bifurcations are seen. The strictures are usually short and annular, alternating with normal or slightly dilated segments, producing a beaded appearance. Coarse nodular mural irregularities are often seen, as well as small eccentric outpouchings and webs.

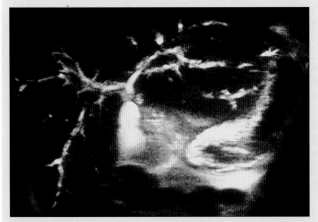

Figure 3. PSC: MRI findings. MR cholangiogram shows characteristic irregular strictures and segmental dilatations involving intrahepatic and extrahepatic ducts.

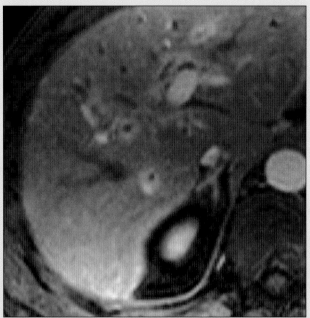

Figure 4. PSC: MRI findings. Abnormal periductal enhancement is identified on this axial image.

- Inflammatory changes of the hilar bile ducts, resulting in a high T2 signal along the porta hepatis
- Other findings: mural irregularities, webs, diverticula, and stones

Utility

- MR cholangiopancreatography is noninvasive and does not require the use of iodinated contrast material or ionizing radiation.
- It correlates with ERCP findings.
- Sensitivity: 80%-90%
- Specificity: 80%-95%
- Accuracy: 87%

CLINICAL PRESENTATION

- Twenty-five percent of patients with PSC are asymptomatic at presentation.
- Patients exhibit fatigue, pruritus, jaundice, right upper quadrant pain, and hepatosplenomegaly when symptomatic.
- Serum alkaline phosphatase level is elevated.
- There are no specific serologic markers of this disorder.

DIFFERENTIAL DIAGNOSIS

- Cholangiocarcinoma
- Primary biliary cirrhosis
- Bile duct injury and bile leak
- Bile duct strictures
- Obstructive cholangitis
- Ascending cholangitis
- AIDS-related cholangitis

PATHOLOGY

- PSC is characterized by fibrosing inflammation of the biliary tract.
- Four histologic stages are portal hepatitis or cholangitis, periportal hepatitis or fibrosis, septal fibrosis or bridging necrosis (or both), and cirrhosis.

INCIDENCE/PREVALENCE AND EPIDEMIOLOGY

- Median age of onset is 40 years; 70% of patients are men.
- PSC is commonly associated with inflammatory bowel disease, ulcerative colitis, and Crohn disease.
- Other associated conditions include sicca complex, Riedel struma, retroperitoneal fibrosis, and mediastinal fibrosis.

Suggested Readings

Bader TR, Beavers KL, Semelka RC: MR imaging features of primary sclerosing cholangitis: Patterns of cirrhosis in relationship to clinical severity of disease. *Radiology* 226:675-685, 2003.

Caoili EM, Paulson EK, Heyneman LE, et al: Helical CT cholangiography with three-dimensional volume rendering using an oral biliary contrast agent: Feasibility of a novel technique. *AJR Am J Roentgenol* 174:487-492, 2000.

Dodd GD, Baron RL, Oliver JH, et al: End-stage primary sclerosing cholangitis: CT findings of hepatic morphology in 36 patients. *Radiology* 211:357-362, 1999.

Ernst O, Asselah T, Sergent G, et al: MR cholangiography in primary sclerosing cholangitis. *AJR Am J Roentgenol* 171:1027-1030, 1998.

Ito K, Mitchell DG, Outwater EK, et al: Primary sclerosing cholangitis: MR imaging features. *AJR Am J Roentgenol* 172:1527-1533, 1999.

Recurrent Pyogenic Cholangitis (Oriental Cholangiohepatitis)

DEFINITION: Pigmented stone formation in the intrahepatic and extrahepatic bile ducts that is commonly accompanied by recurrent gram-negative bacterial infections.

ANATOMIC FINDINGS

Biliary Ducts
- Dilated ducts containing stones and sludge are seen.
- Ductal stones are primarily extrahepatic, are predominantly composed of cholesterol, and most often originate in the gallbladder.
- All segments of biliary tree may be involved, but the lateral segment of the left lobe is most often and extensively involved.

Liver
- Atrophy, fatty metamorphosis, duct wall enhancement, segmental parenchymal enhancement, hepatic abscess, biloma, and pneumobilia

IMAGING

MRI and MR Cholangiopancreatography (MRCP)
Findings
- Dilated ducts containing stone and sludge
- Parenchymal atrophy, hepatic steatosis, hepatic abscess, and bile duct wall enhancement

Utility
- Superior to CT and ultrasound in showing the ductal system

CT
Findings
- Dilated ducts containing stones and sludge
- Parenchymal atrophy, fatty metamorphosis, duct wall enhancement, segmental parenchymal enhancement, hepatic abscess, biloma, and pneumobilia
- Large amounts of nonshadowing and isodense material may mask duct dilation.

Utility
- Superior to MRI and ultrasound in demonstrating stone calcification

Ultrasound
Findings
- Dilated ducts containing stones and sludge
- Parenchymal atrophy, fatty metamorphosis, duct wall enhancement, segmental parenchymal enhancement, hepatic abscess, biloma, and pneumobilia
- Large amounts of nonshadowing and isodense material may mask duct dilation.

DIAGNOSTIC PEARLS
- Dilated ducts containing stones and sludge
- Parenchymal atrophy, fatty metamorphosis, duct wall enhancement, segmental parenchymal enhancement, hepatic abscess, biloma, and pneumobilia
- Strictures suggested by the presence of abruptly tapered ducts

Utility
- Inferior to CT and MRI in the depiction of entire extent of disease

Interventional Radiology
Findings
- Strictures suggested by the presence of abruptly tapered ducts

Utility
- Interventional radiology provides the best detail on duct status.
- It is a necessary component of the radiologic interventional management of stones and strictures.

CLINICAL PRESENTATION
- Patient exhibits right upper quadrant pain, chills, fever, and jaundice.
- Natural history is characterized by exacerbations and remissions of cholangitis, with duct injury and cholestasis, leading to biliary cirrhosis.

DIFFERENTIAL DIAGNOSIS
- Obstructive cholangitis
- Sclerosing cholangitis
- Ascending cholangitis

PATHOLOGY
- Pigmented stone formation in intrahepatic and extrahepatic bile ducts that are commonly accompanied by recurrent gram-negative bacterial infections

---

WHAT THE REFERRING PHYSICIAN NEEDS TO KNOW
- Patients are at risk for developing liver abscesses and cirrhosis.

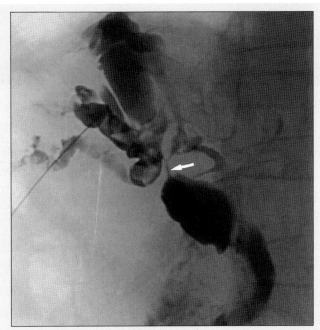

Figure 1. Oriental cholangiohepatitis. Percutaneous transhepatic cholangiography shows severe stricture *(arrow)*, with dilated ducts, multiple filling defects, and abrupt tapering in the right anterior segment. (*From Mi-Suk Park M-S, Yu J-S, Kim KW, et al: Recurrent pyogenic cholangitis: Comparison between MR cholangiography and direct cholangiography.* Radiology *220:677-681, 2001.*)

INCIDENCE/PREVALENCE AND EPIDEMIOLOGY

- Common in certain Asian populations
- Sporadic occurrence in non-Asians

Suggested Readings

Chan FL, Man SW, Leong LLY, et al: Evaluation of recurrent pyogenic cholangitis with CT: Analysis of 50 patients. *Radiology* 170:165-169, 1989.

Kerlan RK Jr, Pogany AC, Goldberg HI, et al: Radiologic intervention in Oriental cholangiohepatitis. *AJR Am J Roentgenol* 145:809-813, 1985.

Kusano S, Okada Y, Endo T, et al: Oriental cholangiohepatitis: Correlation between portal vein occlusion and hepatic atrophy. *AJR Am J Roentgenol* 158:1011-1014, 1992.

Lim JH, Ko YT, Lee DH, et al: Oriental cholangiohepatitis: Sonographic findings in 48 cases. *AJR Am J Roentgenol* 155:511-514, 1990.

Part 44

POSTSURGICAL AND TRAUMATIC LESIONS OF THE BILIARY TRACT

Bile Duct Injury and Bile Leak

DEFINITION: Surgical injury to the bile duct and postoperative bile leak.

IMAGING

CT
Findings
- Free bile in the peritoneal cavity, resulting in sterile or infected biliary ascites
- Loculated fluid collection that may be a sterile biloma or an infected subhepatic or a subdiaphragmatic abscess

Utility
- CT may be used as an initial imaging study in suspected bile leak or biliary sepsis in the early postoperative period.
- It is useful in detecting intra-abdominal fluid collections.
- CT cannot differentiate among lymphocele, hematoma, seroma, and biloma.
- It cannot accurately define the source of the leak.

Ultrasound
Findings
- Intra-abdominal fluid collections

Utility
- Ultrasound may be used as initial imaging test with suspected bile leak or biliary sepsis in the early postoperative period.
- It is useful in detecting intra-abdominal fluid collections.
- It cannot differentiate among lymphocele, hematoma, seroma, and biloma.
- CT is unreliable in detecting bile leaks.
- It cannot accurately define the source of the leak.

Interventional Radiology
Findings
- Bile leaks freely into the peritoneal cavity.

Utility
- Interventional radiology is used to differentiate cystic duct versus common bile duct leak.
- Cholangiography is excellent for the diagnosis and management of biliary complications of laparoscopic cholecystectomy.

DIAGNOSTIC PEARLS

- Bile leaks freely into the peritoneal cavity, demonstrated by cholangiogram, scintigram, or MRCP.
- Free bile may leak into the peritoneal cavity, resulting in sterile or infected biliary ascites.
- Loculated fluid collection may occur, which may be sterile biloma or infected subhepatic or subdiaphragmatic abscess.

Nuclear Medicine
Findings
- Bile leakage with isotope identified outside the biliary and the gastrointestinal tract

Utility
- Nuclear medicine is a good method for diagnosing bile leaks, with an accuracy rate of approximately 85%.
- Anatomic site of the leak and the level of injury cannot be determined.

MRI
Findings
- Intraperitoneal bile has high signal intensity on T2-weighted images and low signal intensity on TI-weighted images.

Utility
- MR cholangiopancreatography (MRCP) is a noninvasive technique that can accurately diagnose postoperative bile duct injuries.

CLINICAL PRESENTATION

- Injury to the bile duct occurs within days to weeks after surgery.
- Obstructive jaundice, progressive elevation of liver function tests, or leakage of bile from the drain may be seen.
- Upper abdominal pain or mass
- Peritonitis
- Sepsis

WHAT THE REFERRING PHYSICIAN NEEDS TO KNOW
- Site of injury or leakage should be assessed as to whether the cystic duct or common bile duct leak is occurring.

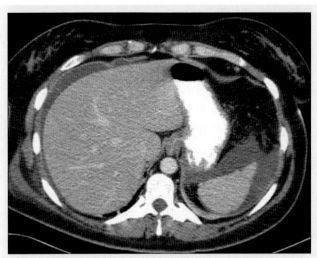

Figure 1. Bile leak inducing bile peritonitis. Ten days after laparoscopic cholecystectomy, CT scan shows free fluid, compatible with bile, surrounding the liver and spleen.

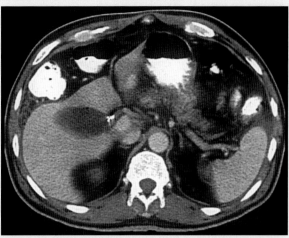

Figure 2. Bile leak resulting in a biloma and biliary ascites. CT several days after laparoscopic cholecystectomy shows a biloma in the gallbladder fossa adjacent to the surgical clips. Free fluid surrounds the spleen.

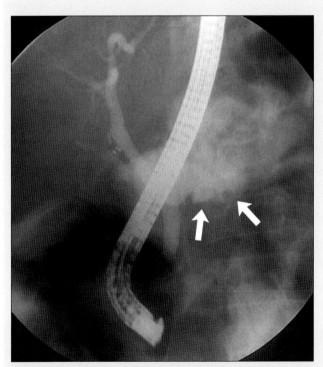

Figure 3. Postoperative bile leak. Endoscopic retrograde cholangiopancreatography after the CT study shows extensive extravasation, probably from the cystic duct remnant *(arrows)*.

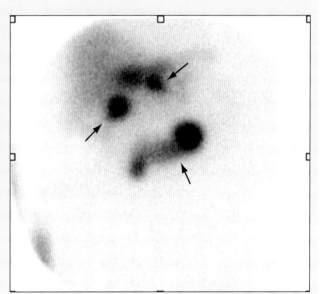

Figure 4. Bile leakage from choledochoduodenostomy. Four days after laparoscopic cholecystectomy, which was converted to open cholecystectomy with subsequent choledochoduodenostomy caused by impacted stones in common bile duct. Tc 99m-iminodiacetic acid scintigraphy 50-minute image shows extravasated tracer activity in the gallbladder fossa and porta hepatis *(upper two arrows)*. Tracer activity is also present in the duodenum *(inferior arrow)*, indicating bile leak but not complete transection. *(Courtesy of M. Cohenpour, MD.)*

DIFFERENTIAL DIAGNOSIS

- Obstructive cholangitis
- Primary sclerosing cholangitis
- Recurrent pyogenic cholangitis (Oriental cholangiohepatitis)
- Primary sclerosing cholangitis
- Acquired immunodeficiency syndrome–related cholangitis
- Biliary ascites
- Infected subhepatic fluid collection
- Sterile biloma
- Subdiaphragmatic abscess

PATHOLOGY

- Iatrogenic injury of bile ducts may be seen.
- Necrosis of the cystic duct after clipping may occur.
- Risk factors include acute or chronic inflammation, inadequate exposure, obesity, and congenital anatomic anomalies of the bile ducts.

INCIDENCE/PREVALENCE AND EPIDEMIOLOGY

- Incidence of bile duct injuries from laparoscopic cholecystectomy is 0.1%-1.3%.
- Incidence after open cholecystectomy is 0.1%-0.2%.

Suggested Readings

Braithwaite BM, Cabanilla LT, Lilly M: Hepatic subcapsular biloma: A rare complication of laparoscopic cholecystectomy and common bile duct exploration. *Curr Surg* 60:196-198, 2003.

Khalid TR, Casillas VJ, Montalvo BM, et al: Using MR cholangiopancreatography to evaluate iatrogenic bile duct injury. *AJR Am J Roentgenol* 177:1347-1352, 2001.

Park MS, Kim KW, Yu JS, et al: Early biliary complications of laparoscopic cholecystectomy: Evaluation on T2-weighted MR cholangiography in conjunction with mangafodipir trisodium-enhanced T1-weighted MR cholangiography. *AJR Am J Roentgenol* 183:1559-1566, 2004.

Ragozzino A, De Ritis R, Mosca A, et al: Value of MR cholangiography in patients with iatrogenic bile duct injury after cholecystectomy. *AJR Am J Roentgenol* 183:1567-1572, 2004.

Ray CE Jr, Hibbeln JF, Wilbur AC: Complications after laparoscopic cholecystectomy: Imaging findings. *AJR Am J Roentgenol* 160:1029-1032, 1993.

Ward EM, LeRoy AJ, Bender CE, et al: Imaging of complications of laparoscopic cholecystectomy. *Abdom Imaging* 18:150-155, 1993.

Bile Duct Strictures

DEFINITION: Stricture of the bile duct after surgery.

ANATOMIC FINDINGS

Bile Duct
- Dilated biliary tract
- Blind-ending distal duct
- Opacified proximal ducts

IMAGING

Ultrasound
Findings
- Dilated biliary tract

Utility
- Ultrasound is important in the initial evaluation of suspected bile duct stricture.

CT
Findings
- Dilated biliary tract

Utility
- CT is important in the initial evaluation of a suspected bile duct stricture.
- Multiplanar reformatted images are useful in detecting the exact site and location of the biliary obstruction.

Interventional Radiology
Findings
- Complete obstruction and stricture is demonstrated on endoscopic retrograde cholangiopancreatography (ERCP).
- Proximal bile ducts are clearly demonstrated on percutaneous transhepatic cholangiography (PTC).

Utility
- PTC is superb for evaluating patients with bile duct strictures.
- PTC is superior to ERCP owing to its ability to demonstrate the proximal biliary tree clearly.
- With high ductal injuries or complete obstruction seen on ERCP, PTC is performed to determine the proximal level of the duct injury.

MRI
Findings
- Stricture

DIAGNOSTIC PEARLS
- Complete obstruction; stricture demonstrated on ERCP, PTC, and MRCP
- Blind-ending distal duct
- Opacified proximal ducts
- Dilated biliary tract

Utility
- MR cholangiopancreatography (MRCP) can accurately diagnose biliary strictures.
- Image quality is dependent on the patient's capacity to breath-hold.

CLINICAL PRESENTATION
- Stricture of the bile duct is recognized months to years after surgery.
- Most common symptom is cholangitis.
- Painless jaundice may occur, with no evidence of sepsis.
- Advanced biliary cirrhosis and its complications may occur.

DIFFERENTIAL DIAGNOSIS
- Cirrhosis
- Obstructive cholangitis
- Primary sclerosing cholangitis
- Primary sclerosing cholangitis (MRCP)
- Recurrent pyogenic cholangitis (Oriental cholangiohepatitis)
- Acquired immunodeficiency syndrome–related cholangitis

PATHOLOGY
- Ischemia of bile duct occuring during dissection
- Intense connective tissue response with fibrosis and scarring after bile duct injury

---

WHAT THE REFERRING PHYSICIAN NEEDS TO KNOW
- With high ductal injuries or complete obstruction seen on ERCP, MRCP or PTC is performed to determine the proximal level of duct injury.
- Gap of several centimeters between the blind-ending distal duct and the proximal bile ducts precludes percutaneous transhepatic stricture dilation.

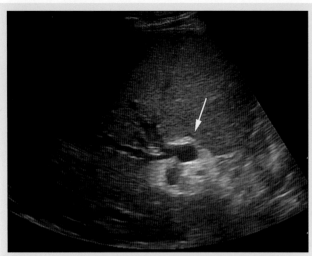

Figure 1. Anastomotic stricture. Ultrasound shows abrupt tapering of dilated common duct within the porta hepatis *(arrow)*.

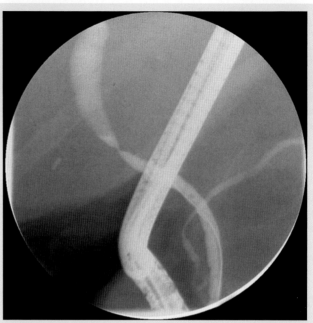

Figure 2. Anastomotic stricture. ERCP confirms an anastomotic stricture. The stricture was successfully stented.

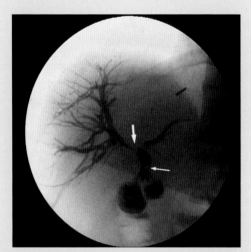

Figure 3. Nonanastomotic biliary stricture. Percutaneous cholangiogram in a patient with hepatic artery stenosis who developed a nonanastomotic stricture at the duct bifurcation *(large arrow)*; an anastomotic stricture is also seen at the choledochojejunostomy *(small arrow)*.

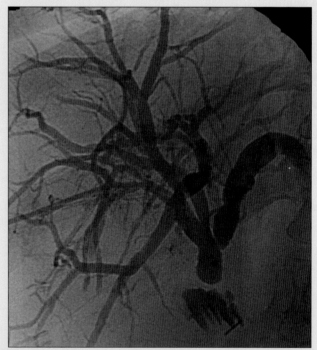

Figure 4. A 44-year-old woman after a hepaticojejunostomy for iatrogenic injury during laparoscopic cholecystectomy. Tight stricture of the hepatojejunostomy and slight dilation of the intrahepatic bile ducts are seen. A small amount of contrast material shows a jejunal afferent loop (Roux-en-Y reconstruction). (*From Köcher M, Cerná M, Havlik R, et al: Percutaneous treatment of benign bile duct strictures. Eur J Radiol 62:170-174, 2007.*)

Suggested Readings

Costamagna G, Shah SK, Tringali A: Current management of postoperative complications and benign biliary strictures. *Gastrointest Endosc Clin North Am* 13:635-648, 2003:ix.

Lillemoe KD: Benign post-operative bile duct strictures. *Baillieres Clin Gastroenterol* 11:749-779, 1997.

Lillemoe KD: Biliary strictures and sclerosing cholangitis. In Greenfield LJ (ed): *Surgery, Scientific Principles and Practice*. Philadelphia, Lippincott Williams & Wilkins, 2001, pp 1046-1061.

Cholecystectomy: Postsurgical Findings

DEFINITION: Nonpathologic and pathologic findings secondary to laparoscopic cholecystectomy.

ANATOMIC FINDINGS

Gallbladder Fossa
- Small fluid collections in the gallbladder fossa are normal.

Abdominal Wall
- Small densities in the subcutaneous fat from trocar insertion are normal.
- Subcutaneous emphysema in first 24-48 hours is normal.

Peritoneal Space
- Small fluid collections in pelvis are normal.
- Small amount of pneumoperitoneum is normal.

IMAGING

CT
Findings
- Subcutaneous emphysema
- Absorbable materials appearing as masses with mixed or low attenuation and with central or, occasionally, peripheral gas collections
- Intraperitoneal free bile or loculated collection that may be a sterile biloma, or an infected subhepatic or a subdiaphragmatic abscess
- Dilated biliary tract, possibly indicating bile duct stricture in the portion proximal to the dilation
- Fluid collection containing small opacities, ranging in density from hypodense to partially or completely calcified nodules (stone nidus)

Utility
- Absorbable surgical materials are confused with a postoperative abscess and fluid collection.
- If differentiation cannot be made, serial CT is performed, because absorbable materials are expected to disappear over a period of weeks.

Ultrasound
Findings
- Highly echogenic foci with posterior acoustic shadowing within the cystic duct remnant or lying free in the abdomen

DIAGNOSTIC PEARLS

- Small fluid collections and subcutaneous emphysema in first 24-48 hours postoperatively are normal.
- Small densities in the subcutaneous fat from the trocar insertion are normal.
- Dilated biliary tract may indicate bile duct stricture in the portion proximal to the dilation.
- Intraperitoneal free bile or loculated collection may be seen, which may be a sterile biloma or an infected subhepatic or subdiaphragmatic abscess.
- Absorbable materials appear as masses with mixed or low attenuation and with central or, occasionally, peripheral gas collections that disappear over a period of weeks.

CLINICAL PRESENTATION

- Fluid collections are usually asymptomatic and resolve spontaneously.
- Majority of complications occur in the early postoperative period, but others may appear weeks and even months after the procedure.
- Complication symptoms include fever, abdominal pain, jaundice, leukocytosis, tachycardia, vomiting, and bile leakage from the drain or wound site.

DIFFERENTIAL DIAGNOSIS

- Cystadenoma and cystadenocarcinoma (cystic bile duct neoplasms)
- Bile duct adenoma
- Hematoma
- Seroma
- Biloma
- Abscess
- Surgicel
- Retained sponge

WHAT THE REFERRING PHYSICIAN NEEDS TO KNOW
- Subcutaneous emphysema is common in first 24-48 hours after surgery.
- Absorbable surgical materials are confused with a postoperative abscess and fluid collections.
- If differentiation cannot be made, serial CT is performed because absorbable materials are expected to disappear over a period of weeks.
- Biliary tract injuries are the most serious complications of cholecystectomy.

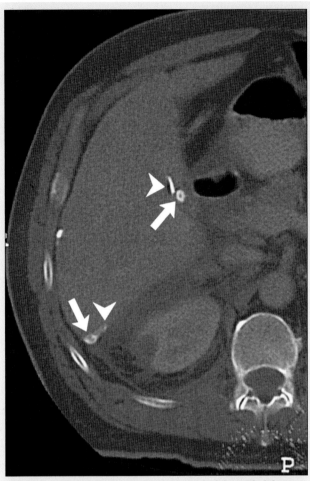

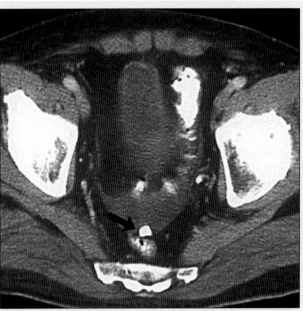

Figure 2. Spilled gallstones. Pelvic CT in a soft-tissue window setting shows a small amount of free fluid with a small calcified focus in the dependent part of the fluid *(arrow)*.

Figure 1. Spilled gallstones. CT at the level of the mid-abdomen in the bone window setting in a patient with jaundice 3 months after laparoscopic cholecystectomy (LC) shows two small calcified foci *(arrows)*, one in the gallbladder fossa and the other posterior to the liver, both adjacent to the surgical clips *(arrowheads)*. The calcified rim, typical of a gallstone, is clearly seen here.

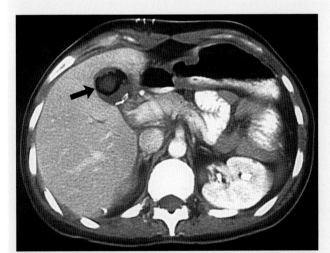

Figure 3. Gelfoam in gallbladder fossa. CT 3 days after LC shows heterogeneous density consisting of fluid and air *(arrow)* in the gallbladder fossa adjacent to the surgical clips. Gelfoam used in this patient for hemostasis accounts for this finding.

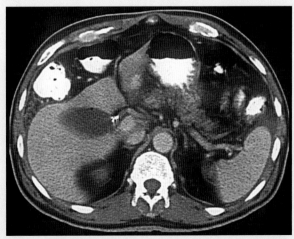

Figure 4. Bile leak resulting in a biloma and biliary ascites. CT several days after LC shows a biloma in the gallbladder fossa adjacent to the surgical clips. Free fluid surrounds the spleen.

PATHOLOGY

- Subcutaneous emphysema results from dissection of insufflated carbon dioxide around the trocars into the soft tissues.
- Laparoscopic procedure complications include abdominal wall or omental bleeding, intraperitoneal or retroperitoneal vessel injury, gastrointestinal perforation, and solid visceral injury.
- Cholecystectomy complications include gallbladder fossa bleeding, bile duct injury, bile leakage, gallbladder perforation, retained stones, *dropped* stones, and biliary strictures.

INCIDENCE/PREVALENCE AND EPIDEMIOLOGY

- Approximately 800,000 people undergo cholecystectomy for gallstones each year in the United States.
- Bile duct injuries occur in up to 1.5% of laparoscopic cholocystectomies.

Suggested Readings

Gayer G, Jonas T, Apter S, et al: Postoperative pneumoperitoneum as detected by CT: Prevalence, duration, and relevant factors affecting its possible significance. *Abdom Imaging* 25:301-305, 2000.

Hakansson K, Leander P, Ekberg O, Hakansson HO: MR imaging of upper abdomen following cholecystectomy. Normal and abnormal findings. *Acta Radiol* 42:181-186, 2001.

Kang EH, Middleton WD, Balfe DM, Soper NJ: Laparoscopic cholecystectomy: Evaluation with sonography. *Radiology* 181:439-442, 1991.

Lillemoe KD: Benign post-operative bile duct strictures. *Baillieres Clin Gastroenterol* 11:749-779, 1997.

McAllister JD, D'Altorio RA, Rao V: CT findings after uncomplicated and complicated laparoscopic cholecystectomy. *Semin Ultrasound CT MR* 14:356-367, 1993.

O'Connor AR, Coakley FV: Retained surgical materials in the postoperative abdomen and pelvis. *Semin Ultrasound CT MR* 25:290-302, 2004.

Ray CE Jr, Hibbeln JF, Wilbur AC: Complications after laparoscopic cholecystectomy: Imaging findings. *AJR Am J Roentgenol* 160:1029-1032, 1993.

Schauer PR, Page CP, Ghiatas AA, et al: Incidence and significance of subdiaphragmatic air following laparoscopic cholecystectomy. *Am Surg* 63:132-136, 1997.

Post-Traumatic Lesions of the Gallbladder and Biliary Tract

DEFINITION: Injury to the gallbladder after blunt-force or penetrating abdominal trauma.

ANATOMIC FINDINGS

Gallbladder
- Pericholecystic fluid is present.
- Dense layering fluid within the gallbladder lumen may be an indication of intraluminal hemorrhage.
- Collapsed gallbladder or thickening or poor definition of the gallbladder wall should raise the possibility of perforation or avulsion.

IMAGING

CT
Findings
- Pericholecystic fluid is present.
- Dense layering fluid within the gallbladder lumen is an indication of intraluminal hemorrhage.
- Collapsed gallbladder in the fasting patient and thickening or poor definition of the gallbladder wall should raise the possibility of gallbladder perforation or avulsion.

Utility
- CT is the most widely used modality in the evaluation of abdominal trauma.
- CT findings of gallbladder injury are largely nonspecific and are often overlooked because of injuries to adjacent organs.
- Sensitivity: 80%-95%
- Specificity: 90%-95%

Ultrasound
Findings
- Pericholecystic fluid is present.
- Dense layering fluid within the gallbladder lumen is an indication of intraluminal hemorrhage.
- Collapsed gallbladder in the fasting patient and thickening or poor definition of the gallbladder wall should raise the possibility of gallbladder perforation or avulsion.

Utility
- Gallbladder injuries can be detected with ultrasound.
- Sensitivity: 70%-90%
- Specificity: 85%-95%

DIAGNOSTIC PEARLS

- Pericholecystic fluid
- Dense layering fluid within the gallbladder lumen
- Collapsed gallbladder in the fasting patient and thickening or poor definition of the gallbladder wall

MRI
Findings
- Pericholecystic fluid is present.
- Dense layering fluid within gallbladder lumen is an indication of intraluminal hemorrhage.
- Collapsed gallbladder in the fasting patient and thickening or poor definition of the gallbladder wall should raise the possibility of gallbladder perforation or avulsion.

Utility
- Gallbladder injuries can be detected with MR cholangiopancreatography.
- Sensitivity: 75%-90%
- Specificity: 85%-95%

Nuclear Medicine
Findings
- Isotope is identified outside of the liver, gallbladder, biliary tract, and gut.

Utility
- Gallbladder injuries can be detected with hepatobiliary scintigraphy.
- Sensitivity: 80%-95%
- Specificity: 85%-95%

CLINICAL PRESENTATION

- Initial symptoms may be minimal, with gradual clinical deterioration related to the spillage of bile into the peritoneal cavity.
- Patient may complain of right upper quadrant pain, peritoneal signs, and abnormal liver function tests.

WHAT THE REFERRING PHYSICIAN NEEDS TO KNOW
- Pericholecystic fluid may also originate from injuries to the liver or right kidney.
- High-density intraluminal fluid represents blood.

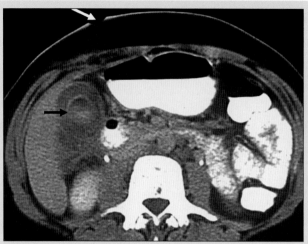

Figure 1. Gallbladder trauma. CT 2 days after a stab wound to the right upper quadrant shows gallbladder wall thickening with an intraluminal bile-blood level and infiltration of the pericholecystic tissue *(black arrow)*. A subcutaneous right upper quadrant *(white arrow)* defect indicates the location of the penetrating knife. At surgery, two lacerations were found in the anterior and posterior aspects of the gallbladder, with mild biliary peritonitis. *(From Zissin R, Osadchy A, Shapiro-Feinberg M, et al: CT of a thickened-wall gall bladder. Br J Radiol 76:137-143, 2003.)*

DIFFERENTIAL DIAGNOSIS

- Acute cholecystitis
- Chronic cholecystitis
- Hematoma
- Seroma
- Biloma
- Abscess

PATHOLOGY

- Injury to the gallbladder occurs after both blunt-force and penetrating abdominal trauma.

INCIDENCE/PREVALENCE AND EPIDEMIOLOGY

- Injury to the gallbladder is found in up to 3% of patients undergoing laparotomy after blunt-force trauma.
- Injury to the gallbladder is associated with injuries to other abdominal organs, most often the liver.

Suggested Readings

Burgess P, Fulton RL: Gallbladder and extrahepatic biliary duct injury following abdominal trauma. *Injury* 23:413-414, 1992.

Carrillo EH, Lottenberg L, Saridakis A: Blunt traumatic injury of the gallbladder. *J Trauma* 57:408-409, 2004.

Erb RE, Mirvis SE, Shanmuganathan K: Gallbladder injury secondary to blunt trauma: CT findings. *J Comput Assist Tomogr* 18:778-784, 1994.

Gupta A, Stuhlfaut JW, Fleming KW, et al: Blunt trauma of the pancreas and biliary tract: A multimodality imaging approach to diagnosis. *RadioGraphics* 24:1381-1395, 2004.

Retained Biliary Stones

DEFINITION: Unremoved biliary stones after a cholecystectomy.

ANATOMIC FINDINGS

Bile Duct
- Small biliary stones may be present within the cystic duct remnant and intrahepatic and extrahepatic ducts, or they may migrate to the common bile duct (CBD).

IMAGING

Ultrasound
Findings
- Highly echogenic foci with posterior acoustic shadowing within the cystic duct remnant

Utility
- Ultrasound fails to demonstrate any abnormality in the absence of the CBD.
- Sensitivity: 65%-95%
- Specificity: 90%-100%
- Accuracy: 88%

Interventional Radiology
Findings
- Small calculus in the distal CBD

Utility
- Endoscopic retrograde cholangiopancreatography (ERCP) offers both diagnostic and therapeutic options.

MRI
Findings
- Defect in biliary system

Utility
- MR cholangiopancreatography (MRCP) can accurately diagnose retained biliary stones.
- Sensitivity: 90%-100%
- Specificity: 90%-100%
- Accuracy: 95%

CT
Findings
- Filling defect in bile duct

Utility
- Sensitivity: 65%-90%
- Specificity: 90%-100%
- Accuracy: 85%

DIAGNOSTIC PEARLS
- Highly echogenic foci with posterior acoustic shadowing within the cystic duct remnant
- Intraductal stone identified on ERCP and MRCP

CLINICAL PRESENTATION
- Symptoms of retained CBD stones include jaundice and right upper quadrant pain.
- Patients may present with abnormal liver function tests and/or cholangitis.

DIFFERENTIAL DIAGNOSIS
- Gas bubbles
- Surgical clips
- Blood vessels
- Sludge
- Bile duct neoplasm
- Parasites

PATHOLOGY
- Stones can migrate distally into the CBD, resulting in biliary obstruction.

INCIDENCE/PREVALENCE AND EPIDEMIOLOGY
- Incidence of retained stones after laparoscopic cholecystectomy is 0.5%.

Suggested Readings
Park MS, Kim KW, Yu JS, et al: Early biliary complications of laparoscopic cholecystectomy: Evaluation on T2-weighted MR cholangiography in conjunction with mangafodipir trisodium-enhanced T1-weighted MR cholangiography. *AJR Am J Roentgenol* 183:1559-1566, 2001.

Ward EM, LeRoy AJ, Bender CE, et al: Imaging of complications of laparoscopic cholecystectomy. *Abdom Imaging* 18:150-155, 1993.

WHAT THE REFERRING PHYSICIAN NEEDS TO KNOW
- Retained stones are more common after laparoscopic than after open cholecystectomy.

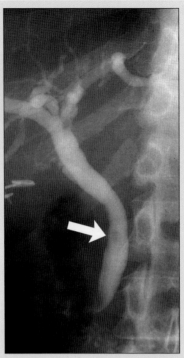

Figure 1. Retained stone in the CBD. ERCP 16 days after laparoscopic cholecystectomy shows a small calculus *(arrow)* in the distal CBD. Sphincterotomy was performed, and the stone was removed.

Spilled Gallstones

DEFINITION: Gallstones spilled from the gallbladder into the abdominal cavity during cholecystectomy.

IMAGING

Ultrasound
Findings
- Spilled stones lying free in the abdomen, mainly around the liver
- Echogenic shadowing foci (stone nidus) within the fluid collection
- Possible nidus for abscess formation

Utility
- Inferior to CT because often it cannot depict the entire abdomen and pelvis
- Sensitivity: 46%
- Specificity: 92%
- Accuracy: 58%

CT
Findings
- Spilled stones lying free in the abdomen, mainly around the liver
- Fluid collection containing small opacities, ranging in density from hypodense to partially or completely calcified nodules (stone nidus)
- Possible nidus for abscess formation

Utility
- Is preferred method of diagnosis because it can visualize the entire abdomen and pelvis
- Sensitivity: 94%
- Specificity: 98%
- Accuracy: 97%

CLINICAL PRESENTATION

- Symptoms include abdominal pain, abdominal swelling, fever or chills (or both), nausea and vomiting, and weight loss.
- Delay between surgery and abscess presentation has a mean of 5.5 months, with the range of 0-36 months.
- Cholelithoptysis (expectoration of gallstones) or pleurolithiasis may be seen.

DIFFERENTIAL DIAGNOSIS

- Milk of calcium bile
- Injuries to the liver or right kidney
- Vicarious excretion of intravenous contrast media from prior imaging studies

DIAGNOSTIC PEARLS

- Spilled stones lying free in the abdomen, mainly around the liver
- Stone within the abscess, as seen on CT and ultrasound

PATHOLOGY

- Unusual locations include the right thorax, the subphrenic space, the abdominal wall at the trocar sites, and the sites of incisional hernias.
- Abscesses are confined to the subhepatic space or retroperitoneum below the subhepatic space.
- Gallbladder perforation and intraperitoneal spillage of gallstones may occur during dissection and gallbladder removal.
- Transdiaphragmatic migration of stones occurs either by gallstone erosion through diaphragm or by formation of a subphrenic abscess connecting to the thorax.

INCIDENCE/PREVALENCE AND EPIDEMIOLOGY

- Spilled gallstones occur in up to one third of patients undergoing laparoscopic cholecystectomy.

Suggested Readings

Bennett AA, Gilkeson RC, Haaga JR, et al: Complications of "dropped" gallstones after laparoscopic cholecystectomy: Technical considerations and imaging findings. *Abdom Imaging* 25: 190-193, 2000.

Brockmann JG, Kocher T, Senninger NJ, Schurmann GM: Complications due to gallstones lost during laparoscopic cholecystectomy. *Surg Endosc* 16:1226-1232, 2002.

Hanna SJ, Barakat O, Watkin S: Cholelithoptysis: An unusual delayed complication of laparoscopic cholecystectomy. *J Hepatobiliary Pancreat Surg* 11:190-192, 2004.

Morrin MM, Kruskal JB, Hochman MG, et al: Radiologic features of complications arising from dropped gallstones in laparoscopic cholecystectomy patients. *AJR Am J Roentgenol* 174:1441-1445, 2000.

Patterson EJ, Nagy AG: Don't cry over spilled stones: Complications of gallstones spilled during laparoscopic cholecystectomy: Case report and literature review. *Can J Surg* 40:300-304, 1997.

WHAT THE REFERRING PHYSICIAN NEEDS TO KNOW
- Location of stones and abscess should be ascertained.

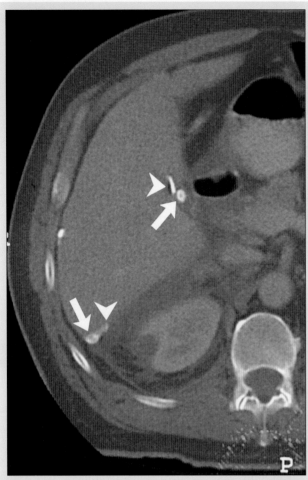

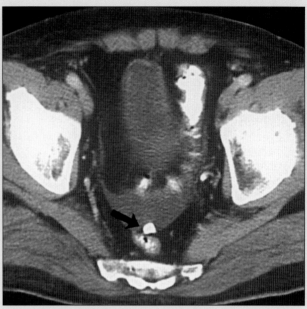

Figure 2. Spilled gallstones. Pelvic CT in the soft-tissue window setting shows a small amount of free fluid with a small calcified focus in the dependent part of fluid *(arrow)*.

Figure 1. Spilled gallstones. CT at the level of the mid-abdomen in the bone window setting in a patient with jaundice 3 months after laparoscopic cholecystectomy shows two small calcified foci *(arrows)*, one in the gallbladder fossa and the other posterior to the liver, both adjacent to surgical clips *(arrowheads)*. The calcified rim, typical of a gallstone, is clearly seen here.

Liver

Part 45 ANOMALIES AND ANATOMIC VARIANTS OF THE LIVER

Riedel's Lobe

DEFINITION: Riedel's lobe is a tongue-like projection from the anterior aspect of the right lobe of the liver that can extend quite far inferiorly in some patients.

IMAGING

CT
Findings
- Inferior extension of the right lobe of the liver below the iliac crest.

Radiography
Findings
- Inferior extension of the right lobe of the liver below the iliac crest

Ultrasound
Findings
- Inferior extension of the right lobe of the liver

MRI
Findings
- Inferior extension of the right lobe of the liver

CLINICAL PRESENTATION

- Riedel's lobe is usually asymptomatic and is discovered incidentally.
- Occasionally, it may be complicated by torsion, with gangrenous changes.

DIFFERENTIAL DIAGNOSIS

- Hepatomegaly
- Renal mass
- Abdominal wall mass

DIAGNOSTIC PEARLS

- Inferior extension of the right lobe of the liver below the iliac crest

PATHOLOGY

- Riedel's lobe is a tongue-like projection from the anterior aspect of the right lobe of the liver that can extend quite far inferiorly in some patients.
- It extends along the right paracolic gutter into the iliac fossa.
- Riedel's lobe results from excessive development of hepatic tissue.
- It is connected to the liver by a pedicle consisting of hepatic parenchyma or fibrous tissue.

INCIDENCE/PREVALENCE AND EPIDEMIOLOGY

- Riedel's lobe is the most common accessory lobe of the liver.
- It is seen most frequently in asthenic women.

Suggested Readings

Kasales CJ, Patel S, Hopper KD: Imaging variants of the liver, pancreas, and spleen. *Crit Rev Diagn Imaging* 35:485-543, 1994.

White M: Hepatic anatomic variations and developmental anomalies. In Ferrucci J (ed): *Radiology*. Philadelphia, Lippincott-Raven, 1997.

WHAT THE REFERRING PHYSICIAN NEEDS TO KNOW
- On physical examination, this anomaly can be mistaken for an enlarged liver or a right renal mass.
- Occasionally, the left lobe can behave as a Riedel's lobe and extend inferiorly in the abdomen.

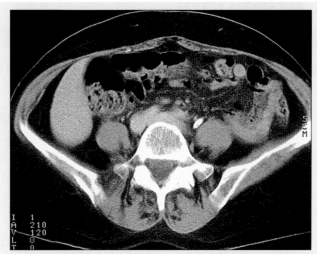

Figure 1. Riedel's lobe. Axial CT image reveals inferior extension of the right lobe of the liver below the iliac crest.

Bile Duct Adenoma

DEFINITION: Benign, solitary, small (<1 cm) mass is composed of small bile ducts.

ANATOMIC FINDINGS

Bile Duct
- Benign, solitary, small (< 1 cm) mass

IMAGING

CT
Findings
- Inhomogeneous mass with areas of low density
- Hypodense mass caused by the presence of fat and glycogen within the tumor

MRI
Findings
- Hemorrhage and low-signal areas corresponding to necrosis
- Loss of signal intensity of the mass, indicating fat

Ultrasound
Findings
- Hyperechoic lesion with central anechoic areas, corresponding to zones of internal hemorrhage if present

CLINICAL PRESENTATION
- These lesions are often found incidentally.
- May present with right upper quadrant pain, jaundice, and cholangitis

DIFFERENTIAL DIAGNOSIS
- Bile duct hamartomas
- Bile duct fibromas

DIAGNOSTIC PEARLS
- Benign, solitary, small (< 1 cm) bile duct mass
- Presence of fat, necrosis, and hemorrhage within the mass

- Granular cell tumors
- Heterotopic gastric mucosa
- Heterotopic pancreatic mucosa

PATHOLOGY
- Benign, solitary, small mass composed of small bile ducts
- Presence of fat, necrosis, and hemorrhage within the mass of cholangiocellular origin

INCIDENCE/PREVALENCE AND EPIDEMIOLOGY
- Discovered incidentally at autopsy
- Composed of small bile ducts

Suggested Readings
Kew MC: Hepatic tumors and cysts. In Feldman M, Scharschmidt BF, Sleisinger MH (eds): *Sleisinger and Fordtran's Gastrointestinal and Liver Disease*, 6th ed. Philadelphia, WB Saunders, 1998, pp 1364–1387.

WHAT THE REFERRING PHYSICIAN NEEDS TO KNOW
- These benign neoplasms are quite rare.
- Occasionally they become large and cause biliary obstruction.

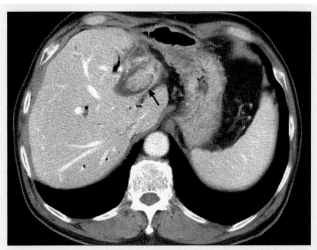

Figure 1. Multiple bile duct adenomas. CT shows an intraluminal polypoid tumor (*arrow*) with homogeneous enhancement in dilated left intrahepatic bile duct.

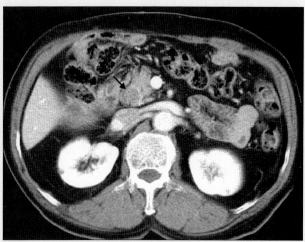

Figure 2. Multiple bile duct adenomas. CT demonstrates similar intraductal mass (*arrow*) in common bile duct.

Bile Duct Hamartoma

DEFINITION: Bile duct hamartoma (BDH) is a focal, disorderly collection of bile ducts that is caused by the failure of involution of the embryonic bile ducts.

ANATOMIC FINDINGS

Bile Duct
- Lesions 1-5 mm in size
- Multiple low-signal-intensity lesions on T1-weighted images and high-signal-intensity lesions on T2-weighted images

IMAGING

CT
Findings
- Cystic lesions less than 5 mm in diameter

Utility
- CT is less sensitive than MR and MR cholangiopancreatography (MRCP) in showing these incidental lesions

MRI
Findings
- Multiple low–signal-intensity lesions on T1-weighted images and high–signal-intensity lesions on T2-weighted images

Utility
- MR and MRCP are the most sensitive means of depicting these incidental lesions.

CLINICAL PRESENTATION
- Bile duct hamartomas are typically asymptomatic.

DIFFERENTIAL DIAGNOSIS
- Multiple metastases
- Multiple microabscesses
- Biliary dilation

DIAGNOSTIC PEARLS
- Multiple low-signal-intensity lesions on T1-weighted images and high-signal-intensity lesions on T2-weighted images
- Cystic lesions less than 5 mm in diameter
- Hyperintense bile duct lesions with bile duct intensity

PATHOLOGY
- Focal disorderly collection of bile ducts resulting from failure of involution of the embryonic bile ducts
- Small bile ductules embedded in a fibrous, sometimes hyalinized, stroma
- Each lumen possibly containing inspissated bile concrements and possibly interconnecting lumina
- Small and multiple ductules located in the subcapsular region and distributed in both lobes

INCIDENCE/PREVALENCE AND EPIDEMIOLOGY
- Nearly all individuals with adult polycystic liver disease (APLD) have multiple BDHs, and 11% of patients with multiple BDHs have APLD.
- BDHs have a 0.69%-5.6% incidence at autopsy.

Suggested Readings

Kew MC: Hepatic tumors and cysts. In Feldman M, Scharschmidt BF, Sleisinger MH (eds): *Sleisinger and Fordtran's Gastrointestinal and Liver Disease*, 6th ed. Philadelphia, WB Saunders, 1998, pp 1364-1387.

Taylor HM, Ros PR: Hepatic imaging: An overview. *Radiol Clin North Am* 36:237-246, 1998.

WHAT THE REFERRING PHYSICIAN NEEDS TO KNOW
- The normal-sized liver can have 50,000-100,000 BDHs.
- Larger cysts of APLD result from the gradual dilation of hamartomas.
- BDHs are usually an incidental finding at autopsy and cross-sectional imaging.

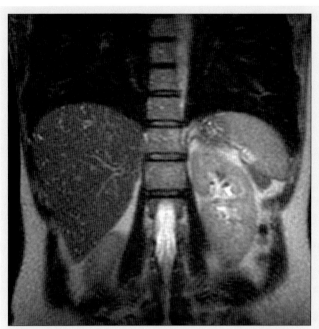

Figure 1. **Multiple bile duct hamartomas (von Meyenberg complexes).** Coronal, T2-weighted MRI scan shows multiple, tiny hyperintense lesions in the liver.

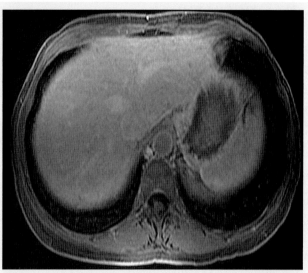

Figure 2. **Multiple bile duct hamartomas (von Meyenberg complexes).** T1-weighted MR image shows these tiny hypointense lesions. They have fluid (bile) signal intensity.

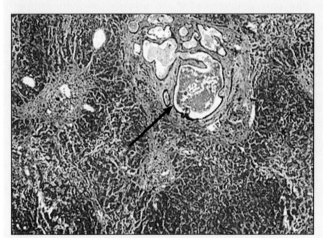

Figure 3. **Multiple bile duct hamartomas (von Meyenberg complexes).** These hamartomas are small bile ductules embedded in a fibrous, sometimes hyalinized, stroma. Each lumen may contain inspissated bile *(arrow)* concretements, and the lumina may interconnect. These findings are usually incidental at autopsy and cross-sectional imaging.

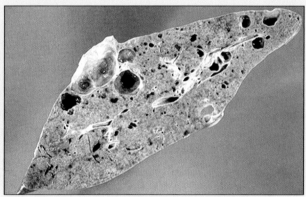

Figure 4. **Multiple bile duct hamartomas (von Meyenberg complexes).** They are usually small and multiple, located in the subcapsular region and distributed in both lobes.

Focal Nodular Hyperplasia

DEFINITION: Tumor-like condition characterized by a central fibrous scar with surrounding nodules of hyperplastic hepatocytes and small bile ductules.

ANATOMIC FINDINGS

Liver
- *Spoke-wheel* pattern
- Isointense tumor on T1-weighted images becoming slightly hyperintense to isointense on T2-weighted images.

IMAGING

Radiography
Findings
- Lesion may project to the liver margin and compress the stomach or hepatic flexure.

Utility
- Plain films are not useful in making the diagnosis.

CT
Findings
- Isodense to liver on noncontrast scans
- Homogeneous flash-filling lesions with the exception of the central scar following contrast administrations
- Lesion rapidly becomes isodense with liver.
- Central scar shows delayed enhancement.

Utility
- Most lesions are found incidentally on CT and in many cases can be characterized by this examination.

Ultrasound with Color Doppler
Findings
- Well-demarcated, hypoechoic mass homogeneous in tissue texture, except for the central scar
- Increased blood flow
- Pattern of blood vessels radiating peripherally from the central feeding artery
- Hyperperfused structure relative to the adjacent liver tissue
- Structure remaining isoechogenic with the portal vein and later with the liver parenchyma
- Increased contrast uptake within the scar relative to the surrounding liver

Utility
- Ultrasound is not as accurate as CT or MRI in establishing the diagnosis.

DIAGNOSTIC PEARLS
- Nodules lacking normal central veins and portal tracts
- *Spoke-wheel* pattern
- Early isotope uptake and late defect

MRI
Findings
- Enhances robustly and homogeneously in the arterial phase, with exception of a late-enhancing central scar
- Persistent lesion enhancement on delayed-phase images (telangiectatic focal nodular hyperplasia)

Utility
- MRI is often diagnostic, and the diagnosis can be further confirmed by giving Eovist contrast agent.
- Central scar is hyperintense on T2-weighted images.

CLINICAL PRESENTATION
- Right upper quadrant or epigastric pain
- The vast majority of these lesions are asymptomatic and incidentally discovered.

DIFFERENTIAL DIAGNOSIS
- Hepatocellular adenoma
- Hepatocellular carcinoma
- Fibrolamellar carcinoma
- Hemangioma
- Giant hemangiomas

PATHOLOGY
- Focal nodular hyperplasia is a tumor-like condition characterized by a central fibrous scar with surrounding nodules of hyperplastic hepatocytes and small bile ductules.
- Nodules lack normal central veins and portal tracts; the bile ductules in the central scar do not connect to the biliary tract.
- Vessels course through the tumor and are most abundant in the fibrous scar.

WHAT THE REFERRING PHYSICIAN NEEDS TO KNOW
- Bile ductules seen within the central scar do not connect to the biliary tract.
- Oral contraceptives have a trophic effect on focal nodular hyperplasia.

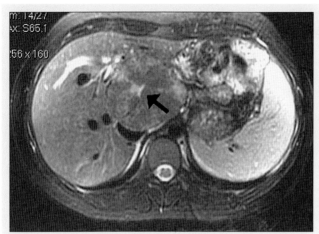

Figure 1. Focal nodular hyperplasia: MRI features. A large lesion is seen on this T2-weighted MR image obtained with fat suppression. The lesion is isointense to the normal liver, and the central scar is hyperintense *(arrow)*.

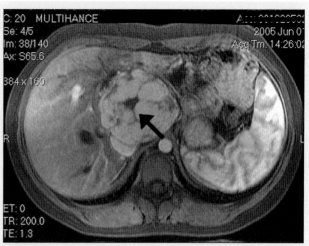

Figure 2. Focal nodular hyperplasia: MRI features. Gadolinium-enhanced early arterial phase demonstrates homogeneous enhancement of the lesion. The central scar *(arrow)* does not enhance early.

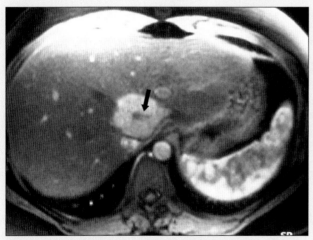

Figure 3. Focal nodular hyperplasia: MRI features. During the arterial phase of enhancement, the lesion shows robust enhancement, with the exception of the central scar *(arrow)*.

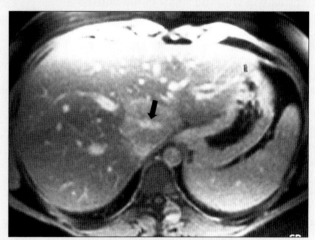

Figure 4. Focal nodular hyperplasia: MRI features. The mass rapidly de-enhances, and delayed enhancement of the central scar is seen *(arrow)*.

- Nodule is a well-circumscribed, solitary mass that is often located on the surface of the liver or pedunculated.
- Majority of these tumors have an obvious central fibrous scar, although the margin is sharp; no capsule is seen.
- Tumors are less than 5 cm, with a mean diameter of 3 cm; consistency is firm to rubbery, and the color is paler than the surrounding liver.

INCIDENCE/PREVALENCE AND EPIDEMIOLOGY

- Focal nodular hyperplasia is the second most common benign hepatic tumor, constituting 8% of primary hepatic tumors.
- It is more common in women, predominating in the third to fifth decades of life.
- Findings are usually incidental at autopsy, elective surgery, or cross-sectional imaging.

- Arteries have hypertrophied muscular media but no intimal proliferation (telangiectatic focal nodular hyperplasia).
- Significant association exists between focal nodular hyperplasia and hemangioma in the liver.

Suggested Readings

Drane WE, Krinsky GA, Johnson DA: Radionuclide imaging of primary tumors and tumor-like conditions of the liver. *Clin Nucl Med* 12:569-582, 1987.

Ishak KG: Benign tumors and pseudotumors of the liver. *Appl Pathol* 6:82-104, 1988.

Kurtaran A, Becherer A, Pfeffel F, et al: ^{18}F-fluorodeoxyglucose (FDG)-PET features of focal nodular hyperplasia (FNH) of the liver. *Liver* 20:487-490, 2000.

Ros PR: Radiologic-pathologic correlation in liver tumors. In Ferrucci JT, Stark DD (eds): *Liver Imaging.* Boston, Andover Medical Publishers, 1990, pp 137-153.

Welch TJ, Sheedy PF II, Johnson CM, et al: Focal nodular hyperplasia and hepatic adenoma: Comparison of angiography, CT, US and scintigraphy. *Radiology* 156:593-595, 1985.

Hemangioma

DEFINITION: Hemangioma is defined microscopically as a tumor composed of multiple vascular channels lined by a single layer of endothelial cells supported by a thin, fibrous stroma.

IMAGING

Radiography
Findings
- Calcification: large and coarse (amorphous calcification within the zones of the fibrosis) or phlebolith-like thrombi within the vascular channels of the hemangioma are commonly seen.

Utility
- Less than 10% of hemangiomas have calcification detectable by plain films.
- Plain radiographs are not useful in making the diagnosis.

MRI
Findings
- Marked hyperintensity containing low-intensity areas correlating with the zones of the fibrosis
- Early or peripheral nodular enhancement progressing centripetally to uniform enhancement
- Peripheral nodular enhancement, whereas the center of the lesion remains hypointense

Utility
- MRI is superior to CT and ultrasound in characterizing hemangiomas.

CT
Findings
- Early, peripheral, globular enhancement that is isodense with the blood pool
- Low-density masses with well-defined, lobulated borders
- Centripetal enhancement progressing to uniform filling that is isodense with blood pool

Utility
- Findings occur in 10%-20% of cases.
- Findings also occur in the arterial phase and portal venous phase.
- Hemangiomas are most commonly found incidentally on CT, and in most cases a specific diagnosis can be made.
- 16% of all hemangiomas and 42% of small ones show immediate homogeneous enhancement at arterial phase.

Nuclear Medicine
Findings
- Defect in the early phases
- Prolonged and persistent *filling-in*

DIAGNOSTIC PEARLS
- Early or peripheral nodular enhancement progressing centripetally to uniform enhancement
- Centripetal enhancement progressing to uniform filling
- *Cotton wool* appearance on angiography

Utility
- Tagged red blood cell pool scans are used.
- Very sensitive and specific for hemangiomas larger than 2 cm away from the cardiac border

Ultrasound
Findings
- Hyperechoic and well demarcated, exhibiting faint acoustic enhancement
- Peripheral nodular contrast enhancement and centripetal filling-in

Utility
- Echogenicity may vary because the tumors may contain cystic and fibrotic regions.
- Ultrasound contrast agents consist of microbubbles of air or perfluorocarbon gas.
- Imaging in first 60 seconds is critical in characterizing hemangiomas on ultrasound.

Ultrasound with Color Doppler
Findings
- Filling vessels in the periphery of the tumor but no significant flow deep within the hemangioma

Utility
- This technique is not generally used to confirm the diagnosis.

Ultrasound with Power Doppler
Findings
- Minimal flow
- Pattern is nonspecific and may be seen in hepatocellular carcinomas and metastases.

Utility
- This technique is not generally used to confirm the diagnosis.

WHAT THE REFERRING PHYSICIAN NEEDS TO KNOW
- Hemangiomas larger than 10 cm are defined as giant hemangiomas.
- Focal liver lesion with the classic appearance of hemangioma on ultrasound, CT, or MRI should be left alone.

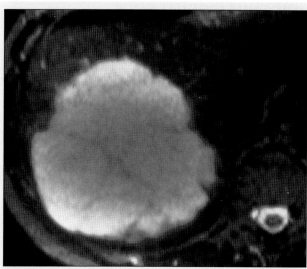

Figure 1. Hepatic hemangioma: MRI findings. Nonenhanced T2-weighted MR image shows a large hyperintense hepatic mass.

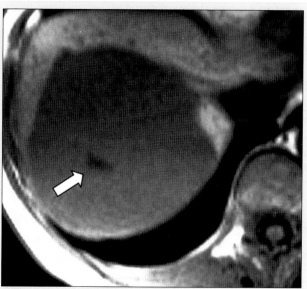

Figure 2. Hepatic hemangioma: MRI findings. Nonenhanced T1-weighted image shows low signal intensity. A central scar *(arrow)* is often seen in large hemangiomas.

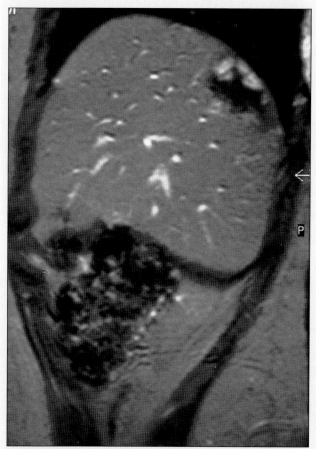

Figure 3. Hepatic hemangioma: MRI features. Sagittal gadolinium-enhanced image shows a lesion with a central scar. Although central scars are generally associated with focal nodular hyperplasia, the contrast retention in this lesion establishes the diagnosis of a hemangioma.

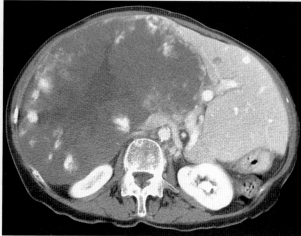

Figure 4. Hepatic hemangioma: CT features. Giant hemangioma, which replaces the right lobe, shows peripheral nodular enhancement, which progresses in a centripetal fashion. The attenuation of the enhanced portions of the mass is isodense with the blood pool. The central portion of the lesion is a low-attenuation region of central fibrosis.

CLINICAL PRESENTATION

- Virtually all hemangiomas are discovered incidentally.
- Very large hemangiomas may present with right upper quadrant pain due to mass effect and/or hemorrhage.

DIFFERENTIAL DIAGNOSIS

- Hepatocellular carcinoma
- Hepatocellular adenoma
- Focal nodular hyperplasia
- Peliosis hepatis

PATHOLOGY

- Hemangiomas are composed of multiple vascular channels lined by a single layer of endothelial cells supported by thin, fibrous stroma.
- Channels are separated by thin fibrous septa, which may form finger-like protrusions into the channels.
- Tumors are frequently solitary, well circumscribed, blood filled, and range in size from a few millimeters to more than 20 cm.

INCIDENCE/PREVALENCE AND EPIDEMIOLOGY

- Hemangioma is the most common benign tumor of the liver, with a reported incidence ranging from 1%-20%.
- Tumors occur primarily in women (female/male ratio of 5:1).
- Hemangioma is seen commonly in postmenopausal women.
- Worldwide prevalence of this tumor is fairly uniform.
- Significant association exists between focal nodular hyperplasia and hemangioma in the liver.

Suggested Readings

Moihuddin M, Allison JR, Montgomery JH, et al: Scintigraphic diagnosis of hepatic hemangioma: Its role in the management of hepatic mass lesions. *AJR Am J Roentgenol* 145:223-228, 1985.

Ros PR: Computed tomography. Pathologic correlations in hepatic tumors. In Ferrucci JT, Mathieu DG (eds): *Advances in Hepatobiliary Radiology*. St. Louis, CV Mosby, 1990, pp 75-108.

Ros PR, Rasmussen JF, Li KCP: Radiology of malignant and benign liver tumors. *Curr Probl Diagn Radiol* 18:95-155, 1989.

Vilgrain V, Uzan F, Brancatelli G, et al: Prevalence of hepatic hemangioma in patients with focal nodular hyperplasia: MR imaging analysis. *Radiology* 229:75-79, 2003.

Hepatocellular Adenoma

DEFINITION: Hepatocellular adenomas (HCAs) are benign lesions composed of neoplastic hepatocytes.

IMAGING

Radiography
Findings
- Right upper quadrant mass

Utility
- Plain radiographs

MRI
Findings
- Predominantly hyperintense relative to the liver
- May contain fat
- Heterogeneous in appearance
- Areas of increased signal intensity
- Peripheral rim corresponding to a fibrous capsule
- Early enhancement during the arterial phase and rapid washout

Utility
- MRI is the most accurate noninvasive imaging test in the characterization of this lesion by virtue of its ability to show fat and hemorrhage.

Ultrasound with Doppler
Findings
- Large hyperechoic lesion with central anechoic areas
- Lesion demonstrating peripheral arteries and veins
- Intratumoral veins
- Complex mass with large cystic components

Utility
- Is the least accurate cross-sectional imaging test in characterizing this lesion

CT
Findings
- Hypodense mass caused by the presence of fat and glycogen within the tumor
- Hyperdense areas: rapidly enhancing lesion
- Peripheral and centripetal enhancement pattern
- Hemorrhage may be seen on noncontrast scans.

Utility
- CT easily depicts the intra- and extra-tumoral hemorrhage that accompanies this lesion.

CLINICAL PRESENTATION

- Abdominal mass
- Abdominal hemorrhage
- Right upper quadrant pain

DIAGNOSTIC PEARLS

- Peripheral rim corresponding to the fibrous capsule
- Complex mass with large cystic components
- Hypodense mass caused by the presence of fat and glycogen within the tumor

DIFFERENTIAL DIAGNOSIS

- Focal nodular hyperplasia
- Hepatocellular carcinoma
- Metastasis

PATHOLOGY

- HCAs are composed of hepatocytes arranged in cords that occasionally form bile.
- They are also composed of neoplastic cells separated by compressed sinusoidal spaces, resulting in a sheet-like pattern.
- Necrosis, hemorrhage, and rupture commonly occur in large tumors.
- Surface is tan and irregular and frequently has large areas of hemorrhage or infarction.
- Sinusoids are lined by endothelial cells and enzymatically active Kupffer cells.

INCIDENCE/PREVALENCE AND EPIDEMIOLOGY

- HCA is related to oral contraceptive use, with overall estimated incidence of four adenomas per 100,000 users.
- HCA is also associated with the use of anabolic steroids.

Suggested Readings

Goodman ZD: Benign tumors of the liver. In Okuda K, Ishak KG (eds): *Neoplasms of the Liver*. Tokyo, Springer-Verlag, 1987, pp 105-125.

Yoshida H, Itai Y, Ohtomo K, et al: Small hepatocellular carcinoma and cavernous hemangioma: Differentiation with dynamic FLASH MR imaging with Gd-DTPA. *Radiology* 171:339-342, 1989.

WHAT THE REFERRING PHYSICIAN NEEDS TO KNOW
- Adenomas rarely undergo malignant transformation to hepatocellular carcinoma.

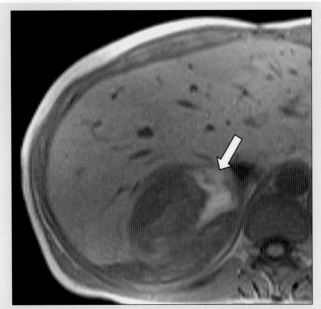

Figure 1. Adenoma: MRI features. In-phase image shows high-signal-intensity hemorrhage *(arrow)* within this mass.

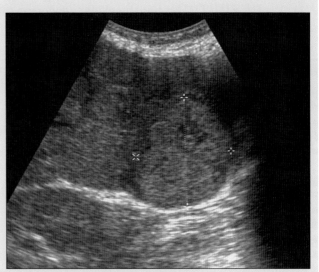

Figure 2. Adenoma: ultrasound findings. A large, solid echogenic mass *(cursors)* can be seen in the right lobe of the liver. Note the fairly well-defined hypoechoic rim.

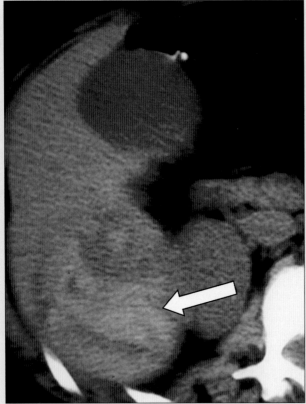

Figure 3. Adenoma: Noncontrast CT features. Hyperdense hemorrhage *(arrow)* is present within the right lobe of the liver.

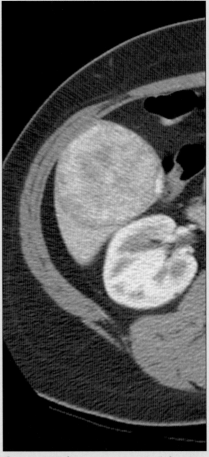

Figure 4. Adenoma: CT features. A mosaic, inhomogeneous enhancement pattern is seen after intravenous contrast administration.

Infantile Hemangioendothelioma

DEFINITION: Infantile hemangioendothelioma (IHE) is a vascular tumor derived from endothelial cells that proliferate and form the vascular channels.

IMAGING

MRI
Findings
- Predominantly hypointense on T1-weighted images and hyperintense on T2-weighted images
- Flow voids on T2-weighted images in tumors with arteriovenous shunting
- Foci of hyperintense or hypointense signal corresponding to areas of hemorrhage and fibrosis
- Enhancement pattern similar to that of multidetector CT
- *Rim-like* enhancement

Utility
- MRI is used to depict the entirety of the tumor and its blood supply.

Radiography
Findings
- Upper abdominal mass or hepatomegaly
- Speckled calcifications

Ultrasound with Doppler
Findings
- Complex liver mass with large, draining hepatic veins
- Lesions that range from hypoechoic to hyperechoic
- Lesions that tend to involute slowly and develop increased echogenicity
- Dilated hepatic vasculature with prominent blood flow

Utility
- Is typically the initial imaging test employed in neonates and infants with hepatic masses.

CT
Findings
- Single or multiple hypodense masses, with or without calcifications
- Nodular peripheral early enhancement and delayed progression to the center of the lesion
- Central portion of the tumor remaining hypodense as a result of fibrosis, hemorrhage, and necrosis

Utility
- CT uses ionizing radiation, so generally ultrasound and MRI are obtained in these young patients.

Interventional Radiography
Findings
- Enlarged tortuous feeding arteries
- Draining vessels and large vascular lakes with prolonged pooling of contrast agent

DIAGNOSTIC PEARLS

- Complex liver mass with large, draining, hepatic veins
- Nodular peripheral early enhancement and delayed progression to the center of the lesion
- Draining vessels and large vascular lakes with prolonged pooling of contrast agent

- Aorta with a decreased caliber distal to the hepatic mass origin

Utility
- Angiography

CLINICAL PRESENTATION

- Hepatomegaly, congestive heart failure, thrombocytopenia, and occasional rupture with hemoperitoneum

DIFFERENTIAL DIAGNOSIS

- Mesenchymal hamartoma
- Hepatic mesenchymal hamartoma (fetal liver)

PATHOLOGY

- IHEs are composed of a proliferation of small vascular channels lined by endothelial cells.
- Vascular tumors are derived from endothelial cells that proliferate and form the vascular channels.
- Nodules of IHEs vary from a few millimeters to 15 cm or more in size.

INCIDENCE/PREVALENCE AND EPIDEMIOLOGY

- IHE is the most common benign vascular tumor of infancy and accounts for 12% of all childhood hepatic tumors.
- IHEs develop in young infants between 1 and 6 months of age.

WHAT THE REFERRING PHYSICIAN NEEDS TO KNOW

- Most tumors grow during the first year of life, then spontaneously regress.
- Tumor may grow to a large size, causing cardiac failure.
- Radiologic findings for IHE are similar to those for multiple hemangiomas of the liver in adults.

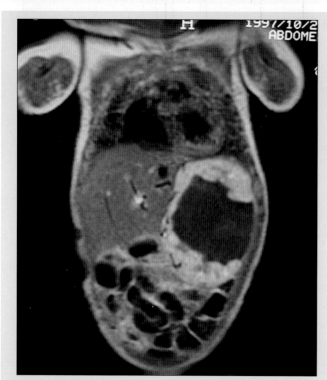

Figure 1. **Infantile hemangioendothelioma: MRI appearance.** Coronal MR image demonstrates peripheral enhancement.

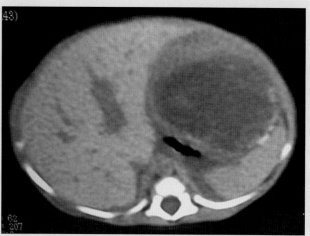

Figure 2. **Infantile hemangioendothelioma: CT appearance.** The nonenhanced CT shows a large hypodense lesion in the left lobe of the liver with some peripheral calcification.

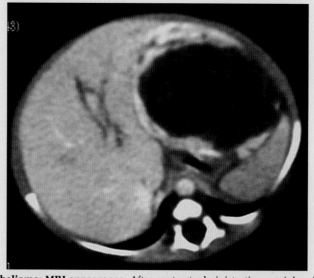

Figure 3. **Infantile hemangioendothelioma: MRI appearance.** After contrast administration, peripheral enhancement is noted, similar to that of a hemangioma identified on this axial MR image.

- Girls are affected more often than boys.
- Cutaneous hemangiomas occur in up to 40% of patients.

Suggested Readings

Helmberger TK, Ros PR, Mergo PJ, et al: Pediatric liver neoplasms: A radiologic-pathologic correlation. *Eur Radiol* 9:1339-1347, 1999.

Pobiel RS, Bisset GS III: Pictorial essay: Imaging of liver tumors in the infant and child. *Pediatr Radiol* 25:495-506, 1995.

O'Neil J, Ros PR: Knowing hepatic pathology aids MRI of liver tumors. *Diagn Imaging* 19:58-67, 1989.

Slovis TL, Berdon WE, Haller JO, et al: Hemangiomas of the liver in infants. *AJR Am J Roentgenol* 123:791-801, 1975.

Lipomatous Tumors

DEFINITION: Lipomatous tumors are benign hepatic tumors composed of fat cells.

IMAGING

Ultrasound
Findings
- Highly echogenic

Utility
- Fatty tumors are indistinguishable from hemangiomas.

CT
Findings
- Well-defined masses with attenuation values of those of fat

Utility
- CT is less sensitive than MRI in detecting fat within hepatic lesions.

MRI
Findings
- Fatty component of angiomyolipomas has high signal on non–fat-suppressed images.
- Fatty areas of angiomyolipomas are well vascularized and enhance early.
- Hypointensity to the liver is seen on fat-suppressed images.
- *Macroaneurysms* are seen.

Utility
- MRI is exquisitely sensitive in the depiction of intralesional fat.

CLINICAL PRESENTATION

- Most lipomatous tumors are asymptomatic and are incidental findings.
- Patients complain of abdominal pain.

DIFFERENTIAL DIAGNOSIS

- Hepatocellular carcinoma
- Hepatocellular adenoma

DIAGNOSTIC PEARLS

- Well-defined masses with attenuation values of those of fat
- Fatty areas that are well vascularized and enhance early
- Hypervascular and may show large aneurysms

PATHOLOGY

- Solitary, well circumscribed, and round and usually occur in noncirrhotic liver
- Microscopic features similar to lipomatous tumors of soft tissues

INCIDENCE/PREVALENCE AND EPIDEMIOLOGY

- No sex predilection has been found, and a broad age range of occurrence (24-70 years) exists.
- Approximately 10% of patients with tuberous sclerosis and renal angiolipomas have hepatic fatty tumors.

Suggested Readings

Goodman ZD, Ishak KG: Angiomyolipomas of the liver. *Am J Surg Pathol* 8:745-750, 1984.

Prayer LM, Schurawitzki HJ, Wimberger DM: Case report: Lipoma of the liver: Ultrasound, CT and MR imaging. *Clin Radiol* 45:353-354, 1992.

Roberts JL, Fishman EK, Hartman DS, et al: Lipomatous tumors of the liver: Evaluation with CT and US. *Radiology* 158:613-617, 1986.

WHAT THE REFERRING PHYSICIAN NEEDS TO KNOW

- Most lipomatous tumors are hepatic lipomas that are found incidentally and typically are of no clinical significance.

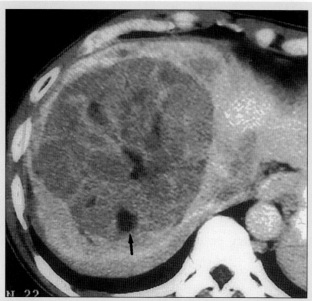

Figure 1. Angiomyolipoma. Contrast-enhanced CT scan shows a well-circumscribed, heterogeneous tumor of the right lobe with foci of fat *(arrow).* (*From Prasad SR, Wang H, Rosas H, et al: Fat-containing lesions of the liver: Radiologic-pathologic correlation,* RadioGraphics *25: 321-331, 2005.*)

Mesenchymal Hamartoma

DEFINITION: Mesenchymal hamartoma is a benign cystic developmental lesion consisting of cysts, remnants of the portal triads, hepatocytes, and fluid-filled mesenchyme.

IMAGING

Radiography
Findings
- Noncalcified right upper quadrant soft-tissue mass

Utility
- Plain radiographs are usually noncontributory.

Ultrasound
Findings
- Large cysts with internal septa (cystic predominance)
- Smaller cyst with thick septa (mesenchymal predominance)

Utility
- Is usually the first examination ordered in an infant with a hepatic mass

CT
Findings
- Well-defined masses with central hypodense areas and internal septa

Utility
- CT with multiplanar reformatted images can depict the lesion better than ultrasound.

Interventional Radiology
Findings
- Hypovascular or avascular mass, causing displacement of vessels
- Hypervascularity described in the solid portions

Utility
- Angiography is seldom used in evaluating these patients.

MRI
Findings
- Lower signal intensity than the normal liver (stromal predominance) on T1-weighted images
- Mesenchymal hamartoma markedly hyperintense (cystic predominance) on T2-weighted images
- Multiple septa transversing the tumor (cystic predominance)

DIAGNOSTIC PEARLS

- Noncalcified right upper quadrant soft-tissue mass
- Well-defined masses with central hypodense areas and internal septa
- Mesenchymal hamartoma that is markedly hyperintense (cystic predominance)

- Stromal components enhancing after the administration of gadolinium-chelate agents

Utility
- MRI is superior to ultrasound in characterizing this lesion.

CLINICAL PRESENTATION

- Slow, progressive, painless abdominal enlargement
- Respiratory distress and lower-extremity edema

DIFFERENTIAL DIAGNOSIS

- Hepatoblastoma (pediatric)
- Infantile hemangioendothelioma

PATHOLOGY

- Composed of gelatinous mesenchymal tissue with cyst formation and remnants of normal hepatic parenchyma
- Large, soft, predominantly cystic mass measuring 15 cm or more in diameter
- Mesenchymal hamartoma that is not neoplastic but rather a failure of normal development
- Either mesenchymal or cystic predominance
- Tumor consisting of cysts, remnants of the portal triads, hepatocytes, and fluid-filled mesenchyme
- Cysts exhibiting grossly in 80% of cases

WHAT THE REFERRING PHYSICIAN NEEDS TO KNOW
- Mesenchymal hamartoma is differentiated in part on cross-sectional imaging from hepatoblastoma and infantile hemangioendothelioma by the predominance of cysts in the mesenchymal hamartoma.
- Mesenchymal hamartoma should not be confused with other cystic-appearing masses that may occur in the liver of toddlers.

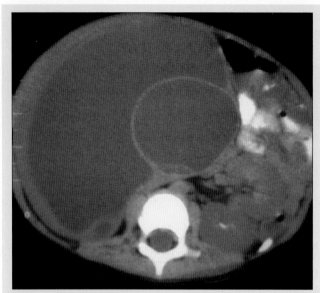

Figure 1. Mesenchymal hamartoma. CT appearance. The lesion is markedly cystic and has septa.

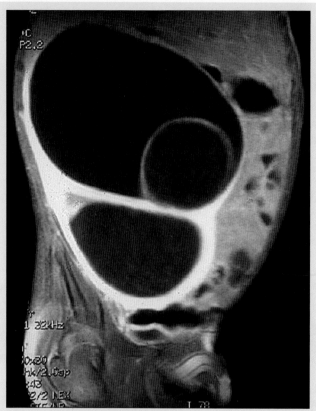

Figure 2. Mesenchymal hamartoma. MRI appearance. The lesion is markedly cystic and has septa.

INCIDENCE/PREVALENCE AND EPIDEMIOLOGY

■ Mesenchymal hamartoma accounts for 8% of all childhood liver tumors.

■ It occurs during the first 3 years of life, and a slight male predominance exists.

Suggested Readings

Dehner LP, Ewing SL, Sumner HW: Infantile mesenchymal hamartoma of the liver. Histologic and ultrastructural observations. *Arch Pathol Lab Med* 99:379-382, 1975.

Kaude JV, Felman AH, Hawkins IF: Ultrasonography in primary hepatic tumors in early childhood. *Pediatr Radiol* 9:77-83, 1980.

Ros PR, Goodman ZD, Ishak KG, et al: Mesenchymal hamartoma of the liver: Radiologic-pathologic correlation. *Radiology* 158:619-624, 1986.

Stanley P, Hall TR, Woolley MM, et al: Mesenchymal hamartomas of the liver in childhood: Sonographic and CT findings. *AJR Am J Roentgenol* 147:1035-1039, 1986.

Stocker JT, Ishak KG: Mesenchymal hamartoma of the liver: Report of 30 cases and review of the literature. *Pediatr Pathol* 1:245-267, 1983.

Nodular Regenerative Hyperplasia

DEFINITION: Nodular regenerative hyperplasia (NRH) is defined as diffuse nodularity of the liver produced by many regenerative nodules that are not associated with fibrosis. This is most often seen in patients with chronic Budd-Chiari syndrome.

IMAGING

Radiography
Findings
- Splenomegaly, ascites, and other signs of portal hypertension

Utility
- Plain radiographs do not demonstrate these lesions.

Ultrasound
Findings
- Focal nodules that vary in echogenicity
- Central hemorrhage within the large nodule

Utility
- Lesions are poorly depicted on ultrasound.

CT
Findings
- Hypervascular lesions
- Focal nodules of varying attenuation that are primarily hypodense
- Complex mass with variable density

Utility
- These lesions are best seen on the arterial phase.

MRI
Findings
- Isointense to the normal liver on T2-weighted images
- Foci of high signal on T1-weighted images
- Lesions possibly showing robust enhancement after intravenous administration of Gd-DTPA (gadolinium diethylenetriaminopentaacetic acid)

Utility
- These lesions are best seen on the arterial phase.

CLINICAL PRESENTATION

- Patient may be asymptomatic or exhibit symptoms from complications (portal hypertension, splenomegaly).

DIFFERENTIAL DIAGNOSIS

- Hypervascular metastases
- Multifocal hepatocellular carcinoma
- Multiple hemangiomas or focal nodular hyperplasia

DIAGNOSTIC PEARLS

- Large nodules composed of abnormal hepatocytes with Kupffer cells, taking up technetium Tc99m-sulfur colloid
- Vascular, peripherally filling nodules
- Focal nodules of varying attenuation that are primarily hypodense on CT

PATHOLOGY

- NRH is characterized by diffuse nodularity of the liver produced by many regenerative nodules that are not associated with fibrosis.
- It is also characterized by multiple bulging nodules on the external surface of the liver.
- Nodules vary in size from few millimeters to several centimeters and are diffusely scattered.
- Nodules are composed of cells resembling normal hepatocytes.

INCIDENCE/PREVALENCE AND EPIDEMIOLOGY

- NRH is rare, although autopsy series have shown the prevalence to be as high as 0.6%.
- It is discovered either incidentally on autopsy or in a workup for portal hypertension and its complications.
- Various systemic diseases and drugs are associated with NRH.

Suggested Readings

Dachman AH, Ros PR, Goodman ZD, et al: Nodular regenerative hyperplasia of the liver: Clinical and radiologic observations. *AJR Am J Roentgenol* 148:717-722, 1987.

Wanless IR, Solt LC, Kortan P, et al: Nodular regenerative hyperplasia of the liver associated with macroglobulinemia. *Am J Med* 170:1203-1209, 1981.

Wanless IR, Todwin TA, Allen F, et al: Nodular regenerative hyperplasia of the liver in hematologic disorders, a possible response to obliterative portal venopathy: A morphometric study of nine cases with an hypothesis on the pathogenesis. *Medicine (Baltimore)* 49:367-379, 1980.

WHAT THE REFERRING PHYSICIAN NEEDS TO KNOW

- NRH is an underdiagnosed disease, frequently related to chronic illnesses or prolonged therapy.
- NRH must be differentiated from other hepatocellular hyperplasias that are seen in post-hepatitis and post alcoholic cirrhosis.

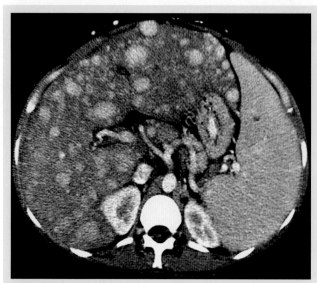

Figure 1. Nodular regenerative hyperplasia. Multiple robustly enhancing hepatic masses are identified on this contrast-enhanced CT scan in this patient with the Budd-Chiari syndrome. (*Courtesy of Michael P. Federle, MD, Pittsburgh, PA.*)

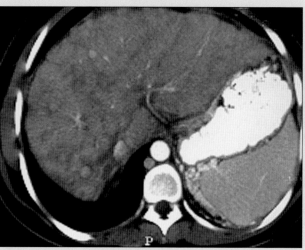

Figure 2. Nodular regenerative hyperplasia. Multiple robustly enhancing hepatic masses are identified on this contrast-enhanced CT scan in this patient with the Budd-Chiari syndrome.

Part 47 MALIGNANT TUMORS OF THE LIVER

Angiosarcoma

DEFINITION: Malignant tumor derived from endothelial lining cells occurring primarily in adults with exposure to a variety of chemical agents and radiation.

IMAGING

Radiography
Findings
- Soft-tissue–density mass in the upper abdomen
- Localized areas of increased density in the liver, spleen, and the mesenteric and celiac lymph nodes
- Circumferential displacement of Thorotrast by nodules of angiosarcoma

Utility
- Findings depend on the presence or absence of prior Thorotrast exposure.
- Plain films typically are noncontributory in establishing the diagnosis.

Nuclear Medicine
Findings
- Solitary or multiple filling defects
- Possibly showing early and late uptake
- Retention of tagged red blood cells not as prolonged as that by hemangiomas

Utility
- Typically not performed in evaluating this lesion

Ultrasound
Findings
- Single or multiple hyperechoic masses
- Heterogeneous echo architecture because of hemorrhage of various ages

Utility
- Typically has a nonspecific sonographic appearance

CT
Findings
- Reticular pattern of deposition of Thorotrast in both the liver and the spleen
- Circumferential displacement of Thorotrast in the periphery of the nodule
- Single or multiple masses that are hypodense on unenhanced CT scans, except for hyperdense areas of fresh hemorrhage

DIAGNOSTIC PEARLS

- Single or multiple masses that are hypodense on unenhanced CT scans, except for hyperdense areas of fresh hemorrhage
- Focal areas of enhancement that show less attenuation than the aorta or peripheral ring-shaped enhancement
- Diffuse puddling of contrast medium that persists into the venous phase
- Low signal intensity on T1-weighted images and of predominantly high signal on T2-weighted images with central areas of low signal

- Centripetal enhancement with contrast material
- Focal areas of enhancement that show less attenuation than the aorta or peripheral ring-shaped enhancement
- Diffuse puddling of contrast medium that persists into the venous phase on angiography
- Centripetal flow on angiography

Utility
- CT angiography is used to establish the vascularity of this neoplasm.

MRI
Findings
- Low signal intensity on T1-weighted images and predominantly high signal on T2-weighted images with central areas of low signal
- Fluid-fluid levels and marked heterogeneity with high-intensity focal areas along with septum-like or rounded areas of low intensity
- Peripheral nodular enhancement that progresses centripetally
- On delayed postcontrast images, peripheral enhancement persisting, whereas the center of the lesion remains unenhanced

Utility
- MR angiography can be used to establish the vascularity of this neoplasm.

WHAT THE REFERRING PHYSICIAN NEEDS TO KNOW
- Angiosarcoma occurs primarily in adults with exposure to a variety of chemical agents (polyvinyl chloride) and radiation (thorium oxide administration).

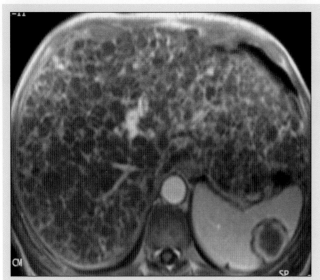

Figure 1. Angiosarcoma. Gadolinium-enhanced MR image obtained in the arterial phase demonstrates the replacement of the liver parenchyma with numerous nodules. An angiosarcoma is also present in the spleen.

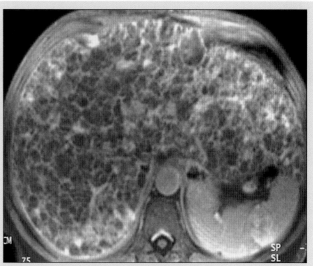

Figure 2. Angiosarcoma. Gadolinium-enhanced MR image obtained in the portal venous phase demonstrates the replacement of the liver parenchyma with numerous nodules. An angiosarcoma is also present in the spleen.

CLINICAL PRESENTATION

- Generalized weakness, weight loss, abdominal pain, hepatomegaly, and ascites
- Thrombocytopenia caused by platelet sequestration within a large angiosarcoma (possible)
- Rupture and acute hemoperitoneum (rare)

DIFFERENTIAL DIAGNOSIS

- Hemangioendothelioma
- Hepatocellular carcinoma
- Hypervascular metastasis
- Peliosis

PATHOLOGY

- Angiosarcoma is a malignant tumor derived from endothelial lining cells, occurring primarily in adults with exposure to chemical agents and radiation.
- Microscopically, the tumor is composed of malignant endothelial cells lining the vascular channels of variable size from cavernous to capillary.
- Thorotrast particles can be found within the malignant endothelial cells in cases of Thorotrast-induced angiosarcoma.
- Grossly, the majority of angiosarcomas are multiple and have areas of internal hemorrhage.
- Tumors may appear as a single, large mass with no capsule and contains large cystic areas filled with bloody debris.
- Angiosarcoma is associated with hemochromatosis and previous exposure to toxins such as Thorotrast, vinyl chloride, arsenicals, and steroids.

INCIDENCE/PREVALENCE AND EPIDEMIOLOGY

- Angiosarcoma is a rare neoplasm that occurs most frequently in men (2:1-4:1 more often than in women) in the seventh decade of life.
- Angiosarcoma is 30 times less common than hepatocellular carcinoma.

Suggested Readings

Azodo MVU, Gutierrez OH, Greer T: Thorotrast-induced ruptured hepatic angiosarcoma. *Abdom Imaging* 18:78-81, 1993.

Buetow PC, Buck JL, Pantongrag-Brown L, et al: Undifferentiated (embryonal) sarcoma of the liver: Pathologic basis of imaging findings in 28 cases. *RadioGraphics* 203:779-783, 1997.

Buetow PC, Buck JL, Ros PR, et al: Malignant vascular tumors of the liver: Radiologic-pathologic correlation. *RadioGraphics* 14:153-166, 1994.

Horowitz ME, Etcubanas E, Webber BL, et al: Hepatic differentiated (embryonal) sarcoma and rhabdomyosarcoma in children. Results of therapy. *Cancer* 59:396-402, 1987.

Klatskin G: Adenocarcinoma of the hepatic duct at its bifurcation within the porta hepatis. *Am J Med* 38:241-256, 1965.

Levy DW, Rindsberg S, Friedman AC, et al: Thorotrast-induced hepatosplenic neoplasia: CT identification. *AJR Am J Roentgenol* 146:997-1004, 1986.

Locker GY, Doroshow JH, Zwelling LA, et al: The clinical features of hepatic angiosarcoma: A report of four cases and a review of the English literature. *Medicine (Baltimore)* 58:48-64, 1979.

Mahony B, Jeffrey RB, Federle MP: Spontaneous rupture of hepatic and splenic angiosarcoma demonstrated by CT. *AJR Am J Roentgenol* 183:965-966, 1982.

Ros PR, Rasmussen JF, Li KCP: Radiology of malignant and benign liver tumors. *Curr Probl Diagn Radiol* 11:95-99, 1989.

Whelan JG Jr, Creech JL, Tamburro CL: Angiographic and radionuclide characteristics of hepatic angiosarcoma in vinyl chloride workers. *Radiology* 118:549-557, 1976.

Worawattanakul S, Semelka RC, Kelekis NL, et al: Angiosarcoma of the liver: MR imaging pre- and post chemotherapy. *Magn Reson Imaging* 15:613-617, 1997.

Fibrolamellar Carcinoma

DEFINITION: Slow-growing tumor that arises in the normal liver composed of neoplastic hepatocytes separated into cords by lamellar fibrous strands.

IMAGING

Radiography
Findings
- Partially calcified upper abdominal mass

Utility
- Plain films are noncontributory in making the diagnosis.

Ultrasound
Findings
- Large, well-defined, lobulated mass with variable echotexture
- Mixed echogenicity (60% of cases) and predominantly containing hyperechoic or isoechoic components
- Central scar and a central area of hyperechogenicity

Utility
- Ultrasound shows a nonspecific appearance of this neoplasm.

CT
Findings
- Hypodense mass with a well-defined contour on unenhanced CT
- Areas of decreased density within the tumor corresponding to the central scar or necrosis and hemorrhage
- Stellate calcification within the central scar
- During arterial and portal phases of dynamic enhanced CT, *nonscar* portion of fibrolamellar carcinoma enhancing heterogeneously
- Central scar: delayed enhancement and appearance of the tumor closely simulating that of focal nodular hyperplasia on delayed enhancement
- Hypervascular tumor with compartmentalization in the capillary phase resulting from multiple fibrous septa on angiography
- Features that determine the resectability of fibrolamellar carcinomas such as portal vein invasion and lymphadenopathy are well seen on CT scans.

Utility
- CT is superior in showing the calcifications that typically accompany this lesion. CT is an excellent technique for staging this tumor.

MRI
Findings
- Hypointense or isointense with normal liver on T1-weighted images and isointense or slightly hyperintense on T2-weighted images

DIAGNOSTIC PEARLS
- Large, well-defined, lobulated mass with variable echotexture
- Hypodense mass with a well-defined contour
- Hypointense or isointense with the normal liver on T1-weighted images and isointense or slightly hyperintense on T2-weighted images

- Scar is hypointense on both T1- and T2-weighted images.
- Heterogeneous enhancement in the arterial and portal phases and progressively becoming more homogeneous on delayed images

Utility
- MRI is excellent for staging this neoplasm but is inferior to CT in detecting intratumoral calcification.

CLINICAL PRESENTATION
- Pain, malaise, and weight loss
- Jaundice occurring when fibrolamellar carcinoma invades the biliary tract
- Palpable mass in two thirds of patients
- Usually normal α-fetoprotein levels

DIFFERENTIAL DIAGNOSIS
- Focal nodular hyperplasia
- Hepatocellular carcinoma
- Hepatocellular adenoma
- Liver metastasis

PATHOLOGY
- Fibrolamellar carcinoma is a slow-growing tumor that arises in the normal liver.
- It is composed of neoplastic hepatocytes separated into cords by lamellar fibrous strands.
- Distinctive microscopic pattern is seen, with eosinophilic, malignant hepatocytes containing prominent nuclei.
- Fibrolamellar carcinoma arises in the normal liver, with only 20% of patients having underlying cirrhosis.

WHAT THE REFERRING PHYSICIAN NEEDS TO KNOW
- Major differential diagnosis with fibrolamellar carcinoma is focal nodular hyperplasia.

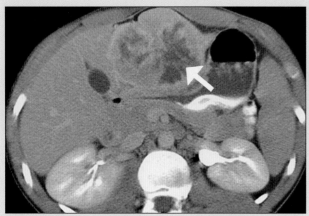

Figure 1. Fibrolamellar carcinoma: imaging features.
Enhanced arterial-phase CT scan improves definition of the
lesion. Note the central low-density area representing necrosis
and scar tissue *(arrow)*.

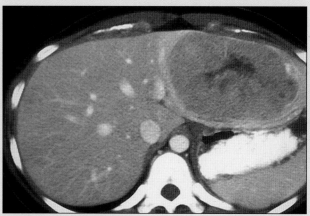

Figure 2. Fibrolamellar carcinoma: CT findings. The central
scar is better appreciated on this contrast-enhanced scan.

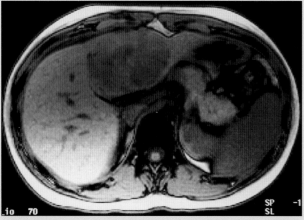

Figure 3. Fibrolamellar carcinoma: MR findings. Unenhanced
scan shows a low-signal-intensity mass that showed striking
enhancement.

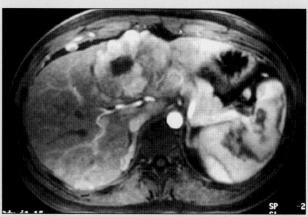

Figure 4. Fibrolamellar carcinoma: MR findings. A low-signal-
intensity mass shows striking enhancement with the exception of
the central scar on this contrast-enhanced image.

■ Fibrous component accounts for one half of the tumor,
distributed in multilamellate strands, except in larger
tumors containing large central scars.

■ Grossly, satellite nodules are present, as well as a central scar and multiple fibrous septa.

INCIDENCE/PREVALENCE AND EPIDEMIOLOGY

■ Fibrolamellar carcinoma occurs in adolescents and
adults younger than age 40 and without underlying
cirrhosis or other predisposing risk factors.

■ No sex predominance has been found.

■ Mean survival is 45-60 months, with a high likelihood
of cure (40%) if the tumor is surgically resectable.

Suggested Readings

Berman MA, Burnham JA, Sheahan DG: Fibrolamellar carcinoma of
the liver: An immunohistochemical study of nineteen cases and a
review of the literature. *Hum Pathol* 19:784-794, 1988.
Buetow PC, Midkiff RB: Primary malignant neoplasms in the adult.
MRI Clin North Am 5:289-318, 1997.

Caseiro-Alves F, Zins M, Mahfouz A-E: Calcification in focal nodular
hyperplasia: A new problem for differentiation from fibrolamellar
hepatocellular carcinoma. *Radiology* 198:889-892, 1996.
Corrigan K, Semelka RC: Dynamic contrast-enhanced MR imaging of
fibrolamellar hepatocellular carcinoma. *Abdom Imaging* 20:122-
125, 1995.
Francis IR, Agha FP, Thompson NW, et al: Fibrolamellar hepatocarcinoma: Clinical, radiologic and pathologic features. *Gastrointest
Radiol* 11:67-72, 1986.
Friedman AC, Lichtenstein JE, Goodman Z, et al: Fibrolamellar hepatocellular carcinoma. *Radiology* 157:583-587, 1985.
Hamrick-Turner JE, Shipkey FH, Cranston PE: Fibrolamellar hepatocellular carcinoma: MR appearance mimicking focal nodular
hyperplasia. *J Comput Assist Tomogr* 18:301-304, 1994.
Mattison GR, Glazer GM, Quint LE, et al: MR imaging of hepatic focal
nodular hyperplasia: Characterization and distinction from primary
malignant hepatic tumors. *AJR Am J Roentgenol* 148:711-715, 1987.
McLarney JK, Rucker PT, Bender GN, et al: Fibrolamellar carcinoma
of the liver: Radiologic-pathologic correlation. *RadioGraphics*
19:453-471, 1999.
Ros PR, Rasmussen JF, Li KCP: Radiology of malignant and benign
liver tumors. *Curr Probl Diagn Radiol* 11:95-99, 1989.
Ross Stevens W, Johnson CD, Stephens DH, et al: Fibrolamellar hepatocellular carcinoma: Stage at presentation and results of
aggressive surgical management. *AJR Am J Roentgenol* 164:
1153-1158, 1995.

Epithelioid Hemangioendothelioma

DEFINITION: Rare malignant hepatic neoplasm of vascular origin.

ANATOMIC FINDINGS

Liver
- Hemangioendothelioma develops in the periphery of the liver and commonly shows calcifications corresponding to the fibrotic nature of this tumor.

IMAGING

Radiography
Findings
- Calcifications

Utility
- May show hepatomegaly

Ultrasound
Findings
- Primarily hypoechoic lesion

Utility
- Ultrasound is typically the first examination obtained in infants with hepatomegaly and suspected hepatic mass.

CT
Findings
- Full spectrum of growth possibly seen from multiple nodules to large confluent masses
- Portions of large, low-attenuation masses becoming isodense after the administration of contrast material
- Compensatory enlargement of the uninvolved portions of the liver seen with extensive involvement
- Hypervascular, hypovascular, or avascular, depending on the extent of hyalinization and sclerosis within the tumor on angiography
- Tumor invasion of hepatic veins

Utility
- CT is useful in diagnosis of the tumor in adults.
- In children, MRI is preferred because it does not use ionizing radiation.

MRI
Findings
- Peripheral nodules or larger confluent lesions
- Hypointense on T1- and hyperintense on T2-weighted images, although hypointense center may be seen on both sequences

DIAGNOSTIC PEARLS
- Portions of large, low-attenuation masses that become isodense after the administration of contrast material
- Hypervascular, hypovascular, or avascular, depending on the extent of hyalinization and sclerosis
- Hypointense on T1- and hyperintense on T2-weighted images, although a hypointense center may be seen on both sequences

- Peripheral enhancement and delayed central enhancement
- In infants these lesions are heterogeneous and hypointense and multinodular on T1-weighted images. There are varying degrees of hyperintensity on T2-weighted images.

Utility
- MRI demonstrates the internal architecture better than CT.
- It also demonstrates tumor invasion of the portal veins in adults.

CLINICAL PRESENTATION
- Usually discovered incidentally in adults
- Jaundice, liver failure, and, occasionally, rupture with hemoperitoneum in adults

DIFFERENTIAL DIAGNOSIS
- Angiosarcoma
- Hepatocellular carcinoma in adults
- Metastases in adults
- Mesenchymal hamartoma

PATHOLOGY
- Grossly, tumors are often multiple and are composed of neoplastic cells that infiltrate the sinusoids and intrahepatic veins.

WHAT THE REFERRING PHYSICIAN NEEDS TO KNOW
- Prognosis is much more favorable than that of angiosarcoma in adults.
- Extrahepatic metastases occur in only one third of the reported cases in adults.
- Biologic behavior of this tumor is related to its matrix, including inflammation, sclerosis, and calcification in adults.

INCIDENCE/PREVALENCE AND EPIDEMIOLOGY

- This is the most common benign hepatic tumor during the first 6 months of life.
- Epithelioid hemangioendothelioma develops in adults with an average age of 45 at presentation with 2:1 female predominance.

Suggested Readings

Van Beers B, Roche A, Mathieu D, et al: Epithelioid hemangioendothelioma of the liver: MR and CT findings. *J Comput Assist Tomogr* 16:420-424, 1992.

Worawattanakul S, Semelka RC, Kelekis NL, et al: Angiosarcoma of the liver: MR imaging pre- and post chemotherapy. *Magn Reson Imaging* 15:613-617, 1997.

Hepatic Cystadenoma and Cystadenocarcinoma

DEFINITION: Locules of mucinous tumors are lined by columnar, cuboidal, or even flattened epithelium.

IMAGING

Interventional Radiology
Findings
- Communication of the tumor with the bile duct
- Large, unilocular or multilocular mass on cross-sectional imaging

Utility
- Endoscopic retrograde cholangiopancreatography

Ultrasound
Findings
- Septa, as well as mural nodules, in the wall of these tumors

Utility
- Good correlation is seen between nodularity and septation on ultrasound scans and gross specimens.

CT
Findings
- Large, unilocular or multilocular, low-attenuation intrahepatic masses with well-defined, thick, fibrous capsules, mural nodules, and internal septa
- Calcification possibly seen within the wall and septa in a minority of cases

CT Angiography
Findings
- Avascular, although a small peripheral vascular blush on angiography

MRI
Findings
- Multiseptated, predominantly high signal on T2-weighted images and mixed or low signal on T1-weighted images

DIAGNOSTIC PEARLS

- Large, unilocular or multilocular mass on cross-sectional imaging
- Avascular characteristics, although a small peripheral vascular blush possibly in a few cases
- Multiseptated and with a predominantly high signal on T2-weighted images and mixed or low signal on T1-weighted images

- Areas of high signal on T1-weighted images, representing hemorrhagic fluid components
- Low signal rim on T2-weighted images possibly caused by hemorrhage in the wall of the lesion
- Variable signal intensity within the locules on both T1- and T2-weighted images

DIFFERENTIAL DIAGNOSIS

- Amebic abscesses

PATHOLOGY

- Microscopically, a mucinous, but serous, variety is also recognized; locules of these tumors are lined by columnar, cuboidal, or even flattened epithelium.
- Polypoid projections and papillary areas are frequently present; a well-formed wall and focal calcification within the wall are rare.
- In cystadenocarcinoma, malignant epithelial cells line the cysts.
- Grossly, locules are solitary, up to 30 cm in size, and have a shiny, smooth, or bosselated surface, with multiple communicating locules of variable size on the cut section.

WHAT THE REFERRING PHYSICIAN NEEDS TO KNOW

- Cystadenocarcinoma is overtly malignant, and cystadenoma has a malignant potential.
- Transformation of cystadenoma to cystadenocarcinoma is a recognized complication.
- Cystadenocarcinoma with ovarian stroma is found in women and has an indolent course and a good prognosis.
- Tumors without an ovarian stroma are found in both sexes and have an aggressive clinical course and a poor prognosis.
- Combination of septation and nodularity is suggestive of cystadenocarcinoma, whereas septation without nodularity is seen only in cystadenoma.
- Presence of distant metastases, adenopathy, or other signs of widespread malignancy is consistent with cystadenocarcinoma.
- Distinguishing among cystadenoma or cystadenocarcinoma, hydatid disease, and abscess is difficult on cross-sectional imaging.

■ Papillary excrescences or mural nodules are seen in the tumor wall.

INCIDENCE/PREVALENCE AND EPIDEMIOLOGY

■ Cystadenomas and cystadenocarcinomas are rare and represent only 5% of all intrahepatic cysts of bile duct origin.
■ They usually occur in middle-aged women.

Suggested Readings

Agildere AM, Haliloglu M, Akhan O: Biliary cystadenoma and cystadenocarcinoma (letter). *AJR Am J Roentgenol* 156:1113, 1991.

Ishak KG: Benign tumors and pseudotumors of the liver. *Appl Pathol* 6:82-104, 1988.

Ishak KG: Mesenchymal tumors of the liver. In Okuda K, Peter RL (eds): *Hepatocellular Carcinoma*. New York, John Wiley & Sons, 1976, pp 228-587.

Ishak KG: In Farber E, Phillips MJ, Kaufman N (eds): *Pathogenesis of Liver Diseases. International Academy of Pathology Monograph*, No. 28. Baltimore, Williams & Wilkins, 1987, pp 314-315.

Mortele KJ, Ros PR: Cystic focal liver lesions in the adult: Differential CT and MR imaging features. *RadioGraphics* 21:895-910, 2001.

Ros PR, Rasmussen JF, Li KCP: Radiology of malignant and benign liver tumors. *Curr Probl Diagn Radiol* 11:95-99, 1989.

Stoupis C, Ros PR, Dolson DJ: Recurrent biliary cystadenoma: MR imaging appearance. *J Magn Reson Imaging* 4:99-101, 1994.

Hepatoblastoma

DEFINITION: Malignant tumor of hepatocyte origin that often contains mesenchymal elements.

IMAGING

Radiography
Findings
- Large solitary tumor
- Large right upper quadrant mass
- Extensive coarse and dense calcification caused by osteoid formation

Utility
- Plain radiographs are insensitive in depicting this and other hepatic neoplasms.

Nuclear Medicine
Findings
- Large defect on sulfur colloid scans
- Possibly taking up gallium and fluorodeoxyglucose and excreting iminodiacetic acid–derivative agents

Utility
- This technique is now seldom used.

Ultrasound
Findings
- Echogenic mass that may have shadowing, echogenic foci corresponding to intratumor calcification
- Hyperechoic or cystic areas, possibly both, corresponding to hemorrhage within the tumor and necrotic areas

Utility
- Ultrasound is the initial test used in evaluating children with suspected liver tumors.

Ultrasound Doppler
Findings
- Associated with high Doppler frequency shifts that correlate with neovascularity, which is typical of this tumor

Utility
- Doppler is useful in assessing tumor vascularity.

CT
Findings
- Solid hypodense mass, with or without calcification, that may occupy large portions of liver on unenhanced CT scans
- Lobulated pattern caused by bands of fibrosis
- Particularly extensive calcification and heterogeneous appearance in mixed hepatoblastoma
- Hyperintense after contrast administration
- Demonstrated invasion of perihepatic vessels or other structures

DIAGNOSTIC PEARLS

- Large right upper quadrant mass with extensive coarse, dense calcification
- Echogenic mass that may have shadowing echogenic foci
- Solid hypodense mass, with or without calcification, that may occupy large portions of the liver
- Hypervascular and, occasionally, a *spoke-wheel* pattern

Utility
- Three-dimensional reconstruction of helical CT data provides important information in the preoperative assessment of patients.
- If shrinkage of the tumor away from the vessel is seen on follow-up three-dimensional CT, then surgery is indicated.
- Advantages over MRI in pediatric abdomen evaluation are shorter scanning times and fewer motion artifacts.

CT Angiography
Findings
- Hypervascular mass, occasionally with *spoke-wheel* pattern, reminiscent of focal nodular hyperplasia
- Hypovascular or avascular zones resulting from hemorrhage possibly occurring within the tumor

Utility
- This technique is useful for surgical planning.

MRI
Findings
- Hyperintense on T2-weighted images and hypointense on T1-weighted images
- Foci of high signal that may be seen on T1-weighted images as a result of hemorrhage
- On T2-weighted images, internal septa corresponding to fibrosis within the tumor appearing as hypointense bands
- Mixed type having a more heterogeneous appearance
- Immediate diffuse (homogeneous or heterogeneous) enhancement followed by rapid washout after intravenous gadolinium administration

Utility
- MRI demonstrates the presence of perihepatic vascular invasion.

WHAT THE REFERRING PHYSICIAN NEEDS TO KNOW
- Hepatoblastoma is associated with Beckwith-Wiedemann syndrome, hemihypertrophy, familial polyposis coli, and Wilms tumor.

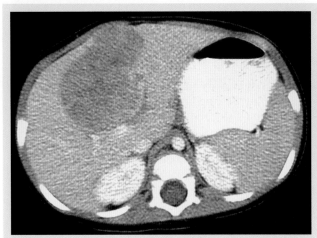

Figure 1. Hepatoblastoma: imaging features. Axial CT image demonstrates a large hypodense mass in the right hepatic lobe.

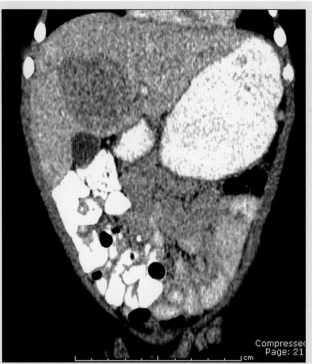

Figure 2. Hepatoblastoma: imaging features. Coronal CT image demonstrates a large hypodense mass in the right hepatic lobe.

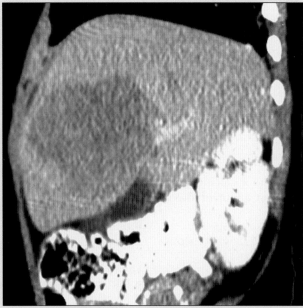

Figure 3. Hepatoblastoma: imaging features. Sagittal CT image demonstrates a large hypodense mass in the right hepatic lobe.

- It is also more accurate than conventional CT in both assessing preoperative tumor extension and in detecting postoperative tumor recurrence.

CLINICAL PRESENTATION

- Abdominal swelling that may be accompanied by anorexia or weight loss
- Rarely, precocious puberty caused by secretion of gonadotropins or testosterone
- Aggressive lung metastases encountered at the time of diagnosis (frequent)
- Markedly elevated serum α-fetoprotein level in most patients

DIFFERENTIAL DIAGNOSIS

- Beckwith-Wiedemann syndrome (fetal syndromes)
- Familial polyposis syndrome (pediatric)
- Wilms tumor (pediatric)
- Mesenchymal hamartoma
- Hepatic mesenchymal hamartoma (fetal liver)
- Meconium peritonitis (neonatal, gastrointestinal)
- Meconium peritonitis (prenatal/neonatal)
- Hemihypertrophy

PATHOLOGY

- Hepatoblastoma is a malignant tumor of hepatocyte origin that often contains mesenchymal elements.
- Microscopically, it can be classified as epithelial or mixed (epithelial-mesenchymal).
- Mixed hepatoblastoma: The epithelial (hepatocyte) component and mesenchymal component consist of primitive mesenchymal tissue and osteoid material or cartilage, or both.
- Epithelial type, particularly if it has fetal hepatocyte predominance, has a better prognosis than other forms.
- Grossly, large, well-circumscribed solitary mass that has nodular or lobulated surface can be seen.
- Epithelial hepatoblastomas are more homogeneous.
- Mixed hepatoblastomas are associated with osteoid and cartilage, large calcifications, fibrotic bands, and an overall more heterogeneous appearance.

INCIDENCE/PREVALENCE AND EPIDEMIOLOGY

- Hepatoblastoma is the most common primary liver neoplasm in childhood.
- It usually develops in the first 3 years of life.
- It may occur at birth or develop in adolescents and young adults.
- Peak incidence is between 18 and 24 months of age.
- Hepatoblastoma is more frequent in boys than in girls.

Suggested Readings

Bates SM, Keller MS, Ramos IM, et al: Hepatoblastoma: Detection of tumor vascularity with duplex Doppler US. *Radiology* 176:505-507, 1990.

Boechat MI, Kangarloo H, Ortega J, et al: Primary liver tumors in children: Comparison of CT and MR imaging. *Radiology* 169:727-732, 1988.

Dachman AH, Parker RL, Ros PR, et al: Hepatoblastoma: A radiologic-pathologic correlation in 50 cases. *Radiology* 164:15-19, 1987.

Davey MS, Cohen MD: Imaging of gastrointestinal malignancy in childhood. *Radiol Clin North Am* 34:717-742, 1996.

Giacomantonio M, Ein SH, Mancer K, et al: Thirty years of experience with pediatric primary malignant liver tumors. *J Pediatr Surg* 19:516-523, 1984.

Helmberger TK, Ros PR, Mergo PJ, et al: Pediatric liver neoplasms: A radiologic-pathologic correlation. *Eur Radiol* 9:1339-1347, 1999.

Kaude JV, Felman AH: Hawkins IF Jr. Ultrasonography in primary hepatic tumors in early childhood. *Pediatr Radiol* 9:77-83, 1980.

Miller JH: The ultrasonographic appearance of cystic hepatoblastoma. *Radiology* 138:141-143, 1981.

Murakami T, Baron RL, Peterson MS, et al: Hepatocellular carcinoma: MR imaging with mangafodipir trisodium (MnDPDP). *Radiology* 200:69-77, 1996.

O'Neil J, Ros PR: Knowing hepatic pathology aids MRI of liver tumors. *Diagn Imaging* 19:58-67, 1989.

Plumley DA, Grosfeld JL, Kopecky KK, et al: The role of spiral (helical) computerized tomography with three-dimensional reconstruction in pediatric solid tumors. *J Pediatr Surg* 30:317-321, 1995.

Powers C, Ros PR, Stoupis C, et al: Primary liver neoplasms: MR imaging with pathologic correlation. *RadioGraphics* 14:459-482, 1994.

Ros PR, Rasmussen JF, Li KCP: Radiology of malignant and benign liver tumors. *Curr Probl Diagn Radiol* 11:95-99, 1989.

Smith WL, Franken EA, Mitros FA: Liver tumors in children. *Semin Roentgenol* 18:136-148, 1983.

Hepatocellular Carcinoma

DEFINITION: Most common primary hepatic tumor.

IMAGING

Radiography
Findings
- Nonspecific upper abdominal mass is seen.
- Calcification is rare.
- Hemochromatosis: Plain films of the extremities demonstrate degenerative changes, with calcium pyrophosphate deposition disease in the cartilages.

Utility
- Plain radiographs are not used to make this diagnosis.

Nuclear Medicine
Findings
- Fluorodeoxyglucose (FDG) *leaking back* to the circulation
- Well-differentiated hepatocellular carcinoma (HCC) tending to show a negative uptake for FDG because of the glucose-6-phosphatase; has uptake of ^{11}C-methionine

Utility
- 30%-50% of HCCs are not FDG avid or are only mildly avid.

Ultrasound
Findings
- Defects are hyperechoic, particularly if a fatty change or a marked sinusoidal dilation is present.
- Small HCCs are seen: hypoechoic and associated with posterior acoustic enhancement.
- Tumors larger than 3 cm more often have a mosaic or mixed pattern.
- Peripheral halo sign is seen.

Utility
- When combined with serum α-fetoprotein assays, it serves as a screening method for high-risk patients with long-standing cirrhosis. This works best in asthenic patients and is very operator dependent.

DIAGNOSTIC PEARLS

- Large, hypodense mass with central areas of lower attenuation is noted.
- Low-intensity, isointensity, and high-intensity patterns are seen on T1-weighted images.
- Presence of internal fibrosis is seen, as well as a dominant histologic pattern.
- Lesions take on a *nodule within a nodule* appearance when small.

- It is capable of demonstrating the capsule in encapsulated HCC.

Ultrasound Doppler
Findings
- Intralesional tangle of vessels, *basket* pattern, in up to 15% of cases, indicating hypervascularity and tumor shunting
- Central pattern of vascularity
- Chaotic vessel dysmorphologic features and washout during the portal venous phase

Utility
- In conjunction with color and duplex Doppler and color Doppler ultrasound, tumor thrombus in the portal and hepatic veins and inferior vena cava can be diagnosed.
- It is also used to assess the vascularity of the HCC.

CT
Findings
- Large, hypodense mass with central areas of lower attenuation
- Early enhancement during arterial phase; relatively hypodense on the delayed-phase images caused by early washout

---

WHAT THE REFERRING PHYSICIAN NEEDS TO KNOW

- Prognosis differs according to the associated condition (e.g., cirrhosis) and the extent of the tumor at the time of diagnosis.
- Encapsulated HCC has a better prognosis because of its greater resectability.
- Tumor cells resemble normal liver cells microscopically, often making it difficult to distinguish normal hepatocytes from cells of HCC.
- Variety of products can be produced by abnormal hepatocytes of HCC: Mallory bodies, α-fetoprotein, α_1-antitrypsin, and other serum proteins.
- Successful treatment of HCCs using any of the available therapies is most likely if the lesion is small.
- Early detection is difficult but critical.
- Most frequent HCC histologic growth pattern is trabecular; tumor cells attempt to recapitulate the cords seen in the normal liver.
- Nonalcoholic steatohepatitis is becoming an important risk factor for the development of hepatocellular carcinoma in obese individuals.

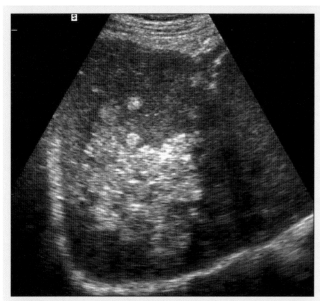

Figure 1. HCC: sonographic features. The neoplasm is strikingly echogenic in this patient. Because of the variable amounts of hemorrhage and necrosis, this tumor can have a variety of sonographic appearances.

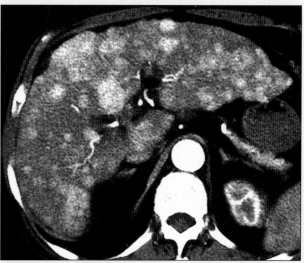

Figure 2. HCC: CT appearance. Contrast-enhanced arterial-phase CT scan of a patient with multifocal HCC. These lesions demonstrate robust enhancement during the hepatic arterial phase. *(Courtesy of Tomoaki Ichikawa, MD, Yamanashi University, Yamanashi, Japan.)*

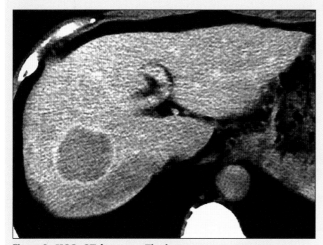

Figure 3. HCC: CT features. The heterogeneous appearance on contrast-enhanced CT scans is suggestive of necrosis. The tumor capsule shows enhancement on the delayed-phase image. *(Courtesy of Tomoaki Ichikawa, MD, Yamanashi University, Yamanashi, Japan.)*

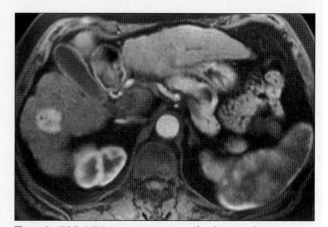

Figure 4. HCC: MRI appearance. A unifocal tumor that is encapsulated is seen in this patient with cirrhosis.

- Small tumors possibly appearing as lesions of different attenuation
- Larger tumor almost always demonstrating central necrosis
- Capsule appearing isodense or hypodense relative to the liver during the hepatic arterial phase, and enhancing on delayed CT images
- Enlarged venous segment that exhibits intraluminal low attenuation, which is highly suggestive of tumor thrombus

Utility
- Multiphasic multidetector CT is an efficient technique for the detection of HCC and preoperative staging of HCC.
- Multiphasic evaluation including noncontrast and arterial scans is essential.
- It depicts complications of HCC, such as hemoperitoneum associated with the rupture of the HCC and vascular invasion.

- It is noninvasive in the evaluation of hepatic arterial anatomy in potential candidates for liver transplantation.

CT Angiography
Findings
- Shows feeding vessels and displays tumor vascularity
- Depicts anatomic variants, which may confound surgery

Utility
- Three-dimensional CT arteriography is comparable to conventional arteriography and surgical findings in the delineation of the major hepatic arteries.
- Three-dimensional CT angiography is safe, convenient, and less invasive than conventional arteriography.

MRI
Findings
- Low-intensity, isointensity, and high-intensity patterns on T1-weighted images
- Hyperintense on T2-weighted images
- *Nodule within a nodule* appearance
- Fibrous capsule that may be demonstrated as a hypointense band on delayed-phase images
- Early enhancement in the hepatic arterial phase, rapidly becoming hypointense as a result of contrast medium washout on delayed phase
- Miliary pattern
- Encapsulated in the homogeneous unifocal tumor

Utility
- MR cholangiopancreatography may occasionally demonstrate that the tumor is causing obstruction or a mass within the biliary tract.
- It can also differentiate small HCCs from regenerative nodules of cirrhosis.
- It depicts vascular invasion.
- Superparamagnetic iron oxide-enhanced MRI is especially helpful in the detection of small HCCs in cirrhotic livers.
- It provides valuable information concerning the internal morphologic features of these lesions.
- Contrast-enhanced MRI is the most sensitive noninvasive imaging test for the diagnosis of hepatocellular carcinoma.

CLINICAL PRESENTATION

- In low-incidence areas, symptoms are insidious in onset and include malaise, fever, and abdominal pain.
- Jaundice is rare.
- Liver function tests are normal, and the results are indistinguishable from those in cirrhosis, except for elevation of the α-fetoprotein level.
- Other proteins produced by HCC give rise to numerous paraneoplastic syndromes, such as erythrocytosis, hypercalcemia, hypoglycemia, hypercholesterolemia, and hirsutism.
- In high-incidence areas, HCC is aggressive and may produce hepatic rupture and massive hemoperitoneum.

DIFFERENTIAL DIAGNOSIS

- Metastases
- Gallbladder carcinoma
- Hemangioma
- Focal nodular hyperplasia
- Lipomatous tumors
- Hepatocellular adenoma
- Fibrolamellar carcinoma

PATHOLOGY

- HCC is the most common primary hepatic tumor and one of the most common visceral malignancies worldwide.
- HCC is a malignant lesion composed of cells that attempt to differentiate into the normal liver, mimicking hepatocyte cords.
- On gross examination, three major patterns of growth are seen: single or massive HCC, nodular or multifocal HCC, and diffuse or cirrhotomimetic HCC.
- Lesion is a soft tumor that frequently undergoes necrosis and hemorrhage because of the lack of stroma; vascular invasion of perihepatic vessels is common.
- Microscopically, HCC cells resemble normal cells, and distinguishing normal hepatocytes from cells of HCC and hepatocellular adenoma is difficult.
- Variety of products produced by the abnormal hepatocytes of HCC are Mallory bodies, α-fetoprotein, α_1-antitrypsin, and other serum proteins.
- Primary etiologic factors in high-incidence areas are hepatitis B and C viruses and exposure to aflatoxins.

INCIDENCE/PREVALENCE AND EPIDEMIOLOGY

- HCC assumes a bimodal geographic distribution in terms of the incidence and clinical presentation.
- It is rare in the Western hemisphere (low-incidence areas) and relatively frequent in sub-Saharan Africa and Asia (high-incidence areas).
- Incidence ranges from 0.9 in 100,000 in women in New York to 30.9 in 100,000 in men of Chinese origin in San Francisco.
- Worldwide, the highest incidence is in Japan, where it is reported to be as high as 4.8%.
- The usual age of presentation in low-incidence areas is 70-80 years, and the male-female ratio is 2.5:1.
- Most patients have a long history of alcoholic cirrhosis, hemochromatosis, or steroid use.
- In high-incidence areas, the age at presentation is 30-45 years, and men are affected eight times more frequently than women.

Suggested Readings

Baron RL, Oliver JH III, Dodd GD III, et al: Hepatocellular carcinoma: Evaluation with biphasic, contrast-enhanced helical CT. *Radiology* 199:505-511, 1996.

Becker CD, Grossholz M, Mentha G, et al: Ablation of hepatocellular carcinoma by percutaneous ethanol injection: Imaging findings. *Cardiovasc Intervent Radiol* 20:204-209, 1997.

Brannigan M, Burns PN, Wilson SR: Blood flow patterns in focal liver lesions at microbubble-enhanced US. *RadioGraphics* 24:921-935, 2004.

Brown JJ, Naylor MJ, Yagan N, et al: Imaging of hepatic cirhosis. *Radiology* 202:1-16, 1997.

Catalano O, Nunziata A, Lobianco R, et al: Real-time harmonic contrast material-specific US of focal liver lesions. *RadioGraphics* 25:333-349, 2005.

Choi BG, Park SH, Byun JY, et al: The findings of ruptured hepatocellular carcinoma on helical CT. *Br J Radiol* 74:142-146, 2001.

Curley SA, Jones DV: Management of hepatocellular carcinoma. In Meyers MA (ed): *Neoplasms of the Digestive Tract: Imaging, Staging, and Management.* Philadelphia, Lippincott-Raven, 1998, pp 347-360.

del Pilar Fernandez M, Redvanley RD: Primary hepatic malignant neoplasms. *Radiol Clin North Am* 36:333-348, 1998.

DeSantis M, Romagnoli R, Cristani A, et al: MRI of small hepatocellular carcinoma: Comparison with US, CT, DSA and Lipiodol-CT. *J Comput Assist Tomogr* 16:189-197, 1992.

Dietrich CF: Characterisation of focal liver lesions with contrast enhanced ultrasonography. *Eur J Radiol* 51(Suppl):S9-S17, 2004.

Earls JP, Theise ND, Weinreb JC, et al: Dysplastic nodules and hepatocellular carcinoma: Thin-section MR imaging of explanted cirrhotic livers with pathologic correlation. *Radiology* 201:207-214, 1996.

Harisinghani MG, Hahn PF: Computed tomography and magnetic resonance imaging evaluation of liver cancer. *Gastroenterol Clin North Am* 31:759-776, 2002.

Ho CL: Clinical PET imaging—an Asian perspective. *Ann Acad Med Singapore* 33:155-165, 2004.

Hussain SM, Zondervan PE, Ijzermans JN, et al: Benign versus malignant hepatic nodules: MR imaging findings with pathologic correlation. *RadioGraphics* 22:1023-1036, 2002.

Jang HJ, Lim JH, Lee SJ, et al: Hepatocellular carcinoma: Are combined CT during arterial portography and CT hepatic arteriography in addition to triple-phase helical CT all necessary for preoperative evaluation. *Radiology* 215:373-380, 2000.

Kanazawa S, Yusui K, Doke T, et al: Hepatic arteriography in patients with hepatocellular carcinoma. *AJR Am J Roentgenol* 147:531-536, 1995.

Kanematsu M, Imaeda T, Yamawaki Y, et al: Rupture of hepatocellular carcinoma: Predictive value of CT findings. *AJR Am J Roentgenol* 158:1247-1250, 1992.

Lencioni R, Pinto F, Armilotta N, et al: Assessment of tumor vascularity in hepatocellular carcinoma: Comparison of power Doppler US and color Doppler US. *Radiology* 201:353-358, 1996.

Mitchell DG, Rubin R, Siegelman ES, et al: Hepatocellular carcinoma within siderotic regenerative nodules: Appearance as a nodule within a nodule on MR images. *Radiology* 178:101-103, 1991.

Nakashima T, Okuda K, Kojiro M, et al: Pathology of HCC in Japan: 232 Consecutive cases autopsied in ten years. *Cancer* 51:863-877, 1983.

Ros PR, Murphy BJ, Buck JL, et al: Encapsulated hepatocellular carcinoma: Radiologic findings and pathologic correlation. *Gastrointest Radiol* 15:233-237, 1990.

Sadek AG, Mitchell DG, Siegelman ES, et al: Early hepatocellular carcinoma that develops within macroregenerative nodules: Growth depicted at serial MR imaging. *Radiology* 195:753-756, 1995.

Shimamoto K, Sakuma S, Ishigaki T, et al: Hepatocellular carcinoma: Evaluation with color Doppler US and MR imaging. *Radiology* 182:149-153, 1992.

Yu SC, Yeung DT, So NM: Imaging features of hepatocellular carcinoma. *Clin Radiol* 59:145-156, 2004.

Intrahepatic Cholangiocarcinoma

DEFINITION: Large, firm mass with large amounts of whitish, fibrous tissue that originates in the small intrahepatic ducts.

IMAGING

Radiography
Findings
- Large upper abdominal mass may be seen.

Utility
- Plain radiographs are not used to establish this diagnosis.

Nuclear Medicine
Findings
- Large defect is seen.
- Signs of cirrhosis are present in 20% of patients with intrahepatic cholangiocarcinoma.
- Defect without late uptake is seen, reflecting the markedly hypovascular nature of this tumor.

Utility
- Nuclear medicine studies are usually not employed in making the diagnosis.

Ultrasound
Findings
- Homogeneous mass that is usually hypoechoic
- Possibly satellite nodules
- Calcified foci demonstrating as high-level echoes with acoustic shadowing
- Slightly hyperperfused on color Doppler ultrasound studies
- In arterial phase of contrast-enhanced sonography, variable perfusion picture but mainly hyperperfused
- In late portal venous phase, tumor contrasting as punched-out defects

Utility
- Sensitivity: 35%-70%
- Specificity: 50%-80%

CT
Findings
- Homogeneous, hypodense mass on unenhanced CT
- After contrast injection, early peripheral enhancement with delayed and persistent central enhancement
- Retraction of overlying liver capsule
- Small areas of necrosis, hemorrhage, mucin, central scar, and calcification within the tumor
- Biliary dilation adjacent to the tumor as another finding in 20% of cases

DIAGNOSTIC PEARLS

- Homogeneous mass that is usually hypoechoic with satellite nodules
- Slightly hyperperfused in color Doppler ultrasound studies
- Early peripheral enhancement with delayed, persistent, central enhancement
- Large mass of decreased signal intensity on T1-weighted images and increased signal on T2-weighted images

- Extension through hepatic capsule and invasion of organs adjacent to liver (common)
- Hypovascular with small, thin vessels corresponding to fibrous nature of the tumor

Utility
- Sensitivity: 70%-90%
- Specificity: 65%-90%

MRI
Findings
- Mass of decreased signal intensity on T1-weighted images and increased signal on T2-weighted images
- Central area of hypointensity in some cases on T2-weighted images corresponding to the central scar
- Larger intrahepatic cholangiocarcinoma (>4 cm) showing peripheral enhancement that slowly progresses centripetally and spares the central scar
- Smaller lesions (2-4 cm) enhancing homogeneously
- Satellite nodules, invasion of portal vein, and dilation of intrahepatic bile ducts distal to the lesion

Utility
- Sensitivity: 75%-85%
- Specificity: 70%-90%

CLINICAL PRESENTATION

- Signs and symptoms are related to site of origin of the tumor.
- Symptoms are vague until the tumor is far advanced.
- Abdominal pain and palpable mass in upper abdomen may occur.

WHAT THE REFERRING PHYSICIAN NEEDS TO KNOW
- Clinical signs and symptoms are related to the site of origin of the tumor.
- Central tumors become symptomatic earlier than more peripheral tumors.

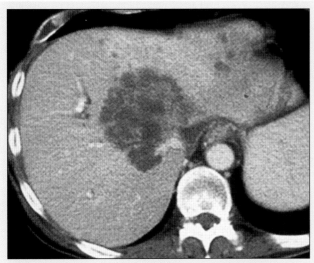

Figure 1. Intrahepatic cholangiocarcinoma: CT features. This lesion does not enhance on the portal-venous-phase image.

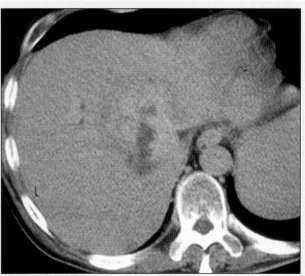

Figure 2. Intrahepatic cholangiocarcinoma: CT features. Significant contrast enhancement, with the exception of the central scar, is present on the 10-minute delayed scan.

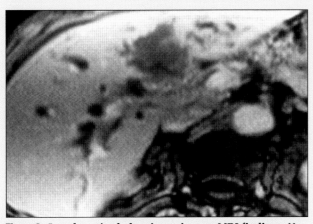

Figure 3. Intrahepatic cholangiocarcinoma: MRI findings. No significant enhancement of the tumor is noted on the early-phase scan.

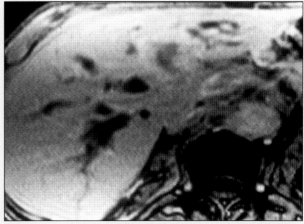

Figure 4. Intrahepatic cholangiocarcinoma: MRI findings. On the 10-minute delayed scan, enhancement of the tumor is seen, with the exception of the central scar.

- Jaundice is rarely a presenting symptom.
- Patients with extrahepatic cholangiocarcinomas typically present earlier with obstructive jaundice.

DIFFERENTIAL DIAGNOSIS

- Metastases
- Fibrolamellar carcinoma
- Hepatocellular carcinoma
- Abscess

PATHOLOGY

- Intrahepatic cholangiocarcinoma is an adenocarcinoma of biliary duct origin.
- It originates in the small intrahepatic ducts.
- Grossly, these neoplasms are large, firm masses.

- Cut section reveals the presence of large amounts of whitish, fibrous tissue, with rare internal areas of necrosis and hemorrhage.
- Microscopically, the adenocarcinoma has a glandular appearance with cells resembling biliary epithelium; mucin and calcification can often be demonstrated.
- Large amount of desmoplastic reaction is typical of cholangiocarcinoma.

INCIDENCE/PREVALENCE AND EPIDEMIOLOGY

- Ten percent of all cholangiocarcinomas
- Second most common primary hepatic malignancy in adults
- Occurring usually in the seventh decade of life, with a slight male predominance

Suggested Readings

Adjei ON, Tamura S, Sugimura H, et al: Contrast-enhanced MR imaging of intrahepatic cholangiocarcinoma. *Clin Radiol* 50:6-10, 1995.

Buetow PC, Buck JL, Pantongrag-Brown L, et al: Biliary cystadenoma and cystadenocarcinoma: Clinical-imaging-pathologic correlation with emphasis on the importance of ovarian stroma. *Radiology* 196:805-810, 1995.

Carr DH, Hadjis NS, Banks LM, et al: Computed tomography of hilar cholangiocarcinoma: A new sign. *AJR Am J Roentgenol* 145:53-56, 1985.

Choi BI, Han JK, Kim TK: Diagnosis and staging of cholangiocarcinoma by computed tomography. In Meyers MA (ed): *Neoplasms of the Digestive Tract: Imaging, Staging, and Management.* Philadelphia, Lippincott-Raven, 1998, pp 503-516.

Fan ZM, Yamashita Y, Harada M, et al: Intrahepatic cholangiocarcinoma: Spin-echo and contrast-enhanced dynamic MR imaging. *AJR Am J Roentgenol* 161:313-317, 1993.

Ishak KG, Willis GW, Cummins SD, et al: Biliary cystadenoma and cystadenocarcinoma. Report of 14 cases and review of the literature. *Cancer* 39:322-338, 1977.

Itai Y, Araki T, Furui S, et al: Computed tomography of primary intrahepatic biliary malignancy. *Radiology* 147:485-490, 1983.

Meyers MA: Cholangiocarcinoma: Imaging, staging, and management. In Meyers MA (ed): *Neoplasms of the Digestive Tract: Imaging, Staging, and Management.* Philadelphia, Lippincott-Raven, 1998, pp 150-183.

Murphy BJ, Casillas J, Ros PR, et al: The CT appearance of cystic masses of the liver. *RadioGraphics* 9:307-322, 1989.

Ros PR, Rasmussen JF, Li KCP: Radiology of malignant and benign liver tumors. *Curr Probl Diagn Radiol* 11:95-99, 1989.

Soyer P, Bluemke DA, Reichle R, et al: Imaging of cholangiocarcinoma: 1. Peripheral cholangiocarcinoma. *AJR Am J Roentgenol* 165:1427-1431, 1995.

Wheeler DA, Edmondson HA: Cystadenoma with mesenchymal stroma (CMS) in the liver and bile ducts. A clinicopathologic study of 17 cases, 4 with malignant change. *Cancer* 56:1434-1445, 1985.

Yu SC, Yeung DT, So NM: Imaging features of hepatocellular carcinoma. *Clin Radiol* 59:145-156, 2004.

Lymphoma (Gastrointestinal)

DEFINITION: Lymphoma can be either primary or secondary and can occur in both Hodgkin disease and non-Hodgkin lymphoma.

IMAGING

Radiography
Findings
- Hepatomegaly is seen.
- Calcifications are not detected in untreated lymphoma.

Utility
- Barium studies may demonstrate other involved areas in the gut.

Ultrasound
Findings
- Tumoral form: hypoechoic mass or masses
- Diffuse form: hepatic parenchyma echogenicity that may be normal or overall liver architecture that may be altered

Utility
- Ultrasound is inferior to CT in showing extent of gastrointestinal and nodal tumor involvement.

CT
Findings
- Multiple well-defined, large, homogeneous low-density masses
- Lymphomatous liver mass that is usually hypovascular or avascular
- Arterial displacement and encasement not noted
- In capillary phase, a relatively hypolucent tumor mass

Utility
- CT is the preferred imaging method for evaluating lymphoma of the liver, with specificity of almost 90% and sensitivity of almost 60%.
- Angiography is used.

MRI
Findings
- Hypointense compared with the normal liver on T1-weighted images and hyperintense on T2-weighted images
- After intravenous contrast administration, transient perilesional enhancement
- Tumors remaining hypointense during the dynamic study as a result of their poor vascularity

Utility
- MRI is more accurate than CT in depicting hepatic and splenic involvement.

PET
Findings
- PET and PET-CT show increased activity in lymphomatous deposits in the liver, other solid parenchymal organs, and lymph nodes.

Utility
- PET-CT has become an important method of staging non-Hodgkin lymphoma and Hodgkin disease.

DIAGNOSTIC PEARLS
- Lymphoma produces multiple well-defined, large, homogeneous low-density masses.
- In the capillary phase, the tumor mass is relatively hypolucent.
- Tumor is hypointense compared with the normal liver on T1-weighted images and hyperintense on T2-weighted images.

CLINICAL PRESENTATION
- Patients may exhibit right upper quadrant pain, hepatomegaly, or tender upper abdominal mass.
- Hepatomegaly may occur in an uninvolved liver, and a diffusely infiltrated liver can be of normal size.

DIFFERENTIAL DIAGNOSIS
- Ménétrier disease
- Antral gastritis
- Malignant gastrointestinal stromal tumors
- *Helicobacter pylori* gastritis
- Hypertrophic gastritis
- Kaposi sarcoma
- Portal hypertensive gastropathy
- Duodenal ulcers
- Zollinger-Ellison syndrome and peptic ulcer disease
- Gastric adenocarcinoma

PATHOLOGY
- Lymphoma can be either primary or secondary and can manifest as either Hodgkin disease (HD) or non-Hodgkin lymphoma (NHL).
- Majority of lymphomas of the liver are secondary; primary lymphoma is rare.
- Secondary lymphoma of the liver is found in more than 50% of patients with NHL.
- Grossly, nodular and diffuse forms of hepatic lymphoma are seen.
- In patients with HD, a Reed-Sternberg variant type of cell is accepted as evidence for liver involvement.
- In NHL, the lymphocytic form tends to be miliary, whether large cell or histiocytic varieties are nodular or tumoral.
- In both HD and NHL, the initial involvement is seen in portal areas because of scant lymphatic tissue of liver.

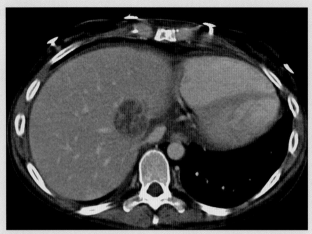

Figure 1. Hepatic lymphoma. Contrast-enhanced CT scan shows a lesion with heterogeneous low attenuation in the right hepatic lobe.

INCIDENCE/PREVALENCE AND EPIDEMIOLOGY

- Primary hepatic lymphoma occurs most commonly in middle-aged white men.
- Organ transplant recipients and patients with acquired immunodeficiency syndrome are at high risk for developing hepatic lymphoma.

Suggested Readings

Ben Haim S, Bar-Shalom R, Israel O, et al: Liver involvement in lymphoma: Role of gallium-67 scintigraphy. *J Nucl Med* 36: 900-904, 1995.

Biemer JJ: Hepatic manifestations of lymphoma. *Ann Clin Lab* 14:252-260, 1984.

Bruneton JN, Schnider M: *Radiology of Lymphoma.* New York, Springer-Verlag, 1986.

Castellino RA, Hoppe RT, Blank N, et al: Computed tomography, lymphography and staging laparotomy in colon correlations in staging of Hodgkin disease. *AJR Am J Roentgenol* 143:37-41, 1984.

Ginaldi S, Bernardino ME, Jing BS: Patterns of hepatic lymphoma. *Radiology* 136:427-431, 1980.

Golding SJ, Fletcher EWL: The radiology of secondary malignant neoplasms of the liver. In Wilkins RA, Nunnerly HB (eds): *Imaging of the Liver, Pancreas and Spleen.* Oxford, Blackwell Scientific Publications, 1990, pp 198-219.

Goodman ZD: Nonparenchymal and metastatic malignant tumors of the liver. In Haubrich WS, Schaffner F, Berk JE (eds): *Bockus Gastroenterology.* Philadelphia, WB Saunders, 1995, pp 2488-2500.

Jaffe ES: Malignant lymphoma. Pathology of hepatic involvement. *Semin Liver Dis* 7:257-268, 1987.

Kelekis NL, Semelka RC, Siegelman ES, et al: Focal hepatic lymphoma: Magnetic resonance demonstration using current techniques including gadolinium enhancement. *Magn Reson Imaging* 15:625-636, 1997.

Shirkhoda A, Ros PR, Farah J, et al: Lymphoma of the solid abdominal viscera. *Radiol Clin North Am* 28:785-799, 1990.

Weiss L, Gilbert HA: *Liver Metastases.* Boston, GK Hall, 1992.

Weissleder R, Stark DD, Elizondo G: MRI of hepatic lymphoma. *Magn Reson Imaging* 6:675-681, 1988.

Wilson MA: Metastatic disease of the liver. In Wilson MA, Ruzicka FF (eds): *Modern Imaging of the Liver.* New York, Marcel Dekker, 1989, pp 631-659.

Yamamoto H, Yamashita Y, Yoshimatsu S, et al: Hepatocellular carcinoma in cirrhotic livers: Detection with unenhanced and iron-oxide enhanced MR imaging. *Radiology* 195:106-112, 1995.

Zornoza J, Ginaldi S: Computed tomography in hepatic lymphoma. *Radiology* 138:405-410, 1981.

Metastases to the Liver

DEFINITION: Most common cause of malignant focal liver lesions.

IMAGING

Radiography
Findings
- Nonspecific findings include hepatomegaly, ascites, and splenomegaly.
- Calcification is a more specific sign but is insensitive.
- Colloid carcinomas of the colon or stomach are the most common cause; calcification is described as stippled, amorphous, flaky, punctate, granular, or poppy seed-like.

Utility
- Plain radiographs of the abdomen in metastatic disease are most commonly normal.

PET
Findings
- ^{18}F-fluorodeoxyglucose (FDG): a glucose analog that is metabolized more rapidly in tumor cells than normal cells, resulting in increased uptake in malignant lesions

Utility
- PET is a very sensitive tool for the detection of liver metastases.
- It yields poor spatial resolution, hence the complementary anatomic information from cross-sectional imaging techniques such as CT is necessary.
- PET and CT combine metabolic imaging and spatial localization; the advantages of PET and CT are a very effective solution.
- ^{18}F-FDG uptake of inflammatory lesion makes clinical correlation necessary to assess the significance of the PET findings.
- Uptake may not be significantly increased in metastatic mucinous tumors.

Ultrasound
Findings
- Hyperechoic metastasis
- Bull's-eye or target pattern
- Hypoechoic metastases
- Cystic metastases
- Calcified metastases
- Diffuse infiltration

Utility
- Intraoperative ultrasound has a diagnostic sensitivity of over 90% in the detection of metastases.

DIAGNOSTIC PEARLS

- *Doughnut, target, halo,* and *light-bulb* signs on MRI
- Hypervascularity or hypovascularity depending on the vascularity of the primary tumor
- Increased FDG uptake on PET scan

- Transabdominal ultrasound has sensitivity, specificity, accuracy.

CT
Findings
- Lesions are seen as hyperdense, isodense, and hypodense, with peripheral enhancement, cystic, complex, calcified, or diffusely infiltrating.
- Majority of metastases are hypodense.
- Some metastases will show hypoattenuating peripheral areas surrounding an enhanced center on delayed image.
- Calcifications are seen.
- Rim enhancement is seen: vascularized viable tumor periphery contrasted with a hypovascular or necrotic center.
- Hypodense lesions are best depicted during the portal phase of enhancement (60 seconds after intravenous contrast).

Utility
- Sensitivity: 75%-95%
- Specificity: 85%-95%
- Accuarcy: 87%

MRI
Findings
- Hypervascular lesions are best seen during the arterial phase of enhancement.
- T1 and T2 relaxation times that are longer than those of normal liver and shorter than those of simple cysts or hemangiomas
- *Doughnut* sign
- *Target* sign
- *Halo* sign

Utility
- MRI is used in the delineation of the precise number and location of metastases and their relationship to adjacent vascular structures.

WHAT THE REFERRING PHYSICIAN NEEDS TO KNOW

- When only a single defect is seen, it must be differentiated from a normal variant, cyst, abscess, or intrahepatic gallbladder.
- Multiple defects make the diagnosis of metastases likely; however, occasionally, multiple cysts, hemangiomas, or abscesses may have the same appearance.
- Imaging is the key to both the diagnosis and serial follow-up of liver metastases.

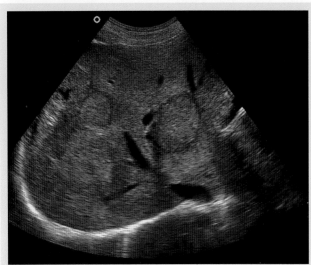

Figure 1. Hepatic metastases: spectrum of sonographic findings. *Bull's-eye* lesions are present on this axial scan in a patient with metastatic lung cancer.

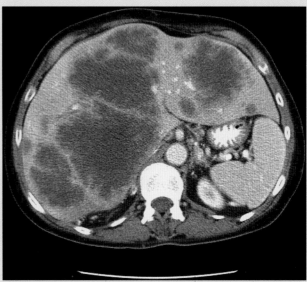

Figure 2. Hypovascular liver metastases on CT. Multiple large, hypodense masses are present in both lobes of the liver. These lesions do show uniform rim enhancement.

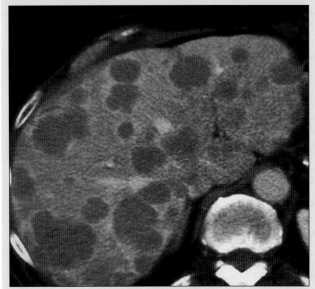

Figure 3. Ring enhancement of liver metastases on CT. Portal-venous-phase image shows a hypervascular ring of enhancement. This complete ring of enhancement is typical of metastases but can also be seen in hepatic abscesses.

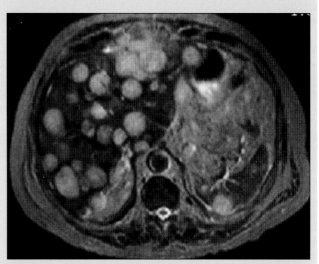

Figure 4. Liver metastases: MRI features. Most metastases have prolonged T1 and T2 relaxation times compared with normal liver. Thus these lesions have high signal intensity on T2-weighted images.

- It is also helpful in assessing tumor vascularity and the degree of necrosis.
- Sensitivity: 80%-100%
- Specificity: 85%-100%
- Accuracy: 92%

CLINICAL PRESENTATION

- Hepatomegaly is the most common finding, followed by ascites, jaundice, and varices.

- Liver function tests are notoriously unreliable for detecting metastases; these tests are normal in 25%-50% of cases.

DIFFERENTIAL DIAGNOSIS

- Multifocal hepatoma
- Focal regions of hepatic steatosis
- Multiple hepatic adenomas, hemangiomas, or focal nodular hyperplasia
- Transient hepatic attenuation differences

PATHOLOGY

- Metastases vary in size, consistency, uniformity of growth, stromal response, and vascularity; they can also be infiltrative or expansive.
- Metastatic adenocarcinomas show a slimy cut surface because of mucin production; expanding and massive tumors with central liquefactive necrosis can also be seen.
- Metastases have significant necrosis or fibrosis (or both) and can umbilicate the surface of the liver capsule.
- Poorly differentiated tumors (seminomas, oat cell carcinomas, undifferentiated sarcomas) are uniformly soft and take on a *fish flesh–like* consistency.
- Squamous cell carcinomas have a granular and caseous central portion that lacks the shiny appearance of most adenocarcinomas.
- Most metastases maintain the microscopic features of the primary tumor, including the degree of stromal growth.
- Metastases that penetrate the large portal veins disseminate throughout the peripheral portal branches; pulmonary metastases develop when the hepatic veins are penetrated.

INCIDENCE/PREVALENCE AND EPIDEMIOLOGY

- Liver metastases are the most common cause of malignant focal liver lesions, outnumbering primary malignant tumors by a factor of 18:1.
- Colon (42%), stomach (23%), pancreas (21%), breast (14%), and lung (13%) are the most common primary neoplasms.
- Liver is second only to the regional lymph nodes as metastatic disease site.
- Highest percentage of liver metastases occurs in primary carcinoma of gallbladder, pancreas, colon, and breast and lowest in prostate cancer.
- Many of these patients have good survival rates of 20%-40% at 5 years if resection of the liver metastases is performed.

Suggested Readings

Abbitt PL: Ultrasonography: Update on liver technique. *Radiol Clin North Am* 36:299-308, 1998.

Baker ME, Pelley R: Hepatic metastases: Basic principles and implications for radiologists. *Radiology* 197:329-337, 1995.

Baker SR: *The Abdominal Plain Film.* East Norwalk, CT, Appleton & Lange, 1990, pp 243–298.

Baron RL, Oliver JH III, Dodd GD III, et al: Hepatocellular carcinoma: Evaluation with biphasic, contrast-enhanced helical CT. *Radiology* 199:505-511, 1996.

Bipat S, van Leeuwen MS, Comans EFI, et al: Colorectal liver metastases: CT, MR imaging, and PET for diagnosis: Meta-analysis. *Radiology* 237:123-131, 2005.

Delbeke D, Vitola JV, Sandler MP, et al: Staging recurrent metastatic colorectal carcinoma with PET. *J Nucl Med* 38:1196-1201, 1997.

Dolan PA: Tumor calcification following therapy. *AJR Am J Roentgenol* 89:166-168, 1963.

Drane WE: Nuclear medicine techniques for the liver and biliary system. *Radiol Clin North Am* 29:1129-1149, 1991.

Federle MP, Filly RA, Moss AA: Cystic hepatic neoplasms: Complementary roles of computed tomography and sonography. *AJR Am J Roentgenol* 136:345-348, 1980.

Findlay M, Young H, Cunningham D, et al: Noninvasive monitoring of tumor metabolism using fluorodeoxyglucose and positron emission tomography in colorectal cancer liver metastases: Correlation with tumor response to fluorouracil. *J Clin Oncol* 14:700-708, 1997.

Friedman AC, Fishman EK, Radecki PD, et al: Focal disease. In Friedman AC (ed): *Radiology of the Liver, Biliary Tract, Pancreas and Spleen.* Baltimore, Williams & Wilkins, 1987, pp 151-264.

Goldberg MA, Lee MJ, Fischman AJ, et al: Fluorodeoxyglucose PET of abdominal and pelvic neoplasms: Potential role in oncologic imaging. *RadioGraphics* 13:1047-1062, 1993.

Goldberg MA, Saini S, Hahn PF, et al: Differentiation between hemangiomas and metastases of the liver with ultrafast MR imaging: Preliminary results with T2 calculations. *AJR Am J Roentgenol.* 157:727-730, 1991.

Gore RM, Goldberg HI: Plain film and cholangiographic findings in liver tumors. *Semin Roentgenol* 18:87-93, 1983.

Hahn PF: Liver specific MR imaging contrast agents. *Radiol Clin North Am* 36:287-298, 1998.

Kinnard MF, Alavi A, Rubin RP, et al: Nuclear imaging of solid hepatic masses. *Semin Roentgenol* 30:375-395, 1995.

Lee MJ, Saini S, Compton CC: MR demonstration of edema adjacent to a liver metastasis: Pathologic correlation. *AJR Am J Roentgenol* 157:499-501, 1991.

Lewis KH, Chezmar JL: Hepatic metastases. *MRI Clin North Am* 5:319-330, 1997.

Marn CS, Bree RL, Silver TM: Ultrasonography of liver: Technique and focal and diffuse disease. *Radiol Clin North Am* 29:1151-1170, 1991.

Niesenbaum HL, Rowling SE: Ultrasound of focal hepatic lesions. *Semin Roentgenol* 30:324-346, 1995.

Oliver JH 3rd, Baron RL, Federle MP, et al: Hypervascular liver metastases: Do unenhanced and hepatic arterial phase CT images affect tumor detection? *Radiology* 205:709-715, 1997.

Pedro MS, Semelka RC, Braga L: *MR imaging of hepatic metastases. Magn Reson Imaging Clin North Am* 10:15-29, 2002.

Semelka RC: Liver. In Semelka RC, Ascher SM, Reinhold C (eds): *MRI of the Abdomen and Pelvis.* New York, Wiley-Liss, 1997, pp 19-136.

Semelka RA, Mitchell DG: Liver and biliary system. In Edelman RR, Hesselink JR, Zlatkin MB (eds): *Clinical Magnetic Resonance Imaging,* 2nd ed. Philadelphia, WB Saunders, 1996, pp 1466-1512.

Seneterre E, Taourel P, Bouvier Y, et al: Detection of hepatic metastases. Ferumoxides-enhanced MR imaging versus unenhanced MR imaging and CT during arterial portography. *Radiology* 200:785-792, 1996.

Sica GT, Ji H, Ros PR: CT and MR imaging of hepatic metastases. *AJR Am J Roentgenol* 174:691-698, 2000.

Amebic Abscesses

DEFINITION: Amebic abscess refers to invasion and destruction of the liver parenchyma infected by *Entamoeba histolytica.*

ANATOMIC FINDINGS

Liver
- Amebic abscesses are most often solitary (85%) and affect the right lobe more often (72%) than the left lobe (13%).

IMAGING

Nuclear Medicine
Findings
- Cold lesion with hot periphery is diagnostic for an amebic abscess.

Utility
- Not routinely used for detection of hepatic amebic abscess
- Sulfur colloid hepatobiliary scintiscans

Ultrasound
Findings
- Round or oval, sharply defined, hypoechoic mass with homogeneous, fine, low-level echoes and distal acoustic enhancement

Utility
- CT and MRI are usually employed to establish the diagnosis.

CT
Findings
- Peripheral, round, or oval areas of low attenuation (10-20 HU)
- Peripheral rim of slightly higher attenuation on non-contrast scans and marked enhancement after the administration of contrast material
- Unilocular or multilocular with nodular margins
- Peripheral zone of edema around the abscess (also common and characteristic for this lesion)

Utility
- Variable and nonspecific
- Sensitivity: 85%-98%

DIAGNOSTIC PEARLS
- Cold lesion with hot periphery on scintigram is diagnostic for amebic abscess.
- Round or oval, sharply defined, hypoechoic mass is seen, with homogeneous, fine, low-level echoes and distal acoustic enhancement on ultrasound.
- Peripheral rim of slightly higher attenuation on noncontrast scans and marked enhancement after the administration of contrast material are seen.

- Specificity: 80%-95%
- Accuracy: 93%

MRI
Findings
- Spherical and usually solitary lesion, with central T2 hyperintensity corresponding to T1 hypointensity
- Diffuse central inhomogeneity and edema on normal surrounding parenchyma on T2-weighted image
- Homogeneously hypointense on T2-weighted image after treatment
- Successful treatment possibly showing concentric rings of different signal intensity surrounding lesion on T2-weighted image
- Abscess wall thick with postgadolinium enhancement pattern, similar to that of pyogenic abscess

Utility
- Sensitivity: 90%-95%
- Specificity: 85%-95%
- Accuracy: 94%

CLINICAL PRESENTATION
- Patients exhibit a tender liver and right upper quadrant pain.
- Diarrhea and hepatomegaly may occur.
- Amebae are not found in the stool of most patients with an amebic liver abscess.

WHAT THE REFERRING PHYSICIAN NEEDS TO KNOW
- If the abscess is not treated, it may rupture into the peritoneum, pleural cavity, lung, or pericardium.
- Primary role of percutaneous aspiration and drainage in these patients is the diagnosis and treatment of superimposed bacterial infection.
- With nonspecific or negative clinical features and stool examination, serologic tests are particularly needed for diagnosis.

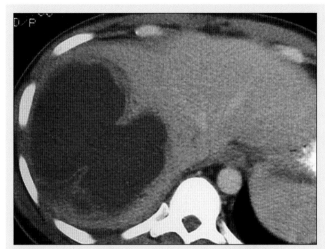

Figure 1. **Amebic abscess: CT features.** A large unilocular mass with an enhancing wall demonstrates a thin peripheral hypoattenuating rim of surrounding edema that is typical of amebic abscesses.

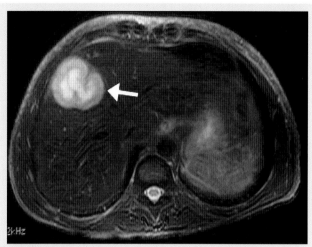

Figure 2. **Amebic abscess: MRI features.** T2-weighted image shows the hyperintense center and the relatively less hyperintense abscess wall *(arrow)*. (*Courtesy of N. Cem Balci, MD, Saint Louis University, St. Louis, MO.*)

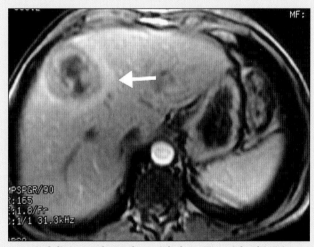

Figure 3. **Amebic abscess: MRI features.** Gadolinium-enhanced arterial-phase T1-weighted MR image shows the hypointense center. In this phase, the wall does not enhance. Note the enhancing inflamed liver parenchyma surrounding the abscess *(arrow)*. (*Courtesy of N. Cem Balci, MD, Saint Louis University, St. Louis, MO.*)

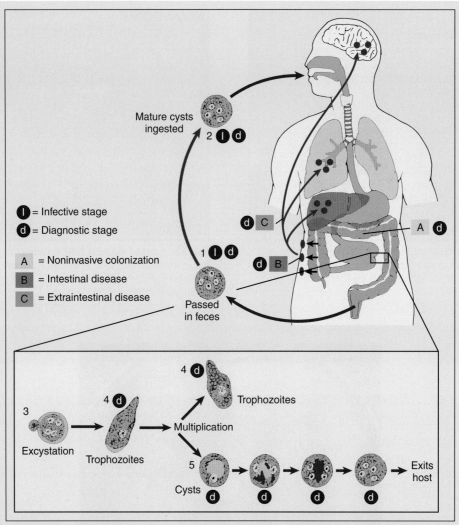

Figure 4. Amebiasis: pathologic findings. Life cycle: Cysts are passed in feces (1). Infection by *E. histolytica* occurs by the ingestion of mature cysts (2) in fecally contaminated food, water, or hands. Excystation (3) occurs in the small intestine, and trophozoites (4) are released, which migrate to the large intestine. The trophozoites multiply by binary fission and produce cysts (5), which are passed in the feces (1). Because of the protection conferred by their walls, the cysts can survive days to weeks in the external environment and are responsible for transmission. (Trophozoites can also be passed in diarrheal stools, but they are rapidly destroyed once outside the body and, if ingested, would not survive exposure to the gastric environment.) In many cases, the trophozoites remain confined to the intestinal lumen (A: noninvasive infection) of individuals who are asymptomatic carriers, passing cysts in their stool. In some patients, the trophozoites invade the intestinal mucosa (B: intestinal disease), through the bloodstream, or extraintestinal sites such as the liver, brain, and lungs (C: extraintestinal disease), with resultant pathologic manifestations. It has been established that the invasive and noninvasive forms represent two separate species, respectively, *E. histolytica* and *E. dispar;* however, not all persons infected with *E. histolytica* will have invasive disease. These two species are morphologically indistinguishable. Transmission can also occur through fecal exposure during sexual contact (in which case not only cysts, but also trophozoites might prove infective). (*From Centers for Disease Control and Prevention. Available at: http://www.cdc.gov/Ncidod/parasites.*)

- Indirect hemagglutination test is positive in more than 90% of these patients.
- Pleuropulmonary amebiasis is characterized by a pulmonary consolidation or abscess, serous effusion, empyema, or hepatobronchial fistula in 20%-35% of patients.

DIFFERENTIAL DIAGNOSIS

- Pyogenic abscess
- Necrotic metastasis
- Necrotic hepatoma
- Necrotic adenoma

PATHOLOGY

- Cystic form of *E. histolytica* gains access to the body via oral ingestion of infected material, usually contaminated water.
- Liver is invaded via the portal vein, through lymphatics, or via direct extension through the colon wall, peritoneum, and liver capsule.

- Thrombosis and infarction of small areas of hepatic parenchyma (amebic hepatitis) occur.
- Coalition of multiple small areas of ischemic necrosis and amebic destruction of hepatic parenchymal cells is seen.

INCIDENCE/PREVALENCE AND EPIDEMIOLOGY

- Ten percent of the world's population is infected with *E. histolytica,* and 3%-7% has amebic liver abscess.
- *E. histolytica* has been isolated in the stool of up to 30% of sexually active homosexual men.
- Eighty-five to ninety percent of amebic liver abscesses occur in men.

Suggested Readings

Elizondo G, Weissleder R, Stark DD, et al: Amebic liver abscess: Diagnosis and treatment evaluation with MR imaging. *Radiology* 165:795-800, 1987.

Fujihara T, Nagai Y, Kuba T, et al: Amebic liver abscess. *J Gastroenterol* 31:659-663, 1996.

Reed SL: Amebiasis: An update. *Clin Infect Dis* 14:385-393, 1992.

Bacterial (Pyogenic) Hepatic Abscesses

DEFINITION: Abscess formation in the liver secondary to bacterial infection.

IMAGING

Ultrasound
Findings
- Spherical or ovoid but possibly lobulated or lentiform, variable mural thickness, irregular and hypoechoic wall
- Anechoic (50%), hyperechoic (25%), or hypoechoic (25%) with septa, fluid-fluid levels, internal debris, and posterior acoustic enhancement
- Echogenic and poorly demarcated early lesions, then evolving into well-demarcated, nearly anechoic lesions
- Gas in abscess appearing as brightly echogenic reflectors with posterior reverberation
Utility
- Ultrasound detects hepatic abscesses as small as 1.5 cm, with a sensitivity of 75%-90%.

CT
Findings
- Hypodense rounded masses on both contrast and non-contrast scans (0-45 HU)
- Enhancing peripheral rim or capsule
- Small, pyogenic abscesses appearing to cluster or aggregate (*cluster* sign)
- Central gas either as air bubbles or air-fluid level
- Large air-fluid or fluid-debris level is often associated with communication with the gut.
- Presence of central gas is a specific sign but is present in fewer than 20% of cases.
Utility
- CT is the single best method for detecting hepatic abscess; sensitivity is 97%.

MRI
Findings
- Abscesses showing rim enhancement (*double target* sign)
- Fast and intense wall enhancement that persists on portal-venous-phase and late-phase images
- Perilesional edema: high signal on T2-weighted images, associated with 50% of abscesses
- Small lesions (< 1 cm) may enhance homogeneously, mimicking hemangiomas.
- Abscess wall enhancement on dynamic postgadolinium images may be considered as a distinctive feature of pyogenic liver abscesses.

DIAGNOSTIC PEARLS
- Hypodense rounded masses on both contrast and noncontrast scans (0-45 HU) on CT
- Postgadolinium showing rim enhancement (*double target* sign) on MRI
- Presence of central gas

- Perilesional edema can be used to differentiate hepatic abscess from benign cystic hepatic lesion.
- Resolution of perilesional edema may indicate response to therapy.
Utility
- Limitations include high cost and lack of easy access for drainage procedures.
- MR cholangiopancreatography is an important tool in diagnosing obstructive biliary tract lesions.
- Sensitivity: 85%-100%
- Specificity: 85%-95%
- Accuracy: 93%

Interventional Radiology
Findings
- An obstructed and/or stone-containing biliary system is identified.
- Communication with an abscess cavity may be visualized.
Utility
- Cholangiography is an important aid in the diagnosis of ascending cholangitis.
- Percutaneous transhepatic cholangiography and endoscopic retrograde cholangiography can define the level and cause of biliary obstruction and biliary anatomy for the surgeon.

CLINICAL PRESENTATION
- Fever, malaise, pain, rigors, nausea and vomiting, and weight loss
- Tender hepatomegaly, leukocytosis, elevated serum alkaline phosphatase levels, hypoalbuminemia, and prolonged prothrombin time

---

WHAT THE REFERRING PHYSICIAN NEEDS TO KNOW
- All imaging findings are nonspecific and require aspiration for diagnosis and treatment.
- Aspiration is sufficient as treatment if the abscess is unilocular, well demarcated, less than 3 cm in diameter, and without extrahepatic communication.

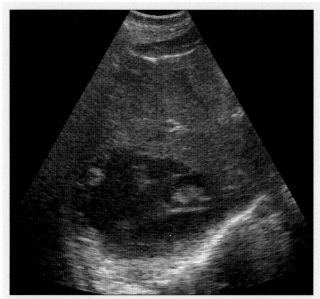

Figure 1. Pyogenic liver abscess: sonographic features. Transverse sonogram of the liver shows a complex, predominantly hypoechoic mass with posterior acoustic enhancement containing coarse, clumpy debris.

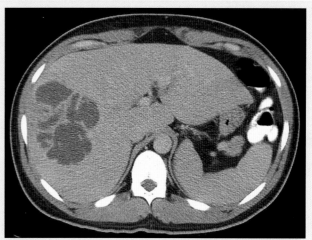

Figure 2. Pyogenic liver abscess: CT findings. Axial image shows the classic *cluster* sign of a multiloculated pyogenic liver abscess. Note the peripheral lobulations and thin enhancing wall.

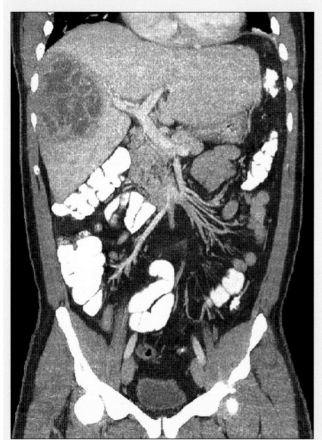

Figure 3. Pyogenic liver abscess: CT findings. Coronal image shows the classic *cluster* sign of a multiloculated pyogenic liver abscess. Note the peripheral lobulations and thin enhancing wall.

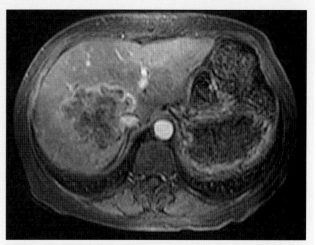

Figure 4. Pyogenic liver abscess: MRI findings. Gd-enhanced, fat-suppressed T1-weighted image shows a predominantly low-signal-intensity mass with an enhancing wall and septations.

DIFFERENTIAL DIAGNOSIS

- Cystadenoma and cystadenocarcinoma (cystic bile duct neoplasms)
- Hepatic cystadenoma and cystadenocarcinoma
- Metastases
- Multifocal hepatocellular carcinoma

PATHOLOGY

- Bacterial (pyogenic) hepatic abscesses develop via five major routes: biliary, portal vein, hepatic artery, direct extension from contiguous organs, and traumatic injury.
- Biliary tract disease is now the most common source of pyogenic liver abscess.
- Facultative gram-negative enteric bacilli, anaerobic gram-negative bacilli, and microaerophilic streptococci are organisms most often responsible for liver abscesses.
- *Escherichia coli* is the organism most commonly isolated in the culture in adults.
- Staphylococci organisms are most often isolated from hepatic abscesses in children.

INCIDENCE/PREVALENCE AND EPIDEMIOLOGY

- Pyogenic hepatic abscesses are uncommon in Western countries, accounting for 0.1% of hospital admissions and a prevalence at autopsy series of nearly 1%.
- Slight female predominance has been seen.
- These abscesses most often affect persons 40-60 years of age.

Suggested Readings

Catalano O, Sandomenico F, Raso MM, Siani A: Low mechanical index contrast-enhanced sonographic findings of pyogenic hepatic abscesses. *AJR Am J Roentgenol* 182:447-450, 2004.

Gerzof SG, Johnson WC, Robbins AH, et al: Intrahepatic pyogenic abscess treatment by percutaneous drainage. *Am J Surg* 149:487-494, 1985.

Huang C-J, Pitt HA, Lipsett PA, et al: Pyogenic hepatic abscess: Changing trends over 42 years. *Ann Surg* 223:600-609, 1996.

Jeffrey RB, Tolentino CS, Chang FC, et al: CT of small pyogenic hepatic abscesses: The cluster sign. *AJR Am J Roentgenol* 151:487-489, 1988.

Johnson RD, Mueller PR, Ferrucci JT, et al: Percutaneous drainage of pyogenic liver abscesses. *AJR* 144:463-467, 1985.

Newlin N, Silver TM, Stuck KJ, et al: Ultrasonic features of pyogenic liver abscesses. *Radiology* 139:155-159, 1991.

Hepatic Candidiasis and Fungal Infections

DEFINITION: Infection with fungus, commonly affecting immunocompromised individuals.

IMAGING

Ultrasound
Findings
- Peripheral zone that surrounds inner echogenic wheel that surrounds the central hypoechoic nidus (a wheel within a wheel)
- 1- to 4-mm lesion with a hyperechoic center that surrounds the hypoechoic rim (bull's eye)
- Uniformly hypoechoic, indicating fibrosis
- After antifungal therapy, lesions increase in echogenicity and decrease in size, often disappearing altogether.
- Inhomogeneity of the liver persists for up to 3 years after treatment.

Utility
- CT and MRI are more sensitive than ultrasound in the detection of these lesions.

CT
Findings
- Multiple small, rounded areas of decreased attenuation
- Areas of scattered increased attenuation (calcification) seen on noncontrast scans
- Periportal areas of increased attenuation
- CT requires both precontrast and postcontrast scans.

Utility
- Sensitivity: 60%-90%
- Specificity: 60%-80%
- Accuracy: 75%

MRI
Findings
- Dark ring is usually seen around these lesions with all sequences.
- Untreated nodules are minimally hypointense on T1-weighted images.
- Pre- and postgadolinium images; markedly hyperintense nodules are seen on T2-weighted images.
- After treatment, mildly to moderately hyperintense nodules are seen on T1- and T2-weighted images, with postcontrast enhancement.
- Completely treated lesions are minimally hypointense on T1-weighted images and isointense to mildly hyperintense on T2-weighted images.

DIAGNOSTIC PEARLS

- Increased attenuation (calcification) is seen on noncontrast CT scans.
- Multiple small, rounded areas of decreased attenuation are also seen.
- Percutaneous needle biopsy achieves a definitive diagnosis in the majority of cases.
- Sonographic findings of a *wheel within a wheel* and bull's-eye lesions are seen.

Utility
- Sensitivity: 75%-95%
- Specificity: 80%-95%
- Accuracy: 90%

CLINICAL PRESENTATION

- Hepatosplenomegaly
- Fever, right upper quadrant pain, and sepsis
- Typically occurs in an immunocompromised patient

DIFFERENTIAL DIAGNOSIS

- Multiple metastases
- Multiple small pyogenic abscesses
- Multifocal hepatocellular carcinoma

PATHOLOGY

- Microabscesses of liver secondary to fungal infection

INCIDENCE/PREVALENCE AND EPIDEMIOLOGY

- Infection with fungus has become more common with the acquired immunodeficiency syndrome epidemic and with increasingly intensive chemotherapy.
- It is seen in 50%-70% of patients with acute leukemia and 50% of those with lymphoma at the time of autopsy.

WHAT THE REFERRING PHYSICIAN NEEDS TO KNOW

- Diagnosis is difficult on clinical grounds because blood cultures are positive in only 50% of affected patients.
- Cross-sectional imaging is necessary for diagnosis.
- Percutaneous needle biopsy achieves a definitive diagnosis in the majority of cases.

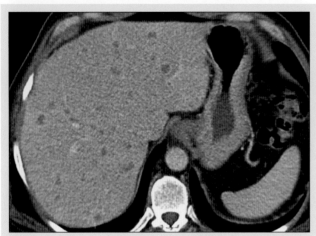

Figure 1. Candidiasis on CT. Contrast-enhanced CT scan of the liver shows multiple hypoattenuating microabscesses less than 1 cm in diameter disseminated throughout the hepatic parenchyma. (*From Mortele KJ, Segatto E, Ros PR: The infected liver: Radiologic-pathologic correlation.* RadioGraphics *24:937-955, 2004.*)

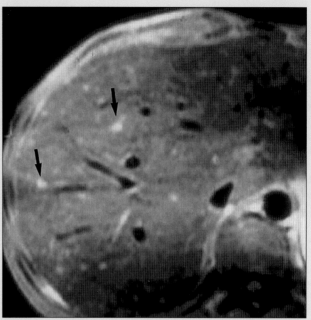

Figure 2. Candidiasis on MRI. Axial T1-weighted MR image reveals relatively hyperintense lesions less than 1 cm in diameter in the liver *(arrows)*. (*From Mortele KJ, Segatto E, Ros PR: The infected liver: Radiologic-pathologic correlation.* RadioGraphics *24:937-955, 2004.*)

Suggested Readings

Berlow ME, Spirt BA, Weil L: CT follow-up of hepatic and splenic fungal microabscesses. *J Comput Assist Tomogr* 8:42-45, 1984.

Francis IR, Glazer GM, Amendola MA, et al: Hepatic abscesses in the immunocompromised patient: Role of CT in detection, diagnosis, management, and follow-up. *Gastrointest Radiol* 11:257-262, 1986.

Gordon SC, Watts JC, Vener RJ, et al: Focal hepatic candidiasis with perihepatic adhesions: Laparoscopic and immunohistologic diagnosis. *Gastroenterology* 88:214-217, 1990.

Hepatic Echinococcal Disease

DEFINITION: Parasitic infection of the liver caused by echinococci.

ANATOMIC FINDINGS

Liver
- Hepatomegaly
- Calcification
- Unilocular or multilocular well-defined cysts

IMAGING

Radiography
Findings
- *Echinococcus multilocularis* can cause faint or dense punctate calcification scattered throughout necrotic and granulomatous tissue.
- Calcification is usually curvilinear or ring-like and lies in the pericyst.

Utility
- Plain radiographs are insensitive in the diagnosis of hepatic echinococcal disease.

Ultrasound
Findings
- Well-defined anechoic cyst and a multiseptate cyst with a daughter cyst (characteristic)
- Cyst with a floating, undulating membrane, the *water lily* sign
- Densely calcified mass
- Infected hydatid cysts, diffusely hyperechoic
- *E. multilocularis* infection: single or multiple echogenic lesions in the right lobe, some with irregular necrotic regions
- Intrahepatic biliary dilation
- Microcalcifications described in approximately 50% of cases

Utility
- Ultrasound is used to monitor the efficacy of medical antihydatid therapy.

DIAGNOSTIC PEARLS
- Multiseptate cyst with a daughter cyst
- Curvilinear ring-like calcifications
- Cyst with a floating, undulating membrane

CT
Findings
- Unilocular or multilocular, well-defined cysts with either thick or thin walls
- Daughter cysts: low-attenuating areas in the periphery of the lesion
- Curvilinear ring-like calcification (a common feature)
- *E. multilocularis:* geographic, infiltrating lesions without sharp margins or high-attenuation rims
- Little if any enhancement with intravenous contrast administration

Utility
- Altering the patient's position may change the position of the free-floating daughter cysts, confirming the diagnosis of echinococcal disease.
- Low-density (14-40 HU) lesions are solid masses rather than cysts.
- Calcification, when present, is usually amorphous rather than ring-like.
- When the alveolar lesion is located centrally, hepatic lobar atrophy may occur.

MRI
Findings
- Pericyst: low signal intensity on T1- and T2-weighted images
- Distinctive features having a thin rim and multiloculated or multicystic appearance
- Hydatid matrix: hypointense on T1-weighted images and markedly hyperintense on T2-weighted images

---

WHAT THE REFERRING PHYSICIAN NEEDS TO KNOW
- Percutaneous therapy should be attempted only with an accessible, dominant cyst that is truly cystic and uncomplicated.
- Infected cysts and cysts that communicate with the biliary system require surgical drainage.
- *E. multilocularis* is fatal within 10-15 years when left untreated.
- Serologic tests are positive in more than 80% of cases and are diagnostic of echinococcosis.

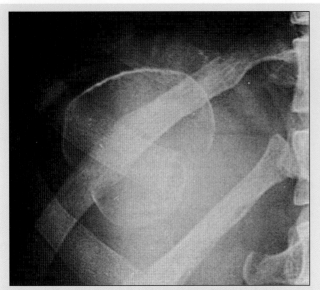

Figure 1. **Hydatid cyst: plain-film radiograph findings.**
Curvilinear calcification of the pericyst is present in 20%-30% of
abdominal radiographs in patients with hydatid cysts.

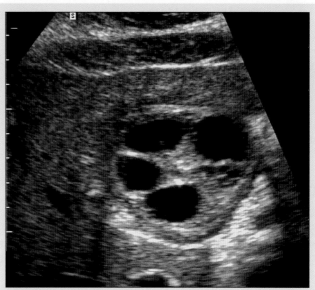

Figure 2. **Hydatid disease: sonographic features.** Longitudinal
scan shows a rounded, well-defined, multilocular hypoechoic
lesion with echogenic internal septa caused by *E. granulosus*.

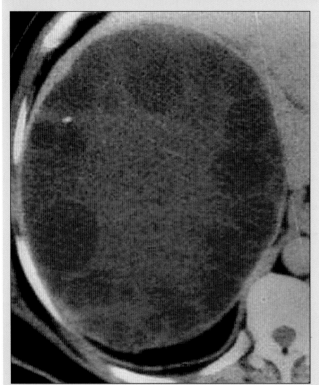

Figure 3. **Hydatid disease: CT findings.** CT scan shows a large
multilocular cyst with a thick wall. Multiple daughter cysts line
the periphery of the mass.

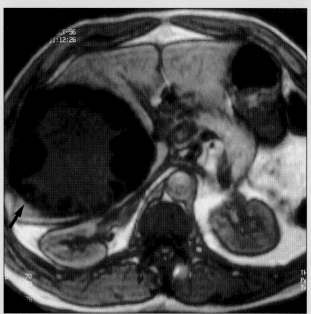

Figure 4. **Hydatid disease: MRI features.** Axial gradient-
echo T1-weighted MR image shows a hydatid cyst with a
hypointense fibrous pericyst *(arrow)*. The hydatid matrix has
intermediate signal intensity; the peripheral daughter cysts that
are hypointense relative to the matrix are seen. (*From Mortele
KJ, Segatto E, Ros PR: The infected liver: Radiologic-pathologic
correlation*. RadioGraphics *24:937-955, 2004.*)

- Daughter cysts: hypointense relative to the matrix on both T1- and T2-weighted images
- Floating membranes with low signal intensity on T1- and T2-weighted images
- Fibrous and parasitic tissue: low signal intensity on T1- and T2-weighted images
- Small cystic extensions: peripheral areas of increased signal on T2-weighted images (active portions)

Utility

- MRI is useful in displaying the extrahepatic extension of *E. multilocularis.*
- Calcifications display a low signal but are more difficult to identify on MRI than on CT.

CLINICAL PRESENTATION

- Patients are initially asymptomatic and remain so until the cysts grow large enough to cause pain, fever, jaundice, allergic reaction, and portal hypertension.
- Clinical manifestations of *E. multilocularis* infection may occur 5-20 years after the inciting event.
- Abdominal discomfort, jaundice, hepatomegaly, and eosinophilia are frequently observed.
- Serum levels of transaminases usually remain normal, whereas alkaline phosphatase and gamma-glutamyl transpeptidase values are elevated.
- Serologic titers are elevated in alveolar echinococcosis.

DIFFERENTIAL DIAGNOSIS

- Cystic biliary neoplasms
- Cystic primary hepatic neoplasms
- Cystic metastases
- Amebic or pyogenic abscess
- Complicated hepatic cyst
- Choledochal cyst
- Caroli disease

PATHOLOGY

- Two main forms that affect humans are *E. granulosus* and *E. multilocularis.*
- Infection occurs by ingesting contaminated, unwashed vegetables or through contact with infected dogs.

- It can also occur through the ingestion of wild fruits contaminated with fox feces or by direct contact with infected animals.
- Larvae reach the liver via the portal vein, where they proliferate and penetrate the surrounding tissue, causing a diffuse and infiltrative process.
- *E. multilocularis* induces a brisk granulomatous reaction with central necrosis, cavitation, and calcification.

INCIDENCE/PREVALENCE AND EPIDEMIOLOGY

- Most patients acquire hydatid disease in childhood but are not diagnosed until the third or fourth decade of life.
- Disease flourishes in rural areas where dogs are used for herding livestock, especially sheep.
- Greece, Uruguay, Argentina, Australia, and New Zealand are countries with the highest incidence of hydatid disease.
- *E. multilocularis (alveolaris)* is endemic in central Europe, Russia, Japan, and central and northern North America.

Suggested Readings

Acunas B, Rozanes I, Acunas G, et al: Hydatid cyst of the liver identification of detached cyst lining on CT scans obtained after cyst puncture. *AJR Am J Roentgenol* 156:751-752, 1991.

Acunas B, Rozanes I, Celik L, et al: Purely cystic hydatid disease of the liver: Treatment with percutaneous aspiration and injection of hypertonic saline. *Radiology* 182:541-543, 1992.

Bezzi M, Teggi A, De Rosa F, et al: Abdominal hydatid disease: US findings during medical treatment. *Radiology* 162:91-95, 1987.

Camunez F, Simo G, Robledo R, et al: Ultrasound diagnosis of ruptured hydatid cyst of the liver with biliary obstruction. *Gastrointest Radiol* 11:330-333, 1986.

Claudon M, Bessieres M, Regent D, et al: Alveolar echinococcosis of the liver: MR findings. *J Comput Assist Tomogr* 14:608-614, 1990.

Didier D, Weiler S, Rohmer P, et al: Hepatic alveolar echinococcosis: Correlative US and CT study. *Radiology* 154:179-186, 1985.

Pneumocystis carinii (jiroveci) Infection

DEFINITION: Opportunistic infection in patients with acquired immunodeficiency syndrome (AIDS) and other causes of immunocompromise caused by *Pneumocystis carinii (jiroveci)*.

IMAGING

Ultrasound
Findings
- Diffuse, tiny, nonshadowing echogenic foci or echogenic clumps of dense calcification
- Multiple, punctate calcifications

Utility
- This pattern has also been reported in *Mycobacterium avium-intracellulare* and cytomegalovirus infection.

CT
Findings
- Hypodense but then becoming characteristically calcified (punctate, nodular, or rim-like calcification)

Utility
- CT is helpful in revealing the presence of calcifications and gas and in detailing enhancement pattern.
- CT is more sensitive than ultrasound in the detection of the calcifications.

CLINICAL PRESENTATION

- Hepatosplenomegaly
- Fevers
- Right or left upper quadrant pain

DIFFERENTIAL DIAGNOSIS

- *Mycobacterium avium-intracellulare* complex
- Cytomegalovirus infection (gastrointestinal)

DIAGNOSTIC PEARLS

- Diffuse, tiny, nonshadowing echogenic foci or echogenic clumps of dense calcification in the liver
- Most common opportunistic infection in patients with AIDS

PATHOLOGY

- *P. carinii (jiroveci)* is the most common cause of opportunistic infection in patients with AIDS.
- The lungs, liver, spleen, and kidneys are the organs most commonly involved.

INCIDENCE/PREVALENCE AND EPIDEMIOLOGY

- The incidence of *Pneumocystis* infection has greatly diminished due to the effectiveness of HAART (highly active anti-retroviral therapy).

Suggested Readings

Gore RM, Miller FH, Yaghmai V: Acquired immunodeficiency syndrome (AIDS) of the abdominal organs: Imaging features. *Semin Ultrasound CT MR* 9:175-189, 1998.

Mathieson JR, Smith FJ: Hepatobiliary and pancreatic ultrasound in AIDS. In Reeders JWAJ, Mathieson JR (eds): *AIDS Imaging: A Practical Approach.* London, WB Saunders, 1998, pp 188-202.

Poles MA, Lew EA, Dieterich DT: Diagnosis and treatment of hepatic disease in patients with HIV. *Gastroenterol Clin North Am* 26: 291-321, 1997.

WHAT THE REFERRING PHYSICIAN NEEDS TO KNOW

- Differential diagnosis includes *M. avium-intracellulare* and cytomegalovirus infections.

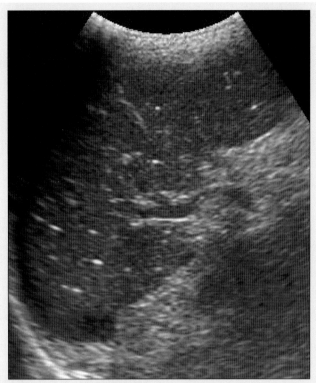

Figure 1. *Pneumocystis carinii (jiroveci)* **pneumonia.** Longitudinal ultrasound image demonstrates multiple, punctate calcifications after successful treatment.

Schistosomiasis

DEFINITION: Schistosomiasis is a parasitic infection caused by schistosomal trematodes.

IMAGING

Radiography
Findings
- Calcification
- Splenomegaly
- Esophageal and gastric varices on barium contrast studies

Utility
- Abdominal plain radiographs and barium studies are usually noncontributory.

Ultrasound
Findings
- Thick (2 cm), densely echogenic bands radiating from the porta hepatis to the periphery
- Round echogenic material with a hypoechoic rim *network* pattern
- *Bird's claw* appearance at the bifurcating points
- Enlarged liver (early stage)
- Progressive periportal fibrosis: contracted liver with features of portal hypertension (varices, splenomegaly, ascites)

Utility
- Ultrasound findings are typically nonspecific in these patients.

CT
Findings
- Peripheral hepatic or capsular calcification, the hallmark of *Schistosoma japonicum* infection
- Gross septations, resulting in bands of calcification, the *turtle back* appearance
- Prominent periportal low-density areas
- Acute schistosomiasis (Katayama syndrome): multiple hypodense nodules
- *Schistosoma mansoni* infection: low-density, rounded foci with linear branching bands that enhance

Utility
- It is the primary imaging test for evaluating suspected hepatic involvement by schistosomiasis.

MRI
Findings
- Low signal on T1-weighted images and hyperdense on T2-weighted images with postgadolinium enhancement

Utility
- Septal calcifications are less well depicted.
- These are better demonstrated with CT.

Interventional Radiology
Findings
- Normal hepatic venous outflow, decreased portal blood flow, and compensatorily increased hepatic arterial flow
- Normal or slightly elevated wedged hepatic venous pressure

Utility
- Angiography
- Hemodynamic changes of presinusoidal portal hypertension
- This technique is seldom used.

CLINICAL PRESENTATION

- Schistosomiasis is insidious and chronic.
- Symptoms of portal hypertension (varices, splenomegaly, ascites) become more apparent later.
- *S. haematobium* infection affects the liver less severely and typically causes hematuria as a result of urinary tract involvement.

DIFFERENTIAL DIAGNOSIS

- Alcohol-induced hepatitis and cirrhosis
- Viral-induced hepatitis and cirrhosis

PATHOLOGY

- Human infection occurs in the course of bathing in or wading through contaminated irrigation canals, streams, and ponds.
- Host responds to the ova with granulomatous inflammation that is replaced by fibrous tissue, leading to periportal fibrosis.
- When trematode infestation is sufficiently chronic and heavy, intrahepatic portal vein occlusion, presinusoidal portal hypertension, varices, and splenomegaly result.
- Hepatocellular necrosis occurs late in the course of the condition.

WHAT THE REFERRING PHYSICIAN NEEDS TO KNOW

- Schistosomiasis is the most common cause of portal hypertension worldwide.
- Incidence of hepatocellular carcinoma is increased in the liver, with prominent periportal low-density areas.

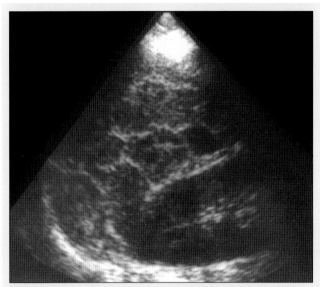

Figure 1. Schistosomiasis on ultrasound. Hepatic *Schistosoma japonicum* infection. Sonogram demonstrates thick and densely echogenic bands producing a network pattern.

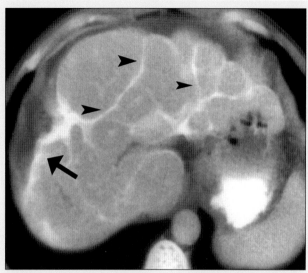

Figure 2. Schistosomiasis on CT. Hepatic *S. japonicum* infection. Contrast-enhanced CT scan demonstrates capsular calcification (*arrow*) and gross septations (*arrowheads*).

INCIDENCE/PREVALENCE AND EPIDEMIOLOGY

- Schistosomiasis is one of the most common and serious parasitic infections of humans.
- It affects 200 million people worldwide; the prevalence in endemic areas is 70%.
- Ten percent of patients in endemic areas exhibit hepatosplenic involvement.
- *S. japonicum* occurs in coastal areas of China, Japan, Taiwan, and the Philippines.
- *S. mansoni* occurs in parts of Africa, the Middle East, the West Indies, and in the northern part of South America.
- *S. haematobium* is seen in North Africa, the Mediterranean, and southwest Asia.

Suggested Readings

Araki T, Hayakawa K, Okada J, et al: Hepatic *Schistosomiasis japonica* identified by CT. *Radiology* 157:757-760, 1985.

Cheung H, Lai YM, Loke TK, et al: The imaging diagnosis of hepatic *Schistosomiasis japonica* sequelae. *Clin Radiol* 51:51-55, 1996.

Monzawa S, Ohtomo K, Oba H, et al: Septa in the liver of patients with chronic hepatic *Schistosomiasis japonica*: MR appearance. *AJR Am J Roentgenol* 162:1347-1351, 1994.

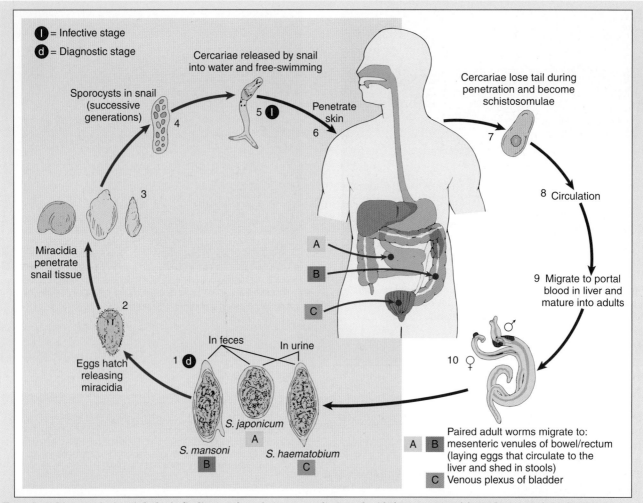

Figure 3. **Schistosomiasis: pathologic findings.** Life cycle. Eggs are eliminated with feces or urine (1). Under optimal conditions, the eggs hatch and release miracidia (2), which swim and penetrate specific snail intermediate hosts (3). The stages in the snail include two generations of sporocysts (4) and the production of cercariae (5). On release from the snail, the infective cercariae swim, penetrate the skin of the human host (6), and shed their forked tail, becoming schistosomulae (7). The schistosomulae migrate through several tissues and stages to their residence in the veins (8, 9). Adult worms in humans reside in the mesenteric venules in various locations, which at times seem to be specific for each species (10). For instance, *S. japonicum* is more frequently found in the superior mesenteric veins draining the small intestine (A), and *S. mansoni* occurs more often in the superior mesenteric veins draining the large intestine (B). However, both species can occupy either location, and they are capable of moving between sites; thus it is not possible to state unequivocally that one species only occurs in one location. *S. haematobium* most often invades the venous plexus of bladder (C), but it can also be found in the rectal venules. The females (size 7-20 mm; males slightly smaller) deposit eggs in the small venules of the portal and perivesical systems. The eggs are moved progressively toward the lumen of the intestine (*S. mansoni* and *S. japonicum*) and of the bladder and ureters (*S. haematobium*) and are eliminated with feces or urine, respectively (1). The pathologic features of *S. mansoni* and *S. japonicum* schistosomiasis include Katayama fever, presinusoidal egg granulomas, Symmers pipe stem periportal fibrosis, portal hypertension, and, occasionally, embolic egg granulomas in the brain or spinal cord. The pathologic features of *S. haematobium* schistosomiasis include hematuria, scarring, calcification, squamous cell carcinoma, and, occasionally, embolic egg granulomas in the brain or spinal cord. (*From Centers for Disease Control and Prevention. Available at: http://www.cdc.gov/Ncidod/parasites.*)

Acquired Immunodeficiency Syndrome

DEFINITION: Hepatic involvement in patients with AIDS consists of superimposed concomitant disease processes.

IMAGING

Ultrasound
Findings
- Hyperechoic parenchymal echo pattern, hepatomegaly, and focal masses
- Periportal hyperechoic and hypoechoic regions
- Kaposi sarcoma: small hyperechoic nodules and dense periportal bands
- Non-Hodgkin lymphoma: hypoechoic lesions compared with the normal liver parenchyma; also possibly anechoic and septate, mimicking fluid
- Adenopathy in the porta hepatis and retroperitoneum
- Irregularity of intrahepatic and extrahepatic bile duct walls with intervening strictures and dilation

Utility
- Sensitivity: 65%-90%
- Specificity: 72%-85%
- Accuracy: 78%

CT
Findings
- Hepatomegaly associated with focal or diffuse fatty infiltration
- Periportal lymphedema: reflecting lymphadenitis, hepatitis, or malnutrition
- Lymphoma: hypodense lesions
- Parenchymal calcifications in the liver, spleen, lymph nodes and kidneys, seen in patients with healed disseminated *Pneumocystis carinii (jiroveci)* infection
- Kaposi sarcoma: small low-attenuation masses located near the portal triads that simulate bile ducts or fungal microabscesses; enhancement on delayed scans
- Cytomegalovirus: mural thickening of the gallbladder, gallbladder distention, and intrahepatic and extrahepatic biliary dilation
- Irregularity of intrahepatic and extrahepatic bile duct walls with intervening strictures and dilation

Utility
- Sensitivity: 80%-95%
- Specificity: 75%-90%
- Accuracy: 85%

DIAGNOSTIC PEARLS
- Hepatomegaly associated with focal or diffuse fatty infiltration
- Kaposi sarcoma: small hyperechoic nodules and dense periportal bands
- Irregularity of intrahepatic and extrahepatic bile duct walls with intervening strictures and dilation

CLINICAL PRESENTATION
- Hepatic involvement may manifest with right upper quadrant pain.
- Weight loss, fevers, and malaise

DIFFERENTIAL DIAGNOSIS
- Hepatic candidiasis
- Hepatic *Pneumocystis* infection
- Hepatic tuberculosis
- Hepatic pyogenic infections

PATHOLOGY
- Nonspecific macrovesicular steatosis and portal inflammation are the most common findings.
- Granulomas are most frequently associated with mycobacterial infection, usually *Mycobacterium avium-intracellulare.*
- Other AIDS-related diseases include lymphoma, Kaposi sarcoma, cytomegalovirus, *Cryptococcus, Histoplasma, Coccidioides,* and *M. avium-intracellulare* infections.

INCIDENCE/PREVALENCE AND EPIDEMIOLOGY
- Hepatic granulomas have been reported in 16%-100% of biopsy and autopsy specimens.
- Virtually all human immunodeficiency virus–positive patients have evidence of prior hepatitis B infection; the latter infection may potentiate the former.

WHAT THE REFERRING PHYSICIAN NEEDS TO KNOW
- Liver biopsy seldom affects therapeutic decisions or leads to improved survival.
- Biopsy should be reserved for patients with unexplained fever, elevated serum alkaline phosphatase, and focal mass lesions on imaging.

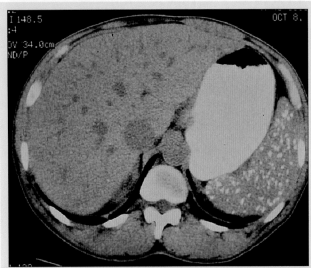

Figure 1. *P. carinii (jiroveci)* **infection of the spleen in a patient with AIDS.** Treated, healed infections typically give these small splenic calcifications, which are demonstrated on the CT.

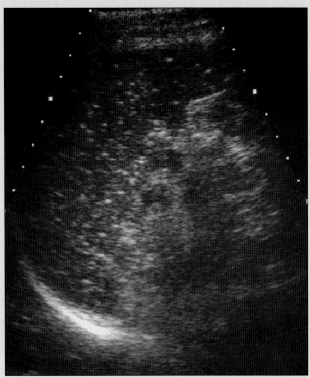

Figure 2. *P. carinii (jiroveci)* **infection of the spleen in a patient with AIDS.** Treated, healed infections typically give these small splenic calcifications, which are demonstrated on this longitudinal ultrasound scan.

Suggested Readings

Carucci LR, Halvorsen RA: Abdominal and pelvic CT in HIV-positive population. *Abdom Imaging* 29:631-642, 2004.

Semelka RC, Braga L, Armao D: Liver. In Semelka RC (ed): *Abdominal-Pelvic MRI.* New York, Wiley-Liss, 2002, pp 33-318.

Wilson SR, Withers CE: The liver. In Rumack C, Wilson SR, Charboneau WR, et al: *Diagnostic Ultrasound*, 3rd ed. Philadelphia, Elsevier-Mosby, 2005.

Amyloidosis (Gastrointestinal)

DEFINITION: A group of heterogeneous disorders caused by interstitial deposits of a protein-polysaccharide in various organs leading to hypoxia, mucosal atrophy, and muscle atrophy.

ANATOMIC FINDINGS

Liver
- Enlargement with amyloid deposition

IMAGING

Radiography
Findings
- Small bowel barium studies show decreased motility, transient intussusceptions, thickened nodular folds, and focal ulceration.
- Thick gastric folds can also be seen.

Utility
- Barium studies are abnormal in 40% of patients with primary amyloidosis.

CT
Findings
- Nonspecific; includes hepatomegaly and low-attenuation regions where amyloid deposits are found
- Delayed-contrast enhancement

Utility
- Abnormalities seen in the spleen are helpful in differentiating amyloid deposition from neoplasms and fatty infiltration.

MRI
Findings
- Decreased T2 values of the spleen and adrenals and increased T2 value of the pancreas in patients with primary amyloidosis
- Not significantly changed T2 values in the liver, subcutaneous fat, bone marrow, or kidney

Utility
- MRI has little role in the assessment of hepatic involvement in amyloidosis.

Ultrasound
Findings
- Liver is enlarged and has inhomogeneous echoes.

Utility
- Ultrasound plays little role in the evaluation of patients with amyloidosis.

DIAGNOSTIC PEARLS

- Nonspecific hepatomegaly and low-attenuation regions are seen where amyloid deposits are found.
- Delayed-contrast enhancement may be seen in involved areas because of vascular and sinusoidal infiltration.
- T2 values of the spleen and adrenals are decreased; T2 value of the pancreas is increased.

CLINICAL PRESENTATION

- Hepatic infiltration and enlargement are found in patients with systemic amyloidosis.
- Severe amyloidosis causes right upper quadrant pain, pruritus, ascites, malaise, weight loss, intrahepatic cholestasis, and portal hypertension.
- Involvement of the gut may cause malabsorption (diarrhea, protein loss), occult gastrointestinal bleeding, obstruction, macroglossia.

DIFFERENTIAL DIAGNOSIS

- Gastric outlet obstruction

PATHOLOGY

- Hepatic infiltration and enlargement are frequently found in patients with systemic amyloidosis, but significant liver disease is rare.
- Amyloids are proteolysis-resistant fibrils derived from monoclonal immunoglobulin light chains.
- Amyloids are deposited in the space of Disse and progressively encroach on adjacent hepatic parenchymal cells and sinusoids.
- Total replacement of large areas of the liver parenchyma may occur, giving the liver a pale, waxy gray, firm appearance.
- Hepatic function is usually preserved despite massive amyloid infiltration.

WHAT THE REFERRING PHYSICIAN NEEDS TO KNOW
- Hepatic infiltration and enlargement are frequently found in patients with systemic amyloidosis, but significant liver disease is rare.

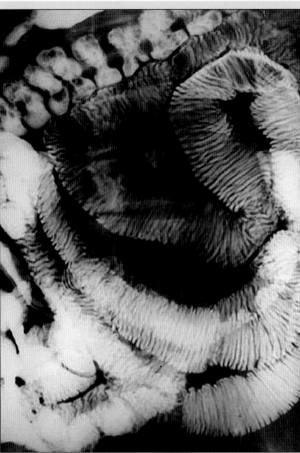

Figure 1. Small bowel follow-through series demonstrates diffuse, regular thickening of the valvulae conniventes of the small bowel. Note the bowel does not appear wet. These findings are typical of amyloidosis of the small bowel.

INCIDENCE/PREVALENCE AND EPIDEMIOLOGY

- The secondary form of amyloidosis is usually secondary to long-standing infections, neoplasms, and inflammatory disorders. It is seen in 20% of patients with rheumatoid arthritis and 10% to 15% of patients with multiple myeloma.
- The primary form is probably of autosomal-dominant inheritance with immumologically determined dysfunction of plasma cells.

Suggested Readings

Georgiades CS, Neyman EG, Fishman EK: Cross-sectional imaging of amyloidosis: An organ system based approach. *J Comput Assist Tomogr* 26:1035-1041, 2002.

Maineti PP, D'Agostino L, Socia E, et al: Hepatic and splenic amyloidosis: Dual-phase spiral CT findings. *Abdom Imaging* 28:688-690, 2003.

Mieli-Vergani G, Thompston R: Genetic and metabolic liver disease. In Weinstein WM, Hawkey CJ, Bosch J (eds): *Clinical Gastroenterology and Hepatology*. Philadelphia, Elsevier-Mosby, 2005, pp 687-692.

Monzawa S, Tsukamoto T, Omata K, et al: A case of primary amyloidosis of the liver and spleen: Radiologic findings. *Eur J Radiol* 41:237-241, 2002.

Palladini G, Perfetti V, Merlini G: Therapy and management of systemic (primary) amyloidosis. *Swiss Med Wkly* 136:715-720, 2006.

Thiele DL: Hepatic manifestations of systemic disease and other disorders of the liver. In Feldman M, Friedman LS, Sleisenger MH (eds): *Gastrointestinal and Liver Disease*, 7th ed. Philadelphia, Saunders, 2002, pp 1603-1619.

Cirrhosis

DEFINITION: Chronic liver disease characterized by diffuse parenchymal necrosis, fibrosis, and nodular regeneration, resulting in disorganization of the lobular and vascular architecture.

IMAGING

Ultrasound

Findings
- Findings are nonspecific.
- Flattening of the hepatic venous waveforms is caused by decreased compliance of the fibrotic liver.
- Segment IV undergoes atrophy in patients with cirrhosis; the mean diameter of segment IV is 28 mm ($\pm$9).
- Regenerating nodules are hypoechoic areas with echogenic borders resulting from fibrous and fatty connective tissue surrounding and separating the nodules.
- Mesenteric, omental, and retroperitoneal edema can be seen in patients with cirrhosis and portal hypertension.
- Siderotic nodules, or Gamna-Gandy bodies, rarely identified as hyperechoic masses in the spleen, are seen in patients with portal hypertension.

Utility
- Reported sensitivity of ultrasound in the diagnosis of cirrhosis is based on hepatic architecture, varying between 65% and 95%.
- Ultrasound has up to 98% positive predictive value in diffuse parenchymal disease diagnosis, but it cannot reliably differentiate fat from fibrosis.
- High-resolution sonography is found to be useful in assessing the severity of hepatic scarring and differentiating macronodular and micronodular cirrhosis.
- Ultrasound is a difficult tool to use for screening in cirrhotic patients for detecting hepatocellular carcinoma.
- Sensitivity: 60%-95%
- Specificity: 85%-95%
- Accuracy: 90%

CT

Findings
- Fatty infiltration, focal confluent fibrosis, and nodularity of liver contour are seen.
- In the later stages of cirrhosis, the overall liver volume is diminished.
- Regenerating nodules, isoattenuating with the liver parenchyma, are seen before and after contrast material administration.
- Siderotic nodules, with a higher attenuation than the liver and other soft-tissue organs, and isoattenuating with the contrast-enhanced liver parenchyma are seen.
- Caudate lobe–right lobe ratio exceeds 0.65.

DIAGNOSTIC PEARLS

- Flattening of the hepatic venous waveforms caused by decreased compliance of the fibrotic liver
- Atrophy of medial segment of left lobe and right lobe with sparing or hypertrophy of the central segments of left lobe and caudate lobe
- Caudate lobe–right lobe ratio exceeding 0.65

- Gallbladder becomes a more lateral and superficial structure.
- Squared or rounded appearance of liver, marked atrophy of right lobe, and lateral segment coupled with marked caudate lobe hypertrophy are seen.

Utility
- CT is the primary noninvasive imaging modality in the evaluation of cirrhosis.
- The advent of multidetector CT has substantially increased the accuracy of CT in screening patients with cirrhosis for hepatocellular carcinoma.
- Sensitivity: 85%-100%
- Specificity: 85%-100%
- Accuracy: 92%

MRI

Findings
- Lace-like hypointense network of abnormal signal intensity
- Linear enhancement and enlargement of the hilar periportal space
- Atrophy of the medial segment of the left lobe and right lobe, with sparing or hypertrophy of the central segments of the left lobe and caudate lobe
- Siderotic nodules: small dark nodules on T2-weighted and gradient-echo images
- Benign regenerating nodules possibly having a high signal intensity on T1-weighted images
- Focal confluent fibrosis: focal mass and wedge-shaped hypointense regions

Utility
- MRI can often detect cirrhosis at an earlier stage than CT and ultrasound.
- It can demonstrate subtle changes such as fine strands of fibrosis and enlargement of the hilar and periportal space.

WHAT THE REFERRING PHYSICIAN NEEDS TO KNOW

- Patients with cirrhosis caused by alcoholism have an increased incidence of developing hepatocellular carcinoma.
- Cirrhosis is the most common cause of intrahepatic portal hypertension.

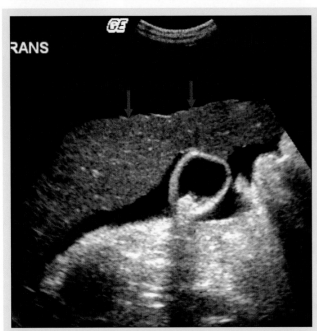

Figure 1. Cirrhosis: sonographic findings. A nodular hepatic surface *(arrows)* is highlighted by the presence of ascites. Note the thick gallbladder wall and gallstones.

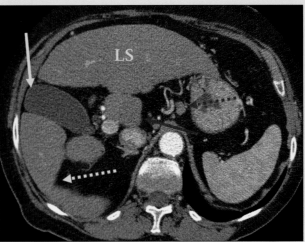

Figure 2. Cirrhosis: CT features. Contrast-enhanced CT demonstrates enlargement of the lateral segment (LS) of the left lobe, atrophy of the medial segment *(solid red arrow)* of the left lobe, and atrophy of the right lobe with a characteristic notch *(broken yellow arrow)* in the right posterior surface of the liver. Note that the gallbladder *(solid yellow arrow)* is in a more superficial and lateral position as a result of these morphologic changes. Several borderline-sized lymph nodes *(broken red arrow)* are present within the gastrohepatic ligament.

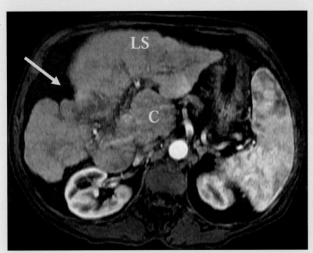

Figure 3. Confluent hepatic fibrosis: MRI features. Contrast-enhanced, T1-weighted MR image shows the classic location of capsular retraction in confluent hepatic fibrosis *(arrow)*. Note the hypertrophy of the caudate (C) lobe and lateral segment (LS) of the left lobe.

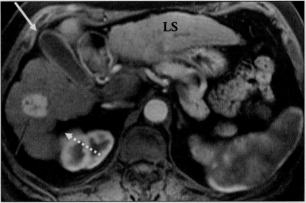

Figure 4. Hepatocellular nodules in cirrhosis: MRI features. Small hepatocellular carcinoma *(red arrow)* is present within a cirrhotic liver showing a nodular hepatic contour, right lobe notch *(broken yellow arrow)*, enlarged lateral segment (LS) of the left lobe, and a superficial gallbladder *(solid yellow arrow)*.

- It can also assess liver size, evaluate the effects of portal hypertension, screen for hepatocellular carcinoma, and better characterize masses detected by other techniques.
- MRI is useful for differentiating dysplastic nodules from hepatocellular carcinoma in patients with cirrhosis.
- It is also useful in the discrimination of alcoholic- and virus-induced cirrhosis.
- MR elastography has shown promise as a noninvasive means of determining the degree of hepatic fibrosis.
- Sensitivity: 85%-100%
- Specificity: 90%-100%
- Accuracy: 96%

CLINICAL PRESENTATION

- Anorexia, weakness, fatigue, weight loss
- Jaundice, low-grade fever
- Anemia, coagulopathy, hypoalbuminemia, diarrhea, hypogonadism

- Bleeding from esophageal varices, hepatic encephalopathy
- Hepatomegaly is seen.
- Ascites is the most common complication of cirrhosis and is associated with nearly 50% of deaths.

DIFFERENTIAL DIAGNOSIS

- Gallbladder carcinoma
- Hepatopulmonary syndrome
- Hepatic infarction
- Wilson disease

PATHOLOGY

- Classification of cirrhosis includes micronodular (Laënnec) cirrhosis, macronodular (postnecrotic) cirrhosis, and mixed cirrhosis.
- Entire parenchymal architecture is disorganized by interconnecting fibrous scars formed in response to hepatocyte injury and loss.
- Fibrosis may appear as delicate portal-central or portal-portal bands (or both), or it may constitute broad scars replacing multiple adjacent lobules.
- Micronodules or macronodules are created by regenerative activity and the network of scars.
- Vascular architecture of the liver is also reorganized by the parenchymal damage and scarring with formation of abnormal arteriovenous interconnections.
- Cirrhosis leads to two major potentially life-threatening complications: hepatocellular failure resulting from hepatocyte damage and portal venous hypertension.
- Incidence of developing hepatocellular carcinoma is increased and 2.5-fold greater in cirrhotic hepatitis B surface antigen–positive than hepatitis B surface antigen–negative patients.

INCIDENCE/PREVALENCE AND EPIDEMIOLOGY

- Alcohol abuse is the most common cause of cirrhosis in the West.
- Cirrhosis is one of the 10 leading causes of death in the Western world and the sixth leading cause in the United States.
- Age-adjusted mortality is 2.3 times higher in men than women and 1.7 times higher in black than white persons.
- Cirrhosis is the third leading cause of death for men 34-54 years of age.

Suggested Readings

Aguirre DA, Behling CA, Alpert E, et al: Liver fibrosis: Noninvasive diagnosis with double contrast material-enhanced MR imaging. *Radiology* 239:425-437, 2006.
Awaya H, Mitchell DG, Kamishima T, et al: Cirrhosis: Modified caudate-right lobe ratio. *Radiology* 224:769-774, 2002.
Baik SKB, Kim JW, Kim HS, et al: Recent variceal bleeding: Doppler US hepatic vein waveform in assessment of severity of portal hypertension and vasoactive drug response. *Radiology* 240:574-580, 2006.
Bass NM, Yao FY: Portal hypertension and variceal bleeding. In Feldman M, Friedman LS, Sleisenger MH (eds): *Gastrointestinal and Liver Disease*, 7th ed. Philadelphia, Saunders, 2002, pp 1487-1516.
Berzigotti A, Casadei A, Magalotti D, et al: Renovascular impedance correlates with portal pressure in patients with cirrhosis. *Radiology* 240:581-586, 2006.
Carlos RC, Kin HM, Hussain HK, et al: Developing a prediction rule to assess hepatic malignancy with cirrhosis. *AJR Am J Roentgenol* 180:893-900, 2003.
Caturelli E, Castellano L, Fusilli S, et al: Coarse nodular US pattern in hepatic cirrhosis: Risk for hepatocellular carcinoma. *Radiology* 226:691-697, 2003.
Colli A, Fraquelli M, Andreoletti M, et al: Severe liver fibrosis or cirrhosis: Accuracy of US for detection: Analysis of 300 cases. *Radiology* 227:89-94, 2003.
D'Amico G, Malizia G: Cirrhosis of the liver. In Weinstein WM, Hawkey CJ, Bosch J (eds): *Clinical Gastroenterology and Hepatology*. Philadelphia, Elsevier-Mosby, 2005, pp 699-706.
Gibo M, Murata S, Kuroki S: Pericaval fat collection mimicking an intracaval lesion on CT in patients with chronic liver disease. *Abdom Imaging* 26:492-495, 2001.
Hussain HK, Syed I, Nghiem HV, et al: T2-weighted MR imaging in the assessment of the cirrhotic liver. *Radiology* 230:637-644, 2004.
Ito K, Mitchell DG, Gabata T, et al: Expanded gallbladder fossa: Simple MR imaging sign of cirrhosis. *Radiology* 211:723-726, 1999.
Kim M, Mitchell DG, Ito K: Portosystemic collaterals of the upper abdomen: Review of anatomy and demonstration on MR imaging. *Abdom Imaging* 25:462-470, 2006.
Lafortune M, Matricardi L, Denys A, et al: Segment 4 (the quadrate lobe): A barometer of cirrhotic liver disease. *Radiology* 206:157-160, 1998.
Lim AKP, Patel N, Eckersley RJ, et al: Can Doppler sonography grade the severity of hepatitis C-related liver disease? *AJR Am J Roentgenol* 184:1848-1853, 2005.
Lipson JA, Qayyum A, Avrin DE, et al: CT and MRI of hepatic contour abnormalities. *AJR Am J Roentgenol* 184:75-81, 2005.
Martinez-Noguera A, Montserrat E, Torrubia S, et al: Doppler in hepatic cirrhosis and chronic hepatitis. *Semin Ultrasound CT MRI* 23:19-36, 2002.
Mortele KJ, Ros PR: MR imaging in chronic hepatitis and cirrhosis. *Semin Ultrasound CT MRI* 23:79-100, 2002.
Nakagawa H, Toda N, Taniguchi M, et al: Prevalence and sonographic detection of Chilaiditi's sign in cirrhotic patients without ascites. *AJR Am J Roentgenol* 187:W589-W593, 2006.
Nicolau C, Bianchi L, Vilana R: Grey-scale ultrasound in hepatic cirrhosis and chronic hepatitis: Diagnosis, screening, and intervention. *Semin Ultrasound CT MRI* 23:3-18, 2002.
Nishura T, Watanabe H, Ito M, et al: Ultrasound evaluation of the fibrosis stage in chronic liver disease by the simultaneous use of low and high frequency probes. *Br J Radiol* 78:189-197, 2005.
Okazaki H, Ito K, Fujita T, et al: Discrimination of alcoholic from virus-induced cirrhosis on MR imaging. *AJR Am J Roentgenol* 175:1677-1681, 2000.
Rouviere O, Yin M, Drsner MA, et al: MR elastography of the liver: Preliminary results. *Radiology* 240:440-673, 2006.
Valls C, Andia E, Roca Y, et al: CT in hepatic cirrhosis and chronic hepatitis. *Semin Ultrasound CT MRI* 23:37-91, 2002.
Van Beers BE, Leconte I, Materne R, et al: Hepatic perfusion parameters in chronic liver disease. *AJR Am J Roentgenol* 176:667-673, 2001.
Vitellas KM, Tzalonikou MT, Bennett WF, et al: Cirrhosis: Spectrum of findings on unenhanced and dynamic gadolinium-enhanced MR imaging. *Abdom Imaging* 26:601-615, 2001.
Wanless IR, Crawford JM: Cirrhosis. In Odze RD, Goldblum JR, Crawford JM (eds): *Surgical Pathology of the GI Tract, Liver, Biliary Tract, and Pancreas*. Philadelphia, Saunders, 2004, pp 863-885.
Yang DM, Kim HS, Cho SW, et al: Various causes of hepatic capsular retraction: CT and MR findings. *Br J Radiol* 75:994-1002, 2002.

Gaucher Disease (Gastrointestinal)

DEFINITION: Deficiency of glucosylceramidase, resulting in glucosylceramide accumulation in reticuloendothelial cells of the body.

ANATOMIC FINDINGS

Abdomen
- Hepatosplenomegaly and, occasionally, multiple well-circumscribed calcifications
- Nonspecific fatty and cirrhotic changes of hepatic parenchyma

Femur
- Bone changes, modeling deformities of lower femoral shafts (*Erlenmeyer flask* appearance), pathologic fractures, and vertebral body collapse
- Pathologic fractures

Vertebral Body
- Vertebral body collapse

IMAGING

Radiography
Findings
- Bone changes and fractures

Utility
- Plain films are useful in evaluating the bony, but not the abdominal, manifestations of this disease.

Ultrasound
Findings
- Hypoechoic nodular lesion in spleen

Utility
- Ultrasound is useful for evaluating hepatic and splenic size.

CT
Findings
- Ill-defined, homogeneous hypodense lesions corresponding to the focal accumulation of Gaucher cells in liver and spleen
- Hepatosplenomegaly

Utility
- CT is useful for evaluating hepatic and splenic size.

CLINICAL PRESENTATION

- Hepatosplenomegaly
- Impaired liver function and ascites

DIAGNOSTIC PEARLS

- Hepatosplenomegaly with occasional multiple well-circumscribed calcifications
- Modeling deformities of the lower femoral shafts (*Erlenmeyer flask* appearance)
- Ill-defined, homogeneous hypodense lesions corresponding to the focal accumulation of Gaucher cells

- Pancytopenia, anemia, leukopenia, and thrombocytopenia
- Dull bone pain

DIFFERENTIAL DIAGNOSIS

- Leukemia
- Lymphoma
- Metabolic bone disease

PATHOLOGY

- Rare, autosomal-recessive lysosomal storage disease
- Deficiency of glucosylceramidase, resulting in glucosylceramide accumulation in the reticuloendothelial cells of the body
- Extensive replacement of the liver by Gaucher cells (lipid-laden macrophages), causing cirrhosis and portal hypertension to develop

INCIDENCE/PREVALENCE AND EPIDEMIOLOGY

- Incidence is 1 in 2500 births.
- Gaucher disease is most common in Ashkenazi Jews.

Suggested Readings

Niederau C, Haussinger D: Gaucher's disease: A review for the internist and hepatologist. *Hepatogastroenterology* 47:984-997, 2000.
Poll LW, Koch JA, vom Dahl S, et al: Extraosseous manifestation of Gaucher's disease type I: MR and histological appearance. *Eur Radiol* 10:1660-1663, 2000.

WHAT THE REFERRING PHYSICIAN NEEDS TO KNOW
- Degree of liver and splenic involvement correlates with the severity of extrahepatic disease.

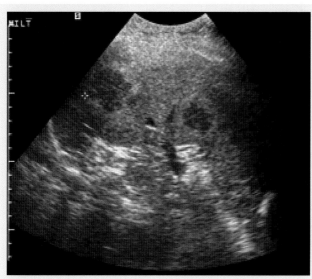

Figure 1. Gaucher disease. Splenomegaly and two irregular, nodular, hypoechoic lesions. (*Courtesy of M. Maas, MD, Amsterdam, Netherlands.*)

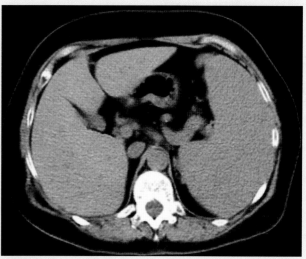

Figure 2. Gaucher disease. Unenhanced CT shows splenomegaly but no focal abnormalities. (*Courtesy of M. Maas, MD, Amsterdam, Netherlands.*)

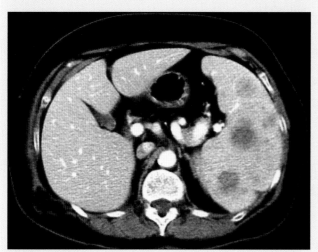

Figure 3. Gaucher disease. Contrast-enhanced CT image shows ill-defined, hypodense lesions. These nodular areas correspond to focal homogeneous clusters of Gaucher cells determined at histopathologic examination. (*Courtesy of M. Maas, MD, Amsterdam, Netherlands.*)

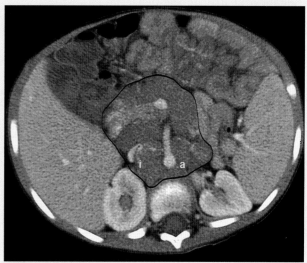

Figure 4. Axial CT image of the abdomen with contrast (patient is 5 years of age). Image demonstrates an extensively enlarged mass (outlined) encasing the aorta (a) and inferior vena cava (i) and mesentery with calcification. (*From Burrow TA, Cohen MB, Bokulic R, et al: Gaucher disease: Progressive mesenteric and mediastinal lymphadenopathy despite enzyme therapy. J Pediatr 150:202-206, 2007.*)

Glycogen Storage Disease

DEFINITION: Inherited disorder of glycogen metabolism affecting the liver, the most common of which is von Gierke disease.

IMAGING

Ultrasound
Findings
- Enlarged liver: demonstrates increased echogenicity and sound attenuation
- Increased sound transmission with refractile shadowing at the tumor margins
- Hepatic adenomas: well-circumscribed and possibly hypoechoic, isoechoic, or hyperechoic in relation to the remainder of the liver

Utility
- CT and MRI are more sensitive in the depiction of focal hepatic lesions associated with this lesion.

CT
Findings
- Glycogen storage increases hepatic density.
- Liver, spleen, and kidneys are typically enlarged.
- Renal cortex may appear dense.
- On noncontrast CT, hepatic adenomas are hypodense compared with the normal liver and spuriously hyperdense in the setting of concomitant fatty infiltration.
- Contrast-enhanced CT may show enhancement of hepatic adenomas.
- Hepatic adenomas may be spuriously hyperdense in the setting of concomitant fatty infiltration.

Utility
- Adenomas should remain stable in size or show slow growth on follow-up examination.
- Malignant degeneration should be suspected if the growth or density change is rapid.

MRI
Findings
- Hepatic adenomas may show fat signal intensity.

Utility
- Is the most sensitive means of diagnosis of complications of these disorders

CLINICAL PRESENTATION

- Patients exhibit failure to thrive, hypoglycemia, hyperlipidemia, hyperuricemia, stunted growth, hepatomegaly, and nephromegaly.

DIAGNOSTIC PEARLS

- Glycogen storage increases hepatic density.
- On sonography, sound transmission is increased, with refractile shadowing at the tumor margins.
- Hepatic adenomas may show fat-signal intensity on MRI.

DIFFERENTIAL DIAGNOSIS

- Amyloidosis
- Primary or secondary hepatic neoplasms

PATHOLOGY

- von Gierke disease is a type 1 glycogen storage disease (glucose-6-phosphatase deficiency in the liver and kidneys).
- Excessive glycogen is deposited in hepatocytes and the proximal renal tubules.
- Intracytoplasmic accumulation of glycogen and small amounts of lipid are found.
- Hepatic adenomas and hepatocellular carcinomas result from chronic hormonal stimulation from chronic hypoglycemia and decreased insulin and increased glucagon levels.

INCIDENCE/PREVALENCE AND EPIDEMIOLOGY

- von Gierke disease is the most common type of glycogen storage disease to affect the liver.
- Eight percent of all patients with glycogen storage disease and up to 40% with type 1 disease have hepatic adenomas.

Suggested Readings

Cobbold JF, Wylezinska M, Cunningham C, et al: Non-invasive evaluation of hepatic fibrosis using magnetic resonance imaging and ultrasound techniques. *Gut* 55:1670-1672, 2006.

Mieli-Vergani G, Thompston R: Genetic and metabolic liver disease. In Weinstein WM, Hawkey CJ, Bosch J (eds): *Clinical Gastroenterology and Hepatology*. Philadelphia, Elsevier-Mosby, 2005, pp 687–692.

WHAT THE REFERRING PHYSICIAN NEEDS TO KNOW

- Imaging of patients is necessary to exclude the development of hepatic adenomas and hepatocellular carcinomas.
- Lesions with a rapidly changing sonographic appearance should be carefully monitored because this circumstance may reflect malignant degeneration or hemorrhagic necrosis.

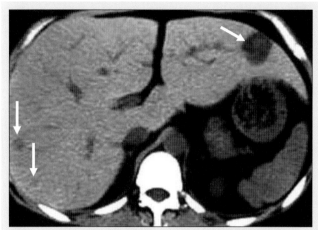

Figure 1. von Gierke disease: imaging findings. Unenhanced CT scan of the liver shows a diffuse increase in the density of the liver caused by glycogen deposition. Three fat-containing adenomas *(arrows)* are present.

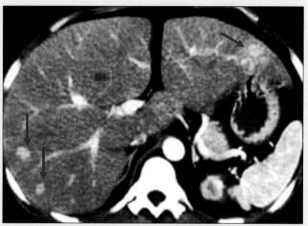

Figure 2. von Gierke disease: imaging findings. Contrast-enhanced CT scan shows that these adenomas *(arrows)* are hypervascular.

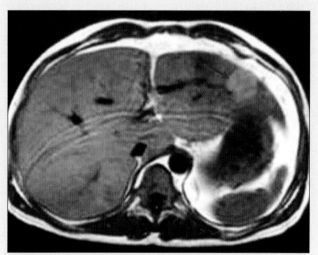

Figure 3. von Gierke disease: imaging findings. Axial T1-weighted MR scan shows high-signal-intensity fat within the adenoma in the left lobe *(arrow)*.

Thiele DL: Hepatic manifestations of systemic disease and other disorders of the liver. In Feldman M, Friedman LS, Sleisenger MH (eds): *Gastrointestinal and Liver Disease*, 7th ed. Philadelphia, Saunders, 2002, pp 1603–1619.

Wilson SR, Withers CE: The liver. In Rumack C, Wilson SR, Charboneau WR, et al: *Diagnostic Ultrasound*, 3rd ed. Philadelphia, Elsevier-Mosby, 2005.

Hemosiderosis and Hemochromatosis

DEFINITION: Excessive iron deposition in various organs, particularly the liver, spleen, and pancreas.

IMAGING

MRI
Findings
- Dramatic reduction is seen in the signal intensity of the liver (90%) and pancreas (20%) in hemochromatosis.
- In parenchymal overload, the liver and pancreas have low signal intensity.
- In reticuloendothelial cell overload, the liver and spleen have low signal intensity, but the pancreas is spared.

Utility
- MRI is the most sensitive and specific imaging test for the demonstration of hepatic iron overload and follow-up of patients under treatment.
- It can distinguish parenchymal overload caused by hemochromatosis from reticuloendothelial cell iron overload in hemosiderosis.
- Serum iron concentrations greater than 300 μmol/g preclude accurate measurement.

CT
Findings
- Homogeneously increased liver density, with an attenuation of 75-135 HU
- On unenhanced CT, diffusely increased liver attenuation highlighting the hepatic and portal veins

Utility
- When liver neoplasms are suspected, obtaining noncontrast images is important.

Ultrasound
Findings
- Liver fibrosis and cirrhosis

Utility
- Ultrasound is nonspecific and has no role in the diagnosis.

Radiography
Findings
- Chondrocalcinosis and degenerative arthritis in the second and third metacarpal heads
- Rarely, diffuse and homogeneously increased density of the liver

Utility
- Plain radiographs have no role in establishing the diagnosis.

DIAGNOSTIC PEARLS

- Dramatic reduction in the signal intensity of the liver (90%) and pancreas (20%)
- Homogeneously increased liver density, with an attenuation of 75-135 HU.
- Diffusely increased liver attenuation highlighting the hepatic and portal veins

CLINICAL PRESENTATION

- Classic triad consists of micronodular pigment cirrhosis, diabetes mellitus, and hyperpigmentation.
- Patients may have hepatomegaly, splenomegaly, arthropathy, cardiac and endocrine involvement, and hyperpigmentation.
- Cirrhosis is irreversible, and approximately one third of patients develop hepatocellular carcinoma as a late sequela.
- Patients with hemosiderosis may present with hemolytic anemias, arthralgias, cirrhosis, and portal hypertension.

DIFFERENTIAL DIAGNOSIS

- Copper overload (on CT)
- Amiodarone overload (on CT)
- Gold therapy (on CT)
- Profound anemia (on CT)

PATHOLOGY

- Classic primary hemochromatosis features principally excessive ferritin and hemosiderin in the liver, pancreas, myocardium, joints, endocrine glands, and skin.
- Because the liver contains up to one third of the total body iron stores, it is the organ most profoundly damaged.
- Pancreas is similarly affected, leading to exocrine deficiency but to a greater extent endocrine deficiency.
- In hemosiderosis the reticuloendothelial cells of the liver (Kupffer cells), spleen, and marrow accumulate too much iron.

WHAT THE REFERRING PHYSICIAN NEEDS TO KNOW

- Early diagnosis and therapy of hemochromatosis can prevent or minimize the damaging effects of iron overload.
- The physician must differentiate parenchymal (hemochromatosis) from reticuloendothelial cell (hemosiderosis) iron overload, given that the former causes severe tissue damage as compared to the latter.

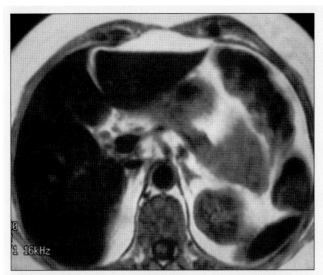

Figure 1. Hemosiderosis: MRI findings. Axial T1-weighted image shows markedly decreased signal intensity of the liver and spleen caused by iron deposition into the Kupffer cells of the liver and the reticuloendothelial cells of the spleen. The absence of iron deposition in the pancreas is a differentiating feature from hemochromatosis.

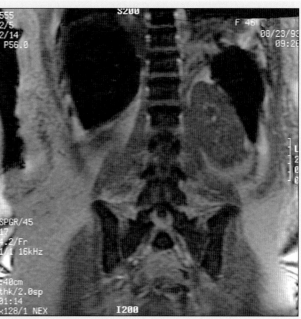

Figure 2. Hemosiderosis: MRI findings. Coronal image shows that the liver, spleen, and bone marrow of the spine have markedly decreased signal intensity caused by the deposition of iron in the reticuloendothelial cells of these organs.

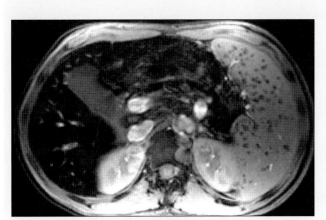

Figure 3. Hemochromatosis: MRI findings. T1-weighted gradient-echo image of the upper abdomen shows marked hypointensity of the liver and spleen caused by the deposition of iron in the hepatocytes of the liver and the acinar cells of the pancreas. Notice the low signal intensity Gamna-Gandy bodies in the spleen, secondary to hemosiderin deposition, a finding seen in portal hypertension with microhemorrhages into the splenic parenchyma.

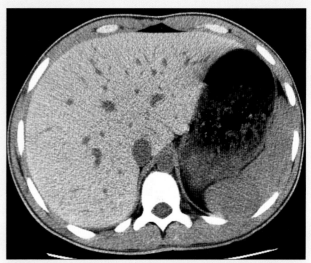

Figure 4. Iron overload: CT findings. The attenuation of the liver is diffusely increased secondary to intraparenchymal iron deposition.

INCIDENCE/PREVALENCE AND EPIDEMIOLOGY

- Hemochromatosis usually occurs in the fourth or fifth decades of life, with a 10:1 male-female predominance.
- Risk of development of hepatoma is increased over 200-fold in patients with hereditary hemochromatosis.
- One in twelve Caucasians carries a recessive gene for hemochromatosis.

Suggested Readings

Alustiza JM, Artetxe J, Agirre A, et al: MR quantification of hepatic iron concentration. *Radiology* 230:479-484, 2004.

Ben Salem D, Cercueil J-P, Ricolfi F, et al: Erythropoietic hemochromatosis. *Radiology* 233:116-119, 2004.

Danet I-M, Semelka RC, Braga L: MR imaging in diffuse liver disease. *Radiol Clin North Am* 41:67-87, 2003.

Kauffman JM, Grace ND: Hemochromatosis. In Weinstein WM, Hawkey CJ, Bosch J (eds): *Clinical Gastroenterology and Hepatology*. Philadelphia, Elsevier-Mosby, 2005, pp 659-664.

Tavill AS, Bacon DR: Hemochromatosis and iron overload syndromes. In Zakim D, Boyer TD (eds): *Hepatology: A Textbook of Liver Disease*. Philadelphia, WB Saunders, 2003, pp 3-31.

Hepatitis

DEFINITION: Hepatitis is a general term used to describe acute or chronic inflammation of the liver.

IMAGING

Ultrasound
Findings
- Acute viral hepatitis: The liver and spleen are frequently enlarged.
- When parenchymal damage is severe, a *starry sky* appearance is seen.
- Centrilobar pattern is seen indicating parenchymal edema.
- Mural thickening of the gallbladder and hepatomegaly are other nonspecific findings in patients with hepatitis.
- Chronic hepatitis produces increased parenchymal echogenicity and loss of mural definition of the portal veins.
- Acute alcoholic hepatitis: The liver is quite echogenic because of fatty infiltration.
- Alcoholic hepatitis: The liver may be enlarged early on but becomes atrophic as cirrhosis ensues.

Utility
- Major role of ultrasound in hepatitis is to exclude biliary obstruction as the cause of the liver disease.

CT
Findings
- Hepatomegaly: gallbladder wall thickening, and hepatic periportal lucency
- Chronic active hepatitis: lymphadenopathy in the porta hepatis, gastrohepatic ligament, and retroperitoneum
- Alcoholic hepatitis: fatty infiltration in a normal-sized, enlarged, or atrophic liver

Utility
- The primary role of CT in patients with hepatitis is to exclude focal masses or a hepatocellular carcinoma.
- It can follow the course of immunosuppression by observing the reduction of lymph node size with therapy.

MRI
Findings
- Acute hepatitis: heterogeneous signal intensity, on T2-weighted sequences and heterogeneous pattern of enhancement on arterial-dominant-phase spoiled gradient-echo images

DIAGNOSTIC PEARLS
- *Starry sky* appearance on ultrasound
- Increased parenchymal echogenicity, with loss of portal-venous wall definition in chronic viral hepatitis
- Echogenic liver caused by fatty infiltration in acute alcoholic hepatitis

- Adenopathy in the lesser omentum
- Early patchy enhancement patterns in patients with chronic hepatitis associated with significant parenchymal inflammatory reaction
- Progressive enhancement on delayed images caused by leakage of gadolinium contrast from the intravascular into the interstitial space
- Cells being more alkaline than normal on phosphorus-31 MR spectroscopy in alcoholic hepatitis

Utility
- MRI depicts hepatic size and morphologic features and can be useful in depicting hepatic fibrosis and steatosis.
- Phosphorus-31 MR spectroscopy uses intracellular pH and an absolute molar concentration of adenosine triphosphate.

CLINICAL PRESENTATION
- Viral hepatitis produces fatigue, anorexia, nausea, vomiting, malaise, mild pyrexia, myalgias, photophobia, pharyngitis, cough, and coryza.
- Symptoms of viral hepatitis precede the onset of jaundice by 1-2 weeks.
- Clinical condition improves when jaundice appears, but the liver becomes enlarged and tender.
- Chronic hepatitis ensues if inflammatory changes persist for more than 6 months.
- Alcoholic hepatitis produces fever, neutrophil leukocytosis, malaise, anorexia, weight loss, upper abdominal pain, tender hepatomegaly, and jaundice.

WHAT THE REFERRING PHYSICIAN NEEDS TO KNOW
- Hepatitis A is self-limited, does not cause chronic hepatitis, and rarely causes fulminant hepatitis; the incubation period is 15-50 days.
- Drug addicts, dialysis patients, and health care workers are at significant risk for contracting hepatitis B infection.
- Hepatitis B virus infection is closely linked to hepatocellular carcinoma.
- Routine blood test for anti–hepatitis C antibody has been developed, improving transfusion safety.
- Repeated acute alcoholic hepatites are associated with a 10%-20% risk of death and a 35% risk of developing cirrhosis.
- Cessation of alcohol consumption and adequate nutrition may ameliorate the symptoms of the patient with alcoholic hepatitis clinically and histologically.

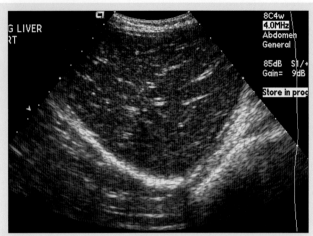

Figure 1. Hepatitis: sonographic features. In a patient with acute hepatitis, a transverse scan of the right lobe of the liver shows diffusely decreased parenchymal echogenicity with accentuated brightness of the portal triads and periportal cuffing, the so-called *starry sky* appearance.

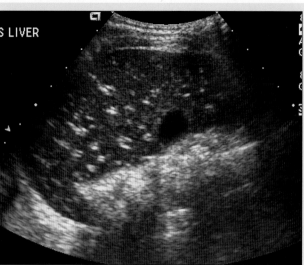

Figure 2. Hepatitis: sonographic features. In a patient with acute hepatitis, a sagittal scan of the right lobe of the liver shows diffusely decreased parenchymal echogenicity with accentuated brightness of the portal triads and periportal cuffing, the so-called *starry sky* appearance.

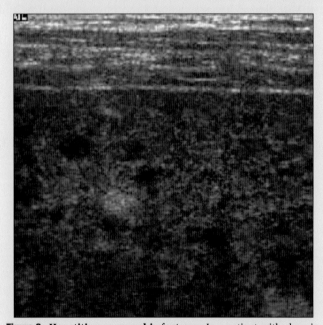

Figure 3. Hepatitis: sonographic features. In a patient with chronic active hepatitis, inhomogeneous parenchymal echogenicity is increased as a result of the inflammatory process surrounding the lobules that abut the portal triads. *(Courtesy of Peter Cooperberg, MD, Vancouver, British Columbia, Canada.)*

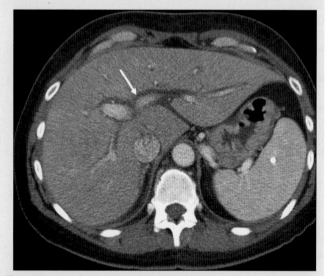

Figure 4. Acute hepatitis: CT findings. CT scan shows periportal edema *(arrow)* highlighting the intrahepatic blood vessels.

DIFFERENTIAL DIAGNOSIS

- Cholecystitis
- Cirrhosis
- Pancreatitis
- Primary and secondary liver neoplasms

PATHOLOGY

- Hepatitis: a term used to describe acute or chronic liver inflammation that may be viral, alcohol, or drug induced

- Inflamed liver: centrilobular necrosis, hepatocyte necrosis, periportal infiltration, reactive changes in Kupffer cells, and sinusoidal lining cells
- Chronic active hepatitis: necrosis and the formation of intralobular septa
- Chronic persistent hepatitis: relatively benign condition characterized histologically by cellular infiltrates in the necrosis
- Alcoholic hepatitis: part of the spectrum of alcoholic liver disease in which a major drinking binge produces acute liver cell necrosis
- Mallory bodies: histologic hallmark of alcoholic hepatitis; eosinophilic cytoplasmic inclusions or *candle droppings* in ballooned, and degenerating hepatocytes
- Alcoholic hepatitis: accompanied by pericellular and perivenular fibrosis, suggesting that this is a precursor of cirrhosis

INCIDENCE/PREVALENCE AND EPIDEMIOLOGY

- Viral hepatitis is responsible for 60% of cases of fulminant hepatic failure in the United States.
- Hepatitis B virus carriers worldwide total 200 million, 1.5 million of whom are in the United States; the incidence is 3.2 cases per 100,000 population.
- Hepatitis C virus (HCV) affects 0.5%-1.0% of normal volunteer blood donors in the United States.
- HCV accounts for 90% of hepatitis cases that develop after blood transfusions.
- Repeated acute alcoholic hepatitis is associated with a 10%-20% risk of death and a 35% risk of developing cirrhosis.

Suggested Readings

Cobbold JF, Wylezinska M, Cunningham C, et al: Non-invasive evaluation of hepatic fibrosis using magnetic resonance imaging and ultrasound techniques. *Gut* 55:1670-1672, 2006.

Danet I-M, Semelka RC, Braga L: MR imaging in diffuse liver disease. *Radiol Clin North Am* 41:67-87, 2003.

Farrell GC: Liver disease caused by drugs, anesthetics, and toxins. In Feldman M, Friedman LS, Sleisenger MH (eds): *Gastrointestinal and Liver Disease*, 7th ed. Philadelphia, Saunders, 2002, pp 1403-1447.

Hoofnagle JH, Heller T: Hepatitis C. In Zakim D, Boyer TD (eds): *Hepatology: A Textbook of Liver Disease*. Philadelphia, WB Saunders, 2003, pp 3-31.

Lamps LW, Washington K: Acute and chronic hepatitis. In Odze RD, Goldblum JR, Crawford JM (eds): *Surgical Pathology of the GI Tract, Liver, Biliary Tract, and Pancreas*. Philadelphia, WB Saunders, 2004, pp 863-885.

Lee V: Can MR imaging replace liver biopsy for the diagnosis of early fibrosis? *Radiology* 239:309-310, 2006.

Lee WM: Drug-induced hepatotoxicity. *N Engl J Med* 349:474-484, 2003.

Ly JN, Miller FH: Periportal contrast enhancement and abnormal signal intensity on state-of-the-art MR images. *AJR Am J Roentgenol* 176:891-897, 2001.

Maher JJ: Alcoholic liver disease. In Feldman M, Friedman LS, Sleisenger MH (eds): *Gastrointestinal and Liver Disease*, 7th ed. Philadelphia, Saunders, 2002, pp 1375-1386.

Martin DR, Semelka RC: Magnetic resonance imaging of the liver: Review of techniques and approach to common diseases. *Semin Ultrasound CT MRI* 26:116-131, 2005.

Mookerjee RP, Jalan R: Alcoholic liver disease. In Weinstein WM, Hawkey CJ, Bosch J (eds): *Clinical Gastroenterology and Hepatology*. Philadelphia, Elsevier-Mosby, 2005, pp 637-646.

Russmann S, Reichen J: Drug-induced and toxic liver disease. In Weinstein WM, Hawkey CJ, Bosch J (eds): *Clinical Gastroenterology and Hepatology*. Philadelphia, Elsevier-Mosby, 2005, pp 677-686.

Semelka RC, Braga L, Armao D: Liver. In Semelka RC (ed): *Abdominal-Pelvic MRI*. New York, Wiley-Liss, 2002, pp 33-318.

Stolz A: Liver physiology and metabolic function. In Feldman M, Friedman LS, Sleisenger MH (eds): *Gastrointestinal and Liver Disease*, 7th ed. Philadelphia, WB Saunders, 2002, pp 1202-1226.

Tchelepi H, Ralls PW, Radin R, et al: Sonography of diffuse liver disease. In Rumack C, Wilson SR, Charboneau WR (eds): *Diagnostic Ultrasound*, 3th ed. Philadelphia, Elsevier-Mosby, 2005.

Thimme R, Spangenberg HC, Blum HE: Acute viral hepatitis. In Weinstein WM, Hawkey CJ, Bosch J (eds): *Clinical Gastroenterology and Hepatology*. Philadelphia, Elsevier-Mosby, 2005, pp 583-594.

Yee HF, Lidofsy SD: Acute liver failure. In Feldman M, Friedman LS, Sleisenger MH (eds): *Gastrointestinal and Liver Disease*, 7th ed. Philadelphia, Saunders, 2002, pp 1202-1226.

Nonalcoholic Steatohepatitis

DEFINITION: Hepatic fatty metamorphosis or steatosis is a metabolic complication of a variety of toxic, ischemic, and infectious insults to the liver.

IMAGING

CT
Findings
- Increased hepatic fat decreases mean hepatic CT attenuation.
- In advanced cases, the liver is less dense than the portal and hepatic veins on nonenhanced CT.
- Mildly prominent lymph nodes are present in the porta hepatis in 58.3% of patients.
- Fatty infiltration may be lobar, segmental, or wedge-shaped.

Utility
- Excellent correlation exists between the hepatic parenchymal attenuation value and the amount of hepatic triglycerides found during a liver biopsy.
- Liver biopsy should be avoided in donors with an unacceptable degree of macrovesicular steatosis.
- Relationship of liver or spleen attenuation is reliably compared using unenhanced CT images.
- Contrast-enhanced images can be suggestive of the diagnosis of fatty infiltration.
- *Skip* areas of spared parenchyma in an otherwise fatty liver can also present a diagnostic challenge.

MRI
Findings
- Lesions containing fat show loss of signal intensity on the opposed-phase images when compared with the in-phase images.
- MR spectroscopy is very sensitive for fat detection.

Utility
- Proton chemical shift or opposed-phase gradient echo imaging is useful in differentiating fatty metamorphosis from neoplasm.
- Caveat: Neoplasms such as hepatocellular carcinoma have macroscopic fat and may show similar changes.
- MRI is useful in screening liver donors for hepatic macrosteatosis.

DIAGNOSTIC PEARLS
- Hepatic fat decreases mean hepatic CT attenuation.
- Lesions containing fat show a loss of signal intensity on opposed-phase MRIs when compared with in-phase images.
- Fatty liver usually appears diffusely echogenic on ultrasound.

Ultrasound
Findings
- Fatty liver appears diffusely echogenic.
- Increased attenuation of the ultrasound beam, with poorer visualization of deep hepatic structures and the hepatic venous system
- Focal fatty infiltration pattern: hyperechoic nodule, multiple confluent hyperechogenic lesions, hypoechoic skip nodules, and irregular hyperechoic and hypoechoic areas
- Liver parenchyma–spared areas from fatty metamorphosis appearing as ovoid, spherical, or sheet-like hypoechoic mass

Utility
- Degree of echogenicity is roughly proportional to the level of steatosis.
- Technical considerations are important in the sonographic diagnosis of focal fat because the operator may erroneously change time-gain-compensation curve.

Radiography
Findings
- Liver may appear hyperlucent and blend with the right properitoneal fat stripe.
- Fat-fluid interface may be present if the patient has ascites.
- Outer wall of the gut and viscus wall sign as soft-tissue density of the bowel wall are contrasted with the fatty liver.

WHAT THE REFERRING PHYSICIAN NEEDS TO KNOW
- With current obesity epidemic in United States, hepatic steatosis has become a major source of hepatic dysfunction.
- Nonalcoholic steatohepatitis may be seen in patients with hyperlipidemia and diabetes and may lead to *cryptogenic* cirrhosis.
- Histologic lesion of fatty infiltration caused by toxins is often reversible with substance abstinence.

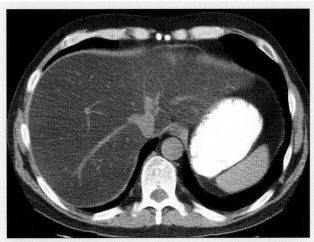

Figure 1. Hepatic steatosis: spectrum of CT findings. Diffuse hepatic steatosis. The density of the liver parenchyma is lower than that of the spleen on this unenhanced CT scan. Note how the intrahepatic blood vessels stand out as hyperattenuating structures.

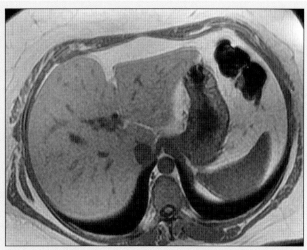

Figure 2. Hepatic steatosis: spectrum of MRI findings. In-phase T1-weighted spoiled gradient-echo image demonstrates normal hepatic signal intensity.

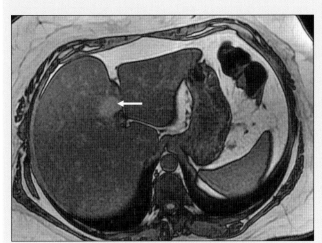

Figure 3. Hepatic steatosis: spectrum of MRI findings. Opposed-phase image shows diffuse loss of hepatic signal intensity, indicating diffuse hepatic steatosis. Note the focal region of sparing *(arrow)* adjacent to the falciform ligament in the medial segment of the left hepatic lobe.

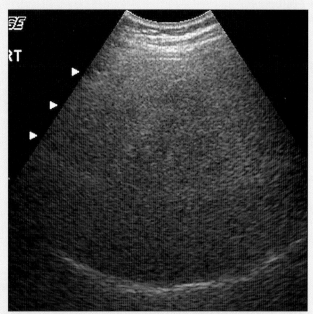

Figure 4. Hepatic steatosis: spectrum of sonographic findings. Sagittal scan of the right lobe of the liver shows an enlarged, echogenic liver with poor sound penetration. The walls of the hepatic veins and portal veins are not defined.

Utility

- Radiography is insensitive to the presence of fat in the liver unless marked degrees of infiltration are present.
- It is not used to establish the diagnosis.

CLINICAL PRESENTATION

- Fatty metamorphosis is clinically silent in most cases, and liver chemistry values are normal.
- Liver may be slightly enlarged in the asymptomatic obese or diabetic patient.
- In alcoholic patients, vague right upper quadrant tenderness and pain with hepatomegaly is associated with abnormal liver function tests.
- Acute fatty liver in pregnancy, carbon tetrachloride exposure, and alcoholic binge patients may have jaundice, acute hepatic failure, or even encephalopathy.

DIFFERENTIAL DIAGNOSIS

- Alcoholic steatohepatitis
- Hepatic infarction
- Hepatic necrosis
- Multiple metastases if focal
- Primary benign or malignant liver tumor if focal

PATHOLOGY

- Hepatic fatty metamorphosis or steatosis is a metabolic complication of a variety of toxic, ischemic, and infectious insults to the liver.
- It is most frequently seen on liver biopsies of alcoholics and is seen in up to 50% of patients with diabetes mellitus.
- Lipid accumulates within the cytoplasm of the hepatocyte in the centrilobular zone.
- Segmental areas of fatty infiltration of the liver culminate in a *metabolic infarct* of the involved region.
- Fatty replacement occurs where glycogen is depleted from the liver.

INCIDENCE/PREVALENCE AND EPIDEMIOLOGY

- Fatty infiltration of liver has been observed in 25% of nonalcoholic, previously healthy adult males meeting accidental deaths.

Suggested Readings

Adams LA, Lymp JF, St. Sauver J, et al: The natural history of nonalcoholic fatty liver disease: A population-based cohort study. *Gastroenterology* 129:113-121, 2005.

Cobbold JF, Wylezinska M, Cunningham C, et al: Non-invasive evaluation of hepatic fibrosis using magnetic resonance imaging and ultrasound techniques. *Gut* 55:1670-1672, 2006.

Day CP: From fat to inflammation. *Gastroenterology* 130:207-210, 2006.

Guha IN, Parkes J, Roderick PR, et al: Non-invasive markers associated with liver fibrosis in non-alcoholic fatty liver disease. *Gut* 55:1650-1660, 2006.

Hamer OW, Aguirre DA, Casola G, et al: Imaging features of perivascular fatty infiltration of the liver: Initial observations. *Radiology* 237:159-169, 2005.

Hamer OW, Aguirre DA, Casola G, et al: Fatty liver: Imaging patterns and pitfalls. *RadioGraphics* 26:1637-1653, 2006.

Hoofnagle JH, Heller T: Hepatitis C. In Zakim D, Boyer TD (eds): *Hepatology: A Textbook of Liver Disease.* Philadelphia, WB Saunders, 2003, pp 3-31.

Hubscher SG: Histological assessment of non-alcoholic fatty liver disease. Histopathology 49:450-465, 2006.

Hussain HK, Chenervert TL, Londy FJ, et al: Hepatic fat fraction: MR imaging for quantitative measurement and display: Early experience. *Radiology* 237:1048-1055, 2005.

Khalili K, Lan FP, Hanbridge AE, et al: Hepatic subcapsular steatosis in response to intraperitoneal insulin delivery: CT findings and prevalence. *AJR Am J Roentgenol* 180:1601-1604, 2003.

Kim SH, Lee JM, Han JK, et al: Hepatic macrosteatosis. *Radiology* 240:116-129, 2006.

Lamps LW, Washington K: Acute and chronic hepatitis. In Odze RD, Goldblum JR, Crawford JM (eds): *Surgical Pathology of the GI Tract, Liver, Biliary Tract, and Pancreas.* Philadelphia, WB Saunders, 2004, pp 863-885.

Merkle EM, Nelson RC: Dual gradient-echo in-phase and opposed-phase hepatic MR imaging: A useful tool for evaluating more than fatty infiltration or fatty sparing. *RadioGraphics* 26:1409-1418, 2006.

Miyake K, Hayakawa K, Nishino M, et al: Effects of oral 5-fluorouracil drugs on hepatic fat content in patients with colon cancer. *Acad Radiol* 12:722-727, 2005.

Moscatiello S, Manini R, Marchesini G: Diabetes and liver disease: An ominous association. *Nutr Metab Cardiovasc Dis* 17:63-70, 2007.

Oliva MR, Mortele KJ, Segatto E, et al: Computed tomography features of nonalcoholic steohepatitis with histopathologic correlation. *J Comput Assist Tomogr* 30:37-46, 2006.

Park SH, Kim PN, Kim KW, et al: Macrovesicular hepatic steatosis in living liver donors: Use of CT for quantitative and qualitative assessment. *Radiology* 239:105-112, 2006.

Tchelepi H, Ralls PW, Radin R, et al: Sonography of diffuse liver disease. In Rumack C, Wilson SR, Charboneau WR, et al (eds): *Diagnostic Ultrasound,* 3rd ed. Philadelphia, Elsevier-Mosby, 2005.

Radiation-Induced Liver Disease

DEFINITION: Hepatic injury in patients receiving radiation therapy.

IMAGING

Ultrasound
Findings
- Hypoechoic regions relative to the remainder of the liver

Utility
- Liver involvement is easily detected sonographically in patients who have fatty livers resulting from chemotherapy or other causes.

CT
Findings
- Sharply defined band of low attenuation corresponding to the treatment port
- Patchy congestion simulating tumor nodules
- In patients with fatty infiltration of liver, irradiated area appearing as a region of increased attenuation
- Over a period of weeks, initially sharp borders of irradiated area that become irregular and indistinct
- Eventually, irradiated area becomes atrophic

Utility
- In patients with fatty infiltration of liver, the irradiated area may appear as region of increased attenuation.

MRI
Findings
- Geographic areas of low signal intensity on T1-weighted images
- High signal intensity on T2-weighted images
- Increased water content

Utility
- MR spectroscopy

CLINICAL PRESENTATION

- Hepatomegaly and ascites are seen.
- If the irradiated area is small, the patient may be asymptomatic.
- If the liver receives a high dose of radiation during childhood, the liver may become atrophic.

DIFFERENTIAL DIAGNOSIS

- Segmental hepatic steatosis
- Transient hepatic attenuation differences
- Transient hepatic intensity differences

DIAGNOSTIC PEARLS

- Hypoechoic regions relative to the remainder of the liver on ultrasound
- Sharply defined band of low attenuation corresponding to the treatment port on CT
- Areas of low signal intensity on T1-weighted images and high signal intensity on T2-weighted MRIs

PATHOLOGY

- Massive panlobar congestion, hyperemia, hemorrhage, and mild proliferative changes in sublobular central veins are seen.
- Stasis secondary to injury of these veins is responsible for most of the acute findings.
- Patient may exhibit permanent hepatocyte loss, fat deposition, fibrosis, and obliteration of central veins.
- These changes are seen within the radiation portal.

INCIDENCE/PREVALENCE AND EPIDEMIOLOGY

- Patients receiving a single 1200-rad dose of external beam radiation or 4000-5500-rad fractionated dose over 6 weeks

Suggested Readings

Friedman SL, Rockey DC, Bissell DM: Hepatic fibrosis 2006: Report of the third AASLD Single Topic Conference. *Hepatology* 45:242-249, 2007.

Lamps LW, Washington K: Acute and chronic hepatitis. In Odze RD, Goldblum JR, Crawford JM (eds): *Surgical Pathology of the GI Tract, Liver, Biliary Tract, and Pancreas.* Philadelphia, WB Saunders, 2004, pp 863-885.

Semelka RC, Braga L, Armao D: Liver. In Semelka RC (ed): *Abdominal-Pelvic MRI.* New York, Wiley-Liss, 2002, pp 33-318.

Wilson SR, Withers CE: The liver. In Rumack C, Wilson SR, Charboneau WR (eds): *Diagnostic Ultrasound*, 3rd ed. Philadelphia, Elsevier-Mosby, 2005.

WHAT THE REFERRING PHYSICIAN NEEDS TO KNOW

- Complete clinical recovery is typically seen within 60 days.
- Nearly 75% of patients receiving whole liver irradiation have abnormal liver function tests.

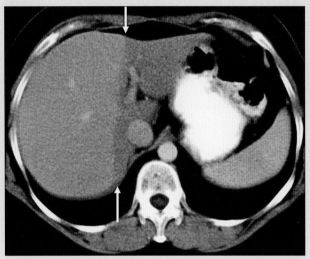

Figure 1. Radiation-induced hepatic injury. Contrast-enhanced CT scan shows a sharply defined *(arrows)* region of hepatic hypoattenuation near the dome of the liver. This patient had received external beam radiation therapy for lung carcinoma.

Sarcoidosis (Gastrointestinal)

DEFINITION: Sarcoidosis is a systemic granulomatous disorder that commonly affects the liver.

ANATOMIC FINDINGS

Liver
- Hepatomegaly
- Nodules within the liver parenchyma

IMAGING

CT
Findings
- Hepatomegaly, splenomegaly, upper abdominal adenopathy, and gastric outlet obstruction
- Hypoattenuating nodules varying in size up to 2 cm

Utility
- Imaging studies depict nodular changes in only one third of affected patients.
- Sensitivity: 35%
- Specificity: 25%
- Accuracy: 28%

Ultrasound
Findings
- Larger granulomas appearing as hypoechoic nodules
- Hepatomegaly, splenomegaly, upper abdominal adenopathy, and gastric outlet obstruction

Utility
- Ultrasound is inferior to CT and MRI in the depiction of these changes.

MRI
Findings
- Nodules appear hypointense on both T1-weighted and T2-weighted sequences when compared with adjacent liver parenchyma.
- Hepatomegaly, splenomegaly, upper abdominal adenopathy, and gastric outlet obstruction

Utility
Sensitivity: 40%
Specificity: 25%
Accuracy: 30%

CLINICAL PRESENTATION

- Clinically apparent liver disease is infrequent in patients with hepatic sarcoidosis.
- Rarely, sarcoidosis can lead to chronic inflammation, chronic hepatitis, and cirrhosis.

DIAGNOSTIC PEARLS

- Most prevalent CT finding of sarcoidosis in liver is hepatomegaly.
- Hypoattenuating nodules varying in size up to 2 cm will be seen on CT.
- Mitochondrial antibody test is negative in sarcoidosis.

- Patients may have cholestatic liver disease with jaundice.
- Jaundice, weight loss, cough, shortness of breath, and right upper quadrant pain

DIFFERENTIAL DIAGNOSIS

- Gastric outlet obstruction (stomach and duodenum)
- Ménétrier disease (stomach and duodenum)
- Duodenal ulcers

PATHOLOGY

- Biopsy of the liver will reveal diffuse, small, noncaseating granulomas, usually less than 2 mm in size.

INCIDENCE/PREVALENCE AND EPIDEMIOLOGY

- Twenty-four to seventy-nine percent of patients with sarcoidosis have liver involvement.

Suggested Readings

Ayyala US, Padilla ML: Diagnosis and treatment of hepatic sarcoidosis. *Curr Treat Options Gastroenterol* 9:475-483, 2006.
Jung G, Brill N, Poll LW, et al: MRI of hepatic sarcoidosis: Large confluent lesions mimicking malignancy. *AJR Am J Roentgenol* 183:171-173, 2004.
Karagiannidis A, Karavalaki M, Koulaouzidis A: Hepatic sarcoidosis. *Ann Hepatol* 5:251-256, 2006.
Koyama T, Ueda H, Togashi K, et al: Radiologic manifestations of sarcoidosis in various organs. *RadioGraphics* 24:87-104, 2004.
Nguyen BD: F-18 FDG PET imaging of disseminated sarcoidosis. *Clin Nucl Med* 32:53-54, 2007.
Warshauer DM, Lee JKT: Imaging manifestations of abdominal sarcoidosis. *AJR Am J Roentgenol* 182:15-28, 2004.

WHAT THE REFERRING PHYSICIAN NEEDS TO KNOW

- Most granulomas are small; imaging studies depict nodular changes in only approximately one third of affected patients.

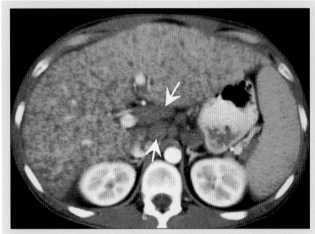

Figure 1. Sarcoidosis: CT findings. Contrast-enhanced CT shows hepatomegaly with innumerable small hypodense nodules. Portal adenopathy is also present *(arrows)*. *(From Warshauer DM, Lee JKT: Imaging manifestations of abdominal sarcoidosis. AJR Am J Roentgenol 182:15-28, 2004. Reprinted with permission from the American Journal of Roentgenology.)*

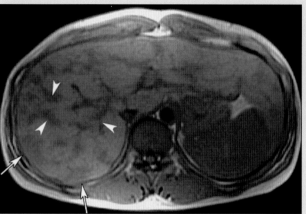

Figure 2. Sarcoidosis: MRI findings. Unenhanced gradient-echo T1-weighted MR image of the upper abdomen demonstrates irregularly shaped, low-signal-intensity nodules peripherally in the liver *(arrows)* and widening of the periportal tract *(arrowheads)*. *(From Koyama T, Ueda H, Togashi K, et al: Radiologic manifestations of sarcoidosis in various organs. RadioGraphics 24:87-104, 2004.)*

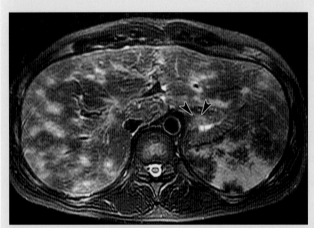

Figure 3. Sarcoidosis: MRI findings. On a T2-weighted MR image of the upper abdomen, the peripheral liver nodules demonstrate increased signal intensity. Multiple hypointense nodules in the spleen create a heterogeneous appearance. The area of focal hyperintensity *(arrowheads)* represents gastric mucosal involvement. *(From Koyama T, Ueda H, Togashi K, et al: Radiologic manifestations of sarcoidosis in various organs. RadioGraphics 24:87-104, 2004.)*

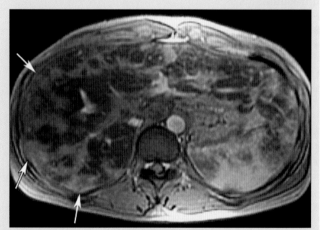

Figure 4. Sarcoidosis: MRI findings. Ferumoxide-enhanced gradient-echo T2-weighted MR image shows multiple hyperintense nodules scattered throughout the periphery of the liver *(arrows)* and a hyperintense, widened periportal tract. *(From Koyama T, Ueda H, Togashi K, et al: Radiologic manifestations of sarcoidosis in various organs. RadioGraphics 24: 87-104, 2004.)*

Secondary Biliary Cirrhosis

DEFINITION: Results from long-standing partial or complete obstruction of the common bile duct or its major branches.

ANATOMIC FINDINGS

Liver
- Lobulation of the liver contour, atrophy of the posterior and lateral segments, and hypertrophy of the caudate lobe are seen.
- Atrophy of the lateral segment of the left lobe is distinctive because, in other forms of cirrhosis, the lateral segment hypertrophies.

Spleen
- Splenomegaly and retrosplenic varices

IMAGING

CT
Findings
- Caudate lobe may have higher attenuation than the remainder of the liver on noncontrast scans, producing a pseudotumor appearance.
- Enlarged lymph nodes in the lesser omentum are also quite common.

Utility
- Inferior to MRI diagnostically
- Sensitivity: 50%-83%
- Specificity: 45%-90%
- Accuracy: 60%-80%

MRI
Findings
- Peripheral wedge-shaped zones of hyperintense signal can be seen on T2-weighted images.
- These triangular areas range in size from 1-5 cm.
- On T1-weighted images, areas of increased signal intensity in the liver that do not correspond to fat may be seen.
- After contrast administration, areas of patchy or segmental increased enhancement are frequently seen.
- Areas often remain mildly or markedly hyperintense on delayed images.
- Large regenerative nodules that cause obstruction of bile ducts and segmental atrophy of peripheral liver may be seen.

Utility
- The best test for noninvasively making the diagnosis
- Sensitivity: 80%-95%

DIAGNOSTIC PEARLS
- Lobulation of the liver contour, atrophy of the posterior and lateral segments, and hypertrophy of the caudate lobe are seen.
- Atrophy of lateral segment of the left lobe is distinctive.
- Peripheral wedge-shaped zones of hyperintense signal are seen on T2-weighted images.

- Specificity: 75%-85%
- Accuracy: 90%

CLINICAL PRESENTATION
- Long-standing history of hepatic dysfunction
- Variceal bleeding
- Liver failure
- Splenomegaly

DIFFERENTIAL DIAGNOSIS
- Viral associated cirrhosis
- Alcohol associated cirrhosis

PATHOLOGY
- Based on the involved areas of inflammatory and fibrotic changes, secondary biliary cirrhosis has four pathologic stages.
- These stages are as follows: stage 1, portal; stage 2, periportal; stage 3, septal; and stage 4, cirrhosis.

INCIDENCE/PREVALENCE AND EPIDEMIOLOGY
- Primary sclerosing cholangitis is the most common cause of secondary biliary cirrhosis.
- It is seen more commonly in patients with ulcerative colitis than Crohn disease.

WHAT THE REFERRING PHYSICIAN NEEDS TO KNOW
- Lobulation of the liver contour, atrophy of posterior and lateral segments, and hypertrophy of caudate lobe are seen.
- Atrophy of the lateral segment of the left lobe is distinctive because, in other forms of cirrhosis, the lateral segment hypertrophies.

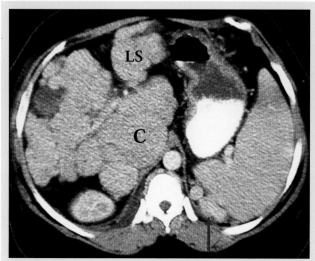

Figure 1. Secondary biliary cirrhosis caused by primary sclerosing cholangitis: CT findings. Advanced cirrhotic changes are present with a markedly lobulated liver, enlargement of the caudate lobe (C), and widening of the fissures. Atrophy of the lateral segment (LS) of the left lobe can be seen, which is a key differentiating feature from alcoholic and posthepatic cirrhosis. Note the splenomegaly and retrosplenic varices (*arrow*).

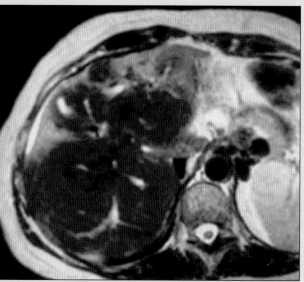

Figure 2. Secondary biliary cirrhosis caused by primary sclerosing cholangitis: CT findings. T2-weighted, single-shot, fat-suppressed image shows a very lobulated liver with caudate lobe enlargement and atrophy of the lateral segment of the left lobe.

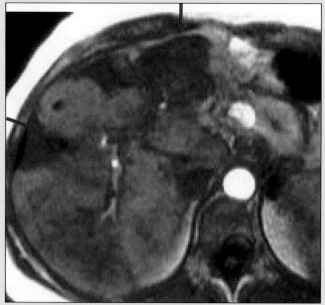

Figure 3. Secondary biliary cirrhosis caused by primary sclerosing cholangitis: CT findings. Early postgadolinium T1-weighted image shows peripheral areas of fibrosis that show contrast accretion on the delayed images (*arrows*).

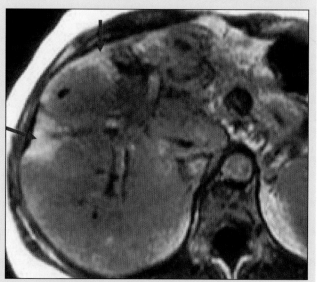

Figure 4. Secondary biliary cirrhosis caused by primary sclerosing cholangitis: CT findings. Delayed postgadolinium T1-weighted image shows peripheral areas of fibrosis that show contrast accretion on the delayed images (*arrows*).

Suggested Readings

Bader TR, Beavers KL, Semelka RC: MR imaging features of primary sclerosing cholangitis: Patterns of cirrhosis in relationship to clinical severity of disease. *Radiology* 226:675-685, 2003.

Berstad AE, Aabakken L, Smith HJ, et al: Diagnostic accuracy of magnetic resonance and endoscopic cetrograde cholangiography in primary sclerosing cholangitis. *Clin Gastroenterol Hepatol* 4:514-520, 2006.

Dodd GD 3rd, Baron RL, Oliver JH 3rd, et al: End-stage primary sclerosing cholangitis: CT findings of hepatic morphology in 36 patients. *Radiology* 211:357-362, 1999.

Dusunceli E, Erden A, Erden I, et al: Primary sclerosing cholangitis: MR cholangiopancreatography and T2-weighted MR imaging findings. *Diagn Interv Radiol* 11:213-218, 2005.

Elsayes KM, Oliveira EP, Narra VR, et al: MR and MRCP in the evaluation of primary sclerosing cholangitis: Current applications and imaging findings. *J Comput Assist Tomogr* 30:398-404, 2006.

Jessurun J, Pambuccian S: Infectious and inflammatory disorders of the gallbladder and extrahepatic biliary tract. In Odze RD, Goldblum JR, Crawford JM (eds): *Surgical Pathology of the GI Tract, Liver, Biliary Tract, and Pancreas*. Philadelphia, Saunders, 2004.

Johnson KJ, Olliff JF, Olliff SP: The presence and significance of lymphadenopathy detected by CT in primary sclerosing cholangitis. *Br J Radiol* 71:1279-1282, 1998.

Mahadevan U, Bass NM: Sclerosing cholangitis and recurrent pyogenic cholangitis. In Feldman M, Friedman LS, Sleisenger MH (eds): *Gastrointestinal and Liver Disease*, 7th ed. Philadelphia, Saunders, 2002.

Mendes FD, Lindor KD: Primary sclerosing cholangitis. In Weinstein WM, Hawkey CJ, Bosch J (eds): *Clinical Gastroenterology and Hepatology*, Philadelphia, Elsevier-Mosby, 2005.

Revelon G, Rashid A, Kawamoto S, et al: Primary sclerosing cholangitis: MR imaging findings with pathologic correlation. *AJR Am J Roentgenol* 173:1037-1042, 1999.

Toxin- and Drug-Induced Liver Disease

DEFINITION: Acute or chronic liver disease caused by certain drugs or chemical agents.

IMAGING

MRI

Findings

- Chemotherapy damage, most prominently in the periportal regions
- High proton signal intensity on T2-weighted images and high sodium signal intensity on spectroscopy

Utility

- MRI is vital in showing diffuse parenchymal disease rather than biliary obstruction or liver metastases as the cause of hepatic dysfunction.
- Carbon tetrachloride produces water and sodium retention, which can be detected by sodium-23 and proton imaging.

Ultrasound

Findings

- Amiodarone toxicity is nonspecific and is related to fatty infiltration or cirrhosis.

Utility

- The findings on ultrasound are nonspecific.

CT

Findings

- Increased parenchymal attenuation simulating hemochromatosis can be identified when amiodarone accumulates in sufficient quantities in the liver.

Utility

- The findings on CT are nonspecific.

CLINICAL PRESENTATION

- Spectrum of hepatotoxicity is varied.
- Hepatotoxicity ranges from acute, dose-related, hepatocellular necrosis to chronic disorders (e.g., mild chronic persistent hepatitis) to severe chronic active hepatitis.
- Jaundice
- Right upper quadrant pain
- Fatigue
- Malaise
- Hepatomegaly

DIAGNOSTIC PEARLS

- Findings are nonspecific and identical to those seen in other liver injuries: hepatomegaly, cirrhosis, and fatty infiltration.
- Increased parenchymal attenuation simulating hemochromatosis is identified when amiodarone accumulates in sufficient quantities in the liver.
- Chemotherapy damage is most prominent in periportal regions on MRI.

DIFFERENTIAL DIAGNOSIS

- Steatohepatitis
- Hepatitis B
- Hepatitis C
- Alcoholic hepatitis

PATHOLOGY

- Methotrexate causes fatty change, portal triad fibrosis, and cirrhosis, whereas corticosteroids and L-asparaginase induce fatty metamorphosis.
- Dacarbazine and 6-thioguanine cause intrahepatic portal vein thrombosis, producing a Budd-Chiari–type of appearance.
- Azathioprine and 6-mercaptopurine therapy induces intrahepatic cholestasis and variable degrees of parenchymal cell necrosis.
- Intra-arterial infusion of floxuridine causes chemical hepatitis and biliary strictures, simulating sclerosing cholangitis.
- Mithramycin, the most hepatotoxic drug used in chemotherapy, is associated with acute parenchymal necrosis.
- Avastin has been associated with hepatic veno-occlusive disease.
- More severe amiodarone toxicity simulates alcoholic liver disease with liver fatty metamorphosis, Mallory bodies, and cirrhosis.

WHAT THE REFERRING PHYSICIAN NEEDS TO KNOW

- Certain drugs and other chemical agents are capable of producing virtually all types of acute and chronic liver disease.
- Findings are nonspecific and identical to those seen in other liver injuries: hepatomegaly, cirrhosis, and fatty infiltration.
- Imaging is vital in showing diffuse parenchymal disease rather than biliary obstruction or liver metastases as the cause of hepatic dysfunction.

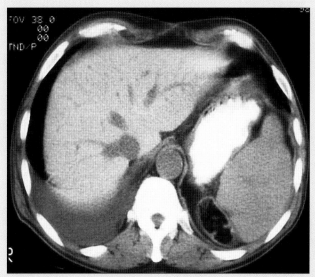

Figure 1. Amiodarone hepatotoxicity. Noncontrast CT scan of a cardiac patient who had been taking amiodarone demonstrates a liver with an abnormally high attenuation when compared with the spleen. Note how the hepatic blood vessels are highlighted by the dense parenchyma. The appearance is indistinguishable from that of hepatic iron overload. A right-sided pleural effusion can be seen.

INCIDENCE/PREVALENCE AND EPIDEMIOLOGY

- Toxin- and drug-induced liver disease accounts for 2%-5% of hospital admissions for jaundice in the United States.
- It accounts for up to 43% of admissions for *acute hepatitis*.
- Drugs such as halothane, acetaminophen, α-methyldopa, and phenytoin account for 20%-50% of cases of fulminant hepatic failure.

Suggested Readings

Farrell GC: Liver disease caused by drugs, anesthetics. In Feldman M, Friedman LS, Sleisenger MH (eds): *Gastrointestinal and Liver Disease*, 7th ed. Philadelphia, Saunders, 2002.

Lee WM: Drug-induced hepatotoxicity. *N Engl J Med* 349:474-484, 2003.

Maher JJ, Feldman M, Friedman LS, Sleisenger MH: Alcoholic liver disease. In *Gastrointestinal and Liver Disease*, 7th ed. Philadelphia, Saunders, 2002.

Semelka RC, Braga L, Armao D: Liver. In Semelka RC (ed): *Abdominal-Pelvic MRI*. New York, Wiley-Liss, 2002.

Wilson Disease

DEFINITION: Rare, autosomal-recessive inherited disorder of copper metabolism.

ANATOMIC FINDINGS

Liver
- Fatty infiltration changes
- Acute hepatitis
- Chronic active hepatitis
- Cirrhosis
- Massive liver necrosis

Bone
- Osteomalacia
- Chondrocalcinosis
- Premature degenerative joint disease with fragmentation
- Cystic changes and sclerosis of subchondral bone
- Anterior compression of dorsal vertebral bodies

IMAGING

Ultrasound
Findings
- Fatty infiltration changes and cirrhosis

Utility
- Indistinguishable from those of other causes

CT
Findings
- Fatty infiltration changes and cirrhosis

Utility
- Indistinguishable from those of other causes

MRI
Findings
- Hypointense nodules may be seen on T2-weighted images.
- Elevation in phosphomonoester (PME) resonance is concurrent with reduction in phosphodiester (PDE) resonance.

Utility
- MR spectroscopy is used.
- Phosphorus-31 MR spectroscopy offers potential in grading and disease monitoring in patients with Wilson disease.

DIAGNOSTIC PEARLS

- Kayser-Fleischer rings are seen.
- Bone changes occur in over 85% of patients.
- Most cases occur in childhood or early adolescence with manifestations of liver disease.

- It provides information about the pathophysiologic features of liver injury.
- It also contributes to the assessment of hepatic functional state in chronic liver disease.
- Specificity: 90%
- Sensitivity: 40%
- Accuracy: 55%

CLINICAL PRESENTATION

- Most cases occur in childhood or early adolescence with manifestations of liver disease before the onset of neurologic changes.
- Nearly one half of untreated patients remain asymptomatic to age 16 years.
- In adults, hepatic injury appears insidiously after the cirrhosis evolves, clinically simulating chronic active hepatitis.
- If hepatic changes remain subclinical, the condition may occur in the patient's late teens or early 20s with a Parkinson-like movement disorder.
- Psychiatric disturbances occur in the late teens or early 20s.
- Kayser-Fleischer rings of green to brown copper deposits occur on the cornea.
- Serum ceruloplasmin value is low (< 20 mg/100 mL) in 95% of cases, and the urinary excretion of copper is elevated (> 100 pg/day).

DIFFERENTIAL DIAGNOSIS

- Cirrhosis

WHAT THE REFERRING PHYSICIAN NEEDS TO KNOW

- Imaging is needed in patients with a normal ceruloplasmin level and high copper content.
- Spectrum of hepatic injury is nonspecific.
- Fatty infiltration, acute hepatitis, chronic active hepatitis, cirrhosis, or massive liver necrosis may be seen.
- Penicillamine and zinc are effective in chelating the copper and in preventing its toxic deposition in the liver and brain.
- Treatment of asymptomatic patients prevents the disease from manifesting.
- Symptomatic patients improve, sometimes dramatically.

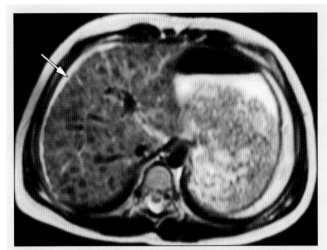

Figure 1. Wilson disease: imaging findings. A 9-year-old girl with Wilson disease. T2-weighted axial MR image (TR/TE, 1800/90) of the liver shows numerous tiny hypointense nodules in the liver at presentation before medical treatment. Note hyperintense ascitic fluid *(arrow)* around edge of liver. *(From Chu WCW, Leung TF, Chan KF, et al: Wilson's disease with chronic active hepatitis: Monitoring by in vivo 31-phosphorus MR spectroscopy before and after medical treatment. AJR Am J Roentgenol 183:1339-1342, 2004. Reprinted with permission from the American Journal of Roentgenology.)*

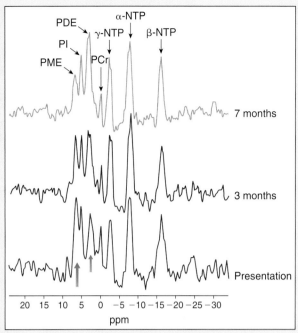

Figure 2. Wilson disease: imaging findings. Graph shows representative serial phosphorus-31 MR liver spectra before and after 3 and 7 months of medical treatment. Elevation in phosphomonoester resonance *(long arrow)* is concurrent with reduction in phosphodiester resonance *(short arrow)* at presentation followed by gradual reversal change in subsequent 3- and 7-month spectra. (*NTP*, nucleotide triphosphate; *PI*, inorganic phosphate; *PCr*, phosphocreatine.) *(From Chu WCW, Leung TF, Chan KF, et al: Wilson's disease with chronic active hepatitis: Monitoring by in vivo 31-phosphorus MR spectroscopy before and after medical treatment. AJR Am J Roentgenol 183:1339-1342, 2004. Reprinted with permission from the American Journal of Roentgenology.)*

PATHOLOGY

- Result of impaired biliary excretion of copper
- Excessive absorption of copper from the gastrointestinal tract
- Initially, copper accumulating in the liver
- Abnormal urinary excretion of copper
- Deposition to toxic levels occurring in the basal ganglia, renal tubules, cornea, bones, joints, and parathyroid glands

INCIDENCE/PREVALENCE AND EPIDEMIOLOGY

- Most cases occur in childhood or early adolescence.

Suggested Readings

Akpinar E, Akhan O: Liver imaging findings of Wilson's disease. *Eur J Radiol* (Epub ahead of print) Dec 7, 2006.

Bean MJ, Horton KM, Fishman EK: Concurrent focal hepatic and splenic lesions: A pictorial guide to differential diagnosis. *J Comput Assist Tomogr* 28:605-612, 2004.

Chu WCW, Leung TF, Chan KF, et al: Wilson's disease with chronic active hepatitis: Monitoring by in vivo 31-phosphorus MR spectroscopy before and after medical treatment. *AJR Am J Roentgenol* 183:1339-1342, 2004.

Ferenci P: Wilson's disease. *Clin Gastroenterol Hepatol* 3:726-733, 2005.

Gitlin JD: Wilson's disease. In Zakim D, Boyer TD (eds): *Hepatology: A Textbook of Liver Disease*. Philadelphia, WB Saunders, 2003.

Kozic D, Svetel M, Petrovic I, et al: Regression of nodular liver lesions in Wilson's disease. *Acta Radiol* 47:624-627, 2006.

Medici V, Trevisan CP, D'Inca R, et al: Diagnosis and management of Wilson's disease: Results of a single center experience. *J Clin Gastroenterol* 40:936-941, 2006.

Mehta A: Epidemiology and natural history of Gaucher's disease. *Eur J Intern Med* 17(Suppl):S2-S5, 2006.

Budd-Chiari Syndrome and Hepatic Veno-Occlusive Disease

DEFINITION: Diverse group of conditions associated with hepatic venous outflow obstruction at the level of either the large hepatic veins or the suprahepatic segment of the inferior vena cava; also, in a subset of cases, nonthrombotic occlusion of small presinusoidal venules (hepatic veno-occlusive disease).

ANATOMIC FINDINGS

Liver
- Gross swelling
- Abnormal shape with enlargement of caudate lobe and right lobe atrophy (in chronic disease)
- Nodularity of hepatic contour
- Nonthrombotic occlusion of presinusoidal venule

Portal Vein
- Slow or reversal of flow
- Intraluminal thrombus
- Membranous webs

Hepatic Veins
- Stenosis
- Absent or reversal of flow
- Intraluminal thrombus
- Membranous webs

Inferior Vena Cava
- Stenosis
- Absent or reversal of flow
- Intraluminal thrombus
- Membranous webs

DIAGNOSTIC PEARLS
- Duplex ultrasound findings of absent or reversed hepatic vein flow with reversed inferior vena cava flow is diagnostic.
- Clinical diagnosis may be inferred from an absent cirrhotic cause, abdominal pain episodes over the preceding month, and, uncommonly, a palpable caudate lobe.
- *Flip-flop* pattern of contrast enhancement is a classic finding.
- Diagnosis is seldom made on clinical grounds alone because clinicians tend to ignore symptoms of cirrhosis.

IMAGING

Ultrasound
Findings
- Thick, echogenic walls and proximal dilation of the hepatic veins (hepatic vein stenosis)
- Echogenic intravenous thrombi
- Intrahepatic collaterals or extrahepatic anastomoses

WHAT THE REFERRING PHYSICIAN NEEDS TO KNOW
- Diagnosis is seldom made on clinical grounds alone because clinicians tend to assume symptoms are due to cirrhosis.
- Correct diagnosis may be inferred from an unknown cause of cirrhosis, abdominal pain episodes over the preceding month, and, uncommonly, a palpable caudate lobe.
- Duplex ultrasound findings of absent or reversed hepatic vein flow with reversed inferior vena cava flow are diagnostic.
- *Flip-flop* pattern of contrast enhancement is a classic finding.
- Treatment and prognosis are based on the rate and degree of hepatic outflow obstruction.
- Most patients require portal decompression to prevent liver failure and relieve ascites.
- Treatment ranges from medical (high-dose steroids or nutritional therapy) to interventional techniques (angioplasty with balloons or lasers or stent insertion).

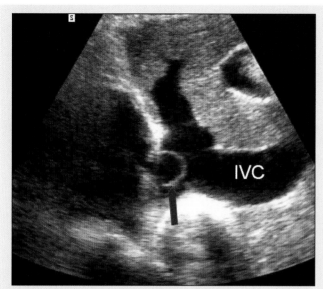

Figure 1. Budd-Chiari syndrome: sonographic findings. Sagittal sonogram shows a thin fibrous web *(arrow)* across the inferior vena cava.

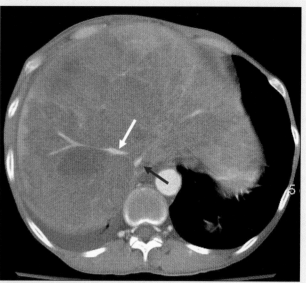

Figure 2. Budd-Chiari syndrome: CT features. The inferior vena cava *(red arrow)* and right hepatic vein *(white arrow)* are narrowed and attenuated in this patient with a swollen, inhomogeneous liver.

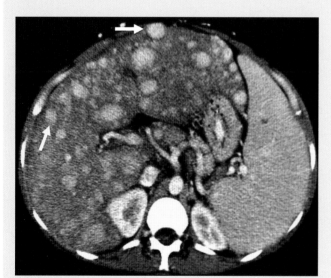

Figure 3. Budd-Chiari syndrome: nodular regenerative hyperplasia. Multiple hypervascular lesions *(arrows)* are identified on CT scan. (*Courtesy of Michael P. Federle, MD, Pittsburgh, PA.*)

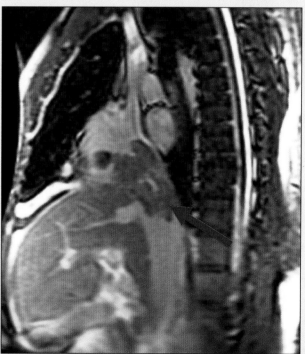

Figure 4. Budd-Chiari syndrome: MRI findings in a patient with hepatocellular carcinoma invading the hepatic veins and inferior vena cava. Parasagittal image shows tumor thrombus *(arrow)* invading the inferior vena cava and right atrium.

- Large infrahepatic inferior vena cava
- Hepatomegaly
- Ascites
- Echogenic or focal luminal obliterations (membranous webs)

Utility
- Ultrasound has excellent sensitivity and is a highly specific, noninvasive, and economic screening tool.
- It obviates the need for angiography and venography.

Ultrasound Power Doppler
Findings
- Absent or reversed hepatic venous flow
- Flat hepatic venous flow with reversed flow in the inferior vena cava
- Slow or reversed portal venous flow
- Arterial type flow possibly present in a malignant thrombus

Utility
- Doppler studies are useful when evaluating flow in the hepatic veins and inferior vena cava.

Ultrasound Color Doppler
Findings
- Reversed flow in the retrohepatic inferior vena cava
- Intrahepatic venous collaterals
- Absent flow or flow status in the thrombosed vessels

Utility
- Rapid, accurate status and flow direction assessment of hepatic veins and inferior vena cava

CT
Findings
- *Flip-flop* contrast pattern and central hepatic hypodensity (contrast washout) compared with slow–contrast-accreting peripheral zones
- Narrowed or compressed inferior vena cava and hepatic veins (in chronic cases)
- Diffuse hepatic hypodensity (congestion) with global enlargement and ascites
- Hyperdense thrombus involving the inferior vena cava and hepatic and portal veins
- Patchy contrast enhancement (portal and sinusoidal stasis)
- Large homogeneously enhancing (arterial phase) and slightly hyperdense (portovenous) regenerative nodules

Utility
- Multidetector CT is useful in detecting regenerative nodules.
- It obviates the need for angiography and venography.

MRI
Findings
- Enhancing tumor thrombus
- Higher water content and longer T2 relaxation (acute congestion)
- Caudate lobe hypertrophy
- Absent vascular flow in the inferior vena cava or hepatic veins with intrahepatic collaterals or extrahepatic anastomoses

- Inhomogeneous and coarsened hepatic parenchyma with ascites (in chronic cases)
- Regenerative nodules: T1-weighted bright and T2-weighted isointense or hypointense relative to the liver
- Inhomogeneous enhancement pattern in the post-contrast phase

Utility
- MRI is a useful screening diagnostic tool with multiplanar capability.
- It obviates the need for angiography and venography.

Interventional Radiology
Findings
- Membranous webs or thrombus obstructing venous structures

Utility
- Hepatic venography and cavography were radiographic gold standards but are now seldom used unless they serve as a prelude to an interventional procedure.
- Interventional radiology is not a suitable screening tool.
- Transcatheter interventions such as stenting are used when there is membranous obstruction of the inferior vena cava.

CLINICAL PRESENTATION

- Acute symptoms include abdominal pain, hepatomegaly, vomiting, ascites, arterial hypotension associated with increased serum bilirubin and transaminase, and decreased clotting factors.
- Chronic symptoms include ascites of insidious onset, right upper quadrant pain, hepatomegaly, normal transaminase, decreased albumin, and decreased clotting factors.
- Patients can exhibit mild jaundice, splenomegaly, or variceal bleeding if cirrhosis develops.
- Clinical diagnosis may be inferred from an unknown cause of cirrhosis, abdominal pain episodes over the preceding month, and, uncommonly, a palpable caudate lobe.

DIFFERENTIAL DIAGNOSIS

- Cirrhosis and portal hypertension
- Right-sided heart failure
- Constrictive pericardial disease
- Carcinomatosis
- Hepatitis

PATHOLOGY

- Budd-Chiari syndrome is classified as either primary or secondary, depending on the cause and pathophysiologic manifestations.
- Primary type is characterized by total or incomplete membranous obstruction of hepatic venous blood.

- Secondary type is based on the hepatic venous obstruction site.
- Simultaneous obstruction of all three hepatic veins or obstruction of the last patent hepatic vein may be present.
- In the acute syndrome, the liver is enlarged and reddish, sinusoidal dilation is evident, and parenchymal damage (atrophy to hemorrhagic necrosis) is seen in the centrilobular areas.
- In the chronic syndrome, the liver is nodular and irregular in shape, is often accompanied by caudate lobe hypertrophy, and the hallmark is centrilobular fibrosis.
- Regenerative nodules are often seen, which are composed of hyperplastic hepatocytes, usually multiple, measuring between 5 and 40 mm.

INCIDENCE/PREVALENCE AND EPIDEMIOLOGY

- Membranous obstruction is uncommon in Europe and North America but is the most common cause of Budd-Chiari syndrome in Japan, India, Israel, and South Africa.

- Inferior vena cava membranous obstruction is complicated by hepatocellular carcinoma in 20%-40% of cases in South Africa and Japan.

Suggested Readings

Kamath PS: Budd-Chiari syndrome: Radiologic findings. *Liver Transpl* 12(11 suppl 2):S21-S22, 2006.

Menon KV, Shah V, Kamath PS: The Budd-Chiari syndrome. *N Engl J Med* 350:578-585, 2004.

Valla DC: The diagnosis and management of the Budd-Chiari syndrome: Consensus and controversies. *Hepatology* 38:793-803, 2003.

Zimmerman MA, Cameron AM, Ghobrial RM: Budd-Chiari syndrome. *Clin Liver Dis* 10:259-273, 2006.

Cavernous Transformation of the Portal Vein

DEFINITION: In patients with portal vein thrombosis, small collateral veins near the edge of the portal vein dilate, expand, and effectively replace the obliterated portal vein as the major hepatopetal venous conduit.

ANATOMIC FINDINGS

Portal Vein
- Narrowing or complete occlusion caused by thrombosis
- Absent or diminished flow caused by thrombosis

Liver
- Periportal venous collateral vessels

IMAGING

Ultrasound Color Doppler
Findings
- Mass of tubular anechoic collaterals
- Slightly turbulent, low-velocity venous signal with little or no respiratory or cardiac variation, hepatopetal direction, and portal venous waveform
- Obliteration of normal portal venous landmarks
- Splenomegaly
- Thickening and varices of the lesser omentum
- Spontaneous splenorenal shunts
- Gallbladder varices

Utility
- The collaterals are well depicted on color-flow Doppler.

CT
Findings
- Contrast enhancement of portal collaterals
- Abnormal enhancement patterns caused by increased hepatic arterial blood flow

Utility
- The collateral vessels are often best appreciated on coronal reformatted images.

MRI
Findings
- Contrast enhancement of portal collaterals
- Abnormal enhancement patterns caused by increased hepatic arterial blood flow

Utility
- Flow-sensitive MR techniques depict the collaterals to best advantage.

DIAGNOSTIC PEARLS
- Cavernous transformation induces morphologic changes in the liver with hypertrophy of liver segment IV and the caudate lobe.
- Compensatory arterial flow may produce a peculiar enhancement pattern in the liver.

CLINICAL PRESENTATION
- Splenomegaly
- Small liver caused by right lobe atrophy
- Hepatic dysfunction
- Right upper quadrant pain

PATHOLOGY
- Cavernous transformation of portal vein develops when collateral veins dilate, expand, and replace the obliterated portal vein.
- Periportal collateral circulation develops after long-standing portal vein thrombosis to maintain hepatopetal portal flow.
- Hepatic segment IV and caudate lobe hypertrophy occur as a result of the close proximity to cavernous transformation sites.
- Degree of collaterals in cavernous transformation is not typical in cirrhosis because of high intrahepatic portal resistance.

INCIDENCE/PREVALENCE AND EPIDEMIOLOGY
- Cavernous transformation develops in long-standing portal vein thrombosis.
- It is usually found as a complication of a benign disease.

WHAT THE REFERRING PHYSICIAN NEEDS TO KNOW
- Cavernous transformation develops in long-standing portal vein thrombosis, requiring 12 months to occur.
- It is usually found as a complication of a benign disease.

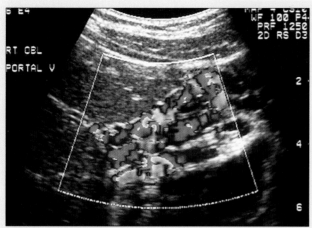

Figure 1. **Cavernous transformation of the portal vein: sonographic features.** Color Doppler scans show multiple collateral vessels in the portal vein in a patient with schistosomiasis.

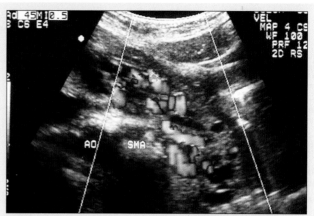

Figure 2. **Cavernous transformation of the portal vein: sonographic features.** Color Doppler scans show multiple collateral vessels in the splenic vein in a patient with schistosomiasis.

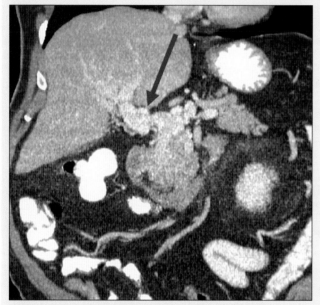

Figure 3. **Cavernous transformation of the portal vein: CT features.** Coronal multidetector CT reformatted image shows multiple enhancing tubular structures *(arrows)* in the hepatoduodenal ligament.

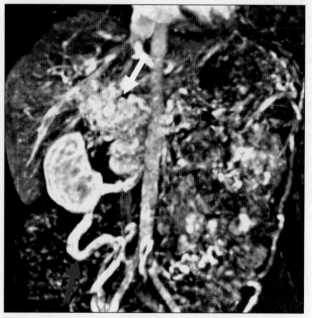

Figure 4. **Cavernous transformation of the portal vein: MRI features.** MR portogram shows multiple dilated peribiliary collaterals *(yellow arrow)* from the superior mesenteric and splenic veins to the intrahepatic portal veins. Note the dilated right gonadal vein *(red arrow)*.

Suggested Readings

Chang CY, Yang PM, Hung SP, et al: Cavernous transformation of the portal vein: Etiology determines the outcome. *Hepatogastroenterology* 53:892-897, 2006.

Song B, Min P, Oudkerk M, et al: Cavernous transformation of the portal vein secondary to tumor thrombosis of hepatocellular carcinoma: Spiral CT visualization of the collateral vessels. *Abdom Imaging* 25:385-396, 2005.

Vilgrain V, Condat B, Bureau C, et al: Atrophy-hypertrophy complex in patients with cavernous transformation of the portal vein. *Radiology* 241:149-155, 2006.

HELLP Syndrome

DEFINITION: HELLP syndrome (hemolysis, elevated liver enzymes, and low platelets) is a variant of toxemia that can occur during pregnancy either before or after delivery.

ANATOMIC FINDINGS

Liver
- Hepatocellular damage, cell necrosis, and hemorrhage

IMAGING

Ultrasound
Findings
- Portions of liver undergoing necrosis have increased echogenicity.
- Appearance is nonspecific and can mimic focal areas of fatty infiltration.

Utility
- Is less accurate than CT and MRI in establishing the diagnosis

CT
Findings
- Well-defined, hypodense, nonenhancing areas or multiple peripheral wedge-shaped areas of low attenuation
- Appearance is nonspecific and can mimic focal areas of fatty infiltration.

Utility
- Sensitivity: 75%-95%
- Specificity: 90%-100%
- Accuracy: 90%

MRI
Findings
- Edema or cellular necrosis shows up as areas of low T1 signal intensity and corresponding high T2 signal intensity.
- Appearance depends on the degree of hemorrhage, necrosis, and steatosis.

Utility
- Sensitivity: 80%-93%
- Specificity: 90%-100%
- Accuracy: 92%

CLINICAL PRESENTATION

- Epigastric or right upper quadrant pain
- Malaise, nausea, vomiting, headache, and nasal bleeding
- Hemolytic anemia (hemoglobin < 11 g/dL), elevated liver enzymes (lactate dehydrogenase > 400 IU/L), and thrombocytopenia (< 100,000/dL)

DIAGNOSTIC PEARLS

- Sonographically, portions of liver undergoing necrosis have increased echogenicity.
- CT scan reveals well-defined, hypodense, nonenhancing areas or multiple peripheral wedge-shaped areas of low attenuation.
- Edema or cellular necrosis is seen as having low signal intensity on T1-weighted MRIs and high signal intensity on T2-weighted images.

DIFFERENTIAL DIAGNOSIS

- Fatty infiltration

PATHOLOGY

- Endothelial damage in the placental bed activates platelets and triggers a coagulation cascade, which leads to disseminated intravascular coagulation.
- Hemolytic anemia is caused by the passage of red blood cells through the small vessels, with damaged endothelium covered by fibrin.
- Fibrin deposition in the liver leads to hepatocellular damage, necrosis, and hemorrhage.

INCIDENCE/PREVALENCE AND EPIDEMIOLOGY

- HELLP syndrome develops in 4%-12% of patients with severe preeclampsia.

Suggested Readings

Harris BM, Kuczkowski KM: Diagnostic dilemma: Hepatic rupture due to HELLP syndrome vs trauma. *Arch Gynecol Obstet* 12:234-238, 2005.

Nunes JO, Turner MA, Fulcher MA: Abdominal imaging features of HELLP syndrome: A 10-year retrospective review. *AJR Am J Roentgenol* 185:1205-1210, 2005.

Van Runnard Heimel PJ, Franx A, Schobben AF, et al: Corticosteroids, pregnancy, and HELLP syndrome: A review. *Obstet Gynecol Surg* 60:57-70, 2005.

Zissin R, Yaffe D, Fejgin M, et al: Hepatic infarction in preeclampsia as part of the HELLP syndrome: CT appearance. *Abdom Imaging* 24:594-596, 1999.

WHAT THE REFERRING PHYSICIAN NEEDS TO KNOW

- Hepatic ischemia, hemorrhage, and infarction are well-known complications of HELLP syndrome.
- Complications include liver cell necrosis, disseminated intravascular coagulation, abruptio placentae, renal failure, pulmonary edema, hypoglycemia, and rupture of a subcapsular hematoma.
- Standard treatment consists of the expeditious delivery of the fetus.

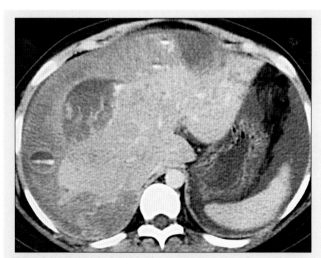

Figure 1. HELLP syndrome. This pregnant patient has acute abdominal pain, hemolysis, elevated liver enzymes, and low platelets. CT scan shows a hepatic hemorrhage with active contrast extravasation from multiple sites. Hypodense areas are also present, suggesting thrombosis.

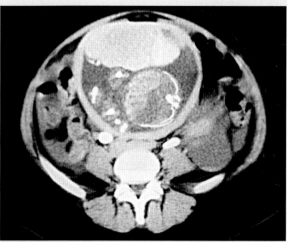

Figure 2. HELLP syndrome. This pregnant patient has acute abdominal pain, hemolysis, elevated liver enzymes, and low platelets. CT scan obtained at a lower level shows the fetus.

Hepatic Infarction

DEFINITION: Insufficient liver blood supply, causing ischemia and infarction.

ANATOMIC FINDINGS

Liver
- Area of infarction appearing as a well-circumscribed, peripheral, wedge-shaped lesion
- Edema
- Necrosis
- Atrophy

IMAGING

Ultrasound
Findings
- Hypoechoic region secondary to edema and round-cell infiltration
- Bile duct lakes or cysts appearing when necrotic tissues are resorbed

Utility
- Hepatic infarction is difficult to detect during its early stages by cross-sectional imaging.
- Sensitivity: 40%-50%
- Specificity: 65%-80%

CT
Findings
- Area of infarction is seen as a well-circumscribed, peripheral, wedge-shaped lesion, but it may be round or oval and centrally located.
- Areas of infarction develop a more distinct margin and may undergo considerable atrophy.
- Gas formation within sterile infarcts has also been described.
- Bile duct lakes may be seen.

Utility
- Hepatic infarction is difficult to detect during its early stages by cross-sectional imaging.
- Sensitivity: 65%-75%
- Specificity: 70%-85%

MRI
Findings
- Edema of infarction is seen as having lower signal intensity on T1-weighted images and higher signal intensity on T2-weighted images.
- Bile duct lakes have low signal intensity on T1-weighted images and higher signal intensity on T2-weighted images.

DIAGNOSTIC PEARLS
- Usually, the diagnosis is based on the characteristic hepatic histopathologic appearance: minimal centrilobular necrosis and seronegativity for viral hepatitis.
- Infarcts are usually well-circumscribed, peripheral, wedge-shaped lesions, but they can be round or oval and centrally located.
- On MRIs, the edema of the infarction lengthens the T1 and T2 relaxation times, causing lower signal intensity on T1-weighted images and higher signal intensity on T2-weighted images.

Utility
- Hepatic infarction is difficult to detect during its early stages by cross-sectional imaging.
- MRI is the most accurate noninvasive means of making the diagnosis.
- Sensitivity: 70%-80%
- Specificity: 75%-90%

CLINICAL PRESENTATION
- Abdominal or back pain
- Fever
- Possibly asymptomatic
- Jaundice
- Sepsis

DIFFERENTIAL DIAGNOSIS
- Cirrhosis
- Decreased portal flow
- Viral hepatitis
- Segmental hepatic steatosis

PATHOLOGY
- Infarction of liver secondary to insufficient blood supply
- Histopathologically seen as minimal centrilobular necrosis

WHAT THE REFERRING PHYSICIAN NEEDS TO KNOW
- Decreased portal flow from thrombus, tumor compression, or segmental hepatic vein obstruction may produce similar CT findings.

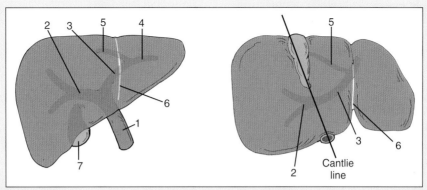

Figure 1. Hepatic blood supply. Normal branching pattern of portal vein. Coronal *(left)* and axial *(right)* diagrams show that the main portal vein (1) divides into the right (2) and left portal veins. The left portal vein first courses horizontally (the horizontal portion [3]) then turns anteriorly (the umbilical portion [4]) toward the ligamentum teres (6). The Cantlie line corresponds to the median fissure and extends from the gallbladder (7) to the inferior vena cava. It is located to the right of the umbilical ligament and divides the liver into the right and left lobes. (*5,* Branch to segment IV.) (*From Gallego C, Velasco M, Marcuello P, et al: Congenital and acquired anomalies of the portal venous system.* RadioGraphics *22:141-159, 2002.*)

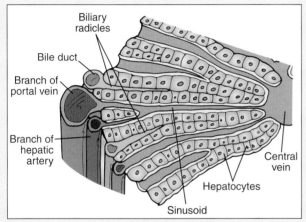

Figure 2. Hepatic blood supply. Diagram shows the anatomic relationship between the hepatic arterial branches and the portal venous branches and bile duct (portal triad), biliary radicals, cords of hepatocytes, intervening sinusoid, and the central draining hepatic vein. Diagram depicting hepatic blood supply at the sinusoidal level. Note that the bile ducts derive their blood supply primarily from the hepatic arteries. (*From Pandharipande PV, Krinsky GA, Rusinek H, Lee VS: Perfusion imaging of the liver: Current challenges and future goals.* Radiology *234:661-673, 2005.*)

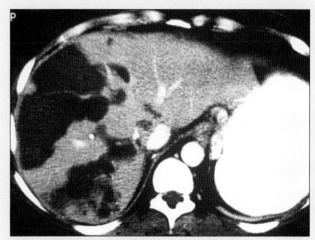

Figure 3. Hepatic infarction: CT features. Multiple areas of decreased attenuation are present within the liver associated with bile duct lakes.

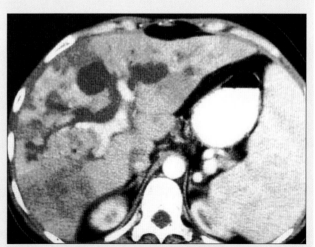

Figure 4. Hepatic infarction: CT features. Multiple areas of decreased attenuation are present within the liver associated with bile duct lakes.

- Area of infarction appearing as a well-circumscribed, peripheral, wedge-shaped lesion but may be round or oval and centrally located
- Areas of infarction developing a more distinct margin and possibly undergoing considerable atrophy

INCIDENCE/PREVALENCE AND EPIDEMIOLOGY

- Hepatic infarction is uncommon.
- It is associated with shock, sepsis, anesthesia, oral contraceptives, sickle cell disease, polyarteritis nodosa, eclampsia, metastasis, bacterial endocarditis, arterial emboli, and trauma.
- Incidence of ischemic hepatitis in cirrhotic patients with variceal bleeding is reported to be as high as 9%.

Suggested Readings

Giovine S, Pinto A, Crispano S, et al: Retrospective study of 23 cases of hepatic infarction: CT findings and pathological correlations. *Radiol Med (Torino)* 111:11-21, 2006.

Khong SY, James M, Smith P: Diagnosis of liver infarction postpartum. *Obstet Gynecol* 105(5 Pt 2):1271-1273, 2005.

Tuvia J, Lebwohl O, Lefkowitz J: Hepatic infarction due to thrombotic angiitis: MR appearance. *Clin Radiol* 55:803-805, 2000.

Hepatopulmonary Syndrome

ANATOMIC FINDINGS

Intrapulmonary Vessels
- Dilated

IMAGING

Ultrasound
Findings
- Delayed appearance (4 to 6 heartbeats after the initial appearance in the right chambers) of contrast material (microbubbles) in the left heart chambers

Utility
- Contrast-enhanced echocardiography is valuable for demonstrating the presence of intrapulmonary vascular dilations in patients with hypoxemia and liver disease.
- Sensitivity: 98%
- Specificity: 95%
- Accuracy: 96%

Nuclear Medicine
Findings
- Presence of isotope in brain or kidneys indicates right-to-left shunt through either the intracardiac or the intrapulmonary shunt.
- Shunt magnitudes ranging from 10%-71% have been documented in patients with hepatopulmonary syndrome (HPS).

Utility
- Perfusion lung scan with technetium-99m (99mTc)-labeled macroaggregated albumin is the second major method for detecting intrapulmonary vascular dilation.
- Shunt magnitude is calculated by taking the ratio of systemic activity to total body activity of the isotope.
- Sensitivity: 88%
- Specificity: 65%
- Accuracy: 74%

CT
Findings
- Enlarged vessels that do not taper normally, extending to the pleural surface and being most numerous at lung bases
- Higher segmental arterial diameter to bronchial diameter ratio in the right lower lobe in HPS than in normoxemic liver cirrhosis

DIAGNOSTIC PEARLS

- Hepatopulmonary syndrome must be excluded in all patients with cirrhosis prior to transplantation.

Utility
- CT is not employed in establishing this diagnosis.

Interventional Radiology
Findings
- Vascular dilations depicted as enlarged vessels that do not taper normally, extending to the pleural surface and being most numerous at lung bases
- Higher segmental arterial diameter to the bronchial diameter ratio in the right lower lobe in HPS than in normoxemic liver cirrhosis

Utility
- Angiography is seldom used to establish the diagnosis.

Radiography
Findings
- Decreased lung volumes
- Pleural effusions
- Increased interstitial and pulmonary vascular markings

Utility
- Findings are not helpful in establishing the diagnosis.
- Findings are nonspecific.
- Same abnormalities may be seen on chest radiograph in all cirrhotic patients.

CLINICAL PRESENTATION

- Hypoxemia at room air
- Severe cirrhosis
- Shortness of breath

DIFFERENTIAL DIAGNOSIS

- Chronic obstructive pulmonary disease
- Cardiac right-to-left shunts

PATHOLOGY

- HPS is characterized by severe parenchymal liver disease and evidence of tortuous, dilated intrapulmonary vessels that lead to right-to-left shunting.

WHAT THE REFERRING PHYSICIAN NEEDS TO KNOW

- Treatment of HPS is liver transplantation. A lung transplant may also be needed.
- Transjugular intrahepatic portosystemic shunt procedure has been used as a temporizing measure in patients awaiting transplant.

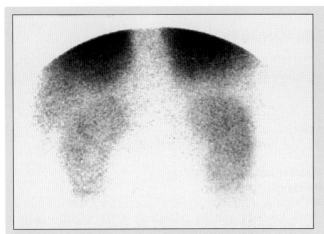

Figure 1. Hepatopulmonary syndrome: scintigraphy.
Pulmonary perfusion image obtained with technetium-99m
(99mTc)-macroaggregated albumin shows extrapulmonary
uptake in the kidneys, indicating right-to-left shunting.

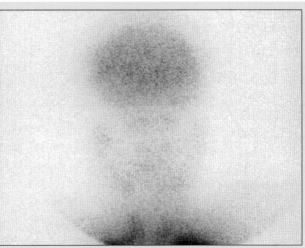

Figure 2. Hepatopulmonary syndrome: scintigraphy.
Pulmonary perfusion image obtained with 99mTc-
macroaggregated albumin shows extrapulmonary uptake in the
brain, indicating right-to-left shunting.

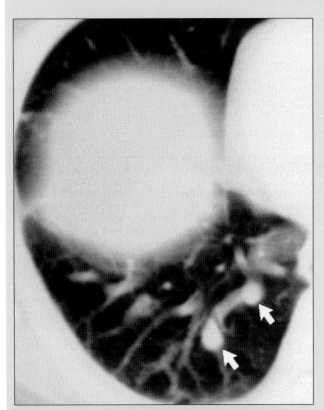

Figure 3. Hepatopulmonary syndrome: CT features. CT scan
obtained in 64-year-old man with hepatopulmonary syndrome
shows tortuous dilated peripheral vessels *(arrows)* 2 cm from
the pleura. (*From Lee K-N, Lee H-J, Shin WW, et al: Hypoxemia
and liver cirrhosis [hepatopulmonary syndrome] in eight patients.*
Radiology *211:549-553, 1999.*)

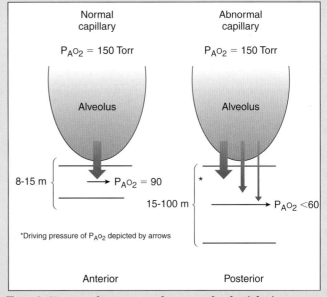

**Figure 4. Hepatopulmonary syndrome: pathophysiologic
features.** Schematic diagram of precapillary vascular abnormality
seen in both acute and chronic liver disorders. The driving pressure
of arterial oxygen is depicted by the *arrows.*

INCIDENCE/PREVALENCE AND EPIDEMIOLOGY

- The hepatopulmonary syndrome occurs in 3%-10% of patients with cirrhosis.

Suggested Readings

Engleke C, Schaefer-Prokop C, Schirg E, et al: High-resolution CT and CT angiography of peripheral pulmonary vascular disorders. *RadioGraphics* 22:739-764, 2002.

Leung AN: Hepatopulmonary syndrome. *Radiology* 229:64-67, 2003.

Mandell MS: The diagnosis and treatment of hepatopulmonary syndrome. *Clin Liver Dis* 10:387-405, 2006.

Meyer CA, White CA, Sherman KE: Diseases of the hepatopulmonary axis. *RadioGraphics* 20:687-698, 2000.

Liver in Cardiac Disease

DEFINITION: Passive hepatic congestion is a common complication of congestive heart failure and constrictive pericarditis.

IMAGING

Ultrasound
Findings
- Hepatic enlargement
- Dilation of the inferior vena cava and hepatic veins. (The mean diameter of the right hepatic vein main trunk is 8.8 mm and increases to 13.3 mm with pericardial effusion.)
- Diminished respiratory variation in the caliber of the inferior vena cava and hepatic veins
- Cirrhosis

Utility
- Ultrasound is an excellent means of quantitating cardiac dysfunction.

Ultrasound Spectral Doppler
Findings
- Patients with other forms of cirrhosis may also show flattening of Doppler waveform in the hepatic veins.
- Loss of normal triphasic flow pattern in the hepatic veins and inferior vena cava
- Spectral signal of hepatic vein having an M shape
- Cardiac cirrhosis: unidirectional and low-velocity continuous flow pattern of hepatic veins
- Severe congestive heart failure: increased pulsatility of the portal venous Doppler signal
- In tricuspid regurgitation, the hepatic vein demonstrating a decrease of antegrade systolic wave and a systolic or diastolic flow velocity ratio of less than 0.6

Utility
- Ultrasound is an excellent means of quantitating cardiac dysfunction.

CT
Findings
- Dilation of inferior vena cava and hepatic veins
- Retrograde opacification and enhancement of the inferior vena cava and hepatic veins
- Inhomogeneous, mottled, reticulated-mosaic pattern of parenchymal contrast enhancement
- Linear and curvilinear regions of poor enhancement
- Larger patchy regions of poor or delayed enhancement in the periphery of the liver

DIAGNOSTIC PEARLS
- Patients exhibit hepatic enlargement and dilation of the inferior vena cava and hepatic veins.
- Spectral Doppler waveform of hepatic vein shows an M shape; ultimately, in cardiac cirrhosis, a unidirectional, low-velocity, continuous flow pattern may be seen.
- Contrast-enhanced CT scans may show an inhomogeneous, mottled, reticulated-mosaic pattern of parenchymal contrast enhancement.

- Ancillary findings: cardiomegaly, hepatomegaly, and intrahepatic periportal lucency resulting from perivascular lymphedema, pleural effusions, ascites, and pericardial effusions

Utility
- Sensitivity: 60%-95%
- Specificity: 72%-90%
- Accuracy: 85%

MRI
Findings
- Early MR contrast-enhanced images show liver enhancement in a mosaic fashion, with a reticulated pattern of low-signal-intensity linear markings.
- Signal intensity of the liver becomes more homogeneous after 1 minute.
- Reflux of contrast into, dilation of hepatic veins, and suprahepatic inferior vena cava may be seen.
- Gradient-echo MRIs may show a slow or even absent antegrade flow within the inferior vena cava.

Utility
- Sensitivity: 75%-95%
- Specificity: 80%-98%
- Accuracy: 90%

CLINICAL PRESENTATION
- Right upper quadrant pain
- Hepatojugular reflux on physical examination

WHAT THE REFERRING PHYSICIAN NEEDS TO KNOW
- Passive hepatic congestion may be transient, and a full recovery follows once the patient's congestive heart failure is corrected.
- In chronic right atrial failure, cardiac cirrhosis may ensue.
- Diagnosis is not usually made clinically because signs and symptoms of cardiac failure overshadow those of the liver disease.

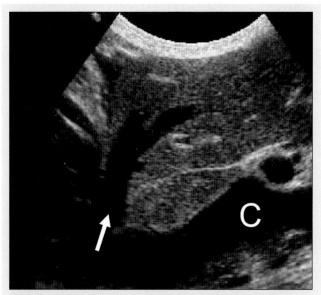

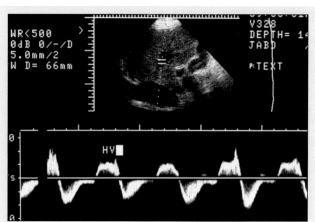

Figure 2. **Passive hepatic congestion: sonographic findings.** In passive hepatic congestion, the normal triphasic pattern is lost.

Figure 1. **Passive hepatic congestion: sonographic findings.** Sagittal sonogram shows dilation of the inferior vena cava (C) and middle hepatic vein *(arrow)*.

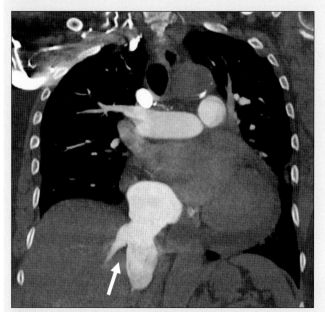

Figure 3. **Passive hepatic congestion: CT features.** Coronal reformatted multidetector CT image demonstrates reflux of contrast into dilated inferior vena cava *(arrow)* and hepatic veins.

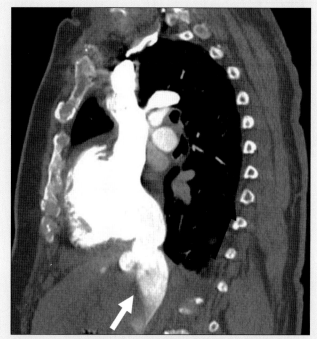

Figure 4. **Passive hepatic congestion: CT features.** Sagittal reformatted multidetector CT image demonstrates reflux of contrast into the dilated inferior vena cava *(arrow)* and hepatic veins.

DIFFERENTIAL DIAGNOSIS

- Other causes of liver cirrhosis
- Constrictive pericardial disease
- Pulmonary artery hypertension

PATHOLOGY

- Elevated central venous pressure is directly transmitted from the right atrium to the hepatic veins.
- Passive hepatic congestion is caused by blood stasis within the liver parenchyma because of compromised hepatic venous drainage.
- Liver becomes tensely swollen as hepatic sinusoids engorge and dilate with blood.
- Histopathologic assessment shows a classic finding of *nutmeg* liver.

INCIDENCE/PREVALENCE AND EPIDEMIOLOGY

- Common complication of congestive heart failure and constrictive pericarditis

Suggested Readings

Barakat M: Non-pulsatile hepatic and portal vein waveforms in patients with liver cirrhosis: Concordant and discordant relationships. *Br J Radiol* 77:547-550, 2004.

Giallourakis CC, Rosenberg PM, Friedman LS: The liver in heart failure. *Clin Liver Dis* 6:947-967, 2002.

Gieling RG, Ruijter JM, Maas AAW, et al: Hepatic response to right ventricular overload. *Gastroenterology* 127:1210-1221, 2004.

Morrin MM, Pedrosa I, Rofsky NM: Magnetic resonance imaging for disorders of liver vasculature. *Top Magn Reson Imaging* 13:177-190, 2002.

Moulton JS, Miller BL, Dodd GD 3rd, et al: Passive hepatic congestion in heart failure: CT abnormalities. *AJR Am J Roentgenol* 151:939-942, 1988.

Osler-Weber-Rendu Disease

DEFINITION: A rare autosomal-dominant disorder characterized by multiple mucocutaneous telangiectasias that may involve most organ systems.

ANATOMIC FINDINGS

Liver
- Telangiectasia
- Cavernous hemangioma
- Intraparenchymal branch of a hepatic artery aneurysm
- Hepatoportal and hepatohepatic arteriovenous fistula
- Left-to-right intrahepatic shunts

IMAGING

Ultrasound Color Doppler
Findings
- Large arteriovenous malformation or tangled masses of enlarged tortuous arteries or multiple aneurysms of the hepatic arterial branches within the liver
- High-velocity flow (153 cm/s) in the dilated and tortuous hepatic artery and its branches
- Pulsatility of portal flow with phasic or continuous reversal

Utility
- The velocity of flow through arterial malformations is nicely depicted with Doppler ultrasound.

CT Angiography
Findings
- Prominent extrahepatic (may also include intrahepatic hepatic artery) artery that is often associated with dilated hepatic or portal veins
- Early filling of the portal venous or hepatic venous trunks
- Other abnormalities: telangiectasias, large confluent vascular masses, and transient hepatic attenuation differences

Utility
- Intrahepatic arteriovenous fistulas are being visualized with increased frequency with the use of multidetector CT.

MR Angiography
Findings
- Prominent extrahepatic (may also include intrahepatic hepatic artery) artery that is often associated with dilated hepatic or portal veins
- Early filling of portal venous or hepatic venous trunks
- Other abnormalities: telangiectasias, large confluent vascular masses, and transient hepatic attenuation differences

DIAGNOSTIC PEARLS

- Color Doppler sonography demonstrates a large arteriovenous malformation or tangled masses of enlarged tortuous arteries or multiple aneurysms of hepatic arterial branches within liver.
- High-velocity flow (153 cm/s) in dilated and tortuous hepatic artery and its branches is seen.
- Early filling of portal venous or hepatic venous trunks is seen.

Utility
- MR angiography can provide a map of anomalous vessels.
- Dynamic gradient-echo imaging obtained after the injection of Gd-DTPA (gadolinium diethylenetriaminopentaacetic acid) allows the analysis of filling kinetics.

Interventional Radiology
Findings
- Tortuous dilated hepatic arteries
- Diffuse angiectases with a diffuse mottled capillary blush
- Hemangiomas
- Early filling of the hepatic or portal veins indicating shunt

Utility
- Angiographic appearance depends on the stage of development of the hepatic arteriovenous shunt.

CLINICAL PRESENTATION

- Hepatic involvement is usually diagnosed 10-20 years after the first appearance of mucocutaneous telangiectasias.
- High-output heart failure occurs as a result of left-to-right intrahepatic shunts.
- Multiple mucocutaneous telangiectasias may involve most organ systems.

DIFFERENTIAL DIAGNOSIS

- Peliosis hepatis
- Cirrhosis
- Post-traumatic arteriovenous malformation
- Nodular regenerative hyperplasia

WHAT THE REFERRING PHYSICIAN NEEDS TO KNOW
- Many patients develop high-output heart failure as a result of left-to-right intrahepatic shunts.

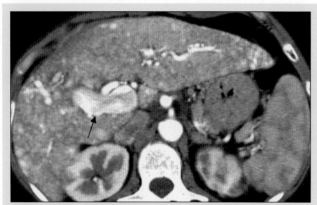

Figure 1. Osler-Weber-Rendu disease: CT features. Dilation and early filling of the main portal vein *(arrow)* during the arterial phase are consistent with an arterioportal shunt. *(From Wu JS, Saluja S, Garcia-Tsao G, et al: Liver involvement in hereditary hemorrhagic telangiectasia. AJR Am J Roentgenol 187:W399-W405, 2006. Reprinted with permission from the American Journal of Roentgenology.)*

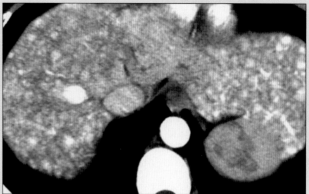

Figure 2. Osler-Weber-Rendu disease: CT features. CT angiogram shows diffuse parenchymal heterogeneity and numerous telangiectasias. *(From Wu JS, Saluja S, Garcia-Tsao G, et al: Liver involvement in hereditary hemorrhagic telangiectasia. AJR Am J Roentgenol 187:W399-W405, 2006. Reprinted with permission from the American Journal of Roentgenology.)*

PATHOLOGY

- Osler-Weber-Rendu disease is an autosomal-dominant disorder characterized by multiple mucocutaneous telangiectasias that may involve most organ systems.
- Angiodysplastic vascular changes may be seen, including telangiectasias, cavernous hemangiomas, and aneurysms of the intraparenchymal branches of the hepatic artery.
- Hepatoportal and hepatohepatic arteriovenous fistula may be seen.

INCIDENCE/PREVALENCE AND EPIDEMIOLOGY

- Osler-Weber-Rendu disease is a rare autosomal-dominant disorder with an incidence of 1-2 per 100,000 population.

Suggested Readings

Guttmacher AE, Marchuk DA, White RI: Hereditary hemorrhagic telangiectasia. *N Engl J Med* 333:918-924, 1995.

Jaskolka J, Wu L, Chan RP, et al: Imaging of hereditary hemorrhagic telangiectasia. *AJR Am J Roentgenol* 183:307-314, 2004.

Proctor DD, Henderson KJ, Dziura JD, et al: Enteroscopic evaluation of the gastrointestinal tract in symptomatic patients with hereditary hemorrhagic telangiectasia. *J Clin Gastroenterol* 39:115-119, 2005.

Ravard G, Soyer P, Boudiaf M, et al: Hepatic involvement in hereditary hemorrhagic telangiectasia. *J Comput Assist Tomogr* 28: 488-495, 2004.

Shovlin CL, Johanns W, Janssen J, et al: Diagnostic criteria for hereditary hemorrhagic telangiectasia (Rendu-Osler-Weber syndrome). *Am J Med Genet* 91:66-67, 2000.

Wu JS, Saluja S, Garcia-Tsao G, et al: Liver involvement in hereditary hemorrhagic telangiectasia: CT and clinical findings do not correlate in symptomatic patients. *AJR Am J Roentgenol* 187: W399-W405, 2006.

Peliosis Hepatis

DEFINITION: A rare disorder characterized by cystic hepatic sinusoidal dilation and the presence of multiple blood-filled lacunar spaces of various sizes (1 mm to 3 cm) throughout the liver.

ANATOMIC FINDINGS

Liver
- Hepatomegaly
- Multiple blood-filled lacunar spaces of various sizes (1 mm to 3 cm) throughout the liver
- Cystic sinusoidal dilation
- Portal tracts within the fibrous stroma of blood spaces

IMAGING

Ultrasound
Findings
- Hepatic echo pattern that is inhomogeneous, with hyperechoic and hypoechoic regions, predominantly in the right lobe
- Sometimes present with hepatomegaly, portal hypertension, esophageal varices, and ascites

Utility
- A high degree of suspicion is required because radiographic and sonographic findings are nonspecific.
- Sensitivity: 30%-50%
- Specificity: 60%-75%
- Accuracy: 54%

CT
Findings
- Lesions may appear hypodense early in disease and isodense with time.

Utility
- Detecting lesions on CT scans is difficult unless fatty infiltration to contrast higher-density aggregation of blood-filled spaces is present.
- Sensitivity: 56%-80%
- Specificity: 80%-87%
- Accuracy: 78%

Interventional Radiology
Findings
- Multiple small accumulations of contrast material on the late arterial phase, which become more prominent on parenchymal and venous phases

DIAGNOSTIC PEARLS

- Hepatic echo pattern is inhomogeneous, with hyperechoic and hypoechoic regions, predominantly in the right lobe.
- Lesions may appear hypodense early and isodense with time on CT.
- Multiple small accumulations of contrast material are seen on the late arterial phase, which become more prominent on the parenchymal and venous phases.

Utility
- Angiography
- Less sensitive and specific in establishing the diagnosis

CLINICAL PRESENTATION

- Possibly asymptomatic
- Hepatic failure and liver rupture, with hemoperitoneum and shock
- Hepatomegaly, portal hypertension, esophageal varices, and ascites

DIFFERENTIAL DIAGNOSIS

- Hemangioma
- Osler-Weber-Rendu disease
- Cirrhosis with arterial-portal shunts

PATHOLOGY

- Cystic hepatic sinusoidal dilation with multiple blood-filled lacunar spaces of various sizes (1 mm to 3 cm) throughout the liver
- Blood-filled spaces freely communicating with sinusoids and lined by a thin band of collagenous tissue and endothelial cells
- Outflow obstruction at the sinusoid wall and hepatocellular necrosis, leading to cyst formation

---

WHAT THE REFERRING PHYSICIAN NEEDS TO KNOW

- Peliosis hepatis can cause hepatic failure or liver rupture, with hemoperitoneum and shock.
- Peliosis lesions can be differentiated from hemangiomas by the presence of portal tracts within the fibrous stroma of the blood spaces.
- Peliotic lesions can also occur in the spleen, bone marrow, lymph nodes, and lungs.

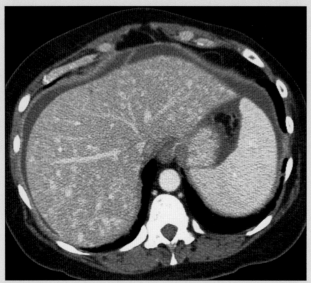

Figure 1. Peliosis hepatis. Multiple small lakes of contrast material are present on this CT scan. The patient also has ascites.

INCIDENCE/PREVALENCE AND EPIDEMIOLOGY

- Peliosis hepatis is a rare disorder.
- It develops from the use of anabolic steroids, cortico-steroids, tamoxifen, oral contraceptives, and diethyl-stilbestrol and after renal or cardiac transplantation.
- Peliosis hepatis is associated with chronic wasting disease (tuberculosis, leprosy, malignancy, sprue, diabetes, necrotizing vasculitis) and exposure to polyvinyl chloride and arsenic.
- It is usually found incidentally at autopsy.

Suggested Readings

Ferrozzi F, Tognini G, Zuccoli G, et al: Peliosis hepatis with pseudo-tumoral and hemorrhagic evolution: CT and MR findings. *Abdom Imaging* 26:197-199, 2001.

Fidelman N, LaBerge JM, Kerlan RK: Massive intraperitoneal hemor-rhage caused by peliosis hepatis. *J Vasc Interv Radiol* 13:542-545, 2002.

Hiorns MP, Rossi UG, Roebuck DJ: Peliosis hepatis using inferior vena cava compression in a 3-year-old child. *Pediatr Radiol* 35:209-211, 2005.

Sandrasegaran K, Hawes DR, Matthew G: Hepatic peliosis (bacillary angiomatosis) in AIDS: CT findings. *Abdom Imaging* 30:738-740, 2005.

Steinke K, Terraciano L, Wiesner W: Unusual cross-sectional imaging findings in hepatic peliosis. *Eur Radiol* 13:1916-1919, 2003.

Portal Vein Thrombosis

DEFINITION: Portal vein may develop a thrombus in its intrahepatic or extrahepatic course, causing occlusion.

ANATOMIC FINDINGS

Portal Vein
- Thrombus
- Portal hypertension

IMAGING

Radiography
Findings
- Calcification in a portal vein thrombus or wall of the portal vein, which may be seen as parallel, discontinuous, and radiodense lines
- Ileus: localized sentinel loop
- Thumbprinting

Utility
- This technique is not used to make this diagnosis.

Ultrasound
Findings
- Nonvisualized portal vein
- Intraluminal echogenic reflector that partially or completely fills the vein, obscuring normal portal vein landmarks
- Portal vein possibly expanded in acute thrombosis or when a neoplasm is present
- Tumor thrombus may present with small sonolucencies.
- Secondary signs of portal vein thrombosis: splenomegaly, ascites, venous collaterals, and mesenteric vein thrombosis

Utility
- Ultrasound is the primary imaging modality for the diagnosis and follow-up of portal vein thrombosis.
- In most cases, a bland thrombus cannot be differentiated from a tumor thrombus.
- Sonography has a sensitivity of 64% and a specificity of 98% as compared with arterial portography.

Ultrasound Doppler
Findings
- Dilated hepatic artery, with increased systolic central streamlined flow in the malignant thrombus
- In chronic thrombosis, typical continuous and low-frequency portal venous flow pattern in the vessels

DIAGNOSTIC PEARLS
- Failure to identify the portal vein on ultrasound is a significant finding and virtually diagnostic of portal vein occlusion.
- Intraluminal echogenic reflector partially or completely fills the vein, obscuring normal portal vein landmarks.
- Hepatic artery is dilated with increased systolic central streamlined flow in a malignant thrombus.

Utility
- Duplex Doppler imaging has a sensitivity of 100% and a specificity of 93% in detecting a thrombus of the main portal vein.
- Diagnosis of intrahepatic portal vein thrombus is more difficult to establish confidently because of the high background echogenicity of the liver.

Ultrasound Color Doppler
Findings
- Tumor thrombus exhibiting color Doppler flow and arterial waveforms (often hepatofugal in direction)

Utility
- Ultrasound color Doppler depicts blood flow in real time.
- It permits a quick diagnosis of abnormal hepatofugal flow.
- It reveals flow and collaterals that are invisible on gray-scale images.
- It allows the diagnosis of potentially confusing helical blood flow.

CT
Findings
- Thrombus within the portal vein
- Low-density central zone surrounded by an intensely enhanced periphery on contrast-enhanced scans
- Transient inhomogeneous enhancement of the periportal hepatic parenchyma
- Enlargement of the occluded vein
- Streaky enhancement of the clot
- In precontrast scan, portal vein contents possibly having high attenuation because of the high protein content of the concentrated red blood cells
- Arterioportal shunting possibly present

WHAT THE REFERRING PHYSICIAN NEEDS TO KNOW
- Medical management is preferred, unless the resulting hemorrhage cannot be controlled or if a repeated life-threatening bleed develops.
- Ultrasound is the primary imaging modality for the diagnosis and follow-up of portal vein thrombosis.
- The diagnosis is most commonly made with multidetector CT.

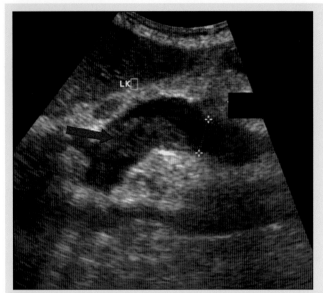

Figure 1. Portal vein thrombosis: sonographic findings.
Sagittal scan through the portal vein shows thrombus *(arrow)*
partially occluding lumen.

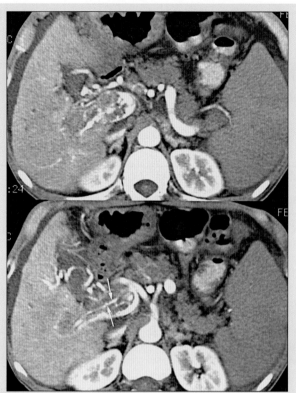

Figure 2. Portal vein thrombosis. Direct visualization of arterial
neovascularity in a tumor thrombus, producing a *streaks-and-
threads (arrows)* appearance. (*Case courtesy of Richard L. Baron,
MD, Chicago,* IL.)

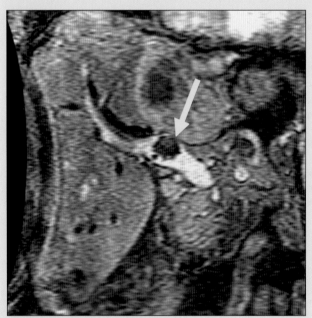

Figure 3. Portal vein thrombosis: MRI findings. Coronal image
shows hepatocellular carcinoma that has invaded the portal vein
(yellow arrow).

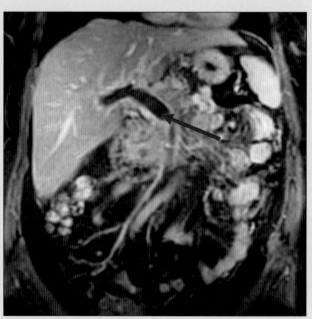

**Figure 4. Portal and superior mesenteric vein thrombosis:
MRI findings.** Coronal image shows a thrombus *(arrow)* in the
main portal vein.

Utility
- CT is the most commonly used means of establishing the diagnosis.
- Sensitivity: 75%-93%
- Specificity: 90%-100%

MRI
Findings
- Nonvisualized portal vein
- Acute thrombus (<5 weeks old) appearing hyperintense relative to the muscle and liver on both T1-weighted and T2-weighted images
- Older thrombi (between 2 and 18 months) appearing hyperintense relative to the liver on T2-weighted images
- Tumor thrombus: higher T2 signal intensity, soft-tissue signal intensity on time-of-flight gradient-echo images, and enhancing with gadolinium
- Bland thrombus: low signal intensity on T2- and time-of-flight gradient-echo images and not enhancing with gadolinium
- Intrahepatic portal vein occlusion possibly showing triangular, wedge-shaped region with the apex seen centrally and the base abutting the liver capsule

Utility
- MRI is another excellent means of demonstrating portal vein thrombosis because of the natural contrast of moving blood.
- Combination of black-blood techniques (e.g., spin-echo sequence with superior and inferior saturation pulses) increases the diagnostic confidence.
- Combination of bright-blood techniques (e.g., time-of-flight gradient-echo or gadolinium-enhanced spoiled gradient-echo) increases the diagnostic confidence.
- Sensitivity: 80%-95%
- Specificity: 85%-100%

Interventional Radiology
Findings
- Filling defect may partially or completely occlude the portal vein on angiography.

Utility
- Portal vein thrombosis can usually be diagnosed angiographically but is better appreciated by direct cross-sectional imaging methods.

CLINICAL PRESENTATION

- Onset may be acute and life threatening in acutely decompensated cirrhotic patients or those with septic pyelophlebitis; more commonly, onset of abdominal pain is insidious.
- Ascites may occur.
- Splenomegaly and hepatomegaly may occur.
- Pyrexia and leukocytosis may occur.
- Varices and hemorrhage may occur.

DIFFERENTIAL DIAGNOSIS

- Flow artifact
- Portal venous gas
- Portal vein parasites

PATHOLOGY

- Myeloproliferative disorders and blood dyscrasias account for 12%-48% of cases.
- Patients with cirrhosis of the liver have portal vein thrombosis because stagnant intrahepatic flow predisposes the patient to thrombus formation.
- Extrahepatic causes of portal vein occlusion include malignancy, pyelophlebitis by contiguous spread from adjacent infected structures, postsurgical thrombosis, and schistosomiasis.

INCIDENCE/PREVALENCE AND EPIDEMIOLOGY

- Portal vein thrombosis is the leading cause of presinusoidal hypertension.
- Incidence of portal vein thrombosis in hepatocellular carcinoma is 26%-34%.
- Ten percent of patients with cirrhosis of the liver have portal vein thrombosis.
- Worldwide, schistosomiasis is the most common cause of portal vein obstruction and the leading cause of portal hypertension.
- Myeloproliferative disorders and blood dyscrasias account for approximately 12%-48% of cases of portal vein thromboses.

Suggested Readings

Jamssen HLA, Wijnhoud A, Iwatsuki S, et al: Extrahepatic portal vein thrombosis: Aetiology and determinants of survival. *Gut* 49:720-724, 2001.

Rossi S, Rosa L, Ravetta V, et al: Contrast-enhanced versus conventional and color Doppler sonography for the detection of thrombosis of the portal and hepatic venous systems. *AJR Am J Roentgenol* 186:763-773, 2006.

Sheen CL, Lamparelli H, Milne A, et al: Clinical features, diagnosis, and outcome of acute portal vein thrombosis. *Q J Med* 93:531-534, 2000.

Valla DC, Condat B: Portal vein thrombosis in adults: Pathophysiology, pathogenesis, and management. *J Hepatol* 32:865-871, 2000.

Webster GJ, Burroughs AK, Riordan SM: Review article: Portal vein thrombosis—New insights into aetiology and management. *Aliment Pharmacol Ther* 21:1-9, 2005.

Splanchnic Vein Aneurysm

DEFINITION: Aneurysms of the portal venous system.

IMAGING

Ultrasound
Findings
- Dilated portal or other splanchnic vein
- Vessel diameter larger at one point (usually 2 cm) than in the remainder of the vessel
- Anechoic aneurysm

Utility
- Gray-scale ultrasound requires the addition of Doppler ultrasound for complete evaluation.

Ultrasound Doppler
Findings
- Constantly swirling blood
- Aneurysm of splenic vein possibly simulating a cystic mass

Utility
- Ultrasound Doppler is necessary for confirming the presence of a thrombus.
- Sensitivity: 85%
- Specificity: 98%
- Accuracy: 95%

CT
Findings
- Dilated portal or other splanchnic vein
- Vessel diameter larger at one point (usually 2 cm) than in the remainder of the vessel

Utility
- Bolus dynamic CT scanning is necessary for the correct diagnosis.
- Sensitivity: 95%
- Specificity: 100%
- Accuracy: 98%

MRI
Findings
- Dilated portal or other splanchnic vein
- Vessel diameter larger at one point (usually 2 cm) than in the remainder of the vessel

Utility
- Dilated portal or other splanchnic vein is best appreciated on a contrast-enhanced examination.
- Sensitivity: 90%
- Specificity: 100%
- Accuracy: 94%

DIAGNOSTIC PEARLS

- On ultrasound and CT studies, a dilated portal vein can usually be identified and distinguished from other lesions.
- Aneurysm is anechoic; however, if a thrombus is present, Doppler studies are necessary for confirmation.
- Constantly swirling blood and an aneurysm in the splenic vein and superior mesenteric vein may simulate a cystic mass and a bolus; dynamic CT scanning and Doppler sonography are necessary for the correct diagnosis.

CLINICAL PRESENTATION

- Duodenal compression
- Common bile duct obstruction
- Chronic portal hypertension
- Abdominal hemorrhage

DIFFERENTIAL DIAGNOSIS

- Caroli disease
- Pseudoaneurysm

PATHOLOGY

- Usually secondary to pancreatitis and trauma
- Possibly congenital in origin
- Occurring in patients with cirrhosis and portal hypertension

INCIDENCE/PREVALENCE AND EPIDEMIOLOGY

- Aneurysms of portal venous system are uncommon.
- Splanchnic vein aneurysms represent only 3% of all aneurysms of the venous system.
- They are the most common visceral aneurysm.

WHAT THE REFERRING PHYSICIAN NEEDS TO KNOW

- Patients who have no symptoms and no signs of portal hypertension should be monitored by serial MR or ultrasound scans.
- Complications include rupture, thrombosis, complete occlusion of the portal vein, portosystemic shunts, or biliary tract compression.

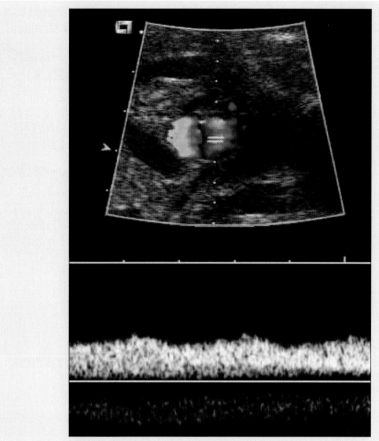

Figure 1. Umbilical vein aneurysm. Color Doppler ultrasound shows flow in this venous aneurysm.

Suggested Readings

De Gaetano AM, Andrisani MC, Gui B, et al: Thrombosed portal vein aneurysm. *Abdom Imaging* 31(5):545-548, 2006.

Laumonier H, Montaudon M, Corneloup O, et al: CT angiography of intrahepatic portal aneurysm. *Abdom Imaging* 30:755-757, 2005.

Okur N, Inal M, Akgul E, et al: Spontaneous rupture and thrombosis of an intrahepatic portal vein aneurysm. *Abdom Imaging* 28:675-677, 2003.

Splenic Vein Thrombosis

DEFINITION: Bland or septic thrombus present in the splenic vein. The splenic vein may also be thrombosed by invasion of tumor from adjacent organs, such as pancreas or stomach.

ANATOMIC FINDINGS

Splenic Vein
- Thrombus and occlusion

Gastric Vessels
- Bleeding varices in the cardia and fundus

Spleen
- Splenomegaly

IMAGING

CT
Findings
- Identical to that observed in portal or superior mesenteric vein thrombosis
- Broad, serpentine, redundant filling defects or clusters of polypoid defects, simulating thickened rugal folds
- Dilation of the gastroepiploic vein

Utility
- Best seen on contrast-enhanced scans
- Sensitivity: 90%-100%
- Specificity: 85%-100%
- Accuracy: 97%

MRI
Findings
- Identical to that observed in portal or superior mesenteric vein thrombosis
- Broad, serpentine, redundant filling defects or clusters of polypoid defects, simulating thickened rugal folds
- Dilation of the gastroepiploic vein

Utility
- Best seen on contrast-enhanced scans
- Sensitivity: 85%-100%
- Specificity: 80%-100%
- Accuracy: 95%

Ultrasound
Findings
- Identical to that observed in portal or superior mesenteric vein thrombosis

DIAGNOSTIC PEARLS

- The splenorenal ligament should be carefully evaluated in all patients who have had a splenectomy or have pancreatitis, or carcinoma of the stomach and pancreas.

- Broad, serpentine, redundant filling defects or clusters of polypoid defects, simulating thickened rugal folds
- Dilation of gastroepiploic vein

Utility
- Best seen on Doppler studies
- Sensitivity: 70%-90%
- Specificity: 80%-95%
- Accuracy: 84%

CLINICAL PRESENTATION

- Often clinically silent
- Left-sided portal hypertension caused by splenic vein occlusion
- Gastric varices in the cardia and fundus that may bleed
- Splenomegaly
- Left upper quadrant pain

DIFFERENTIAL DIAGNOSIS

- Splenic vein gas
- Splenic vein parasites

PATHOLOGY

- Splenic vein thrombosis is usually the result of pancreatitis, pancreatic carcinoma, lymphoma, or propagation of a clot from the portal vein.
- Splenic vein occlusion produces rerouting of venous flow through the short gastric veins and the gastroepiploic vein, causing *left-sided* portal hypertension.

WHAT THE REFERRING PHYSICIAN NEEDS TO KNOW

- Gastric varices in the cardia and fundus are seen in 74%-83% of patients with splenic vein occlusion.
- Splenic vein thrombosis is often clinically silent, but it may cause localized venous hypertension that can result in splenomegaly and bleeding gastric varices.
- Splenic vein thrombosis should be suspected in patients with splenomegaly and those with a history of gastrointestinal hemorrhage with normal liver function tests.
- Splenectomy and gastrotomy with oversewing of bleeding varices is sufficient treatment.

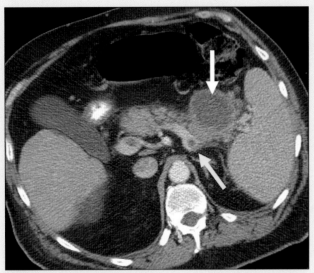

Figure 1. Splenic vein thrombosis. A small thrombus *(yellow arrow)* is present in this patient with pancreatitis and a pseudocyst *(white arrow)*.

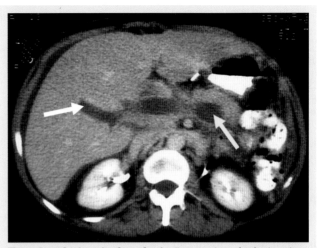

Figure 2. Splenic vein thrombosis. Propagation of splenic vein thrombus *(yellow arrow)* into the intrahepatic portal vein *(white arrow)* after a splenectomy.

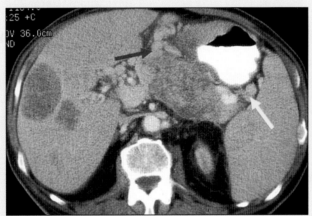

Figure 3. Splenic vein thrombosis. Thrombus is present within the splenic vein in this patient with pancreatitis and a pseudocyst. The pancreas and splenic vein have been invaded by gastric carcinoma. Note the collateral blood vessels in the gastrohepatic *(red arrow)* and gastrosplenic *(yellow arrow)*, as well as two liver metastases.

■ Other causes include sclerotherapy, splenectomy, and causes of portal vein and superior mesenteric artery thrombosis.

INCIDENCE/PREVALENCE AND EPIDEMIOLOGY

■ Chronic pancreatitis accounts for 65% of all cases of splenic vein thrombosis.

Suggested Readings

Hiraiwa K, Morozumi K, Miyazaki H, et al: Isolated splenic vein thrombosis secondary to splenic metastasis: A case report. *World J Gastroenterol* 12:6561-6563, 2006.

Ikeda M, Sekimoto M, Takiguchi S, et al: Total splenic vein thrombosis after laparoscopic splenectomy: A possible candidate for treatment. *Am J Surg* 193:21-25, 2007.

Mortele KJ, Mergo PJ, Taylor HM, et al: Peripancreatic vascular abnormalities complicating acute pancreatitis: Contrast-enhanced helical CT findings. *Eur J Radiol* 52:67-72, 2004.

Mortele KJ, Mergo PJ, Taylor HM, et al: Splenic and perisplenic involvement in acute pancreatitis: Determination of prevalence and morphologic helical CT features. *J Comput Assist Tomogr* 25:50-54, 2001.

Superior Mesenteric Vein Thrombosis

DEFINITION: Thrombus formation in superior mesenteric vein (SMV).

IMAGING

Radiography
Findings
- Complications such as ileus, pneumatosis intestinalis, and ascites

Utility
- Usually noncontributory

CT
Findings
- Low-density intraluminal mass with a hyperdense periphery
- Mural thickening of the gut
- Pneumatosis
- Mesenteric hemorrhage and edema

Utility
- Similar findings to those of portal vein thrombosis
- Sensitivity: 82%-98%
- Specificity: 85%-100%
- Accuracy: 92%

MRI
Findings
- Thrombus within superior mesenteric vein

Utility
- Sensitivity: 75%-98%
- Specificity: 90%-100%
- Accuracy: 90%

Interventional Radiology
Findings
- Spasm of the superior mesenteric artery and no opacification of affected veins in the venous phase

Utility
- Angiography
- Similar findings to those of portal vein thrombosis

Ultrasound Doppler
Utility
- Sensitivity: 65%-85%
- Specificity: 90%-100%
- Accuracy: 82%

DIAGNOSTIC PEARLS
- Low-density intraluminal mass with a hyperdense periphery, as in portal vein thrombosis
- Mural thickening of the gut
- Spasm of superior mesenteric artery and no opacification of affected veins in the venous phase

CLINICAL PRESENTATION
- Acute thrombosis produces symptoms that are less than 4 weeks including pain and nausea and vomiting, with or without bloody diarrhea.
- Most cases have associated acidosis and mild to moderate leukocytosis.
- Chronic thrombosis is usually asymptomatic until late complications occur, such as variceal bleeding caused by portal hypertension.
- SMV thrombosis may cause weight loss, food avoidance, and postprandial pain or distention.

DIFFERENTIAL DIAGNOSIS
- Mesenteric venous gas
- Mesenteric invasion by neoplasm
- Parasites

PATHOLOGY
- Thrombus formation in the SMV, commonly associated with portal vein thrombosis
- Secondary to myeloproliferative disorders, peritonitis, inflammatory disorder of the abdomen, tumor compression, portal hypertension, postoperative state, and hypercoagulable states

INCIDENCE/PREVALENCE AND EPIDEMIOLOGY
- SMV thrombosis constitutes 5%-15% of all intestinal vascular thromboses.
- It is most common in patients 50-60 years of age.

WHAT THE REFERRING PHYSICIAN NEEDS TO KNOW
- Conservative management is recommended in cases with no evidence of ischemia or infarction.
- Angiographically guided direct infusion of fibrinolytic agents into the mesenteric portal system is an alternative treatment.

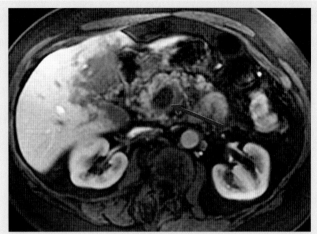

Figure 1. Portal and superior mesenteric vein thrombosis: MRI findings. The thrombus continues into the superior mesenteric vein on this axial MR scan.

Suggested Readings

Bradbury MS, Kavanagh PV, Bechtold RE, et al: Mesenteric venous thrombosis: Diagnosis and noninvasive imaging. *RadioGraphics* 22:527-541, 2002.

Hatoum OA, Spinelli KS, Abu-Hajir M, et al: Mesenteric venous thrombosis in inflammatory bowel disease. *J Clin Gastroenterol* 39:27-31, 2005.

Ibukuro K, Ishii R, Fukuda H, et al: Collateral venous pathways in the transverse mesocolon and greater omentum in patients with pancreatic disease. *AJR Am J Roentgenol* 182:1187-1225, 2004.

Joh JH, Kim DL: Mesenteric and portal vein thrombosis: Treated with early initiation of anticoagulation. *Eur J Vasc Endovasc Surg* 29:204-208, 2005.

Transient Hepatic Attenuation Differences and Transient Hepatic Intensity Differences

DEFINITION: Areas of parenchymal enhancement caused by a compensatory increase in arterial flow secondary to a decrease in portal flow.

ANATOMIC FINDINGS

Liver
- Compromised flow in the portal vein
- Increased arterial flow
- Communication between the main vessels and sinusoids; dilating peribiliary venules
- Masses, abscesses, portal vein or hepatic thrombus formation, anomalous blood supply, or biliary dilation possibly seen

IMAGING

CT
Findings
- Mass-associated lobar multisegmental transient hepatic attenuation differences and transient hepatic intensity differences (THADs/THIDs) cause surrounding parenchyma perfusion; it does not assume a triangular shape; a straight border may be present.
- Mass-associated segmental THADs/THIDs exhibit triangular areas.
- Non–mass-associated sectorial THADs/THIDs assume a globular shape, especially when adjacent to the Glisson capsule.
- Polymorphous THADs/THIDs are associated with external compression, an anomalous blood supply, inflammation of adjacent organs, and post-traumatic causes.
- Diffuse THADs/THIDs are associated with abnormal attenuation and signal intensity adjacent to the portal triads in Budd-Chiari syndrome and right-sided heart failure.
- Liver segment IV hyperenhancement in patients with superior vena cava obstruction may be seen.

Utility
- Areas of parenchymal enhancement are visible during the hepatic arterial phase after the intravenous administration of contrast media.

MRI
Findings
- Mass-associated lobar multisegmental THADs/THIDs cause surrounding parenchymal perfusion; they do not assume a triangular shape; a straight border may be present.

DIAGNOSTIC PEARLS
- Segmental THADs/THIDs appear as triangular areas.
- THIDs/THADs can have a globular shape, especially when they are adjacent to the Glisson capsule.
- In lobar multisegmental THADs/THIDs, a straight border may be present between the arterial phenomenon and the adjacent parenchyma.

- Mass-associated segmental THADs/THIDs exhibit triangular areas.

Utility
- These defects can be confused with true hepatic masses on arterial phase imaging.

DIFFERENTIAL DIAGNOSIS
- Hypervascular metastases
- Hepatocellular carcinoma
- Focal nodular hyperplasia
- Hepatocellular adenoma
- Nodular regenerative hyperplasia

PATHOLOGY
- If portal vein flow is compromised, a segment of liver will derive its blood supply almost exclusively from the hepatic artery.
- Masses produce THADs/THIDs via a direct siphoning effect, by portal branch compression or infiltration, by thrombus, or by flow diversion.
- Lobar multisegmental THADs/THIDs: A benign hypervascular lesion or abscess ensues, and primary arterial inflow increases (the siphoning effect).
- Segmental THADs/THIDs follow the hepatic vessel dichotomy and are seen in benign and malignant tumors, as well as abscesses.
- Non–mass-associated sectorial THIDs/THADs are caused by portal hypoperfusion from thrombosis, long-standing biliary obstruction, or an arterioportal shunt.

WHAT THE REFERRING PHYSICIAN NEEDS TO KNOW
- Diffuse THADs/THIDs can be seen in right-sided heart failure, Budd-Chiari syndrome, and biliary obstruction.
- These masses should not be confused with true hepatic masses.

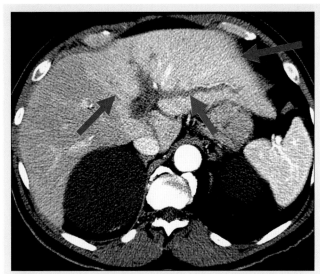

Figure 1. THADs and THIDs: malignant causes. Multidetector CT shows THAD *(red arrows)* in the lateral segment of the left hepatic lobe caused by portal vein thrombosis *(blue arrow)* secondary to hepatocellular carcinoma (not shown).

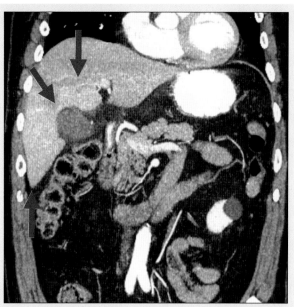

Figure 2. THADs and THIDs: benign causes. In a patient with acute cholecystitis, coronal reformatted CT image shows hyperenhancement of liver *(arrows)* adjacent to the gallbladder fossa.

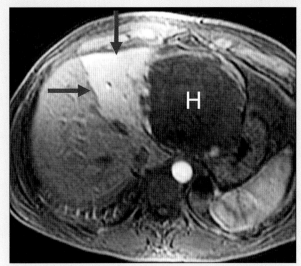

Figure 3. THADs and THIDs resulting from hemangioma. MR image in the same patient shows early peripheral nodular enhancement of hemangioma (H) and THID *(arrows)* during an arterial-dominant image.

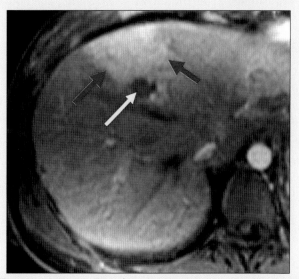

Figure 4. THIDs resulting from hemangiomas. Early-phase MRI shows THID *(red arrows)*. The *yellow arrow* points to the hemangioma.

- Polymorphous THADs/THIDs major causes are external compression, an anomalous blood supply, inflammation of adjacent organs, and post-traumatic, postbiopsy, or postradiofrequency ablation.

INCIDENCE/PREVALENCE AND EPIDEMIOLOGY

- These defects are becoming increasingly common with technical improvements in breath-hold MRI and multi-detector CT.

Suggested Readings

Choi SH, Lee JM, Lee KH, et al: Relationship between various patterns of transient hepatic attenuation on CT and portal vein thrombosis related to acute cholecystitis. *AJR Am J Roentgenol* 183:437-442, 2004.

Colagrande S, Centi N, La Villa G, et al: Transient hepatic attenuation differences. *AJR Am J Roentgenol* 183:459-464, 2004.

Kim HJ, Kim AY, Kim TK, et al: Transient hepatic attenuation differences in focal hepatic lesions: Dynamic CT features. *AJR* 184: 83-90, 2005.

Lee KH, Han JK, Jeong JY, et al: Hepatic attenuation differences associated with obstruction of the portal or hepatic veins in patients with hepatic abscesses. *AJR Am J Roentgenol* 185:1015-1023, 2005.

Visceral Artery Aneurysms (Liver and Splanchnic Circulation)

DEFINITION: Aneurysms of visceral arteries primarily involve the splenic, hepatic, and superior mesenteric arteries.

IMAGING

Radiography
Findings
- Curvilinear calcification at the right upper quadrant is seen.
- When large, it produces a mass effect on the adjacent viscera on barium studies or in the bile ducts on cholangiograms.

Utility
- Only seen when vessel is densely calcified

Ultrasound Color Doppler
Findings
- Pulsatile, cystic mass with arterial flow or sonolucent or mixed echogenic mass with dilation of the ducts proximally

Utility
- Ultrasound is the noninvasive screening method of choice for hepatic artery aneurysm.
- Sensitivity: 85%-90%
- Specificity: 95%-100%

CT
Findings
- Aneurysm wall calcification is seen.
- After bolus administration of contrast material, residual lumen demonstrates intense enhancement.
- Low-density thrombus is seen peripherally.

Utility
- Use of multidetector CT has resulted in increased detection of post-traumatic false aneurysms of the intrahepatic arterial branches.
- Sensitivity: 90%-95%
- Specificity: 95%-100%

MRI
Findings
- Tubular structure has flow void or strong signal intensity, depending on the imaging sequence used.

DIAGNOSTIC PEARLS
- Hepatic artery aneurysms is suggested by a pulsatile, cystic mass with arterial flow or a sonolucent or mixed echogenic mass and dilation of the ducts proximally.
- Curvilinear calcification at right upper quadrant may occur.
- Tubular structure has flow void or strong signal intensity on MRI.

Utility
- Vascular calcification may interfere with detection.
- Sensitivity: 85%-95%
- Specificity: 95%-100%

Interventional Radiology
Findings
- Aneurysm

Utility
- Angiography is primarily used prior to endovascular repair or embolization.
- Sensitivity: 95%-100%
- Specificity: 95%-100%

CLINICAL PRESENTATION
- Left upper quadrant pain in splenic artery aneurysm
- Epigastric or right upper quadrant pain, hemobilia, and obstructive jaundice appearing in hepatic artery aneurysms
- Acute colicky upper abdominal pain, nausea, and vomiting
- Abdominal bruit or pulsatile mass

WHAT THE REFERRING PHYSICIAN NEEDS TO KNOW
- Enlarging aneurysm and those larger than 2.5-3.0 cm typically require treatment.
- Hepatic artery aneurysm has high incidence of rupture, with associated mortality of up to 82%.
- It can be treated via open surgical or endovascular approaches.
- Rupture of a splenic artery aneurysm is most common during the third trimester, with high maternal and fetal mortality rates.

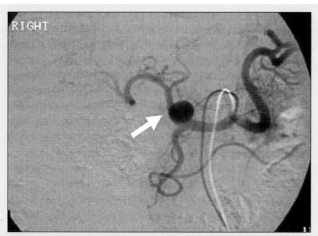

Figure 1. **Visceral artery aneurysm.** Digital subtraction angiogram shows an aneurysm *(arrow)* of the proximal proper hepatic artery just after the origin of the gastroduodenal artery.

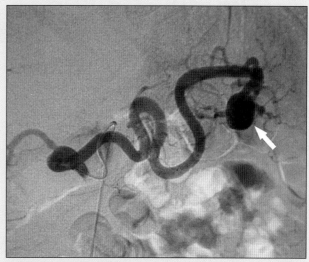

Figure 2. **Visceral artery aneurysm.** Aneurysm *(arrow)* of the distal portion of the splenic artery is evident on this angiogram.

PATHOLOGY

- Female predilection in splenic artery aneurysm relates to the hormonal effects of estrogen and progesterone.
- Superior mesenteric artery (SMA) aneurysms may be mycotic in origin and secondary to inflammation, vasculitis, trauma, arterial dissection, dysplasia, or degeneration.
- Hepatic artery aneurysms may be caused by trauma, iatrogenic injury, infection, or vasculitis; they may be degenerative or dysplastic.
- Gastroduodenal and pancreaticoduodenal artery aneurysms are often complications of acute and chronic pancreatitis and pancreatic surgery.

INCIDENCE/PREVALENCE AND EPIDEMIOLOGY

- Splenic artery aneurysms account for 60% of visceral artery aneurysms, hepatic artery aneurysms (20%), and SMA aneurysms (5.5%).
- Splenic artery aneurysm is four times more common in women.

- Twofold male dominance is seen in hepatic artery aneurysm.
- SMA aneurysm occurs mostly in men in the fifth decade of life.
- Celiac artery aneurysm is present mostly in the fifth decade.

Suggested Readings

Carr SC, Mahvi DM, Hoch JR, et al: Visceral artery aneurysm rupture. *J Vasc Surg* 33:806-811, 2001.

Chiesa R, Astore D, Guzzo G, et al: Visceral artery aneurysms. *Ann Vasc Surg* 11:440-445, 2005.

Kalko Y, Ugurlucan M, Basaran M, et al: Visceral artery aneurysms. *Heart Surg Forum* 10:E24-E29, 2007.

Sessa C, Tinelli G, Poren P, et al: Treatment of visceral artery aneurysm: Description of a retrospective series of 42 aneurysms in 34 patients. *Ann Vasc Surg* 18:695-703, 2004.

Hepatic Trauma

DEFINITION: Blunt or penetrating trauma to the liver.

IMAGING

CT
Findings
- Immediately after injury, hematomas on noncontrast scans are hyperdense relative to the normal hepatic parenchyma.
- Sentinel clot is the highest density blood collection seen and usually lies adjacent to the injured organ.
- Lacerations appear as branching or linear low-attenuation areas; they may be superficial (< 3 cm from liver surface) or deep (> 3 cm from surface).
- Subcapsular hematomas are distinguished from free hemoperitoneum by the mass effect on the liver surface, creating a contour deformity.
- Active extravasation has very high attenuation approximating that of the aorta, as compared with the density of clotted blood.
- Bilomas and intrahepatic and perihepatic abscesses are major post-traumatic complications.

Utility
- Multidetector CT (MDCT) is the imaging of choice for hepatic trauma, with enormous impact on the detection and management of liver injuries.
- Significant hepatic and extrahepatic injuries can be detected reliably.
- MDCT documents the interval healing of hepatic injuries and detects early and delayed complications.
- It also detects associated and unsuspected injuries to other organs.
- Sensitivity: 90%-100%
- Specificity: 95%-100%

Ultrasound
Findings
- Subcapsular hematoma is a lentiform or curvilinear fluid collection with echogenic properties that vary with the age of the lesion.

DIAGNOSTIC PEARLS

- The sentinel clot is the highest density blood collection seen and usually lies adjacent to the injured organ.
- Lacerations are associated with branching or linear low-attenuation areas.
- Subcapsular hematomas are distinguished from free hemoperitoneum by the mass effect on the liver surface, creating a contour deformity.

- Parenchymal contusions are normally hypoechoic on the initial presentation, transiently becoming hyperechoic and then hypoechoic.
- Parenchymal tears, with or without a hematoma, are characterized by irregular defects with an abnormal echotexture relative to the surrounding normal tissue.
- Intraparenchymal hematomas as small as 3.5 mL can be visualized as rounded, echogenic foci.
- Bilomas are rounded or ellipsoid, anechoic, loculated structures with sharply defined margins close to the liver and bile ducts.

Utility
- Ultrasound is more frequently performed in the emergency room by surgeons, radiologists, and emergency room physicians.
- Advantages of sonography include portability, the ability to detect intraperitoneal blood rapidly, and the relatively low cost.
- Problems include the operator-dependent nature of ultrasound and limitations in demonstrating the extent of the injury.
- Focused abdominal sonogram for trauma can demonstrate many traumatic lesions: subcapsular hematomas, parenchymal tears, contusions, bilomas, and hemoperitoneum.
- Sensitivity: 70%-80%
- Specificity: 95%-100%

WHAT THE REFERRING PHYSICIAN NEEDS TO KNOW
- Majority of patients with blunt-force hepatic trauma and some with penetrating liver injuries are managed nonoperatively if they are hemodynamically stable.
- Three main surgical principles of management are (1) achieve control of the hemorrhage, (2) drain the infection, and (3) repair the biliary system.
- Injuries to the hepatic veins are a major cause of immediate death from hepatic trauma; they are also difficult to repair.
- Biliary injury must be recognized and repaired, given that it will not heal spontaneously.

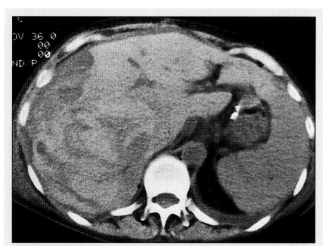

Figure 1. **Noncontrast appearance of hepatic laceration and hematoma.** Noncontrast CT demonstrates a heterogeneous mass-like region in the right hepatic lobe with central hyperdensity consistent with a hematoma.

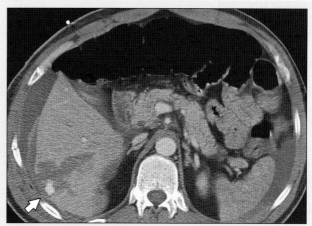

Figure 2. **Hepatic laceration with active extravasation.** CT shows a low-density laceration in the posterior segment of the right hepatic lobe. Focal hyperdensity consistent with active extravasation of contrast and active hemorrhage is seen *(arrow)*.

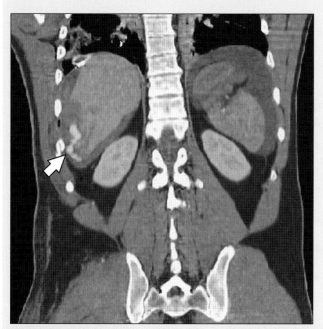

Figure 3. **Hepatic laceration with active extravasation.** A coronal reformatted image further reveals the extent of active extravasation *(arrow)*. High-density fluid in the peritoneal cavity is consistent with hemoperitoneum.

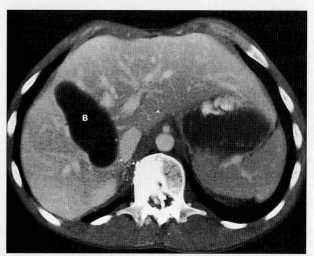

Figure 4. **Biloma.** Biloma (B) after a gunshot wound to the liver. The large low-attenuation (5 HU) collection in the liver was aspirated and proved to be a biloma.

Nuclear Medicine

Findings

- With bile leakage, the tracer appears as a subcapsular collection or may pool freely in the peritoneal cavity.
- Parenchymal injuries such as lacerations and hematomas are easily identified on early hepatic-phase images.

Utility

- Hepatobiliary scan is the most sensitive means of detecting bile leakage, allowing the diagnosis before the onset of clinical symptoms.

MRI

Findings

- Bile leaks
- Injuries
- Bleeding
- Bilomas
- Hematomas

Utility

- Gadolinium-enhanced MRI can depict complex hepatic injuries in patients with contraindications to iodinated contrast material.
- Contrast-enhanced MRI has been shown to demonstrate traumatic hepatic injuries equal to, and occasionally better than, contrast-enhanced CT.
- Longer imaging time is required, and it cannot accommodate metallic life support and monitoring equipment.
- MR imaging can help differentiate bilomas from subacute hematomas.
- Sensitivity: 90%-100%
- Specificity: 95%-100%

Interventional Radiology

Findings

- Bile leak

Utility

- Endoscopic retrograde cholangiopancreatography can be used to guide the insertion of a biliary endoprosthesis.

Radiography

Findings

- Associated fractures are seen, and lung involvement is noted.
- Hepatomegaly, irregularity of liver margin, and caudal displacement of hepatic flexure all suggest liver injury.

Utility

- Plain radiography findings are neither sensitive nor specific in patients with hepatic trauma.

CLINICAL PRESENTATION

- Patient may exhibit right upper quadrant pain and tenderness with guarding and rebound tenderness, as well as falling hematocrit and hypotension.

- Delayed manifestations of biliary trauma, such as bilomas, are usually accompanied by right upper quadrant pain and jaundice.
- Hepatic trauma is characterized by hematemesis or melena associated with right upper quadrant pain.

PATHOLOGY

- Severe compressive trauma to the liver from a steering wheel injury or direct blow produces stellate fractures that often involve the entire lobe.
- Rapid deceleration in motor vehicle accidents produces shearing forces that cause different degrees of parenchymal tears.
- Acute penetrating trauma caused by a stabbing, gunshot, or shotgun injury may involve the liver.
- Liver can be damaged by external cardiac compression during the course of resuscitation and by an inappropriately low insertion of a chest tube.
- Diagnostic and interventional procedures include liver capsule tear, subcapsular hematoma, bile leak, arteriovenous fistula, arteriobiliary or venobiliary fistula, hepatic hematoma, hemoperitoneum, and biloma.
- Spontaneous rupture may result from hemolysis, elevated liver enzymes, and low platelets (known as HELLP syndrome).

INCIDENCE/PREVALENCE AND EPIDEMIOLOGY

- Reported prevalence of liver injury in patients who have sustained blunt-force trauma ranges from 1%-8%.
- In large city hospitals, penetrating injuries from firearms and stabbings predominate.
- Liver is the most frequently injured viscus, owing to its anterior and partially subcostal location.
- Liver biopsy is most common cause of subcapsular hematoma in the United States today.
- High incidence of associated extrahepatic injury occurs, including splenic rupture, head injuries, and rib, facial, and pelvic fractures.

Suggested Readings

Cushing BM, Clark DE, Cobean R, et al: Blunt and penetrating trauma: Has anything changed. *Surg Clin North Am* 77:1321-1332, 1997.
Eiseman B, Rainer W: Liver trauma: An old friend revisited. In Najarian JS, Delaney JP (eds): *Progress in Hepatic, Biliary and Pancreatic Surgery*. Chicago, Year Book Medical, 1990, pp 98-107.
Feliciano DV, Lewis CA: Hepatic trauma. In Pitt HA, Carr-Locke DL, Ferrucci JT (eds): *Hepatobiliary and Pancreatic Disease*. Boston, Little, Brown, 1995, pp 107-124.
Shanmuganathan K, Mirvis SE: CT evaluation of blunt hepatic trauma. *Radiol Clin North Am* 36:399-412, 1998.
Shanmuganathan K, Mirvis SE: CT evaluation of the liver with acute blunt trauma. *Crit Rev Diagn Imaging* 36:73-113, 1995.

SECTION XI

Pancreas

Part 52

ANOMALIES AND ANATOMIC VARIANTS OF THE PANCREAS

Annular and Semiannular Pancreas

DEFINITION: Band of pancreatic tissue partially or completely encircling the duodenum.

ANATOMIC FINDINGS

Stomach
- Dilation

Duodenum
- Usually in second portion of duodenum
- Dilation of the proximal duodenum
- Partially or completely encircling flat band of pancreatic tissue

Pancreas
- Pancreatic head and associated duct encircle the duodenum.
- Body and tail have a normal main pancreatic duct.

IMAGING

Radiography
Findings
- *Double-bubble sign:* dilated stomach and duodenal bulb on plain radiography
- Periampullary stenosis with extrinsic-eccentric defect on the medial margin of the second portion of the duodenum on barium study
- Intact duodenal mucosa, unless with associated peptic ulcer

Utility
- Maximal duodenal distention helps optimize the demonstration of characteristic barium study findings.
- Sensitivity: 30%-50%
- Specificity: 90%

Interventional Radiology
Findings
- Normally located main pancreatic duct communicates with small duct encircling the duodenum.
- Encircling duct originates from the right anterior surface of the duodenum, goes around, then enters the main pancreatic or the common bile duct.
- Biliary obstruction may be seen.

DIAGNOSTIC PEARLS
- Encircling duct originates from the right anterior surface of the duodenum, goes around, then enters the main pancreatic or common bile duct.
- Normal-appearing pancreatic tissue encircling duodenum is seen on fat-suppressed T1-weighted MR sequences.
- Periampullary stenosis with extrinsic-eccentric defect may be seen.

- Celiac angiography shows an anomalous branch from the posterior pancreaticoduodenal artery supplying annular moiety.

Utility
- Endoscopic retrograde cholangiopancreatography (ERCP) shows typical features in approximately 85% of cases.
- Celiac angiography is used.
- Sensitivity: 80%-85%
- Specificity: 100%

Ultrasound
Findings
- Nonspecific enlargement of the pancreatic head

Utility
- Endoscopic ultrasound is more accurate than an abdominal scan.
- Sensitivity: 40%-55%
- Specificity: 90%-95%

CT
Findings
- Enlargement of pancreatic head
- Central region of high attenuation representing contrast material within the narrowed duodenum
- Apparent circumferential thickening of duodenal wall with an enlarged pancreatic head

WHAT THE REFERRING PHYSICIAN NEEDS TO KNOW
- Annular and semiannular pancreas may be associated with other congenital anomalies.
- If associated with a periampullary ulcer, Zollinger-Ellison syndrome is also considered.
- Malignancy should be ruled out in cases with obstructive jaundice.

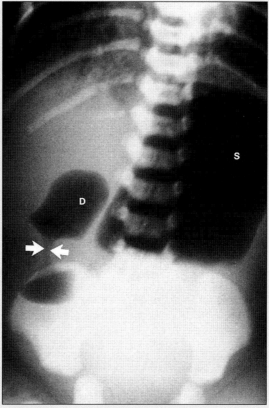

Figure 1. **Annular pancreas.** Annular pancreas in the neonatal period with narrowing *(arrows)* of the descending duodenum. Duodenal bulb (D) and stomach (S) are dilated, producing the classic *double-bubble sign.*

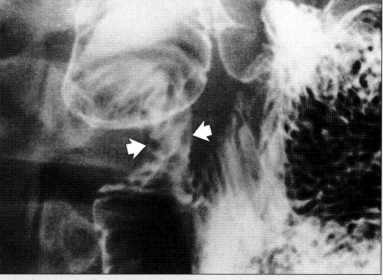

Figure 2. **Annular pancreas.** Annular pancreas demonstrated as concentric duodenal narrowing *(arrows)* in this adult patient who had nondescript epigastric pain.

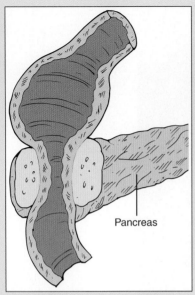

Figure 3. **Annular pancreas.** Diagram illustrates the pathologic process shown on the barium study.

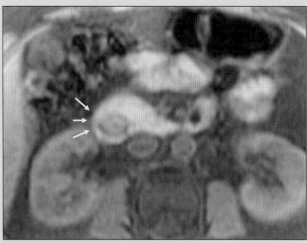

Figure 4. **Annular pancreas: MRI features.** Axial fat-saturation T1-weighted image shows the duodenum surrounded by pancreatic tissue *(arrows)*. *(Courtesy of Carmen DeJuan, MD, Department of Radiology Hospital Clinic, University of Barcelona, Spain.)*

Utility
- Findings are often nonspecific.
- Sensitivity: 60%-80%
- Specificity: 90%-95%

MRI
Findings
- Normal-appearing pancreatic tissue encircling the duodenum on fat-suppressed T1-weighted sequence
- MR cholangiopancreatography (MRCP) shows similar findings as ERCP.

Utility
- MRI is used to discriminate the pancreas from the duodenum clearly.
- Sensitivity: 75%-85%
- Specificity: 90%-95%

CLINICAL PRESENTATION
- Abnormal pancreatic tissue may occur clinically in neonates or in adulthood.
- Symptoms are usually related to duodenal obstruction.
- Neonates have vomiting on first day of life with a history of fetal gastrointestinal obstruction.
- Older patients have nausea, vomiting, and epigastric pain.

DIFFERENTIAL DIAGNOSIS
- Post-traumatic sequelae

PATHOLOGY
- Annular pancreas and semiannular pancreas are bands of pancreatic tissue completely or partially encircling the duodenum.
- It may result from hypertrophy of the dorsal and ventral ducts.
- Alternatively, adherence of the ventral duct to the duodenum may be present before rotation.
- Third possibility is hypertrophy or adherence of the left bud of the paired ventral primordia.

INCIDENCE/PREVALENCE AND EPIDEMIOLOGY
- Incidence is 1 in 12,000-15,000 live births.
- It occurs clinically in the third to fifth decade of life.

Suggested Readings
Desai MB, Mitchell DG, Munoz SJ: Asymptomatic annular pancreas: Detection by magnetic resonance imaging. *Magn Reson Imaging* 12:683-685, 1994.
Godil A, McCracken GA: Images in clinical medicine. Annular pancreas. *N Engl J Med* 336:1794, 1997.
Schneck CD, Dabezies MA, Friedman AC: Embryology, histology, gross anatomy, and normal imaging of the pancreas. In Friedman AC, Dachman AH (eds): *Radiology of the Liver, Biliary Tract, and Pancreas*. St. Louis, Mosby, 1994, pp 715–742.
Ueki T, Yao T, Beppu T, et al: Three-dimensional computed tomography pancreatography of an annular pancreas with special reference to embryogenesis. *Pancreas* 32:426-429, 2006.
Urayama S, Kozarek R, Ball T, et al: Presentation and treatment of annular pancreas in an adult population. *Am J Gastroenterol* 90:995-999, 1995.

Heterotopic Pancreatic Tissue

DEFINITION: Pancreatic tissue found outside of the pancreas.

ANATOMIC FINDINGS

- Ectopic rests of pancreatic tissue most commonly occur in the gastric antrum (25.5%) or the proximal portion of the duodenum (27.7%).
- Less frequent sites include the jejunum (15.9%), ileum, Meckel diverticulum, colon, appendix, mesentery, omentum, liver, gallbladder, spleen, bile ducts, and esophagus.

IMAGING

Radiography
Findings
- Broad-based, smooth, extramucosal or intramural lesion with a central niche or umbilication is diagnostic.
- Niche is absent in approximately one half of cases.

Utility
- Barium contrast study is used.
- If no central niche is present, the lesion cannot be differentiated from other submucosal tumors.

CT
Findings
- Broad-based, smooth, extramucosal or intramural lesion is seen.
- Rarely, large intramural cystic collections are seen.

Utility
- CT features of this disorder are nonspecific.
- CT is insensitive for the depiction of heterotopic pancreatic tissue.

CLINICAL PRESENTATION

- Majority of cases are asymptomatic and are found incidentally.
- Heterotopic pancreas may simulate a duodenal ulcer, gallbladder disease, or even appendicitis.
- It may cause pyloric or biliary obstruction.

DIFFERENTIAL DIAGNOSIS

- Hyperplastic polyp
- Adenoma
- Leiomyoma

DIAGNOSTIC PEARLS

- Broad-based, smooth, extramucosal or intramural lesion with a central niche or umbilication is diagnostic.

- Lipoma
- Gastrointestinal stromal tumor

PATHOLOGY

- Heterotopic pancreas usually results from heteroplastic differentiation of parts of the embryonic entoderm that do not normally produce pancreatic tissue.
- Heterotopic pancreas with glandular acinar ducts and well-differentiated islets is seen in organs derived from the entoderm.
- In the duodenum and stomach, heterotopic pancreas is usually composed of normal pancreatic tissue, including islet cells and a pancreatic duct.
- Islet cells are usually absent at other sites.
- Ectopic pancreatic tissue usually lies submucosally (73%), although it can be located in the muscularis mucosae or on the serosal surface of the gut.

INCIDENCE/PREVALENCE AND EPIDEMIOLOGY

- Heterotopic pancreas is found in the duodenum in nearly 14% of autopsies.
- It is also found in 14.1% of postmortem studies of the biliary system.

Suggested Readings

Claudon M, Verain AL, Bigard MA, et al: Cyst formation in gastric heterotopic pancreas: Report of two cases. *Radiology* 169:659-660, 1988.

Eklof O: Accessory pancreas in the stomach and duodenum: Clinical features, diagnosis, and therapy. *Acta Chir Scand* 121:19-20, 1961.

Eklof O, Lassrich A, Stanley P, et al: Ectopic pancreas. *Pediatr Radiol* 1:24-27, 1973.

Mortele KJ, Rocha TC, Streeter JL, et al: Multimodality imaging of pancreatic and biliary congenital anomalies. *RadioGraphics* 26:715-731, 2006.

Schneck CD, Dabezies MA, Friedman AC: Embryology, histology, gross anatomy, and normal imaging of the pancreas. In Friedman AC, Dachman AH (eds): *Radiology of the Liver, Biliary Tract, and Pancreas*. St. Louis, Mosby, 1994, pp 715-742.

WHAT THE REFERRING PHYSICIAN NEEDS TO KNOW

- No treatment is necessary unless complications are present.

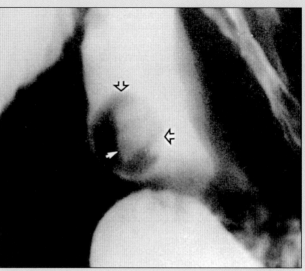

Figure 2. Ectopic pancreas: barium contrast studies. Ectopic rests of pancreatic tissue are present in the duodenal bulb. The mound of pancreatic tissue is signified by the *open arrows*. The *solid arrow* shows the draining duct.

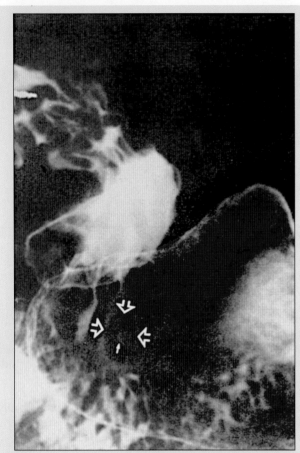

Figure 1. Ectopic pancreas: barium contrast studies. Ectopic rests of pancreatic tissue are present in the gastric antrum. The mound of pancreatic tissue is signified by the *open arrows*. The *solid arrow* shows the draining duct.

Pancreas Divisum

DEFINITION: Anatomic variant wherein the ducts of the dorsal and ventral anlagen fail to merge.

ANATOMIC FINDINGS

- Pancreas divisum is an anatomic variant wherein the pancreas is divided into two separate parts as a result of absent or incomplete fusion of ventral and dorsal anlagen.
- It has separate ductal systems: The head and uncinate process are drained by the duct of Wirsung, the body and tail by the duct of Santorini.
- It may have an anatomic variant of the pancreatic duct, which includes fusion variants (pancreas divisum and functional divisum) and a duplication variant.
- Small duct of Santorini results in chronic stasis of pancreatic fluid, increasing the risk of pancreatitis.
- Association with pancreatic tumors, multiple neuroendocrine tumors of pancreas, and intestinal malrotation has been reported.

IMAGING

Interventional Radiology
Findings
- Injection of contrast material into the duct of Wirsung is met with resistance (and pain on the patient's part).
- Duct of Wirsung is short and tapers gradually from the orifice, with acinarization.
- Duct of Santorini is not visualized by the injection of the major papilla or is seen without communication.
Utility
- Interventional radiology is an effective modality for confirming a diagnosis of pancreas divisum.
- Endoscopic retrograde cholangiopancreatography (ERCP) is used.
- Sensitivity: 95%-100%
- Specificity: 100%

Ultrasound
Findings
- Excluded if the portal vein, common bile duct, and main pancreatic duct are demonstrated in one image.
- Excluded if the main pancreatic duct passes from the major papilla to the body and tail.
- Excluded if the main pancreatic duct crosses the border separating the ventral and dorsal anlagen.
- Secretin-induced dilation of the main pancreatic duct is seen.

DIAGNOSTIC PEARLS

- Two separate moieties with normal pancreatic tissue
- No connection between separate ductal systems
- Fat cleft between moieties

Utility
- Endoscopic ultrasound allows detailed imaging of the parenchyma and ductal system.
- It also allows the direct visualization and biopsy of pancreatic masses that cause pseudodivisum.
- Sonographic secretin test is controversial; dilation can be a normal finding.
- Sensitivity: 5%-10%
- Specificity: 90%-95%

CT
Findings
- Contour abnormalities of the pancreatic head and neck or pancreatic head enlargement is seen.
- Two distinct pancreatic moieties or an unfused ductal system are identified.
- Deep fat cleft separating the two moieties can be identified.
Utility
- Multidetector CT with high-resolution oblique coronal image reconstruction for pancreatic ducts
- Sensitivity: 50%-90%
- Specificity: 90%-95%

MRI
Findings
- Identification of two separate moieties and ductal systems.
Utility
- MRI uses heavily T2-weighted, two-dimensional, fast spin-echo sequences with body coil.
- MR cholangiopancreatography (MRCP) is superior to ERCP for visualizing pancreatic ducts.
- MRI also uses a half-Fourier acquisition single-shot turbo spin-echo sequence or a single-shot rapid acquisition with relaxation enhancement.
- T1-weighted sequences with fat suppression show the ducts and pancreatic parenchyma around the duodenum.

WHAT THE REFERRING PHYSICIAN NEEDS TO KNOW

- Presence of pancreatitis and ductal dilation or imaging findings should raise suspicion for malignancy.

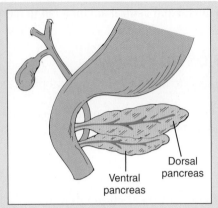

Figure 1. Pancreatic duct development. The final stage of pancreatic duct maturation entails fusion of the two systems. (*From Taylor AJ, Bohorfoush AG:* Interpretation of ERCP: With Associated Digital Imaging Correlation. *Philadelphia, Lippincott-Raven, 1996, pp 209-210.*)

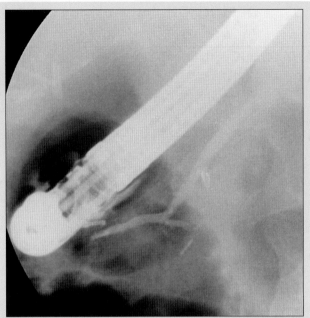

Figure 2. Pancreas divisum in a 36-year-old patient with recurrent pancreatitis. ERCP was able to demonstrate the dorsal pancreatic duct by cannulation of the minor papilla. (*From Fulcher AS, Turner MA: MR pancreatography: A useful tool for evaluating pancreatic disorders.* RadioGraphics *19:5-24, 1999.*)

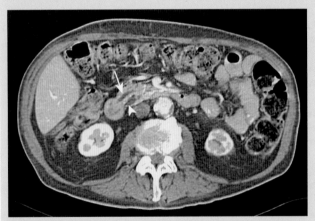

Figure 3. Pancreas divisum: CT findings. The axial contrast-enhanced CT study through the head of the pancreas reveals two separate pancreatic ducts draining into the duodenum. Other images prove the separate nature of these ducts, the upper one (*arrow*) draining the head and body of the pancreas into the minor papilla and the lower one (*arrowhead*) only from the inferior head and the uncinate process draining into the major papilla.

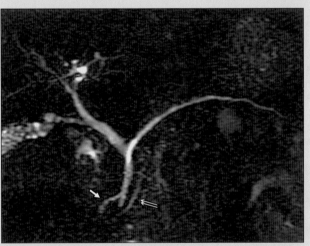

Figure 4. Pancreas divisum: MRCP findings. Coronal oblique thick-slab MRCP image reveals that the pancreatic duct drains through the minor papilla (*single arrow*). The duct of Wirsung is also depicted (*double arrows*) without connection between the two systems. The findings are consistent with complete pancreas divisum. This image was obtained after secretin injection. (*Courtesy of Carmen DeJuan, MD, Department of Radiology Hospital Clinic, University of Barcelona, Spain.*)

- Sensitivity: 85%-90%
- Specificity: 95%-100%

CLINICAL PRESENTATION

- Most cases are asymptomatic.
- Pancreas divisum is associated with recurrent episodes of pancreatitis.

INCIDENCE/PREVALENCE AND EPIDEMIOLOGY

- Pancreas divisum is seen in 4%-11% of autopsy series.
- It is also seen in 3%-4% of ERCP series.
- Age at presentation is between 30 and 50 years.

Suggested Readings

Itoh S, Takada A, Satake H, et al: Diagnostic value of multislice computed tomography for pancreas divisum: Assessment with oblique coronal reconstruction images. *J Comput Assist Tomogr* 29:452-460, 2005.

Laghi A, Catalano C, Panebianco V, et al: Pancreas divisum: Demonstration of a case with cholangiopancreatography with magnetic resonance. *Radiol Med (Torino)* 93:648-650, 1997.

Lai R, Freeman ML, Cass OW, et al: Accurate diagnosis of pancreas divisum by linear-array endoscopic ultrasonography. *Endoscopy* 36:705-709, 2004.

Schneck CD, Dabezies MA, Friedman AC: Embryology, histology, gross anatomy, and normal imaging of the pancreas. In Friedman AC, Dachman AH (eds): *Radiology of the Liver, Biliary Tract, and Pancreas*. St. Louis, Mosby, 1994, pp 715-742.

Zeman RK, McVay LV, Silverman PM, et al: Pancreas divisum: Thin section CT. *Radiology* 169:395-398, 1988.

Acute Pancreatitis

DEFINITION: Acute pancreatitis is an acute inflammation of the pancreas secondary to a variety of causes, most commonly gallstones or alcoholism.

ANATOMIC FINDINGS

- Grade A: normal pancreas
- Grade B: focal or diffuse enlargement of the gland, including contour irregularities and inhomogeneous attenuation
- Grade C: intrinsic pancreatic abnormalities associated with inflammatory changes in the peripancreatic fat
- Grade D: small and usually single, ill-defined fluid collection
- Grade E: two or more large fluid collections or the presence of gas in the pancreas or retroperitoneum

IMAGING

Radiography
Findings
- Abnormal abdominal gas pattern: gasless abdomen, ileus pattern (small bowel ileus, adynamic sentinel loop, *colon cutoff sign*)
- Elevated diaphragms, pleural and pericardial effusions, basal atelectasis, pulmonary infiltrates, and adult respiratory distress syndrome
- Thickening and spiculation of mucosal folds in the stomach and duodenum, which can be seen on barium studies
- Varying degrees of atony associated with spastic segments of the duodenum, jejunum, and transverse colon also possibly present
Utility
- Plain abdominal radiographs and barium studies are insensitive in the diagnosis and staging of pancreatitis.

CT
Findings
- *Colon cutoff sign* can also be seen on CT.
- Mild disease is characterized by a normal-sized gland or a slight to moderate increase in gland size, with

DIAGNOSTIC PEARLS

- Mild disease is characterized by a normal-sized gland or a slight to moderate increase in gland size, with mild inflammation surrounding an otherwise normal-appearing gland.
- Pancreas may be diffusely enlarged, with a shaggy, irregular contour and slightly hypoenhancing heterogeneous parenchyma.
- In more advanced cases, extravasation of pancreatic fluid leads to the formation of intrapancreatic and extrapancreatic fluid collections.

mild inflammation surrounding an otherwise normal-appearing gland.
- In more advanced cases, extravasation of pancreatic fluid leads to the formation of intrapancreatic and extrapancreatic fluid collections.
- In severe forms of necrotizing pancreatitis, the gland may become enlarged, enveloped by high-attenuation heterogeneous fluid collections.
- Pancreatic necrosis is associated with nonenhancement in the arterial phase, which is a poor prognostic sign.
- Patchy areas of absence of enhancement, fragmentation, and liquefaction necrosis are seen.
- Complications include pseudocyst, hemorrhage, abscess, and infection.
Utility
- Best diagnostic images are obtained with multidetector CT (MDCT), achieving optimal vascular and parenchymal enhancement while avoiding respiratory motion.
- CT is the premier imaging test in the diagnosis and management of patients with acute pancreatitis.

WHAT THE REFERRING PHYSICIAN NEEDS TO KNOW

- Segmental pancreatitis should be carefully evaluated to exclude adenocarcinoma simulating pancreatitis or a mass causing pancreatitis.
- Endoscopic ultrasound, endoscopic retrograde cholangiopancreatography, biopsy, follow-up CT, or MRI is appropriate for suspected carcinoma.
- Cystic masses should be scrutinized with Doppler ultrasound studies to exclude pancreatic pseudoaneurysms.
- Fat necrosis and hemorrhage are poor prognostic signs.
- Prompt detection of complications is essential because they are responsible for more than 50% of mortality in acute pancreatitis.
- Complications include pseudocyst, infected necrosis, abscess, and hemorrhage.

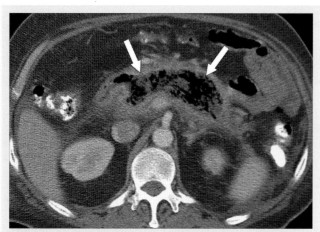

Figure 1. Infected necrosis. Axial contrast-enhanced MDCT image shows an absence of normal enhancing pancreatic parenchyma. Air bubbles and debris *(arrows)* are seen in the pancreatic bed, suggesting infected necrosis. The patient underwent pancreatic débridement.

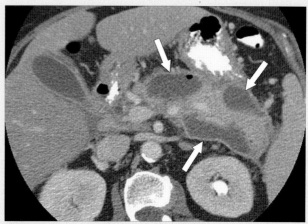

Figure 2. Pancreatic abscess. Axial contrast-enhanced MDCT image shows fluid collection *(arrows)* containing an air bubble involving the pancreas consistent with an abscess. The patient underwent surgical drainage of the abscess and pancreatic débridement.

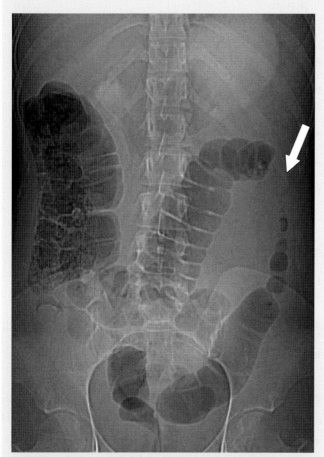

Figure 3. Colon cutoff sign on MDCT. Scout topogram for abdominal MDCT shows abrupt interruption *(arrow)* of colonic gas at the splenic flexure in a patient with acute pancreatitis.

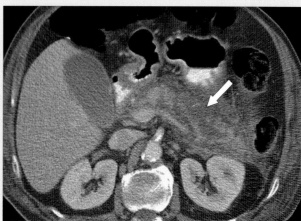

Figure 4. Grade E pancreatitis with necrosis evolving into pseudocyst. Axial contrast-enhanced MDCT image shows patchy, confluent, necrotic areas *(arrow)* in the pancreatic body and tail. Note the peripancreatic inflammatory stranding.

- Radiation dose delivered by CT may be a significant factor for young patients with pancreatitis who will require multiple examinations.
- Sensitivity: 85%-90%
- Specificity: 90%-95%

Interventional Radiology
Findings
- Compression and obstruction of the distal common bile duct are seen as a smooth and symmetric narrowing on cholangiography.
- Multiple gallstones as a cause of pancreatitis are demonstrated with cholangiography.
- Cholangiography also demonstrates pancreas divisum, choledochocele, choledochal cyst, perivaterian duodenal diverticulum, pancreatic or bile duct carcinoma, and ampullary carcinoma.
- Angiography demonstrates vascular causes of the pancreatitis.
- In edematous pancreatitis, vessels are stretched and displaced, with increased parenchymal staining.
- Vessels may be beaded with an irregular caliber or may show thrombosis or pseudoaneurysm formation.
- If a parenchymal hemorrhage is present, the parenchymal stain will be mottled.

Utility
- Angiography is not performed in patients with acute pancreatitis unless a pseudoaneurysm is suspected, which can be treated with transcatheter embolization.
- Elucidating vascular causes of pancreatitis can also be helpful.

MRI
Findings
- Pancreas may be diffusely enlarged, with a shaggy, irregular contour and a slightly hypoenhancing heterogeneous parenchyma.
- Mild disease is characterized by a normal-sized gland or a slight to moderate increase in gland size, with mild inflammation surrounding an otherwise normal-appearing gland.
- In more advanced cases, extravasation of pancreatic fluid leads to the formation of intrapancreatic and extrapancreatic fluid collections.
- In severe forms of necrotizing pancreatitis, the gland may become enlarged, enveloped by high-attenuation heterogeneous fluid collections.
- Decreased pancreatic signal intensity is seen on T1-weighted fat-suppressed sequences and on pre- and post-gadolinium administration, depending on the degree of inflammation and edema.
- Peripancreatic high signal intensity may be seen on T1-weighted fat-suppressed sequences related to fat necrosis and hemorrhage.
- Complications include pseudocyst, hemorrhage, abscess, and infection.

Utility
- MR cholangiopancreatography can determine the cause of the pancreatitis; it is accurate and noninvasive and prevents complications associated with endoscopic retrograde cholangiopancreatography (ERCP).
- MRI can be helpful in determining the cause of the pancreatitis, including choledocholithiasis, pancreas divisum, and underlying tumors.
- Advantages include high soft-tissue contrast resolution, as well as the ability to evaluate the common bile duct, pancreatic duct, and parenchyma in a single examination.
- It does not use ionizing radiation, which is a consideration in younger patients who may need serial examinations.
- It does not require iodinated contrast and is preferred in patients with renal insufficiency or severe pancreatitis with increased renal disease risk.
- MRI is limited in the acute setting when the patient is very ill because patient cooperation and breath-holding may be compromised during a longer examination.
- Sensitivity: 90%-95%
- Specificity: 95%-100%

Ultrasound
Findings
- Classic sonographic appearance of pancreatitis is a diffusely enlarged, hypoechoic pancreas.
- Less commonly, a focal enlargement is present.
- Echogenicity of the pancreas in acute pancreatitis is extremely variable and depends on numerous factors.
- Similarly, size changes are difficult to assess without a baseline scan.
- Pancreatic duct may dilate, particularly if the inflammation is confined to the pancreatic head.
- Focal intrapancreatic masses may be seen, and fluid collection may be acute; also seen is hemorrhage or an ill-defined, hypoechoic, pancreatic enlargement that may sonographically simulate carcinoma.
- Lesser sac fluid collections are often seen and may produce a *butterfly* appearance.

Utility
- Abnormal findings are seen on sonography in 33%-90% of patients with acute pancreatitis.
- Ultrasound is a good screening test in patients with suspected biliary pancreatitis.
- In acute pancreatitis, bowel gas and other factors will limit the visualization of the gland in one fourth to one third of patients.
- Ultrasound is unable to define completely the complex extrapancreatic spread of infection along the fascial planes and within the peripancreatic compartments.
- Ultrasound cannot specifically reveal areas of pancreatic necrosis in patients with severe pancreatitis.
- Tissue-harmonic imaging improves image quality, the delineation of the pancreatic tail, lesion conspicuity,

and fluid-solid differentiation relative to B-mode sonography.
- Sensitivity: 75%-80%
- Specificity: 93%-97%

CLINICAL PRESENTATION

- Patients' symptoms range from mild abdominal pain, nausea, vomiting, fever, tachycardia, and abdominal distention to severe abdominal pain and shock.
- Most patients have abdominal tenderness and guarding.
- In very severe cases, flank ecchymosis (Grey-Turner sign) or periumbilical hematoma (Cullen sign) may be present.

DIFFERENTIAL DIAGNOSIS

- Pancreatic carcinoma
- Peptic ulcer disease
- Diverticulitis (stomach and duodenum)
- Gastric outlet obstruction (stomach and duodenum)
- Peritoneal carcinomatosis

PATHOLOGY

- Alcoholic pancreatitis mechanisms include a necrosis-fibrosis sequence, duct obstruction, and leakage of enzymes from pancreatic duct.
- Activated pancreatic enzymes are extravasated, causing pancreatic autodigestion and necrosis.
- Cholelithiasis-induced pancreatitis is associated with an obstruction of the common biliopancreatic channel by a stone, with resultant bile reflux into the pancreatic duct, and with pancreatic enzyme activation.
- Pseudocysts cause localized collections of pancreatic fluid confined by a capsule of fibrous or granulation tissue.
- Abscess is an encapsulated collection of pus in proximity to the pancreas without associated pancreatic necrosis.

- Pseudoaneurysm is a focal area of dilation of the splanchnic artery.
- Pancreatic ascites is an outpouring of pancreatic fluid from the disrupted pancreatic duct into the peritoneal cavity by way of a fistula.

INCIDENCE/PREVALENCE AND EPIDEMIOLOGY

- Incidence of acute pancreatitis is 0.005%-0.01% in the general population.
- Alcoholism and biliary tract disease (gallstones) account for approximately 90% of cases of acute pancreatitis in the United States.
- Alcoholic pancreatitis is more common in urban Veterans Administration hospitals, whereas gallstone pancreatitis is seen in suburban and rural hospitals.
- Cause is idiopathic in 10%-30% of cases.
- Prevalence is increased in patients with acquired immunodeficiency syndrome.

Suggested Readings

Balthazar EJ, Freeny PC, vanSonnenberg E: Imaging and intervention in acute pancreatitis. *Radiology* 193:297-306, 1994.
Banks PA: Acute and chronic pancreatitis. In Feldman M, Scharschmidt BF, Sleisenger MH (eds): *Sleisenger and Fordtran's Gastrointestinal and Liver Disease.* Philadelphia, WB Saunders, 1998, pp 809-862.
Bradley EL III: A clinically based system for acute pancreatitis. *Arch Surg* 128:586-590, 1993.
Dervenis C, Johnson CD, Bassi C, et al: Diagnosis, objective assessment of severity, and management of acute pancreatitis. *Int J Pancreatol* 25:195-210, 1999.
Karne S, Gorelick FS: Etiopathogenesis of acute pancreatitis. *Surg Clin North Am* 79:699-710, 1999.
May G, Gardiner R: *Clinical Imaging of the Pancreas.* New York, Raven, 1987, pp 57-114.
McKay CJ, Imrie CW: Staging of acute pancreatitis. Is it important? *Surg Clin North Am* 79:733-743, 1999.
Radecki PD, Friedman AC, Dabezies MA: Pancreatitis. In Friedman AC, Dachman AH (eds): *Radiology of the Liver, Biliary Tract, and Pancreas.* St. Louis, Mosby, 1994, pp 763–806.
Ranson JH: Etiological and prognostic factors in human acute pancreatitis: A review. *Am J Gastroenterol* 77:633-638, 1982.

Chronic Pancreatitis

DEFINITION: Chronic pancreatitis is prolonged pancreatic inflammation characterized by irreversible morphologic and functional damage to the pancreas.

ANATOMIC FINDINGS

Pancreas
- Size abnormality and contour irregularity
- Ductal dilation and obstruction
- Calcification

IMAGING

Radiography
Findings
- Most pancreatic calculi are small, irregular calcifications that may be diffuse or confined to a specific region of the pancreas.
- Typical pancreatic calcifications are diagnostic of chronic pancreatitis.

Utility
- This exam is insensitive in the depiction of chronic pancreatitis.

Ultrasound
Findings
- Gland size abnormality, irregular margins, inhomogeneous or heterogeneous echogenicity of the parenchyma, and dilation of the pancreatic duct are seen.
- Calcifications are recognized as shadowing echogenic foci within the parenchyma or main pancreatic duct.
- Pseudocysts are often present in chronic pancreatitis; they are usually unilocular, anechoic, and sharply defined.
- Other complications of chronic pancreatitis such as biliary dilation and splenic vein thrombosis can also be detected with sonography.
- Decreased echogenicity occurs in the setting of acute exacerbations, with parenchymal edema.

DIAGNOSTIC PEARLS

- MR cholangiopancreatography (MRCP) findings include fluid-filled structures such as pseudocysts, pancreatic duct dilation, irregularity, stones, and obstructions.
- EUS findings include parenchymal calcifications, hyperechoic foci or strands, pseudocysts, heterogeneous echotexture, and lobular contour of gland.
- ERCP findings include dilation, contour irregularity, clubbing, stenosis, and opacification of small cavities of the side branches of the pancreatic duct.

Utility
- Sonography has a 60%-80% diagnostic accuracy rate and provides a noninvasive, inexpensive, and rapid method of evaluating morphologic changes.
- Similar to CT, transabdominal sonography is insensitive in diagnosing early chronic pancreatitis.
- Abnormalities in size and the contour of the pancreas are the least sensitive indicators of chronic pancreatitis on ultrasound studies.
- Pancreatic parenchymal echogenicity is also unreliable in the diagnosis of chronic pancreatitis because it can be normal, increased, or decreased.

Interventional Radiology
Findings
- Endoscopic retrograde cholangiopancreatography (ERCP) findings include dilation, contour irregularity, clubbing, stenosis, and opacification of the small cavities of the side branches of the pancreatic duct.
- In mild disease, the main pancreatic duct is normal, but at least three side branches are abnormal.

WHAT THE REFERRING PHYSICIAN NEEDS TO KNOW

- Some changes can be seen in elderly normal patients and must be interpreted with caution in this age group.
- Calculi develop in 40%-60% of patients with alcoholic pancreatitis.
- If solitary stricture is seen in main pancreatic duct, differential considerations include neoplasm or pseudocyst.
- ERCP and MRCP help evaluate the pancreatic duct for chronic pancreatitis in patients with abdominal pain refractory to medical therapy.
- Pancreatic or bile duct strictures or obstructions are the major cause of pain and the main surgical indications in chronic pancreatitis.
- Imaging features of adenocarcinoma and focal pancreatitis overlap; ERCP and EUS with fine-needle aspiration biopsy may be required.
- Smooth-tapering duct through the mass, calcifications, and lower duct caliber/gland width ratio favor the diagnosis of an inflammatory mass over adenocarcinoma.

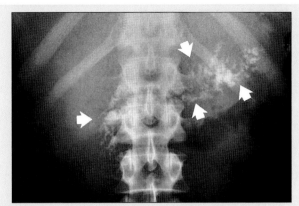

Figure 1. Pancreatic calcifications on plain abdominal radiographs. The entire gland contains numerous small calcifications located in the main pancreatic duct and its radicles *(arrows).*

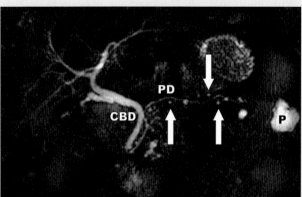

Figure 2. Early chronic pancreatitis. Coronal T2-weighted thick-slab RARE MRI shows mild dilation of the secondary branches of the pancreatic duct *(arrows)* and pseudocyst (P) in the pancreatic tail. The main pancreatic duct (PD) and the common bile duct (CBD) have normal caliber. (*RARE,* Rapid acquisition with relaxation enhancement.) (*From Miller FH, Keppke AL, Wadhwa A, et al: MRI of pancreatitis and its complications: Part 2. Chronic pancreatitis.* AJR Am J Roentgenol *183:1645-1652, 2004. Reprinted with permission from the* American Journal of Roentgenology.)

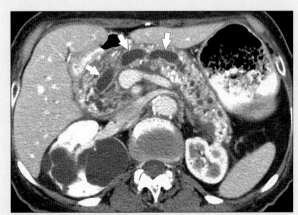

Figure 3. Chronic pancreatitis. Axial contrast-enhanced multidetector CT (MDCT) image shows diffuse calcifications in the pancreas with a dilated main pancreatic duct *(arrows)* measuring 9 mm and dilated side branches.

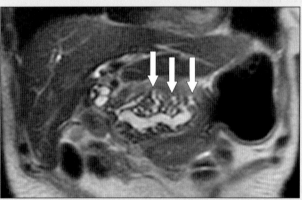

Figure 4. Chronic pancreatitis. Coronal T2-weighted MR image shows the dilated pancreatic duct and secondary radicles *(arrows)* associated with chronic pancreatitis. (*From Miller FH, Keppke AL, Wadhwa A, et al: MRI of pancreatitis and its complications: Part 2. Chronic pancreatitis.* AJR Am J Roentgenol *183:1645-1652, 2004. Reprinted with permission from the* American Journal of Roentgenology.)

- In moderate disease, abnormalities are seen in the main pancreatic duct and in more than three side branches.
- In severe disease, abnormalities of moderate disease are seen plus one of following: a large cavity, ductal obstruction, filling defects, severe dilation, or an irregularity.
- Endoscopic ultrasound (EUS) detects small pancreatic tumors and microlithiasis, which are causes of chronic pancreatitis.
- EUS findings include parenchymal calcifications, hyperechoic foci or strands, pseudocysts, heterogeneous echotexture, and lobular contour of the gland.

- Ductal abnormalities include dilation and irregularity, hyperechoic walls, intraductal stones, and visible branches.

Utility

- Because of its invasiveness and potentially serious complications, ERCP is ideally reserved for patients who need intervention.
- ERCP is able to detect early chronic pancreatitis before morphologic abnormalities can be seen on CT.
- Chronic pancreatitis is likely when more than two EUS findings are present.

- With more than six findings, the disease is probably moderate to severe.
- Good correlation of EUS with ERCP exists in patients with moderate or severe chronic pancreatitis but not with mild disease.
- Disadvantages of EUS include its cost, limited availability, and long learning curve; it is also very operator-dependent.

MRI

Findings

- MRCP findings include fluid-filled structures such as pseudocysts, pancreatic duct dilation, irregularity, stones, and obstructions.
- Abnormalities in size and contour of the gland, dilation and shape of pancreatic duct, and the presence of ductal calcifications are seen.
- Decreased signal intensity is best visualized on nonenhanced T1-weighted fat-suppressed images.
- Decreased and heterogeneous enhancement are seen during the arterial phase; later phases show relative increased enhancement on gadolinium-enhanced T1-weighted fat-suppressed images.

Utility

- Advantages of MRCP include lack of ionizing radiation; it does not require iodinated contrast material, and it is noninvasive.
- MRCP is also helpful in patients with anatomic abnormalities that impede the cannulation of the common bile duct or pancreatic duct.
- MRCP has advantage of showing ductal segments proximal and distal to the obstruction.
- Sensitivity of MRCP for ductal abnormalities and dilation ranges from 56%-100%, and the specificity ranges from 86%-100%.
- Administration of secretin during MRCP allows for the evaluation of exocrine function of the pancreas and improves delineation of the pancreatic duct.
- Pancreatic duct abnormalities are better demonstrated on MRI than on CT.

CT

Findings

- Abnormalities in size and contour of the gland, dilation and shape of the pancreatic duct, and the presence of ductal calcifications are seen.
- Dilation of the pancreatic duct and its secondary radicles (>2-3 mm in size) are characteristic for chronic pancreatitis.
- In advanced disease, the main duct appears beaded, irregular, or smooth, often containing stones.
- CT demonstrates pancreatic calcifications in approximately 50% of patients with chronic pancreatitis.

Utility

- CT is the most specific, accurate imaging modality for depicting pancreatic calcifications.
- CT has reported sensitivities of 50%-90% and specificities of 55%-85% in the detection of chronic pancreatitis.
- Although CT correctly detects morphologic alterations of chronic pancreatitis, its ability to evaluate disease severity is more limited.

CLINICAL PRESENTATION

- Pain is the predominant clinical finding in 95% of patients.
- Pain radiates from the epigastrium through the back and can be constant or intermittent.
- Weight loss often accompanies pain.
- Diabetes and malabsorption with steatorrhea eventually develop.

DIFFERENTIAL DIAGNOSIS

- Pancreatic carcinoma
- Diverticula (stomach and duodenum)

PATHOLOGY

- Disease of prolonged pancreatic inflammation characterized by irreversible morphologic and functional damage to pancreas
- Continued heavy consumption of alcohol for 5- to 12-year period
- Hyperlipidemia, hyperparathyroidism, trauma, and pancreas divisum all have been implicated as risk factors for developing chronic pancreatitis.

INCIDENCE/PREVALENCE AND EPIDEMIOLOGY

- Chronic pancreatitis is a relatively uncommon disease that has been increasing in frequency in the Western world.
- Incidence of pancreatic cancer is significantly elevated in patients with chronic pancreatitis.
- Approximately 90% of calcific pancreatitis is caused by alcoholism.
- In the United States, approximately 75% of cases of chronic pancreatitis are caused by alcoholism.

Suggested Readings

Alpern MB, Sandler MA, Kellman GM, et al: Chronic pancreatitis: Ultrasonic features. *Radiology* 155:215-219, 1985.

Atri M, Finnegan PW: The pancreas. In Rumack CM, Wilson SR, Charboneau JW (eds): *Diagnostic Ultrasound*, 2nd ed. St. Louis, Mosby, 1998, pp 225-278.

Bolondi L, Gaiani S, Casanova P, et al: Critical evaluation and controversial points of ultrasound findings in chronic pancreatitis. In Malfertheiner P, Ditschuneit H (eds): *Diagnostic Procedures in Pancreatic Disease*. Berlin, Springer-Verlag, 1986, pp 149-154.

Catalano MF, Geenen JE: Diagnosis of chronic pancreatitis by endoscopic ultrasonography. *Endoscopy* 30:A111-A115, 1998.

May G, Gardiner R: *Clinical Imaging of the Pancreas*. New York, Raven, 1987, pp 57-114.

Radecki PD, Friedman AC, Dabezies MA: Pancreatitis. In Friedman AC, Dachman AH (eds): *Radiology of the Liver, Biliary Tract, and Pancreas*. St. Louis, Mosby, 1994, pp 763-806.

Pancreatic Ductal Adenocarcinoma

DEFINITION: Pancreatic adenocarcinoma with scant cellular elements and eliciting an intense desmoplastic response and encasing blood vessels.

ANATOMIC FINDINGS

Main Pancreatic Duct
- Obstructed (The surrounding parenchyma is atrophic.)

IMAGING

CT
Findings
- Tumor appears hypodense compared with the background parenchyma and borders; poorly defined lesions may be isoattenuating.
- Dilation of the upstream pancreatic duct and common bile duct is seen when the tumor is located within the pancreatic head.
- Obliteration of normal fat is seen between the pancreatic margin and the adjacent vessel.
- Morphologic changes in the artery are seen that include narrowing or encasement of the affected artery.
- When the superior mesenteric vein is involved with the tumor, it may display a *teardrop* configuration.

Utility
- Multidetector CT (MDCT) is the primary imaging test for patients with suspected pancreatic adenocarcinoma.
- It can detect lesions of small size before they deform the contour of the gland.
- CT angiography is more accurate in detecting arterial involvement from pancreatic adenocarcinoma than by looking at traditional axial images alone.
- Use of curved-multiplanar reformatting or three-dimensional volume rendering can improve the detection of a ductal dilation.

DIAGNOSTIC PEARLS
- Mass is hypodense compared with the background parenchyma and borders, and poorly defined lesions may be isoattenuating.
- Obliteration of normal fat is noted between the pancreatic margin and the adjacent vessel.
- *Teardrop* configuration may be seen.

MRI and MR Cholangiopancreatography (MRCP)
Findings
- Pancreatic mass is hypovascular and elicits a dense desmoplastic response.
- Pancreatic enhancement is maximal approximately 40-50 seconds after intravenous contrast administration (pancreatic phase).

Utility
- MRI can provide superb evaluation of pancreatic cancer rivaling MDCT evaluation.
- Multisequence approach is used for a comprehensive evaluation.
- Multiphasic gadolinium-enhanced sequences using fat suppression are most valuable for lesion detection and for the assessment of resectability.
- Pancreatic phase is the most valuable for mass detection.
- It is obtained to assess bile and pancreatic duct involvement.
- MRCP can superbly depict combined pancreatic duct and bile duct obstruction and dilation, the so-called double duct sign.

WHAT THE REFERRING PHYSICIAN NEEDS TO KNOW
- CT angiography is more accurate for detecting arterial involvement from pancreatic adenocarcinoma than by looking at traditional axial slices alone.
- Assessing for the presence of the small posterior pancreaticoduodenal veins is important.
- When these collaterals are present, the likelihood that the tumor has involved the superior mesenteric vein is high.
- MRI can provide superb evaluation of pancreatic cancer rivaling MDCT evaluation.
- Distant lymph node disease is a contraindication to resection.

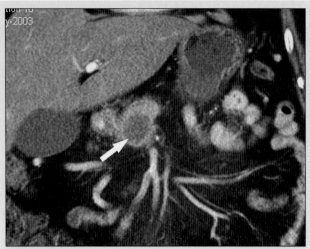

Figure 1. Pancreatic adenocarcinomas. A three-dimensional volume-rendered MDCT image in a 68-year-old woman reveals a low-attenuation mass *(arrow)* in the head of the pancreas. Most pancreatic adenocarcinoma is lower attenuating than the background pancreas on intravenous contrast-enhanced CT imaging.

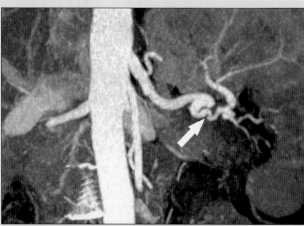

Figure 2. Pancreatic adenocarcinoma: CT angiography. Maximum intensity projection–rendered image of the splenic artery. Notice the encasement *(arrow)* of the splenic artery, typical of pancreatic adenocarcinoma. This image was helpful in establishing the presence of a pancreatic neoplasm, which was subsequently confirmed by fine-needle aspiration.

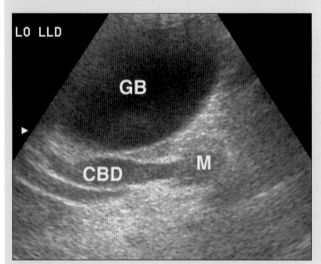

Figure 3. Pancreatic adenocarcinoma: ultrasound evaluation. Longitudinal image reveals a distended gallbladder (GB) and common bile duct (CBD). The CBD can be traced to a mass (M) in the pancreatic head.

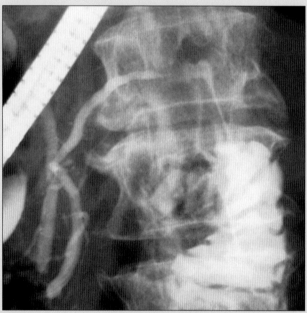

Figure 4. Pancreatic adenocarcinoma: ERCP. A normal pancreatic duct can be traced from the ampulla upstream to an abrupt termination over the mid-portion of the L1 vertebral body. The main pancreatic duct must be visualized at least 2 cm past the left lateral border of the vertebral column. An obstructing stricture in an otherwise normal-appearing pancreatic duct must be considered a neoplasm.

Transabdominal Ultrasound and Endoscopic Ultrasound
Findings
- Hypoechoic irregular mass and hypoechoic enlarged nodes
- Vascular invasion suspected when there is loss of the normal vessel border
- Echogenic mass obstructing either the pancreatic or common bile ducts possibly depicted

Utility
- Endoscopic ultrasound is excellent for the detection of tumors less than 2 cm and provides an excellent guide for a fine-needle aspiration biopsy.
- It is superb for local staging of a neoplasm; the utility decreases in evaluating distant metastases.
- Endoscopic ultrasound is used in cases in which ductal obstruction is visualized without a mass visible on a cross-sectional study.
- It is the best method for obtaining tissue biopsy to confirm malignancy.
- Transabdominal ultrasound is used in patients with jaundice to identify a dilated biliary tract and to evaluate the gallbladder.

PET
Findings
- Increased uptake may be present in the primary pancreatic tumor.

Utility
- Fluorodeoxyglucose-PET produces widely disparate results in the differentiation of pancreatic masses caused by pancreatic adenocarcinoma from those caused by chronic pancreatitis.

Radiography
Findings
- Obstruction or stricture in an otherwise normal main pancreatic duct is indicative of ductal adenocarcinoma.

Utility
- Endoscopic retrograde cholangiopancreatography (ERCP) has no role in preoperative assessment of pancreatic adenocarcinoma when the diagnosis is established by other imaging modalities.
- ERCP is used preoperatively to place a drainage stent within an obstructed common bile duct.

CLINICAL PRESENTATION

- Weight loss, anorexia, and fatigue
- Epigastric pain radiating to back
- Obstructive jaundice
- New-onset diabetes
- Steatorrhea
- Thrombophlebitis

DIFFERENTIAL DIAGNOSIS

- Cholangiocarcinoma
- Ampullary carcinoma
- Pancreatitis
- Gallbladder carcinoma

PATHOLOGY

- Serum CA 19-9 is elevated, which is the only clinically available blood test to suggest the presence of pancreatic malignancy.
- Pancreatic adenocarcinoma has scant cellular elements and elicits an intense desmoplastic response, encasing the intrapancreatic blood vessels.
- It rapidly grows through lymphatics.
- Progression of microscopic epithelial dysplastic change is correlated with specific genetic mutations and alterations.
- Risk factors include cigarette smoking, African-American male, *BRCA2* gene positivity, hereditary pancreatitis, cirrhosis, chronic pancreatitis, diabetes mellitus, hypercholesterolemia, obesity, and exposure to carcinogens.

INCIDENCE/PREVALENCE AND EPIDEMIOLOGY

- Estimated frequency of ductal adenocarcinoma of the pancreas is 9 per 100,000 patients, eleventh among all cancers.
- American Cancer Society estimates 32,800 new cases, equally divided between men and women in the United States, in 2009.
- From 80%-90% of patients with newly diagnosed pancreatic cancer will have advanced disease at the time of discovery.
- Ductal adenocarcinoma accounts for 85%-90% of all pancreatic tumors.
- Up to 22% of tumors can affect multiple regions of the gland (diffuse).

Suggested Readings

Cubilla A, Fitzgerald PJ: Pancreas cancer. I. Duct adenocarcinoma. A clinical-pathologic study of 380 patients. *Pathol Annu* 1:241-289, 1978.

Prokesch RW, Schima W, Chow LC, et al: Multidetector CT of pancreatic adenocarcinoma: Diagnostic advances and therapeutic relevance. *Eur Radiol* 13:2147-2154, 2003.

Roche CJ, Hughes ML, Garvey CJ, et al: CT and pathologic assessment of prospective nodal staging in patients with ductal adenocarcinoma of the head of the pancreas. *AJR Am J Roentgenol* 180:475-480, 2003.

Intraductal Papillary Mucinous Neoplasm

DEFINITION: Neoplasms that involve either the main pancreatic duct or the branch ducts.

ANATOMIC FINDINGS

Pancreas
- Two morphologic forms
- Involving the main pancreatic duct, with or without side branch involvement
- Exclusively involving the branch ducts

IMAGING

CT
Findings
- Communication of a cystic lesion with the pancreatic duct
- Low-attenuation lesion in the uncinate process of the pancreas, which is highly suggestive of branch duct intraductal papillary mucinous neoplasm (IPMN)

Utility
- Multidetector CT
- Lesions are best visualized by the use of three-dimensional techniques, including CT cholangiopancreatography.

MRI
Findings
- Communication of a cystic lesion with the pancreatic duct

Utility
- MR cholangiopancreatography (MRCP) is used.
- Lesions are best visualized by the use of three-dimensional techniques, including MRCP.

Ultrasound
Findings
- Intensely echogenic mucin

Utility
- Endoscopic ultrasound is useful for evaluating main duct tumors, particularly the longitudinal extent of main duct involvement, aiding surgical planning.

Interventional Radiography
Findings
- Thick mucin may block the neck of the branch duct, which will then not fill at the time of cannulation.

DIAGNOSTIC PEARLS
- Diffuse or segmental dilation of the main or branch pancreatic ducts (or both)
- Intraductal growth of the mucin-producing epithelial lining cells
- Protrusion and dilation of the major and minor papilla, with mucus excretion

Utility
- Endoscopic retrograde cholangiopancreatography (ERCP) is useful for aspirating mucin and confirming the diagnosis.
- Cross-sectional techniques are more sensitive than ERCP in visualizing branch duct involvement.
- ERCP aspiration of duct contents aids in the differentiation of main duct IPMN from chronic pancreatitis.

CLINICAL PRESENTATION
- Small tumors (less than 3 cm) confined to branch ducts follow an indolent course.
- Those lesions are typically asymptomatic.

DIFFERENTIAL DIAGNOSIS
- Serous cystadenoma
- Mucinous cystadenocarcinoma
- Cystic adenocarcinoma
- Cystic islet cell tumor

PATHOLOGY
- Diffuse or segmental dilation of the main or branch pancreatic ducts (or both) is seen.
- Intraductal growth of the mucin-producing epithelial lining cells is seen.
- Protrusion and dilation of the major and minor papilla, with mucus excretion, are seen.
- Main ducts involved have a significantly higher likelihood of harboring more malignant epithelium than do those restricted to the branch ducts.

WHAT THE REFERRING PHYSICIAN NEEDS TO KNOW
- Careful attention to protocol will demonstrate a bulging papilla into the duodenal lumen, a finding that allows distinction from chronic pancreatitis.

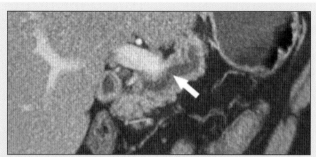

Figure 1. IPMN, combined type. Three-dimensional volume-rendered multidetector CT image from a 48-year-old man. Dilated main pancreatic duct *(arrow)* is seen within the body and tail of the gland.

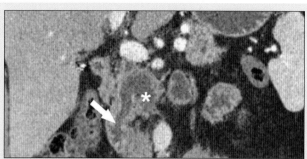

Figure 2. IPMN, combined type. Dilated duct can be followed into the duodenal lumen *(arrow)*, giving the bulging appearance seen on endoscopy. An extension of the mass into a branch duct can be seen *(asterisk)*.

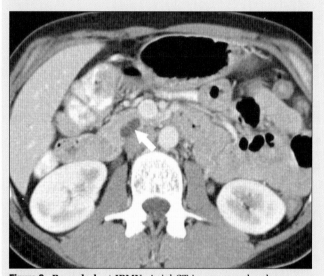

Figure 3. Branch duct IPMN. Axial CT image reveals a low-attenuation lesion in the region of the uncinate process of the pancreas *(arrow)*. The lesion was an incidental finding in this 48-year-old woman. The appearance is highly suggestive of a side branch duct IPMN.

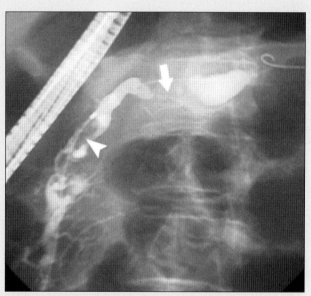

Figure 4. Main duct IPMN. Single view from an ERCP examination in a 75-year-old woman reveals stent catheter traversing a distended main pancreatic duct. Filling defects within the duct represent mucin deposits *(arrowhead)*. A localized stricture is seen in the mid pancreatic duct *(arrow)* that must be considered suspicious for a superimposed neoplasm.

- Branch duct IPMNs can arise anywhere within the pancreas, although the head, neck, and uncinate process are the most common locations.
- Factors include advanced age, main duct involvement, concurrent diabetes or other pancreas-related abdominal symptoms, lesion size (> 3 cm), and multiplicity.

INCIDENCE/PREVALENCE AND EPIDEMIOLOGY

- In more than 50% of cases, the pancreatic duct bulges into the ampulla of Vater, with marked mucus hypersecretion seen in the duodenum.
- As opposed to serous cystadenoma and mucinous cystic tumor, IPMN occurs with a slightly increased frequency in male patients.

Suggested Readings

Fukukura Y, Fujiyoshi F, Sasaki M, et al: Intraductal papillary mucinous tumors of the pancreas: Thin-section helical CT findings. *AJR Am J Roentgenol* 174:441-447, 2000.

Procacci C, Megibow AJ, Carbognin G, et al: Intraductal papillary mucinous tumor of the pancreas: A pictorial essay. *RadioGraphics* 19:1447-1463, 1999.

Sugiyama M, Izumisato Y, Abe N, et al: Predictive factors for malignancy in intraductal papillary-mucinous tumours of the pancreas. *Br J Surg* 90:1244-1249, 2003.

Terris B, Ponsot P, Paye F, et al: Intraductal papillary mucinous tumors of the pancreas confined to secondary ducts show less aggressive pathologic features as compared with those involving the main pancreatic duct. *Am J Surg Pathol* 24:1372-1377, 2000.

Islet Cell Tumors

DEFINITION: Pancreatic endocrine tumors (islet cell tumors) are tumors that derive from embryonic neuroectoderm and are derivatives of the aminoprecursor uptake and decarboxylation cell line arising from the islets of Langerhans.

IMAGING

CT
Findings
- Functioning tumors: hypervascular focus
- Nonfunctioning islet cell tumors: hyperdense pancreatic mass with hypervascular hepatic metastases

Utility
- Current imaging techniques detect up to 90% of functioning endocrine neoplasms.

MRI
Findings
- Functioning tumors: hypervascular focus
- Low signal intensity on fat-suppressed TI-weighted images
- Hyperintense on T2-weighted images, contrast-enhanced scans, and fat-suppressed inversion recovery images

Utility
- Fat-suppressed, gadolinium-enhanced T1-weighted MRI and contrast-enhanced sequences show this neoplasm to best advantage.

CLINICAL PRESENTATION

- Nonfunctioning endocrine tumors may be clinically silent.
- Insulin and proinsulin production is extremely high in patients with insulinoma.
- Gastrin production is excessive in patients with gastrinoma.
- Glucagonoma gives rise to a syndrome: migratory necrolytic erythema, angular stomatitis, cheilitis, and atrophic glossitis.
- Vasoactive intestinal peptide tumors (VIPomas) produce watery diarrhea, hypokalemia, hypochlorhydria, and metabolic acidosis—Verner-Morrison syndrome.

DIAGNOSTIC PEARLS

- Nonfunctioning tumors: The most common appearance is that of a hyperdense pancreatic mass.
- Malignant insulinomas are large and produce extremely high levels of insulin or proinsulin.
- Excessive gastrin production of gastrinoma leads to Zollinger-Ellison syndrome.

DIFFERENTIAL DIAGNOSIS

- Pancreatic metastases
- Primary pancreatic neoplasm

PATHOLOGY

- Malignant insulinomas are large and produce extremely high levels of insulin or proinsulin.
- Pancreatic endocrine tumors (islet cell tumors) are divided into either nonfunctioning (nonsecreting, inactive) or functioning (secreting, active) types.
- They arise from multipotent cells that have retained the ability to differentiate into various endocrine cell types.
- Functioning islet cell tumors include insulinoma, gastrinoma, glucagonoma, VIPoma, and somatostatinoma.
- Nonfunctioning endocrine tumors are clinically silent but do secrete hormones in tiny amounts that are rapidly degraded and biologically inactive.
- Excessive gastrin production leads to Zollinger-Ellison syndrome either as a sporadic entity or as a manifestation of type 1 multiple endocrine neoplasia (MEN I).
- Nonfunctioning tumors are sporadic and are seen in MEN I or von Hippel-Lindau syndrome; masses are usually larger than functioning tumors

---

WHAT THE REFERRING PHYSICIAN NEEDS TO KNOW

- When the lesion is solitary and localized, simple excision or enucleation is sufficient for treatment.
- In advanced cases, surgery must attempt to remove the tumor completely and debulk metastases for adequate control of hypoglycemia.
- In patients with Zollinger-Ellison syndrome or MEN I, the second portion of the duodenum must be carefully evaluated.
- Knowledge of the distinguishing characteristics of both functioning and nonfunctioning islet cell tumors aids in making a more accurate diagnosis of the disease.
- Surgery is the recommended therapy, with attempts to debulk the lesion completely as the major therapeutic goal in nonfunctional tumors.

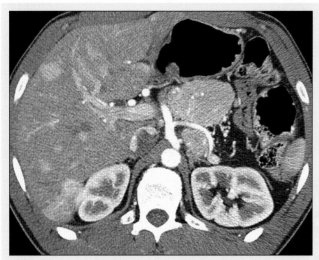

Figure 1. Nonfunctioning islet cell tumor. A hyperdense mass is seen in the pancreatic body. Arterial-phase MDCT also reveals multiple hypervascular liver metastases.

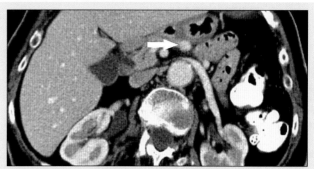

Figure 2. Insulinoma. Arterial-phase CT reveals a brightly enhancing mass in the body of the pancreas *(arrow)*. The patient is an 85-year-old woman with seizures.

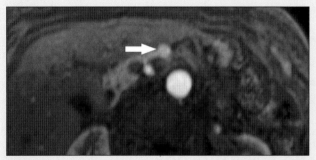

Figure 3. Insulinoma. Arterial-phase gadolinium-enhanced fat-suppressed VIBE MRI reveals a brightly enhancing mass in the body of the pancreas *(arrow)*. The patient is an 85-year-old woman with seizures. (*VIBE,* Volumetric interpolated breath-hold examination.)

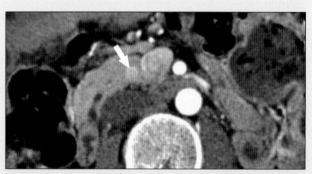

Figure 4. Multiple islet cell neoplasms in a patient with MEN I syndrome. Enhancing mass *(arrow)* in the uncinate process of the pancreas.

INCIDENCE/PREVALENCE AND EPIDEMIOLOGY

- Islet cell tumors account for only 1%-2% of all pancreatic neoplasms.
- They occur with equal frequency in men and women, peak age being in the 50s and 60s, and can be located anywhere within the gland.
- Islet cell tumors can occur sporadically or can be inherited, as in patients with autosomal-dominant MEN I syndrome
- Insulinoma, the most common islet cell tumor, occurs with an incidence of approximately 1:100,000 population.
- Gastrinoma is the second most common islet cell tumor.
- Glucagonoma is a malignant tumor in over 60% of patients at the time of diagnosis; it is usually found in the tail of the pancreas.
- Nonfunctioning tumors: 60%-83% of lesions are malignant at the time of diagnosis.

Suggested Readings

Cirillo F, Falconi M, Bettini R: Clinical manifestations and therapeutic management of hyperfunctioning endocrine tumors. In Procacci C, Megibow AJ (eds): *Imaging the Pancreas: Cystic and Rare Tumors.* Berlin/New York, Springer, 2003.

Noone TC, Hosey J, Firat Z, et al: Imaging and localization of islet-cell tumours of the pancreas on CT and MRI. *Best Pract Res Clin Endocrinol Metab* 19:195-211, 2005.

Procacci C, Carbognin G, Accordini S, et al: Nonfunctioning endocrine tumors of the pancreas: Possibilities of spiral CT characterization. *Eur Radiol* 11:1175-1183, 2001.

Stabile BE, Morrow DJ, Passaro E Jr: The gastrinoma triangle: Operative implications. *Am J Surg* 147:25-31, 1984.

Mucinous Cystic Tumor of the Pancreas

DEFINITION: Tumor formed from variably atypical epithelial cells that produce mucin and are supported by ovarian-type stroma.

IMAGING

CT
Findings
- Large cysts with thin septa are present, best seen after intravenous contrast administration.
- When calcification occurs, it is lamellated and is located in the periphery of the lesion.
- Nodules on the wall are characterized by peripheral calcification and a more disorganized internal architecture.
- Malignant lesions tend to be larger than benign lesions.

Utility
- Multidetector CT is used.
- Lesions are best seen after intravenous contrast administration.
- Lesions are to be compared with a *starburst* pattern and central location of calcification of a serous cystadenoma (SCA).

MRI
Findings
- Bright on T2-weighted sequences
- On T1-weighted sequences, intravenous gadolinium is necessary to image septations that become more apparent the longer the imaging sequence is carried out.

Utility
- Mucin within the lesion produces a decreased signal within the center of the lesion and should not be confused with radiating septae seen in an SCA.

Ultrasound
Findings
- Mural nodularity is easily recognized and differentiated from honeycomb appearance of an SCA.

Utility
- Endoscopic ultrasound is valuable for aspirating cyst fluid.
- Carcinoembryonic antigen (CEA) in cyst fluid has a high predictive value for mucinous cystic tumors.

CLINICAL PRESENTATION

- Often asymptomatic and found incidentally
- Weight loss, epigastric or back pain

DIAGNOSTIC PEARLS

- Large cysts with thin septa are seen.
- When calcification occurs, it is lamellated and in the periphery of the lesion.
- Mural nodularity is easily recognized.

DIFFERENTIAL DIAGNOSIS

- Pseudocysts
- Serous cystadenoma
- Intraductal papillary mucinous neoplasm
- Cystic adenocarcinoma
- Cystic islet cell tumor

PATHOLOGY

- Rare neoplasms thought to be potentially malignant are more properly called mucinous cystic tumors (MCTs).
- They are formed from atypical epithelial cells producing mucin and are supported by ovarian-type stroma that does not communicate with pancreatic duct system.
- Stromal component stains for cytokeratin markers indicative of cellular luteinization.

INCIDENCE/PREVALENCE AND EPIDEMIOLOGY

- MCTs account for 2%-6% of all exocrine pancreatic neoplasms.
- They occurs almost exclusively in women, with peak incidence in the fifth decade.

Suggested Readings

Buetow PC, Rao P, Thompson LD: From the Archives of the AFIP Radiologic-pathologic correlation: Mucinous cystic neoplasms of the pancreas. *RadioGraphics* 18:433-449, 1998.

Itai Y, Ohhashi K, Nagai H, et al: Duct ectatic mucinous cystadenoma and cystadenocarcinoma of the pancreas. *Radiology* 161:697-700, 1986.

Procacci C, Carbognin G, Accordini S, et al: CT features of malignant mucinous cystic tumors of the pancreas. *Eur Radiol* 11:1626-1630, 2001.

Zamboni G, Capelli A, Pesci A, et al: Pathology of cystic tumors. In Procacci C, Megibow AJ (eds): *Imaging of the Pancreas: Cystic and Rare Tumors*. Berlin/New York, Springer, 2003.

WHAT THE REFERRING PHYSICIAN NEEDS TO KNOW

- Rare neoplasms are thought to be potentially malignant; the terms *mucinous cystadenoma* and *mucinous cystadenocarcinoma* should not be used.
- Diagnosis of MCT should not be considered in a male patient.
- Its characteristic features should be differentiated from an SCA.
- Presence of CEA has a high predictive value for the presence of an MCT.

Secondary Pancreatic Neoplasm

DEFINITION: Neoplasm that metastasizes to the pancreas.

IMAGING

CT
Findings
- Hypervascular or hypovascular foci within the pancreatic parenchyma

Utility
- Multidetector CT (MDCT) is less sensitive than MRI in the depiction of these metastases.

MRI
Findings
- Hypervascular or hypovascular masses within the pancreatic parenchyma

Utility
- MRI is more sensitive than MDCT in detecting these metastases.

CLINICAL PRESENTATION

- Usually asymptomatic
- Pancreatitis, jaundice, and pancreatic insufficiency

DIFFERENTIAL DIAGNOSIS

- Ductal pancreatic carcinoma
- Lymphoma

PATHOLOGY

- Pancreas can be secondarily involved via direct extension from a contiguous primary tumor, invasion from local metastatic lymph nodes, or hematogenous metastases.

DIAGNOSTIC PEARLS

- Pancreas can be secondarily involved by a neoplasm via direct extension from a contiguous primary tumor.
- Invasion from local metastatic lymph nodes occurs.
- Hematogenous spread occurs.

INCIDENCE/PREVALENCE AND EPIDEMIOLOGY

- Renal cell carcinoma is the most common primary neoplasm to metastasize to the pancreas.
- Other common sources of metastases to the pancreas include melanoma and lung cancer.
- Seen in 3%-10% of cases at autopsy.

Suggested Readings

Ghavamian R, Klein KA, Stephens DH, et al: Renal cell carcinoma metastatic to the pancreas: Clinical and radiological features. *Mayo Clin Proc* 5:581-585, 2007.

Solcia E, Capella C, Kloppel G (eds): *Tumors of the Pancreas*. Washington, DC, Armed Forces Institute of Pathology, 1997.

WHAT THE REFERRING PHYSICIAN NEEDS TO KNOW
- Metastases to the pancreas can originate from virtually any primary neoplasm.
- Renal cell carcinoma is most common primary neoplasm to metastasize to the pancreas.

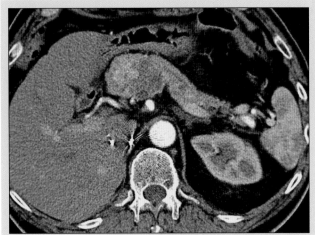

Figure 1. Metastatic renal cell carcinoma to the pancreas.
A heterogeneous mass is seen in the pancreatic neck. Several
hyperdense foci are seen in the mass. The patient is status post–
right nephrectomy. Renal cell carcinoma is the most common
primary tumor to metastasize to the pancreas.

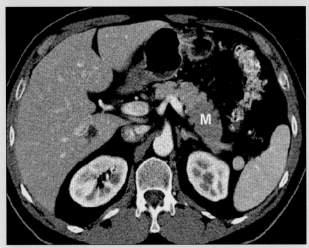

**Figure 3. Metastatic lung carcinomas to the pancreatic tail:
FDG-PET/CT findings.** Arterial-phase multidetector CT image
reveals an infiltrating mass (M) in the tail of the pancreas. Note
the liver lesion is PET negative, representing a hemangioma.

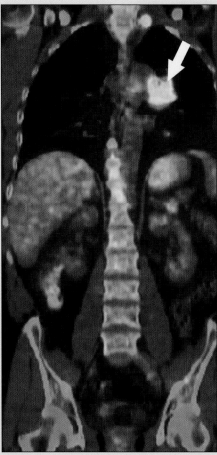

**Figure 2. Metastatic lung carcinomas to the pancreatic tail:
FDG-PET/CT findings.** Uptake by the patient's central lung mass
is increased *(arrow)*. *(FDG,* 18F-Fluorodeoxyglucose.)

Serous Cystadenoma of the Pancreas

DEFINITION: Tumor that contains glycogen-rich, periodic acid-Schiff (PAS)–positive epithelial cells, delimiting cysts.

ANATOMIC FINDINGS

Pancreas
- Classic type: solitary mass that displays central calcification and stellate arrangement of dense tissue, delimiting varying numbers of cysts
- Oligocystic: unilocular nonenhancing cystic mass in the pancreatic head with a lobulated contour

IMAGING

CT
Findings
- Cysts are near water density, and the surrounding fibrous network may appear dense.
- Tumors may encase vessels and obstruct the pancreatic or biliary duct systems, or both.

Utility
- Multidetector CT (MDCT) imaging features reflect the morphologic appearance of the mass.
- Presence of central calcification is best detected by MDCT.
- It establishes the diagnosis of serous cystadenoma (SCA) but is present in fewer than 30% of cases.

MRI and MR Cholangiopancreatography (MRCP)
Findings
- On T1-weighted fat-suppressed images, the fluid component is darker than the fibrous matrix.
- On T2-weighted acquisitions, the fluid component becomes more conspicuous, appearing bright as a result of a longer T2 relaxation time.
- Oligocystic type should be suspected in the setting of unilocular nonenhancing cystic mass in the pancreatic head with a lobulated contour.

Utility
- MRCP shows relationship of lesion to the pancreatic duct.

Ultrasound
Findings
- Honeycombed internal structure in lesions less than 2 cm

DIAGNOSTIC PEARLS
- Microcystic type produces a sponge-like lesion formed from innumerable cysts containing clear, watery fluid.
- Macrocystic type produces scant locules that are unilocular, with no central scar, and the cyst fluid may be clear but is often hemorrhagic.
- Tumor occurs more frequently in women than men, with a mean age of 57 years, most often occurring in the pancreatic head.

Utility
- Endoscopic ultrasound provides an excellent means to sample cyst fluid.
- This is the single best way to evaluate this lesion.

CLINICAL PRESENTATION
- May be incidentally found in asymptomatic patient
- Pain, weight loss, and jaundice
- Palpable midabdominal mass

DIFFERENTIAL DIAGNOSIS
- Serous cystadenocarcinoma
- Intraductal papillary mucinous neoplasm
- Pancreatic pseudocyst
- Cystic pancreatic adenocarcinoma
- Cystic islet cell tumor
- Cystic pancreatic metastasis

PATHOLOGY
- Benign lesion
- Glycogen-rich, PAS-positive epithelial cells, delimiting cysts separated by varying amounts of fibrous septations
- Two morphologic appearances: microcystic (or classic) type and oligocystic type

---

WHAT THE REFERRING PHYSICIAN NEEDS TO KNOW
- Notably, because of the recognition of the oligocystic type, the term *microcystic serous cystadenoma* is no longer used to describe these lesions.
- The imaging features of SCA reflect the morphologic appearance of the mass.
- Is associated with von Hippel-Lindau syndrome

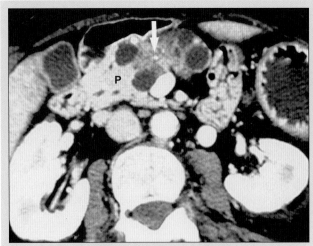

Figure 1. Serous cystadenoma: MDCT findings. MDCT in an 89-year-old woman reveals a mass in the pancreatic neck (P). Several larger, more cystic lobules are seen in the periphery, whereas the central portion displays soft-tissue attenuation secondary to the dense fibrous component. Multiple calcifications are seen within the center of the lesion *(arrow)*. These findings are characteristic of serous cystadenoma.

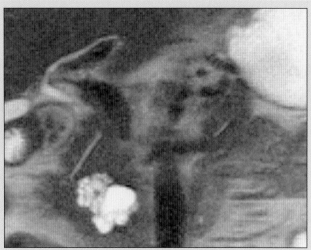

Figure 2. Serous cystadenoma: MRI. T2-weighted coronal MR image reveals a multiloculated hyperintense mass in the pancreatic head. The peripheral cysts are larger than the more central cysts. A low-signal central focus represents dense fibrous stroma. The mass is adjacent to the main pancreatic duct but does not communicate with it.

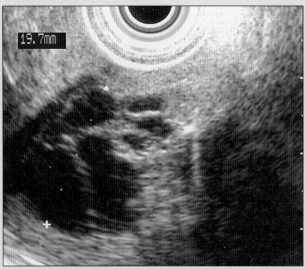

Figure 3. Serous cystadenoma. Endoscopic ultrasound in same patient as in Figure 2 reveals the complex multiseptated morphologic features delimiting cystic spaces of varying sizes. During this examination, serous fluid was obtained by direct transmural aspiration.

- Microcystic form (two thirds of SCAs): a sponge-like lesion formed from innumerable cysts containing clear, watery fluid
- Central fibrous stellate nidus, frequently calcifying, giving rise to radially oriented fibrous bands
- Macrocystic type: scant locules (or unilocular), no central scar, and cyst fluid clear but hemorrhagic

INCIDENCE/PREVALENCE AND EPIDEMIOLOGY

- SCAs account for approximately 1%-2% of all exocrine pancreatic neoplasms.
- From 25%-50% of patients will be symptomatic at the time of diagnosis.
- Tumor occurs more frequently in women than men, with a mean age of 57 years, most often occurring in the pancreatic head.

- SCAs occur sporadically; 60%-80% of patients with von Hippel-Lindau syndrome have pancreatic SCA.

Suggested Readings

Bassi C, Salvia R, Molinari E, et al: Management of 100 consecutive cases of pancreatic serous cystadenoma: Wait for symptoms and see at imaging or vice versa? *World J Surg* 27:319-323, 2003.

Brugge WR: Approach to cystic pancreatic lesions. *Gastrointest Endosc Clin North Am* 15:485-496, 2005.

Cohen-Scali F, Vilgrain V, Brancatelli G, et al: Discrimination of unilocular macrocystic serous cystadenoma from pancreatic pseudocyst and mucinous cystadenoma with CT: Initial observations. *Radiology* 228:727-733, 2003.

Procacci C, Graziani R, Bicego E, et al: Serous cystadenoma of the pancreas: Report of 30 cases with emphasis on the imaging findings. *J Comput Assist Tomogr* 21:373-382, 1997.

Pancreatic Trauma

DEFINITION: Trauma involving the pancreas.

ANATOMIC FINDINGS

Pancreas
- Pancreatic fractures traverse the gland, generally involving the neck of the pancreas perpendicular to its long axis.

IMAGING

CT
Findings
- Pancreatic laceration or fracture: thin linear lucency, well-demarcated lucent defects traversing the gland
- Focal (or diffuse) pancreatic enlargement: diminished or heterogeneous enhancement
- Pancreatic contusion or hematoma possibly isodense, hyperdense (caused by intraparenchymal hemorrhage), or hypodense (caused by edema)
- Fluid between the splenic vein and pancreas, peripancreatic fat, mesocolon, mesentery, anterior and posterior pararenal spaces or lesser sac
- Peripancreatic, mesenteric fat stranding, fluid collections, pseudocyst formation, abscess or fistula formation, left anterior pararenal fascia thickening
- Dilation or discontinuity of the pancreatic duct
- Injuries to adjacent structures, including the duodenum, liver, and spleen

Utility
- CT is the preferred means of evaluating patients with blunt abdominal trauma.
- Pancreatic lacerations, often subtle relative to liver, spleen, or kidney injuries, are difficult to visualize on imaging immediately after trauma.

DIAGNOSTIC PEARLS
- Pancreatic laceration or fracture: thin linear lucency and well-demarcated lucent defects traversing the gland
- Pancreatic contusion or hematoma: possibly isodense and hyperdense (caused by intraparenchymal hemorrhage) or hypodense (caused by edema)
- Fluid between the splenic vein and the pancreas, peripancreatic fat, mesocolon, mesentery, and anterior and posterior pararenal spaces or lesser sac
- Dilation or discontinuity of the pancreatic duct

- Radiologist must rely on secondary findings.
- Major limitation of CT in pancreatic injury is that it often cannot reliably assess the integrity of the pancreatic duct.
- Pancreas may appear relatively normal on initial examinations, showing abnormalities only on later examination.
- Dynamic scanning after bolus injection of contrast medium is important in fracture detection.
- Multidetector CT (MDCT) has greatly improved the ability to identify pancreatic injuries.

Ultrasound
Findings
- Sonographic findings may be relatively subtle, usually demonstrating nonspecific gland enlargement caused by pancreatitis or contusion.

WHAT THE REFERRING PHYSICIAN NEEDS TO KNOW
- Pancreas appears relatively normal on initial examinations, with injuries being apparent only on later examinations.
- Thin sections and repeat scanning in 12-24 hours can be helpful when a pancreatic fracture is suspected, despite negative initial CT scans.
- When the CT scan or MR pancreatography (MRP) study is equivocal or technically inadequate, emergent endoscopic retrograde cholangiopancreatography (ERCP) is useful in identifying pancreatic duct disruption.
- Pseudocysts may form within a few days after pancreatic duct laceration and on CT appear similar to pseudocysts from pancreatitis.
- MRP may also reveal ductal abnormalities such as pancreas divisum, which is important to know before ERCP evaluation.
- Ductal injury is the single most important factor in late morbidity and mortality.

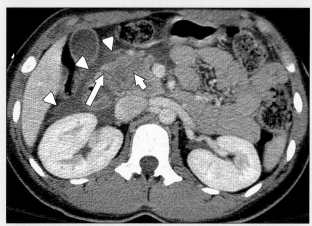

Figure 1. CT findings in pancreatic contusion. Axial MDCT scan of a 44-year-old woman involved in a motor-vehicle accident shows a contusion of the pancreatic head *(short arrow)* and a subtle laceration of the head of the pancreas *(long arrow)*. Note the presence of fluid outlining the duodenum and portion of the pancreatic head *(arrowheads)*.

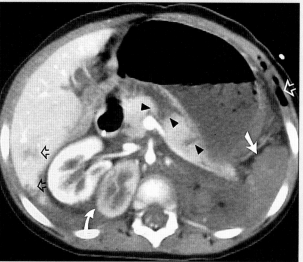

Figure 2. Pancreatic lacerations and multiorgan injury. A 16-month-old toddler was involved in a minivan accident. Contrast-enhanced CT demonstrates multiple pancreatic lacerations *(black arrowheads)*, devitalized spleen *(white arrow)*, vascular injury of an ectopic unfused kidney *(curved white arrow)*, right hepatic laceration *(open black arrows)*, and subcutaneous emphysema *(open arrow)* from a pneumothorax. Patient also had a spinal compression fracture. *(Courtesy of Andrew J. Fisher, MD, Mallinckrodt Institute of Radiology, St. Louis, MO.)*

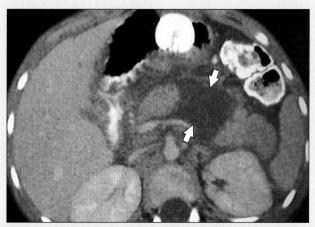

Figure 3. CT findings in pancreatic transection. CT scan of a pediatric patient, a victim of child abuse, shows a very large well-demarcated lucent defect representing a pancreatic fracture with transection of the pancreas *(arrows)*. *(Courtesy of Christine Menias, Mallinckrodt Institute of Radiology, St. Louis, MO.)*

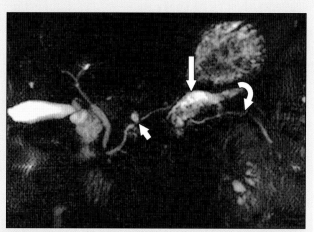

Figure 4. Pancreatic duct injury and subsequent pseudocyst formation. The initial CT scan showed no abnormality in the pancreas but the patient returned with severe abdominal pain. Thick slab (RARE) MR cholangiopancreatographic (MRCP) image shows the disrupted duct *(short arrow)* and the resulting peripancreatic fluid collection *(long arrow)*. Note how, with MRCP, it is feasible to evaluate the pancreatic duct distal to the site of injury and extravasation *(curved arrow)*. *(RARE, Rapid acquisition with relaxation enhancement.)*

Utility
- Although ultrasound is very sensitive in demonstrating intra-abdominal fluid (hemoperitoneum), it has very limited value for demonstrating pancreatic injuries.
- Ultrasound in pancreatic injury can miss an associated hemorrhage because of the retroperitoneal location of the pancreas.
- Actual pancreatic parenchymal injury may be difficult to visualize sonographically.
- In addition, many patients have an associated ileus, limiting sonographic evaluation of the pancreas.
- ERCP is the most sensitive means of diagnosing pancreatic duct injury.

Interventional Radiology
Findings
- Ductal transection appears as a duct obstruction or extravasation of contrast material from the pancreatic duct on endoscopic retrograde cholangiopancreatography (ERCP).
- Post-traumatic ductal stricture and pseudocyst communication may be seen.

Utility
- Ductal disruption can be missed on surgical exploration, leading some surgeons to advocate routine intraoperative or preoperative pancreatography.
- When a CT or MRI study is equivocal or technically inadequate, emergent ERCP is useful in identifying pancreatic duct disruption.
- Patients must be clinically stable for the examination.

MRI
Findings
- MR pancreatography (MRP) may identify fluid collections and the presence of any additional post-traumatic abnormalities upstream from the site of the duct disruption or transection.
- MRP may also reveal ductal abnormalities such as pancreas divisum.

Utility
- MRP has emerged as an attractive alternative for direct imaging of the pancreatic duct.
- Main advantages of MRP include its noninvasive nature, decreased cost, and wider availability; it is also faster than ERCP.
- More studies and clinical experience are needed to establish the exact role of MRP in acute pancreatic injury.

Radiography
Findings
- When coexisting duodenal injuries are suspected, water-soluble agents can disclose the duodenal perforation.
- Mass effect involving duodenum from acute pancreatitis and pseudocysts may be seen.

Utility
- Gastrointestinal study is not useful in specifically evaluating the pancreas.

CLINICAL PRESENTATION
- Clinical triad of upper abdominal pain, leukocytosis, and hyperamylasemia is diagnostic of pancreatic injury.
- *Seat-belt* sign indicates erythema, ecchymoses, and abrasions across abdominal wall from vehicle's seat-belt restraint.

DIFFERENTIAL DIAGNOSIS
- Pancreatic cleft
- Focal pancreatic fat
- Pancreatitis

PATHOLOGY
- Pancreatic injury occurs secondary to blunt-force or penetrating trauma, such as a gunshot or stab wound.
- Blunt-force trauma is caused by sudden localized force to the upper abdomen resulting from a direct blow from a fall, kick, or steering wheel.
- Forces compress the neck or body of the pancreas against the spine, causing a crushing injury or transection.
- Blows to the left of the midline may injure the pancreatic tail or distal body.
- Blows to the right of the midline may injure the pancreatic head or uncinate process along with the bile ducts.

INCIDENCE/PREVALENCE AND EPIDEMIOLOGY
- Pancreatic injuries are rare, found in 72 of 16,000 trauma patients (0.4%).
- Pancreas is involved in 2% of penetrating injuries and 5%-12% of blunt-force abdominal injuries.
- Three quarters of pancreatic injuries are caused by penetrating trauma by gunshot or stab wounds.

Suggested Readings

Cirillo RL Jr, Koniaris LG: Detecting blunt pancreatic injuries. *J Gastrointest Surg* 6:587-598, 2002.

Ilahi O, Bochicchio GV, Scalea TM: Efficacy of computed tomography in the diagnosis of pancreatic injury in adult blunt trauma patients: A single-institutional study. *Am Surg* 68:704-707, 2002.

Jobst MA, Canty TG, Lynch FP: Management of pancreatic injury in pediatric blunt abdominal trauma. *J Pediatr Surg* 34:818-823, 1999.

Jordan GL: Pancreatic trauma. In Howard JM, Jordan FL, Reber HA (eds): *Surgical Diseases of the Pancreas.* Philadelphia, Lea & Febiger, 1987, pp 3-10.

Jurkovich GJ, Carrico CJ: Pancreatic trauma. *Surg Clin North Am* 70:575-593, 1990.

Jurkovich GJ: The duodenum and pancreas. In Mattox KL, Feliciano DV, Moore EE (eds): *Trauma,* 4th ed. New York, McGraw-Hill, 2000, pp 735-762.

Wilson RH, Moorehead RJ: Current management of trauma to the pancreas. *Br J Surg* 78:1196-1202, 1991.

Pancreatic Graft Complications, Including Infection

DEFINITION: Post–pancreatic transplantation complications.

ANATOMIC FINDINGS

Pancreatic Graft
- Pseudocyst formation occurring in various sizes
- Pseudoaneurysm formation
- Edematous pancreatitis
- Fistula formation

Duodenum
- Leakage of the duodenal stump
- Small-bowel obstruction

IMAGING

CT
Findings
- Self-limited edematous pancreatitis is characterized by contrast enhancement and increasing size of the pancreatic graft in the early post-transplant period.
- Necrotizing pancreatitis is associated with contrast-enhanced pancreatic graft.
- Pseudocyst formation occurs in various sizes; contours and septations are seen inside or outside the pancreatic graft.
- Pseudoaneurysm is a small fluid collection with thin-walled contrast-enhanced membrane formation in the arteries.
- Fistula formation is seen with communication to the peritoneal cavity, retroperitoneum, gut, or skin.
- Leakage of a duodenojejunostomy or duodenal stump is seen, with ensuing abscess and peritonitis.

Utility
- Focal swelling of the donor's remaining mesenteric fat attached to the arterial stump should not be misdiagnosed as focal edematous pancreatitis.

Ultrasound
Findings
- Pseudocysts

DIAGNOSTIC PEARLS
- Self-limited edematous pancreatitis: edema and contrast enhancement in the early post-transplant period
- Necrotizing pancreatitis: contrast-enhanced pancreatic graft surrounded by fluid
- Pseudocyst formation occurring in various sizes; contours and septations inside or outside the pancreatic graft
- Pseudoaneurysm: artery surrounded by a small fluid collection with the thin-walled contrast-enhanced membrane
- Other complications: fistula, thrombosis, and abscess

Utility
- Imaging modality of choice for large pseudocysts

Radiography
Findings
- Fistula formation
Utility
- Is not a sensitive technique in diagnosing complication

CLINICAL PRESENTATION
- Signs of local infection
- Sepsis
- Pancreatic dysfunction
- Pain, weight loss

DIFFERENTIAL DIAGNOSIS
- Graft vascular thrombosis

WHAT THE REFERRING PHYSICIAN NEEDS TO KNOW
- Complications of pancreatic graft itself are important causes of morbidity in the early post-transplant period.

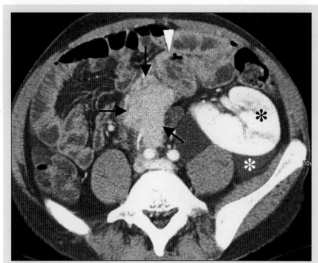

Figure 1. **A 40-year-old man after simultaneous pancreas-kidney transplantation (16 days after the operation) and graft pancreatitis.** Contrast-enhanced multidetector CT (MDCT) shows homogeneous contrast enhancement of pancreatic graft *(arrows)*.

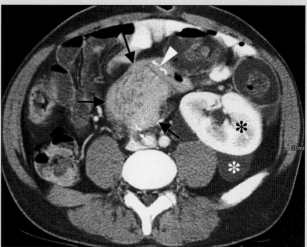

Figure 2. **A 40-year-old man after simultaneous pancreas-kidney transplantation (16 days after the operation) and graft pancreatitis.** Contrast-enhanced MDCT performed 5 days after the initial CT displays inhomogeneous contrast enhancement and increasing size of the pancreatic graft *(arrow)*, indicating edematous pancreatitis. Pancreatic graft *(arrow)*, donor's duodenum *(arrowhead)*, renal graft *(black asterisk)*, and perirenal fluid *(white asterisk)*.

PATHOLOGY

- Pancreatitis, pseudocyst formation, infection with abscess formation, and pseudoaneurysm formation
- Self-limited edematous pancreatitis occurring in the early post-transplant period caused by reperfusion injury and typically involving the entire graft
- Focal edematous swelling of the donor's remaining mesenteric fat, condition that results from the ligature of the donor's lymphatic vessels

INCIDENCE/PREVALENCE AND EPIDEMIOLOGY

- One-year patient survival rate of greater than 95%

Suggested Readings

Dachmann AH, Newmark GM, Thistlethwaite JR, et al: Imaging of pancreatic transplantation using portal venous and enteric exocrine drainage. *AJR Am J Roentgenol* 171:157-163, 1998.

Fernandez NP, Bernadino ME, Neylan JF, et al: Diagnosis of pancreatic transplant dysfunction: Value of gadopentate dimeglumine-enhanced MR imaging. *AJR Am J Roentgenol* 156:1171-1176, 1991.

Freund MC, Steurer W, Gassner EM, et al: Spectrum of imaging findings after pancreas transplantation with enteric exocrine drainage: Part 1, post transplantation anatomy. *AJR Am J Roentgenol* 182:911-917, 2004.

Meador TL, Krebs TL, Wong-You-Cheong JJ, et al: Imaging features of posttransplantation lymphoproliferative disorder in pancreas transplant recipients. *AJR Am J Roentgenol* 174:121-124, 2000.

Moulton JS, Munda R, Weiss MA, et al: Pancreatic transplants: CT with clinical and pathologic correlation. *Radiology* 172:21-26, 1989.

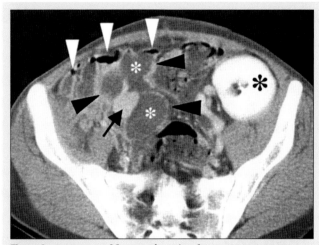

Figure 3. A 27-year-old man after simultaneous pancreas-kidney transplantation (4 weeks after the operation) with an infected peripancreatic pseudocyst requiring percutaneous drainage and a pancreatic-cutaneous fistula. Contrast-enhanced helical CT shows homogeneous contrast enhancement of the pancreatic graft *(arrow)* surrounded by a septated, peripancreatic fluid collection *(white asterisks)* combined with air-fluid level *(white arrowheads)* and a thin, contrast-enhanced wall *(black arrowheads)* consistent with an infected pseudocyst. Annotation: renal graft *(black asterisk)*.

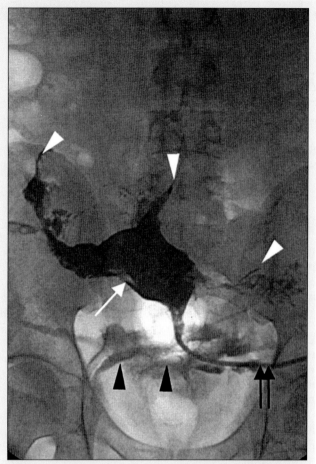

Figure 4. A 29-year-old man after simultaneous pancreas-kidney transplantation (3 weeks after the operation) with an infected peripancreatic pseudocyst and a complex pancreatic-cutaneous fistula. A drainage catheter *(arrows)* was placed through the cutaneous fistula opening, and a sinugram displays a large central cavity *(arrow)* with communication to the peritoneal cavity *(black arrowheads)* and sinus tracts *(white arrowheads)* in the retroperitoneal location.

Pancreatic Vascular Graft Complications, Including Rejection

DEFINITION: Venous and arterial graft thrombosis, resulting in pancreatic graft necrosis.

ANATOMIC FINDINGS

Systemic Vein
- Intraluminal filling defect in the vein graft

Systemic Artery
- Complete occlusion with nonenhancement of the parenchymal arterial graft

IMAGING

CT
Findings
- Intraluminal filling defect in larger graft veins
- Arterial thrombosis appearing as complete occlusion of the vessel with nonenhancement of parenchymal graft, indicating graft necrosis
- Emphysematous transformation of pancreatic graft

Utility
- Sensitivity: 80%-95%
- Specificity: 90%-100%
- Accuracy: 92%

Interventionasl Radiology
Findings
- Arterial thrombosis

Utility
- Angiogram
- Sensitivity: 85%-98%
- Specificity: 90%-100%
- Accuracy: 96%

CLINICAL PRESENTATION

- Signs of local infection
- Sepsis
- Pancreatic dysfunction
- Weight loss

DIFFERENTIAL DIAGNOSIS

- Graft infection

DIAGNOSTIC PEARLS

- Intraluminal filling defect in larger graft veins
- Arterial thrombosis appearing as complete occlusion of the vessel with nonenhancement of the parenchymal graft, indicating graft necrosis
- Emphysematous transformation of the pancreatic graft

PATHOLOGY

- Early graft loss caused by arterial occlusion relates to technical complications involving back-table preparation, particularly the vascular anastomosis in the recipient.
- Late graft loss is usually caused by arterial occlusion resulting from graft rejection secondary to autoimmune vasculitis.

INCIDENCE/PREVALENCE AND EPIDEMIOLOGY

- One-year patient survival rate of greater than 95%

Suggested Readings

Dachmann AH, Newmark GM, Thistlethwaite JR, et al: Imaging of pancreatic transplantation using portal venous and enteric exocrine drainage. *AJR Am J Roentgenol* 171:157-163, 1998.

Fernandez NP, Bernadino ME, Neylan JF, et al: Diagnosis of pancreatic transplant dysfunction: Value of gadopentate dimeglumine-enhanced MR imaging. *AJR Am J Roentgenol* 156:1171-1176, 1991.

Freund MC, Steurer W, Gassner EM, et al: Spectrum of imaging findings after pancreas transplantation with enteric exocrine drainage: Part 1: Post transplantation anatomy. *AJR Am J Roentgenol* 182:911-917, 2004.

Meador TL, Krebs TL, Wong-You-Cheong JJ, et al: Imaging features of posttransplantation lymphoproliferative disorder in pancreas transplant recipients. *AJR Am J Roentgenol* 174:121-124, 2000.

Moulton JS, Munda R, Weiss MA, et al: Pancreatic transplants: CT with clinical and pathologic correlation. *Radiology* 172:21-26, 1989.

WHAT THE REFERRING PHYSICIAN NEEDS TO KNOW

- Risk factors for early graft loss caused by arterial occlusion after pancreas transplantation relate to technical complications.
- Image-guided biopsy of pancreatic graft still represents the gold standard for the diagnosis of graft rejection.

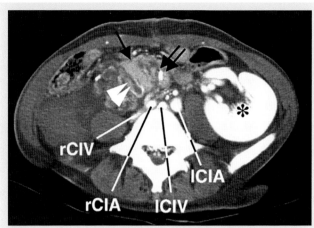

Figure 1. A 43-year-old woman 12 days after simultaneous pancreas-kidney transplantation who had abdominal discomfort. Contrast-enhanced multidetector CT (MDCT) displays acute thrombosis of the superior mesenteric vein *(arrowheads)* and splenic vein *(arrowhead in Fig. 2)* but homogeneous contrast enhancement of the pancreatic graft *(solitary black arrow)* with the donor's duodenum *(double arrows)* and the renal graft *(asterisk)*. Right (r), left (l), common iliac artery (CIA), common iliac vein (CIV).

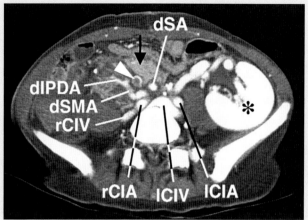

Figure 2. A 43-year-old woman with abdominal discomfort after simultaneous pancreas-kidney transplantation (12 days after the operation). Contrast-enhanced MDCT displays acute thrombosis of the superior mesenteric vein *(arrowheads in Fig. 1)* and splenic vein *(arrowhead)* but homogeneous contrast enhancement of the pancreatic graft *(solitary black arrow)* with the donor's duodenum *(double arrows in Fig. 1)* and the renal graft *(asterisk)*. Right (r), left (l), donor (d), common iliac artery (CIA), common iliac vein (CIV), splenic artery (SA), inferior pancreaticoduodenal artery (IPDA), superior mesenteric artery (SMA).

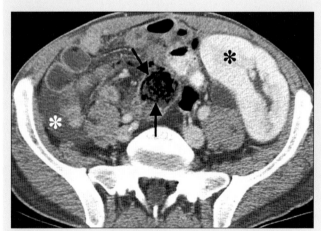

Figure 3. A 44-year-old man after simultaneous pancreas-kidney transplantation (9 months after the operation) with graft necrosis but without local infection or sepsis and subsequent graft extirpation. Contrast-enhanced MDCT shows absent parenchymal enhancement and emphysematous transformation of the pancreatic graft *(arrow)* consistent with innocuous gas collection. Renal graft *(black asterisk)* and ascites *(white asterisk)*.

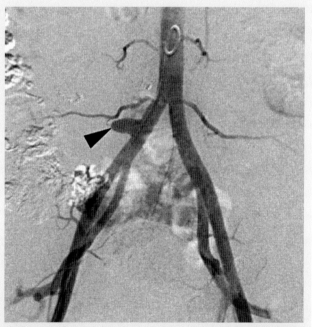

Figure 4. A 36-year-old woman after pancreas transplantation alone (8 months after the operation) with newly developed hyperglycemia, graft necrosis, and subsequent graft pancreatectomy. Angiogram verifies CT findings with residual enhancement of the donor's arterial conduit *(arrowhead)* but no visualization of graft arteries and absent parenchymal enhancement of pancreatic graft.

Spleen

Part 57

ANOMALIES AND ANATOMIC VARIANTS OF THE SPLEEN

Accessory Spleen

DEFINITION: Ectopic spleen of congenital origin.

IMAGING

CT
Findings
- Same density and enhancement as the normal spleen

Utility
- Splenules and accessory spleens are often found incidentally on CT.

Ultrasound
Findings
- Same tissue texture as the main spleen
- Parenchymal bridges between the main spleen and the accessory spleens

Utility
- Relationship of the accessory spleen to the splenic artery and vein can be established in 90% of cases.

MRI
Findings
- Same T1 and T2 characteristics as the normal spleen (ie, dark on T1- and bright on T2-weighted images)

Utility
- Splenules and accessory spleens are often found incidentally on MR.

CLINICAL PRESENTATION

- Symptoms may be produced by the compression of adjacent organs.
- Most patients are asymptomatic with an accessory spleen found incidentally during surgery, autopsy, or radiologic examination.
- Complications are rare but may cause acute symptoms, including spontaneous rupture, infarction, or torsion.
- Torsion of the accessory spleen may be intermittent, causing recurrent pain.

DIAGNOSTIC PEARLS

- Same texture and enhancement as the normal spleen
- Parenchymal bridges between the main spleen and the accessory spleens
- Size, shape, and location of the accessory spleen that do not change on sequential scintigrams

- Accessory spleen with long vascular pedicle can mimic acute appendicitis clinically.

DIFFERENTIAL DIAGNOSIS

- Splenosis
- Splenules surrounding the spleen

PATHOLOGY

- Accessory spleen probably results from the failure of the embryonic splenic buds to unite or extreme lobulation of the spleen.
- Morphologic appearance is identical to that of the normal spleen.
- Accessory spleen is usually supplied by a branch of the splenic artery and drains into the splenic veins.

INCIDENCE/PREVALENCE AND EPIDEMIOLOGY

- Incidence of accessory spleens in autopsy series ranges from 10%-30%.

WHAT THE REFERRING PHYSICIAN NEEDS TO KNOW

- If a therapeutic splenectomy is performed for thrombocytopenic purpura, hypertrophy of accessory spleens may cause recurrence of the disease.
- Splenic neoplasms may also involve the accessory tissue, especially recurrent lymphoma.
- After a splenectomy, the accessory tissue hypertrophies.
- Diagnostic studies are indicated if the tissue simulates a neoplasm or if a therapeutic splenectomy is planned in patients with hematologic disorders.

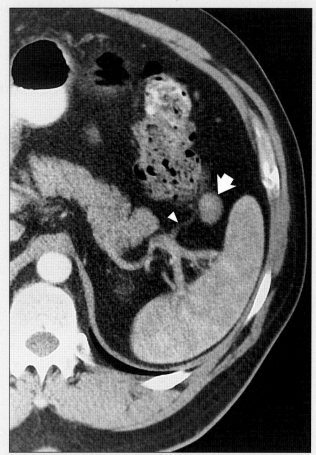

Figure 1. **Accessory spleen: CT findings.** An accessory spleen *(arrow)* is seen with a feeding vessel *(arrowhead)*.It has the same attenuation and enhancement as the main spleen.

Suggested Readings

Harris GN, Kase DJ, Bradnock H, et al: Accessory spleen causing a mass in the tail of the pancreas: MR imaging findings. *AJR Am J Roentgenol* 163:1120-1121, 1994.

Mortele KJ, Mortele B, Silverman SG: CT features of the accessory spleen. *AJR Am J Roentgenol* 183:1653-1657, 2004.

Olsen WR, Beaudoin DE: Increased incidence of accessory spleens in hematologic disease. *Arch Surg* 98:762-763, 1969.

Voet D, Arschrift M, Nachtegaele P, et al: Sonographic diagnosis of an accessory spleen in recurrent idiopathic thrombocytopenic purpura. *Pediatr Radiol* 13:39-41, 1983.

Asplenia

DEFINITION: Congenital absence of the spleen that is virtually always accompanied by a variety of congenital malformations, particularly cardiovascular.

IMAGING

Radiography
Findings
- Abdominal aorta and inferior vena cava are on same side (usually the right side) of the abdomen, a virtually pathognomonic finding.
- Plain radiographs may show situs solitus, situs ambiguus, or situs inversus.
- Right-sided bronchial pattern and minor fissure may be present bilaterally.
- Both pulmonary arteries project anterior to the trachea on lateral chest radiographs.
- Bilateral superior venae cavae may widen the superior mediastinum.
- Liver may be symmetric, with no distinct splenic contour visible.
- Bronchography shows a bilateral, epiarterial, right-sided pattern.

Utility
- Useful in showing anomalies that may accompany asplenia

Ultrasound
Findings
- Locates the inferior vena cava and inferior vena cava–right atrial communications
- Spleen is absent.
- Abdominal aorta and inferior vena cava are located on same side.

Utility
- Sonography is particularly useful in the acutely ill infant.
- Sonography is also useful in demonstrating abnormalities of the situs by the location of the heart, liver, gallbladder, or bowel.
- Diagnosis of asplenia may be missed sonographically in some patients because the left lobe of the liver can simulate the spleen.
- Ultrasound should not be the sole modality used to establish or exclude the diagnosis of asplenia.

CT
Findings
- Aorta and inferior vena cava are seen on the same side of the spine.
- Spleen is absent.

Utility
- Vascular anatomy is well seen on CT with intravenous contrast enhancement.
- CT is useful in demonstrating abnormalities of the situs by the location of the heart, liver, gallbladder, or bowel.

Nuclear Medicine
Findings
- Absence of spleen and hepatic symmetry or prominent left lobe

Utility
- Asplenia can be diagnosed with technetium 99m (99mTc)-sulfur colloid, iminodiacetic acid agents, and tagged red blood cell scans.
- Asplenia may be difficult to prove on 99mTc-sulfur colloid scans when the large, left lobe of liver is present.
- 99mTc-labeled, heat-damaged, red blood cell scan may be needed because it is more sensitive for detection of the spleen.

CLINICAL PRESENTATION

- Majority of patients have cardiopulmonary disease.
- Others have intestinal obstruction.
- Some patients may be asymptomatic.

DIFFERENTIAL DIAGNOSIS

- Prominent left lobe of the liver

PATHOLOGY

- Absence of the spleen with accompanying cardiac, pulmonary, and genital abdominal visceral malformations is noted.

WHAT THE REFERRING PHYSICIAN NEEDS TO KNOW

- Ultrasound should not be the sole modality used to establish or exclude the diagnosis of asplenia.

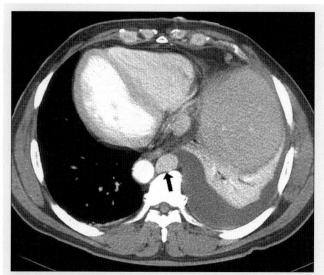

Figure 1. Situs ambiguus with asplenia. Transverse, contrast-enhanced CT scan of the lower chest of a 48-year-old man shows dextrocardia and azygous continuation of the inferior vena cava. The aorta is located to the right of the enlarged azygous vein *(arrow)*. The scan also shows left lower lobe collapse and a left pleural effusion. (*From Fulcher AS, Turner MA: Abdominal manifestations of situs anomalies in adults. RadioGraphics 22:1439-1456, 2002.*)

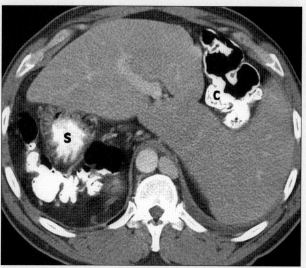

Figure 2. Situs ambiguus with asplenia. CT scan obtained 15 mm caudad to Figure 1 shows the stomach (S) and colon (C) in the expected location of the spleen. The hypoplasia of the anterior segment of the right hepatic lobe allows cephalic migration of the colon. (*From Fulcher AS, Turner MA: Abdominal manifestations of situs anomalies in adults. RadioGraphics 22:1439-1456, 2002.*)

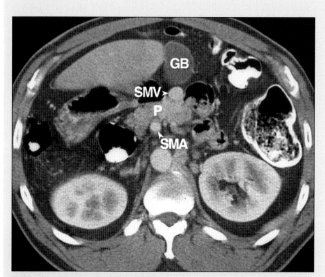

Figure 3. Situs ambiguus with asplenia. On another CT scan obtained caudad to Figure 2, the gallbladder (GB) lies in the midline. The superior mesenteric vein (SMV) lies anterior to the truncated pancreas (P), whereas the superior mesenteric artery (SMA) lies posterior to it. (*From Fulcher AS, Turner MA: Abdominal manifestations of situs anomalies in adults. RadioGraphics 22:1439-1456, 2002.*)

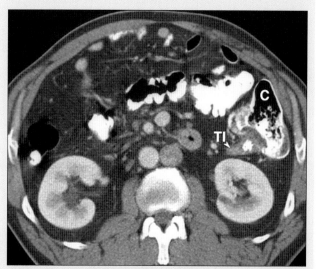

Figure 4. Situs ambiguus with asplenia. CT scan obtained at the level of the right renal hilum reveals that the cecum (C) is located in the left lower quadrant. Notice the terminal ileum (TI) entering the colon. (*From Fulcher AS, Turner MA: Abdominal manifestations of situs anomalies in adults. RadioGraphics 22:1439-1456, 2002.*)

- Delayed curvature of embryonic body has been postulated to explain asplenia and visceroatrial situs abnormalities.
- Pressure of adjacent structures may interfere with the splenic blood supply.
- Cardiac abnormalities are present in approximately 50% of patients with asplenia.
- Pulmonary anomalies include abnormal distribution of the lobes.
- Gastrointestinal abnormalities include situs inversus (total or partial) and symmetric liver.
- Genitourinary anomalies are seen in approximately 15% of cases, which include horseshoe kidney, double collecting system, bilobed urinary bladder, and hydroureter.

INCIDENCE/PREVALENCE AND EPIDEMIOLOGY

- Incidence of asplenia syndrome is 1 case per 40,000 live births.
- It occurs predominantly in boys.

Suggested Readings

Biggar WD, Ramirez RA, Rose V: Congenital asplenia: Immunologic assessment and a clinical review of eight surviving patients. *Pediatrics* 67:548-551, 1981.

Hutchins GM, Morre GW, Lipford EH, et al: Asplenia and polysplenia malformation complexes explained by abnormal embryonic body curvature. *Pathol Res Pract* 177:60-76, 1983.

Ivemark BI: Implications of agenesis of the spleen on the pathogenesis of cono-truncus anomalies in childhood. An analysis of the heart malformations in the splenic agenesis syndrome with fourteen new cases. *Acta Paediatr* 44:1-110, 1955.

Polysplenia

DEFINITION: Polysplenia syndrome is a multisystem congenital abnormality characterized by multiple, small splenic masses and features of bilateral left-sidedness.

ANATOMIC FINDINGS

Thorax
- Absence of the inferior vena cava between the renal and hepatic veins
- Independent drainage of the hepatic veins into the right atrium
- Prominent azygos or hemiazygos vein
- Bilateral morphologic left lung

Abdomen
- Multiple spleens (2-16)
- Abdominal heterotaxy, usually with asymmetric liver and midgut malrotation of various degrees

IMAGING

Radiography
Findings
- Absence of the inferior vena cava and paratracheal soft-tissue prominence is noted on the lateral view.
- Venous prominence caused by interruption of inferior vena cava mimics a mediastinal mass.
- Bilateral epiarterial bronchi project posterior to the trachea on the lateral view.

Utility
- Plain radiographs are useful in showing the heterotaxy.

CT
Findings
- Absent inferior vena cava between the renal and hepatic veins
- Independent drainage of the hepatic veins into the right atrium and a prominent azygos or hemiazygos vein
- Intrahepatic vena cava or crossing of the vena cava in front of the aorta to enter the common atrium on the right
- Termination of the vena cava at the confluence of the hepatic veins, with the hepatic veins entering the atrium independently
- Size, position, and number of spleens and their relationship to the liver and bowel

Utility
- Is useful in depicting the constellation of abnormalities but does use ionizing radiation

DIAGNOSTIC PEARLS

- Multiple, small splenic masses and features of bilateral left-sidedness
- Bilateral morphologic left lung
- Abdominal situs ambiguus
- Intrahepatic interruption of the inferior vena cava

Ultrasound
Findings
- Absent inferior vena cava between the renal and hepatic veins
- Independent drainage of the hepatic veins into the right atrium and a prominent azygos or hemiazygos vein
- Intrahepatic vena cava or crossing of the vena cava in front of the aorta to enter the common atrium on the right
- Termination of the vena cava at the confluence of the hepatic veins, with the hepatic veins entering the atrium independently
- Size, position, and number of spleens and their relationship to the liver and bowel

Utility
- Is usually the test first performed in infants with suspected polysplenia

Nuclear Medicine
Findings
- Liver-spleen sulfur colloid scintigraphy may show multiple spleens.

Utility
- False-negative examinations may occur, or resolution may be insufficient to show the individual splenuli.

MRI
Findings
- Size, position, and number of the spleens and their relationship to the liver and bowel

Utility
- Is useful in showing the multiple anomalies and does not use ionizing radiation

CLINICAL PRESENTATION

- Clinical presentation is usually related to associated cardiac disease.

WHAT THE REFERRING PHYSICIAN NEEDS TO KNOW

- Unlike the treatment for asplenia, prophylactic antibiotics are not needed in polysplenia.
- MRI, ultrasound, and CT are the best noninvasive studies for showing multiple features of polysplenia syndrome.

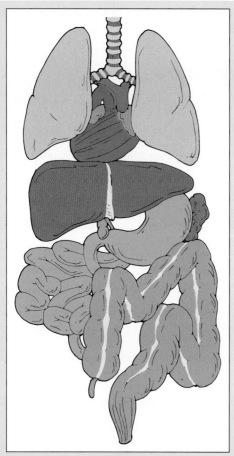

Figure 1. Polysplenia: associated anomalies. Diagram shows the organ position in situs ambiguus with asplenia. (*From Fulcher AS, Turner MA: Abdominal manifestations of situs anomalies in adults. RadioGraphics 22:1439-1456, 2002.*)

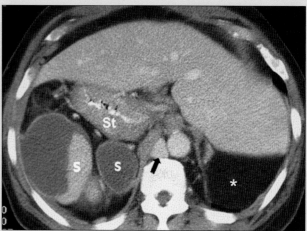

Figure 2. Situs ambiguus with polysplenia in a 67-year-old man. Transverse, contrast-enhanced CT scan of the abdomen shows a midline liver, multiple spleens (S) in the right upper quadrant adjacent to the collapsed stomach (St), and inferior vena cava interruption with azygous continuation (*arrow*). The low attenuation of the spleens is related to infarctions, which cause liquefaction and subcapsular hematomas. Notice the absence of splenic tissue in the left upper quadrant (*asterisk*). (*From Fulcher AS, Turner MA: Abdominal manifestations of situs anomalies in adults. RadioGraphics 22:1439-1456, 2002.*)

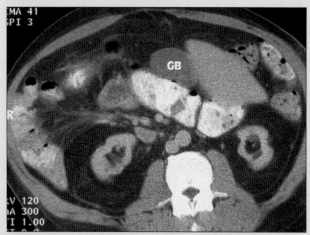

Figure 3. Situs ambiguus with polysplenia in a 67-year-old man. Transverse CT scan through the mid-abdomen reveals a midline gallbladder (GB). (*From Fulcher AS, Turner MA: Abdominal manifestations of situs anomalies in adults. RadioGraphics 22:1439-1456, 2002.*)

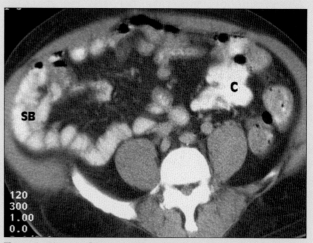

Figure 4. Situs ambiguus with polysplenia in a 67-year-old man. Transverse CT scan through the lower abdomen reveals the small bowel (SB) in the right lower quadrant and the colon in the left lower quadrant. The cecum (C) lies near the midline, a finding that indicates incomplete fixation. (*From Fulcher AS, Turner MA: Abdominal manifestations of situs anomalies in adults. RadioGraphics 22:1439-1456, 2002.*)

- Bowel malrotation may cause obstruction and pain because of infarction.
- Only 25% of patients live to 5 years, and only 10% survive to middle adolescence.

PATHOLOGY

- Polysplenia is a multisystem congenital abnormality characterized by multiple, small splenic masses and features of bilateral left-sidedness.
- Accelerated curvature of the embryonic body is postulated to be a cause of polysplenia.
- Associated abnormalities are bilateral left lung, inferior vena cava course variations, cardiac septal defects, and abdominal situs ambiguus.

INCIDENCE/PREVALENCE AND EPIDEMIOLOGY

- Female predilection

Suggested Readings

Hatayama C, Wells TR: Syndrome of externally bilobed lungs with normal bronchial pattern, congenital heart disease, multiple spleens, intestinal malrotation and short pancreas, an apparently hitherto undefined malrotation complex. *Pediatr Pathol* 2:127-133, 1984.

Paddock RJ, Arensman RM: Polysplenia syndrome: Spectrum of gastrointestinal congenital anomalies. *J Pediatr Surg* 17:563-566, 1982.

Polga JP, Spencer RP: Interesting images: Hepatobiliary imaging as an aid in determining situs in a case of polysplenia. *Clin Nucl Med* 9:159-160, 1984.

Vossen PG, Van Hedent EF, Degryse HR, et al: Computed tomography of the polysplenia syndrome in the adult. *Gastrointest Radiol* 2:209-211, 1987.

Winer-Muram HT, Tonkin IL, Gold RE: Polysplenia syndrome in the asymptomatic adult: Computed tomography evaluation. *J Thorac Imaging* 6:69-71, 1991.

Wandering Spleen: Splenic Torsion

DEFINITION: Ligamentous laxity may result in splenic hypermobility, a condition known as wandering spleen.

ANATOMIC FINDINGS

Wandering Spleen
- A mobile mass in the left or central abdomen, which may be confused with a renal or bowel mass

Colon
- Splenic flexure, often medial and anterior to its usual location, which may be an indication of early ligamentous laxity

Splenic Artery
- Demonstrated absence of blood flow in the spleen and a high resistive index in the splenic artery caused by torsion of a wandering spleen

Portion of or the Entire Spleen
- If torsion leads to infarction, a portion of the spleen or the entire organ may become hypodense.

IMAGING

Radiography
Findings
- Supine and erect positions depict the spleen as mobile mass in the left or central abdomen.
- Normal splenic contour in left upper quadrant is absent, which is filled by bowel loops.
- Torsion of the spleen may appear as a notched mass, with the notch pointing medially and upward.
- Left kidney may be elevated and lack the usual splenic impression or hump.
- Mass is seen anterior to the kidney, which may cause extrinsic compression on the colon.
- Splenic flexure is often medial and anterior to its usual location, which may be an indication of early ligamentous laxity.
- Elongated pedicle of the spleen may cause a linear defect across the bowel in the region of the splenic flexure.

Utility
- Is not used to establish the diagnosis

DIAGNOSTIC PEARLS
- Change in splenic location or apparent changes in shape because of mobility or torsion, as detected by cross-sectional imaging or scintigraphy
- Aberrant location, with the demonstration of the origin of the splenic vasculature in the left upper quadrant
- Abnormal location of spleen, which may migrate on sequential studies

Ultrasound
Findings
- Absence of the spleen in its usual location is noted, and an echogenic mass (the spleen) is found in the left mid-abdomen or flank.
- Splenic infarction with necrosis may cause the spleen to appear less echogenic than normal.
- Superimposed infection in the infarcted spleen with torsion appears as a thick-walled, complex mass.

Utility
- Useful only if spleen visualized

Ultrasound Color Doppler
Findings
- Demonstrates blood flow or absence of blood flow, in the case of torsion

Utility
- Useful only if spleen visualized

CT
Findings
- Change is seen in the splenic location or apparent changes in the shape because of mobility or torsion.
- Torsion may produce a whirled appearance of the splenic pedicle.
- If torsion leads to infarction, a portion of the spleen or the entire organ may become hypodense.
- With intermittent or chronic torsion, a thick, enhancing pseudocapsule develops, presumably representing omental and peritoneal adhesions.

WHAT THE REFERRING PHYSICIAN NEEDS TO KNOW
- When wandering spleen is suspected, sulfur colloid scintiscan or sonogram is the study of choice.
- If no uptake at all is noted, ultrasound and CT can identify the spleen.
- With recognition of postsplenectomy sepsis, splenopexy is now advocated for all cases.
- Splenectomy should be performed only if the splenic torsion has led to splenic infarction.

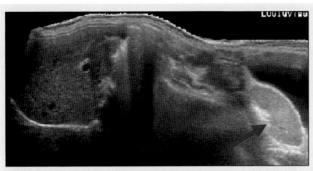

Figure 1. Wandering spleen: sonographic features. Sagittal sonogram shows the spleen *(arrow)* lying superiorly to the bladder. (*Courtesy of Edward Lyons, MD, Winnipeg, Manitoba, Canada.*)

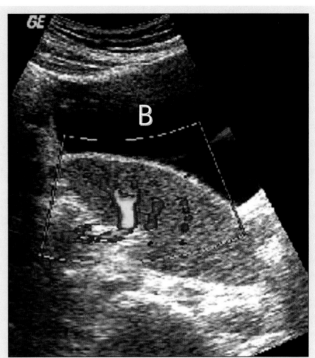

Figure 2. Wandering spleen: sonographic features. Color Doppler image shows blood flow in the splenic hilus. (*Courtesy of Edward Lyons, MD, Winnipeg, Manitoba, Canada.*)

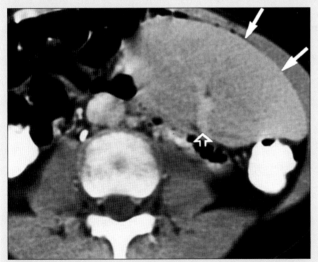

Figure 3. Wandering spleen: CT findings. Contrast-enhanced CT reveals an abdominal mass *(solid arrows)* with vessels entering posteromedially *(open arrow)*. (*From Paterson A, Frush DP, Donnelly LF, et al: A pattern-oriented approach to splenic imaging in infants and children.* RadioGraphics *19:1465-1485, 1999.*)

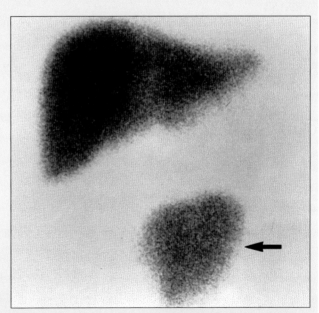

Figure 4. Wandering spleen: scintigraphic findings. Anterior 99mTc-sulfur colloid scintigram shows the mass to be an abnormally located spleen *(arrow)*. The liver also demonstrates radiotracer uptake *(top)* (see Fig. 3). (*From Paterson A, Frush DP, Donnelly LF, et al: A pattern-oriented approach to splenic imaging in infants and children.* RadioGraphics *19:1465-1485, 1999.*)

- Secondary findings, such as ascites or necrosis of the pancreatic tail, may be present.

Utility
- CT is particularly useful if bowel gas obscures the spleen on sonograms.
- Is the best means of quickly establishing the diagnosis.

Nuclear Medicine
Findings
- Abnormal location of the spleen is noted, which may migrate on sequential studies.
- Absence of uptake in the previously demonstrated wandering spleen indicates torsion.

Utility
- Technetium-99m (99mTc)-sulfur colloid scintigraphy is a time-honored method for diagnosing a wandering spleen.
- Decubitus view may be added to show splenic motion.
- Diminished uptake on nuclear scan suggests torsion.

CT Angiography
Utility
- CT shows the exact site of the torsion, defines the abdominal vasculature preoperatively, and may demonstrate gastric varices in chronic torsion.
- Angiography should be reserved for cases in which the diagnosis is uncertain.

MRI
Findings
- Aberrant location, with the demonstration of the origin of the splenic vasculature in the left upper quadrant

Utility
- Scans of the entire abdomen and pelvis are necessary to locate the spleen.

CLINICAL PRESENTATION

- Patient may be asymptomatic.
- Firm, notched mass is found on physical examination or radiography.
- Mild discomfort is noted from splenic congestion.
- Location of symptoms in part related to location of spleen.

- Initial clinical impression in torsion of the wandering spleen is often a twisted ovarian cyst, appendicitis, or cholecystitis.
- Chronic torsion with venous congestion causes fundal gastric varices, further causing acute gastrointestinal hemorrhage.

DIFFERENTIAL DIAGNOSIS

- Adenopathy
- Lymphoma
- Extramedullary hematopoeisis

PATHOLOGY

- Ligamentous laxity may result in splenic hypermobility, but the cause is controversial.
- Most investigators favor a congenital origin related to factors such as abnormal fusion of posterior mesogastrium.
- Splenic torsion has also been called ectopic spleen, aberrant spleen, splenic ptosis, and floating spleen.

INCIDENCE/PREVALENCE AND EPIDEMIOLOGY

- This entity is rare; the incidence is estimated at less than 0.2%.
- Incidence of wandering spleen is higher among multiparous women.
- Most cases are diagnosed in adults, usually multiparous women, between 20 and 40 years of age.

Suggested Readings
Allen KB, Gay BB, Skandalakis JF: Wandering spleen: Anatomic and radiologic considerations. *South Med J* 85:976-984, 1992.

Ben Ely A, Zissin R, Copel L, et al: The wandering spleen: CT findings and possible pitfalls in diagnosis. *Clin Radiol* 61:954-958, 2006.

Sheflin JR, Chung ML, Kretchmar KA: Torsion of the wandering spleen and distal pancreas. *AJR Am J Roentgenol* 142:100-101, 1984.

Vermylen C, Lebecque P, Claus D, et al: The wandering spleen. *Eur J Pediatr* 140:112-115, 1983.

Part 58

BENIGN AND MALIGNANT LESIONS OF THE SPLEEN

Acquired Immunodeficiency Syndrome–Related Lymphoma

DEFINITION: Lymphomas related to AIDS include Hodgkin disease and non-Hodgkin lymphoma (NHL).

IMAGING

Radiography
Findings
- Elevation of the left hemidiaphragm
- Deviation of the stomach and splenic flexure of the colon
- Displacement of the left kidney

Utility
- Noncontributory in establishing the diagnosis

Ultrasound
Findings
- Splenomegaly with normal echotexture
- Enlarged spleen containing multiple, ill-defined, hypoechoic lesions
- Anechoic cystic masses, with or without septations
- Focal masses: more common in AIDS-related lymphoma than in sporadically occurring lymphoma

Utility
- Poor sensitivity in detecting diffuse involvement

CT
Findings
- Splenomegaly with hypodense lesions
- Hypodense mass with capsular invasion
- Rim-enhancing lesions with central necrosis
- Splenic calcifications
- Focal masses: more common in AIDS-related lymphoma than in sporadically occurring lymphoma

Utility
- CT is the established radiologic technique for staging lymphomas.

DIAGNOSTIC PEARLS
- Enlarged spleen containing multiple, ill-defined, and hypoechoic lesions
- Splenomegaly with hypodense lesions
- Increased uptake of radiopharmaceutical in the affected tissue

MRI
Findings
- Splenomegaly with irregularly enhancing regions of high and low signal intensity
- Focal, hypointense lesions relative to the surrounding spleen
- Low-signal intensity splenic masses
- Focal masses: more common in AIDS-related lymphoma than in sporadically occurring lymphoma

Utility
- MRI with contrast agents such as ferumoxide is sensitive in the depiction of hepatosplenic lymphoma.

PET
Findings
- Increased uptake of ^{18}F-fluorodeoxyglucose (FDG) in the affected tissue

Utility
- FDG-PET has a higher sensitivity and specificity than CT and other imaging modalities.

WHAT THE REFERRING PHYSICIAN NEEDS TO KNOW
- Definitive diagnosis of malignant lymphoma requires histopathologic analysis.
- Accurate diagnosis of NHL subtypes usually requires evaluation of tissue's architecture through a core-needle biopsy and, often, an excisional biopsy.
- Accurate staging is essential for patients with lymphoma in guiding management and optimizing outcomes.
- Splenic size correlates with the risk of lymphomatous involvement.
- Splenectomy may still be beneficial for patients with primary splenic lymphoma to provide diagnosis and partial treatment.

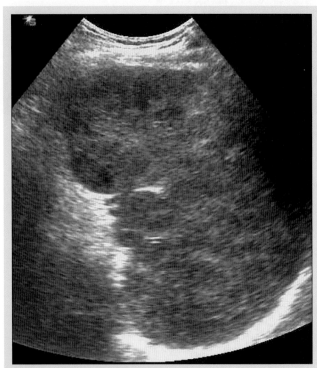

Figure 1. Hodgkin lymphoma in a 42-year-old man. The sagittal sonogram reveals an enlarged spleen containing multiple, ill-defined, hypoechoic lesions.

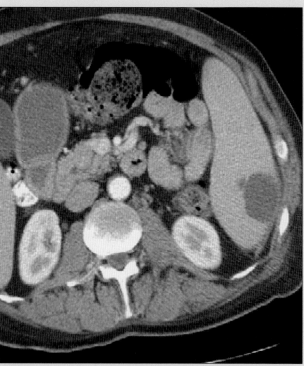

Figure 2. Malignant B-cell lymphoma in a 46-year-old man with subacute abdominal pain in the left upper abdomen. The enhanced helical CT scan during the portal venous phase shows a hypodense peripheral lesion and splenomegaly. Similar lesions were demonstrated in the liver (not shown).

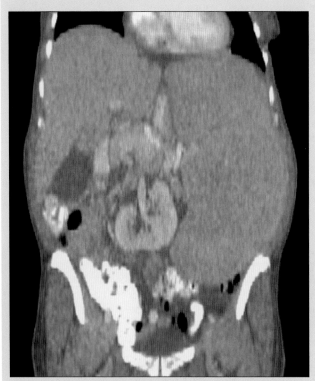

Figure 3. Mantle-cell lymphoma in a 70-year-old woman. Coronal, multiplanar reformatted reconstruction CT scan during the late venous phase demonstrates massive splenomegaly displacing the surrounding organs. The spleen has an inhomogeneous, miliary appearance.

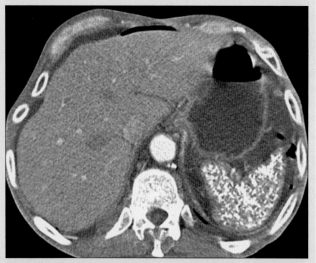

Figure 4. Punctate calcifications throughout the spleen 5 years after successful treatment of NHL. Calcified lymph nodes (not shown) were also demonstrated in other locations. (*Courtesy of M. de Jonge, MD, Amsterdam, Netherlands*).

CLINICAL PRESENTATION

- Splenomegaly and lymphadenopathy
- Left upper quadrant pain
- Highly aggressive behavior

DIFFERENTIAL DIAGNOSIS

- Hepatic infections
- Hepatic abscess
- Hepatic neoplasm
- Kaposi sarcoma (stomach and duodenum)
- Splenic infections
- Splenic abscess
- Splenic neoplasm

PATHOLOGY

- AIDS-related lymphomas are typically aggressive B-cell NHLs.
- Lymphomatous involvement of the spleen is usually confined within the splenic capsule, but extracapsular extension can occur.

INCIDENCE/PREVALENCE AND EPIDEMIOLOGY

- Risk of lymphoma is increased in immunocompromised patients.
- Lymphoma is most common malignancy involving the spleen.

Suggested Readings

Fishman EK, Kuhlman JE, Jones RJ: CT of lymphoma: Spectrum of disease. *RadioGraphics* 11:647-669, 1991.

Guppy AE, Tebbutt NC, Norman A, Cunningham D: The role of surveillance CT scans in patients with diffuse large B-cell non-Hodgkin's lymphoma. *Leuk Lymphoma* 44:123-125, 2003.

Hicks RJ, Mac Manus MP, Seymour JF: Initial staging of lymphoma with positron emission tomography and computed tomography. *Semin Nucl Med* 35:165-175, 2005.

Rini JN, Leonidas JC, Tomas MB, Palestro CJ: ^{18}F-FDG PET versus CT for evaluating the spleen during initial staging of lymphoma. *J Nucl Med* 44:1072-1074, 2003.

Vinnicombe SJ, Reznek RH: Computerised tomography in the staging of Hodgkin's disease and non-Hodgkin's lymphoma. *Eur J Nucl Med Mol Imaging* 30(Suppl 1):S42-S55, 2003.

Leukemia and Other Myeloproliferative Disorders

DEFINITION: Leukemia and other myeloproliferative disorders affect mainly the red pulp, although the white pulp may eventually be infiltrated. They are autonomous clonal disorders initiated by pluripotential hematopoietic stem cells.

IMAGING

Ultrasound
Findings
- Splenomegaly
- Focal lesions that are often hyperechoic

Utility
- Ultrasound is primarily used in children with known or suspected leukemia.

CT
Findings
- Splenomegaly
- Multiple hypoechoic areas of subcapsular and pericapsular dense fluid, and free fluid around the liver
- Extramedullary hematopoiesis

Utility
- CT is less sensitive than MRI in showing splenic involvement.

MRI
Findings
- Splenomegaly
- Multiple masses
- Extramedullary hematopoiesis

Utility
- Most sensitive noninvasive means of detecting focal splenic involvement

CLINICAL PRESENTATION

- Splenomegaly
- Anemia, reticulocytosis, low platelet count

DIFFERENTIAL DIAGNOSIS

- Lymphoma
- Brucellosis and other infections

DIAGNOSTIC PEARLS

- Focal lesions that are often hyperechoic
- Splenomegaly and multiple hypoechoic areas
- Free fluid around the liver

PATHOLOGY

- Myeloproliferative and leukemic disorders affect mainly the red pulp, although the white pulp may eventually be infiltrated.
- Splenic rupture is an uncommon manifestation of leukemic disorders caused by the infiltration of the splenic capsule and trabecular framework or infarction.

INCIDENCE/PREVALENCE AND EPIDEMIOLOGY

- Spleen is often involved in myeloproliferative disorders and in acute and chronic leukemias.

Suggested Readings

Anttila VJ, Lamminen AE, Bondestam S, et al: Magnetic resonance imaging is superior to computed tomography and ultrasonography in imaging infectious liver foci in acute leukaemia. *Eur J Haematol* 56:82-87, 1996.

Chen CY, Chen YC, Tang JL, et al: Hepatosplenic fungal infection in patients with acute leukemia in Taiwan: Incidence, treatment, and prognosis. *Ann Hematol* 82:93-97, 2003.

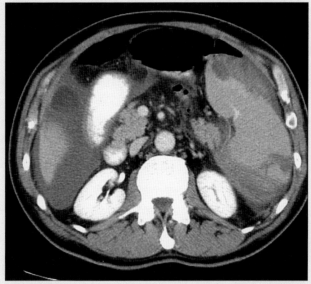

Figure 1. Spontaneous splenic rupture. A 69-year-old man had acute lymphoblastic leukemia. The enhanced helical CT scan demonstrates splenomegaly and multiple hypoechoic areas, subcapsular and pericapsular dense fluid, and free fluid around the liver. Laparotomy and splenectomy revealed a ruptured subcapsular hematoma and diffuse leukemic involvement of the spleen.

Lymphangioma

DEFINITION: Splenic lymphangiomas are typically subcapsular, multicystic lesions filled with watery pink proteinaceous fluid.

IMAGING

Radiography
Findings
- Splenomegaly with mass effect on adjacent viscera
- Curvilinear calcifications

Utility
- Plain radiographs are usually normal.

Ultrasound with Color Doppler
Findings
- Multiple cysts from a few millimeters to several centimeters in diameter and divided by thin septations
- Possibly calcifications
- Internal echoes, depending on the presence of proteinaceous or hemorrhagic fluid
- Vascularity within the walls and septa

Utility
- Ultrasound is more accurate than CT in establishing the cystic nature of these lesions.

CT
Findings
- Subcapsular, low-density, nonenhancing, sharply marginated, thin-walled cysts
- Small, curvilinear or punctate calcifications
- Septal postcontrast enhancement

Utility
- After the administration of intravenous contrast, the septa may demonstrate enhancement.

MRI
Findings
- Multiple, well-defined cysts, hypointense on T1- and hyperintense on T2-weighted images
- Presence of proteinaceous or hemorrhagic fluid, resulting in T1 hyperintensity

Utility
- MRI is the most sensitive means of establishing the diagnosis

DIAGNOSTIC PEARLS

- Multiple cysts from a few millimeters to several centimeters in diameter and divided by thin septations
- Subcapsular, low-density, nonenhancing, sharply marginated, thin-walled cysts
- *Swiss-cheese* appearance in the venous phase of the angiogram

CLINICAL PRESENTATION

- Patients are often asymptomatic.
- Symptoms include left upper quadrant pain, nausea, and abdominal distention.

DIFFERENTIAL DIAGNOSIS

- Klippel-Trenaunay-Weber syndrome

PATHOLOGY

- Lesions are typically subcapsular, multicystic, and filled with watery pink proteinaceous fluid.
- They are composed of multiple, thin-walled cysts of various sizes lined with flat endothelium.
- Lymphangiomas can be isolated solitary lesions within the spleen, or the entire spleen may be replaced.

INCIDENCE/PREVALENCE AND EPIDEMIOLOGY

- Splenic lymphangiomas are rare, benign, slow-growing, congenital neoplasms.

WHAT THE REFERRING PHYSICIAN NEEDS TO KNOW

- Management varies from conservative treatment for small, asymptomatic lesions to partial or total splenectomy for large, symptomatic lesions.
- When the lymphatic spaces are small, lesions have a solid appearance on radiologic imaging techniques, making the correct preoperative radiologic diagnosis difficult.
- Splenic lymphangioma may be part of rare congenital malformation of lymphatics called *lymphangiomatosis.*

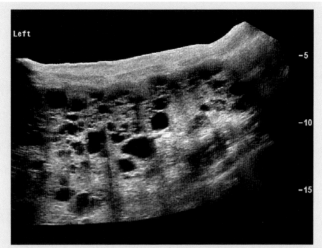

Figure 1. Lymphangiomatosis in a young female patient involving multiple organs, including the spleen. Longitudinal ultrasound image demonstrates an enlarged spleen with numerous cystic lesions, with sizes ranging from a few millimeters to several centimeters.

- They are typically seen in childhood, with few reported cases in adults.
- Lymphangiomas of the spleen are associated with Klippel-Trenaunay-Weber syndrome.

Suggested Readings

Komatsuda T, Ishida H, Konno K, et al: Splenic lymphangioma: US and CT diagnosis and clinical manifestations. *Abdom Imaging* 24:414-417, 1999.

Solomou EG, Patriarheas GV, Mpadra FA, et al: Asymptomatic adult cystic lymphangioma of the spleen: Case report and review of the literature. *Magn Reson Imaging* 21:81-84, 2003.

Wunderbaldinger P, Paya K, Partik B, et al: CT and MR imaging of generalized cystic lymphangiomatosis in pediatric patients. *AJR Am J Roentgenol* 174:827-832, 2000.

Metastatic Disease (Spleen)

DEFINITION: Secondary malignant lesion spread usually seen in patients with advanced disease and widespread involvement of other organs.

IMAGING

CT

Findings
- Indentation and scalloping of the surface of the spleen, with solid and cystic components
- Ill-defined, hypodense, rounded lesions
- Ill-defined mass containing a few small calcifications invading the hilum of the spleen
- Tumor conspicuity is best in the portal-venous phase, 60-70 seconds after intravenous administration of contrast.

Utility
- Sensitivity: 80%-93%
- Specificity: 90%-100%
- Accuracy: 87%

Ultrasound

Findings
- *Target* or *halo* appearance
- Ill-defined, hyperechoic area centrally

Utility
- Ultrasound is less sensitive than CT, MRI, and PET in the depiction of splenic metastases.

MRI

Findings
- Isointense or slightly hypointense lesions on T1-weighted images
- Slightly hyperintense lesions on T2-weighted images
- Melanoma metastases demonstrating high signal intensity on T1-weighted images caused by the T1-shortening effect of melanin
- Necrotic, cystic components

Utility
- MRI can easily detect necrotic or cystic components.
- Sensitivity: 85%-100%
- Specificity: 85%-98%
- Accuracy: 93%

PET

Findings
- Focal increased uptake in affected locations

Utility
- Fluorodeoxyglucose-PET is becoming the imaging modality of choice.

DIAGNOSTIC PEARLS

- Indentation and scalloping of surface of spleen with solid and cystic components
- Ill-defined mass containing few small calcifications invading the hilum of the spleen
- *Target* or *halo* appearance

CLINICAL PRESENTATION

- Most splenic metastases do not cause symptoms and are found incidentally during routine staging.
- Patients exhibit an abdominal mass and left upper quadrant discomfort caused by splenomegaly, which is rare.
- Acute pain is caused by splenic infarcts from tumor emboli.
- Anorexia and cachexia
- Splenic rupture

DIFFERENTIAL DIAGNOSIS

- Lymphoma and other lymphoproliferative disorders
- Leukemia and other myeloproliferative disorders

PATHOLOGY

- Hematogenous spread through splenic artery is considered most probable origin of metastases.
- Spread is through the splenic vein in patients with portal hypertension.
- Retrograde lymphatic spread occurs from the nodes in the splenic hilum.
- Psammomatous or dense calcifications can be seen in cases of metastatic mucinous adenocarcinoma.
- Tumors that most commonly metastasize to the spleen are melanomas and breast, ovary, colon, and lung lesions.

INCIDENCE/PREVALENCE AND EPIDEMIOLOGY

- Splenic involvement by metastases is relatively uncommon and occurs with frequency of 0.6%-7.1% of cases.

WHAT THE REFERRING PHYSICIAN NEEDS TO KNOW

- Isolated splenic metastases are unusual. They usually manifest as part of widespread metastatic disease.

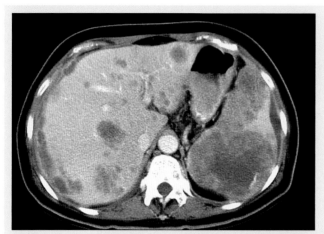

Figure 1. Splenic metastasis from colon cancer. In a 56-year-old woman, enhanced helical CT scan shows large splenic lesions with capsular invasion and subcapsular and intrahepatic metastases. CT also demonstrated diffuse tumor infiltration of the abdomen, as well as peritoneal and omental nodules and subcapsular and intrahepatic metastases. Laparotomy confirmed these findings and showed a cecal adenocarcinoma. (*Courtesy of C. Keogh, MD, Vancouver, British Columbia, Canada.*)

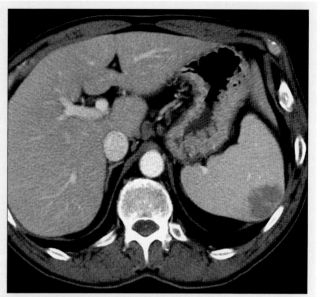

Figure 2. Splenic metastasis from lung cancer. The enhanced CT scan of the upper abdomen during the portal venous phase reveals an ill-defined, hypodense mass in the spleen 6 months after resection of a lung cancer (i.e., confirmed squamous cell cancer).

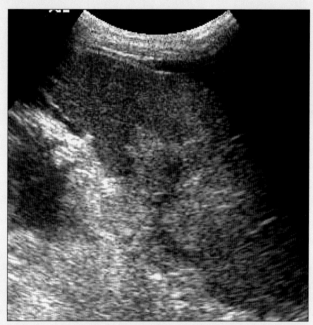

Figure 3. Hyperechoic splenic metastasis from melanoma. The sagittal sonogram shows an ill-defined, hyperechoic area centrally in the spleen and some ascites. Many similar lesions were present throughout the liver (not shown).

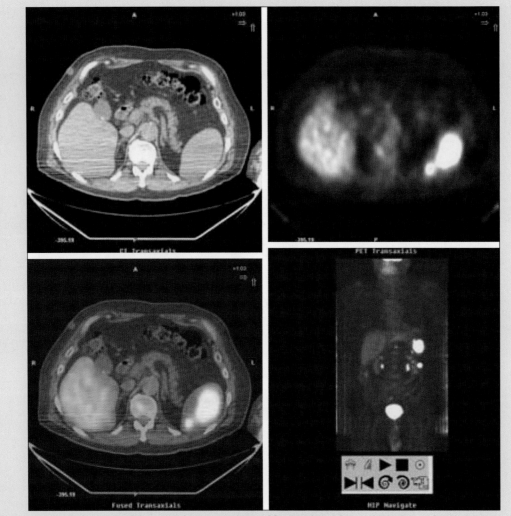

Figure 4. Splenic metastases from a malignant melanoma as imaged by PET/CT. The axial PET image demonstrates two areas of increased ^{18}F-fluorodeoxyglucose activity.

- Isolated metastases to spleen are rare.
- Frequency of splenic metastases is comparable to that of kidney metastases.

Suggested Readings

Hadjileontis C, Amplianitis I, Valsamides C, et al: Solitary splenic metastasis of endometrial carcinoma ten years after hysterectomy. Case report and review of the literature. *Eur J Gynaecol Oncol* 25:233-235, 2004.

Lee SS, Morgenstern L, Phillips EH, et al: Splenectomy for splenic metastases: A changing clinical spectrum. *Am Surg* 66:837-840, 2000.

Siniluoto T, Paivansalo M, Lahde S: Ultrasonography of splenic metastases. *Acta Radiol* 30:463-465, 1989.

Wan YL, Cheung YC, Lui KW, et al: Ultrasonographic findings and differentiation of benign and malignant focal splenic lesions. *Postgrad Med J* 76:488-493, 2000.

Peliosis of the Spleen

DEFINITION: Splenic peliosis is a rare condition characterized by sinusoidal dilation and the formation of multiple, cyst-like, blood-filled cavities within the parenchyma.

IMAGING

Ultrasound
Findings
- Multiple, poorly defined, hypoechoic lesions

Utility
- Ultrasound is insensitive in the diagnosis of splenic peliosis.

CT
Findings
- Multiple areas of low attenuation
- Multiple, small, well-defined, hypoattenuating, cyst-like lesions
- High-attenuation lesions and fluid-fluid levels
- Thought to reflect the hematocrit effect

Utility
- Lesions are best depicted comparing contrast-enhanced and precontrast scans.

MRI
Findings
- Variable postgadolinium enhancement
- Variable signal intensity
- Signal intensities of the lesions on MR examination depend on age and status of blood components.

Utility
- Lesions are best depicted comparing contrast-enhanced and precontrast scans.

CLINICAL PRESENTATION

- Patients are usually asymptomatic.
- Some may experience spontaneous splenic rupture.

DIFFERENTIAL DIAGNOSIS

- Peliosis hepatis

DIAGNOSTIC PEARLS

- Multiple, small, well-defined, hypoattenuating, cyst-like lesions
- High-attenuation lesions and fluid-fluid levels
- Multiple areas of low attenuation

PATHOLOGY

- Splenic peliosis is characterized by sinusoidal dilation and the formation of multiple, cyst-like, blood-filled cavities within the parenchyma.
- Pathogenesis of splenic peliosis is unclear.
- Multiple, blood-filled cavities are round to oval and 1 mm to several centimeters in diameter.
- Cysts located within red pulp are lined with flattened, sinusoidal endothelium; they may lack a clear cell lining.

INCIDENCE/PREVALENCE AND EPIDEMIOLOGY

- Splenic peliosis is rare.
- It is usually associated with hepatic peliosis.

Suggested Readings
Iannaccone R, Federle MP, Brancatelli G, et al: Peliosis hepatis: Spectrum of imaging findings. *AJR Am J Roentgenol* 187:W43-W52, 2006.

Maves CK, Caron KH, Bisset GS III, et al: Splenic and hepatic peliosis: MR findings. *AJR Am J Roentgenol* 158:75-76, 1992.

Shimono T, Yamaoka T, Nishimura K, et al: Peliosis of the spleen: Splenic rupture with intraperitoneal hemorrhage. *Abdom Imaging* 23:201-202, 1998.

WHAT THE REFERRING PHYSICIAN NEEDS TO KNOW

- If the lesions rupture, perisplenic hematoma, splenic laceration, and intraperitoneal hemorrhage may be evident.

Sickle Cell Disease

DEFINITION: Sickle cell disease is an autosomal-recessive disorder affecting red blood cells.

IMAGING

Ultrasound
Findings
- Hypoechoic foci
- Heterogeneous spleen with multiple hypoechoic areas

Utility
- Ultrasound is useful in assessing splenic size but is less sensitive than CT and MRI in showing focal abnormalities.

CT
Findings
- Small and densely calcified spleen
- Enlarged spleen with heterogeneous enhancement and hypodense areas interspersed with areas of higher attenuation

Utility
- CT is the most sensitive technique in detecting splenic calcifications.

MRI
Findings
- Diffuse, diminished signal intensity of the spleen relative to the skeletal musculature
- High signal intensity compatible with hemorrhage

Utility
- MRI is useful in detecting hemorrhage and other focal splenic abnormalities.

Nuclear Medicine
Findings
- Diminished or no uptake of radiotracer

Utility
- Technetium-99m (99mTc)-sulfur colloid scans of the liver and spleen

CLINICAL PRESENTATION

- Splenomegaly exacerbated by stressful conditions such as illness, fever, cold temperature, and high altitude

DIFFERENTIAL DIAGNOSIS

- Leukemia
- Lymphoma
- Myeloproliferative disorder

DIAGNOSTIC PEARLS

- Spleen is heterogeneous, with multiple hypoechoic areas.
- Spleen is enlarged, with heterogeneous enhancement and hypodense areas interspersed with areas of higher attenuation.
- Diffuse, diminished signal intensity of the spleen relative to skeletal musculature is seen.

PATHOLOGY

- Sickle cell disease is an autosomal-recessive disorder affecting red blood cells.
- Mutation in the hemoglobin A gene leads to the formation of an abnormal hemoglobin molecule (HbS).
- Deoxygenated, abnormal hemoglobin molecules form viscous polymers, aggregating with other hemoglobin molecules and distorting red blood cells into an abnormal (sickle) shape.
- Sickle shape results in less-flexible red blood cells that obstruct microcirculation, causing tissue hypoxia and infarction.

INCIDENCE/PREVALENCE AND EPIDEMIOLOGY

- Carrier frequency of sickle cell disease varies worldwide, with high rates in areas with a high incidence of malaria.
- High frequency of the HbS variant is maintained in these populations by increased resistance to malaria infection in heterozygous carriers.
- Sickle cell disease is the most common inherited blood disorder in the United States.
- Eight percent of African Americans are carriers.
- Homozygous form of sickle cell disease affects approximately 1 in every 396 African Americans.

Suggested Readings

Adler DD, Glazer GM, Aisen AM: MRI of the spleen: Normal appearance and findings in sickle-cell anemia. *AJR Am J Roentgenol* 147:843-845, 1986.

WHAT THE REFERRING PHYSICIAN NEEDS TO KNOW

- Acute splenic sequestration is a life-threatening complication of sickle cell disease and occurs in children with homozygous sickle cell disease.

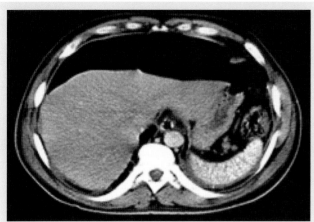

Figure 1. **End-stage spleen in a patient with homozygous sickle cell disease.** Unenhanced CT shows a small and densely calcified spleen. (*Courtesy of R. Attariwala, MD, PhD, Vancouver, British Columbia, Canada.*)

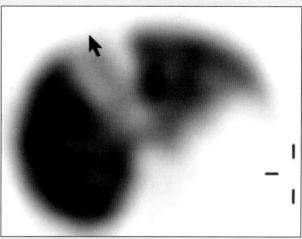

Figure 2. **End-stage spleen in a patient with homozygous sickle cell disease.** 99mTc-sulfur colloid scan of the liver and spleen demonstrates no uptake of the radiotracer, which is consistent with functional asplenia. (*Courtesy of R. Attariwala, MD, PhD, Vancouver, British Columbia, Canada.*)

Gorg C, Zugmaier G: Chronic recurring infarction of the spleen: Sonographic patterns and complications. *Ultraschall Med* 24:245-249, 2003.

Levin TL, Berdon WE, Haller JO, et al: Intrasplenic masses of "preserved" functioning splenic tissue in sickle cell disease: Correlation of imaging findings (CT, ultrasound, MRI, and nuclear scintigraphy). *Pediatr Radiol* 26:646-649, 1996.

Lonergan GJ, Cline DB, Abbondanzo SL: Sickle cell anemia. *RadioGraphics* 21:971-994, 2001.

Roshkow JE, Sanders LM: Acute splenic sequestration crisis in two adults with sickle cell disease: US, CT, and MR imaging findings. *Radiology* 177:723-725, 1990.

Splenic Cysts

DEFINITION: Round, thin-walled lesions with fluid or mixed content.

IMAGING

Radiography
Findings
- Splenic cysts: curvilinear calcifications
- Round mass with a normal, intact, splenic tip
- Hydatid cyst: curvilinear or ring-like calcifications and splenomegaly or a soft-tissue mass

Utility
- Cross-sectional imaging is more useful in delineating splenic cysts.

Ultrasound
Findings
- Splenic cysts: anechoic lesions having smooth borders and demonstrating increased through-transmission
- Epidermoid and pseudocyst: septations, thick walls, trabeculations, internal echoes, and calcified walls
- Hydatid cysts: *snowflake sign, water lily sign* (hydatid disease), daughter cysts filling the mother cyst, and tiny to massive calcifications

Utility
- Ultrasound is the most popular and readily available technique worldwide for evaluating abdominal echinococcal disease.
- Ultrasound is used for diagnosis, therapeutic decision-making, and follow-up of a hydatid cyst.

CT
Findings
- Splenic cysts: homogeneous, well-defined, round, low-enhancing, hypodense lesions, which may be partially calcified and have septations and a thick wall
- Hydatid cyst: well-defined, cystic lesion with varied attenuation, distinguishable wall, coarse calcifications, and wall and septal postcontrast enhancement

Utility
- Attenuation values typically range from 0-15 HU.
- CT is indicated for patients who are unsuited for ultrasound and for the evaluation of widespread or complicated hydatid disease.

DIAGNOSTIC PEARLS
- Splenic cysts: anechoic lesions having smooth borders and demonstrating increased through-transmission
- Hydatid cysts: *snowflake sign* or *water lily sign* (hydatid disease); daughter cysts filling the mother cyst; from tiny to massive calcifications
- Epidermoid and pseudocyst: septations, thick walls, trabeculations, internal echoes, and calcified walls

- CT attenuation of daughter cysts is typically lower than the mother cyst's attenuation.

MRI
Findings
- Splenic cyst: nonenhancing lesion with low T1 signal intensity and high uniform T2 signal intensity
- Presence of proteinaceous fluid or hemorrhage, possibly demonstrating high T1 and mixed T2 signal intensities
- Hydatid cyst: *rim sign, serpent sign* or *snake sign*, wall and septal postgadolinium enhancement
- Daughter hydatid cysts possibly appearing hypointense or isointense relative to the maternal matrix

Utility
- MRI is indicated for patients who are unsuited for ultrasound and for evaluation of widespread or complicated hydatid disease.
- *Rim sign* is characteristic of hydatid cyst.

CLINICAL PRESENTATION
- Most splenic cysts are asymptomatic.
- Left upper quadrant discomfort, fullness, and pain are rare clinical findings.
- If the cyst is large, physical examination may reveal splenomegaly or a palpable mass, with or without tenderness.

WHAT THE REFERRING PHYSICIAN NEEDS TO KNOW
- Correct diagnosis can usually be suggested by analyzing the clinical findings and the symptoms, medical history, and appearance of the cyst.
- Presence of a cystic lesion in a patient from an endemic area and positive serologic tests most likely indicate hydatid disease.
- In almost all cases of splenic hydatid cystic disease, hydatid liver disease coexists.
- Treatment of large and symptomatic cysts includes percutaneous aspiration, with or without sclerotherapy and (partial) splenectomy.
- Splenic hydatid cysts can be treated percutaneously with cyst aspiration and injection of hypertonic saline solution or alcohol.

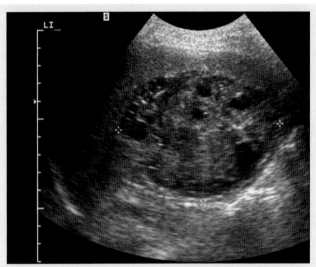

Figure 1. Echinococcal cyst: cystic echinococcosis type 3.
Longitudinal ultrasound image of the spleen demonstrates
a complex lesion with central hyperechoic areas and small
peripheral daughter cysts. (*Courtesy of M. de Jonge, MD,*
Amsterdam, Netherlands.)

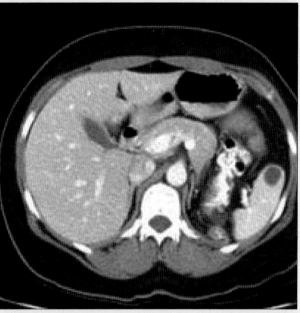

Figure 2. Congenital cyst: small, simple asymptomatic cyst in
a young female patient. Contrast-enhanced CT demonstrates a
well-defined, round, nonenhancing, hypodense lesion.

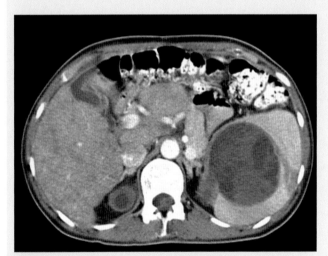

Figure 3. Echinococcal cyst: cystic echinococcosis type 3.
Contrast-enhanced CT during the arterial phase demonstrates
an oval mass involving the medial portion of the spleen
with relatively high central attenuation and a few peripheral
hypodense daughter cysts. Associated involvement of the right
adrenal is seen. (*Courtesy of M. de Jonge, MD, Amsterdam,*
Netherlands.)

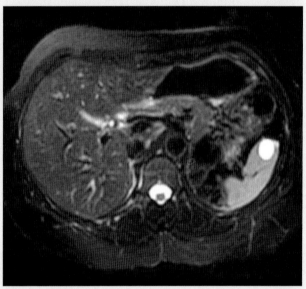

Figure 4. Congenital cyst: small, simple asymptomatic cyst in
a young female patient. Axial, fast spin-echo, fat-saturation MR
image demonstrates small, round lesion with uniform high signal
intensity on the T2-weighted images.

- Complications such as spontaneous hemorrhage, rupture, or secondary infection are rare.
- Hydatid cyst rupture into the abdominal cavity may result in an anaphylactic reaction.

DIFFERENTIAL DIAGNOSIS

- Hematoma
- Metastases (musculoskeletal)
- Cystic metastases
- Splenic abscess
- Splenic lymphoma

PATHOLOGY

- Congenital cysts have epithelial or mesothelial cell lining and are thought to be developmental in origin.
- Congenital cysts result from embryonic inclusions of splenic capsular mesothelial cells into the splenic parenchyma, with subsequent gradual growth.
- Pseudocysts do not have an epithelial lining, are unilocular, and have a smooth inner surface.
- True cysts are typically unilocular and have a trabeculated, shiny, pearly white lining.
- *Echinococcus granulosus* larvae incite an inflammatory response, forming an outer layer of inflammatory cells and a fibrous tissue called a *pericyst* (hydatid disease).

- Hydatid cyst wall is composed of an outer laminated membrane lined by an inner germinal layer made of daughter cysts.
- Pseudocysts result from intrasplenic hematoma, infarct, and infection.

INCIDENCE/PREVALENCE AND EPIDEMIOLOGY

- Incidence of splenic cysts at autopsy is approximately 7.6 per 10,000 people.
- Most common splenic cysts in the Western world are congenital or traumatic in origin.
- Worldwide, parasitic cysts (most are echinococcal) are more common and account for approximately 70% of splenic cysts.
- Congenital cysts are often discovered in children and young adults and have female predominance.

Suggested Readings

Burrig KF: Epithelial (true) splenic cysts. Pathogenesis of the mesothelial and so-called epidermoid cyst of the spleen. *Am J Surg Pathol* 12:275-281, 1988.
Fowler RH: Nonparasitic benign cystic tumors of the spleen. *Int Abstr Surg* 96:209-227, 1953.
Martin JW: Congenital splenic cysts. *Am J Surg* 96:302-308, 1958.
WHO Informal Working Group: International classification of ultrasound images in cystic echinococcosis for application in clinical and field epidemiological settings. *Acta Trop* 85:253-261, 2003.

Splenic Hamartoma

DEFINITION: Splenic hamartomas are composed of disorganized red-pulp elements, with reticuloendothelial cell proliferation.

IMAGING

Ultrasound with Color Doppler
Findings
- Well-defined, homogeneous masses
- Mass, possibly containing cystic areas or coarse calcifications
- Mass often demonstrating an increased blood flow

Utility
- Sonography is more sensitive than CT in depicting hamartomas of spleen.

CT
Findings
- Contour abnormality
- May contain minute speckled calcifications, a central scar, or cystic areas

Utility
- CT is less sensitive than ultrasound or MRI in diagnosing splenic hamartomas.

MRI
Findings
- Well-defined, isointense masses on T1-weighted image
- Prolonged postgadolinium enhancement
- May contain minute speckled calcifications, a central scar, or cystic areas

Utility
- MRI is more sensitive than CT in depicting hamartomas of the spleen.

CLINICAL PRESENTATION

- Large hamartoma may produce a palpable mass or splenomegaly.
- Growth retardation and recurrent infections are seen.

DIFFERENTIAL DIAGNOSIS

- Splenic malignancy

DIAGNOSTIC PEARLS

- Well-defined, isointense masses are seen on T1-weighted images, with prolonged gadolinium enhancement.
- Mass often demonstrates increased blood flow.
- Mass may contain cystic areas or coarse calcifications.

PATHOLOGY

- Lesions are well-circumscribed, solid lesions that compress the surrounding parenchyma.
- They are composed of disorganized red-pulp elements, with reticuloendothelial cell proliferation.
- Normal white pulp is usually absent.
- Splenic hamartomas are considered to be congenital in origin.

INCIDENCE/PREVALENCE AND EPIDEMIOLOGY

- Splenic hamartoma is a rare, benign tumor.
- Reported incidence in large autopsy and splenectomy series varies from 0.12%-0.17%.
- No gender predilection is noted, and they can be found in any age group.
- Splenic hamartoma is associated with hematologic disorders, tuberous sclerosis, malignancies, and Wiskott-Aldrich–like syndrome.

Suggested Readings

Silverman ML, LiVolsi VA: Splenic hamartoma. *Am J Clin Pathol* 70:224-229, 1978.

Zissin R, Lishner M, Rathaus V: Case report: Unusual presentation of splenic hamartoma: Computed tomography and ultrasonic findings. *Clin Radiol* 45:410-411, 1992.

WHAT THE REFERRING PHYSICIAN NEEDS TO KNOW

- Definitive diagnosis of splenic hamartoma is rarely made based on imaging.
- Diagnosis is often confirmed by pathologic evaluation after a splenectomy.
- Definitive diagnosis may be established with percutaneous biopsy.

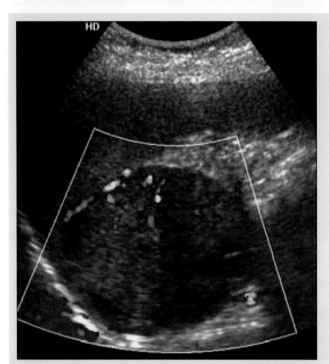

Figure 1. Hamartoma. Longitudinal ultrasound image demonstrates a mildly hypoechoic mass medial to the spleen with some internal color flow.

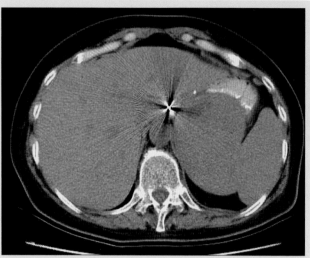

Figure 2. Hamartoma. Unenhanced CT shows a round mass involving the medial portion of the spleen, and it is isodense with the splenic parenchyma. (A metallic artifact from a surgical clip from remote gastric surgery is seen.)

Splenic Infarction

DEFINITION: Splenic infarction is the result of splenic arterial or venous compromise.

IMAGING

CT
Findings
- Wedge-shaped area with the base at the splenic capsule and the apex pointing toward the hilum
- Multinodular or mottled appearance and a mass-like appearance, with irregular margins
- Heterogeneously hypodense, ill-defined, mass-like lesion
- Areas of mottled, increased attenuation

Utility
- Contrast-enhanced CT markedly improves visualization.
- Is the preferred means of establishing the diagnosis

Ultrasound
Findings
- Single or multiple wedge-shaped or round, hypoechoic, anechoic, or hyperechoic lesions

Utility
- Is less accurate than MRI and CT in making the diagnosis

MRI
Findings
- Diffuse low T1 signal intensity
- Inhomogeneously high T2 signal intensity

Utility
- Signal intensity of the infarcted areas depends on the age of the infarct and the degree of the hemorrhagic component.

Nuclear Medicine
Findings
- Focal area of diminished activity on splenic scintigraphy
- No uptake of radiotracer in the spleen observed with massive infarction

Utility
- Technetium-99m (99mTc)-labeled, heat-denatured, red blood cell scan may be used to demonstrate viable splenic tissue.

Interventional Radiology
Findings
- Wedge-shaped regions of decreased perfusion or non-visualization of the spleen on angiography

DIAGNOSTIC PEARLS

- Wedge-shaped area with the base at the splenic capsule and the apex pointing toward the hilum
- Multinodular or mottled appearance and mass-like appearance, with irregular margins
- No uptake of radiotracer in spleen observed with massive infarction

CLINICAL PRESENTATION

- Patient may complain of pain in left upper abdomen and fever.
- Pleuritic chest pain and referred pain to left shoulder and leukocytosis may be seen.
- Thirty to fifty percent of patients remain asymptomatic.

DIFFERENTIAL DIAGNOSIS

- Splenic rupture

PATHOLOGY

- Splenic infarction results from arterial or venous compromise.
- All infarcts are initially hemorrhagic; over time, they become pale with hyperemic borders and, finally, fibrotic.
- Infarcts caused by emboli have a wedge-shaped, pale appearance, with the base at the capsular surface.

INCIDENCE/PREVALENCE AND EPIDEMIOLOGY

- Patients younger than age 40 have an associated hematologic disorder; those older than age 41 often have had an embolic event.
- Most cases are associated with hematologic disorders, including sickle cell disease.

WHAT THE REFERRING PHYSICIAN NEEDS TO KNOW

- Intraparenchymal splenic gas may be found after therapeutic splenic embolization.
- Complicated splenic infarction includes progressive liquefaction necrosis, subcapsular hemorrhage, splenic rupture, and intraparenchymal gas, indicating superimposed infection.
- Vegetations on cardiac valves need to be excluded with echocardiography.
- Synchronous renal infarcts need to be excluded as well.

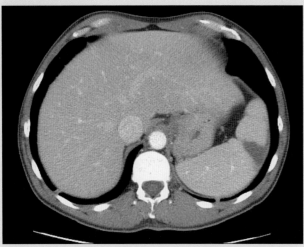

Figure 1. Chronic splenic infarct. Contrast-enhanced CT demonstrates a classic wedge-shaped, peripherally nonenhancing, hypodense area. The base of the infarct is at the splenic capsule, and the apex points toward the hilum. Some volume loss and capsular retraction indicates a chronic infarct.

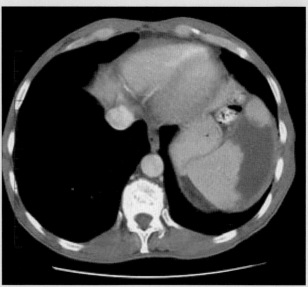

Figure 2. Subacute splenic infarct. Contrast-enhanced CT at a comparable level demonstrates a nonenhancing, hypodense area.

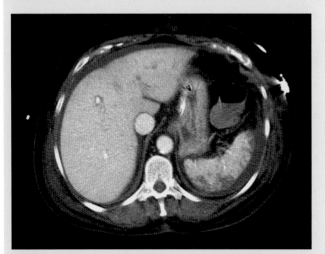

Figure 3. Acute splenic infarct. Contrast-enhanced CT demonstrates a mottled appearance of the splenic infarcts with associated perisplenic fluid.

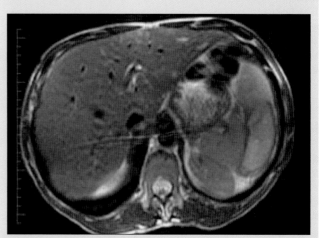

Figure 4. Subacute splenic infarct. Axial view, T2-weighted MR image shows a predominantly high-signal-intensity area in the same patient.

Suggested Readings

Balcar I, Seltzer SE, Davis S, et al: CT patterns of splenic infarction: A clinical and experimental study. *Radiology* 151:723-729, 1984.
Goerg C, Schwerk WB: Splenic infarct: Sonographic patterns, diagnosis, follow-up, and complications. *Radiology* 74:803-807, 1990.

Miller LA, Mirvis SE, Shanmuganathan K, Ohson AS: CT diagnosis of splenic infarction in blunt trauma: Imaging features, clinical significance and complications. *Clin Radiol* 59:342-348, 2004.
Nores M, Phillips EH, Morgenstern L, et al: The clinical spectrum of splenic infarction. *Am Surg* 64:182-188, 1998.

Splenic Infections

DEFINITION: Inflammation and infection of the spleen are recognized by three distinct patterns: (1) generalized splenomegaly without discerning focal lesions, (2) solitary lesions, and (3) a diffuse, miliary, or macronodular pattern, with or without splenomegaly.

IMAGING

Ultrasound
Findings
- Candidiasis: multiple, small, hypoechoic nodules and a *wheel-within-a-wheel* appearance (i.e., *target sign*)
- Tuberculosis: hypoechoic pattern in the spleen
- *Mycobacterium avium-intracellulare* complex: splenomegaly with multiple, small, hypoechoic nodules
- *Pneumocystis jiroveci*: pneumonia, splenomegaly with small, hypoechoic lesions with cystic components or tiny, highly reflective, nonshadowing foci
- Sarcoidosis: hypoechoic to slightly hyperechoic or inhomogeneous nodules
- Splenic abscess: complex cystic lesions with septa, debris, and acoustic shadowing caused by gas

Utility
Sensitivity: 75%-92%
Specificity: 85%-90%
Accuracy: 86%

CT
Findings
- Fungal microabscess: 5- to 10-mm, hypodense, nodular lesions
- Tuberculosis: cat-scratch disease, Gamna-Gandy bodies, and multiple, hypodense nodules
- Sarcoidosis: hypodense nodules relative to the adjacent normal spleen after intravenous contrast
- Splenic abscess: unilocular or multilocular, hypodense collection or complex cystic lesion with an enhancing rim after intravenous contrast
- In the arterial phase (25-35 seconds), most lesions demonstrate a hyperdense peripheral ring that disappears in portal-venous phase.

Utility
Sensitivity: 70%-95%
Specificity: 60%-80%
Accuracy: 74%

DIAGNOSTIC PEARLS
- *Wheel-within-a-wheel* appearance (i.e., *target sign*) (candidiasis)
- Complex cystic lesion with septa, debris, and acoustic shadowing caused by gas (splenic abscess)
- Hypodense nodules relative to the adjacent normal spleen after intravenous contrast (sarcoidosis)

MRI
Findings
- Hepatosplenic fungal disease: peripheral ring of very low signal intensity
- Central region of the lesion may demonstrate enhancement after gadolinium administration.
- It is best seen on early-phase gadolinium-enhanced T2-weighted fat-suppressed images or on T1-weighted sequences.

Utility
Sensitivity: 80%-95%
Specificity: 75%-90%
Accuracy: 82%

PET
Findings
- Increased ^{18}F-fluorodeoxyglucose (FDG) uptake (fungal microabscess)

Utility
- PET cannot differentiate tumor from infection within the spleen.

Radiography
Findings
- Splenic abscess: left pleural effusion, left lung base infiltrate, extraluminal gas or air-fluid levels in the left upper quadrant

---

WHAT THE REFERRING PHYSICIAN NEEDS TO KNOW
- Generalized splenomegaly is nonspecific and found in various diseases, including infections and inflammatory diseases.
- Multiple splenic nodular lesions are commonly associated with nonbacterial infections such as fungal and granulomatous infections.
- Metastatic disease to the spleen may be recognized as solitary or multiple nodules or, rarely, as a miliary pattern.
- For larger abscesses, percutaneous drainage procedures have become the treatment of choice, allowing for the preservation of the spleen.

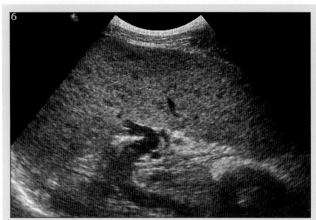

Figure 1. *Mycobacterium avium* **complex.** Longitudinal sonogram demonstrates splenomegaly with multiple, small, hypoechoic nodules.

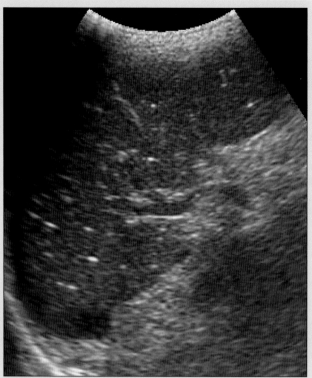

Figure 2. *Pneumocystis jiroveci* **pneumonia.** Longitudinal ultrasound image demonstrates multiple punctate calcifications after successful treatment.

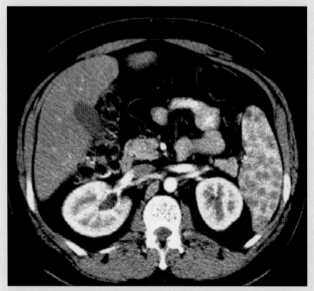

Figure 3. Sarcoidosis. Contrast-enhanced CT obtained in the portal-venous phase shows numerous hypodense nodules.

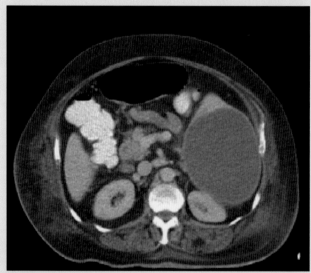

Figure 4. Splenic abscess (methicillin-resistant *Staphylococcus aureus*) in a patient with endocarditis. Contrast-enhanced CT shows a large, unilocular, hypodense collection with a mildly enhancing rim.

Utility

- Plain radiography is typically noncontributory in the diagnosis of splenic infections.

CLINICAL PRESENTATION

- Common manifestation of systemic candidiasis is persistent fever that is unresponsive to conventional antibiotics.
- Fever of unknown origin and abdominal pain may be seen.
- Sarcoidosis-splenomegaly, typically associated with hepatomegaly, abdominal lymphadenopathy, abdominal pain, fatigue, and malaise may be seen.
- Splenic abscess produces fever, left upper abdominal pain, leukocytosis, left pleural effusion, and splenomegaly.

DIFFERENTIAL DIAGNOSIS

- Pancreatic inflammation
- Splenic infarction
- Splenic subcapsular hemorrhage
- Splenic metastases
- Primary splenic neoplasm

PATHOLOGY

- Colonization of gastrointestinal tract is thought to be the main origin of disseminating *Candida* infection.
- Extrapulmonary involvement causes necrotizing granulomas (*P. jiroveci* pneumonia).

INCIDENCE/PREVALENCE AND EPIDEMIOLOGY

- Most patients with multiple splenic nodules have an established diagnosis such as lymphoma, metastases, or tuberculosis.
- Splenic fungal infections typically occur in immunocompromised patients with neutropenia.
- *M. avium-intracellulare* infections are typically seen in immunocompromised patients, such as those with AIDS.
- *P. jiroveci* pneumonia is the most common opportunistic infection in patients with AIDS.
- Cat-scratch disease is a self-limiting infection by *Bartonella henselae* that occurs after being scratched by a domestic cat.
- Sarcoidosis is a systemic disease of unknown cause.
- Splenic abscesses are becoming more common as the result of an increasing number of immunosuppressed patients.

Suggested Readings

Masood A, Sallah S: Chronic disseminated candidiasis in patients with acute leukemia: Emphasis on diagnostic definition and treatment. *Leuk Res* 29:493-501, 2005.

Metser U, Haider MA, Dill-Macky M, et al: Fungal liver infection in immunocompromised patients: Depiction with multiphasic contrast-enhanced helical CT. *Radiology* 235:97-105, 2005.

Murray JG, Patel MD, Lee S, et al: Microabscesses of the liver and spleen in AIDS: Detection with 5-MHz sonography. *Radiology* 197:723-727, 1995.

Rudolph J, Rodenwaldt J, Ruhnke M, et al: Unusual enhancement pattern of liver lesions in hepatosplenic candidiasis. *Acta Radiol* 45:499-503, 2004.

Vasquez TE, Evans DG, Schiffman H, et al: Fungal splenic abscesses in the immunosuppressed patient: Correlation of imaging modalities. *Clin Nucl Med* 12:36-38, 1987.

Splenic Rupture

DEFINITION: Rupture of spleen, which may or may not be associated with trauma.

IMAGING

CT

Findings
- Linear, hypodense parenchymal defect
- Multiple hypoechoic areas, subcapsular and pericapsular dense fluid, and free peritoneal fluid

Utility
- Sensitivity: 90%-100%
- Specificity: 95%-100%
- Accuracy: 97%
- CT is the single best imaging test for evaluating splenic rupture and trauma.

CLINICAL PRESENTATION

- Life-threatening hemorrhage
- Splenomegaly
- Hypotension and shock
- Left upper quadrant pain

DIFFERENTIAL DIAGNOSIS

- Small-bowel trauma
- Splenic infarction

PATHOLOGY

- Pathologic spleen is more prone to rupture because of altered consistency and splenomegaly that extends below the rib cage.
- Splenic rupture is an uncommon manifestation of leukemic disorders caused by infiltration of the splenic capsule and trabecular framework or infarction.

DIAGNOSTIC PEARLS

- Subcapsular hematoma
- Linear, hypodense parenchymal defect
- Free peritoneal fluid

INCIDENCE/PREVALENCE AND EPIDEMIOLOGY

- Rupture of spleen typically occurs in patients with diseased and enlarged spleen, without apparent trauma.
- Spontaneous rupture of the normal spleen is even more uncommon.

Suggested Readings

Choudhury AK: Spontaneous rupture of a normal spleen. *Injury* 35:325-326, 2004.
Stites TB, Ultmann JE: Spontaneous rupture of the spleen in chronic lymphocytic leukemia. *Cancer* 19:1587-1590, 1966.

WHAT THE REFERRING PHYSICIAN NEEDS TO KNOW
- All patients with splenomegaly are at increased risk for spontaneous and traumatic splenic rupture.

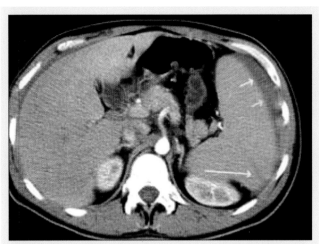

Figure 1. Spontaneous splenic rupture in a patient with malaria. Contrast-enhanced CT demonstrates a subcapsular hematoma *(short arrows)* and a linear, hypodense parenchymal defect *(long arrow)*.

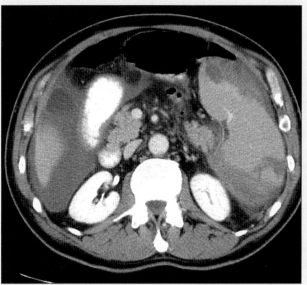

Figure 2. Spontaneous splenic rupture. A 69-year-old man had acute lymphoblastic leukemia. Enhanced helical CT scan demonstrates splenomegaly and multiple hypoechoic areas, subcapsular and pericapsular dense fluid, and free fluid around the liver. Laparotomy and splenectomy revealed a ruptured subcapsular hematoma and diffuse leukemic involvement of the spleen.

Splenosis

DEFINITION: Splenosis results from autotransplantation of splenic tissue after disruption of the splenic capsule by trauma or surgery.

IMAGING

MRI
Findings
- Signal intensity and enhancement are similar to those of normal spleen on all sequences outside of the spleen.

Utility
Sensitivity: 83%-95%
Specificity: 90%-100%
Accuracy: 92%

CT
Findings
- Multiple or single soft-tissue masses with the same attenuation

Utility
Sensitivity: 90%-100%
Specificity: 85%-98%
Accuracy: 96%

CLINICAL PRESENTATION

- History of splenectomy after trauma
- Incidental abdominal mass seen on imaging studies

DIFFERENTIAL DIAGNOSIS

- Accessory spleen
- Splenunculi
- Adenopathy

PATHOLOGY

- Splenosis is an autotransplantation of splenic tissue after disruption of the splenic capsule by trauma or surgery.
- Masses are numerous and variable in size and shape, histologically indistinguishable from the normal spleen.

DIAGNOSTIC PEARLS

- Signal intensity and enhancement are similar to those of normal spleen on all sequences.
- Area is supplied by small perforating vessels arising at the site of implantation.
- Masses are typically located in the abdomen but may be found in various locations, including the pelvis, thorax, and scars.

- They are typically located in the abdomen but may be found in various locations, including the pelvis, thorax, and scars.
- Masses are supplied by small perforating vessels arising at the site of implantation.

INCIDENCE/PREVALENCE AND EPIDEMIOLOGY

- Splenosis is seen in up to 74% of patients who undergo splenectomy after trauma.

Suggested Readings

Normand JP, Rioux M, Dumont M, et al: Thoracic splenosis after blunt trauma: Frequency and imaging findings. *AJR Am J Roentgenol* 161:739-741, 1993.

Yeh CJ, Chuang WY, Kuo TT: Unusual subcutaneous splenosis occurring in a gunshot wound scar: Pathology and immunohistochemical identification. *Pathol Int* 56:336, 2006.

WHAT THE REFERRING PHYSICIAN NEEDS TO KNOW

- Splenosis is of little clinical significance except in cases when the spleen is involved in diseases for which a splenectomy is indicated.

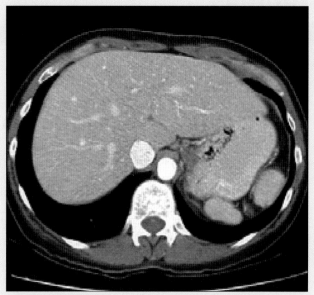

Figure 1. Accessory spleen and splenosis. Contrast-enhanced CT shows two nodular lesions (i.e., splenosis) in the left upper abdomen in a patient with a remote history of splenectomy after a traumatic splenic injury.

Splenic Trauma

DEFINITION: Blunt-force or penetrating trauma to the spleen.

ANATOMIC FINDINGS

Spleen
- Parenchymal hematoma with an intact capsule
- Venous bleeding along the segmental lines
- Stellate fracture with arterial and venous bleeding

IMAGING

CT
Findings
- Splenic hematomas: hyperdense relative to the splenic parenchyma on unenhanced CT and usually hypodense on contrast-enhanced CT
- Intrasplenic hematomas typically appearing as hypodense areas within the splenic parenchyma after the administration of contrast
- Splenic lacerations: linear, low-attenuation foci that may not extend completely across the spleen; single, multiple, or stellate
- Splenic fractures: lacerations that extend completely across the splenic parenchyma and commonly involve the splenic hilum
- Subcapsular hematomas: crescentic fluid collections along the lateral aspect of the spleen that are difficult to distinguish from perisplenic fluid
- Severe disruption of the splenic parenchyma that results in a *shattered* spleen
- Sentinel clot: perisplenic, high-attenuation fluid or clot; a useful indicator of splenic injury

Utility
- Multidetector CT (MDCT) has become the gold standard for the diagnosis of splenic injuries after trauma.
- CT has an accuracy exceeding 95% in the detection of splenic injuries.
- Contrast-enhanced MDCT is the method of choice for the evaluation of trauma patients with suspected abdominal injury.
- MDCT scanning with the bolus technique is preferred to optimize injury detection and minimize delay.

DIAGNOSTIC PEARLS

- Sentinel clot
- Splenic lacerations: linear, low-attenuation foci that may not extend completely across the spleen
- Splenic fractures: lacerations that extend completely across the splenic parenchyma and commonly involve the splenic hilum

- Multislice scanners with fast tube rotation minimize scanning time and motion artifacts.
- CT can reveal commonly associated chest, diaphragmatic, and intra-abdominal injuries.

Ultrasound
Findings
- In the acute setting, lacerations and hematomas appear echogenic because of the presence of clotted blood.
- Fresh and chronic hemorrhage can appear hypoechoic.
- Hemorrhage can be detected by blood surrounding the gastrosplenic ligament (the left butterfly sign).

Utility
- Ultrasound is the primary imaging modality for trauma patients in many centers outside the United States.
- Focused abdominal sonography for trauma (FAST) is performed at the bedside with handheld devices; it uses no ionizing radiation.
- The primary goal of FAST is the detection of free intraperitoneal fluid.
- Ultrasound has limited sensitivity for the detection of retroperitoneal injuries.
- Patient obesity, subcutaneous emphysema, a limited acoustic window, and an isoechoic clot can also limit its sensitivity.
- Scanning should also include a general survey to detect hemoperitoneum within the abdomen.
- Color Doppler may help in the detection of intrasplenic pseudoaneurysm.

WHAT THE REFERRING PHYSICIAN NEEDS TO KNOW
- Signs of persistent intraperitoneal hemorrhage or hemodynamic instability are clear indications for surgery.
- Nonoperative management of splenic injury in pediatric patients is the norm and is successful in more than 90% of appropriately selected patients.
- Major criticisms of nonoperative management include failure to detect associated injuries (bowel perforation or diaphragmatic disruption) and an increase in transfusion requirements.
- Splenic artery embolization has been shown to improve the outcome of nonoperative management.
- CT after embolization is indicated in the setting of abdominal pain, hypotension, or signs of infection.

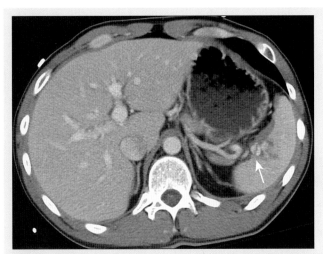

Figure 1. Splenic laceration. Laceration *(arrow)* extends to the hepatic hilum and is associated with traumatic pseudoaneurysm with dissection. Notice the small perisplenic hematoma.

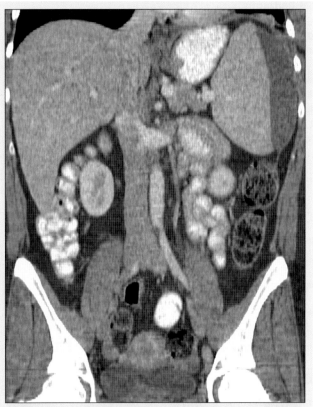

Figure 2. Subcapsular hematoma. The low-attenuation fluid collection is located along the lateral surface of the spleen and causes straightening of the lateral margin. The subcapsular hematoma follows the contour of the spleen. Coronal re-formations can be particularly helpful for the assessment of the location of intra-abdominal free fluid in the setting of trauma.

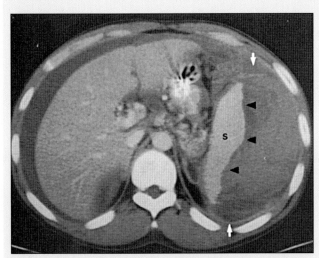

Figure 3. Larger subcapsular hematoma. Distinction between subcapsular and perisplenic fluid can be difficult. In this case, the large subcapsular component *(arrowheads)* is compressing the splenic (S) parenchyma, but it is difficult to separate from perisplenic hematoma *(arrows)*. Notice the blood lateral to the liver.

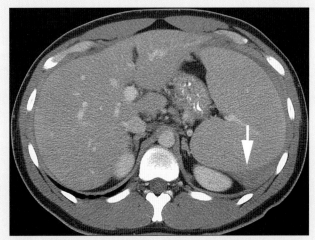

Figure 4. The sentinel clot sign. Isolated, perisplenic, high-attenuation hematoma *(arrow)* indicates a high likelihood of splenic injury. The splenic laceration was not apparent.

Radiography

Findings
- Nonspecific
- Posterior left rib or upper lumbar transverse process fractures
- Medial displacement of a gastric air bubble
- Elevation of the left hemidiaphragm
- Signs of hemoperitoneum

Utility
- Lack of abnormal findings on chest or abdominal radiographs does not obviate the need for further diagnostic evaluation.

CLINICAL PRESENTATION

- Left upper quadrant tenderness or referred left shoulder pain (Kehr sign) is elicited best by placing patients in the Trendelenburg position.
- Rib fractures are found in 7%-10% of patients with multiple trauma.
- Hypotension and overt shock occur in approximately 30%-40% of patients with splenic injuries.

DIFFERENTIAL DIAGNOSIS

- Lateral segment of left lobe of liver extending to left mid-axillary line
- Ascites
- Splenic flow artifact
- Congenital splenic cleft

PATHOLOGY

- Patient has been injured by sudden compression or countercoup mechanisms during rapid deceleration.
- In deceleration injuries, stomach and transverse colon mobility is transferred to the spleen; ligamentous-capsular avulsions or vascular injury occurs to the pedicle or short gastric vessels.
- In blunt compression, a direct blow or transmitted shock wave occurs, resulting in parenchymal injuries and venous bleeding along the segmental anatomic lines.

- Penetrating trauma does not respect the segmental anatomy and tends to have a more vascular disruption and a higher incidence of associated organ injury.
- Enlarged spleen is more prone to blunt-force injury and is exposed beneath the rib cage.
- Splenomegaly can result from a variety of disease states, including portal hypertension, blood dyscrasias, infection, and lymphoproliferative disorders.

INCIDENCE/PREVALENCE AND EPIDEMIOLOGY

- Splenic trauma accounts for 25% of all solid abdominal organ injuries.
- Motor-vehicle accidents and motor sports produce most splenic injuries, followed by direct blows and falls.
- Associated injury of the central nervous system, liver, kidney, and hollow viscera is seen in 10%-40% of cases of blunt-force splenic injuries.
- Up to 40% of all splenectomies are performed for iatrogenic injury; the risk of splenic injury is highest during a left hemicolectomy.
- Most iatrogenic injuries result from excessive retraction and disruption of ligamentous attachments.

Suggested Readings

Cathey KL, Brady WJ, Butler K, et al: Blunt splenic trauma: Characteristics of patients requiring urgent laparotomy. *Am Surg* 64:450-454, 1998.

Gralla J, Spycher F, Pignolet C, et al: Evaluation of a 16-MDCT scanner in an emergency department: Initial clinical experience and workflow analysis. *AJR Am J Roentgenol* 185:232-238, 2005.

Poletti PA, Mirvis SE, Shanmuganathan KM, et al: Blunt abdominal trauma patients: Can organ injury be excluded without performing computed tomography. *J Trauma* 57:1072-1081, 2004.

Rhea JT, Garza DH, Novelline RA: Controversies in emergency radiology. CT versus ultrasound in the evaluation of blunt abdominal trauma. *Emerg Radiol* 10:289-295, 2004.

Salim A, Sangthong B, Martin M, et al: Whole body imaging in blunt multisystem trauma patients without obvious signs of injury: Results of a prospective study. *Arch Surg* 141:468-475, 2006.

Peritoneal Cavity

Biliary Spread

DEFINITION: Spread of infection or tumor through the biliary tract.

ANATOMIC FINDINGS

Bile Duct
- Parasite, neoplasm, stone, or stricture obstructing the duct

IMAGING

Radiography
Findings
- Patients with acquired immunodeficiency syndrome: Infection produces a radiologic appearance similar to that of sclerosing cholangitis, papillary stenosis, or acute cholecystitis.

Utility
- Endoscopic retograde cholangiopancreatography (ERCP) and percutaneous transhepatic cholangiography (PTC) are accurate and invasive means of making the diagnosis.
- Can be used therapeutically

CT
Findings
- Duct wall thickening with increased enhancement
- Hypodense or hyperdense filling defects in bile ducts
- Biliary dilation or stricture

Utility
- Inferior to MRI but superior to ultrasound in depicting associated hepatic abnormalities

MRI
Findings
- Filling defects in bile ducts
- Biliary dilation or stricture
- Abnormal mural thickening and enhancement of bile ducts

Utility
- Best noninvasive means of detecting ductal defects and associated liver findings

DIAGNOSTIC PEARLS
- Obstructive jaundice may be seen.
- Biliary system is the major conduit for infectious disease.

Ultrasound
Findings
- Echogenic filling defects in bile ducts

Utility
- Inferior to MRI and MR cholangiopancreatography (MRCP) in lesion detection

CLINICAL PRESENTATION
- *Ascaris lumbricoides* infection may produce acute cholecystitis or biliary obstruction.
- Established liver infections (hydatid cysts) erode through and rupture into the biliary system; expelled contents cause obstructive jaundice.
- Ascending cholangitis occurs in the clinical setting of obstruction and biliary stasis proximal to the obstructing stone, stricture, or neoplasm.

DIFFERENTIAL DIAGNOSIS
- Acute cholecystitis
- Primary sclerosing cholangitis

PATHOLOGY
- Biliary system is the major conduit for infectious disease.
- Affected persons harbor *Clonorchis sinensis* or *Fasciola hepatica* parasites; the entity obstructs the bile ducts

---

WHAT THE REFERRING PHYSICIAN NEEDS TO KNOW
- Biliary system is a major conduit for infectious disease.
- Patients with *Ascaris* infection may exhibit cholecystitis or biliary obstruction.
- Biliary tract infections are now the most common cause of liver abscess.

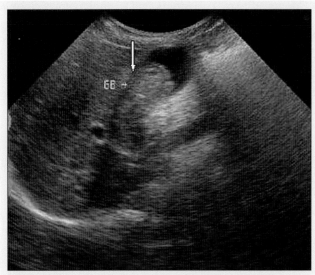

Figure 1. Ultrasound image of upper abdomen showing a poorly defined, echogenic, soft-tissue mass in the gallbladder extending within the cystic duct. Multiple calculi or echogenic foci with posterior acoustic shadowing are also seen. (*From Maheshwari PR: Gallbladder ascariasis.* Clin Radiol 59:8-10, 2004.)

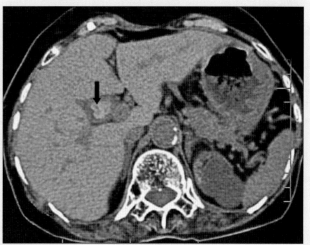

Figure 2. CT image at the level of the cystic duct, showing disk-like lesions with central areas of low attenuation suggestive of worms in cross-section (*arrow*). Incidentally seen is a simple cyst in the left kidney. (*From Maheshwari PR: Gallbladder ascariasis.* Clin Radiol 59:8-10, 2004.)

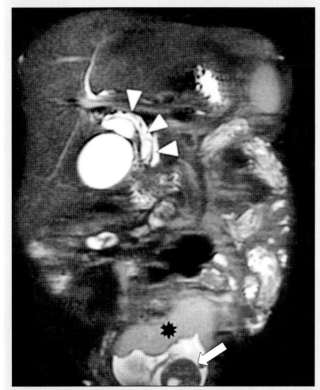

Figure. 3. MR cholangiopancreatography showing hypointense linear filling defects inside dilated bile ducts. The common bile duct is entirely filled with *Ascaris* worms (*arrowheads*). (*Asterisk,* Placenta; *arrow,* fetus.) (*From Alper F, Kantarci M, Bozkurt M, et al: Acute biliary obstruction caused by biliary ascaris in pregnancy: MR cholangiography findings.* Clin Radiol 58:896-898, 2003.)

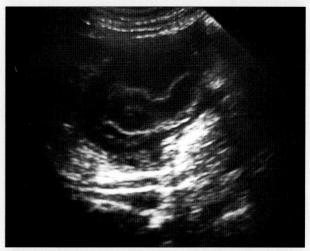

Figure 4. Sonographic image of 50-year-old male patient with separation of the cyst wall from the surrounding liver parenchyma, floating internal membranes, and intraperitoneal fluid revealing intraperitoneal rupture of a hydatid cyst located in the left liver lobe. (*From Turgut AT, Altin L, Topcus S, et al: Unusual imaging characteristics of complicated hydatid diseases.* Eur J Radiol 63:84-93, 2007.)

and acts as a nidus for stone formation and chronic inflammation.

- Liver flukes migrate from the duodenum through ampulla of Vater and on to any part of the biliary tract.
- *A. lumbricoides* worms often migrate from the duodenum through the ampulla of Vater to lodge in the gallbladder, biliary tract, and pancreatic duct.
- Patients with acquired immunodeficiency syndrome are subject to biliary and pancreatic duct abnormalities, with direct involvement by *Cryptococcus* and *Cryptosporidium* organisms.
- Hepatocellular carcinoma and cholangiocarcinoma uncommonly seed the biliary tract.

INCIDENCE/PREVALENCE AND EPIDEMIOLOGY

- Asian cholangiohepatitis is the most common biliary tract disease in parts of China, Japan, and other Far East countries.
- *A. lumbricoides* affects one fourth of world's population.
- Ascending cholangitis is the most common cause of liver abscess in the Western world.

- Hepatocellular carcinoma and cholangiocarcinoma uncommonly seed the biliary tract.
- Ascending cholangitis (a pyogenic infection of the biliary tract) is the most common cause of liver abscess in the Western world.

Suggested Readings

Bass NM: Sclerosing cholangitis and recurrent pyogenic cholangitis. In Feldman M, Scharschmidt BF, Sleisenger MH (eds): *Gastrointestinal Liver Disease*, 6th ed. Philadelphia, WB Saunders, 1998, pp 1275-1283.

Federle MP, Cello JP, Laing FC, et al: Recurrent pyogenic cholangitis in Asian immigrants. Use of ultrasonography, computed tomography and cholangiography. *Radiology* 143:151-156, 1982.

Fullerton JK, Vitale M, Vitale GC: Therapeutic endoscopic retrograde cholangiopancreatography for the treatment of *Fasciola hepatica* presenting as biliary obstruction. *Surg Innov* 13:179-182, 2006.

Grumbach K, Coleman BG, Gal AA, et al: Hepatic and biliary tract abnormalities in patients with AIDS. *J Ultrasound Med* 8:247-254, 1989.

Macris GJ, Galanis NN: Rupture of *Echinococcus* cyst of the liver into the biliary ducts. *Am Surg* 32:36-39, 1966.

Schulman A: Non-Western patterns of biliary stones and the role of ascariasis. *Radiology* 162:425-430, 1987.

Shah OJ, Zargar SA, Robbani I: Biliary ascariasis: A review. *World J Surg* 30:1500-1506, 2006.

Zeman RK, Burrell MI: *Gallbladder and Bile Duct Imaging*. New York, Churchill Livingstone, 1987.

Part 61

ASCITES AND PERITONEAL FLUID COLLECTIONS

Pathways of Fluid Distribution

DEFINITION: Spread of intraperitoneal fluid.

IMAGING

Ultrasound
Findings
- Simple fluid collections tend to be anechoic; more complex collections show septations, masses, and/or internal echoes.

Utility
- Ultrasound is the most sensitive means of diagnosing small amounts of intraperitoneal fluid.

MRI
Findings
- Simple fluid collections tend to be homogeneous in intensity, bright on T2-, and dark on T1-weighted images.
- Complex collections are usually inhomogeneous and may show masses and septations.
- Malignant fluid may be seen distending the pouch of Douglas.

Utility
- MRI is useful in delineating the full extent of larger fluid collections and suggesting their etiology.

CT
Findings
- Simple fluid collections tend to be homogeneous and have an attenuation ≤ 20 HU.
- Complex fluid collections often are inhomogeneous and have a high density, internal septations, and/or masses.
- Gas-containing pouch of Douglas abscess may be seen.

Utility
- CT is useful in depicting the complete extent of larger peritoneal and retroperitoneal fluid collections and suggesting their etiology.

PATHOLOGY

- Factors that determine the distribution of fluid in the peritoneal cavity include volume, peritoneal pressures, the patient's position, and the region of origin.

DIAGNOSTIC PEARLS

- Fluid in the inframesocolic space seeks the pelvis: on the right, through the leaves of the small bowel mesentery; on the left, through the medial side of the rectosigmoid.
- After fluid fills the pouch of Douglas, it fills the lateral paravesical recesses and then ascends the paracolic gutters.
- On the left side, its cephalad extent is limited by the phrenicocolic ligament.
- Fluid in the right paracolic gutter reaches the Morison pouch and subsequently the right subphrenic space.

- Rate of fluid accumulation is determined by the presence of adhesions, fluid density, and peritoneal, mesenteric, and omental ligaments and reflections.
- Pathways of intraperitoneal fluid distribution may be seen.
- Fluid in inframesocolic space seeks the pelvis: on the right, through the leaves of the small bowel mesentery; on the left, through the medial side of the rectosigmoid.
- After fluid fills the pouch of Douglas, it fills the lateral paravesical recesses and then ascends the paracolic gutters.
- On the left, its cephalad extent is limited by the phrenicocolic ligament.
- Fluid in right paracolic gutter reaches the Morison pouch and subsequently the right subphrenic space.

Suggested Readings
Proto AV, Lane EJ, Marangola JP: A new concept of ascitic fluid distribution. *AJR Am J Roentgenol 126*:974-980, 1976.
Raval B, Lakmi N: CT demonstration of preferential routes of the spread of pelvic disease. *Crit Rev Diagn Imaging* 26:17-48, 1987.
Wahl RL, Gyves J, Gross BH, et al: SPECT of the peritoneal cavity: Method of delineating intraperitoneal fluid distribution. *AJR Am J Roentgenol* 152:1205-1210, 1989.
Wojtowicz L, Rzymski K, Czarnecki R: A CT evaluation of intraperitoneal fluid distribution. *Rofo* 137:95-99, 1982.

WHAT THE REFERRING PHYSICIAN NEEDS TO KNOW
- Infectious, inflammatory, hemorrhagic processes tend to spread along preexisting pathways provided by the various abdominal and pelvic ligaments, mesenteries, and omenta.

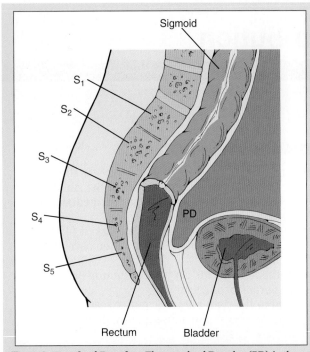

Figure 1. Pouch of Douglas. The pouch of Douglas (PD) is the most dependent portion of the peritoneal cavity and a common site for abscess formation and drop metastases. This sagittal diagram shows the anatomic relationship of this space and indicates the positions of the sacral segments of the spine (S1 through S5). (*From Meyers MA: Distribution of intra-abdominal malignant fluid. AJR Am J Roentgenol 111:198-206, 1973.*)

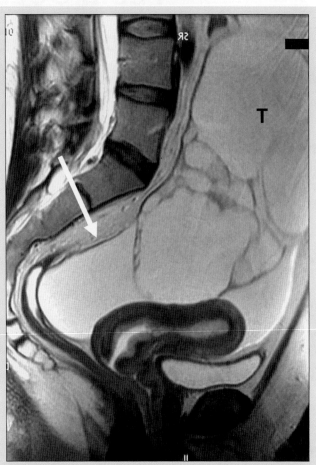

Figure 2. Pouch of Douglas. Sagittal, T2-weighted MR image shows malignant fluid (*arrow*) distending the pouch of Douglas resulting from a large ovarian neoplasm (T). (*Courtesy of Rodney H. Reznek, MD, London, UK.*)

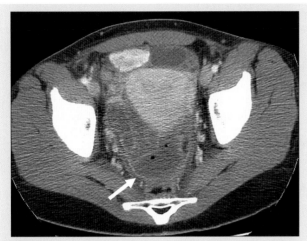

Figure 3. **Pouch of Douglas abscess.** A gas-containing pouch of Douglas abscess *(arrow)* is demonstrated on this CT scan of a patient 10 days after an appendectomy.

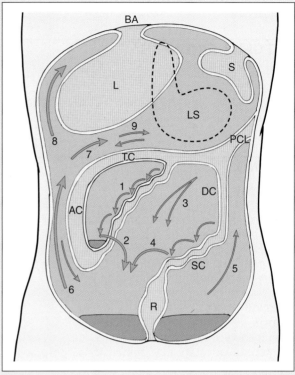

Figure 4. **Common pathways of intraperitoneal fluid spread.** Fluid in the right inframesocolic space (1) cascades down the leaves of the small-bowel mesentery, pools at the medial aspect of the cecum, and then overflows into the pelvis (2). Fluid in the left inframesocolic space (3) seeks the pelvis directly or is deposited on the superior aspect of the sigmoid mesocolon and then flows into the pelvis (4). Fluid in the pelvis may ascend the left paracolic gutter (5) but is stopped by the phrenicocolic ligament (PCL). Fluid in the right paracolic gutter (6) ascends to the Morison pouch (7) and then to the subphrenic space (8), where it is stopped at the bare area (BA) of the liver (L). Potential communication exists with the lesser sac (LS) through the foramen of Winslow (9). (*AC,* Ascending colon; *DC,* descending colon; *R,* rectum; *S,* spleen; *SC,* sigmoid colon; *TC,* transverse colon.)

Peritoneal Fluid Collections

DEFINITION: Ascites is the pathologic accumulation of fluid in the peritoneal cavity.

ANATOMIC FINDINGS

- Fluid in the supramesocolic space usually first accumulates in Morison pouch.
- Fluid in the inframesocolic space usually first accumulates in the cul-de-sac or pouch of Douglas.

IMAGING

Radiography
Findings
- Chylous effusions: Superior mediastinal mass with tracheal deviation may be seen.

Utility
- More than 500 mL of fluid is required for ascites to be diagnosed on abdominal radiographs.

Ultrasound
Findings
- Homogeneous, freely mobile, anechoic collection in the peritoneal cavity that demonstrates deep acoustic enhancement
- Exudate: coarse internal echoes (blood), fine internal echoes (chyle), and multiple septa (tuberculous peritonitis or pseudomyxoma peritonei)
- Pseudomyxoma peritonei: varied appearance; highly echogenic masses containing scattered cystic spaces and multiple rounded, echo-dense masses; liver edge scalloping
- Cerebrospinal fluid ascites: a nonspecific, localized fluid collection in association with a shunt tube tip (pathologic); implies malfunction of shunt
- Hemorrhage (highly variable)

Utility
- Ultrasound is the most sensitive means of detecting a small amount of intraperitoneal fluid.

CT
Findings
- Low-density fluid collection
- Chylous ascites: the presence of intraperitoneal and extraperitoneal water-density fluid in trauma patients
- Urine ascites and cerebrospinal fluid ascites: nonspecific appearance
- Characterizing the nature of peritoneal fluid collection is difficult based on CT density.

DIAGNOSTIC PEARLS

- Exudate: coarse internal echoes (blood), fine internal echoes (chyle), and multiple septa (tuberculous peritonitis or pseudomyxoma peritonei)
- Cerebrospinal fluid ascites: nonspecific; localized fluid collection in association with a shunt tube tip (pathologic); implies malfunction of shunt
- Chylous ascites: the presence of intraperitoneal and extraperitoneal water-density fluid in trauma patients

- Density of ascitic fluid increases with increasing protein content and with exudates.

Utility
- CT is superior to ultrasound in showing the full extent of ascites and determining its cause.

MRI
Findings
- Exudates: intermediate to short T1 values and long T2 values
- T1 relaxation time of fluid decreases with increasing protein content.

Utility
- MRI is superior to CT in depicting the full extent of ascites and determining its cause.

CLINICAL PRESENTATION

- Small amount of ascites is often asymptomatic.
- As the amount of fluid increases, the patient develops a sense of fullness, discomfort, and abdominal distention.
- Weight gain usually accompanies fluid accumulation.
- With massive, tense ascites the patient may present with the abdominal compartment syndrome.

DIFFERENTIAL DIAGNOSIS

- Pleural effusion

WHAT THE REFERRING PHYSICIAN NEEDS TO KNOW

- Paracentesis should be performed in patients who develop ascites for the first time and patients with chronic ascites, with fever, encephalopathy, and abdominal pain.
- Fluid should be analyzed for protein, lactate dehydrogenase, amylase, a blood cell count with differential, bacteriologic and cytologic tests, and assessment of pH and triglycerides.

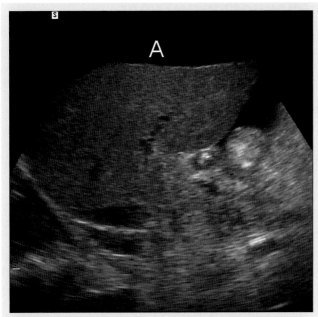

Figure 1. Ascites: sonographic findings. Sonogram of transudative ascites in a patient with cirrhosis of the liver shows anechoic fluid and an echogenic liver.

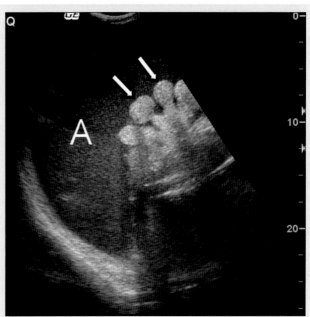

Figure 2. Ascites: sonographic findings. Sonogram shows malignant ascites in a patient with carcinomatosis caused by gastric cancer. Notice the echogenic fluid (A) and bowel loops that are tethered posteriorly. Normally, these loops should be freely flowing.

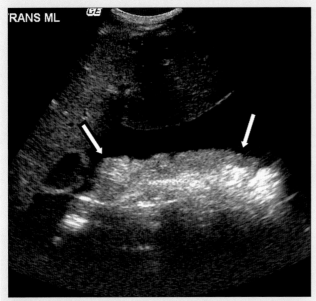

Figure 3. Ascites: sonographic findings. Peritoneal implants *(arrows)* are present in this patient with carcinomatosis.

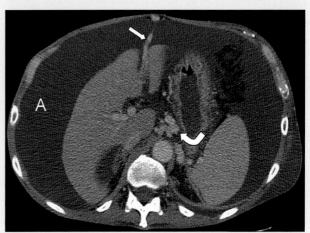

Figure 4. Ascites: CT features. Benign, transudative ascites (A) in a patient with cirrhosis and portal hypertension. The recanalized umbilical vein *(straight arrow)* and varices in the gastrohepatic ligament *(curved arrow)* can be seen.

PATHOLOGY

- Transudates: clear and colorless fluid collections with a protein content of less than 2.5 g/dL and a specific gravity of less than 1.016
- Exudates: yellowish fluid collections with a density greater than 1.016 and protein content greater than 2.5 g/dL; possibly hemorrhagic
- Hemorrhagic ascites: hepatic or splenic trauma resulting from an accident, surgery, or biopsy
- Pus: present in the peritoneal cavity in patients with acute peritonitis
- Chylous ascites: yellowish white, milky fluid from obstruction or disruption of lymph flow through the cisterna chyli and thoracic duct
- Pseudomyxoma peritonei: a massive accumulation of gelatinous, mucinous material in the peritoneal cavity, mesentery, and omentum
- Cerebrospinal fluid ascites: peritoneal cavity failing to absorb fluid or lymphatic diminishing the return of fluid to the bloodstream

INCIDENCE/PREVALENCE AND EPIDEMIOLOGY

- Transudates are most commonly seen in patients with cirrhosis, long-standing heart failure, constrictive pericarditis, chronic renal failure, hypoproteinemia, or anasarca.
- Pus is most often seen in young patients with pneumococcal or hemolytic streptococcal peritonitis.

Suggested Readings

Cattau EL, Benjamin SB, Knuff TE, et al: The accuracy of the physical examination in the diagnosis of suspected ascites. *JAMA* 247:1164-1166, 1966.

Lipsky MS, Sternbach MR: Evaluation and initial management of patients with ascites. *Am Fam Physician* 54:1327-1333, 1996.

Rosner MH, Gupta R, Ellison D, Okusa MD: Management of cirrhotic ascites: Physiological basis of diuretic action. *Eur J Intern Med* 17:8-19, 2006.

Runyon BA: Ascites and spontaneous bacterial peritonitis. In Feldman M, Friedman LS, Sleisenger MH (eds): *Gastrointestinal and Liver Disease*, 7th ed. Philadelphia, WB Saunders, 2002, pp 1154-1517.

Thoeni RF: The role of imaging in patients with ascites. *AJR Am J Roentgenol* 165:16-18, 1995.

Part 62 MESENTERIC AND OMENTAL LESIONS

Small Bowel Carcinoid Tumor

DEFINITION: Tumors derived from the endocrine amine precursor uptake and decarboxylation (APUD) cells.

IMAGING

MRI
Findings
- Mesenteric mass: low T1 signal intensity and intermediate T2 signal intensity; demonstrates evidence of contrast enhancement
- Focus of calcification
- Radiating strands from mesenteric mass, indicative of thickened neurovascular bundles

Utility
- MRI is inferior to CT in showing the calcification that often accompanies this neoplasm.

CT
Findings
- Increased stranding in the mesentery
- Mesenteric mass
- Mesenteric calcification

Utility
- CT is the best cross-sectional imaging test for depicting this neoplasm.

CLINICAL PRESENTATION

- Vague abdominal discomfort
- Small bowel obstruction
- Carcinoid syndrome

DIFFERENTIAL DIAGNOSIS

- Mesenteric panniculitis
- Retractile mesenteritis
- Crohn disease
- Mesenteric metastases

PATHOLOGY

- Rare tumors
- Derived from endocrine APUD cells

DIAGNOSTIC PEARLS

- Mesenteric mass: low T1 signal intensity and intermediate T2 signal intensity, demonstrating evidence of contrast enhancement
- Focus of calcification
- Radiating strands from the mesenteric mass

- Most frequently found in the appendix (50%) and ileum
- Metastatic adenopathy involving mesenteric nodes seen with small bowel carcinoids
- Intense desmoplastic reaction surrounding a mesenteric mass, causing radiating strands from the mesenteric mass, rigidity, and small bowel loop fixation and kinking
- Calcification within mesenteric mass in 70% of cases

INCIDENCE/PREVALENCE AND EPIDEMIOLOGY

- Two percent of all gastrointestinal tumors
- Second most common small bowel neoplasm
- Eighty-five percent of all carcinoid tumors in gastrointestinal tract

Suggested Readings

Bader TR, Semelka RC, Chiu VC, et al: MRI of carcinoid tumors: Spectrum of appearances in the gastrointestinal tract and liver. *J Magn Reson Imaging* 14:261-269, 2001.

Pelage JP, Soyer P, Boudiaf M, et al: Carcinoid tumors of the abdomen: CT features. *Abdom Imaging* 24:240-245, 1999.

Wallace S, Ajanai JA, Charnsangavej C, et al: Carcinoid tumors: Imaging procedures and interventional radiology. *World J Surg* 20:147-156, 1996.

WHAT THE REFERRING PHYSICIAN NEEDS TO KNOW

- Mesenteric fibrosis may also involve mesenteric vasculature and potentially cause mesenteric ischemia.

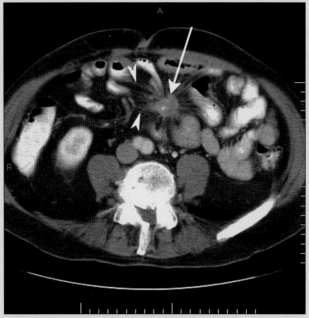

Figure 1. Carcinoid. Carcinoid tumor lymph node metastasis in the mesentery with a focus of calcification *(arrow)* and with adjacent radiating strands is indicative of thickened neurovascular bundles *(arrowheads)*.

Peritoneal Carcinomatosis

DEFINITION: Intra-abdominal metastatic disease resulting from tumors arising from the gastrointestinal tract, pancreas, breast, lung, and ovary or from melanoma.

IMAGING

CT
Findings
- Nodularity, which can progress to peritoneal masses
- Mass effect on organs adjacent to them
- Scalloping of the liver and spleen
- Mesenteric infiltration and thickening, leading to a stellate mesentery
- Involves the surface of the bowel, causing bowel wall thickening and possible obstruction

Utility
- CT is very useful in demonstrating malignant ascites and peritoneal, omental, and mesenteric tumors.

MRI
Findings
- Ascites
- Peritoneal, omental, and mesenteric nodules and masses
- Scalloping of the liver and spleen
- Mass effect on organs next to ascites and nodules

Utility
- MRI is very useful in suggesting malignant ascites and showing the full extent of peritoneal omental and mesenteric tumors.

CLINICAL PRESENTATION

- Abdominal distention
- Bowel obstruction
- Weight loss, fatigue, and malaise
- Abdominal compartment syndrome

DIFFERENTIAL DIAGNOSIS

- Acute cholecystitis
- Acute pancreatitis
- Eosinophilic gastroenteritis (small bowel)
- Inflammatory bowel disease

DIAGNOSTIC PEARLS

- Fluid exists in the peritoneal cavity.
- Peritoneal nodules are seen, which can progress to peritoneal masses.
- Nodules involve the surface of the bowel, causing bowel wall thickening and possible obstruction.

- Pancreatic carcinoma
- Gastric carcinoma (stomach and duodenum)
- Tuberculous peritonitis

PATHOLOGY

- Peritoneal carcinomatosis results from tumors arising from the gastrointestinal tract, pancreas, breast, lung, and ovary, as well as from melanoma.
- Peritoneal nodules can often mimic unopacified small-bowel loops.

INCIDENCE/PREVALENCE AND EPIDEMIOLOGY

- Common sites of involvement include the right hemi-diaphragm, right paracolic gutter, cul-de-sac, and omentum.

Suggested Readings

Meyers MA, Mindelzun RE: Peritoneal reflections, ligaments, recesses, and mesenteries. In Margulis AR (ed): *Modern Imaging of the Alimentary Tube.* Berlin, Springer-Verlag, 1998, pp 247-256.

Meyers MA, Oliphant M, Berne AS, Feldberg MA: The peritoneal ligaments and mesenteries: Pathways of intraabdominal spread of disease. *Radiology* 163:593-604, 1987.

Pannu HK, Bristow RE, Montz FJ, Fishman EK: Multidetector CT of peritoneal carcinomatosis from ovarian cancer. *RadioGraphics* 23:687-701, 2003.

WHAT THE REFERRING PHYSICIAN NEEDS TO KNOW

- Detection of peritoneal carcinomatosis is difficult in the absence of ascites, especially when the nodules are smaller than 1 cm in diameter.
- Accurate assessment for peritoneal carcinomatosis requires adequate bowel opacification and the administration of intravenous contrast.

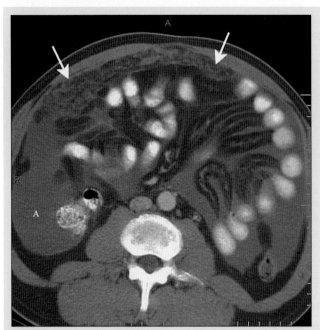

Figure 1. Ovarian carcinomatosis. CT demonstrates subtle nodularity and stranding of the mesentery and more apparent nodularity along the greater omentum *(arrows)* in a patient with ovarian cancer. A small amount of ascites (A) also can be seen.

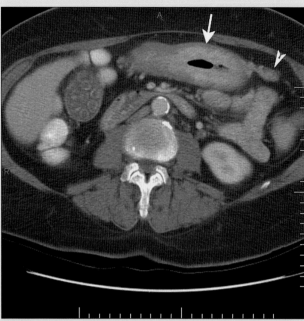

Figure 2. Carcinoma of the stomach. Gastric carcinoma with diffuse gastric wall thickening has a linitis plastica appearance on CT *(arrow)*. Notice the adjacent peritoneal involvement of the gastrocolic ligament *(arrowhead)*.

Primary Neoplasms of the Mesentery

DEFINITION: Primary tumors of the mesentery, usually of mesenchymal origin.

IMAGING

CT

Findings
- Desmoid tumors: nonenhancing to partly enhancing solid lesions; lack of mass effect of fibrosis
- Peritoneal mesothelioma: large peritoneal masses, diffuse peritoneal nodules, and peritoneal thickening, including omental caking and mesenteric infiltration (stellate, fixed appearance)
- Benign cystic peritoneal mesothelioma: well-defined, noncalcified, multiloculated cystic mass with enhancing internal septations
- Desmoplastic small round cell tumor: multiple, large, solid, intraperitoneal mass without an apparent primary site
- Benign lipoma: well-defined, homogeneous lesion containing tissue of fat attenuation
- Liposarcomas: ill-defined, heterogeneous lesions with a variable soft-tissue component; fat interspersed with the soft-tissue component or areas of enhancement

Utility
- Multidetector CT is an excellent means of evaluating desmoid tumors and their relation to surrounding structures.
- It is also used as part of the follow-up of patients who undergo conservative medical therapy.

Ultrasound

Findings
- Desmoid tumors: well-demarcated, solid masses containing low- to mid-level echoes
- Benign cystic peritoneal mesothelioma: multiloculated lesion containing anechoic cystic spaces separated by septations

Utility
- Ultrasound is inferior to CT and MRI in showing the full extent of primary neoplasms of the mesentery.

MRI

Findings
- Desmoid tumors: low T1 and T2 signal intensity, with no or poor enhancement
- Benign cystic peritoneal mesothelioma: well-defined, multiloculated cystic mass with enhancing septations

DIAGNOSTIC PEARLS

- Desmoid tumors produce locally aggressive fibroblast proliferation or fibromatosis.
- Malignant mesothelioma produces an aggressive tumor and mesenteric infiltration.
- Benign cystic peritoneal mesothelioma produces a multiloculated cystic mass and internal septations.
- Desmoplastic small round cell tumors are intraperitoneal masses.

Utility
- MRI is the best noninvasive technique for characterizing neoplasms of the mesentery.

CLINICAL PRESENTATION

- Desmoid tumor: progressive growth may lead to bowel, ureteric, or vascular obstruction and, occasionally, fistulas.
- Malignant mesothelioma: symptoms are nonspecific and include abdominal pain, distention, weight loss, and malaise.
- In primary papillary serous carcinoma, multicentric involvement of peritoneum is associated with omental caking and ascites.
- Desmoplastic small round cell tumor produces abdominal distention, ascites, and hepatic metastases.

DIFFERENTIAL DIAGNOSIS

- Mesenteric metastases
- Mesenteric panniculitis
- Mesenteric hemorrhage
- Mesenteric adenopathy
- Crohn disease involving mesentery

PATHOLOGY

- Primary tumors arising from peritoneum are rare, usually of mesenchymal origin.

WHAT THE REFERRING PHYSICIAN NEEDS TO KNOW

- Desmoid tumors are associated with prior surgery such as colectomy and often recur at the surgical site.
- Fifty-five percent of patients fail to demonstrate evidence of asbestosis on chest radiographs.
- In primary papillary serous carcinoma, calcification seen with this tumor can help differentiate it from malignant mesothelioma.
- In primary papillary serous carcinoma, assessment for primary ovarian masses should be performed to exclude peritoneal carcinomatosis from ovarian cancer.

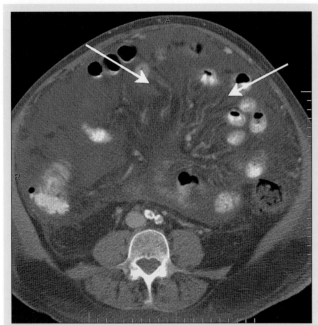

Figure 1. Malignant mesothelioma with splayed and fixed mesenteric leaves *(arrows)*. Each is encased by a thin layer of soft tissue, representing the tumor, and is surrounded by ascites.

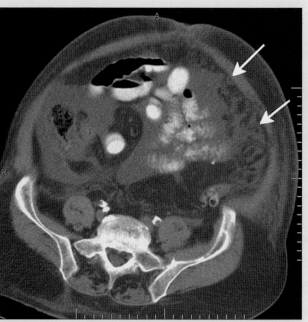

Figure 2. CT scan in the same patient at a more caudal level demonstrates soft-tissue nodules involving the greater omentum *(arrows)*.

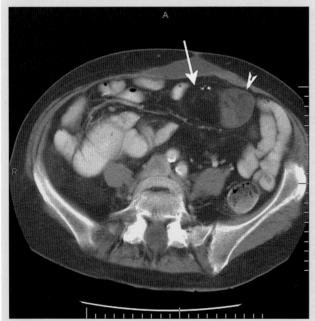

Figure 3. Mesenteric liposarcoma. Liposarcoma with a fatty portion of the tumor *(arrow)* and a soft-tissue portion *(arrowhead)*.

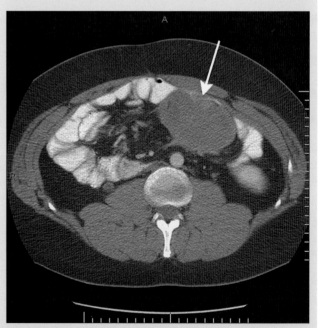

Figure 4. Mesenteric desmoid tumor. The mass displaces the surrounding small bowel loops *(arrow)* and has well-defined margins laterally and slightly irregular margins medially.

- Abdominal desmoids can involve the abdominal wall, mesentery, or retroperitoneum.
- Desmoids are pseudoencapsulated lesions despite their relatively well-defined gross appearance; microscopically, margins are infiltrated.
- Malignant mesothelioma is a rare but aggressive tumor that arises from the serosa lining the pleura and peritoneum.
- Benign cystic peritoneal mesothelioma is a rare but benign multilocular malignancy, producing a cystic neoplasm arising from the peritoneum.
- Primary papillary serous carcinoma is a rare malignancy that typically occurs in postmenopausal women.
- Primary tumors can arise from mesenchymal structures, and they may be of fatty, vascular, lymphatic, or neurogenic tissue origin.

INCIDENCE/PREVALENCE AND EPIDEMIOLOGY

- Desmoid tumors occur in 9%-18% of patients, with familial adenomatous polyposis accounting for approximately 45% of fibrous lesions.
- The most common site for mesenteric desmoids is at the base of the small-bowel mesentery.
- Malignant mesotheliomas account for 30%-45% of all mesotheliomas; a male predilection has been found.
- Malignant mesothelioma has a dismal prognosis, with a median survival time of 8-12 months after diagnosis.
- Benign cystic peritoneal mesothelioma occurs in women of reproductive age and tends to recur locally in 25%-50% of cases.
- Primary papillary serous carcinoma is seen in patients who have had a bilateral salpingo-oophorectomy and even in men.

- Desmoplastic small round cell tumor is an extremely aggressive tumor occurring in male adolescents and young adults, with poor median survival rates.

Suggested Readings

Antman KH: Malignant mesothelioma. *N Engl J Med* 303:200-202, 1980.

Brooks AP, Reznek RH, Nugent K, et al: CT appearances of desmoid tumors in familial adenomatous polyposis: Further observations. *Clin Radiol* 49:601-607, 1994.

Chopra S, Laurie LR, Chintapalli KN, et al: Primary papillary serous carcinoma of the peritoneum: CT-pathologic correlation. *J Comput Assist Tomogr* 24:395-399, 2000.

Chouli M, Viala J, Dromain C, et al: Intra-abdominal desmoplastic small round cell tumors: CT findings and clinicopathological correlations in 13 cases. *Eur J Radiol* 54:438-442, 2005.

Guest PJ, Reznek RH, Selleslag D, et al: Peritoneal mesothelioma: The role of computed tomography in diagnosis and follow-up. *Clin Radiol* 45:79-84, 1992.

Gupta S, Gupta RK, Gujral RB, et al: Peritoneal mesothelioma simulating pseudomyxoma peritonei on CT and sonography. *Gastrointest Radiol* 17:129-131, 1992.

Healy JC, Reznek RH, Clark SK, et al: MR appearances of desmoid tumors in familial adenomatous polyposis. *AJR* 169:465-472, 1997.

Jones IT, Jagelman DG, Fazio VW, et al: Desmoid tumors in familial polyposis coli. *Ann Surg* 204:94-97, 1986.

O'Neil JD, Ros PR, Storm BL, et al: Cystic mesothelioma of the peritoneum. *Radiology* 170:333-337, 1989.

Ozgen A, Akata D, Akhan O, et al: Giant benign cystic peritoneal mesothelioma: US, CT, and MRI findings. *Abdom Imaging* 23:502-504, 1998.

Pickhardt PJ, Fisher AJ, Balfe DM, et al: Desmoplastic small round cell tumor of the abdomen: Radiologic-histopathologic correlation. *Radiology* 210:633-638, 1999.

Primary Neoplasms of the Omentum

DEFINITION: Neoplasms, found primarily in the omentum, can include tumors of mesenchymal origin.

IMAGING

CT

Findings
- Soft tissue mass in greater omentum

Utility
- CT is the most commonly used imaging modality in the assessment of omental or peritoneal disease.
- Optimal bowel contrast opacification is critical in the imaging of patients with suspected omental or peritoneal disease.
- Lack of intra-abdominal fat may make the visualization of omental disease difficult.

Radiography

Findings
- Indirect evidence of omental infiltration may be inferred by the mass effect, tethering of folds, or luminal narrowing on barium studies.

Utility
- Plain abdominal radiographs rarely depict omental disease.
- In cases of large omental masses, secondary signs related to the displacement of the bowel loops may help determine the diagnosis.

Ultrasound

Findings
- Soft tissue mass in greater omentum

Utility
- Ultrasound may be of help in patients with large omental masses; distinguishing a smaller mass from the bowel loops is difficult.
- Ultrasound is operator dependent, making reproducibility and assessment of response challenging.

CLINICAL PRESENTATION

- Symptoms occur late in the course of disease, are nonspecific, and may be related to abdominal bloating and pain.
- Abdominal mass

DIAGNOSTIC PEARLS

- Omental infiltration
- Tethering of folds
- Luminal narrowing
- Optimal bowel contrast opacification

DIFFERENTIAL DIAGNOSIS

- Omental infarction
- Omental metastases
- Omental abscess
- Omental hematoma
- Omental tuberculosis

PATHOLOGY

- Primary omental neoplasms are rare; they include tumors of mesenchymal origin, such as lipoma or liposarcoma, lipoblastoma, fibroma or fibrosarcoma, and leiomyoma or leiomyosarcoma.
- Omentum is affected secondarily in diseases such as peritoneal carcinomatosis and is involved in inflammatory processes affecting the peritoneum and adjacent organs.

INCIDENCE/PREVALANCE AND EPIDEMIOLOGY

- Primary omental neoplasms are quite rare. More commonly the omentum is affected by metastases in Western countries and tuberculosis in Asian countries.

Suggested Readings

Cooper C, Jeffrey RB, Silverman PM, et al: Computed tomography of omental pathology. *J Comput Assist Tomogr* 10:62-66, 1986.

Sompayrac SW, Mindelzun RE, Silverman PM, et al: Greater omentum. *AJR Am J Roentgenol* 168:683-688, 1997.

Takahashi T, Kuwao S, Yanagihara M, et al: A primary solitary tumor of the omentum with immunohistochemical features of gastrointestinal stromal tumors. *Am J Gastroenterol* 93:2269-2273, 1998.

WHAT THE REFERRING PHYSICIAN NEEDS TO KNOW

- The presence of an omental mass should prompt a search for a primary extraomental malignancy.
- If no extraomental tumor is found, a primary neoplasm of the omentum should be considered.

Part 63

HERNIAS AND ABDOMINAL WALL PATHOLOGY

Abdominal Wall Fluid Collections

DEFINITION: Includes hematoma, urinoma, abscess, and cellulitis.

ANATOMIC FINDINGS

Abdominal Wall
- Hematomas of the anterior abdominal wall frequently involve the rectus sheath, although lateral collections do occur.

IMAGING

Ultrasound
Findings
- Cellulitis and phlegmon have ill-defined margins, with the exception of any margin sharply defined by the fascial plane.
Utility
- Ultrasound is used to differentiate cellulitis or phlegmon from a frank abscess.
- Ultrasound appearances of blood vary with the age of the clot and the hematocrit of the patient.

CT
Findings
- Hematoma: hyperdensity within areas of the clot and surrounded by lower-attenuation collections of serum
- Urinomas: intraperitoneal fluid
- Smaller abdominal wall abscesses: usually ovoid or spindle shaped; more mass-like when large
- Cellulitis and phlegmon: ill-defined margins, with the exception of any margin sharply defined by the fascial plane
Utility
- CT is used to differentiate cellulitis or phlegmon from a frank abscess.
- It is the imaging procedure of choice for inflammatory lesions of the abdominal wall.
- CT appearances of blood vary with the age of the clot and the hematocrit of the patient.

DIAGNOSTIC PEARLS
- Hematoma: hyperdensity within the areas of the clot and surrounded by lower-attenuation collections of serum
- Smaller abdominal wall abscesses: usually ovoid or spindle shaped; more mass-like when large
- Cellulitis and phlegmon: ill-defined margins, with the exception of any margin sharply defined by the fascial plane

MRI
Findings
- Hematoma: highly variable and frequently indistinguishable from a tumor or abscess
- Cellulitis and phlegmon: ill-defined margins, with the exception of any margin sharply defined by the fascial plane
Utility
- MRI is used to differentiate cellulitis or phlegmon from a frank abscess.
- It can help characterize the nature of the abdominal wall fluid collection.

Radiography
Findings
- Necrotizing fasciitis: soft-tissue gas
Utility
- Cystography is required whenever bladder rupture or a urethral injury is suspected.

CLINICAL PRESENTATION
- Pain, blood loss, ecchymosis, and abdominal mass may suggest hematoma, but clinical signs are often absent or nonspecific.
- Pain or fever may suggest abscess or other acute intra-abdominal process.

WHAT THE REFERRING PHYSICIAN NEEDS TO KNOW
- Evidence for underlying causative factors of abscess should be sought.
- Urinomas, abscesses, or lymphoceles starting in the prevesical space can mimic rectus sheath hematoma if they track cranially.
- Arterial puncture in the femoral sheath with subsequent hematoma formation has the potential to involve the anterior abdominal wall.
- Subcutaneous abscess may respond to a simple incision and drainage; deeper lesions may require more aggressive therapy.

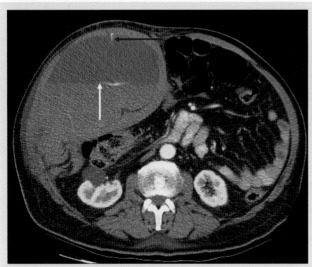

Figure 1. Lateral abdominal wall hematoma. A hematocrit effect *(arrow)* is identified. Notice the active extravasation of contrast *(red arrow)*.

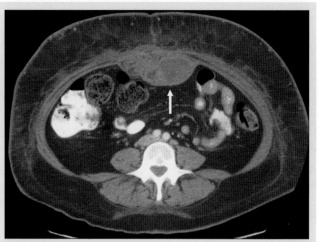

Figure 2. Abdominal wall abscess. An abscess *(arrow)* involves the rectus abdominis muscles in this postoperative patient. Notice the inflammatory changes in the subcutaneous fat.

DIFFERENTIAL DIAGNOSIS

- Abdominal wall primary neoplasm
- Abdominal wall metastatic neoplasm
- Ventral hernia
- Caput medusae

PATHOLOGY

- Hematomas originate from tears in muscle fibers or blood vessels and may be spontaneous or related to trauma.
- Abscess of the anterior abdominal wall can be postoperative, post-traumatic, or spontaneous.
- Necrotizing fasciitis arises spontaneously or from blunt-force or penetrating trauma, surgery, venous stasis, or decubitus ulcers.

INCIDENCE/PREVALENCE AND EPIDEMIOLOGY

- Abscess often occurs in postoperative or critically ill patients, with concomitant sepsis.
- Necrotizing fasciitis is a rare form of aggressive, soft-tissue infection usually seen in diabetics or alcoholics.

Suggested Readings

Goodman P, Balachandran S: CT evaluation of the abdominal wall. *Crit Rev Diagn Imaging* 33:461-493, 1992.
Wechsler RJ (ed): *Cross-Sectional Analysis of the Chest and Abdominal Wall*. St. Louis, CV Mosby, 1989, pp 126-202.

Abdominal Wall Hernias

DEFINITION: Herniations through the walls of the abdominal cavity.

ANATOMIC FINDINGS

Abdominal Wall
- Spigelian hernias occur in the anterolateral aspect of the lower abdomen, along the semilunar line.
- Umbilical hernias occur at the umbilicus.
- Lumbar hernias are located at the flank, more frequently on the left side.
- In an incisional hernia, the most common sites of involvement are along the midline and paramedian incisions.

IMAGING

Ultrasound
Findings
- Umbilical hernia: bowel protruding through an umbilical defect
- Ventral hernia: ventral herniation of omental fat
- Incisional hernia: visualization of the bowel loop, causing acoustic shadowing within the disrupted abdominal wall layers beneath the healed scar

Utility
- Hernias are often best detected with the patient standing and straining.

CT
Findings
- Umbilical hernia: bowel protruding through an umbilical defect
- Ventral hernia: herniated small bowel and mesentery
- Spigelian hernia: herniated small bowel through a peritoneal defect at the lateral border of the right rectus muscle
- Lumbar hernia: colon and mesentery herniating posterolaterally through the left inferior lumbar space or Petit triangle
- Incisional hernia: as with many hernias, ischemic changes, possibly resulting from strangulated bowel loops

Utility
- CT is used to show the precise anatomic site of the hernia sac, shape of the sac, connections, and contents, as well as the hernia cuff and surrounding wall.

DIAGNOSTIC PEARLS

- Bowel loop or mesentery herniating through the abdominal wall defect, as seen through CT, MRI, or radiography
- Bowel loop causing acoustic shadowing within the disrupted abdominal wall layers

- CT also shows complications of the intestinal, vascular, omental, and mesenteric wall and the cavity of the hernia sac.
- It offers exquisite detail of the anterior abdominal and pelvic wall.
- It can also detect postoperative complications and characterize hematomas, abscesses, and neoplasms.

MRI
Findings
- Bowel and fat are seen in hernia sacs.

Utility
- MRI shows the origin and extent of these lesions.
- It can also reveal a defect and associated herniation in the ventral wall of the abdomen.

Radiography
Findings
- Umbilical hernia: distended bowel loops and soft tissue-like density
- Ventral hernia: distended bowel loops proximal to a narrowing or obstruction close to the locally tender part of the abdominal wall
- Spigelian hernia: small-bowel hernia through the semilunar line

Utility
- Coned-down lateral or cross-table view can be helpful in detecting omental fat or bowel loops in umbilical hernias.
- Barium studies of the small or large intestine can show obstruction or protrusion of the gut in the umbilical region.
- CT is now the primary means of evaluating suspected abdominal wall hernias.

WHAT THE REFERRING PHYSICIAN NEEDS TO KNOW

- Most herniations involving the anterior abdominal wall or groin can be easily diagnosed by inspection and palpation.
- Ventral hernia: Incarceration and strangulation of contents may occur frequently and produce symptoms that are out of proportion to the objective findings.
- Lumbar hernia: Bowel incarceration occurs in approximately 25% and may lead to strangulation in approximately 10% of cases.

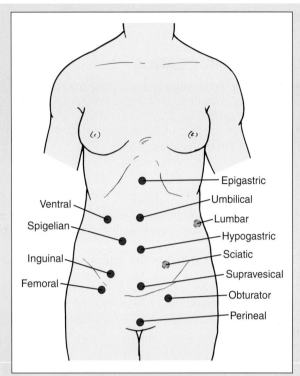

Figure 1. Types and locations of hernias. Herniations through the walls of the abdominal cavity usually involve specific sites of congenital weakness or a previous surgical incision.

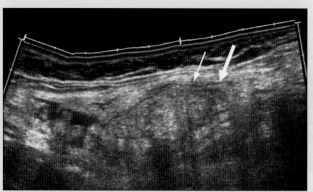

Figure 2. Ventral hernia. The longitudinal sonogram shows a ventral herniation of omental fat *(arrows)*.

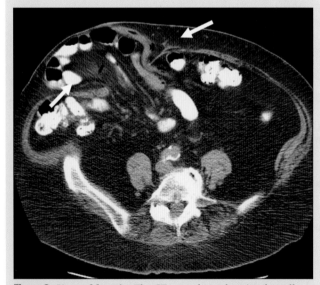

Figure 3. Ventral hernia. The CT scan shows herniated small bowel and mesentery *(arrow)*.

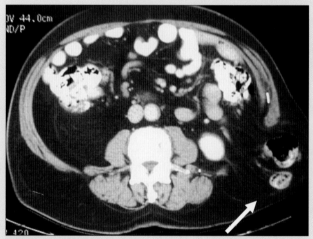

Figure 4. Lumbar hernia. CT shows the descending colon and mesentery herniating *(arrow)* posterolaterally through the left inferior lumbar space or Petit triangle.

CLINICAL PRESENTATION

- Umbilical hernia is a soft, often asymptomatic, bulge that tends to disappear spontaneously.
- Incarcerated umbilical hernia should be suspected in the patient with intestinal obstruction and umbilical tenderness, even if no obvious bulge is noted on the surface.
- Ventral hernia causes pain that is aggravated by exertion and is associated with focal tenderness of the abdominal wall.
- Spigelian hernia is characterized by a prolonged history of intermittent lower abdominal pain and intestinal obstruction associated with a vanishing anterolateral mass.
- Lumbar hernia causes chronic low back pain and intestinal obstruction, as well as a soft, bulging mass in the flank.

DIFFERENTIAL DIAGNOSIS

- Abdominal wall hematoma
- Abdominal wall abscess
- Primary abdominal wall neoplasm
- Metastatic abdominal wall neoplasm

PATHOLOGY

- Results from congenital or acquired weakness in the abdominal wall, with or without increased intra-abdominal pressure

INCIDENCE/PREVALENCE AND EPIDEMIOLOGY

- Abdominal wall hernias account for approximately 750,000 operations per year in the United States.
- They develop in approximately 1.5% of the population and usually involve specific sites of congenital weakness or a previous surgical incision.
- Adult umbilical hernias occur in women with multiple pregnancies, in obese patients, or patients with increased abdominal pressure.
- Spigelian hernias occur with equal frequency in men and women; they are bilateral and are associated with other ventral or inguinal hernias.
- Lumbar hernias occur in middle-aged men.
- Incisional hernias occur in approximately 5% of patients during the first 4 months after surgery.

Suggested Readings

Aguirre DA, Casola G, Sirlin C: Abdominal wall hernias: MDCT findings. *AJR Am J Roentgenol* 183:681-690, 2004.

Aguirre DA, Santosa AC, Casola G, et al: Abdominal wall hernias: Imaging features, complications, and diagnostic pitfalls at multidetector row CT. *RadioGraphics* 25:1501-1520, 2005.

Baker ME, Weinerth JL, Andriani JL, et al: Lumbar hernia: Diagnosis by CT. *AJR Am J Roentgenol* 148:565-567, 1987.

Balthazar EJ, Subramanyam BR, Megibow A: Spigelian hernia: CT and ultrasonography diagnosis. *Gastrointest Radiol* 9:81-84, 1984.

Abdominal Wall Neoplasms

DEFINITION: Neoplastic masses in the abdominal wall, which may be primary malignancies, metastases, or benign tumors.

ANATOMIC FINDINGS

Abdominal Wall
- Gastric cancer has a peculiar predilection to produce isolated metastasis near the umbilicus.
- Desmoid tumors are usually well defined.
- Urachal carcinoma usually arises in the juxtavesical segment of the urachus.

IMAGING

Ultrasound
Findings
- Desmoid tumor: hypoechoic masses are seen.
- Metastases are usually well visualized because of the naturally homogeneous background provided by subcutaneous fat.

Utility
- Ultrasound is inferior to CT and MRI in depicting these neoplasms.

CT
Findings
- Desmoid tumors are hyperdense compared with the muscle, particularly on postcontrast scans.
- Metastases are usually well visualized because of the naturally homogeneous background provided by subcutaneous fat.
- Urachal carcinoma tumors are usually calcified.

Utility
- CT with sagittal and coronal reformatted images can show the complete extent of these tumors.

MRI
Findings
- Desmoid tumor reveals a low signal intensity of fibrous tissue on T1- and T2-weighted images.
- Metastases are usually well visualized because of the naturally homogeneous background provided by subcutaneous fat.

Utility
- MRI shows the origin and extent of the lesions.

DIAGNOSTIC PEARLS
- Desmoid tumors are seen as hypoechoic masses on ultrasound.
- Metastases are usually well visualized.
- Urachal carcinoma tumors are usually calcified.

CLINICAL PRESENTATION
- Urachal carcinoma can cause the passage of blood or mucus in the urine.
- Hormonally responsive endometriomas can be painful at the time of menses.
- Benign lesions produce soft-tissue masses that are discovered incidentally.
- Patients present with abdominal wall mass or bulge that may or may not be painful.

DIFFERENTIAL DIAGNOSIS
- Hematoma
- Seroma
- Hernia
- Muscular atrophy of the contralateral side

PATHOLOGY
- Primary neoplasms of abdominal wall include sarcomas, desmoid tumors (i.e., tumors of mesenchymal origin), and urachal carcinoma.
- Desmoid tumors represent a low-grade, nonmetastasizing variant of fibrosarcoma, with a tendency to arise in the musculoaponeurotic planes.
- Benign tumors include lipomas, neurofibromas, and other mesenchymal tumors.
- Typical primary lesions that cause subcutaneous metastases include melanoma and lung, renal, and ovarian cancer.

WHAT THE REFERRING PHYSICIAN NEEDS TO KNOW
- Desmoid tumor is locally aggressive and may involve the nearby bowel loops, bladder, or adjacent ribs and pelvic bones.
- Differentiating desmoid tumors from various sarcomas is often not possible unless distant metastatic disease is present.

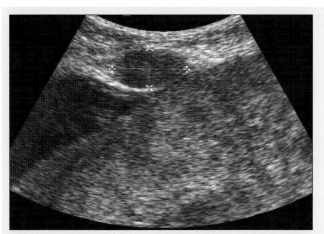

Figure 1. **Abdominal wall metastatic malignancy.** Longitudinal sonogram demonstrates a hypoechoic metastasis *(cursors)* within the subcutaneous fat of the anterior abdominal wall from a gastric carcinoma.

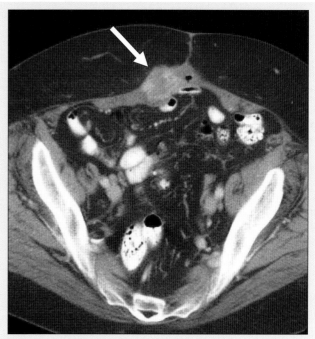

Figure 2. **Abdominal wall metastatic malignancy.** Enhancing abdominal wall metastasis *(arrow)* from colon cancer.

- Direct spread of a variety of intra-abdominal malignancies to the abdominal wall is also common.
- Gastric cancer has a peculiar predilection to produce isolated metastases near the umbilicus.

INCIDENCE/PREVALENCE AND EPIDEMIOLOGY

- Primary malignancies of the anterior abdominal wall are uncommon.
- Endometriomas can occur incorporated in a surgical scar, typically in the setting of a prior cesarean section.
- Urachal carcinoma is a rare lesion, usually occurring in men (75%).
- Desmoid tumors arise frequently in colectomy scars of patients with Gardner syndrome; they are associated with mesentery or paraspinous musculature tumors.

Suggested Readings

Amato MA, Levitt R: Abdominal wall endometrioma: CT findings. *J Comput Assist Tomogr* 8:1213-1214, 1984.

Dunnick NR, Schaner EG, Doppman JL: Detection of subcutaneous metastases by computed tomography. *J Comput Assist Tomogr* 2:275-279, 1978.

Einstein DM, Tagliabue JR, Desai RK: Abdominal desmoids: CT findings in 25 patients. *AJR Am J Roentgenol* 157:275-279, 1991.

Kwok-Liu JP, Zikman JM, Cockshott WP: Carcinoma of the urachus: The role of computed tomography. *Radiology* 137:731-734, 1980.

Shiu MH, Weinstein L, Hajdu SI, et al: Malignant soft-tissue tumors of the anterior abdominal wall. *Am J Surg* 158:446-451, 1989.

Wechsler RJ (ed): *Cross-Sectional Analysis of the Chest and Abdominal Wall*. St. Louis, CV Mosby, 1989, pp 126-202.

Yeh HC, Rabinowitz JG, Rosenblum PJ: Complementary role of CT and ultrasonography in the diagnosis of desmoid tumor of abdominal wall. *Comput Radiol* 6:275-280, 1982.

Diaphragmatic Hernias

DEFINITION: Defect in the diaphragm through which abdominal or retroperitoneal contents pass through to the thoracic cavity.

IMAGING

CT

Findings

- Intrathoracic herniation of abdominal contents
- Foramen of Morgagni hernia: retrosternal diaphragmatic defect
- Foramen of Bochdalek hernia: communication between the thoracic cavity and the retroperitoneal space through a diaphragmatic defect
- Collar or hourglass sign
- Elevated abdominal organs: dependent viscera sign
- Absent diaphragm sign
- Traumatic hernia: active contrast extravasation at the level of the diaphragm; hemoperitoneum and hemothorax; asymmetric thickening of the diaphragm
- Dependent viscera sign

Utility

- CT has a sensitivity ranging between 61% and 100% and a specificity between 77% and 100%.
- Coronal and sagittal reformatting of multidetector CT data may be helpful in establishing the diagnosis.

CLINICAL PRESENTATION

- Traumatic hernias of the diaphragm may present with chest and/or abdominal pain and dysfunction of herniated organs.
- Patients may present as a surgical emergency or may present days, weeks, months, or years later.

DIFFERENTIAL DIAGNOSIS

- Pericardial cyst
- Atelectasis

PATHOLOGY

- Bochdalek hernia is characterized by a pleuropulmonary hiatus defective closure in adults that results from lumbocostal muscle hypoplasia surrounding the Bochdalek foramen.
- Morgagni hernia is a natural weakness of the sternocostal muscular bundles.

DIAGNOSTIC PEARLS

- Foramen of Bochdalek hernia: communication between the thoracic cavity and the retroperitoneal space through a diaphragmatic defect
- Foramen of Morgagni hernia: retrosternal diaphragmatic defect
- Traumatic hernia: active contrast extravasation at the level of the diaphragm; hemoperitoneum and hemothorax; and asymmetric thickening of the diaphragm
- Collar or hourglass sign

- Traumatic hernia develops from blunt force or penetrating trauma.
- Ninety percent of cases of a Morgagni foramen hernia occur on the right side.
- Bochdalek foramen hernia is more common on left than on the right side.
- Left hemidiaphragm is injured three times more often than the right hemidiaphragm in traumatic diaphragmatic hernias.

INCIDENCE/PREVALENCE AND EPIDEMIOLOGY

- Organ herniation occurs in 32%-58% of cases.
- The most frequent injuries associated with diaphragm rupture in motor vehicle accidents include liver and spleen laceration, rib and pelvic fractures, and pulmonary contusion.

Suggested Readings

Bergin D, Ennis R, Keogh C, et al: The "dependent viscera" sign in CT diagnosis of blunt traumatic diaphragmatic rupture. *AJR Am J Roentgenol* 177:1137-1140, 2001.

Eren S, Ciris F: Diaphragmatic hernia: Diagnostic approaches with review of the literature. *Eur J Radiol* 54:448-459, 2005.

Killeen KL, Mirvis SE, Shanmuganathan K, et al: Helical CT of traumatic diaphragmatic rupture secondary to blunt trauma. *AJR Am J Roentgenol* 173:1611-1616, 1999.

Killeen KL, Shanmuganathan K, Mirvis SE: Imaging of traumatic diaphragmatic injuries. *Semin Ultrasound CT MRI* 23:184-192, 2002.

WHAT THE REFERRING PHYSICIAN NEEDS TO KNOW

- Traumatic diaphragmatic ruptures may be an immediate surgical emergency or present days, weeks, months, or years later.
- The most frequent injuries associated with diaphragm rupture in motor vehicle accidents include liver and spleen laceration, rib and pelvic fractures, and pulmonary contusion.
- Bergqvist triad includes rib fractures, spine and/or pelvic fractures, and diaphragmatic rupture.

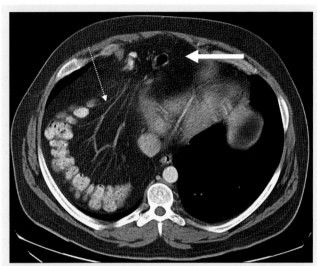

Figure 1. Foramen of Morgagni hernia. CT shows a retrosternal hernia that includes the omentum and colon *(large arrow)*. Notice the fanlike disposition of the mesenteric vessels *(small arrow)* from the front backward.

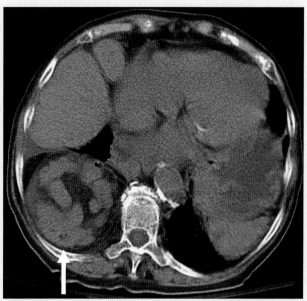

Figure 2. Foramen of Bochdalek hernia. Small bowel *(arrow)* is seen herniated in the right foramen of this Bochdalek hernia.

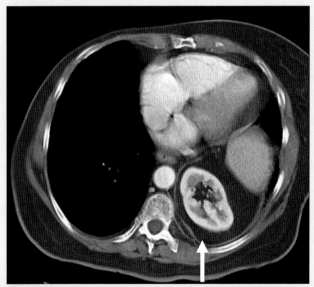

Figure 3. Foramen of Bochdalek hernia. The left kidney and perinephric fat are contained in the left foramen of this Bochdalek hernia *(arrow)*.

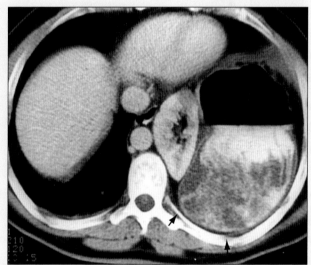

Figure 4. Traumatic diaphragmatic hernia: the dependent viscera sign. In a 32-year-old man with left-sided diaphragmatic rupture, an axial CT scan shows discontinuity of the left hemidiaphragm *(arrows* indicate the extent of the diaphragmatic tear) with gastric and left renal herniation. The stomach lies dependent on the left posterior ribs, which is a positive dependent viscera sign. *(From Bergin D, Ennis R, Keogh C, et al: The "dependent viscera" sign in CT diagnosis of blunt traumatic diaphragmatic rupture. AJR Am J Roentgenol177:1137-1140, 2001. Reprinted with permission from the American Journal of Roentgenology.)*

Internal Abdominal Hernias

DEFINITION: Protrusion of the gut through the peritoneal or mesenteric aperture of the omentum, mesentery, or peritoneal ligament, leading to its encapsulation within another compartment of an otherwise intact abdominal cavity.

ANATOMIC FINDINGS

Peritoneal Cavity

- Paraduodenal fossa of Landzert is located lateral to the ascending or fourth segment of the duodenum beneath the peritoneal fold.
- Fossa of Waldeyer is a pocket in the jejunal mesentery located behind the superior mesenteric artery and inferior to the transverse segment of the duodenum.
- Foramen of Landzert hernia: The small bowel loops enter the sac and herniate into the descending mesocolon and transverse mesocolon.
- Foramen of Waldeyer hernia is a small-bowel herniation into the ascending mesocolon.
- Foramen of Winslow hernia is a protrusion of the viscera into the lesser sac.
- Seventy-five percent of paraduodenal hernias occur on the left side.
- In transmesosigmoid hernias, the small bowel herniates toward the left lower abdomen through a defect between both layers of the sigmoid mesentery.

IMAGING

Radiography

Findings

- Paraduodenal hernias: circumscribed jejunal loops; ovoid mass occupying the left upper quadrant immediately lateral to the ascending or descending duodenum
- Separation of loops from the remaining small intestine; dilation and stasis of barium appearing in the herniated bowel segments
- Foramen of Winslow hernia: bowel loops within the lesser sac medial and posterior to the anteriorly displaced stomach; dilated proximal segment
- Volvulus: distended closed loop in a transmesenteric hernia and constriction around the closely approximated afferent and efferent limbs of the herniated intestine

DIAGNOSTIC PEARLS

- Paraduodenal hernias: circumscribed, ovoid mass of the jejunal loops occupying the left upper quadrant immediately lateral to the ascending or descending duodenum
- Separation of loops from the remaining small intestine and dilation and stasis of barium seen in the herniated bowel segments
- Encapsulation and crowding together of several small bowel loops within the confines of the peritoneal cavity
- Volvulus: distended closed loop in a transmesenteric hernia and constriction around the closely approximated afferent and efferent limbs of the herniated intestine
- Apparent fixation of herniated loops, preventing their separation or dislodgment during fluoroscopic manipulations or by changing position of patient

- Retroanastomotic hernia: herniated jejunal segments appearing clumped or fixed in the left upper abdomen, with dilation and stasis

Utility

- Lateral radiographs are particularly useful for demonstrating retroperitoneal displacement of the hernia contents in a paraduodenal hernia.
- Contrast examinations of gastrointestinal tract are most likely to provide the correct diagnosis during symptomatic periods.
- After the hernia is reduced spontaneously, however, results of barium studies tend to be negative.

CT

Findings

- Foramen of Winslow hernia: aberrant position of the bowel loops among the liver, stomach, and pancreas
- Pericecal hernia: small bowel loops lateral to the proximal ascending colon

---

WHAT THE REFERRING PHYSICIAN NEEDS TO KNOW

- Internal hernias are now among the most comman causes of closed-loop bowel obstruction and strangulation.
- Correct diagnosis can be made if barium studies or CT of the abdomen is performed during symptomatic periods.
- Preoperative diagnosis and the demonstration of radiographic anatomy assist the surgeon in better understanding the extremely confusing laparotomy findings.
- Blind division of the paraduodenal hernial sac should be prevented because it carries the risk of injury to vital mesenteric vessels contained within the wall.
- Clinical and radiologic findings of transomental hernias are almost identical to those of transmesenteric hernias.
- Superior mesenteric arteriogram showing as an abrupt angulation and displacement of visceral branches as they pass through mesenteric defect constitutes an emergency.

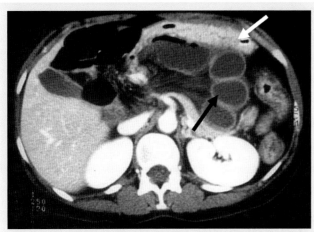

Figure 1. Foramen of Winslow hernia. CT scan shows the small bowel *(arrows)* herniated into the lesser sac, causing a closed loop obstruction.

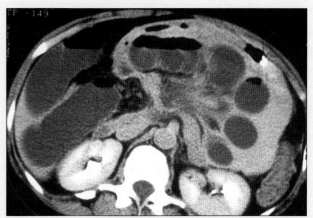

Figure 2. Foramen of Winslow hernia. Scan obtained several hours later from patient in Figure 1 shows that these loops have become ischemic and hemorrhagic.

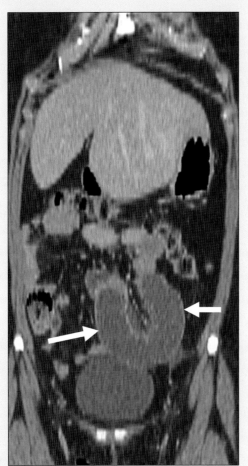

Figure 3. Transmesenteric hernia. Coronal, reformatted CT scan shows closed-loop obstruction *(arrows)* caused by a transmesenteric hernia.

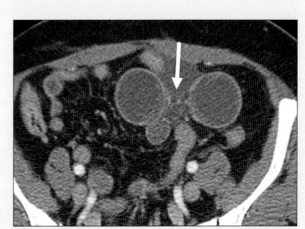

Figure 4. Transmesenteric hernia. Axial CT image of the patient shows the obstructed loops converging at the mesenteric defect *(arrow)*. Mesenteric fluid is also present.

- Portion of the jejunum or ileum encapsulated between the sigmoid loops
- Closed loop obstruction in transmesenteric hernia
- Retroanastomotic hernia involving the afferent loop showing a fluid-filled and markedly distended tubular structure

Utility
- CT scans of the upper abdomen may help demonstrate hernias before the operation.
- CT is the optimal imaging technique for demonstrating the presence and the content of herniations involving the lesser sac.
- CT is the preferred means of making the diagnosis in both acute and nonacute settings.

Interventional Radiology
Findings
- Transmesenteric hernia: superior mesenteric arteriogram showing abrupt angulation and displacement of visceral branches as they pass through the mesenteric defect

Utility
- Superior mesenteric arteriogram
- This technique is now seldom used.

CLINICAL PRESENTATION
- Patients may have from intermittent and mild digestive complaints to acute intestinal obstruction.
- Recurrent periumbilical cramps or postprandial epigastric pain and distention are frequently experienced before the onset of incarceration.
- Volvulus of herniated bowels causes severe periumbilical cramps, hyperactive bowel sounds, progressive distention, and a tender abdominal mass.
- Retroanastomotic hernia causes cramping abdominal pain, a tender mass in the left upper abdomen, nonbilious vomiting, and an elevated serum amylase level.

DIFFERENTIAL DIAGNOSIS
- Adhesive small bowel obstruction
- Volvulus
- Postoperative fossae

PATHOLOGY
- Foramen of Winslow hernia: Predisposing factors include an enlarged foramen of Winslow and a long mesentery or persistence of the ascending mesocolon.
- Herniation into the foramen of Winslow may be provoked by a sudden increase in intra-abdominal pressure, such as during weight lifting.
- Defects causing a transmesenteric hernia in adults are probably caused by previous operations, abdominal trauma, or intraperitoneal inflammation.
- Retroanastomotic hernia usually develop after a partial gastrectomy and gastrojejunostomy.

INCIDENCE/PREVALENCE AND EPIDEMIOLOGY
- Paraduodenal hernias are the most common type of intra-abdominal herniation, accounting for 53% of reported cases.
- Paraduodenal hernias are more common in women than men, with a 3:1 ratio.
- Foramen of Winslow hernia represents 8% of all internal hernias, usually affecting middle-aged patients.
- Intersigmoid fossa is seen in 65% of autopsies.
- Transmesenteric hernia comprises 5% to 10% of all internal hernias.
- Thirty-five percent of transmesenteric hernias affect the pediatric age group, constituting the most common internal hernia at this age.

Suggested Readings
Blachar A, Federle MP, Brancatelli G, et al: Radiologist performance in the diagnosis of internal hernia by using specific CT findings with emphasis on transmesenteric hernia. *Radiology* 221:422-428, 2001.
Gale ME, Gerzof SG, Kiser LC, et al: CT appearance of afferent loop obstruction. *AJR Am J Roentgenol* 138:1085-1088, 1982.
Inoue Y, Nakamura H, Mizumoto S, et al: Lesser sac hernia through the gastrocolic ligament: CT diagnosis. *Abdom Imaging* 21:145-147, 1996.
Martin LC, Merkle EM, Thompson WM: Review of internal hernias: Radiographic and clinical findings. *AJR Am J Roentgenol* 186:703-717, 2006.

Pelvic and Groin Hernias

DEFINITION: Defect in the muscular wall of the pelvis and groin through which abdominal contents may herniate.

IMAGING

CT
Findings
- Obturator hernia: soft-tissue mass or opacified loop protruding through the obturator foramen and extending between the pectineus and obturator muscles
- Sciatic hernia: bowel loop herniating through the sciatic foramen and extending laterally into the subgluteal region
- Perineal hernia: hernia sac and its contents in the ischiorectal fossa
- Inguinal hernia: peritoneal sac containing bowel loops protruding through the inguinal canal
- Femoral hernia: neck below the inguinal ligament and lateral to the pubic tubercle

Utility
- CT provides diagnostic information on the hernia contents and helps differentiate a hernia from other masses.
- CT is the best means of diagnosing complications of hernias, such as obstruction, ischemia, and strangulation.
- Occult hernias are sometimes seen only with a scan obtained while the patient performs the Valsalva maneuver.

Ultrasound
Findings
- Bowel loops are identified in the hernia sac.

Utility
- Ultrasound provides diagnostic information on the hernia contents and helps differentiate a hernia from other masses.
- Having the patient strain in a variety of positions during the examinitation is useful diagnostically.

Radiography
Findings
- Inguinal hernia: convergence of distended intestinal loops toward the inguinal region
- Inguinal hernia: barium examination showing tapered narrowing or obstruction of the intestinal segment as it enters the hernia orifice
- Obturator hernia: bowel obstruction together with a fixed loop containing some gas or contrast medium in the obturator region
- Sciatic hernia: curlicue appearance of the ureter on excretory urogram

DIAGNOSTIC PEARLS

- Tapered narrowing or obstruction of the intestinal segment
- Soft-tissue mass or an opacified loop that protrudes through the obturator foramen
- Bowel loop herniating through the foramen

- Sciatic hernia: barium examination showing the bowel loop herniated through the sciatic foramen and extending laterally into the subgluteal region
- Perineal hernia: protruding loop adjacent to the anus or in one of the buttocks

Utility
- This is an insensitive test in making the diagnosis of hernias without intraluminal contrast material.

CLINICAL PRESENTATION

- Inguinal hernia: bowel distention associated with painful and often tense swelling in a groin or scrotum
- Obturator hernia: acute or recurrent bowel obstruction and a tender mass in the obturator region, as detected on rectal or vaginal examination
- Sciatic hernia: lower abdominal cramps, urinary symptoms, pain radiating to the dorsal thigh or leg, and a palpable, tender gluteal mass
- Perineal hernia: perineal or gluteal mass, causing discomfort when sitting

DIFFERENTIAL DIAGNOSIS

- Abdominal wall neoplasms

PATHOLOGY

- Inguinal hernia: congenital, patent processus vaginalis
- Obturator hernia: enlargement of the obturator canal after pregnancies and as a consequence of aging
- Perineal hernia: defects in the levator ani or coccygeus muscle and an acquired weakness of the pelvic floor

WHAT THE REFERRING PHYSICIAN NEEDS TO KNOW

- Signs of bowel strangulation should be investigated.
- Radiologic studies are performed for preoperative delineation of the herniated viscera and associated complications or when clinical findings are equivocal.

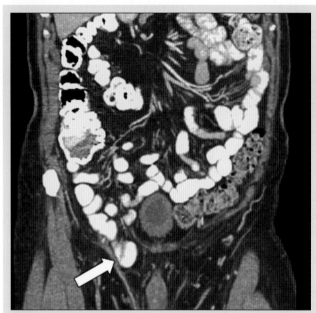

Figure 1. Inguinal hernia. Coronal, reformatted CT image shows a nonobstructing, right inguinal hernia containing the small bowel (*arrow*).

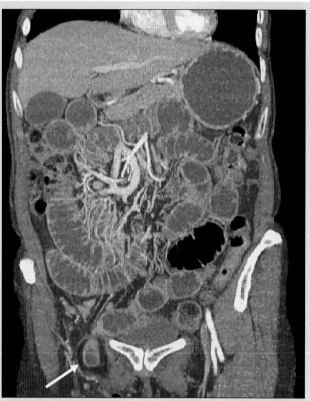

Figure 2. Femoral hernia. An obstructing right femoral hernia (*arrow*) is identified on this coronal CT image. Notice the relationship to the inguinal canal.

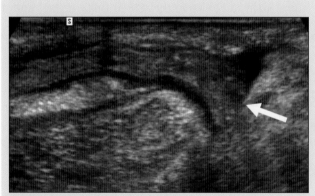

Figure 3. Inguinal hernia. Sagittal sonogram demonstrates an inguinal hernia containing fat, fluid, and gut (*arrow*).

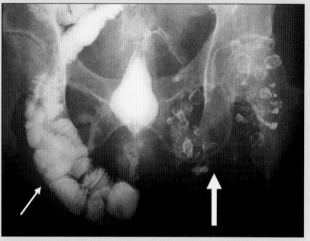

Figure 4. Inguinal hernia. Barium enema examination demonstrates herniation of the distal ileum into the right scrotum (*small arrow*). Herniation of the sigmoid colon into a left inguinal hernia is seen (*large arrow*).

- Sciatic notch herniation of pelvic or abdominal viscera into subgluteal region involving the distal ureter or loop of the small bowel

INCIDENCE/PREVALENCE AND EPIDEMIOLOGY

- Pelvic and groin hernias comprise 75% of all abdominal hernias.
- Inguinal hernia is most common type (indirect inguinal hernia) and more common in men than in women.
- Femoral hernia occurs predominantly in women and accounts for approximately one third of groin hernias in women.
- Obturator hernia: 80%-90% occur in elderly women.
- Perineal hernia typically occurs in women older than 50 years of age.

Suggested Readings

Aguirre DA, Casola G, Sirlin C: Abdominal wall hernias: MDCT findings. *AJR Am J Roentgenol* 183:681-690, 2004.

Arat A, Haliloglu M, Cila A, et al: Demonstration of ureterosciatic hernia with spiral CT. *J Comput Assist Tomogr* 20:816-818, 1996.

Balthazar EJ, Subramanyam BR, Megibow A: Spigelian hernia: CT and ultrasonography diagnosis. *Gastrointest Radiol* 9:81-84, 1984.

Bernardy MO, Umer MA, Flanigan RC: Computed tomography of hydrocele of the tunica vaginalis. *J Comput Assist Tomogr* 9: 203-204, 1985.

Epner SL, Rozenblit A, Gentile R: Direct inguinal hernia containing bladder carcinoma: CT demonstration. *AJR Am J Roentgenol* 161:97-98, 1993.

Ghahremani GG, Michael AS: Sciatic hernia with incarcerated ileum: CT and radiographic diagnosis. *Gastrointest Radiol* 16:120-122, 1991.

Harrison LA, Keesling CA, Martin NL, et al: Abdominal wall hernias: Review of herniography and correlation with cross-sectional imaging. *RadioGraphics* 15:315-332, 1995.

Urachal Abnormalities

DEFINITION: Four congenital lesions of the urachus are known: patent urachus, urachal cyst, urachal sinus, and vesicourachal diverticulum.

IMAGING

Radiography
Findings
- Patent urachus is demonstrated.
- Fistulogram delineates the course of the urachal sinus.

Utility
- Voiding cystourethrogram may demonstrate communication and excludes a lower obstruction.

CT
Findings
- Detects cyst

Utility
- Cyst puncture and drainage for diagnostic purposes

Ultrasound
Findings
- Detects cyst

Utility
- Cyst puncture and drainage for diagnostic purposes

CLINICAL PRESENTATION

- Patent urachus is evident in the first moments or days of life; the umbilical cord may be thickened and tense from urine reflux.
- Urachal cyst produces an enlarging mass, the sensation of fullness, or infection.
- Infected urachal abnormalities may present with pain and erythema.
- Peritonitis may result from rupture.
- Umbilical mass

DIFFERENTIAL DIAGNOSIS

- Abdominal wall neoplasm
- Abdominal wall hematoma
- Abdominal wall infection

DIAGNOSTIC PEARLS

- Patent urachus is demonstrated by a cystourethrogram.
- Urachal cyst is detected by CT and ultrasound.
- Urachal sinus is demonstrated by a fistulogram.

PATHOLOGY

- Four congenital lesions of the urachus are known: patent urachus, urachal cyst, urachal sinus, and vesicourachal diverticulum.

INCIDENCE/PREVALENCE AND EPIDEMIOLOGY

- Patent urachus is present in 1:200,000 live births.
- Urachal cysts are found in 1:5000 at autopsy.
- Urachal carcinoma accounts for 0.2%-0.34% of all bladder cancers and 20%-40% of all primary bladder adenocarcinomas.

Suggested Readings

Bauer SB, Retik AB: Urachal anomalies and related umbilical disorders. *Urol Clin North Am* 5:195-211, 1978.

Blichert-Toft M, Nielsen OV: Congenital patent urachus and acquired variants. *Acta Chir Scand* 137:807-814, 1971.

DiSantis DJ, Siegel MJ, Katz ME: Simplified approach to umbilical remnant abnormalities. *RadioGraphics* 11:59-66, 1991.

Holten I, Lomas F, Mouratidis B, et al: Ultrasonic diagnosis of urachal abnormalities. *Australas Radiol* 40:2-8, 1996.

Khati NJ, Enquist EG, Javitt MC: Imaging the umbilicus and peri-umbilical region. *RadioGraphics* 18:413-429, 1998.

Sarno RC, Klauber G, Carter BL: Computer assisted tomography of urachal abnormalities. *J Comput Assist Tomogr* 7:674-676, 1983.

WHAT THE REFERRING PHYSICIAN NEEDS TO KNOW

- Percutaneous drainage and antibiotic therapy are beneficial preoperatively to reduce infectious complications at surgery.
- Untreated infected cysts usually drain to the anterior abdominal wall, but they may spontaneously rupture into the peritoneal cavity.
- Definitive therapy requires complete excision with resection of the cuff of the bladder dome.

Pediatric Disease

Pediatric Abdominal Masses

DEFINITION: Mass in the abdomen of various causes.

IMAGING

Radiography
Findings
- Obstruction or displacement of the bowel
- Calcifications that suggest meconium peritonitis, teratoma, and hepatoblastoma
- Spinal anomalies that suggest anterior sacral meningocele, obstructed cloacal deformity, or sacrococcygeal teratoma with an internal component

Utility
- Plain radiography most often cannot characterize the mass.

Ultrasound
Findings
- Solid, cystic, or septate mass
- Wall, membrane, or capsule surrounding a mass
- Effect on displacement of surrounding structures
- Ascites
- Spread or extension of a mass

Utility
- Ultrasound is the premier imaging technique for abdominal and pelvic masses in neonates.

CT
Findings
- Findings vary as to the cause of the mass.

Utility
- Multiplanar capabilities of multidetector CT can depict the precise anatomic location of masses.

MRI
Findings
- Findings vary as to the cause of the mass.

DIAGNOSTIC PEARLS
- Solid, cystic, or septate mass detected on ultrasound
- Wall, membrane, or capsule surrounding the mass
- Obstruction or displacement of the bowel
- Calcifications that suggest meconium peritonitis, teratoma, and hepatoblastoma

Utility
- MRI depicts anatomic relationships of the mass to other intra-abdominal structures without using ionizing radiation.

CLINICAL PRESENTATION
- Mass may be detected by prenatal sonography or by abdominal palpation after birth.
- In some neonates, the mass is sufficiently large to distend or distort the abdominal wall and cause respiratory distress.
- Ascites may be present or simulated.
- Pain or obstruction results if the mass is producing pressure on an adjacent structure or if torsion is present.
- Bruit over the liver in an infant with congestive heart failure suggests a hepatic hemangioma.
- Abdominal mass with a mass over the buttocks may represent internal extension of a sacrococcygeal teratoma.

WHAT THE REFERRING PHYSICIAN NEEDS TO KNOW
- From what compartment or organ does mass originate?
- Is the mass solid, cystic, or septate?
- Is there a wall, membrane, or capsule around it?
- Do the structures surrounding the mass look normal?
- Is there ascites?
- Are there any sites of spread or extension within the abdomen or retroperitoneum?
- Differential diagnosis is extensive and includes ovarian mass, alimentary tract duplication, lymphangioma, spleen or liver mass, choledochal cyst, cystic meconium peritonitis, and retroperitoneal masses.

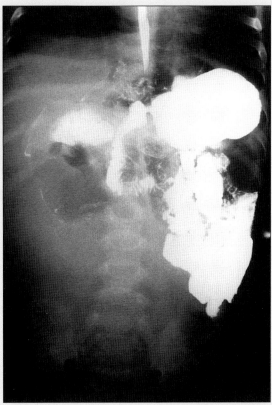

Figure 1. **Neonatal abdominal mass: mesenteric lymphangioma.** Barium is present in the stomach, duodenum, and small bowel. Gastroesophageal reflux is filling the distal esophagus. The duodenal sweep is displaced to the left. Upwardly displaced, compressed, and opacified bowel loops are seen in the right upper quadrant.

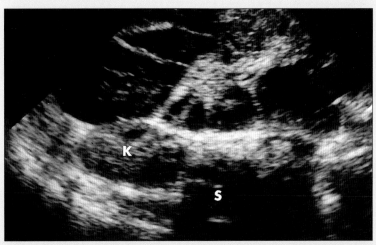

Figure 2. **Neonatal abdominal mass: mesenteric lymphangioma.** Transverse abdominal sonogram to the right of the midline demonstrates multiple, fluid-filled structures. None of these structures had visible peristalsis because they were portions of the lymphangioma. (*K*, kidney; *S*, spine.)

DIFFERENTIAL DIAGNOSIS

- Dilated bladder
- Dilated bowel
- Hydronephrosis
- Multicystic dysplastic kidney
- Dilated ureter
- Enteric duplication cyst
- Lymphangioma
- Ovarian cyst
- Persistent cloaca
- Splenic cyst
- Urachal cyst
- Urinoma
- Hepatomegaly, splenomegaly
- Neuroblastoma

INCIDENCE/PREVALENCE AND EPIDEMIOLOGY

- Most neonatal abdominal masses originate in the kidney, such as ureteropelvic junction obstruction and multicystic dysplastic kidneys.
- Gastrointestinal lesions account for 8%-15% of neonatal abdominal masses.

Suggested Readings

Effmann EL, Griscom NT, Colodny AH, et al: Neonatal gastrointestinal masses arising late in gestation. *AJR Am J Roentgenol* 135:681-686, 1980.

Heling KS, Chaoui R, Kirchmair F, et al: Fetal ovarian cysts: Prenatal diagnosis, management, and postnatal outcome. *Ultrasound Obstet Gynecol* 20:47-50, 2002.

Kassarjian A, Zurakowski D, Dubois J, et al: Infantile hepatic hemangiomas: Clinical and imaging findings and their correlation with therapy. *AJR Am J Roentgenol* 182:785-795, 2004.

Kirkinen P, Partanen K, Merikanto J, et al: Ultrasonic and magnetic resonance imaging of fetal sacrococcygeal teratoma. *Acta Obstet Gynecol Scand* 76:917-922, 1997.

Sbargia L, Paek BW, Feldstein VA, et al: Outcome of prenatally diagnosed solid fetal tumors. *J Pediatr Surg* 36:1244-1247, 2001.

White KS: Imaging of abdominal masses in children. *Semin Pediatr Surg* 1:269-276, 1992.

Wooten-Gorges SL, Thomas KB, Harned RK, et al: Giant cystic abdominal masses in children. *Pediatr Radiol* 35:1277-1288, 2005.

Abnormal Neonatal Bowel Gas

DEFINITION: Too much or too little or unevenly distributed bowel gas in the neonate.

IMAGING

Radiography
Findings
- Initially, a gasless stomach may be caused by esophageal atresia.
- Initial normal bowel finding that becomes gasless suggests an electrolyte imbalance, gastric suctioning, or paralysis with curariform agents for ventilation.
- Paucity or malposition of gas may confirm a suspected diaphragmatic hernia.
- Abdominal mass may displace the bowel loops.
- With a proximal bowel obstruction, few loops of the bowel in the upper abdomen are distended with air and fluid.
- With a distal obstruction, the dilated bowel loops fill the abdomen.

Utility
- Differentiating the small bowel from the large bowel may be difficult because haustral markings are poorly developed in the neonate.
- Distended small bowel may fill the space usually occupied by the colon or even simulate a distended stomach.
- The most distal extent of the air is important because the differential diagnosis depends on the level of the obstruction.
- Prone lateral rectal views may be useful if an extremely distal lesion is suspected.
- Contrast study of the colon may be performed to determine the presence of obstruction and to identify the level and nature of the obstruction.

CLINICAL PRESENTATION

- Abdominal distention
- Abdominal mass
- Vomiting
- Failure to pass flatus
- Failure to pass meconium
- Bowel gas pattern should be carefully scrutinized in any neonate with respiratory or gastrointestinal symptoms.

DIAGNOSTIC PEARLS

- With a high bowel obstruction, a few loops of bowel in upper abdomen are distended with air and fluid.
- Initially, a gasless stomach may be caused by esophageal atresia.
- Paucity or malposition of gas may confirm a suspected diaphragmatic hernia.
- With distal obstruction, dilated bowel loops fill the abdomen.
- It is difficult to distinguish dilated colon from small bowel in neonates.

DIFFERENTIAL DIAGNOSIS

- Congenital diaphragmatic hernia
- Duodenal atresia or stenosis, annular pancreas
- Esophageal atresia without tracheoesophageal fistula
- Esophageal web
- Pyloric, duodenal, or proximal jejunal obstruction

PATHOLOGY

- Delaying of the passage of air into the gastrointestinal tract may be caused by a mechanical obstruction and a depressed swallowing mechanism.
- Abdominal mass may displace the bowel loops and, through pressure on the diaphragm, cause respiratory distress.

INCIDENCE/PREVALENCE

- Seen in up to 50% of neonates

Suggested Readings
Cohen MD, Jansen R, Lemons J, et al: Evaluation of the gasless abdomen in the newborn and young infant with metrizamide. *AJR Am J Roentgenol* 142:393-396, 1984.

WHAT THE REFERRING PHYSICIAN NEEDS TO KNOW
- Determining the most distal extent of the air is important because the correct diagnosis depends on the level of the obstruction.
- Bowel gas pattern should be carefully scrutinized in any neonate with respiratory or gastrointestinal symptoms.
- Additional views may be necessary for detecting air within the colon.

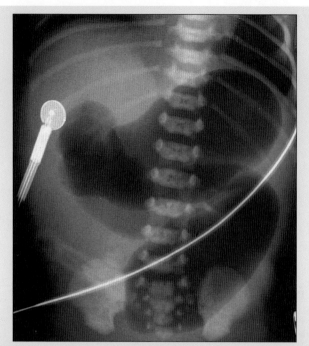

Figure 1. High obstruction. Anteroposterior abdominal radiograph in a child with jejunal atresia shows several markedly distended bowel loops that fill the abdomen. The calcification along the anterior abdominal wall indicates prior bowel perforation and meconium peritonitis.

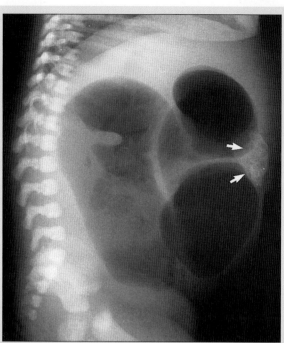

Figure 2. High obstruction. Lateral abdominal radiograph in a child with jejunal atresia shows several markedly distended bowel loops that fill the abdomen. The calcification along the anterior abdominal wall *(arrows)* indicates prior bowel perforation and meconium peritonitis.

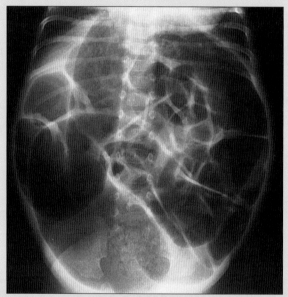

Figure 3. Low obstruction. Colonic obstruction from Hirschsprung disease has produced dilation of multiple bowel loops throughout the abdomen. Because discrete haustral markings cannot be identified, it is difficult to appreciate that, in addition to the entire small bowel, the colon is dilated.

Colonic Atresia

DEFINITION: Congenital absence or closure of the colon.

IMAGING

Ultrasound
Findings
- Prenatal sonography frequently demonstrates polyhydramnios and a dilated, fluid-filled bowel loop.

Utility
- Sonography is useful for excluding the presence of ascites or a mass lesion.

Radiography
Findings
- Postnatal plain radiographs indicate low obstruction; dilated bowel loops may have air-fluid levels or a bubbly appearance because of meconium.
- Contrast column ends abruptly and may taper or have a rounded, *cobra-head* or club deformity if the membrane is present.
- Colon may be normal or small in caliber, depending on when the luminal occlusion occurred.
- If a transition zone is observed, Hirschsprung disease also may be present.

Utility
- Diagnosis by plain radiography is difficult because air may not have reached the most distal bowel segment.
- Contrast enema with nonionic, water-soluble contrast agent is the diagnostic study of choice.
- Examination should be performed with great caution because of the increased incidence of colonic rupture in patients with atresia.

CLINICAL PRESENTATION

- Patients with colonic atresia are more likely to be born at term.
- Colonic atresia causes vomiting and abdominal distention.
- Meconium might have passed normally.
- Vomiting and abdominal distention

DIFFERENTIAL DIAGNOSIS

- Meconium plug
- Hirschprung disease

DIAGNOSTIC PEARLS

- Prenatal sonography frequently demonstrates polyhydramnios and the dilated, fluid-filled bowel loop.
- Contrast column ends abruptly and may taper or have rounded, *cobra-head* or club deformity if the membrane is present.
- Colon may be normal or small in caliber, depending on when the luminal occlusion occurred. If a transition zone is observed, Hirschsprung disease may also be present.

- Duplication
- Intussusception
- Ileal stenosis

PATHOLOGY

- Transverse colon is the most frequently involved site.
- Usually secondary to vascular accidents often related to volvulus or gastroschisis

INCIDENCE/PREVALENCE AND EPIDEMIOLOGY

- Incidence of atresia is lower in the colon than elsewhere in the gut.
- It occurs in approximately 1 of 40,000 live births.
- A slight female predominance is noted.

Suggested Readings

Cox SG, Numanoglu A, Millar AJ, et al: Colonic atresia: Spectrum of presentation and pitfalls in management. A review of 14 cases. *Pediatr Surg Int* 21:813-818, 2005.

Kim PC, Superina RA, Ein S: Colonic atresia combined with Hirschsprung's disease: A diagnostic and therapeutic challenge. *J Pediatr Surg* 30:1216-1217, 1995.

Landes A, Shuckett B, Skarsgard E: Non-fixation of the colon in colonic atresia: A new finding. *Pediatr Radiol* 24:167-169, 1994.

WHAT THE REFERRING PHYSICIAN NEEDS TO KNOW

- Differential diagnosis includes other low obstruction causes: Hirschsprung disease, duplication, meconium plug, intussusception, and distal ileal processes.
- Contrast enema should be performed to narrow the diagnostic possibilities; direct additional testing and therapy should be considered.

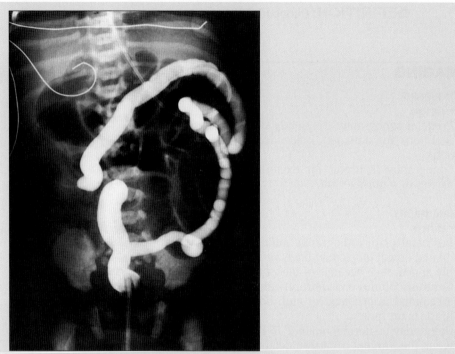

Figure 1. Colonic atresia. Multiple dilated small bowel loops are present. Water-soluble contrast fills a small-caliber colon. The contrast did not pass proximal to the hepatic flexure, the site of the atresia.

Diaphragmatic Hernia

DEFINITION: Hernias of the diaphragm are Bochdalek hernias and hernias of the foramen of Morgagni.

IMAGING

Ultrasound
Findings
- Prenatal diagnosis of a Bochdalek hernia: Heart and other mediastinal contents are shifted from the midline, and the abdominal organs are in the thorax.

Utility
- Prenatal ultrasound can forewarn the managing physicians of this disorder so that it can be promptly treated following delivery.

Radiography
Findings
- On early radiographs, the herniated bowel loops may appear as a soft-tissue mass.
- With time and air swallowing, chest radiographs reveal a more typical bubbly appearance.
- Diaphragmatic hernias that contain the liver may appear more solid and may be accompanied by a pleural fluid collection.
- Mediastinum remains shifted to the side opposite the hernia on immediate postoperative chest radiographs.
- Anteroposterior chest radiographs may show soft tissue or air density along the heart border in a foramen of Morgagni hernia.
- On lateral projection, the anterior location of the hernia and the visualization of bowel markings establish the diagnosis of a foramen of Morgagni hernia.

Utility
- Abdominal radiographs can determine the amount of bowel present in the abdomen.
- If the nature of the thoracic contents is uncertain, a nasogastric tube is inserted to define the stomach and introduce air into the bowel.
- Contrast studies are rarely needed to visualize the upper or lower gastrointestinal tract before surgery.

DIAGNOSTIC PEARLS

- Heart and other mediastinal contents are shifted from the midline, and the abdominal organs are in the thorax on prenatal ultrasound.
- On lateral radiograph, the anterior location of a foramen of Morgagni hernia and the visualization of bowel markings establish the diagnosis of a foramen of Morgagni hernia.
- Chest radiographs initially show bowel loops appearing as a soft-tissue mass but reveal a more typical bubbly appearance.

- Chest radiographs can exclude other causes of neonatal respiratory distress: pulmonary immaturity, congenital cystic adenomatoid malformation, and pneumonia.

CLINICAL PRESENTATION

- Bochdalek hernia: The affected infant exhibits respiratory distress shortly after birth; a scaphoid abdomen is also seen.
- Foramen of Morgagni hernia: Respiratory and gastrointestinal complaints are common but not necessarily related to the hernia; patients may be asymptomatic.

DIFFERENTIAL DIAGNOSIS

- Varicella pneumonia (pediatric lungs)
- Atelectasis
- Congenital anomalies: congenital cystic adenomatoid malformation (congenital pulmonary airway malformation)
- Abscess

WHAT THE REFERRING PHYSICIAN NEEDS TO KNOW

- Most critical factor in determining the infant's outcome is the degree of pulmonary hypoplasia caused by lung compression by the herniated bowels.
- All children are carefully examined for midline defects and cardiac lesions.
- Cardiac, cranial, and abdominal ultrasound studies are performed to identify who can receive extracorporeal membrane oxygenation (ECMO) treatment.
- Infants on ECMO receive a daily chest radiograph for the evaluation of line placement.
- Differential diagnosis of air-containing Morgagni hernias includes pneumonia, atelectasis, pneumatocele, abscess, and cystic adenomatoid malformation.
- If the liver is herniated, a solid appearance may simulate a tumor of the diaphragm, a pericardial mass, or an anterior mediastinal mass.
- Morgagni hernias are corrected even in asymptomatic children because of the potential for incarceration and strangulation.

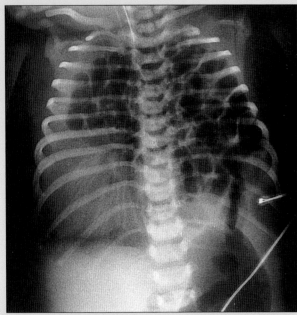

Figure 1. Left Bochdalek hernia. Multiple, air-filled bowel loops fill the left thorax and right apex. The mediastinum is shifted to the right, and the soft-tissue densities of the heart and the hypoplastic right lung merge.

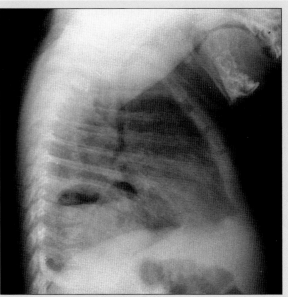

Figure 2. Right Bochdalek hernia. Lateral radiograph shows a posterior soft-tissue density with a focal air collection. This feature simulates a cystic adenomatoid malformation or pneumatocele.

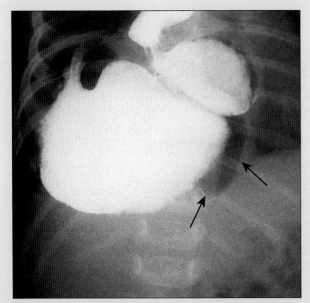

Figure 3. Right Bochdalek hernia. Upper gastrointestinal study reveals that the stomach has herniated into the right thorax. Air-filled small bowel is also in the hernia *(arrows)*.

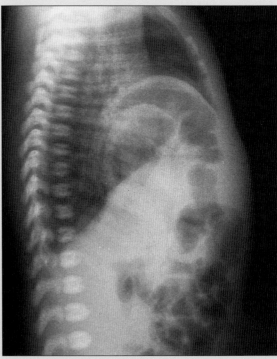

Figure 4. Foramen of Morgagni hernia. On the lateral view, the bowel is seen extending from the abdomen to the retrosternal space.

- Anterior mediastinal mass
- Pericardial masses
- Pneumatocele
- Tumor of the diaphragm

PATHOLOGY

- Some diaphragmatic hernias may be acquired after trauma or infection.
- During neonatal period, diaphragmatic hernias can develop in association with group B streptococcal infection.
- Congenital diaphragmatic hernia occurs six to nine times more often on the left than on the right.
- Regardless of the side on which the hernia occurs, the ipsilateral and contralateral lungs are compressed.
- Such hernias develop if the bowel returns to the abdomen prematurely or if the diaphragm develops late or incompletely during early fetal life.
- Affected children have malrotation of the bowel because the normal rotation that occurs as the bowel returns to the abdomen is interrupted.

- In contrast to Bochdalek hernias, Morgagni hernias are usually right sided and have a covering or sac.

INCIDENCE/PREVALENCE AND EPIDEMIOLOGY

- Posterolateral or Bochdalek hernia occurs in approximately 1 of 3000 live births.
- Foramen of Morgagni hernia accounts for approximately 2%-4% of all diaphragmatic hernias.

Suggested Readings

Baglaj M, Dorobisz U: Late-presenting congenital diaphragmatic hernia in children: A literature review. *Pediatr Radiol* 35:478-488, 2005.

Gorincour G, Bouvenot J, Mourot MG, et al: Prenatal prognosis of congenital diaphragmatic hernia using magnetic resonance imaging of fetal lung volume. *Ultrasound Obstet Gynecol* 26:738-744, 2005.

Lally KP: Congenital diaphragmatic hernia. *Curr Opin Pediatr* 14:486-490, 2002.

Metkus AP, Filly RA, Stringer MD, et al: Sonographic predictors of survival in fetal diaphragmatic hernia. *J Pediatr Surg* 31:148-151, 1996.

Esophageal Atresia

DEFINITION: Atresia of the esophagus.

ANATOMIC FINDINGS

Esophagus
- Distal esophagus is connected to the trachea by a congenital tracheoesophageal fistula (TEF) in more than 80% of cases.
- Complete esophageal atresia (EA) occurs in approximately 10% of cases.
- Proximal fistula is present in 3%-4% of cases.
- H-type fistula is seen in 5% of cases.

IMAGING

Ultrasound
Findings
- Polyhydramnios with absent fluid in the stomach suggests esophageal atresia (EA) without a tracheoesophageal fistula (TEF).
- Fluid-filled upper pouch may be detected with ultrasound.
Utility
- Postnatally, sonography is performed to search for kidney malformations included in vertebral, anorectal, cardiac, tracheoesophageal, renal, and limb anomalies (VATER/VACTERL).

Radiography
Findings
- Presence of bowel gas differentiates pure EA from EA with a TEF.
- Contrast study defines the upper pouch.
- In pure EA, a barium study performed through a gastrostomy tube defines the length of the lower esophageal segment before surgery.
- Barium esophagogram demonstrates an H-type fistula with an N shape as it passes superiorly and anteriorly from the esophagus to the trachea.
Utility
- Evaluation for possible fistula is performed with lateral fluoroscopy of the upper esophagus with the child supported in semiupright position.

DIAGNOSTIC PEARLS
- Contrast study defines the upper pouch.
- Barium esophagogram demonstrates an H-type fistula with an N shape as it passes superiorly and anteriorly from the esophagus to the trachea.
- Polyhydramnios with absent fluid in the stomach suggests EA without a TEF on prenatal ultrasound.

- Chest and abdominal radiographs should be scrutinized for vertebral segmentation and limb anomalies, tetralogy of Fallot, and right-sided aortic arch (VACTERL).
- Because an H-type TEF is not always patent, it may be difficult to demonstrate.

CLINICAL PRESENTATION
- Difficulty in handling secretions at birth is seen.
- Respiratory distress is noted on the first feeding.
- Attempts to pass a nasogastric tube are usually unsuccessful.
- Presence of a distal fistula is evident by a rounded abdomen and bowel sounds.
- Neonates with EA without a distal fistula have a scaphoid abdomen and absent bowel sounds.

DIFFERENTIAL DIAGNOSIS
- Pharyngeal pseudodiverticulum due to traumatic perforation of the posterior pharynx from finger or tube insertion into the oropharynx during delivery

INCIDENCE/PREVALENCE AND EPIDEMIOLOGY
- EA occurs in approximately 1 in 5000 live births; boys and girls are equally affected.

WHAT THE REFERRING PHYSICIAN NEEDS TO KNOW
- The physician should perform a physical examination and obtain imaging before surgery to find anomalies that need emergent correction and those that might influence the surgical correction or affect mortality.
- Virtually all children with EA have disordered esophageal motility.
- Respiratory tract symptoms may persist throughout life.
- Approximately 5 days after surgery, an esophagogram is obtained to detect anastomotic leakage.
- When the eating pattern deteriorates, a barium esophagogram should be obtained to exclude narrowing at the anastomosis or the distal esophagus.
- In an H-type TEF, a second or third study may be necessary to see the fistula.

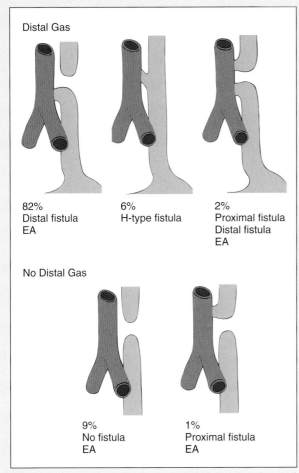

Figure 1. Types of esophageal atresia (EA). Common forms of EA are depicted.

Distal Gas

82%
Distal fistula
EA

6%
H-type fistula

2%
Proximal fistula
Distal fistula
EA

No Distal Gas

9%
No fistula
EA

1%
Proximal fistula
EA

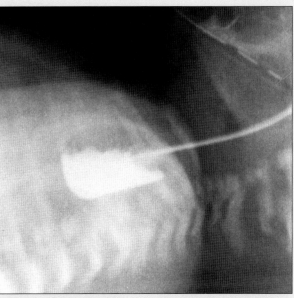

Figure 2. Esophageal atresia without tracheoesophageal fistula. The upper pouch is filled with a small amount of contrast. No fistula is identified. This study was performed with the patient in the supine rather than the preferred upright position.

- It is associated with trisomy 21 and VATER/VACTERL.
- In approximately 50% of infants, EA is an isolated anomaly.

PATHOLOGY

- Incomplete division of the primitive foregut into respiratory and digestive tracts
- Failure of formation of tubular esophagus and abnormal communication between trachea and esophagus
- Occurs during the third and fifth weeks of intrauterine life

Suggested Readings

Griscom NT, Martin TR: The trachea and esophagus after repair of esophageal atresia and distal fistula: Computed tomographic observations. *Pediatr Radiol* 20:447-450, 1990.

Kovesi T, Rubin S: Long-term complications of congenital esophageal atresia and/or tracheoesophageal fistula. *Chest* 126:915-925, 2004.

Stringer MD, McKenna KM, Goldstein RB, et al: Prenatal diagnosis of esophageal atresia. *J Pediatr Surg* 30:1258-1263, 1995.

Usui N, Kamata S, Ishikawa S, et al: Anomalies of the tracheobronchial tree in patients with esophageal atresia. *J Pediatr Surg* 31:258-262, 1996.

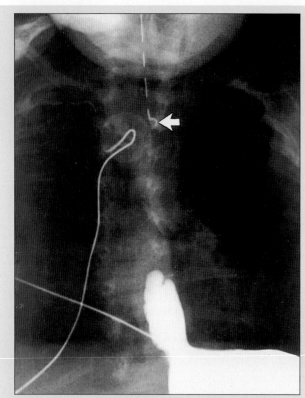

Figure 3. Gastrostomy injection of an esophageal atresia without a tracheoesophageal fistula. A feeding tube is in the upper esophageal pouch *(arrow)*. Contrast injected into the stomach through a gastrostomy has refluxed into the short distal esophageal segment. The distance between the distal aspect of the upper pouch and the proximal aspect of distal esophagus is approximately the height of five vertebral bodies.

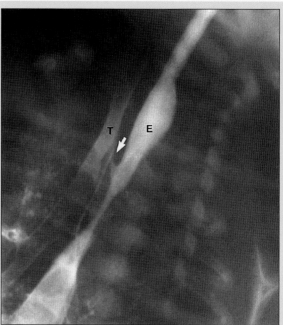

Figure 4. H-type tracheoesophageal fistula. The contrast agent injected into the upper esophagus fills the esophagus (E), the fistula *(arrow)*, and the trachea (T).

Gastroschisis

DEFINITION: Congenital parasagittal abdominal wall defect through which the bowel herniates.

IMAGING

Ultrasound
Findings
- Anterior abdominal wall defect through which the bowel herniation is seen.
- No membrane covers the bowel.
- Thickening of exteriorized bowel loops strongly suggests gastroschisis.
- Amniotic fluid volume is usually normal.
- Bowel caliber greater than 17 mm suggests that atresia is present.
- Bowel of smaller diameter is usually associated with bowel continuity.

Utility
- Prenatal sonographic diagnosis is performed.
- If fetal ascites or a covering membrane is present or the liver is detected in the herniated viscera, omphalocele is more likely.

Radiography
Findings
- Normally positioned umbilical clamp is separated from the herniated bowel loops, which are outlined by air.

Utility
- Postnatal plain abdominal radiographs are obtained.

CLINICAL PRESENTATION

- Prenatally, a rise in maternal serum α-fetoprotein level is noted.
- At birth, the defect and herniated bowel are apparent and are not easily confused with other abdominal wall defects.
- Postsurgically, problems of gastrointestinal motility may be seen (ileus, prolonged transit, gastroesophageal reflux).

DIAGNOSTIC PEARLS

- No membrane covers the bowel.
- Thickening of the exteriorized bowel loops strongly suggests gastroschisis.
- On radiograph, a normally positioned umbilical clamp is separated from the herniated bowel loops, which are outlined by air.

DIFFERENTIAL DIAGNOSIS

- Omphalocele

PATHOLOGY

- Gastroschisis is a parasagittal defect, usually to the right of the normally positioned and normal-appearing umbilical cord, through which the bowel herniates.
- Malrotation or nonrotation of bowel is seen.
- Bowel atresia, present in 20% of cases, is usually the only associated anomaly.
- Antenatal exposure to amniotic fluid produces bowel wall edema and inflammatory thickening of the serosa, which interferes with peristaltic function.

INCIDENCE/PREVALENCE AND EPIDEMIOLOGY

- Gastroschisis occurs in approximately 1 of 10,000 live births.
- Bowel atresia is present in 20% of cases.
- Even though patients are usually term infants, necrotizing enterocolitis (NEC) occurs in 23% of cases 1-4 months after repair.

WHAT THE REFERRING PHYSICIAN NEEDS TO KNOW

- Type of surgical correction depends on the size of the defect and on the presence of other complications, such as atresia and short gut.
- In addition to covering the herniated bowel, creating a stoma may be necessary to decompress the dilated bowel proximal to an atresia.
- Postsurgical barium studies detect gastroesophageal reflux, bowel loop dilation, adhesions and abnormalities of position, peristalsis, and transit time.
- Postoperative radiographs should be scrutinized to detect radiographic changes of NEC: ileus, dilated bowel loops, and intramural air.

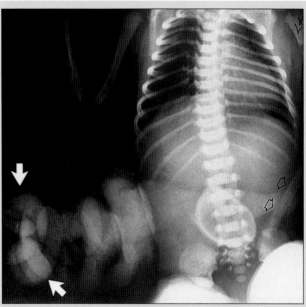

Figure 1. Gastroschisis. Exteriorized bowel loops *(white arrows)* extend lateral to the abdominal wall in this neonate with gastroschisis. Because the loops lack a covering membrane, each is clearly outlined by air. The normally inserted umbilical cord is in the midline, defined by the umbilical clamp to the left of midline *(open arrows)*.

Suggested Readings

Barisic I, Clementi M, Hausler M, et al: Evaluation of prenatal ultrasound diagnosis of fetal abdominal wall defects by 19 European registries. *Ultrasound Obstet Gynecol* 18:309-316, 2001.

Durfee SM, Downard CD, Benson CB, et al: Postnatal outcome of fetuses with the prenatal diagnosis of gastroschisis. *J Ultrasound Med* 21:269-274, 2002.

Hwang PJ, Kouseff BG: Omphalocele and gastroschisis: An 18-year review study. *Genet Med* 6:232-236, 2004.

Saada J, Oury JF, Vuillard E, et al: Gastroschisis. *Clin Obstet Gynecol* 48:964-972, 2005.

Imperforate Anus

DEFINITION: Anus without communication to the rectum.

ANATOMIC FINDINGS

Anus
- High or supralevator imperforate anus is present when the rectum ends above the levator ani muscles.
- Low or infralevator imperforate anus is present when the rectum ends below these muscles.
- Varied congenital anorectal malformations with or without associated anomalies are seen.

IMAGING

Radiography
Findings
- Rectal air stops proximal to the pubococcygeal line in a high imperforate anus.
- Rectal air stops below the pubococcygeal line in a low imperforate anus.
- Intraluminal calcification is reported in a small number of infants.

Utility
- Radiography is used to delineate the distal extent of the rectum because it determines whether the infant needs a neonatal colostomy and the probability of other malformations.
- It is also used to look for an associated spinal deformity, scimitar sacrum, Fallot tetralogy, and a ventricular septal defect.
- Cross-table lateral radiograph of rectum obtained with the infant's knees tucked beneath the prone or knee-chest position is better than an invertogram.
- Radiograph is more accurate when obtained after the first 24 hours of life.
- Voiding cystourethrography is routinely performed to exclude vesicoureteral reflux and a rectourinary fistula.
- Water-soluble contrast agents should be used to fill the unused segment to prevent barium from entering the urinary tract.
- Pressure-augmented antegrade cologram or a repeat voiding cystourethrogram precedes corrective surgery if the initial result is normal.

DIAGNOSTIC PEARLS
- Rectal air stops proximal to the pubococcygeal line in a high imperforate anus.
- Prenatal ultrasound findings suggesting an imperforate anus include dilated bowel and intraluminal enteroliths.
- Echogenic meconium in the distal rectal pouch defines the anomaly as a high or low lesion.

Ultrasound
Findings
- Prenatal ultrasound findings suggesting an imperforate anus include a dilated bowel and intraluminal enteroliths.
- Echogenic meconium in the distal rectal pouch defines the anomaly as a high or low lesion.
- When the pouch cannot be easily classified, it is usually a high imperforate anus.

Utility
- Transperineal sonography has also been used to assess the distal pouch and the puborectalis muscle around it.
- Renal sonography should be routine.
- Spinal ultrasound is commonly performed even when plain radiographs do not demonstrate the spinal anomaly.

CT
Findings
- On direct sagittal imaging, the distal colon can be seen in relation to midline bony structures.
- Preoperative evaluation of the levator sling can be performed with CT but is not routine.

Utility
- CT provides better delineation of the anatomy than do plain radiographs, but it is not commonly used.

MRI
Findings
- Impacted meconium produces an intense signal.

WHAT THE REFERRING PHYSICIAN NEEDS TO KNOW
- Radiologic and clinical data are used to differentiate high from low lesions.
- Incidence of cardiovascular malformations, especially Fallot tetralogy and ventricular septal defect, is increased in children with an otherwise isolated imperforate anus.
- Postoperative studies are performed when clinical suspicion exists of an anastomotic leak, fecal soiling, or severe constipation.
- CT and MRI are occasionally used to assess the position of colon pull-through in relation to the sphincteric muscle complex.
- Postsurgery, the child that evacuates well initially but later develops incontinence should be evaluated for a spinal cord lesion that produces tethering.

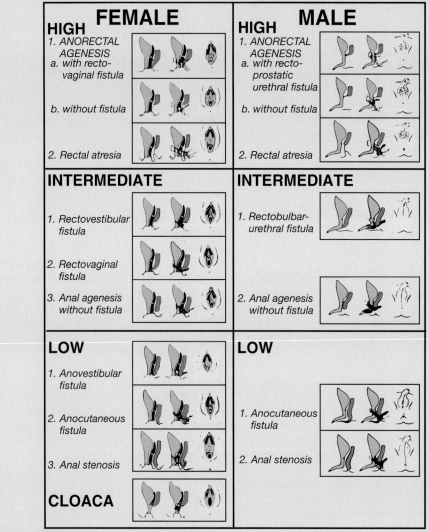

Figure 1. Classification of imperforate anus. This diagram shows many of the possible relationships of the imperforate anus to the internal organs in children of both sexes. *(Adapted from Grosfeld JL, Ballantine TVN, Shoemaker R: Operative management of intestinal atresia and stenosis based on pathologic findings.* J Pediatr Surg 3:368-375, 1979.)

Utility

- Preoperative evaluation of the levator sling can be performed with MRI, but it is not routine.
- MRI displays the sphincteric muscle complex better than CT.
- Muscles are best imaged in the coronal or sagittal planes.
- MRI is useful in evaluating the spinal cord.

CLINICAL PRESENTATION

- High lesions should be suspected when no fistula is seen, when the perineum is smooth, or when the girl has a cloacal anomaly.
- Low lesion is suggested when a fistula, perineal pearls, an extrinsic sphincter corrugated appearance, or a normal-appearing female urethra and vagina are seen.
- Presence of meconium on the perineum or in the urine suggests a low lesion.

PATHOLOGY

- Imperforate anus is a varied congenital anorectal malformation with or without associated anomalies.

INCIDENCE/PREVALENCE AND EPIDEMIOLOGY

- Imperforate anus occurs in approximately 1 of 5000 live births, with a slight male predominance.
- Boys are more likely to have enterourinary fistulas than girls because boys lack the interposed genital structures.
- Girls have a high incidence of enterovaginal fistulas and cloacal anomalies.
- Imperforate anus is associated with genitourinary abnormalities, vertebral, anorectal, cardiac, tracheoesophageal, renal, and limb anomalies (VACTERL), as well as cardiovascular malformations.

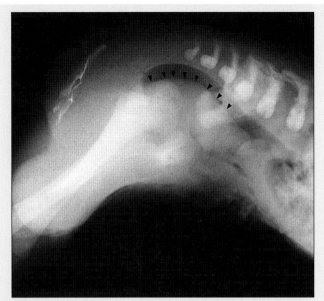

Figure 2. Trendelenburg position invertogram demonstrating an imperforate anus. The child is positioned prone with the hips elevated on a cloth roll. Barium paste marks the anus. Meconium *(arrowheads)* in the rectal pouch is outlined by air.

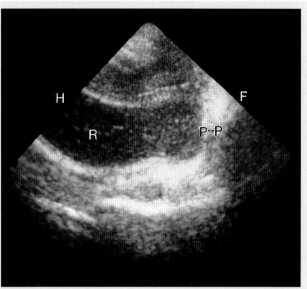

Figure 3. Imperforate anus. On a longitudinal sonogram of the rectal pouch in an infant with an imperforate anus, the echogenic meconium distends and defines the distal rectal (R) pouch. The pouch-to-perineum distance (P-P) is only a few millimeters. (*F,* Inferior; *H,* superior.)

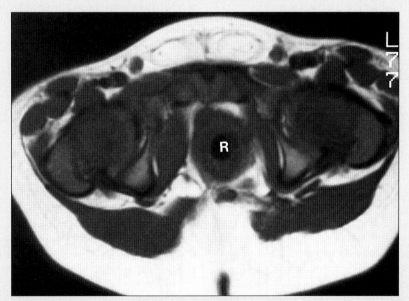

Figure 4. Imperforate anus: MRI of pull-through. Axial MRI shows the anal pull-through in a good position. The rectum (R) is centrally placed within a well-developed sphincteric muscle complex.

■ Renal anomalies (e.g., absence, agenesis, ectopia, horseshoe kidney) are more common and severe in children with a high imperforate anus.

Suggested Readings

Donaldson JS, Black CT, Reynolds M, et al: Ultrasound of the distal pouch in infants with imperforate anus. *J Pediatr Surg* 24:465-468, 1989.

Gross GW, Wolfson PJ, Peña A: Augmented-pressure colostogram in imperforate anus with fistula. *Pediatr Radiol* 21:560-562, 1991.

Han TI, Kim IO, Kim WS: Imperforate anus: US determination of the type with infracoccygeal approach. *Radiology* 228:220-226, 2003.

Metts JC 3rd, Kotkin L, Kasper S, et al: Genital malformations and coexistent urinary tract or spinal anomalies in patients with imperforate anus. *J Urol* 158:1298-1300, 1997.

Narasimharao KL, Prasad GR, Katariya S, et al: Prone cross-table lateral view: An alternative to the invertogram in imperforate anus. *AJR Am J Roentgenol* 140:227-229, 1983.

Shaul DB, Harrison EA: Classification of anorectal malformations: Initial approach, diagnostic test, and colostomy. Semin Pediatr Surg 6:187-195, 1987.

Meconium Ileus

DEFINITION: Narrowed lumen of the distal ileum is impacted with meconium pellets, and the dilated segment above contains thick meconium.

IMAGING

Radiography
Findings
- Multiple, dilated, small-bowel loops
- Small-caliber colon that is malrotated in 33%-50% of patients

Utility
- Contrast enema is used both diagnostically and therapeutically.

Ultrasound
Findings
- Inspissated meconium or meconium in the dilated proximal bowel loops

Utility
- Prenatal or postnatal sonography can demonstrate this echogenic material within dilated small bowel.

CLINICAL PRESENTATION
- No passage of meconium or stool in the neonate
- Abdominal distention and vomiting

DIFFERENTIAL DIAGNOSIS
- Hirschprung disease
- Small bowel atresia with meconium ileus
- Meconium plug syndrome
- Small left colon syndrome
- Obstruction due to duplication cyst
- Imperforate anus

DIAGNOSTIC PEARLS
- Small-caliber colon is malrotated in 33%-50% of patients.
- Inspissated meconium or meconium is seen in the dilated proximal bowel loops.
- Neonate does not pass meconium or stool.

PATHOLOGY
- Narrowed lumen of the distal ileum is impacted with meconium pellets, and the dilated segment above contains thick meconium.

INCIDENCE/PREVALENCE AND EPIDEMIOLOGY
- Meconium ileus indicates cystic fibrosis in approximately 80% of patients.
- The first-year mortality rate for affected infants has diminished markedly but remains approximately 10%.

Suggested Readings

Ein SH, Shandling B, Reilly BJ, et al: Bowel perforation with nonoperative treatment of meconium ileus. *J Pediatr Surg* 22:146-147, 1987.

Kao SC, Franken EA Jr: Nonoperative treatment of simple meconium ileus: A survey of the Society for Pediatric Radiology. *Pediatr Radiol* 25:97-100, 1995.

Neal MR, Seibert JJ, Vanderzalm T, et al: Neonatal ultrasonography to distinguish between meconium ileus and ileal atresia. *J Ultrasound Med* 16:263-266, 1997.

WHAT THE REFERRING PHYSICIAN NEEDS TO KNOW
- Cleansing enemas of hypertonic, water-soluble contrast agents have long been used for diagnosis and treatment.
- The necessity of refluxing contrast into the obstructed terminal ileum may result in the perforation of the unused microcolon.
- To prevent perforation, the physician should not attempt to fill the entire obstructed segment with the first contrast enema.

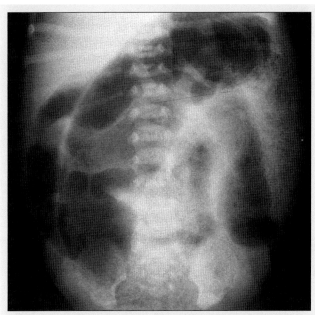

Figure 1. Meconium ileus. Air-filled, dilated bowel loops are present throughout the abdomen. Multiple loops of meconium-filled gut are seen above the distal meconium impaction.

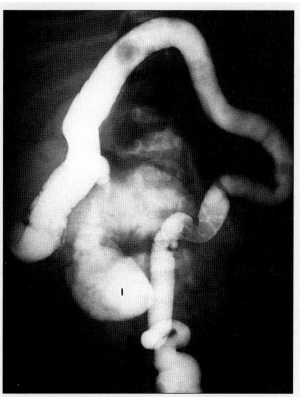

Figure 2. Meconium ileus. The caliber of the colon is slightly diminished on contrast enema. As contrast refluxes into the dilated and obstructed terminal ileum (I), it is diluted by the intraluminal meconium.

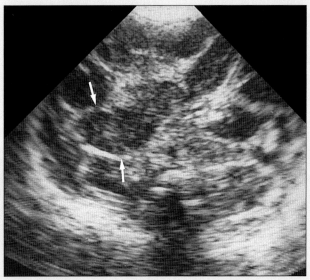

Figure 3. Ultrasound appearance of meconium ileus. Rounded loops of bowel *(arrows)* full of echogenic meconium are visualized on this transverse scan.

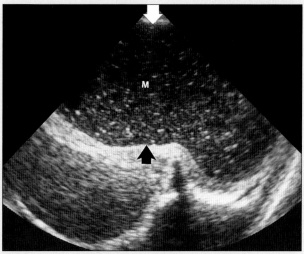

Figure 4. Ultrasound appearance of meconium ileus. Echogenic meconium (M) fills the dilated bowel loop *(arrow)*.

Meconium Peritonitis

DEFINITION: When bowel perforation occurs in utero, sterile meconium leaks into the peritoneal cavity and creates chemical peritonitis.

IMAGING

Ultrasound
Findings
- Fetal ascites may have echogenic debris; echogenicity along the peritoneal surfaces, abnormal cystic abdominal masses, and bowel dilation.
- Ascites alone may be a sign of meconium peritonitis, which, in utero, may simulate fetal hydrops.

Utility
- Ultrasound is used if ascites or a palpable pelvic or abdominal mass is noted.
- It can define the size of the mass and exclude other masses or obstructive lesions.
- It can also differentiate usual ascites from meconium peritonitis with *dirty* ascites.

Radiography
Findings
- Generalized abdominal haziness, bulging flanks, and bowel-loop centralization
- Peritoneal calcifications, intestinal obstruction, mass effect, and, uncommonly, pneumoperitoneum
- Metaphyseal dense bands

Utility
- Often the initial study obtained following delivery

CLINICAL PRESENTATION

- Many children with meconium peritonitis are diagnosed prenatally.
- Abdominal distention and bilious vomiting occur within the first 24 hours of life; also seen are adhesive bands, small bowel atresia, and meconium ascites.

DIFFERENTIAL DIAGNOSIS

- Neuroblastoma
- Hepatoblastoma
- Adrenal hemorrhage
- Renal vein thrombosis
- Teratoma
- Fetal gallstones

DIAGNOSTIC PEARLS

- Fetal ascites may have echogenic debris; also seen is echogenicity along the peritoneal surfaces, in addition to abnormal cystic abdominal masses and bowel dilation.
- Generalized abdominal haziness, bulging flanks, and centralization of bowel loops are seen.
- Peritoneal calcifications are seen.

PATHOLOGY

- When bowel perforation occurs in utero, sterile meconium leaks into the peritoneal cavity and creates chemical peritonitis.
- Perforation may be caused by any process producing bowel ischemia: volvulus, internal hernia, intussusception, and meconium ileus with or without cystic fibrosis.
- Peritonitis is associated with atresia, adhesions, intraabdominal cystic masses, ascites, scrotal masses, and, in many cases, intraperitoneal or scrotal calcifications.
- Meconium peritonitis is categorized as several distinct forms: fibroadhesive, cystic, and generalized.
- In fibroadhesive meconium peritonitis, dense bands and membranes form around and across the bowel loops in response to the peritoneal process.
- In cystic meconium peritonitis, perforation is contained by inflammatory tissue and adjacent loops of bowel that are matted together.
- In the generalized form of meconium peritonitis, loosely adherent or free-floating plaques of calcium are scattered throughout the peritoneal cavity.

INCIDENCE/PREVALENCE AND EPIDEMIOLOGY

- Meconium peritonitis occurs in 1 of 35,000 live births.
- The prognosis for those with meconium peritonitis is good, with a survival rate of approximately 90% of cases.

WHAT THE REFERRING PHYSICIAN NEEDS TO KNOW
- Children with meconium peritonitis should undergo a sweat chloride test to exclude cystic fibrosis.

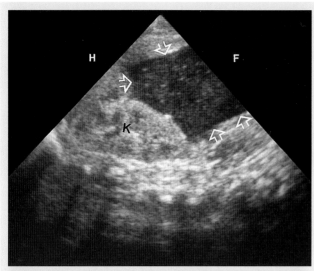

Figure 1. Meconium peritonitis. Longitudinal sonogram reveals a peritoneal collection of meconium *(arrows)* anterior to the echogenic neonatal kidney (K). The meconium is less echogenic than the solid structures, but it contains more echoes than simple transudative ascites. (*H,* Cephalic; *F,* caudal.)

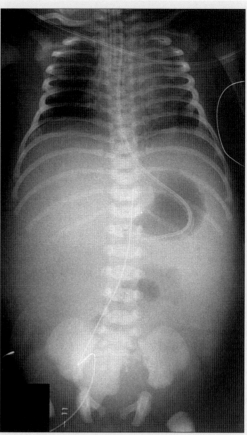

Figure 2. Meconium peritonitis. *Babygram* shows a paucity of abdominal gas, perhaps because the infant is undergoing suction and artificial ventilation. Meconium peritonitis causes generalized abdominal haziness, bulging flanks, and centralization of bowel loops.

Suggested Readings

Chan KL, Tang MH, Tse HY, et al: Meconium peritonitis: Prenatal diagnosis, postnatal management and outcome. *Prenat Diagn* 25:676-682, 2005.

Dirkes K, Crombleholme TM, Craigo SD, et al: The natural history of meconium peritonitis diagnosed in utero. *J Pediatr Surg* 30:979-982, 1995.

Eckoldt F, Heling KS, Woderich R, et al: Meconium peritonitis and pseudocyst formation: Prenatal diagnosis and postnatal course. *Prenat Diagn* 23:904-908, 2003.

Pan EY, Chen LY, Zang JZ, et al: Radiographic diagnosis of meconium peritonitis. *Pediatr Radiol* 13:199-205, 1983.

Wolfson JJ, Engel RR: Anticipating meconium peritonitis from metaphyseal bands. *Radiology* 92:1055-1060, 1969.

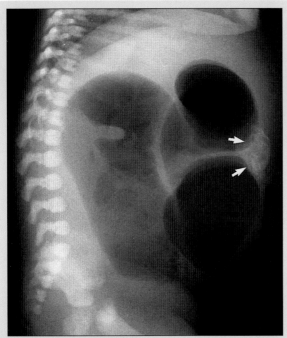

Figure 3. High obstruction. Lateral abdominal radiograph in a child with jejunal atresia shows several markedly distended bowel loops that fill the abdomen. The calcification along the anterior abdominal wall *(arrows)* indicates prior bowel perforation and meconium peritonitis.

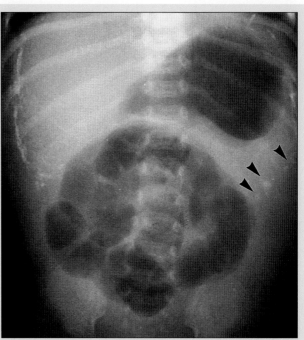

Figure 4. Ileal atresia. Dense calcifications *(arrowheads)* rim the lateral aspect of the upper abdomen. Notice the dilated bowel loops proximal to a surgically proven high ileal atresia.

Meconium Plug Syndrome

DEFINITION: Local inspissation of meconium, delayed passage of meconium, abdominal distention, and low colonic obstruction.

IMAGING

Radiography
Findings
- Multiple, dilated bowel loops are seen.
- Contrast enema, performed with water-soluble agent, outlines the adherent plug, which fills the lumen.
- Colon may be normal in caliber or have diminished caliber up to the splenic flexure.

Utility
- Contrast enema is used diagnostically and therapeutically in this disorder.

CLINICAL PRESENTATION

- Delayed passage of meconium and abdominal distention are the presenting findings in neonates with meconium plug syndrome.
- Most children are promptly and completely relieved by contrast enema, which stimulates passage of the plug.
- Abdominal distention and vomiting.

DIFFERENTIAL DIAGNOSIS

- Hirschprung disease
- Colonic atresia
- Duplication causing colonic obstruction

PATHOLOGY

- Factors associated with a meconium plug include prematurity or maternal treatment with magnesium sulfate.

DIAGNOSTIC PEARLS

- Contrast enema, performed with a water-soluble agent, outlines the adherent plug, which fills the lumen.
- Multiple, dilated bowel loops are seen.
- Delayed passage of meconium and abdominal distention are seen.

INCIDENCE/PREVALENCE AND EPIDEMIOLOGY

- Meconium plug syndrome occurs in approximately 1 of 500-1000 neonates.
- Twenty-five percent of patients have cystic fibrosis, and another 5%-10% have Hirschsprung disease.
- Boys are affected with milk curd syndrome approximately five times more often than girls.

Suggested Readings

Berdon WE, Slovis TL, Campbell JB, et al: Neonatal left colon syndrome: Its relationship to aganglionosis and meconium plug syndrome. *Radiology* 125:457-462, 1977.

Burge D, Drewett M: Meconium plug obstruction. *Pediatr Surg Int* 20:108-110, 2004.

De Backer AI, De Schepper AM, Deprettere A, et al: Radiographic manifestations of intestinal obstruction in the newborn. *JBR-BTR* 82:159-166, 1999.

Konvolinka CW, Frederick J: Milk curd syndrome in neonates. *J Pediatr Surg* 24:497-498, 1990.

Rosenstein BJ: Cystic fibrosis presenting with the meconium plug syndrome. *Am J Dis Child* 132:167-169, 1978.

WHAT THE REFERRING PHYSICIAN NEEDS TO KNOW

- In most instances, the obstruction spontaneously resolves within a few days.
- When obstructive symptoms develop after an uneventful perinatal period, contrast enema may be performed to exclude Hirschsprung disease.
- If the obstruction recurs, excluding Hirschsprung disease by rectal biopsy is necessary.
- If the biopsy shows filling defects in the terminal ileum, milk curd syndrome should be considered and treated with hypertonic contrast enema.

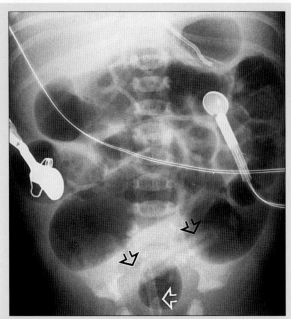

Figure 1. **Meconium plug in Hirschsprung disease.** Multiple dilated bowel loops fill the abdomen. None can be specifically identified as the colon. The umbilical clamp projects *(open black arrows)* over the lower abdomen. A rectal enema tip is in place *(open white arrow)*.

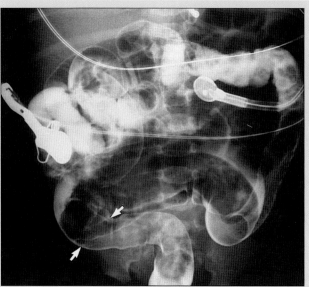

Figure 2. **Meconium plug in Hirschsprung disease.** An intraluminal tubular defect *(arrows)* extends from the descending colon to the rectum. A subtle change is noted in the caliber of the colon, with the sigmoid colon being larger than the rectum.

Megacystis-Microcolon–Intestinal Hypoperistalsis Syndrome

DEFINITION: Megacystis-microcolon–intestinal hypoperistalsis syndrome (MMIHS) is a congenital abnormality producing a small nonfunctioning colon and an enlarged urinary bladder.

ANATOMIC FINDINGS

Colon
- Small, nonfunctioning

Urinary Bladder
- Enlarged

IMAGING

Ultrasound
Findings
- Markedly dilated bladder and upper urinary tract in the female infant not associated with a decreased amount of amniotic fluid

Utility
- Prenatal ultrasound excludes other causes of the abdominal mass.

Radiography
Findings
- Dilated upper urinary tract without any site of mechanical obstruction is seen.
- Contrast enema easily fills the microcolon, which has tendency to be abnormally rotated or fixed.

Utility
- Contrast studies of the genitourinary tract are routinely performed to exclude vesicoureteral reflux.

CLINICAL PRESENTATION

- Patients exhibit abdominal distention and vomiting shortly after birth.
- Wrinkled appearance of the abdomen may not be appreciated until the huge bladder is catheterized and drained.
- All children with MMIHS die in infancy.

DIAGNOSTIC PEARLS

- Small, nonfunctioning colon and a markedly dilated bladder and upper urinary tract
- Not associated with a decreased amount of amniotic fluid
- Abdominal distention and vomiting shortly after birth

DIFFERENTIAL DIAGNOSIS

- Colonic atresia
- Malrotation
- Hirschprung disease
- Imperforate anus
- Hypoplastic left colon syndrome

PATHOLOGY

- Most cases are sporadic, but some have shown a pattern of autosomal-recessive inheritance.
- MMIHS is a congenital abnormality producing a small nonfunctioning colon and an enlarged urinary bladder.

INCIDENCE/PREVALENCE AND EPIDEMIOLOGY

- Rare condition that occurs almost exclusively in girls

Suggested Readings

Carlsson SA, Hokegard KH, Mattsson LA: Megacystis-microcolon-intestinal hypoperistalsis syndrome: Antenatal appearance in two cases. *Acta Obstet Gynecol Scand* 71:645-648, 1992.
Goulet O, Jobeer-Giraud A, Michel JL, et al: Chronic intestinal pseudo-obstruction syndrome in pediatric patients. *Eur J Pediatr Surg* 9:83-89, 1999.

WHAT THE REFERRING PHYSICIAN NEEDS TO KNOW

- Although hyperalimentation improves nutritional status, it is a temporary measure because bowel function is never corrected.
- Neither pharmacologic stimulation nor an ileostomy or colostomy improves gastrointestinal tract function.
- In some children, biopsy of the colon may be necessary to exclude Hirschsprung disease.

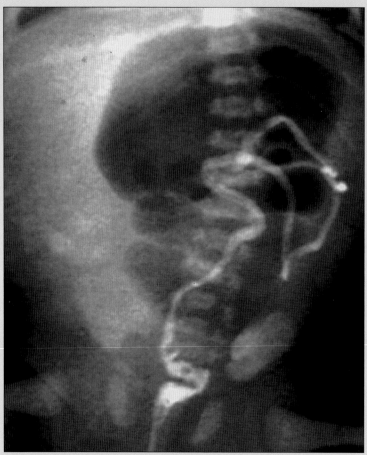

Figure 1. A contrast enema showing microcolon in a patient with MMIHS. *(From Puri P, Shinkai M: Megacystis microcolon intestinal hypoperistalsis syndrome.* Semin Pediatr Surg *14:58-63, 2005.)*

Kubota M, Ikeda K, Ito Y: Autonomic innervation of the intestine from a baby with megacystis microcolon intestinal hypoperistalsis syndrome. II. Electrophysiological study. *J Pediatr Surg* 24:1267-1270, 1989.

Kubota M, Ikeda K, Shono T, et al: Autonomic innervation of the intestine from a baby with megacystis microcolon intestinal hypoperistalsis syndrome. I. Immunohistochemical study. *J Pediatr Surg* 24:1264-1266, 1989.

Manco LG, Osterdahl P: The antenatal diagnosis of megacystis-microcolon-intestinal hypoperistalsis syndrome. *J Clin Ultrasound* 12:595-598, 1984.

Young LW, Yunis EJ, Girdany BR, et al: Megacystis-microcolon-intestinal hypoperistalsis syndrome: Additional clinical, radiological, surgical, and histopathologic aspects. *AJR Am J Roentgenol* 137:749-755, 1981.

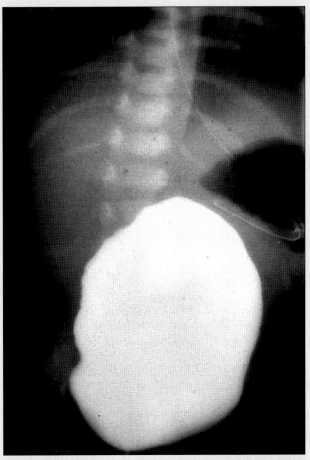

Figure 2. Voiding cystourethrogram showing a massively enlarged bladder in a patient with MMIHS. *(From Puri P, Shinkai M: Megacystis microcolon intestinal hypoperistalsis syndrome. Semin Pediatr Surg 14:58-63, 2005.)*

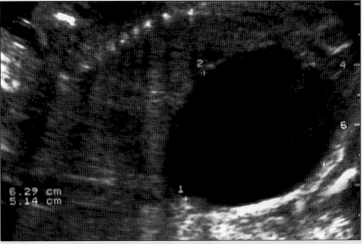

Figure 3. Large fetal bladder seen on a longitudinal view of abdominal ultrasound at 22 weeks' gestation. The fetus is in prone position. *(From Puri P, Shinkai M: Megacystis microcolon intestinal hypoperistalsis syndrome. Semin Pediatr Surg 14:58-63, 2005.)*

Necrotizing Enterocolitis

DEFINITION: Necrotizing enterocolitis (NEC) is a life-threatening process that affects primarily the gastrointestinal tracts of premature infants.

IMAGING

Radiography

Findings

- Gastric dilation, persistently dilated bowel loop, or an unchanging bowel gas pattern is seen.
- Pneumatosis intestinalis produces intramural gas, creating a linear, streaky pattern that parallels the bowel wall; circular lucency is seen around the bowel lumen.
- Gas enters the mesenteric veins and intrahepatic branches of the portal vein, producing streaky lucencies radiating to the periphery of the liver.
- Bowel perforation and free intraperitoneal air are seen; a diffuse lucency appears over the liver or mid-abdomen.
- Air outlines the falciform ligament; the inverted V sign is seen in the pelvis; a triangular lucency is seen in the Morison pouch.
- Strictures are seen.

Utility

- When the presence of free air is suspected, supine abdominal radiographs are supplemented by cross-table lateral radiographs.
- Contrast enema should be used to evaluate the entire colon and terminal ileum.

Ultrasound

Findings

- Mural thickening of the affected loops and portal venous gas are seen before their detection on plain radiographs.
- Intrahepatic portal venous gas is seen as bright reflectors bubbling through the liver.
- Hepatic parenchyma develops unusually bright echoes in a patchy distribution.
- Severely affected (gangrenous) bowel loops may demonstrate diminished or absent blood flow when color Doppler imaging is used.

DIAGNOSTIC PEARLS

- Pneumatosis intestinalis
- Bowel perforation, free intraperitoneal air, and diffuse lucency appearing over the liver or mid-abdomen
- Inverted V sign in the pelvis and triangular lucency in the Morison pouch

Utility

- This diagnosis is generally made with plain abdominal radiographs.

CLINICAL PRESENTATION

- Signs and symptoms of NEC usually develop in the first 2 weeks of life.
- Rising gastric residual volume, abdominal distention, bloody stools, lethargy, and even changing respiratory status are seen.
- Erythema of the abdominal wall, a positive result of paracentesis, or palpation of an abdominal mass suggests bowel perforation.
- Blood-streaked stools in 50%, explosive diarrhea
- Generalized sepsis
- Mild respiratory distress

PATHOLOGY

- NEC is a life-threatening process that affects primarily the gastrointestinal tracts of premature infants.
- Ulceration begins in mucosa and extends to the submucosa; inflammatory cells are present in multiple bowel layers.

WHAT THE REFERRING PHYSICIAN NEEDS TO KNOW

- Timing of surgery is crucial; ideally, surgery should take place when gangrene is present but before bowel perforation.
- Erythema of the abdominal wall, positive results of paracentesis, or palpation of abdominal mass suggests bowel perforation and mandates surgical treatment.
- Specific plain radiographic changes considered to be good indications for surgery are pneumoperitoneum and portal venous gas.
- When NEC is suspected clinically, the infant is treated accordingly, even in the absence of radiographic findings.
- Although some of the strictures may spontaneously regress, most are resected surgically or dilated with balloon catheters.
- To exclude stricture, children with NEC undergo antegrade contrast study of the entire gastrointestinal tract before feeding is resumed.
- Medical management of infants with suspected NEC includes parenteral nutrition and antibiotic therapy.

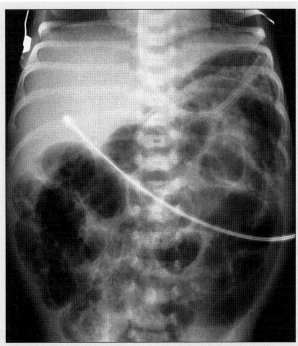

Figure 1. Necrotizing enterocolitis with pneumatosis intestinalis. The bubbly appearance of the abdomen is caused by air within the bowel wall. In some segments, the intramural air clearly parallels the lumen; in other segments, it is seen as a circular pattern surrounding the lumen.

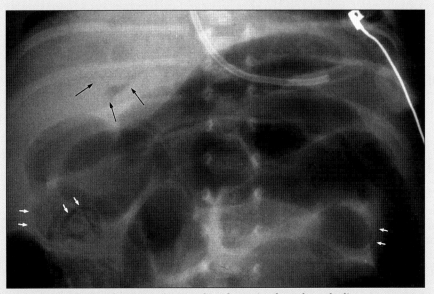

Figure 2. Necrotizing enterocolitis with portal venous air. Branching lucencies throughout the liver represent gas within the portal venous system *(black arrows)*. Intramural air is also present *(white arrows)*.

- Pneumatosis intestinalis is seen in the submucosa and subserosa; in 50% of cases, normal areas of the bowel are interposed between the diseased segments.
- Occasional epidemic nature of NEC indicates that a viral or bacterial agent may play a role in some cases.

- NEC is associated with bowel ischemia of any cause: abnormal gut hormones, immunoglobulins, or peristalsis, as well as enteral feedings and maternal cocaine use.
- Complications include gangrene, perforation with peritonitis or enterocyst formation or stricture formation, enteric fistulas, and sepsis.

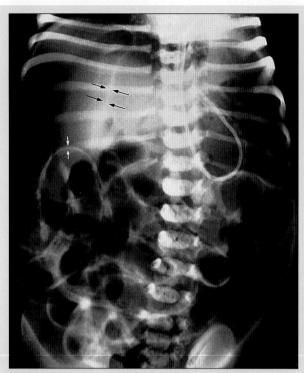

Figure 3. Necrotizing enterocolitis with perforation: the football sign. A large amount of free peritoneal air outlines the falciform ligament *(black arrows)*. The air has also given the entire right upper quadrant an unusual lucent appearance. The inner and outer walls *(white arrows)* of multiple bowel loops are visible, another sign of free peritoneal air.

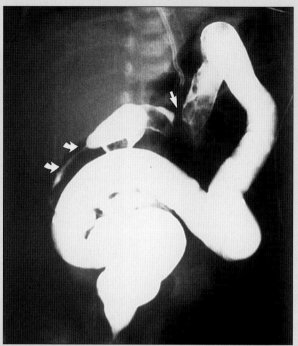

Figure 4. Colonic stricture from necrotizing enterocolitis. Water-soluble enema depicts an area of minor narrowing in the mid transverse colon *(straight arrow)* and a more severely narrowed segment at the hepatic flexure *(curved arrows)*.

- Late complications include short gut syndrome, sepsis, abdominal abscess, recurrent NEC, and stricture formation, as well as some extragastrointestinal problems.

INCIDENCE/PREVALENCE AND EPIDEMIOLOGY

- Strictures are late findings that develop in approximately 9%-35% of children with NEC.
- Seventy-five percent of strictures occur in the colon, in the region of the splenic flexure; 15% are multiple; the terminal ileum is involved in 15% of affected infants.

Suggested Readings

Brill PW, Olson SR, Winchester P: Neonatal necrotizing enterocolitis: Air in Morison pouch. *Radiology* 174:469-471, 1990.

Engum SA, Grosfeld JL: Necrotizing enterocolitis. *Curr Opin Pediatr* 10:123-130, 1998.

Faingold R, Daneman A, Tomlinson G, et al: Necrotizing enterocolitis: Assessment of bowel viability with color Doppler US. *Radiology* 235:587-594, 2005.

Hartman GE, Drugas GT, Sochat SJ: Post-necrotizing enterocolitis strictures presenting with sepsis or perforation: Risk of clinical observation. *J Pediatr Surg* 23:562-566, 1988.

Horwitz JR, Lally KP, Cheu HW, et al: Complications after surgical intervention for necrotizing enterocolitis: A multicenter review. *J Pediatr Surg* 30:994-999, 1995.

Hsueh W, Caplan MS, Qu XW, et al: Neonatal necrotizing enterocolitis: Clinical considerations and pathogenetic concepts. *Pediatr Dev Pathol* 6:6-23, 2003.

Kosloske AM: Indications for operation in necrotizing enterocolitis revisited. *J Pediatr Surg* 5:663-666, 1994.

Martinez-Tallo E, Claure N, Bancalari E: Necrotizing enterocolitis in full-term or near-term infants: Risk factors. *Biol Neonate* 71:292-298, 1997.

Merritt CRB, Goldsmith JP, Sharp MJ: Sonographic detection of portal venous gas in infants with necrotizing enterocolitis. *AJR Am J Roentgenol* 143:1059-1062, 1984.

Morrison SC, Jacobson JM: The radiology of necrotizing enterocolitis. *Clin Perinatol* 21:347-363, 1994.

Neu J: Neonatal necrotizing enterocolitis: An update. *Acta Pediatr Suppl* 94:100-105, 2005.

Rencken IO, Sola A, Al-Ali F, et al: Necrotizing enterocolitis: Diagnosis with CT examination of urine after enteral administration of iodinated water-soluble contrast material. *Radiology* 205:87-90, 1997.

Rescorla FJ: Surgical management of pediatric necrotizing enterocolitis. *Curr Opin Pediatr* 7:335-341, 1995.

Seibert JJ, Parvey LS: The telltale triangle: Use of the supine cross-table lateral radiograph of the abdomen in early detection of pneumoperitoneum. *Pediatr Radiol* 5:209-210, 1977.

Sharma R, Tepas JJ, Hudak ML, et al: Portal venous gas and surgical outcome of neonatal necrotizing enterocolitis. *J Pediatr Surg* 40:371-376, 2005.

Stringer MD, Cave E, Puntis JW, et al: Enteric fistulas and necrotizing enterocolitis. *J Pediatr Surg* 31:1268-1271, 1996.

Tonkin ILD, Bjelland JC, Hunter TB, et al: Spontaneous resolution of colonic strictures caused by necrotizing enterocolitis: Therapeutic implications. *AJR Am J Roentgenol* 130:1077-1081, 1978.

Omphalocele

DEFINITION: Midline defect of variable size through which the bowel, liver, spleen, pancreas, and uterus may protrude, usually covered by a membrane or sac.

IMAGING

Ultrasound
Findings
- Visualization of the umbilical cord inserting into membrane covering structures anterior to the abdominal wall of fetus
- Fetal ascites, abnormal amounts of amniotic fluid, and associated congenital defects
Utility
- Prenatal sonographic diagnosis is easily made.

Radiography
Findings
- Soft-tissue density and margins well-defined by adjacent air are seen.
- Bowel loops are not individually seen unless the omphalocele sac has ruptured.
- Malrotation of bowel and malposition of other organs are identified on postoperative imaging studies.
Utility
- Postnatal plain radiographs of the abdomen show extra-abdominal bowel loops.

CLINICAL PRESENTATION

- Midline defect of variable size through which the bowel, liver, spleen, pancreas, and uterus may protrude
- Beckwith-Weidemann syndrome, large at birth, large tongue, and hypoglycemia
- Small anterior abdominal defects and a normally developed thorax
- Giant omphaloceles, small thorax, increased incidence of pulmonary hypoplasia and respiratory insufficiency (may require ventilatory support after surgery)

DIFFERENTIAL DIAGNOSIS

- Gastroschisis (neonatal gastrointestinal)
- Limb-body wall complex

DIAGNOSTIC PEARLS

- Visualization of umbilical cord inserting into the membrane covering the structures anterior to the abdominal wall of the fetus
- Soft-tissue density and well-defined margins by adjacent air
- Bowel loops not individually seen unless the omphalocele sac has ruptured

PATHOLOGY

- Membrane or sac covers herniated organs but it can be ruptured at birth; the umbilical cord inserts into the apex of the sac, and the bowel is malrotated.
- Maternal α-fetoprotein levels are elevated and tend to be less than those found with gastroschisis defects because of the covering sac.

INCIDENCE/PREVALENCE AND EPIDEMIOLOGY

- Omphalocele is present in approximately 1 of 5000 live births.
- Eight to twenty percent of these children have Meckel diverticulum.
- Associated anomalies are seen in 50%-80% of infants with omphalocele.
- Children with Beckwith-Wiedemann syndrome account for almost 12% of the population with omphalocele.
- Down syndrome (i.e., trisomy 21), trisomy 13, and trisomy 18 are associated with an increased incidence of omphalocele.

Suggested Readings
Barisic I, Clementi M, Hausler M, et al: Evaluation of prenatal ultrasound diagnosis of fetal abdominal wall defects by 19 European registries. *Ultrasound Obstet Gynecol* 18:309-316, 2001.
Blazer S, Zimmer EZ, Gover A, et al: Fetal omphalocele detected early in pregnancy: Associated anomalies and outcomes. *Radiology* 232:191-195, 2004.

WHAT THE REFERRING PHYSICIAN NEEDS TO KNOW
- The diagnosis of omphalocele can be made with prenatal ultrasound.
- Defect is corrected by primary skin closure or closure with a Silastic halo.
- Procedure is determined by the size of the defect, and larger defects may require a staged reduction.

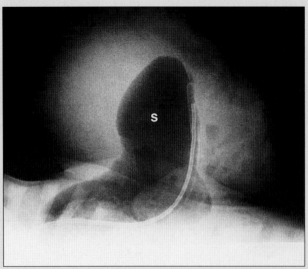

Figure 1. Omphalocele. Lateral plain radiograph of the abdomen reveals a membrane-covered omphalocele. The sac of the omphalocele is outlined by air and clearly seen, but individual bowel loops cannot be identified because they are not exposed to air, unlike the situation in gastroschisis. The air-filled stomach (S) protrudes into the omphalocele.

Brantberg A, Blaas HGK, Haugens SE, et al: Characteristics and outcome of 90 cases of fetal omphalocele. *Ultrasound Obstet Gynecol* 26:527-537, 2005.

Cyr DR, Mack LA, Schoenecker SA, et al: Bowel migration in the normal fetus: US detection. *Radiology* 161:119-121, 1986.

Getachew MM, Goldstein RB, Edge V, et al: Correlation between omphalocele contents and karyotypic abnormalities: Sonographic study in 37 cases. *AJR Am J Roentgenol* 158:133-136, 1992.

Hwang PJ, Kouseff BG: Omphalocele and gastroschisis: An 18-year review study. *Genet Med* 6:232-236, 2004.

Parulekar SG: Sonography of normal fetal bowel. *J Ultrasound Med* 10:211-220, 1991.

Stoll C, Alembik Y, Dott B, et al: Risk factors in congenital abdominal wall defects (omphalocele and gastroschisis): A study in a series of 265,858 consecutive births. *Am Genet* 44:201-208, 2001.

Tsakayannis DE, Zurakowski D, Lillehei CW: Respiratory insufficiency at birth: A predictor of mortality for infants with omphalocele. *J Pediatr Surg* 31:1088-1090, 1996.

Zaccara A, Iacobelli BD, La Sala E, et al: Sonographic biometry of liver and spleen size long after closure of abdominal wall defects. *Eur J Pediatr* 162:490-492, 2003.

Small Left Colon Syndrome

DEFINITION: Congenital reduction of colon caliber in neonates of diabetic mothers.

IMAGING

Radiography
Findings
- Rectum is large, but the descending colon and sigmoid colon are much smaller than normal.
- Abrupt change in caliber at level of splenic flexure is a classic finding for this syndrome.
Utility
- The diagnosis is usually established with a retrograde contrast enema.

DIFFERENTIAL DIAGNOSIS

- Meconium plug syndrome
- Hirschprung disease
- Colonic atresia

PATHOLOGY

- Functional obstruction is noted due to immaturity of myenteric plexus.
- Abrupt change in the caliber at the level of the splenic flexure is a classic finding for this syndrome.
- Rectum is large, but the descending colon and sigmoid colon are much smaller than normal.

DIAGNOSTIC PEARLS

- Rectum is large.
- Descending colon and sigmoid colon are much smaller than normal.
- Abrupt change in caliber is seen at the level of the splenic flexure.

INCIDENCE/PREVALENCE AND EPIDEMIOLOGY

- Small left colon syndrome occurs in infants of diabetic mothers.

Suggested Readings

Davis WS, Allen RP, Favara BE, et al: Neonatal small left colon syndrome. *AJR Am J Roentgenol* 120:322-329, 1974.

WHAT THE REFERRING PHYSICIAN NEEDS TO KNOW

- Colon with diminished caliber up to splenic flexure is also seen in neonates with meconium plug syndrome.
- There is gradual resolution of functional immaturity over days to weeks.

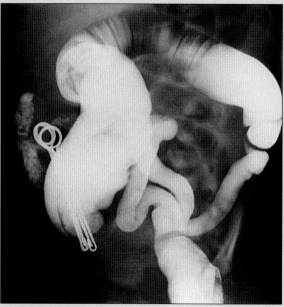

Figure 1. Small left colon syndrome. The rectum is large, but the descending colon and sigmoid colon are much smaller than normal. An abrupt change in caliber is seen at the level of the splenic flexure, a classic finding.

Foreign Bodies and Caustic Ingestions (Pediatric Esophagus)

DEFINITION: Ingestion of a foreign body or caustic agents.

IMAGING

Radiography
Findings
- Severe injury: Retention of contrast material within the esophageal wall and persistent gaseous dilation of the esophagus are seen.
- Caustic-induced dysmotility may be associated with the appearance of transverse folds in the esophagus and the development of strictures.
- Plain radiographs of the airway or chest may be entirely normal despite the presence of an esophageal foreign body.
- Thickening of soft tissues between esophagus and trachea is a sign of esophageal edema.
- Thickening or anterior bowing of the esophagus may result from mediastinitis, which develops after esophageal perforation.

Utility
- After caustic ingestion, airway and chest radiographs should be obtained.
- Barium studies are not useful in the diagnosis or management immediately after caustic ingestion.
- In the early recuperative period, contrast studies may show abnormalities of predictive value.
- Barium studies are of value in detecting late changes of the esophagus, such as stricture, or abnormalities in the sites not visualized during endoscopy.
- Barium study is recommended in the healthy-appearing child with drooling or dysphagia to exclude a non-opaque foreign body, congenital lesion, or acquired inflammatory lesion.
- Mediastinum should be carefully analyzed on the lateral projection.

DIAGNOSTIC PEARLS
- Swelling of epiglottis or edema of airway
- Mediastinal air
- Thickening or anterior bowing of the esophagus

CLINICAL PRESENTATION
- Acids and other low-pH corrosive agents may injure the gastric antrum and can produce burns and scars in the esophagus.
- Contact between the acid and the upper airway can produce life-threatening epiglottitis in some children.
- Bleaches have a neutral pH of 7 and generally cause only transient irritation of the esophagus without long-term complications.
- Children with dysphagia or prolonged drooling are likely to have developed esophageal strictures or scars.
- Dysphagia, odynophagia, and vomiting

PATHOLOGY
- In the young infant, caustic ingestion should raise the specter of child abuse; in the older child, caustic ingestion may indicate a suicide attempt.
- Caustic agents (lye and laundry detergents) have a high pH and cause most of the damage in the mouth and upper esophagus.
- An impacted battery can cause severe focal tissue damage in several ways, often within a few hours.

WHAT THE REFERRING PHYSICIAN NEEDS TO KNOW
- The type and location of mucosal injury depend on the pH of the ingested material.
- Most children recover without sequelae.
- Contact between acid and the upper airway can produce life-threatening epiglottitis in some children.
- Clinical findings do not correlate with the extent of the injury found endoscopically, but they do correlate with the degree of mucosal damage.
- Radiologic diagnosis is coupled with treatment if the radiologist is skillful in removing foreign bodies with the combined balloon catheter and fluoroscopic technique.
- In asymptomatic children, a recently swallowed coin lodged in the esophagus below the thoracic inlet may be allowed to pass without intervention.
- Any swelling of the epiglottis or edema of the airway should prompt measures to ensure airway patency.

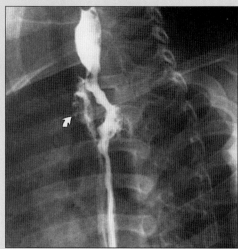

Figure 1. Battery-induced tracheoesophageal fistula.
Esophagogram. Water-soluble contrast material passes from the normal cervical esophagus into the irregular-appearing region where the battery was previously seen. The anterior collection *(arrow)* of contrast material indicates that perforation occurred.

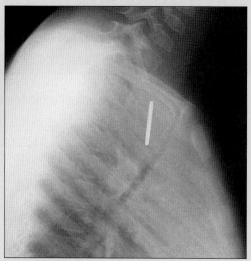

Figure 2. Coin ingestion. The coin is seen in the upper esophagus. The trachea is bowed anteriorly and is narrowed.

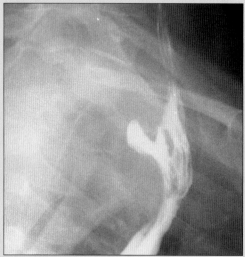

Figure 3. Coin ingestion. After removal of the coin, the contrast study demonstrates that the coin had perforated the esophagus posteriorly and that the esophagus was pushed anteriorly by the inflammatory process surrounding the site of perforation.

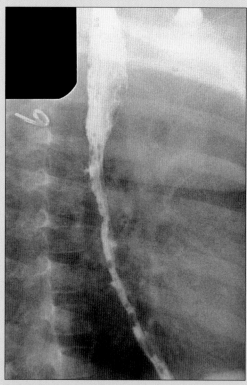

Figure 4. Lye ingestion and surgical correction. Irregularity of the distal esophagus and lack of distensibility indicate the degree of damage done by the ingestion of lye.

- The esophagus may be damaged by pressure necrosis, fluid leaking from the battery, or a low-voltage electrical injury.
- If tissue necrosis ensues, traumatic tracheoesophageal fistula or a lethal fistula to the aorta may develop.
- Physiologic sites of narrowing trap ingested foreign bodies: the thoracic inlet, the level of aortic knob, and the gastroesophageal junction.
- Foreign-body impaction at any other level should raise suspicion of an intrinsic stricture or vascular ring.

INCIDENCE/PREVALENCE AND EPIDEMIOLOGY

- Most caustic and foreign-body ingestions occur in children younger than 5 years of age.
- Perforation or stricture formation occurs in approximately 3% of patients.

Suggested Readings

Cadranel S, Di Lorenzo C, Rodesch P, et al: Caustic ingestion and esophageal function. *J Pediatr Gastroenterol Nutr* 10:164-168, 1990.

Eggli KD, Potter BM, Garcia V, et al: Delayed diagnosis of esophageal perforation by aluminum foreign bodies. *Pediatr Radiol* 16:511-516, 1986.

Gundogdu HZ, Tanyel FC, Buyukpamukcu N, et al: Colonic replacement for the treatment of caustic esophageal strictures in children. *J Pediatr Surg* 27:771-774, 1992.

Harned RK, Strain JD, Hay TC, et al: Esophageal foreign bodies: Safety and efficacy of Foley catheter extraction of coins. *AJR Am J Roentgenol* 168:443-446, 1997.

Macpherson RI, Hill JG, Othersen HB, et al: Esophageal foreign bodies in children: Diagnosis, treatment, and complications. *AJR Am J Roentgenol* 166:919-924, 1996.

Reeder JD, Kramer SS, Dudgeon DL: Transverse esophageal folds: Association with corrosive injury. *Radiology* 155:303-304, 1985.

Sharieff GQ, Brousseau TJ, Bradshaw JA, et al: Acute esophageal coin ingestions: Is immediate removal necessary? *Pediatr Radiol* 33:359-363, 2003.

Pediatric Swallowing Disorders

DEFINITION: Derangement of the oral stage of swallowing caused by congenital anomalies.

IMAGING

Fluoroscopy
Findings
- As barium passes over the tongue, the palate does not close off the nasopharynx, which is filling with barium.
- Cricopharyngeal spasm may be seen.

Utility
- All stages of the swallowing process (oral, pharyngeal, and esophageal) should be observed as part of the swallowing examination.
- Modified barium swallow, a rehabilitative swallow study, or a cookie swallow may be attempted.
- Older children are given age-appropriate foods to assess the completeness of mastication and the ability to centralize food within the oral cavity.
- Modified barium swallow, performed with the child supported in the semiupright position, simulating the way the child usually eats, may be attempted.

CLINICAL PRESENTATION

- Absence of tongue
- Macroglossia
- Cleft palate
- Micrognathia
- Dysphagia
- Odynophagia

DIFFERENTIAL DIAGNOSIS

- Familial dysautonomia
- Developmental delay
- Prematurity
- Retardation
- Beckwith-Wiedemann syndrome

PATHOLOGY

- Patients may exhibit derangement of the oral portion of swallowing caused by congenital anomalies (absence of the tongue, macroglossia, cleft palate, and micrognathia).

DIAGNOSTIC PEARLS

- Cricopharyngeal spasm
- Derangement of the oral stage of swallowing
- Neuromuscular disorders

- Acquired swallowing problems result from neurologic disorders such as cerebral palsy, cranial trauma, meningomyelocele, or central nervous system tumors.
- Sucking motions for each swallow persist in children with neuromuscular disorders.
- Neuromuscular disorders affect the tongue (causing poor bolus formation), the palate (causing nasopharyngeal aspiration), and the epiglottis, with secondary tracheal penetration or aspiration.
- In the pharynx, poor emptying and *laryngeal spill* are seen despite relatively normal epiglottic function; the cricopharyngeal muscle is seen interfering with the passage of the bolus.
- Failure of the cricopharyngeal muscle relaxation is called cricopharyngeal spasm or cricopharyngeal bar and occurs transiently in some normal children.

Suggested Readings

Arvedson JC: Dysphagia in pediatric patients with neurologic damage. *Semin Neurol* 16:371-386, 1996.

Jolley SG, McClelland KK, Mosesso-Rousseau M: Pharyngeal and swallowing disorders in infants. *Semin Pediatr Surg* 4:157-165, 1995.

Miller CK, Willging JP: Advancement in the evaluation and management of pediatric dysphagia. *Curr Opin Otolaryngol Head Neck Surg* 11:442-446, 2003.

Pollack IF, Pang D, Kocoshis S, et al: Neurogenic dysphagia resulting from Chiari malformations. *Neurosurgery* 30:709-712, 1992.

Taniguchi MH, Moyer RS: Assessment of risk factors for pneumonia in dysphagic children: Significance of videofluoroscopic swallowing evaluation. *Dev Med Child Neurol* 36:495-502, 1994.

Zerilli KS, Stefans VA, DiPietro MA: Protocol for the use of videofluoroscopy in pediatric swallowing dysfunction. *Am J Occup Ther* 44:441-446, 1990.

WHAT THE REFERRING PHYSICIAN NEEDS TO KNOW

- Swallowing studies are performed in conjunction with a speech or occupational therapist who determines optimal food volume and feeding implements.
- The patient may perform compensatory maneuvers that assist in swallowing.
- Examination should be videotaped to allow immediate and repeated review.
- Structural abnormalities should also be recorded on videotape or radiographs.

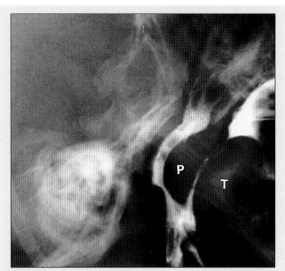

Figure 1. Abnormal swallowing. Nasopharyngeal aspiration. As barium passes over the tongue (T), the palate (P) does not close off the nasopharynx, which is filling with barium.

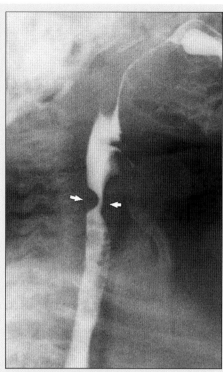

Figure 2. Abnormal swallowing. Cricopharyngeal spasm. Narrowing of the esophagus is seen at the C5 level at the upper esophageal sphincter, which is the cricopharyngeal muscle.

Vascular Rings (Pediatric)

DEFINITION: Vascular rings occur when the esophagus and trachea are encircled, displaced, or compressed by the aorta, its branches, or the remnants of fetal circulation.

IMAGING

Radiography
Findings
- Double aortic arch or right aortic arch with an aberrant left subclavian artery and the presence of the right aortic arch in the child
- Double aortic arch: indentation of the anterior wall of the airway in the lateral view
- Pulmonary sling: anterior displacement of the trachea in the lateral view
- Double aortic arch: indented trachea by the anterior portion of the arch and the esophagus by the posterior portion
- Aberrant subclavian artery: trachea of normal appearance and an esophagus indented posteriorly by an anomalous vessel
- Anomalous innominate artery: trachea flattened anteriorly by the innominate artery and the esophagus of normal appearance
- Vascular sling: displaced trachea anteriorly and esophagus posteriorly by the left pulmonary artery

Utility
- Plain radiographs can often suggest the diagnosis.
- On the frontal view of the airway or chest, the position of the aortic arch and trachea should be carefully evaluated.
- Barium esophagogram was once routinely used to establish this diagnosis.

CT
Findings
- Double aortic arch
- Right aortic arch
- Left aortic arch
- Aberrant pulmonary artery or pulmonary artery slings

Utility
- Contrast-enhanced CT or MRI scans are more commonly used than angiography or echocardiography for the diagnosis and preoperative planning.

MRI
Findings
- Right aortic arch
- Aberrant left subclavian artery
- Pulmonary sling

DIAGNOSTIC PEARLS
- Stridor because of transient esophageal dilation
- Reflex apnea prompts urgent surgery
- Anomaly of pulmonary artery

Utility
- Contrast-enhanced CT or MRI scans are more commonly used than angiography or echocardiography for the diagnosis and preoperative planning.
- MRI provides multiplanar images of the great vessels, which greatly enhances preoperative planning.

CLINICAL PRESENTATION
- Asymptomatic rings are incidentally discovered on chest radiographs.
- In childhood, vascular rings commonly cause stridor during feeding because the transient esophageal dilation produces additional tracheal compression.
- Adults instead tend to have dysphagia as a presenting symptom.
- Reflex apnea is another presentation and may prompt urgent surgery.
- Chronic stridor
- Wheezing
- Recurrent pneumonias

DIFFERENTIAL DIAGNOSIS
- Mediastinal adenopathy
- Mediastinal tumor

PATHOLOGY
- Vascular rings occur when the esophagus and trachea are encircled, displaced, or compressed by the aorta, its branches, or the remnants of fetal circulation.
- Some rings are incomplete, but others, such as double aortic arch, completely surround and frequently compress the esophagus and trachea.

WHAT THE REFERRING PHYSICIAN NEEDS TO KNOW
- Severely symptomatic children may respond to innominopexy, a surgical procedure that elevates and fixes the artery from the trachea.

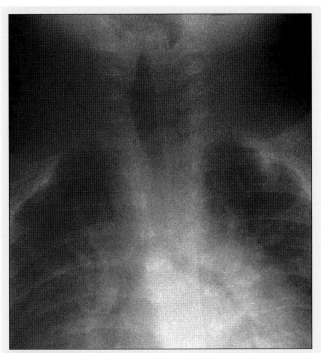

Figure 1. Double aortic arch. The larger and higher right arch is indenting and displacing the trachea toward the left.

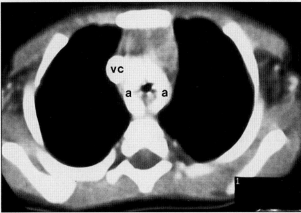

Figure 2. Double aortic arch. During the bolus injection of contrast medium, the CT scan demonstrates both segments of the double aortic arch (a), which encircle the trachea and esophagus. The superior vena cava (vc) is opacified.

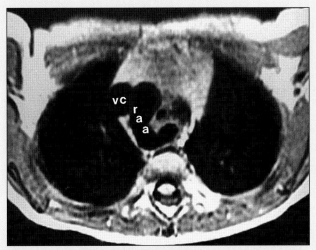

Figure 3. Right aortic arch and aberrant left subclavian artery. The right aortic arch (raa) is medial to the superior vena cava (vc) on this axial MR scan. The anomalous subclavian artery courses posteriorly and to the left and is close to the spine.

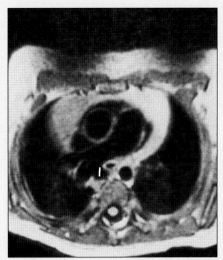

Figure 4. Pulmonary sling: MRI findings. The anomalous left pulmonary artery (l) arises from the right.

- Double aortic arch, the most common vascular ring, is formed by a larger, more cephalad right aortic arch and a smaller, more caudad left aortic arch.
- Vascular sling, an anomaly of the pulmonary artery, increases the incidence of intracardiac and bronchial anomalies, including ventricular septal defects.

INCIDENCE/PREVALENCE AND EPIDEMIOLOGY

- Twenty percent of children with vascular rings have congenital heart disease.

Suggested Readings

Backer CL, Mavroudis C, Rigsby CK, et al: Trends in vascular surgery. *J Thorac Cardiovasc Surg* 129:1339-1347, 2005.

Berdon WE, Baker DH: Vascular anomalies and the infant lung: Rings, slings, and other things. *Semin Roentgenol* 7:39-64, 1972.

Hernanz-Schulman M: Vascular rings: A practical approach to imaging diagnosis. *Pediatr Radiol* 35:961-979, 2005.

Pickman PJ, Siegel MJ, Gutierrez FR: Vascular rings in symptomatic children: Frequency of chest radiographic findings. *Radiology* 203:423-426, 1997.

van Son JA, Julsrud PR, Hagler DJ, et al: Surgical treatment of vascular rings: The Mayo Clinic experience. *Mayo Clin Proc* 68:1056-1063, 1993.

Duodenal Atresia, Stenosis, and Annular Pancreas

DEFINITION: Atresia and stenosis are related anomalies of the proximal duodenum that are attributed to failed canalization of the duodenum during the eighth to tenth weeks in utero.

IMAGING

Ultrasound
Findings
- Dilated, fluid-filled stomach and proximal duodenum

Utility
- Obstruction of the fetal gastrointestinal tract can be diagnosed with ultrasonography in the fetus.

Radiography
Findings
- Classic double bubble, with gas filling the distended stomach and proximal duodenum
- Accompanied by gas in the distal bowel
- Duodenal diaphragm (windsock duodenum): stretched diaphragm and a fine linear filling defect within the barium-filled duodenum

Utility
- Radiograph may be nondiagnostic if the stomach and duodenum are decompressed by vomiting or a nasogastric tube.
- If plain radiographs are not diagnostic, air or barium can be injected through the nasogastric tube.

CLINICAL PRESENTATION
- The newborn usually has bilious vomiting.
- Partial obstruction may not become clinically evident until later in life.
- Rapid clinical deterioration due to loss of fluids and electrolytes

DIFFERENTIAL DIAGNOSIS
- Choledochal cyst
- Peritoneal bands
- Intestinal duplication

DIAGNOSTIC PEARLS
- Classic double bubble
- Distended stomach and proximal duodenum
- Paucity of distal gas

PATHOLOGY
- Atresia and stenosis, related anomalies of the proximal duodenum, and failed canalization of duodenum during eighth to tenth week in utero are seen.
- Partial duodenal obstruction occurs in patients who have duodenal stenosis, duodenal diaphragm, and annular pancreas.
- Partial obstruction may not become clinically evident until later in life.
- Small lumen may become plugged with food after the infant graduates from a liquid to a solid diet.
- Children with trisomy 21 and significant mental retardation ingest foreign bodies; duodenal narrowing is recognized after the duodenum becomes completely obstructed.
- Malrotation is associated with duodenal obstruction.
- Association between duodenal stenosis and annular pancreas should be considered when a duodenal obstruction is identified.

INCIDENCE/PREVALENCE AND EPIDEMIOLOGY
- One third of infants who have atresia or stenosis have trisomy 21.
- Atresia is located distal to the ampulla of Vater in 75% of patients.
- Occurs in 1:10,000 births with equal gender frequency

WHAT THE REFERRING PHYSICIAN NEEDS TO KNOW
- Surgical approach to duodenal stenosis does not differ significantly when an annular pancreas is present; extensive preoperative evaluation is unnecessary.

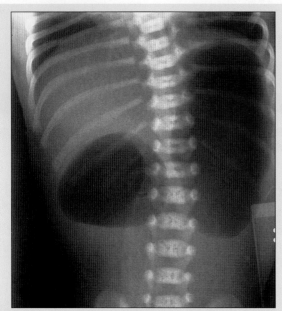

Figure 1. Duodenal atresia. Upright abdominal radiograph of this 2-day-old neonate shows the classic double bubble of duodenal atresia.

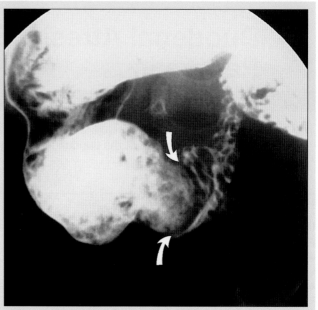

Figure 2. Windsock duodenum. Corn kernels, which had been ingested the evening before the contrast study, filled the duodenum proximal to an obstructive duodenal web in this 18-month-old boy. Intermittent vomiting was the only symptom. Oblique view of the transverse duodenum demonstrates the thin duodenal web *(arrows)*.

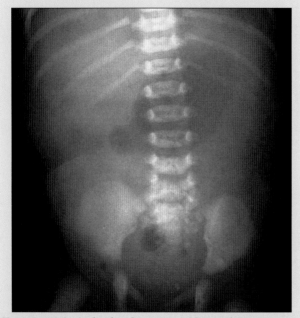

Figure 3. Intrinsic duodenal stenosis with annular pancreas. Abdominal radiograph of a 3-day-old infant shows gas in the stomach, with a paucity of distal gas. The dilated duodenal bulb is filled with fluid.

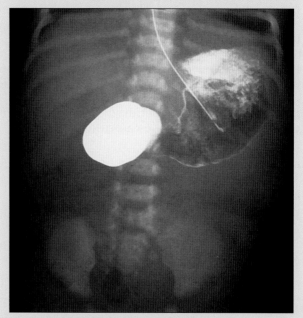

Figure 4. Intrinsic duodenal stenosis with annular pancreas. Contrast administered through an esophagogastric catheter demonstrates high-grade obstruction of the postbulbar duodenum. The infant had been vomiting since birth. Although annular pancreas cannot be diagnosed from this study, the association between duodenal stenosis and annular pancreas should always be considered.

Suggested Readings

Grosfeld JL, Rescoria FJ: Duodenal atresia and stenosis: Reassessment of treatment and outcome based on antenatal diagnosis, pathologic variance, and long-term follow-up. *World J Surg* 17:301-309, 1993.

Samuel M, Wheeler RA, Mami AG: Does duodenal atresia and stenosis prevent midgut volvulus in malrotation. *Eur J Pediatr Surg* 7:11-12, 1997.

Gastric and Duodenal Hematomas (Pediatric Stomach)

DEFINITION: Hematoma in the duodenum resulting from abdominal trauma that may cause obstruction.

IMAGING

CT

Findings
- Retroperitoneal air; a sign of transmural leakage

Utility
- CT is the preferred method of imaging in severe upper abdominal trauma, especially crush injuries, because it can image all organs well.
- It can miss subtle cases of duodenal rupture.

Radiography

Findings
- Gastric distention: a soft-tissue mass in the right hemi-abdomen, and sparse distal gas
- Retroperitoneal air: a sign of transmural leakage
- Duodenal obstruction

Utility
- Upper gastrointestinal study with contrast material shows intramural mass effect of the hematoma.
- It may not demonstrate perforation if the hematoma is plugging the mural rent.

Ultrasound

Findings
- Mural thickening of the bowel
- Intraperitoneal fluid

Utility
- Ultrasound is used to demonstrate and monitor hematoma resolution and adjacent pancreatic injury that are commonly present, but it cannot reliably demonstrate a perforation.

CLINICAL PRESENTATION

- Abdominal pain
- Gastric or duodenal outlet obstruction
- Vomiting
- Hypotension

DIFFERENTIAL DIAGNOSIS

- Peptic ulcer disease
- Gastric or duodenal mass
- Gastritis

DIAGNOSTIC PEARLS

- Blunt-force abdominal trauma
- Adjacent pancreatic injury
- Perforation

- Duodenitis
- Henoch-Schönlein purpura

PATHOLOGY

- Duodenal hematoma results when a child falls onto the handlebars of bicycle or is struck in the abdomen during play or an athletic event.
- Child abuse should be considered when any child has a history of suspicious injuries.
- Other risk factors include Henoch-Schönlein purpura, bleeding associated with leukemia, coagulopathies, idiopathic thrombocytopenia purpura, endoscopic biopsy, and anticoagulant therapy.

INCIDENCE/PREVALENCE AND EPIDEMIOLOGY

- Gastric hematoma from blunt-force abdominal trauma is unusual.
- Duodenal hematoma is more common.

Suggested Readings

Bechtel K, Moss RL, Leventhal JM, et al: Duodenal hematoma after upper endoscopy and biopsy in a 4-year-old girl. *Pediatr Emerg Care* 22:653-654, 2006.

Hernanz-Schulman M, Genieser NB, Ambrosino M: Sonographic diagnosis of intramural duodenal hematoma. *J Ultrasound Med* 8:273-276, 1989.

Iuchtman M, Steiner T, Faierman T, et al: Post-traumatic intramural duodenal hematoma in children. *Isr Med Assoc J* 8:95-97, 2006.

Jewett TC Jr, Caldarola V, Karp MP, et al: Intramural hematoma of the duodenum. *Arch Surg* 123:54-58, 1988.

Megremis S, Segkos N, Andrianaki A, et al: Sonographic diagnosis and monitoring of an obstructing duodenal hematoma after blunt trauma: Correlation with computed tomographic and surgical findings. *J Ultrasound Med* 23:1679-1683, 2004.

Sidhu MK, Weinberger E, Healey P: Intramural duodenal hematoma after blunt abdominal trauma. *AJR Am J Roentgenol* 170:38, 1998.

WHAT THE REFERRING PHYSICIAN NEEDS TO KNOW

- Surgery is mandatory when a perforation is present.
- As the hematoma resolves, perforation and duodenal diastasis may become apparent.
- Every child with duodenal hematoma must be carefully watched during the first 7-10 days after trauma.

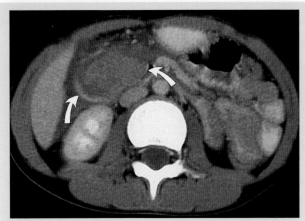

Figure 1. Duodenal hematoma. Axial CT scan shows the duodenal hematoma *(arrows)* sustained when the child fell on bicycle handlebars. CT is the imaging procedure of choice for children who have sustained significant blunt injury to the abdomen. *(Courtesy of Sally Vogel, MD, Starship Children's Hospital, Auckland, New Zealand.)*

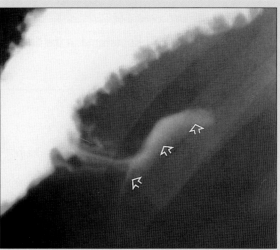

Figure 2. Duodenal hematoma. Prone oblique view from an upper gastrointestinal series shows duodenal obstruction with barium *(arrows)* outlining a duodenal mass.

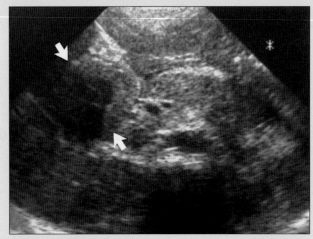

Figure 3. Duodenal hematoma. Transverse sonogram of the upper abdomen demonstrates the mass to be a duodenal hematoma *(arrows)* in this 10-year-old child who sustained a bicycle handlebar injury to the upper abdomen. The complete sonographic study also demonstrated pancreatic swelling and peripancreatic fluid from the injury (not shown).

Gastric or Duodenal Distention (Pediatric Stomach)

DEFINITION: Bloating of the stomach or duodenum, seen in several disorders, particularly in the pediatric population.

IMAGING

Radiography

Findings
- Distention of the stomach predisposes it to volvulus.
- Superior mesenteric artery syndrome: Distention of the stomach and proximal duodenum and sharp cutoff in the mid transverse portion of the duodenum are seen.
- Cystic fibrosis: Thickened mucosal folds, nodular mucosa, and increased intraluminal fluid are seen.

Utility
- Plain radiography is the initial study performed in these patients.

CLINICAL PRESENTATION

- Gastric or duodenal distention
- Vomiting, nausea, and weight loss

DIFFERENTIAL DIAGNOSIS

- Hypertrophic pyloric stenosis
- Antropyloric membrane
- Peptic ulcer disease
- Duplication cysts
- Pyloric stenosis
- Annular pancreas
- Ladd bands
- Volvulus
- Superior mesenteric artery syndrome

DIAGNOSTIC PEARLS

- Tracheoesophageal fistula
- Volvulus
- Idiopathic megaduodenum

PATHOLOGY

- Many children swallow air when crying or nervous; overt aerophagia is seen in some groups of mentally retarded youngsters.
- Gastric distention with air may be caused by a tracheoesophageal fistula, with or without esophageal atresia, after an endotracheal tube is inadvertently placed in the esophagus.
- Diabetes mellitus and prior starvation are causes of gastric dilation that probably results from atony.
- Idiopathic megaduodenum: Dilation of sections of the gastrointestinal tract without anatomic obstruction is characteristic.

Suggested Readings

Chang SW, Lee HC, Yeung CY, et al: Gastric volvulus in children. *Acta Paediatr Taiwan* 47:18-24, 2006.

Eaves ER, Schmidt GT: Chronic idiopathic megaduodenum in a family. *Aust N Z J Med* 15:1-6, 1985.

Elhalaby EA, Mashaly EM: Infants with radiologic diagnosis of gastric volvulus: Are they over-treated? *Pediatr Surg Int* 17:596-600, 2001.

Phelan MS, Fine DR, Zentler-Munro PL, et al: Radiographic abnormalities of the duodenum in cystic fibrosis. *Clin Radiol* 34:573-577, 1983.

WHAT THE REFERRING PHYSICIAN NEEDS TO KNOW

- Operative treatment is rarely necessary.
- Feeding in the prone position, hyperalimentations, or nasojejunal feeding alleviates the symptoms in most patients.

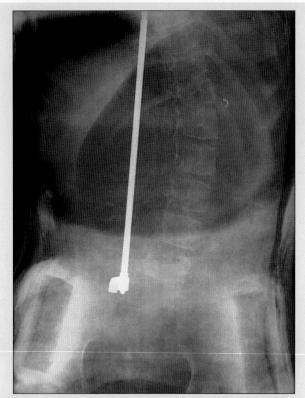

Figure 1. Gastric volvulus. Abdominal radiograph taken 11 days after posterior spinal fusion in a patient who complained of nausea shows marked gastric distention. The patient is in a body cast.

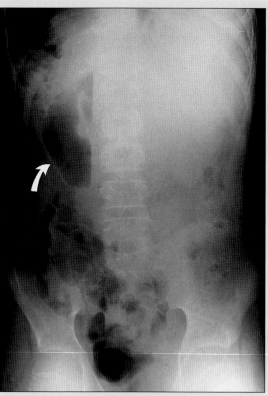

Figure 2. Superior mesenteric artery syndrome. A child had had resection of a primary hepatic tumor and had lost weight on chemotherapy. Gastric and duodenal dilation resulted from partial obstruction of the transverse portion of the duodenum by the root of the mesentery. The gas-filled, dilated duodenum *(arrow)* is demonstrated on this decubitus radiograph. (*Courtesy of Russell Metcalfe, MD, Starship Children's Hospital, Auckland, New Zealand.*)

Malrotation (Pediatric Stomach)

DEFINITION: Malrotation is an incomplete rotation resulting in the formation of abnormal mesenteric attachments (i.e., Ladd bands) and shortening of the mesenteric base.

IMAGING

Radiography

Findings

- Normal or possibly showing an unusual position of an air-filled stomach or intestinal loops; paucity of distal bowel gas
- Dilation of the duodenal bulb or grossly distended air-filled loops with mural thickening if ischemia from a volvulus
- Ladd bands typically causing a Z-type configuration of the duodenum and proximal jejunum
- Abnormal dilation of the duodenum and multiple dilated loops of the small bowel, with thickened walls
- Beaking of barium caused by a twisted bowel
- Corkscrew appearance of the duodenum and jejunum, with proximal dilation of the duodenum from the twist

Utility

- Upper gastrointestinal series with barium delivered through a nasogastric tube is the gold standard in establishing the diagnosis.

Ultrasound

Findings

- Superior mesenteric vein lies to the left of the superior mesenteric artery, and malrotation is likely.
- Preduodenal portal vein can be diagnosed, which often coexists with malrotation and duodenal stenosis.

Utility

- Ultrasound assesses the relative location of the superior mesenteric artery and vein.
- Results may be falsely negative and delay the diagnosis.
- Ultrasound is worthwhile in identifying the superior mesenteric vasculature in children and is part of an evaluation for nonspecific abdominal pain.

CLINICAL PRESENTATION

- Bilious vomiting is the classic presentation.
- Child may be able to tolerate obstruction from an intermittent volvulus, but should be brought to medical attention if episodic pain or malabsorption symptoms are present.

DIAGNOSTIC PEARLS

- Corkscrew appearance of the duodenum and jejunum may be seen.
- Beaking of barium may occur.
- Ladd bands typically produce a Z-type configuration of the duodenum and proximal jejunum.

DIFFERENTIAL DIAGNOSES

- Pyloric stenosis
- Annular pancreas
- Antral web

PATHOLOGY

- Patients may exhibit incomplete rotation, resulting in the formation of abnormal mesenteric attachments and shortening of the mesenteric base.
- Obstruction may result from Ladd bands across the duodenum or from a midgut volvulus around a narrow vascular pedicle.
- Chronic, intermittent volvulus is a cause of secondary lymphangiectasia and chylous ascites.

INCIDENCE/PREVALENCE AND EPIDEMIOLOGY

- Malrotation occurs in 1 in 500 births; however, the true incidence is unknown because asymptomatic patients do not present.
- No gender or racial predilection
- 60% present by 1 month of age, 20%-30% present between 1 and 12 months.

Suggested Readings

Applegate KE, Anderson JM, Klatte EC: Intestinal malrotation in children: A problem-solving approach to the upper gastrointestinal series. *RadioGraphics* 26:1485-1500, 2006.

WHAT THE REFERRING PHYSICIAN NEEDS TO KNOW

- Volvulus is a life-threatening emergency.
- Controlled upper gastrointestinal series with contrast through a nasogastric tube is the best diagnostic approach to a suspected midgut volvulus.
- Contrast should be aspirated through a nasogastric tube if the obstruction is identified.

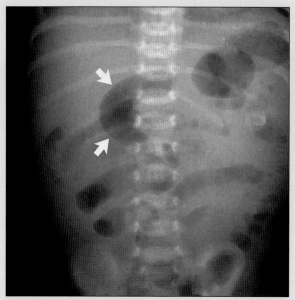

Figure 1. Malrotation with a midgut volvulus. Abdominal radiograph of a 3-week-old boy with bilious vomiting, lethargy, and bloody stools shows abnormal dilation of the duodenum *(arrows)* and multiple dilated loops of small bowel with thickened walls.

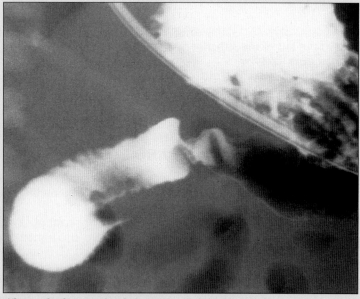

Figure 2. Malrotation with a midgut volvulus. Duodenal obstruction with beaking of the barium is caused by the twisted bowel.

Berdon WE, Baker DH, Bull S, et al: Midgut malrotation and volvulus. Which films are most helpful? *Radiology* 96:375-383, 1970.

Firor HV, Harris VJ: Rotational anomalies of the gut. Re-emphasis of a neglected facet, isolated incomplete rotation of the duodenum. *AJR Am J Roentgenol* 120:315-321, 1974.

Jit I: The development and the structure of the suspensory muscle of the duodenum. *Anat Rec* 113:395-407, 1952.

Long FR, Kramer SS, Markowitz RI, et al: Radiographic patterns of intestinal malrotation in children. *RadioGraphics* 16:547-556, 1996.

Palmas G, Maxia L, Fanos V: Volvulus and intestinal malrotation in the newborn. *Pediatr Med Chir* 27:62-66, 2005.

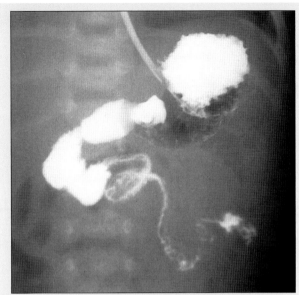

Figure 3. Malrotation with a midgut volvulus. Radiograph taken a few minutes later (same patient as Figure 2) shows the typical corkscrew appearance of the duodenum and proximal jejunum associated with malrotation and midgut volvulus.

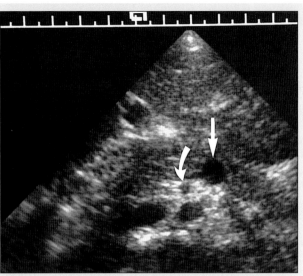

Figure 4. Malrotation with reversal of the position of the superior mesenteric vein and artery. A transverse sonogram demonstrates the superior mesenteric vein *(straight arrow)* at the one-o'clock position relative to the superior mesenteric artery *(curved arrow)*, a reversal of the normal relationship.

Pyloric and Antral Atresias (Pediatric Stomach)

DEFINITION: Complete obstruction of the pylorus.

IMAGING

Radiography
Findings
- Abdomen is gasless except for a single bubble of air.
- Complete obstruction at the pylorus is seen.

Utility
- These examinations are often diagnostic.

Ultrasound
Findings
- Normal canal or muscle is not seen.

Utility
- Initial cross-sectional imaging examination performed in neonates with vomiting

CLINICAL PRESENTATION

- Neonate is unable to feed without vomiting.

DIFFERENTIAL DIAGNOSIS

- Pyloric stenosis
- Antral diaphragm
- Annular pancreas
- Ladd bands

DIAGNOSTIC PEARLS

- The abdomen is gasless except for a single bubble of air.
- Complete obstruction at the pylorus is seen.
- Sonograms performed on infants with pyloric atresia do not show a normal canal or muscle.

PATHOLOGY

- An association exists between pyloric atresia and epidermolysis bullosa.
- In affected patients, minimal skin trauma results in blisters and erosions; pyloric obstruction begins in utero or develops postnatally.

INCIDENCE/PREVALENCE AND EPIDEMIOLOGY

- Pyloric and antral atresias are rare anomalies.

Suggested Readings

Lin AN: Pyloric atresia and epidermolysis bullosa. *Pediatr Dermatol* 14:406-408, 1997.

Orense M, Garcia Hernandez JB, Celorio C, et al: Pyloric atresia associated with epidermolysis bullosa. *Pediatr Radiol* 17:435, 1987.

WHAT THE REFERRING PHYSICIAN NEEDS TO KNOW

- Differentiation between atresia and the membrane usually rests with the surgeon.
- Plain radiographs showing complete obstruction in first day of life mandate an operation.

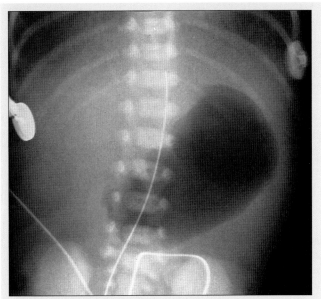

Figure 1. Pyloric atresia. Abdominal radiograph obtained 48 hours after birth shows gas in the stomach and no air distally. (*Courtesy of Michael DiPietro, MD, Ann Arbor, MI.*)

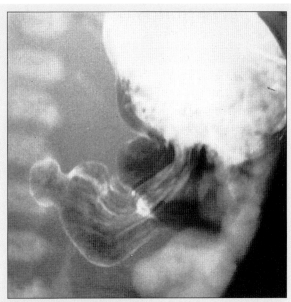

Figure 2. Pyloric atresia. Contrast given orally demonstrates complete obstruction at the pylorus. The intraluminal contrast-highlighted area to the left of the stomach is in the colon, which was opacified during a previous barium enema. Maternal polyhydramnios developed prenatally. (*Courtesy of Michael DiPietro, MD, Ann Arbor, MI.*)

Pyloric Stenosis (Pediatric Stomach)

DEFINITION: Narrowing of the pylorus.

IMAGING

Ultrasound
Findings
- Some surgeons rely primarily on measurements of muscle thickness; others depend on channel length.
- Muscle thickness of more than 3.5 mm and channel length of 17 mm or longer is seen.
- Findings show little or no passage of gastric contents and gastric peristalsis that stops abruptly at the pyloric muscle.
- Distention of antrum with fluid is seen.

Utility
- Ultrasound is part of the established examination for the diagnosis of pyloric stenosis.
- Questionable cases can be rescanned in 24-36 hours or investigated with an upper gastrointestinal series.
- Turn the infant to the right posterior oblique position, and give glucose water through the nipple if the infant's stomach has been emptied by vomiting.

Radiography
Findings
- Partial or complete gastric outlet obstruction
- Hyperperistalsis of the stomach or, if a prolonged history exists, gastric atony
- Elongation of pyloric channel
- Single (string sign) or double (train track sign) streaks of barium within the compressed lumen
- Shoulder sign of pyloric mass indenting the barium-filled stomach, with peristalsis abutting the mass
- Indentation of the base of the duodenal bulb from a pyloric mass

Utility
- Contrast studies can be used if the ultrasound examination is indeterminant.

CLINICAL PRESENTATION
- Projectile and bile-free emesis in a previously healthy 6-week-old infant is the classic presentation.

DIFFERENTIAL DIAGNOSIS
- Ulcers (pyloric channel)
- Duodenal atresia

DIAGNOSTIC PEARLS
- Single (*string sign*) or double (*train-track sign*) streaks of barium
- Partial or complete gastric outlet obstruction
- Shoulder sign of a pyloric mass indenting the barium-filled stomach, with peristalsis abutting the mass
- Muscle thickness of more than 3.5 mm and a channel length of 17 mm or longer

- Annular pancreas
- Ladd band
- Antropyloric membrane
- Duplication cyst of antrum

PATHOLOGY
- Thickened pyloric muscle leads to hypertrophic pyloric narrowing or stenosis.

INCIDENCE/PREVALENCE AND EPIDEMIOLOGY
- Hypertrophic pyloric stenosis is the most common indication for surgery in infants.
- It has a 5:1 male-female predominance and randomly occurs in 3 of 1000 infants.
- Parental history increases the offspring's chance to 6.9%.

Suggested Readings

Blumhagen JD, Maclin L, Krauter D, et al: Sonographic diagnosis of hypertrophic pyloric stenosis. *AJR Am J Roentgenol* 150: 1367-1370, 1988.

Finkelstein MS, Mandell GA, Tarbell KV: Hypertrophic pyloric stenosis: Volumetric measurement of nasogastric aspirate to determine the imaging modality. *Radiology* 177:759-761, 1990.

Hernanz-Schulman M: Infantile hypertrophic pyloric stenosis. *Radiology* 227:319-331, 2003.

Hernanz-Schulman M, Lisa H, Lowe LH, et al: In vivo visualization of pyloric mucosal hypertrophy in infants with hypertrophic pyloric stenosis: Is there an etiologic role? *AJR Am J Roentgenol* 177: 843-848, 2001.

WHAT THE REFERRING PHYSICIAN NEEDS TO KNOW
- Increasing reliance exists on imaging to detect pyloric stenosis.
- Pyloric stenosis is diagnosed earlier, with less metabolic disturbance than in the past; most patients have imaging (ultrasonography) before surgery.

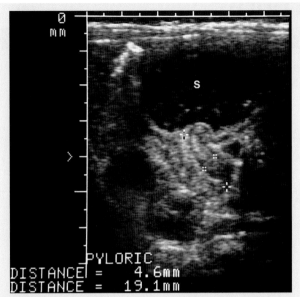

Figure 1. Pyloric stenosis: ultrasonography. Sonography of the pylorus showed no peristalsis during the examination. Echogenic material in the stomach (S) represents retained gastric contents in this 3-week-old boy with a 48-hour history of projectile vomiting. The thickness of one wall of the pyloric muscle is 4.6 mm; the length of the channel is 19.1 mm.

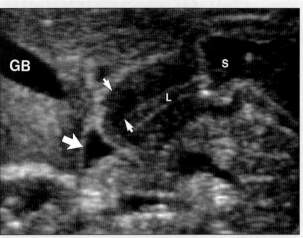

Figure 2. Pyloric stenosis: ultrasonography. This infant was given glucose water before the scans. Enough fluid passed through the pylorus to outline the duodenal bulb *(large arrow).* The thickened pyloric wall *(small arrows)* is also visible, along with the gallbladder (GB), pyloric lumen (L), and stomach (S).

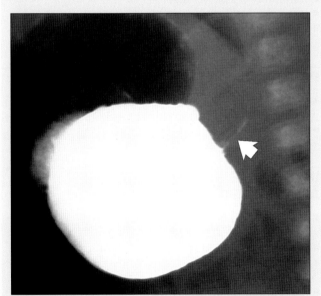

Figure 3. Pyloric stenosis: upper gastrointestinal series. The contrast study shows a single streak of barium (i.e., string sign *[arrow]*) within the narrowed, elongated pyloric channel.

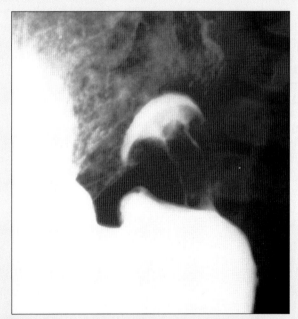

Figure 4. Pyloric stenosis: upper gastrointestinal series. Upper gastrointestinal series in a patient with pyloric stenosis shows double streaks of barium (i.e., train track sign) within the abnormal pyloric channel and indentation on the barium-filled stomach and duodenal bulb from the thickened pyloric muscle.

Henoch-Schönlein Purpura

DEFINITION: A vasculitis affecting multiple organs, including the bowel and gut, producing complications from acute abdominal symptoms to intussusception.

ANATOMIC FINDINGS

Small Bowel
- Bowel perforation
- Intussusception, ileoileal type

Colon
- Bowel perforation
- Intussusception, ileocolic type

IMAGING

Radiography
Findings
- Usually normal unless complicated
- Small-bowel obstruction if with intussusception
- Bowel wall or mucosal thickening (thumbprinting of bowel segments)
- Submucosal edema
Utility
- Contrast enemas are both diagnostic and therapeutic for intussusception reduction but are usually unsuccessful.

Ultrasound
Findings
- Mural thickening of the affected bowel, often distended by fluid
Utility
- Ultrasound is a useful diagnostic tool for excluding intussusception and evaluating acute abdominal pain and tenderness.

CLINICAL PRESENTATION

- Intense abdominal pain
- Acute or surgical abdomen
- Gastrointestinal bleeding
- Purpuric skin rash on legs and extensor surfaces of arms

DIAGNOSTIC PEARLS

- Radiographic films are usually normal unless the abnormality is complicated by perforation or intussusception.
- Thumbprinting of the bowel segments that are distended with air reflects substantial bowel wall thickening.

- Microscopic hematuria
- Proteinuria
- Arthralgias
- Upper respiratory infection

DIFFERENTIAL DIAGNOSIS

- Glomerulonephritis
- Inflammatory bowel disease
- Infectious colitis
- Behçet disease

PATHOLOGY

- Vasculitis serves as the main underlying abnormality, commonly affecting the skin, bowel, gut, and kidneys.
- Granulocytes surround the arterioles and venules.

INCIDENCE/PREVALENCE AND EPIDEMIOLOGY

- Henoch-Schönlein purpura is common in children ages between 3 and 10 years.
- Slight male predominance has been found.
- Thirty percent of affected patients may be older than 20 years.
- It occurs more in winter than other seasons.

WHAT THE REFERRING PHYSICIAN NEEDS TO KNOW

- Surgery may be needed in 3%-5% of children who have complications of bowel perforation or irreducible intussusception.
- Most children recover completely without residua of an acute process.
- Gastrointestinal bleeding occurring in approximately one half of pediatric patients; a blood transfusion is unlikely.

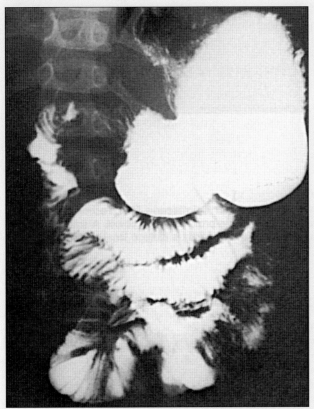

Figure 1. Upper gastrointestinal series: Henoch-Schönlein purpura. The valvulae conniventes are thickened in the jejunum. Contrast medium is diluted as it passes into the more distal, fluid-filled loops.

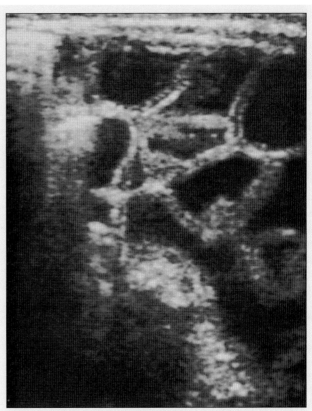

Figure 2. Longitudinal ultrasound: Henoch-Schönlein purpura. The bowel loops are distended with fluid, and the walls are thickened.

- It is the most common systemic allergic vasculitis in children.
- It is precipitated by bacterial and viral infections, allergies, insect stings, and drugs.

Suggested Readings

Chang WL, Yang YH, Lin YT, et al: Gastrointestinal manifestations in Henoch-Schönlein purpura: A review of 261 patients. *Acta Paediatr* 93:1427-1431, 2004.

Connolly B, O'Halpin D: Sonographic evaluation of the abdomen in Henoch-Schönlein purpura. *Clin Radiol* 49:320-323, 1994.

Mills JA, Michel BA, Bloch DA, et al: The American College of Rheumatology 1990 criteria for the classification of Henoch-Schönlein purpura. *Arthritis Rheum* 33:1114-1121, 1990.

Saulsbury FT: Henoch-Schönlein purpura. *Curr Opin Rheumatol* 13:35-40, 2001.

Schwab J, Benya E, Lin R, et al: Contrast enema in children with Henoch-Schönlein purpura. *J Pediatr Surg* 40:1221-1223, 2005.

Sonmez K, Turkyilmaz Z, Demirogullari B, et al: Conservative treatment for small intestinal intussusception associated with Henoch-Schönlein purpura. *Surg Today* 32:1031-1034, 2002.

Intestinal Lymphangiectasia (Pediatric)

DEFINITION: Congenital or acquired disorder of the small-bowel lymphatics, producing symptoms caused by an anatomic abnormality or protein-losing enteropathy.

ANATOMIC FINDINGS

Small Bowel
- Dilated lymphatic channels
- Mucosal inflammatory changes

IMAGING

Radiography
Findings
- Thickening of valvulae conniventes
- Mucosal nodularity
- Excessive secretions if accompanied by malabsorption
- Normal gut caliber
- Thickening of the affected colonic folds

Utility
- Double-contrast small bowel studies show greater extent of bowel involvement.
- Barium enema shows colonic affectation.

Ultrasound
Findings
- Abnormal, dilated lymphatics
- Ascites
- Thickened bowel and mesentery caused by hypoproteinemia

Utility
- Ultrasound shows nonspecific mural thickening of the small bowel.

CT
Findings
- Mural thickening of small bowel with submucosal edema
- Ascites

Utility
- CT shows nonspecific mural thickening of the small bowel.

CLINICAL PRESENTATION
- Protein loss or wasting and failure to thrive in children; also lymphopenia
- Diarrhea

DIAGNOSTIC PEARLS
- Thickened bowel and mesentery caused by hypoproteinemia
- Hypoplasia or atresia of normal lymphatics in the extremities
- Halo sign in the affected bowel loops

- Decreased immunoglobulin levels
- Nausea and abdominal pain
- Lymphatic abnormalities in other organs
- Limb swelling caused by lymphedema or hypoalbuminemia

DIFFERENTIAL DIAGNOSIS
- Nephrotic syndrome
- Hypoproteinemia
- Portal hypertension
- Celiac disease
- Giardiasis
- Protein-losing gastroenteritis
- Eosinophilic gastroenteritis

PATHOLOGY
- Intestinal lymphangiectasia can be congenital or acquired.
- Histologic changes include dilated lymphatics in all bowel layers accompanied by villous changes and infiltration of the mucosa by inflammatory cells.
- Process can involve large segments of the bowel, or it can be focal.
- Segmental enlargement of the lymphatic channels of the bowel and mesentery is a different entity that tends to exhibit as a mass.

INCIDENCE/PREVALENCE AND EPIDEMIOLOGY
- Intestinal lymphangiectasia affects both pediatric and adult groups.

WHAT THE REFERRING PHYSICIAN NEEDS TO KNOW
- Small-bowel biopsy allows differentiation of intestinal lymphangiectasia from intestinal lymphatic hypoplasia.
- Segmental enlargement of the bowel and mesenteric lymphatics is caused mainly by lymphangioma and tends to show as a mass.
- Intestinal lymphangiectasia is recognized as part of Noonan and Hennekam syndromes.

Suggested Readings

Abramowsky C, Hupertz V, Kilbridge P, et al: Intestinal lymphangiectasia in children: A study of upper gastrointestinal endoscopic biopsies. *Pediatr Pathol* 9:289-297, 1989.

Aoyagi K, Iida M, Yao T, et al: Intestinal lymphangiectasia: Value of double-contrast radiographic study. *Clin Radiol* 49:814-819, 1994.

Bloomfield FH, Hadden W, Gunn TR: Lymphatic dysplasia in a neonate with Noonan's syndrome. *Pediatr Radiol* 27:321-323, 1997.

Dorne HL, Jequier S: Sonography of intestinal lymphangiectasia. *J Ultrasound Med* 5:13-16, 1986.

Forzano F, Faravelli F, Loy A, et al: Severe lymphedema, intestinal lymphangiectasia, seizures and mild mental retardation: Further case of Hennekam syndrome with a severe phenotype. *Am J Med Genet* 111:68-70, 2002.

Olmsted WW, Madewell JE: Lymphangiectasia of the small intestine: Description and pathophysiology of roentgenographic signs. *Gastrointest Radiol* 1:241-243, 1976.

Puri AS, Aggarwal R, Gupta RK, et al: Intestinal lymphangiectasia: Evaluation by CT and scintigraphy. *Gastrointest Radiol* 17:119-121, 1991.

Stevens RL, Jones B, Fishman EK: The CT halo sign: A new finding in intestinal lymphangiectasia. *J Comput Tomogr* 21:1005-1007, 1997.

Yang DM, Jung DH: Localized intestinal lymphangiectasia: CT findings. *AJR Am J Roentgenol* 180:213-214, 2003.

Meckel Diverticulum (Pediatric)

DEFINITION: Failure of the normal complete regression of the omphalomesenteric (vitelline) duct, producing a true diverticulum along the course of the duct.

ANATOMIC FINDINGS

Small Bowel
- Diverticulum in an antimesenteric location
- Obstruction if complicated by intussusception or in symptomatic mesodiverticular bands
- Ulceration and bleeding of adjacent normal small bowel if containing extopic gastric mucosa
- Focal volvulus in the left upper quadrant (a complication of the giant form)
- Stasis leading to malabsorption caused by bacterial overgrowth

IMAGING

Radiography
Findings
- Usually normal
- Barium- or air-filled structure in contrast study
- Dilated small-bowel loops
- Mucosal triangular plateau or triradiate fold pattern in the right lower quadrant

Utility
- Diverticulum may opacify with high-pressure enteroclysis or in delayed contrast studies.
- Compression increases the diagnostic yield by displacing the overlying bowel loops.

Ultrasound
Findings
- Tubular structure with thickened but irregular walls
- Inverted Meckel diverticulum (the lead point of intussusception)
- Inflammatory bowel changes

Utility
- Ultrasound is a routine diagnostic tool for symptomatic pediatric patients.
- Doppler and color Doppler depict better delineation of findings.

DIAGNOSTIC PEARLS
- Diverticulum may opacify with high-pressure enteroclysis or in delayed contrast studies.
- CT and ultrasound can demonstrate inverted Meckel diverticulum, which is the lead point of intussusception.
- Pentagastrin-enhanced scintigraphy stimulates diverticular gastric mucosal uptake and is used if study findings are negative or equivocal and if a high index of suspicion exists.

CT
Findings
- Tubular structure with thickened walls
- Inflammatory changes in the bowel or adjacent mesentery
- Air- or fluid levels
- Inverted Meckel diverticulum (the lead point of intussusception)

Utility
- CT is quite useful in differentiating appendiceal and Meckel diverticular abnormalities.

Nuclear Medicine
Findings
- Isotope localization in right lower quadrant or hypochondrium

Utility
- Technetium 99m-pertechnetate scintigraphy is the most widely used diagnostic tool for bleeding cases, with a sensitivity of 85%.
- Pentagastrin-enhanced scintigraphy stimulates diverticular gastric mucosal uptake and is used after negative or equivocal study findings in the setting of a high index of suspicion.
- False-negative and false-positive studies occur, but the latter are easier to recognize.

WHAT THE REFERRING PHYSICIAN NEEDS TO KNOW
- Meckel diverticulum serves as most common lead point of irreducible intussusception.
- Giant form of Meckel diverticulum can serve as the lead point for a focal volvulus.
- Initial radiographic studies are usually normal, unless the abnormality is complicated by intussusception.
- Meckel diverticulum rarely fills on routine barium studies.
- Additional imaging may be performed before surgery to exclude other acute abdominal processes.
- Technetium 99m-pertechnetate scintigraphy is the most widely used and sensitive diagnostic tool for bleeding cases of Meckel diverticulum.
- Pentagastrin-enhanced scintigraphy can be performed after a negative or equivocal study but with a high index of suspicion.

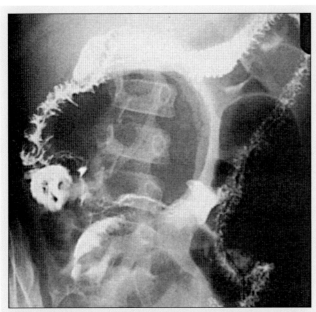

Figure 1. Giant Meckel diverticulum. Radiograph obtained after a barium enema demonstrates residual contrast material within the colon and several small-bowel loops. The large, rounded gas collection in the mid-abdomen, causing proximal small-bowel obstruction, is a giant Meckel diverticulum.

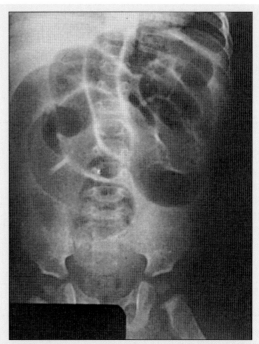

Figure 2. Omphalomesenteric band. Multiple, dilated small-bowel loops suggest a low obstruction on the plain abdominal radiograph of an infant.

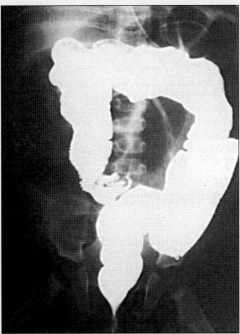

Figure 3. Omphalomesenteric band. The colon was normal, except that the right colon was displaced from the lateral abdominal wall, and distending the cecum was impossible. At surgery, the small bowel that had herniated beneath the omphalomesenteric duct was found to be entrapped.

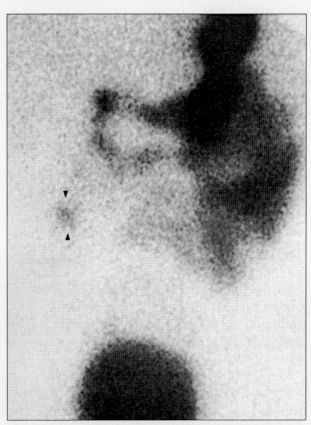

Figure 4. Nuclear scintiscan: Meckel diverticulum. Technetium 99m-pertechnetate has passed from the stomach into the proximal small bowel. A small region of activity in the right lower quadrant *(arrowheads)* is isotope localizing within the Meckel diverticulum.

CLINICAL PRESENTATION

- Painless lower gastrointestinal bleeding
- Intussusception
- Bowel obstruction
- Malabsorption states

DIFFERENTIAL DIAGNOSIS

- Appendicitis
- Intussusception
- Small bowel obstruction
- Crohn disease
- Omental infarction
- Small bowel tumor
- Celiac disease

PATHOLOGY

- Failure of the normal complete regression of omphalo-mesenteric (vitelline) duct, producing a true diverticulum along the course of the duct

INCIDENCE/PREVALENCE AND EPIDEMIOLOGY

- Almost one half of cases occur before the age of 2 years.
- Male predominance in symptomatic cases has been seen.
- Approximately 90% of cases with bleeding are complicated with gastric mucosa.

Suggested Readings

Daneman A, Lobo E, Alton DJ, et al: The value of sonography, CT, and air enema for detection of complicated Meckel diverticulum in children with nonspecific clinical presentation. *Pediatr Radiol* 28:928-932, 1998.

Emamian SA, Shalaby-Rana E, Majd M: The spectrum of heterotopic gastric mucosa in children detected by Tc-99m pertechnetate scintigraphy. *Clin Nucl Med* 26:529-535, 2001.

Galifer RB, Noblet D, Ferran JL: "Giant Meckel's diverticulum": Report of an unusual case in a child with preoperative x-ray diagnosis. *Pediatr Radiol* 11:217-218, 1981.

Rossi P, Gourtsoyiannis N, Bezzi M, et al: Meckel's diverticulum: Imaging diagnosis. *AJR Am J Roentgenol* 166:567-573, 1996.

Rutherford RB, Akers DR: Meckel's diverticulum: A review of 148 pediatric patients with special reference to the pattern of bleeding and to mesodiverticular bands. *Surgery* 59:618-626, 1966.

Society of Nuclear Medicine: Procedure guideline for gastrointestinal bleeding and Meckel's diverticulum scintigraphy. *J Nucl Med* 40:1226-1232, 1999.

St. Vil D, Brandt ML, Panic S, et al: Meckel's diverticulum in children: A 20-year review. *J Pediatr Surg* 26:1289-1292, 1991.

Appendicitis (Pediatric)

DEFINITION: Infection of the appendix.

IMAGING

Ultrasound

Findings

- Normal appendix identified in up to 50% of children who do not have appendicitis
- Dilated, incompressible appendix
- Widened appendix
- Acutely ruptured appendix: decompressed appendix with a diameter of less than 6 mm; appendix not identified because of overlying bowel gas

Utility

- When cross-sectional imaging is indicated, sonography and CT have more than 90% specificity and sensitivity.
- In thin children, ultrasound is a reasonable first-line choice.
- Sonography and CT are helpful in differentiating *Yersinia* enterocolitis (frequently associated with right lower quadrant pain) from appendicitis.
- In addition to imaging the appendicitis, radiologists can percutaneously drain the appendiceal abscesses.

CT

Findings

- Appendicolith
- Appendiceal abscess: a complex mass that compresses the right ureter

Utility

- In heavier children, or when ultrasound is not readily available, CT is successful in diagnosing or excluding appendicitis or detecting alternate disease processes.
- Sonography and CT are helpful in differentiating *Yersinia* enterocolitis from appendicitis.
- In addition to imaging the appendicitis, radiologists can percutaneously drain appendiceal abscesses.
- CT is considered the gold standard in the noninvasive imaging of appendicitis. It has an accuracy of 95%.

DIAGNOSTIC PEARLS

- Dilated, incompressible appendix
- Widened appendix
- Acutely ruptured appendix: decompressed appendix with a diameter of less than 6 mm; appendix not identified because of overlying bowel gas

Radiography

Findings

- Ileus
- Appendicolith
- Appendiceal abscess

Utility

- Radiography is insensitive in the diagnosis of appendicitis.

CLINICAL PRESENTATION

- Symptoms include abdominal pain, vomiting, and low-grade fever.
- Signs include pain on palpation of the right lower quadrant and rebound tenderness.
- Laboratory data include low-grade leukocytosis and the absence of urinary tract infection.
- After rupture, the abdominal symptoms may temporarily diminish, which obscures the diagnosis.
- Phlegmon or periappendiceal abscess may be palpated as a right lower quadrant mass.

DIFFERENTIAL DIAGNOSIS

- Crohn disease
- Meckel diverticulum

WHAT THE REFERRING PHYSICIAN NEEDS TO KNOW

- Imaging is performed in persons whose atypical presentation suggests the possibility of other, even nonsurgical, diagnoses.
- Rupture or perforation occurs more commonly in children than in adults.
- Appendicitis needs to be excluded in any child presenting with small bowel obstruction.
- CT is useful diagnostically and as an imaging guide to percutaneous drainage of appendiceal abscesses.

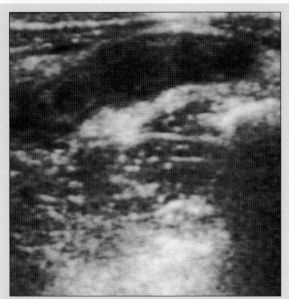

Figure 1. Sonography of appendicitis. A dilated, incompressible appendix lies beneath the abdominal musculature on this longitudinal scan.

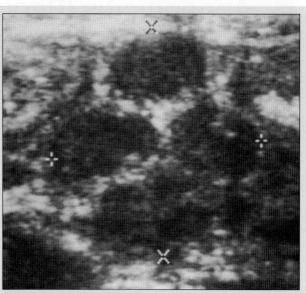

Figure 2. *Yersinia* **enterocolitis.** Several enlarged lymph nodes *(cursors)* are seen on this sagittal sonogram of a child whose appendix appeared normal.

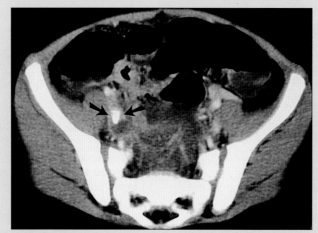

Figure 3. Appendicitis. CT demonstrates an appendicolith *(arrows)* in the dilated appendix.

- Intussusception
- Parasitic infections
- Omental infarction
- Epiploic appendagitis

PATHOLOGY

- If rupture has occurred, the inflammation of the local soft tissues (e.g., bowel, omentum) is called a phlegmon.
- Phlegmon or periappendiceal abscess occurs in 7% of children with acute appendicitis and is common in those whose symptoms are of longer duration.

- Appendicoliths are more common in children than in adults with appendicitis; when present, they are more likely to be associated with appendiceal rupture.

INCIDENCE/PREVALENCE AND EPIDEMIOLOGY

- The most common indication for emergency laparotomy in children is an inflamed or ruptured appendix.
- In pediatric patients who have had preoperative imaging studies, the perforation rate at surgery is as high as 50%.

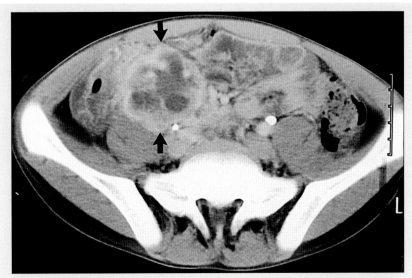

Figure 4. CT of appendiceal abscess. CT reveals a complex mass *(arrows)*, which compresses the right ureter.

Suggested Readings

Emil S, Mikhail P, Laberge JM, et al: Clinical versus sonographic evaluation of acute appendicitis in children: A comparison of patient characteristics and outcomes. *J Pediatr Surg* 36:780-783, 2001.

Friedland JA, Siegel MJ: CT appearance of acute appendicitis in childhood. *AJR Am J Roentgenol* 168:439-442, 1997.

Hernandez JA, Swischuk LE, Angel CA, et al: Imaging of acute appendicitis: US as the primary imaging modality. *Pediatr Radiol* 35:392-395, 2005.

Patriquin HB, Garcier J-M, Lafortune M, et al: Appendicitis in children and young adults: Value of sonography in detecting perforation. *AJR Am J Roentgenol* 166:629-633, 1996.

Ramachandran P, Sivit CJ, Newman KD, et al: Ultrasonography as an adjunct in the diagnosis of acute appendicitis: A 4-year experience. *J Pediatr Surg* 31:164-169, 1996.

Sivit CJ, Applegate KE, Stallion A, et al: Imaging evaluation of suspected appendicitis in a pediatric population: Effectiveness of sonography versus CT. *AJR Am J Roentgenol* 175:980-997, 2002.

Hemolytic-Uremic Syndrome (Pediatric)

DEFINITION: Infection with a specific *Escherichia coli* bacterium, causing symptoms of acute microangiopathic hemolytic anemia, oliguric renal failure, and thrombocytopenia.

IMAGING

Radiography
Findings
- Disordered bowel gas pattern and thickening or thumbprinting of the affected bowel loops
- Colon: spasm, thumbprinting, ulceration, straightening, and narrowing of edematous segments
- Strictures possibly forming

Utility
- Conventional radiographs are often abnormal but nondiagnostic.
- Barium enema is used.

Ultrasound Doppler
Findings
- Peritoneal fluid, bowel wall thickening, and increased echogenicity of the renal parenchyma
- During periods of oliguria or anuria, profound abnormalities of systolic and diastolic blood flow on Doppler studies
- Return of normal blood flow heralding impending diuresis

Utility
- Ultrasound is useful in excluding causes of surgical abdomen and showing changes that suggest the diagnosis.
- It also provides useful information in children undergoing dialysis.

CLINICAL PRESENTATION

- Patients exhibit acute microangiopathic hemolytic anemia, oliguric renal failure, and thrombocytopenia.
- Also included are influenza-like illness, gastroenteritis, and bloody diarrhea that precedes striking renal and hematologic manifestations by several days or weeks.
- Acute surgical abdomen may be seen.
- Diagnosis is often delayed until anemia, thrombocytopenia, or renal failure appears.
- Urinalysis provides vital information because most patients have proteinuria, hemoglobinuria, or hematuria early in the course of the disease.

DIAGNOSTIC PEARLS

- Disordered bowel gas pattern and thickening or thumbprinting of the affected bowel loops
- Colon demonstrating spasm, thumbprinting, ulceration, straightening, and narrowing of edematous segments
- Peritoneal fluid, bowel wall thickening, and increased echogenicity of the renal parenchyma

- Patients without diarrhea have a worse prognosis for renal disease than those who have diarrhea at presentation.

DIFFERENTIAL DIAGNOSIS

- Crohn disease
- Ulcerative colitis
- Infectious colitis
- Behçet disease

PATHOLOGY

- Hemolytic-uremic syndrome is a pathologic entity with two different groups of affected patients: those who are infected with a specific *E. coli* bacterium and those who have a genetic component.
- Dialysis is necessary until renal function resumes.
- Most patients recover without sequelae.
- Death from hemolytic-uremic syndrome is more frequent in children with anuria, attributable to the manner in which the thrombotic process affects organs other than the kidneys.

INCIDENCE/PREVALENCE AND EPIDEMIOLOGY

- A genetic component may exist.
- Hemolytic-uremic syndrome occurs in toddlers and children between 2 and 10 years of age.

WHAT THE REFERRING PHYSICIAN NEEDS TO KNOW
- Vigorous fluid therapy given to children with active peritoneal signs results in overhydration and can cause peripheral and pulmonary edema.
- Prompt diagnosis averts an unwarranted laparotomy and contributes to the proper management of fluid needs.
- Dialysis is necessary until renal function resumes.

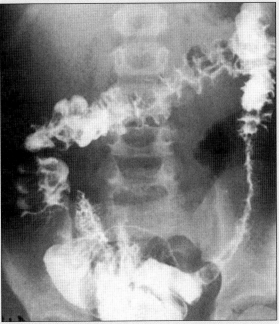

Figure 1. Hemolytic-uremic syndrome. Spasm and ulceration are present in the descending colon, and mild thumbprinting deforms the transverse colon on this barium enema study.

Suggested Readings

Gianviti A, Tozzi AE, De Petris L, et al: Risk factors for poor renal prognosis in children with hemolytic uremic syndrome. *J Pediatr Nephrol* 18:1229-1235, 2003.

Patriquin HB, O'Reagan S, Robitalle P, et al: Hemolytic-uremic syndrome: Intrarenal arterial Doppler patterns as a useful guide to therapy. *Radiology* 172:625-628, 1989.

Petermann A, Offermann G, Distler A, et al: Familial hemolytic-uremic syndrome in three generations. *Am J Kidney Dis* 32: 1063-1067, 1998.

Seror D, Szold A, Udassin R, et al: Surgical complications in hemolytic-uremic syndrome: Gangrenous appendicitis. *Pediatr Surg Int* 5:214-215, 1990.

Siegler RL: The hemolytic uremic syndrome. *Pediatr Clin North Am* 42:1505-1529, 1995.

Siegler R, Oakes R: Hemolytic uremic syndrome: Pathogenesis, treatment, and outcome. *Curr Opin Pediatr* 17:200-204, 2005.

Hirschsprung Disease (Pediatric)

DEFINITION: Hirschsprung disease (HD) is the absence of ganglion cells in the Auerbach plexus and the Meissner plexus in the affected bowel.

IMAGING

Radiography
Findings
- Changes of distal bowel obstruction are seen.
- Rarely, calcifications are seen in the bowel lumen.
- Small-caliber enema tip should be used to prevent dilating the rectum.
- In infants, a funnel- or cone-shaped appearance is seen.
- Aganglionosis is a crinkled appearance of the distal colon and corrugated rectum.
- HD-induced colitis produces a spastic and difficult-to-distend colon, with spiculated or saw-toothed mucosa.

Utility
- Early diagnosis of HD can be lifesaving.
- Radiologic diagnosis is more difficult in the neonatal period than in later life.
- Contrast enema examination is performed for the diagnosis and to exclude other causes of distal obstruction.
- Reconstituted powdered barium prevents the retention and absorption of tap water above the aganglionic segment, which can cause serious electrolyte disturbances.
- Enema performed in the left lateral decubitus position improves visualization of segments that are most likely to be abnormal.
- Filling of the colon proximal to an abnormal configuration is not recommended in case the barium becomes impacted.

CLINICAL PRESENTATION

- Neonates exhibit delayed passage of meconium, abdominal distention, vomiting, and abnormal stooling.
- Older children with undiagnosed HD usually have an abnormal neonatal stooling history and unremitting constipation.
- Delayed diagnosis (second and third decades of life) leads to chronic constipation, chronic laxative abuse, and colonic distention.

DIAGNOSTIC PEARLS

- Delayed passage of meconium
- In infants, a funnel- or cone-shaped appearance
- Aganglionosis: a crinkled appearance of the distal colon and a corrugated rectum

- On physical examination, the rectal ampulla is empty in those with HD.

DIFFERENTIAL DIAGNOSES

- Psychogenic constipation
- Imperforate anus (neonate)
- Hypoplastic left colon syndrome (neonate)
- Meconium plug syndrome (neonate)

PATHOLOGY

- HD is characterized by the absence of ganglion cells in the Auerbach plexus and the Meissner plexus in the affected bowel.
- It is caused by the arrest of the usual craniocaudal migration of primitive neuroblasts and is associated with other abnormalities of the neural crest.
- Children with central hypoventilation syndrome have an increased incidence of HD.
- Involved segment is of variable length and is always distal.
- Total colonic aganglionosis, with or without small-bowel involvement, is seen in 8% of affected children.
- Extensive aganglionosis is rare and a lethal variant in which the entire small bowel and stomach lack normal ganglion cells.
- Zonal aganglionosis is rare and may be an acquired lesion or have a different embryologic basis.

WHAT THE REFERRING PHYSICIAN NEEDS TO KNOW

- Delay in diagnosis can lead to bowel perforation or potentially fatal enterocolitis.
- Pseudomembranous colitis may also occur in these children, even without recent exposure to antibiotics, and it can lead to perforation of the appendix and proximal colon in 5% of cases.
- Suction biopsy of the rectal mucosa excludes the diagnosis of HD by histologic demonstration of ganglion cells.
- Definitive or corrective surgery usually delayed until the child is 1 year of age.
- Early diagnosis can be lifesaving.

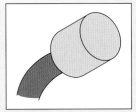

Figure 1. Hirschsprung disease. The diagram (lateral view) depicts the varied appearance of the transition zone in the rectum in HD. A discrete change in caliber is more typical, with the radiologic transition zone more clearly defined.

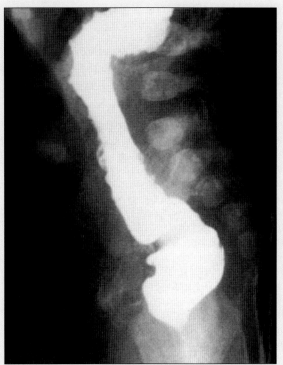

Figure 2. Total colonic Hirschsprung disease. Frontal view from a barium enema study shows that the rectum is larger than the more proximal colon. Intense spasm from colitis prevents colonic distention. Spiculation and mucosal ulcerations are present throughout, except in the rectum.

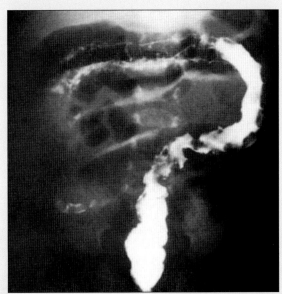

Figure 3. Total colonic Hirschsprung disease. Lateral view from a barium enema study shows that the rectum is larger than the more proximal colon. Intense spasm from colitis prevents colonic distention. Spiculation and mucosal ulcerations are present throughout, except in the rectum.

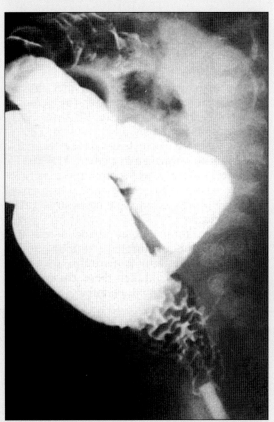

Figure 4. Hirschsprung disease. On this lateral view from a barium enema study, the rectum is smaller than the sigmoid colon. The corrugated appearance of the rectum has also been described in HD.

INCIDENCE/PREVALENCE AND EPIDEMIOLOGY

- Two thirds to three fourths of children with classic HD are boys; total colonic aganglionosis affects boys and girls equally.
- HD is the most common cause of neonatal obstruction of the colon, and more than 70% of cases are diagnosed in this period.
- Incidence is increased among children with trisomy 21, Waardenburg syndrome, Smith-Lemli-Opitz syndrome, and several other syndromes
- Initial treatment of HD is directed toward decompressing the colon to prevent enterocolitis.
- More common treatment is a colostomy above the aganglionic segment, with intraoperative pathologic guidance to define the true transition zone.
- All operations (Swenson, Soave, and Duhamel procedures) attempt to restore normal function by removing or bypassing the aganglionic segment.
- Postoperative complications include leakage at the anastomosis, continued obstruction, and, rarely, the development of secondary aganglionosis in a previously normal segment.

Suggested Readings

Amiel J, Lyonnet S: Hirschsprung disease, associated syndromes, and genetics: A review. *J Med Genet* 38:729-739, 2001.

Arliss J, Holgerson LO: Neonatal perforation and Hirschsprung's disease. *J Pediatr Surg* 25:694-695, 1990.

Filston HC, Kirks DR: The association of malrotation and Hirschsprung's disease. *Pediatr Radiol* 12:6-10, 1982.

Foster P, Cowan G, Wrenn EL Jr: Twenty-five years' experience with Hirschsprung's disease. *J Pediatr Surg* 25:531-534, 1990.

Ghosh A, Griffiths DM: Rectal biopsy in the investigation of constipation. *Arch Dis Child* 79:266-268, 1998.

Jasonni V, Martucciello G: Total colonic aganglionosis. *Semin Pediatr Surg* 7:174-180, 1998.

Moore SW, Rode H, Millar AJW, et al: Intestinal atresia and Hirschsprung's disease. *Pediatr Surg Int* 5:182-184, 1990.

Newman B, Nussbaum A, Kirkpatrick JA Jr: Bowel perforation in Hirschsprung's disease. *AJR Am J Roentgenol* 148:1195-1197, 1987.

Pochaczevsky R, Leonidas JC: The "recto-sigmoid index." A measurement for the early diagnosis of Hirschsprung's disease. *AJR Am J Roentgenol* 123:770-777, 1975.

Suita S, Taguchi T, Kamimura T, et al: Total colonic aganglionosis with or without small bowel involvement: A changing profile. *J Pediatr Surg* 32:1537-1541, 1997.

Intussusception (Pediatric)

DEFINITION: Proximal segment of bowel passes into the lumen of the more distal segment; the proximal segment is the intussusceptum, and the distal segment is the intussuscipiens.

IMAGING

Radiography
Findings
- Subnormal amount of intestinal gas, displaced bowel loops from the right hypochondrium
- Soft-tissue mass
- Barium dissecting between the intussusceptum and the intussuscipiens, a sign of nonreduction, and a coil spring appearance
- Suspicion of intussusception: contrast enema with barium, air, or water-soluble agents for diagnosis and treatment

Utility
- Therapeutic enema examination is performed only in the medically stable child.
- Barium or water-soluble contrast is suspended above the table, and flow of contrast continues until the colon is filled and free reflux into small bowel or intussusceptum is encountered.
- Contrast bag remains open throughout the study to maintain constant pressure, and an attempt is made to push the gut to its original place.
- Delayed abdominal radiograph is helpful in identifying a residual cecal mass that may represent lymphoma or another lead point.

Ultrasound
Findings
- Target or doughnut appearance on transverse scans
- Pseudokidney or *sandwich sign* on longitudinal scans

Utility
- False-positive results are produced when the bowel is thickened for other reasons, such as lymphoma or Crohn disease.
- False-negative results occur when the amount of bowel gas present precludes a complete abdominal examination.
- Ultrasound may be diagnostic or therapeutic.

DIAGNOSTIC PEARLS
- Barium dissecting between the intussusceptum and the intussuscipiens is a sign of nonreduction, with a coil spring appearance.
- Target or doughnut appearance is seen on transverse scans.
- Pseudokidney or sandwich sign is seen on longitudinal scans.

CT
Findings
Target or sausage sign
Utility
- CT is not useful because it is expensive and cannot be used to treat intussusception when found.

CLINICAL PRESENTATION
- Patients exhibit colicky abdominal pain.
- Stools may test positive for occult blood or have the classic, but infrequent, currant jelly appearance.
- Vomiting, diarrhea, and abdominal mass may be seen.
- A few children are lethargic or dehydrated.
- Rectal bleeding is also more common in the neonate with intussusception than in the older child.

DIFFERENTIAL DIAGNOSIS
- Cystic fibrosis (pediatric gastrointestinal)
- Hernia
- Crohn disease
- Meckel diverticulum
- Polyp or mass in stomach, duodenum, small bowel, or colon

WHAT THE REFERRING PHYSICIAN NEEDS TO KNOW
- Surgery reduces intussusceptions that do not respond to barium enema and treats children whose clinical status precludes radiologic intervention.
- Perforated bowel or a gangrenous gut is suggested by fever, elevated white blood cell count, peritoneal signs, and marked systemic toxicity, which requires immediate surgery.
- Analgesia and sedation may be given if the first reduction attempt is unsuccessful; they make the patient more comfortable and aid in spontaneous reduction.
- Success rate for reduction decreases with evidence of small-bowel obstruction or the presence of symptoms for greater than 24 hours.
- Children with Henoch-Schönlein purpura, recent abdominal surgery, or cystic fibrosis have an increased incidence of intussusception.

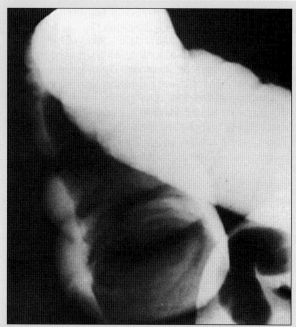

Figure 1. Dissection sign of intussusception on barium enema study. Contrast medium is seen along the sides of the intussusception, which has a coil-spring appearance. When this sign is observed, the likelihood of successful reduction is diminished, although reduction is still possible.

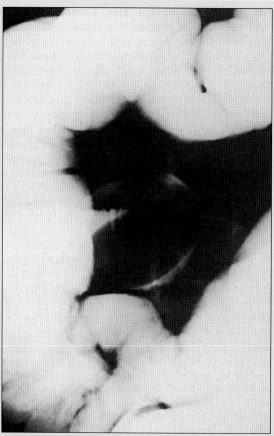

Figure 2. Intussusception. A persistent filling defect is seen on barium enema examination in the ileum in this child who had a normal-appearing colon. Because the sonogram that preceded this study showed the intussusception, it was necessary to reflux into more ileal loops than usual to confirm and treat the problem.

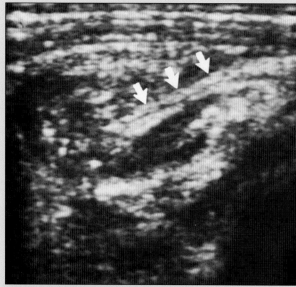

Figure 3. Sonography of intussusception. Transverse scan shows the parallel echogenic mucosa *(arrows)* of the intussuscipiens and intussusceptum.

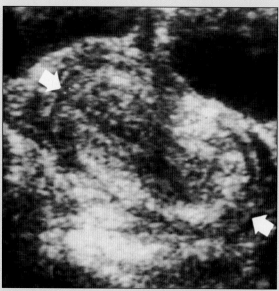

Figure 4. Sonography of intussusception. The pseudokidney *(arrows)* sign of intussusception is demonstrated on this longitudinal sonogram. The sonolucent structures anteriorly are dilated bowel loops.

PATHOLOGY

- Proximal segment of the bowel passes into the lumen of the more distal segment, and, through peristalsis, it is propelled distally.
- Proximal segment is termed the *intussusceptum*, and the distal segment is called the *intussuscipiens*.
- Most common form is ileocolic; less common types of intussusceptions are ileoileocolic, ileoileal, and jejuno-ileal.
- No prodrome or discernible cause has been found.
- Only 3%-10% of children have an intrinsic bowel abnormality (the lead point for intussusception): duplication, hemangioma, polyp, Meckel diverticulum, or lymphoma.

INCIDENCE/PREVALENCE AND EPIDEMIOLOGY

- Most intussusceptions occur in children between 3 months and 3 years of age, with a 2:1 male/female predominance.

Suggested Readings

Barr LL, Stansberry SD, Swischuk LE: Significance of age, duration, obstruction and the dissection sign in intussusception. *Pediatr Radiol* 20:454-456, 1990.

Bramson RT, Blickman JG: Perforation during hydrostatic reduction of intussusception: Proposed mechanism and review of the literature. *J Pediatr Surg* 27:589-591, 1992.

Collins DL, Pickney LE, Miller KE, et al: Hydrostatic reduction of ileocolic intussusception: A second attempt in the operating room with general anesthesia. *J Pediatr* 115:204-207, 1989.

Daneman A, Alton DJ, Ein S, et al: Perforation during attempted intussusception reduction in children—A comparison of perforation with barium and air. *Pediatr Radiol* 25:81-86, 1995.

del-Pozo G, Albillos JC, Tejedor D, et al: Intussusception in children: Current concepts in diagnosis and enema reduction. *RadioGraphics* 19:299-319, 1999.

Devred PH, Faure F, Padovani J: Pseudotumoral cecum after hydrostatic reduction of intussusception. *Pediatr Radiol* 14:295-298, 1984.

Gu L, Zhu H, Wang S, et al: Sonographic guidance of air enema for intussusception reduction in children. *Pediatr Radiol* 30:339-340, 2000.

Hernandez JA, Swischuk LE, Angel CA: Validity of plain films in intussusception. *Emerg Radiol* 10:323-326, 2004.

Ong NT, Beasley SW: The lead point in intussusception. *J Pediatr Surg* 25:640-643, 1990.

Stephenson CA, Seibert JJ, Strain JD, et al: Intussusception: Clinical and radiographic factors influencing reducibility. *Pediatr Radiol* 20:57-60, 1989.

Touloukian RJ, O'Connell JB, Markowitz RI, et al: Analgesic premedication in the management of ileocolic intussusception. *Pediatrics* 79:432-434, 1987.

Typhlitis (Pediatric)

DEFINITION: Acute inflammation of the cecum that occurs in immunosuppressed patients.

ANATOMIC FINDINGS

Colon
- Inflammatory changes with submucosal edema
- Mural thickening

IMAGING

Radiography
Findings
- Abnormal amount of bowel gas or soft-tissue mass in the right lower quadrant, ascites, or pneumatosis intestinalis
- Free intraperitoneal air
- Contrast enema: demonstrates changes in appearance of inflammatory changes in the cecum but may lead to perforation

Utility
- Contrast enema is not recommended in patients with suspected typhlitis.

Ultrasound
Findings
- Mural thickening of cecum, ascending colon, and ileum
- Increased transmural blood flow

Utility
- Ultrasound is useful in identifying abscesses and in excluding appendiceal inflammation.
- Color Doppler is used.

CT
Findings
- CT shows mural thickening of the cecum associated with submucosal edema.
- In severe cases, low-density abscesses or frank pneumatosis intestinalis may develop.

Utility
- CT is the most useful noninvasive means of making the diagnosis.
- CT used to assess the efficacy of antibiotic therapy and the need for surgery

DIAGNOSTIC PEARLS
- Abnormal amount of bowel gas or a soft-tissue mass in the right lower quadrant, ascites, or pneumatosis intestinalis
- Free intraperitoneal air
- Mural thickening of the cecum, ascending colon, and ileum

CLINICAL PRESENTATION
- Right lower quadrant pain
- Leukopenia
- Fever
- Peritoneal signs
- Occasionally with an inflammatory mass
- Uncommonly with lower gastrointestinal hemorrhage
- Possible perforation of the cecum

DIFFERENTIAL DIAGNOSIS
- Appendicitis
- Infectious colitis
- Inflammatory bowel disease
- Mesenteric adenitis
- Meckel diverticulitis

PATHOLOGY
- Acute inflammation of the cecum that occurs in immunocompromised patients

INCIDENCE/PREVALENCE AND EPIDEMIOLOGY
- Typhlitis or neutropenic fever is a common complication of profound neutropenia found in immunocompromised patients caused by acute lymphocytic (lymphoblastic) leukemia, acquired immunodeficiency syndrome, or chemotherapy.

WHAT THE REFERRING PHYSICIAN NEEDS TO KNOW
- Granulocyte transfusions, antibiotics, and surgical resection of the affected bowel stop the progress of inflammation.
- Diagnostic delay may lead to perforation, sepsis, and death.
- The differential diagnosis includes appendicitis, right-sided diverticulitis, Crohn disease, and pseudomembranous colitis.

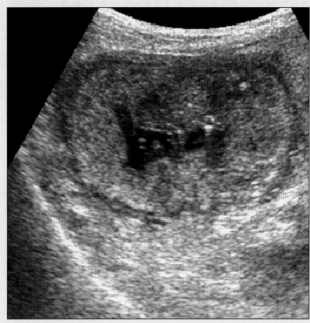

Figure 1. Pediatric typhlitis. Marked mural thickening of the cecum is demonstrated sonographically in this 8-year-old boy with profound neutropenia secondary to acute lymphocytic leukemia.

Suggested Readings

Hobson MJ, Carney DE, Molik KA, et al: Appendicitis in childhood hematologic malignancies: Analysis and comparison with typhlitis. *J Pediatr Surg* 40:214-219, 2005.

McCarville MB, Adelman CS, Li C, et al: Typhlitis in childhood cancer. *Cancer* 104:380-387, 2005.

McCarville MB, Thompson J, Li C, et al: Significance of appendiceal thickening in association with typhlitis in pediatric oncology patients. *Pediatr Radiol* 34:245-249, 2004.

Schlatter M, Snyder K, Freyer D: Successful nonoperative management of typhlitis in pediatric oncology patients. *J Pediatr Surg* 37:1151-1155, 2002.

Teefey SA, Montana MA, Goldfogel GA, et al: Sonographic diagnosis of neutropenic typhlitis. *AJR Am J Roentgenol* 149:731-733, 1987.

Part 69

DISEASES INVOLVING MULTIPLE AREAS OF THE GASTROINTESTINAL TRACT

Cystic Fibrosis (Pediatric Gastrointestinal)

DEFINITION: Cystic fibrosis (CF) is a congenital genetic disorder in which mucus-producing glands exhibit an abnormality of exocrine function.

ANATOMIC FINDINGS

Small Bowel
- Meconium ileus: impaction of thick meconium or pellets of meconium at the distal ileum
- Dilation, prolonged transit time, and prominent valvulae conniventes

Colon
- Fibrosing colonopathy manifests as a colonic stricture of varying severity extending proximally from the cecum.
- The rectum is usually spared.
- The colon is foreshortened and the haustra are obliterated in the affected segment.

Peritoneum
- Peritoneal calcifications

Pancreas
- Pancreatic calcifications

IMAGING

Radiography
Findings
- Bowel obstruction findings in cases of intussusception or meconium ileus are seen.
- Meconium ileus equivalents are likely to have large amounts of bubbly fecal debris visible on abdominal radiographs.
- Benign pneumatosis intestinalis and peritoneal or pancreatic calcifications are seen.
- Oral contrast studies of the duodenum and small bowel demonstrate dilation, prolonged transit time, and prominent valvulae conniventes.

DIAGNOSTIC PEARLS
- Prenatal sonogram findings include polyhydramnios, meconium peritonitis, intra-abdominal cyst, ascites, and dilated bowel filled with echogenic material.
- Oral contrast studies of the duodenum and small bowel demonstrate dilation, prolonged transit time, and prominent valvulae conniventes.
- Bubbly fecal debris with signs of bowel obstruction in cases of meconium ileus–equivalent syndrome may be seen.

- Duodenal filling defects or irregular and spiculated appearance can also result from enlarged Brunner glands or paraduodenal varices.
- Esophagograms reveal esophagitis and a stricture from gastroesophageal reflux.
- Enlarged spleen is seen in patients with portal hypertension.

Utility
- Plain radiographs of abdomen are taken.
- Intussusception may be difficult to differentiate from meconium ileus–equivalent syndrome.
- Pneumatosis intestinalis may simulate meconium ileus equivalent.

Ultrasound
Findings
- Prenatal sonogram findings: polyhydramnios, meconium peritonitis, intra-abdominal cyst, ascites, or dilated bowel filled with echogenic material
- Small or indistinguishable gallbladder, gallstones, and sludge

---

WHAT THE REFERRING PHYSICIAN NEEDS TO KNOW
- Prenatal testing should be performed when both parents are known carriers of the CF gene or when a sibling has been diagnosed with CF.
- Children with rectal prolapse without an underlying abnormality (e.g., constipation, diarrhea) should undergo sweat chloride analysis for the exclusion of CF.
- Correlation of sonographic findings with biochemical studies of liver function may allow early identification of a patient whose liver needs more careful monitoring.
- Children with CF and meconium ileus have a more severe phenotype.

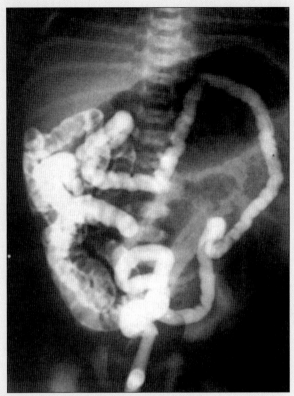

Figure 1. Meconium ileus demonstrated by water-soluble enema. The colon is small in caliber, similar in diameter to the small bowel, which is impacted with multiple, small, rounded pellets of meconium.

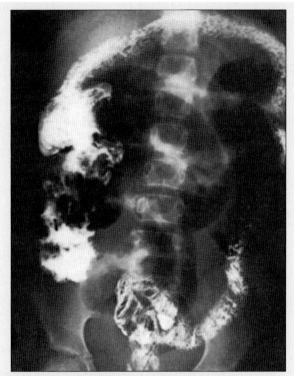

Figure 2. Meconium ileus–equivalent syndrome. The postevacuation radiograph demonstrates residual fecal material in the dilated ascending colon. The colonic mucosa has an abnormal, spiculated appearance.

- Pancreas possibly becoming replaced with fat or possibly developing a single or multiple macrocysts

Utility
- Prenatal sonogram findings take on a particular significance when cystic fibrosis has been diagnosed in a sibling.

Ultrasound Doppler
Utility
- Portal venous flow can be evaluated by Doppler sonography when portal hypertension is suspected.

CT
Findings
- Varices
- Pancreas possibly becoming replaced with fat or possibly developing a single or multiple macrocysts

Nuclear Medicine
Findings
- Abnormalities of bile flow
Utility
- Hepatobiliary scintigraphy

MRI
Findings
- Pancreas possibly becoming replaced with fat or possibly developing a single or multiple macrocysts

CLINICAL PRESENTATION
- Symptoms related to a gastrointestinal abnormality include abdominal pain and distention, retrosternal pain, diarrhea, malabsorption, and rectal prolapse.

DIFFERENTIAL DIAGNOSIS
- Intussusception

PATHOLOGY
- CF is a congenital defect caused by a mutated, recessive CF gene *(F508)*.
- All mucus-producing glands exhibit an abnormality of exocrine function, resulting in unusually thick secretions.
- Diminished exocrine function of the pancreas produces malabsorption and failure to thrive unless enzyme supplements are taken.

INCIDENCE/PREVALENCE AND EPIDEMIOLOGY
- CF is the most common lethal genetic abnormality in the white population.

- Recessive CF gene is carried by approximately 3% of this group.
- CF occurs in 1 of 3000 live births.

Suggested Readings

Accurso FJ, Sontag MK, Wagener JS: Complications associated with symptomatic diagnosis in infants with cystic fibrosis. *J Pediatr* 147:S37-S41, 2005.

Hudson VL, Guill MF: New developments in cystic fibrosis. *Pediatr Ann* 27:515-520, 1998.

Mushtaq I, Wright VM, Drake DP, et al: Meconium ileus secondary to cystic fibrosis. The East London experience. *Pediatr Surg Int* 13:365-369, 1998.

Nadel HR: Hepatobiliary scintigraphy in children. *Semin Nucl Med* 26:25-42, 1996.

Wilschanski M, Fisher D, Hadas-Halperin I, et al: Findings on routine abdominal ultrasonography in cystic fibrosis patients. *J Pediatr Gastroenterol Nutr* 28:182-185, 1999.

Gastrointestinal Duplications (Pediatric)

DEFINITION: Duplications of any portion of the gastrointestinal tract, from tongue to rectum.

ANATOMIC FINDINGS

Abdomen
- Duplications are located on the mesenteric side of the bowel.
- Noncommunicating duplications tend to be rounded and cystic, but they may be dumbbell shaped.
- Elongated, tubular duplications are more likely to communicate with the adjacent bowel.
- Typically, colonic duplication is a segmental, noncommunicating mass but can be complex.
- Duplications are located in continuity with or in close apposition to the gut.

Thorax
- Esophageal duplications are five times more frequent on the right than on the left.
- Approximately 15% of esophageal duplications straddle the esophageal hiatus.

IMAGING

Ultrasound
Findings
- Prenatal ultrasound reveals a fluid-filled structure in the abdominal cavity.
- Many duplications have a signature sonolucent muscular rim peripheral to the echogenic mucosa.
- Fluid within the duplication may become echogenic if hemorrhage or communication with adjacent bowel exists.

Utility
- Perform postnatal scanning to assess any change in size and echogenicity and to detect secondary characteristics that can assist in the diagnosis.
- When an extraluminal mass is detected on radiography, sonography should be performed to look for the muscular rim of the duplication.

DIAGNOSTIC PEARLS
- Many duplications have the signature sonolucent muscular rim peripheral to the echogenic mucosa.
- Duplications are located on mesenteric side of the bowel.
- Noncommunicating duplications tend to be rounded and cystic, but they may be dumbbell shaped.
- Elongated, tubular duplications are more likely to communicate with the adjacent bowel.

Radiography
Findings
- Esophageal duplications are seen as soft-tissue masses on chest radiographs.

Utility
- Esophageal duplications simulate adenopathy or mediastinal tumors.
- Barium esophagogram is rarely performed as part of the evaluation.
- Abdominal plain radiographs are of little value in the diagnosis of duplication because calcification and mass effect are rarely present.

CT
Findings
- Density of fluid within the duplication depends on the protein content and the presence of hemorrhage and communication with the gut.

Utility
- When chest radiographs demonstrate a mediastinal mass, chest CT should be the next examination.
- CT shows the full extent of the duplication, excludes noncystic masses, and detects any additional anomalies.

WHAT THE REFERRING PHYSICIAN NEEDS TO KNOW
- Esophageal duplications and bronchogenic cysts have a shared presentation and location but are differentiated by microscopic examination of the mucosal lining.
- Management of the duplication is based on the location, size, presenting symptoms, and the presence of communication with adjacent structures.
- Drainage of gastric mucosa–lined duplications is potentially dangerous because acidic gastric secretions can ulcerate the mucosa of the adjacent bowel.
- Choledochal cysts are excluded by hepatobiliary scan; sonography identifies renal duplication, and sonography helps differentiate choledochal cysts from ovarian cysts.
- MRI and CT scans are performed in cases of associated vertebral changes.

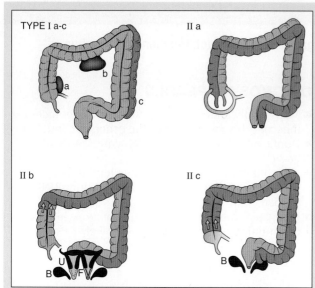

Figure 1. Types of colonic duplication. Type I: segmental colonic duplication without other caudal duplication: **a,** noncommunicating spherical duplication; **b,** noncommunicating tubular duplication; **c,** communicating tubular duplication. Type II: complete or segmental colonic duplication with genitourinary duplication: **a,** duplication with two perineal openings; **b,** duplication with one or both segments ending as a fistula to the vagina, bladder, or perineum; **c,** duplication with one or both segments imperforate and no fistula. (*B*, Bladder; *F*, fistula; *U*, uterus; *V*, vagina.) (*From Carr SL, Shaffer HA, de Lange EE: Duplication of the colon: Varied presentations of a rare congenital anomaly. Can Assoc Radiol J 39:29-32, 1988.*)

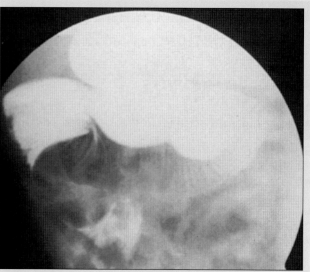

Figure 2. Jejunal duplication. Upper gastrointestinal series performed on a neonate with vomiting shows a filling defect in the jejunum that was only intermittently observed. For this reason, sonography was performed.

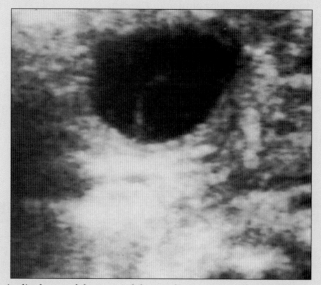

Figure 3. Jejunal duplication. Longitudinal scan of the upper abdomen demonstrates a fluid-filled structure with a muscular rim that could be identified only in the deepest portion of the duplication.

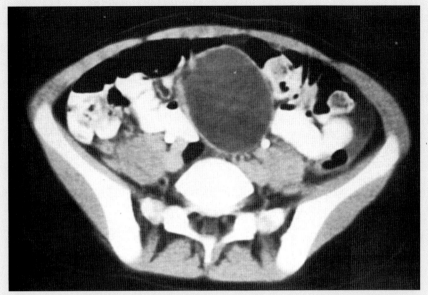

Figure 4. Ileal duplication. CT shows a spherical cystic mass with a perceptible wall that enhances to the same degree as adjacent muscular structures.

- CT may be required if the patient has atypical symptoms or if the diagnosis remains uncertain after ultrasound.
- CT depicts vertebral structural bone abnormalities to the best advantage.

MRI
Findings
A solid and/or cystic mass may be demonstrated.
Utility
- MRI shows the full extent of the duplication, excludes noncystic masses, and detects any additional anomalies.
- MRI is superior in demonstrating associated spinal cord disease.
- Imaging of the spinal canal and cord is recommended when vertebral changes associated with a suspected duplication occur.

Nuclear Medicine
Findings
- Gastric mucosa
Utility
- Technetium 99m-pertechnetate scintigraphy is used for suspected duplication with bleeding.

CLINICAL PRESENTATION

- In neonates, manifestations are small-bowel obstruction, intussusception, mass, or bleeding.
- In later childhood, duplications are often recognized by a mass or hemorrhage.
- Oral or esophageal duplications may cause airway narrowing and respiratory symptoms, or they may be an incidental finding on chest radiograph.

- Clinically, pyloric duplications may simulate hypertrophic pyloric stenosis.
- Intrapancreatic or duodenal duplications can obstruct pancreatic drainage and cause pancreatitis or perforation of the adjacent bowel.
- Results of the physical examination are often unremarkable.
- If duplication causes tracheal or bronchial compression, abnormal air exchange or wheezing may be detected.

DIFFERENTIAL DIAGNOSIS

- Omental and mesenteric cysts
- Congenital anomalies: bronchogenic cyst
- Choledochal cysts
- Renal duplication
- Ovarian cysts
- Adenopathy
- Mediastinal mass

PATHOLOGY

- Duplication may contain mucosa of any segment of the gastrointestinal tract and even the pancreas, regardless of its location.
- It can also contain more than one type of mucosa.
- Although stomach duplications account for less than 10% of all duplications, heterotopic gastric mucosa is found in 20%-50% of cases.
- Communicating duplication shares the wall or lumen with the adjacent gastrointestinal tract.
- Noncommunicating duplication is adjacent to the segment of the gastrointestinal tract but does not share the lumen.

- Neurenteric cysts are a rare form of duplication in which a gastrointestinal abnormality is associated with a vertebral anomaly, usually spinal dysraphism.

INCIDENCE/PREVALENCE AND EPIDEMIOLOGY

- Up to 15% of children have multiple duplications.
- Multiple duplications are associated with additional congenital malformations.
- Noncommunicating duplications are four times more common than communicating ones.
- Vertebral anomalies are seen more frequently in children with thoracic duplications than those with abdominal duplications, even in the absence of a neurenteric cyst.

Suggested Readings

Carachi R, Azmy A: Foregut duplications. *Pediatr Surg Int* 18:371-374, 2002.

Fitch SJ, Tonkin ILD, Tonkin AK: Imaging of foregut duplication cysts. *RadioGraphics* 6:189-201, 1986.

Iyer CP, Mahour GH: Duplications of the alimentary tract in infants and children. *J Pediatr Surg* 30:1267-1270, 1995.

Macpherson RI: Gastrointestinal tract duplications: Clinical, pathologic, etiologic, and radiologic considerations. *RadioGraphics* 13:1063-1080, 1993.

Puliganda PS, Nguyen LT, St-Vil D, et al: Gastrointestinal duplications. *J Pediatr Surg* 38:740-744, 2003.

Stringer MD, Spitz L, Abel R, et al: Management of alimentary tract duplication in children. *Br J Surg* 82:74-78, 1995.

Pediatric Small-Bowel and Colonic Infections

DEFINITION: Infections of the small bowel and colon.

IMAGING

Radiography
Findings
- Barium studies may show changes in the terminal ileum reminiscent of Crohn disease.

Utility
- Barium studies are seldom used to establish the diagnosis.

Ultrasound
Findings
- *Yersinia* infection is often accompanied by enlarged lymph nodes.
- Mural thickening of bowel
- Hyperperistalsis
- Intraperitoneal fluid

Utility
- Ultrasound helps exclude appendicitis.
- It does not use ionizing radiation.

CT
Findings
- Mural thickening of the affected gut
- Submucosal edema
- Pericolonic or small bowel fluid
- Intraperitoneal fluid

Utility
- CT provides the most comprehensive look at abdominal infectious and inflammatory disorders.
- Does employ ionizing radiation

CLINICAL PRESENTATION

- Patients exhibit fever, diarrhea, bleeding, and abdominal pain.
- *Helicobacter pylori* organism is associated with a peptic ulcer and diarrheal illness and may produce lactose intolerance.

DIAGNOSTIC PEARLS

- Barium studies may show changes in the terminal ileum reminiscent of Crohn disease.
- *Yersinia* infection is often accompanied by enlarged lymph nodes.
- Clinical pattern and serologic or stool cultures are often enough to make the diagnosis.

- *Yersinia* enterocolitis may produce symptoms that simulate appendicitis or Crohn disease.

DIFFERENTIAL DIAGNOSIS

- Crohn disease
- Appendicitis
- Ulcerative colitis
- Behçet disease
- Vasculitis
- Hemolytic-uremic syndrome
- Henoch-Schönlein purpura

PATHOLOGY

- Symptoms of intestinal infection result from enterotoxin release, mucosal invasion, and damage to enterocytes.

INCIDENCE/PREVALENCE AND EPIDEMIOLOGY

- Bacterial, viral, and parasitic forms of gastroenteritis are major causes of pediatric morbidity and mortality worldwide.
- Children with an *H. pylori*–associated peptic ulcer disease have an increased incidence of gastric body adenocarcinoma in later life.

WHAT THE REFERRING PHYSICIAN NEEDS TO KNOW

- Imaging is not needed when the clinical pattern is typical or when the diagnosis is made based on serologic or stool cultures.
- Imaging is useful when symptoms persist and suggest a complication or secondary process.
- Most children are successfully treated with oral rehydration.
- Medications to decrease gut motility or antibiotics to control infections are used in specific settings and are contraindicated in others.

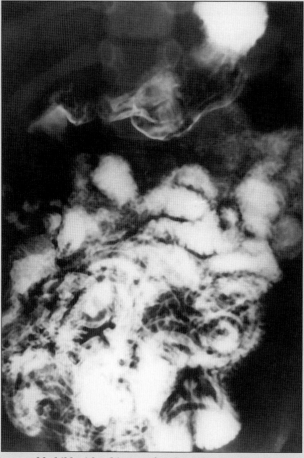

Figure 1. Intestinal ascariasis in a 4-year-old child with a history of malnutrition. A frontal supine abdominal radiograph from a small-bowel examination shows barium-filling loops of small bowel in which long, smooth, filling defects (worms) are noted. Sometimes the worm ingests the barium, thus revealing a long, thin line within the worm that represents its own intestinal tract (not shown here).

Suggested Readings

Amieva MR: Important bacterial gastrointestinal pathogens in children: A pathogenesis perspective. *Pediatr Clin North Am* 52:749-777, 2005.

Elliot EJ, Dalby-Payne JR: Acute infectious diarrhea and dehydration in children. *Med J Aust* 181:565-570, 2004.

Goodgame RW: Viral causes of diarrhea. *Gastrointest Clin North Am* 30:779-795, 2001.

O'Ryan M, Prado V, Pickering LK: A millennium update on pediatric diarrheal illness in the developing world. *Semin Pediatr Infect Dis* 16:125-136, 2005.

Zetterstrom R: The Nobel Prize in 2005 for the discovery of *Helicobacter pylori:* Implications for child health. *Acta Pediatr* 95:3-5, 2006.

Part 70

DISEASES OF THE GALLBLADDER AND BILIARY TRACT

Alagille Syndrome

DEFINITION: A rare autosomal-dominant disease characterized by chronic cholestasis caused by a paucity of interlobular bile ducts relative to the number of portal areas within the liver.

IMAGING

Ultrasound
Findings
- Liver size and echogenicity may be normal or increased; intrahepatic bile ducts are typically not visualized.

Utility
- Sonographic findings of Alagille syndrome are similar to those of neonatal hepatitis.

Nuclear Medicine
Findings
- Poor hepatic uptake of the isotope
- Typically failing to show normal excretion of the radioisotope into the bowel

Utility
- Nuclear hepatobiliary scintigraphy findings initially resemble biliary atresia.

Radiography
Findings
- Cholangiography
- Demonstrated patency of the extrahepatic bile ducts

Utility
- Provides the best spatial resolution in the depiction of biliary anatomy

CLINICAL PRESENTATION

- For the diagnosis, at least three of five typical features of the disease are exhibited:
- Chronic cholestasis from interlobular bile duct paucity
- Congenital heart disease, typically involving hypoplasia or stenosis of the peripheral pulmonary arteries
- *Butterfly* vertebrae
- Posterior embryotoxon (an ocular abnormality)
- Peculiar facies

DIAGNOSTIC PEARLS

- Liver size and echogenicity may be normal or increased, and intrahepatic bile ducts are typically not visualized.
- Poor hepatic uptake of the isotope on hepatobiliary scintigraphy is seen.
- Paucity of interlobular bile ducts is seen on biopsy.

- Children with this abnormality may have findings of cirrhosis at an older age.

DIFFERENTIAL DIAGNOSIS

- Bile plug syndrome
- Biliary atresia
- Byler syndrome

PATHOLOGY

- Arteriohepatic dysplasia
- Rare autosomal-dominant disease
- Chronic cholestasis caused by a paucity of interlobular bile ducts relative to the number of portal areas within the liver
- Pulmonary artery stenosis at various levels, one of the most common manifestations of Alagille syndrome
- Vascular anomalies: basilar or middle cerebral artery aneurysms, internal carotid artery anomalies, aortic coarctation or aneurysm, and moyamoya disease
- Benign lesions such as nodular hyperplasia also described in children with Alagille syndrome and cirrhosis

---

WHAT THE REFERRING PHYSICIAN NEEDS TO KNOW

- Neonatal presentation mimics biliary atresia; treatment with the Kasai procedure may be performed before a pathologic diagnosis is made.
- Liver transplant may ultimately be required.

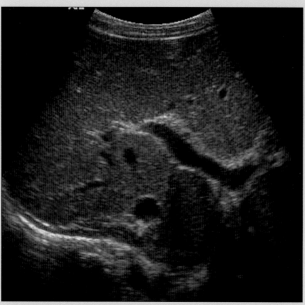

Figure 1. Nonsyndromic intrahepatic bile duct paucity: ultrasound and hepatobiliary scintigram. The cholestatic infant has a lack of a sonographically identifiable gallbladder or intrahepatic bile ducts.

INCIDENCE/PREVALENCE AND EPIDEMIOLOGY

- Alagille syndrome usually occurs in neonates but may present later.
- Intracranial vascular anomalies account for up to 34% of the mortality in these patients.
- Biliary cirrhosis occurs in 12% of children with Alagille resulting from chronic cholestasis.

Suggested Readings

Kamath BM, Spinner NB, Emerick KM, et al: Vascular anomalies in Alagille syndrome: A significant cause of morbidity and mortality. *Circulation* 109:1354-1358, 2004.

Lykavieris P, Hadchouel M, Chardot C, Bernard O: Outcome of liver disease in children with Alagille syndrome: A study of 163 patients. *Gut* 49:431-435, 2001.

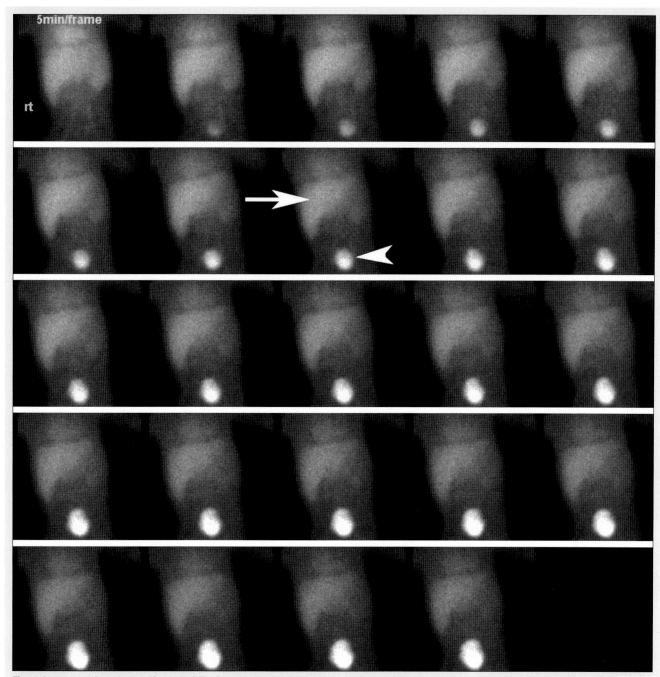

Figure 2. Nonsyndromic intrahepatic bile duct paucity: ultrasound and hepatobiliary scintigram. Nuclear scintigraphy demonstrates poor hepatic extraction *(arrow)* of the radiopharmaceutical. Some of the radiopharmaceutical is seen in the urinary bladder *(arrowhead)*.

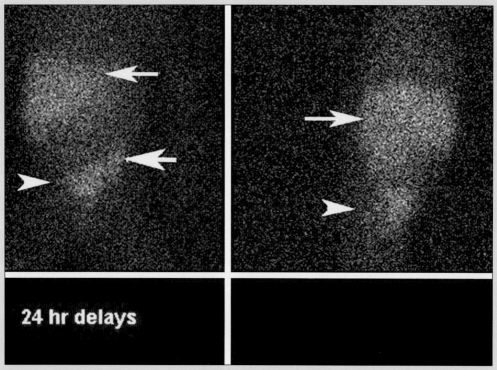

Figure 3. **Nonsyndromic intrahepatic bile duct paucity: ultrasound and hepatobiliary scintigram.** Minimal small-bowel activity is seen at 24 hours *(gray arrow)*. These findings can be seen in the setting of neonatal hepatitis or paucity of intrahepatic bile ducts with cholestasis. Liver biopsy confirmed a paucity of intrahepatic ducts. This child lacked other clinical abnormalities that are associated with Alagille syndrome.

Bile Plug Syndrome

DEFINITION: A dilated common bile duct with a normal-appearing gallbladder occluding the bile plug is evident sonographically.

ANATOMIC FINDINGS

Common Bile Duct
- Dilated

Gallbladder
- Normal appearing

IMAGING

Ultrasound
Findings
- Dilated common bile duct with a normal-appearing gallbladder
- Slightly hyperechoic, inspissated bile that causes no acoustic shadowing
- Fluid-debris level possibly seen in the dilated, obstructed bile duct
- Sludge isoechoic with the liver
- Hepatic echotexture possibly increased because of cholestasis

Utility
- An occluding bile plug is evident sonographically in 30% of children.
- A postprocedural follow-up sonogram shows a return of the bile ducts to a normal caliber.
- If sludge fills the gallbladder lumen, it may make gallbladder difficult to visualize.

CLINICAL PRESENTATION

- Jaundice, icterus, and clay-colored stools
- Cholangitis

DIAGNOSTIC PEARLS

- Surgically treatable neonatal jaundice may be seen.
- A fluid-debris level may be seen in the dilated obstructed bile duct.
- Sludge can be isoechoic with the liver, which may make the gallbladder difficult to visualize.

DIFFERENTIAL DIAGNOSIS

- Biliary atresia
- Byler syndrome
- Alagille syndrome

INCIDENCE/PREVALENCE AND EPIDEMIOLOGY

- Bile plug syndrome is the second most common cause of surgically treatable neonatal jaundice after biliary atresia.
- It is slightly more common than a choledochal cyst.

Suggested Readings

Desmet VJ: Ludwig symposium on biliary disorders. Part I. Pathogenesis of ductal plate abnormalities. *Mayo Clin Proc* 73:80-89, 1998.
Matos C, Avni EF, Van Gansbeke D, et al: Total parenteral nutrition (TPN) and gallbladder diseases in neonates. Sonographic assessment. *J Ultrasound Med* 6:243-248, 1987.

WHAT THE REFERRING PHYSICIAN NEEDS TO KNOW
- Percutaneous transhepatic cholangiography confirms the diagnosis.
- It is treated with therapeutic saline lavage of the biliary tree during the procedure.

Biliary Atresia

DEFINITION: Biliary atresia is an obliterative process of unknown origin that affects the bile ducts antenatally or during the newborn period and is characterized by cholestasis and persistent conjugated hyperbilirubinemia, ultimately leading to hepatic fibrosis and cirrhosis.

ANATOMIC FINDINGS

Common Bile Duct
- Extremely hypoplastic but patent common bile duct (CBD)
- Triangular cord sign (TCS), fibrotic, and obliterated common bile duct in infants with biliary atresia
- Focal hyperechoic area cephalad to the main portal vein bifurcation, measured as the echogenic anterior wall of the right portal vein

Common Hepatic Duct
- No filling of the common hepatic duct or intrahepatic ducts

Pancreatic Duct
- Patent

Gallbladder
- A small gallbladder with an irregular wall identified

IMAGING

Ultrasound
Findings
- Variable sonographic findings; lack of identifiable bile ducts and homogeneous liver parenchyma; lack of CBD visualization
- TCS: focal echogenic triangular or tubular echogenic area just cephalad to the main portal vein bifurcation
- No flow on color Doppler examination
- Associated round, linear, or tubular hypoechoic or cystic lesions within the triangular cord
- TCS masked by diffuse periportal hyperechogenicity or possibly being difficult to appreciate if the fibrotic cord is small
- Gallbladder ghost triad: atretic gallbladder; thinned mucosa or lack of smooth, complete echogenic mucosal lining with indistinct walls; knobby, irregular, or lobular contour

DIAGNOSTIC PEARLS
- No intestinal activity occurs by 24 hours, and hepatocyte clearance is relatively preserved.
- Gallbladder ghost triad may occur.
- TCS may be seen.

Utility
- Preoperative definition of the patient's anatomy with Doppler ultrasound is used in the technical planning of the surgical procedure.
- Ultrasound is the initial imaging modality for children with cholestatic jaundice.
- Infants should fast for 3-4 hours before the ultrasound examination in an attempt to maximize gallbladder distention.
- False-negative findings occur.
- Repeat, short-term follow-up sonograms are warranted if the initial examination appears to be normal or suggests neonatal hepatitis but worsening jaundice.
- Normal gallbladder does not exclude the diagnosis of biliary atresia.

CT
Findings
- Absent or atretic bile ducts
- Atretic gallbladder
Utility
- Preoperative definition of the patient's anatomy with CT is used in the technical planning of the surgical procedure.

Radiography
Findings
- Absent or atretic bile ducts
- Atretic gallbladder

WHAT THE REFERRING PHYSICIAN NEEDS TO KNOW
- Ovarian, greater saphenous, and the external iliac or internal jugular vein from living and related donors can be used for transplants.
- If untreated, biliary atresia is fatal, with an average survival of 18 months.
- Untreated biliary atresia results in progressive intrahepatic ductopenia during infancy, leading to cirrhosis.
- Children with biliary atresia are treated with portoenterostomy (i.e., the Kasai procedure).

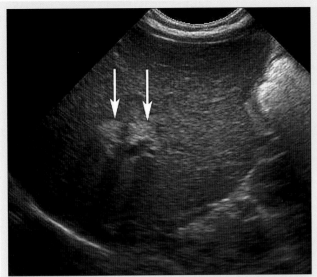

Figure 1. Biliary atresia: triangular cord sign on ultrasound. The *triangular cord sign* is a term used to describe the fibrotic, obliterated common bile duct in infants with biliary atresia. It is seen as a focal hyperechoic area just cephalad to the main portal vein bifurcation, or it can be measured as the echogenic anterior wall of the right portal vein *(arrows)*. The hypoechoic area within this is a branch of the right hepatic artery. *(Courtesy of Myung-Joon Kim, MD, Yonsei University College of Medicine, Severance Hospital, Seoul, Korea.)*

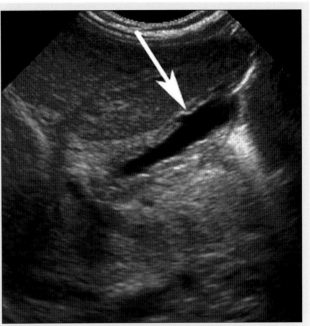

Figure 2. Biliary atresia: gallbladder ghost triad on ultrasound. The combination of an atretic gallbladder with irregular mucosa and wall contour *(arrow)* has been called the gallbladder ghost triad. It is associated with biliary atresia. *(Courtesy of Myung-Joon Kim, MD, Yonsei University College of Medicine, Severance Hospital, Seoul, Korea.)*

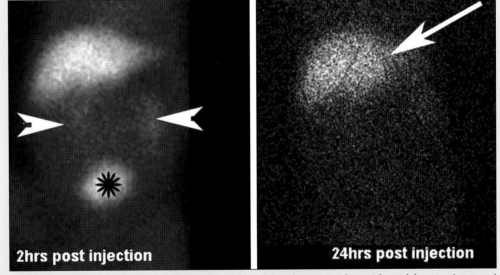

Figure 3. Biliary atresia: hepatobiliary nuclear scintigram. Anterior delayed images. After a 2-hour delay, persistent activity is seen within the liver, as well as continued clearance by the kidneys *(arrowheads)* with excreted radiopharmaceutical detected within the urinary bladder *(asterisk)*. The 24-hour image also demonstrates some activity in the liver *(arrow)* but no evidence of biliary excretion into the small intestine.

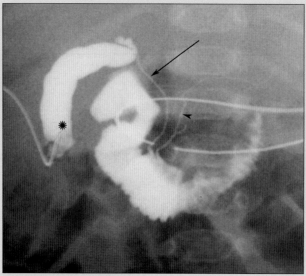

Figure 4. Biliary atresia, type B: cholangiographic features. Intraoperative cholangiography is performed by catheterization of the gallbladder *(asterisk)* and injection of contrast. This infant has an extremely hypoplastic but patent common bile duct *(arrow)*. No filling of the common hepatic duct or intrahepatic ducts is seen. This is consistent with type B biliary atresia. The pancreatic duct *(arrowhead)* is opacified.

Utility
- Preoperative definition of the patient's anatomy with angiography is used in the technical planning of the surgical procedure.
- Angiography is necessary to demonstrate the location and size of the portal trunk when not seen by CT or MRI examination.

Nuclear Medicine
Findings
- Biliary atresia likely when no intestinal activity occurs by 24 hours and hepatocyte clearance is relatively preserved
- If radiopharmaceutical is excreted into the bowel by 24 hours, the diagnosis of biliary atresia is essentially excluded.

Utility
- Scintigraphy is used if ultrasonography is not diagnostic of biliary atresia.
- Nuclear scintigraphy performed with technetium-99m (99mTc) and an iminodiacetic acid derivative.
- Babies are prepared for examination with a 3-7 day course of phenobarbital then administered 1 mCi of 99mTc-DISIDA intravenously.
- Reported diagnostic accuracy in biliary atresia is 56%-81.6%, sensitivity is 91.7%-100%, and specificity is 35%-76.9%.
- Anastomosis patency in the Kasai procedure is confirmed by nuclear scintigraphy.

MRI and MR Cholangiopancreatography (MRCP)

Findings
- Nonvisualization of the main bile ducts, small or absent gallbladder, and periportal fibrosis

- Periportal fibrosis: high-signal-intensity triangular area anterior to the porta hepatis on T2-weighted images
- Hypointense signal paralleling the portal vein branches on echo-gradient turbo field-echo T1-weighted sequences, becoming isointense with the liver after gadolinium administration
- T2-weighted images: focal hyperintensity within high-signal-intensity periportal fibrosis in some children with biliary atresia
- Cystic clefts also seen as triangular areas of increased signal intensity on T2-weighted, thick-slab, single-shot MR cholangiography images

Utility
- MRCP can demonstrate the extrahepatic bile ducts in neonates without biliary atresia in 96% of cases.
- Gadolinium administration distinguishes enhancing periportal fibrosis from nonenhancing, dilated periportal ducts seen in other disease processes.
- MRCP relies on bile production and excretion into bile ducts to image the biliary tract.

CLINICAL PRESENTATION
- Children may exhibit icterus and clay-colored stool.
- Bacterial cholangitis produces fever and acholic stools or fever and jaundice, with elevated direct bilirubin level, resulting in positive C-reactive protein.

DIFFERENTIAL DIAGNOSIS
- Bile plug syndrome
- Alagille syndrome
- Byler syndrome

PATHOLOGY

- Biliary atresia is an obliterative process of unknown origin that affects the bile ducts antenatally or during the newborn period.
- It is characterized by cholestasis and persistent conjugated hyperbilirubinemia, ultimately leading to hepatic fibrosis and cirrhosis.
- Three types of extrahepatic biliary atresia: type A, complete fibrous obliteration of extrahepatic bile ducts; type B, which has an extremely hypoplastic but patent CBD with atretic intrahepatic ducts; and type C, which has cystic dilation of the common hepatic duct with an atretic common bile duct
- The CBD is hypoplastic but patent; hepatic ducts are atretic; cystic dilation of the common hepatic duct occurs with an atretic CBD.
- Biliary atresia splenic malformation syndrome is biliary atresia associated with polysplenia and situs inversus.
- Bacterial cholangitis is a serious complication in biliary atresia survivors, which leads to sudden cessation of bile drainage after the Kasai procedure.
- Untreated biliary atresia results in progressive intrahepatic ductopenia during infancy, leading to cirrhosis.

INCIDENCE/PREVALENCE AND EPIDEMIOLOGY

- Biliary atresia occurs in 1 of 8000-16,700 live births, with an increased incidence in Asian populations.
- Obliteration of the ducts is at or above the porta hepatis in 75%-80% of cases.

Suggested Readings

Azuma T, Nakamura T, Nakahira M, et al: Pre-operative ultrasonographic diagnosis of biliary atresia—With reference to the presence or absence of the extrahepatic bile duct. *Pediatr Surg Int* 19:475-477, 2003.

Caffey's: *Pediatric Diagnostic Imaging*, 10th ed. Philadelphia, Mosby, 2004.

Coleman R: Duke University, Standard Operating Procedure, Nuclear Medicine Department: In *Hepatobiliary Scan Biliary Atresia*. Duke University, Durham, NC, 2002.

Han SJ, Kim MJ, Han A, et al: Magnetic resonance cholangiography for the diagnosis of biliary atresia. *J Pediatr Surg* 37:599-604, 2002.

Hussein A, Wyatt J, Guthrie A, Stringer MD: Kasai portoenterostomy—new insights from hepatic morphology. *J Pediatr Surg* 40:322-326, 2005.

Park WH, Choi SO, Lee HJ, et al: A new diagnostic approach to biliary atresia with emphasis on the ultrasonographic triangular cord sign: Comparison of ultrasonography, hepatobiliary scintigraphy, and liver needle biopsy in the evaluation of infantile cholestasis. *J Pediatr Surg* 32:1555-1559, 1997.

Pediatric Caroli Disease

DEFINITION: Caroli disease is a rare, congenital disease of the intrahepatic bile ducts characterized by multiple cystic dilations of the ducts.

ANATOMIC FINDINGS

Intrahepatic Bile Duct
- Dilated

IMAGING

Ultrasound
Findings
- Dilated intrahepatic bile ducts
- Echogenic septa that completely or incompletely traverse the dilated duct lumen
- Small portal venous branches that are partly or completely surrounded by the dilated bile ducts

Utility
- Usually initial test obtained in child with suspected biliary tract pathology

CT
Findings
- Centrally enhancing portal vein branch surrounded by low-attenuation, dilated bile ducts, called the *central dot sign*

Utility
- Not the primary imaging test in this disorder

MRI and MR Cholangiopancreatography (MRCP)
Findings
- Diffuse intrahepatic bile duct dilation with scattered areas of saccular dilation

Utility
- MRCP best depicts the communicating cavernous ectasia of the intrahepatic bile ducts.

CLINICAL PRESENTATION

- Patients have periportal fibrosis that leads to the development of cirrhosis and portal hypertension.
- Fever, recurrent or crampy abdominal pain, and transient jaundice may be seen.
- Recurrent abdominal pain, pruritus, acholic stools, and intermittent jaundice may be seen.
- Liver may be enlarged.

DIFFERENTIAL DIAGNOSIS

- Splanchnic vein aneurysm
- Polycystic liver disease
- Multiple hepatic abscesses

DIAGNOSTIC PEARLS

- Multiple cystic dilations of the ducts
- Congenital hepatic fibrosis
- Central dot sign
- Bile stasis and stone formation
- Intermittent jaundice

PATHOLOGY

- Also known as Todani type V choledochal cystic disease and as communicating cavernous ectasia
- A rare congenital disease of intrahepatic bile ducts characterized by multiple cystic dilations of the ducts
- Arrest of remodeling of the embryonic ductal plate, resulting in ductal plate malformation
- Congenital segmental intrahepatic bile duct dilation, intraductal calculi formation, cholangitis in the absence of periportal fibrosis, cirrhosis, and portal hypertension
- Associated with renal tubular ectasia and other renal cystic diseases
- Associated with a variety of congenital anomalies, predominantly hepatic and renal

INCIDENCE/PREVALENCE AND EPIDEMIOLOGY

- Most cases occur during childhood or young adulthood.
- Cholangiocarcinoma has been reported in up to 7% of people with congenital cystic dilation of intrahepatic bile ducts.
- Rare, probably autosomal recessive disorder characterized by congenital segmental saccular cystic dilation of major intrahepatic bile ducts
- Present in childhood and second and third decades of life; occasionally occurs in infancy
- Male-to-female ratio of 1:1

Suggested Readings

Dayton MT, Longmire WP Jr, Tompkins RK: Caroli's disease: A premalignant condition. *Am J Surg* 145:41-48, 1983.
Fulcher AS, Turner MA, Sanyal AJ: Case 38: Caroli disease and renal tubular ectasia. *Radiology* 220:720-723, 2001.

WHAT THE REFERRING PHYSICIAN NEEDS TO KNOW

- Early diagnosis of malignant transformation is difficult because the symptoms may mimic cholangitis.

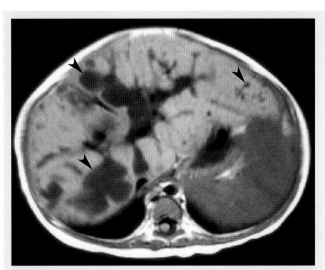

Figure 1. Caroli disease: MRI features. Axial-view T1-weighted MR image demonstrates diffuse intrahepatic bile duct dilation with scattered areas of saccular dilation *(arrowheads)*.

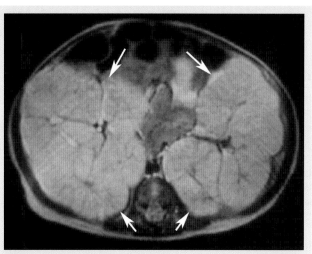

Figure 2. Caroli disease: MRI features. Axial-view T2-weighted MR image of the kidneys. The kidneys *(arrows)* are diffusely enlarged, without hydronephrosis. The constellation of findings is consistent with Caroli disease with associated autosomal-recessive polycystic kidney disease.

Pediatric Choledochal Cysts

DEFINITION: Choledochal cysts are dilated bile ducts that may be extrahepatic or intrahepatic or both, with a morphologic abnormality and no clear mechanical obstruction.

IMAGING

Ultrasound
Findings
- Large, lobular, right upper quadrant cyst extending to the porta hepatis and communicating with the biliary ductal system

Utility
- Ultrasound is useful in making the diagnosis.
- Incidental findings are seen on routine prenatal sonograms.

Nuclear Medicine
Findings
- Cyst can usually be seen as separate from the gallbladder.

Utility
- Nuclear scintigraphy using technetium-99m iminodiacetic acid (IDA) or an analog of IDA
- Biliary nuclear scintigraphy usually confirms the biliary origin of the cyst.
- Choledochal cyst does not fill with radiopharmaceutical but causes a photopenic defect in the liver that correlates with the sonographic findings.

MRI and MR Cholangiopancreatography (MRCP)
Findings
- Tubular cystic dilation of intrahepatic and/or extrahepatic bile ducts

Utility
- Cholangiography or MRCP is a useful adjunct to sonography for preoperative planning.
- MRCP's lower success in children younger than 4 years reflects the patient's small size and maximal resolution of 1 mm.
- MRCP can depict intrahepatic duct stenosis, associated Caroli disease, or the presence of a hepatic biliary duct anomaly.

CLINICAL PRESENTATION

- Patients may exhibit a large abdominal mass, jaundice, and acholic stool.
- Vomiting, pain or discomfort, and fever may also be seen.

DIAGNOSTIC PEARLS

- Dilated bile ducts
- Large, lobular, right upper quadrant cyst extending to the porta hepatis and communicating with the biliary ductal system

- Children older than 12 months have more variable symptoms.
- Abdominal pain and hyperamylasemia are not typically seen in children younger than 2 years old.
- Pruritus, weight loss, and chills

DIFFERENTIAL DIAGNOSIS

- Gallbladder hydrops
- Hydronephrotic right kidney
- Mesenteric, omental, hepatic, renal, adrenal, or pancreatic cyst

PATHOLOGY

- Choledochal cysts are classified as cystic, cylindrical, fusiform, or spindle shaped.
- Choledochal cysts are dilated bile ducts.
- Infants tend to have a palpable, large, cystic dilation that may extend into the liver.
- Children older than 1 year of age may have cystic or a more diffuse dilation of the extrahepatic bile ducts.

INCIDENCE/PREVALENCE AND EPIDEMIOLOGY

- Choledochal cysts are uncommon, with an incidence of 1 case in 750,000 live births.
- The abnormality is four to six times more common in girls than boys.
- It is associated with intraductal calculi, intrahepatic biliary dilation, Caroli disease, anomalous hepatic biliary ducts, recurrent pancreatitis, and extrahepatic bile duct perforation.

WHAT THE REFERRING PHYSICIAN NEEDS TO KNOW

- Cyst excision followed by a Roux-en-Y hepaticojejunostomy is the treatment for choledochal cysts in children with persistent or intermittent jaundice.
- In the newborn period, choledochal cysts are drained externally, followed by cyst excision and biliary reconstruction when the child is 5 months of age.

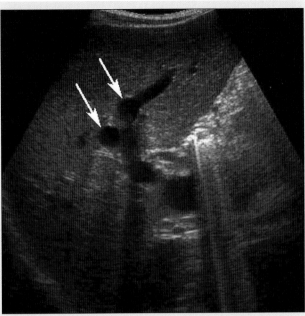

Figure 1. Fusiform choledochal cyst. Sonogram of a 4-year-old child with recurrent pancreatitis. The image demonstrates fusiform dilation of the intrahepatic bile ducts *(arrows)*.

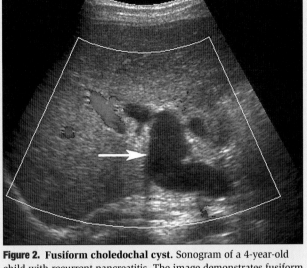

Figure 2. Fusiform choledochal cyst. Sonogram of a 4-year-old child with recurrent pancreatitis. The image demonstrates fusiform dilation of the intrahepatic-extrahepatic bile ducts *(arrows)*.

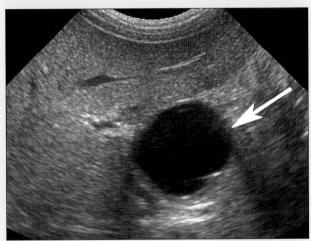

Figure 3. Choledochal cyst: cystic type. Ultrasound image obtained on the third day of life shows the small gallbladder that empties into the choledochal cyst *(white arrow)*.

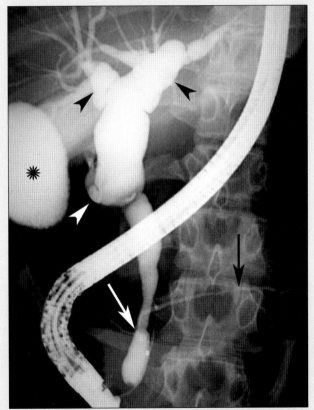

Figure 4. Choledochal cyst: fusiform type on endoscopic retrograde cholangiopancreatography. Fusiform dilation of the right and left hepatic ducts *(black arrowheads)* and their primary intrahepatic branches are seen. The cystic duct *(white arrowhead)* joins the dilated common hepatic duct to form the common bile duct, and an anomalous union of the common bile duct *(white arrow)* and the pancreatic duct *(black arrow)* is seen. The gallbladder is distended with contrast *(asterisk)*. No stones are identified.

- The risk of developing a malignancy in the cyst or nearby bile or pancreatic duct is approximate 4%.
- This cancer risk is approximately 80 times greater than in the general population.

Suggested Readings

Irie H, Honda H, Jimi M, et al: Value of MR cholangiopancreatography in evaluating choledochal cysts. *AJR Am J Roentgenol* 171:1381-1385, 1998.

Lam WW, Lam TP, Saing H, et al: MR cholangiography and CT cholangiography of pediatric patients with choledochal cysts. *AJR Am J Roentgenol* 173:401-405, 1999.

Todani T, Urushihara N, Morotomi Y, et al: Characteristics of choledochal cysts in neonates and early infants. *Eur J Pediatr Surg* 5:143-145, 1995.

Todani T, Watanabe Y, Fujii T, Uemura S: Anomalous arrangement of the pancreatobiliary ductal system in patients with a choledochal cyst. *Am J Surg* 147:672-676, 1984.

Todani T, Watanabe Y, Narusue M, et al: Congenital bile duct cysts: Classification, operative procedures, and review of thirty-seven cases including cancer arising from choledochal cyst. *Am J Surg* 134:263-269, 1997.

Neonatal Jaundice

DEFINITION: Cholestasis is diagnosed when the direct bilirubin is greater than 1.0 mg/dL and the total bilirubin concentration is less than 5 mg/dL or when the direct fraction is greater than 20% of a total bilirubin concentration that is more than 5.0 mg/dL.

IMAGING

Ultrasound
Findings
- Search for biliary stones, sludge, and pericholecystic fluid
- Biliary duct abnormality (e.g., biliary atresia, choledochal cyst, inspissated bile syndrome)
- Hepatic parenchymal abnormality (hepatitis)

Utility
- Ultrasound is the initial imaging study of a child with neonatal jaundice.
- A complete sonographic examination of the abdomen and pelvis, particularly the right upper quadrant, is performed.
- The liver vasculature and parenchyma are evaluated, assessing the size, echotexture, and architecture.
- The size of the intrahepatic and extrahepatic bile ducts is evaluated; the presence and size of the gallbladder length and wall thickness are also assessed.
- The spleen and pancreas are evaluated.

Nuclear Medicine
Findings
- Possibly show decreased radiotracer uptake

Utility
- Nuclear hepatobiliary scintigraphy is used to evaluate hepatocyte function and biliary drainage.

CLINICAL PRESENTATION

- Jaundice
- Dark urine and light stools in breast-fed infants

DIFFERENTIAL DIAGNOSIS

- Bacterial infection
- Viral infection
- Biliary atresia
- Bile plug syndrome
- Idiopathic neonatal hepatitis
- Choledochal cyst
- Cholestasis due to total parenteral nutrition
- Cystic fibrosis

DIAGNOSTIC PEARLS

- Elevated bilirubin during the first 3 weeks of life
- Dark urine
- Light stools

- α_1-A-antitrypsin deficiency
- Alagille syndrome

PATHOLOGY

- Cholestasis is diagnosed when the direct bilirubin is greater than 1.0 mg/dL and the total bilirubin concentration is less than 5 mg/dL or when the direct fraction is greater than 20% of a total bilirubin concentration that is more than 5.0 mg/dL.
- Transient jaundice is associated with hemolysis, hepatic infection, sepsis, metabolic diseases, bile plug syndrome, adrenal hemorrhage, and medications or total parenteral nutrition.
- Persistent neonatal jaundice is associated with neonatal hepatitis, biliary atresia, and choledochal cyst.
- Alagille syndrome and spontaneous perforation of the bile duct are less common.
- Caroli disease is a congenital abnormality of the intrahepatic bile ducts; clinical presentation typically occurs in childhood or adolescence.

INCIDENCE/PREVALENCE AND EPIDEMIOLOGY

- Normal physiologic neonatal jaundice occurs in term and preterm infants.
- Hepatitis and biliary atresia comprise 70%-80% of persistent neonatal jaundice cases.

Suggested Readings
Jaw TS, Kuo YT, Liu GC, et al: MR cholangiography in the evaluation of neonatal cholestasis. *Radiology* 212:249-256, 1999.
Norton KI, Glass RB, Kogan D, et al: MR cholangiography in the evaluation of neonatal cholestasis: Initial results. *Radiology* 222:687-691, 2002.

WHAT THE REFERRING PHYSICIAN NEEDS TO KNOW

- Surgically amenable causes of persistent neonatal jaundice include biliary atresia, inspissated bile syndrome, choledochal malformation, and spontaneous perforation of the bile ducts.

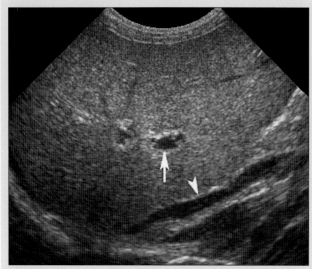

Figure 1. Biliary atresia: sonographic features. Longitudinal sonogram of a 22-day-old girl with cholestatic jaundice. The liver has a normal, uniform echotexture. The intrahepatic inferior vena cava *(arrowhead)*, hepatic veins, and portal veins *(arrow)* are seen, but bile ducts are not identified.

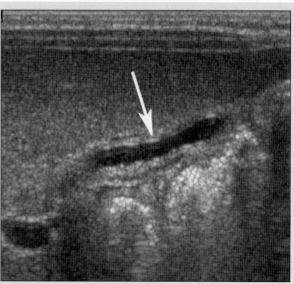

Figure 2. Biliary atresia: sonographic features. A small gallbladder *(arrow)* with an irregular wall is identified. No bile duct dilation is seen. Biliary atresia was confirmed with nuclear scintigraphy, liver biopsy, and intraoperative cholangiogram before treatment with the Kasai procedure.

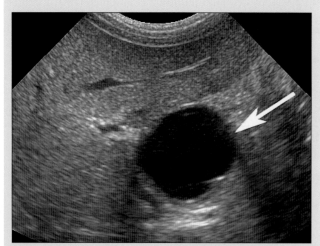

Figure 3. Choledochal cyst: cystic type. Ultrasound image obtained on the third day of life shows the small gallbladder that empties into the choledochal cyst *(white arrow)*.

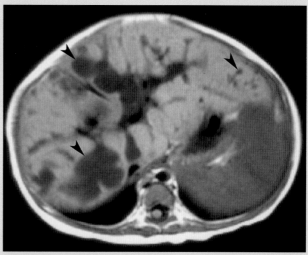

Figure 4. Caroli disease: MRI features. Axial-view T1-weighted MR image demonstrates diffuse intrahepatic bile duct dilation with scattered areas of saccular dilation *(arrowheads)*.

Congenital Hepatic Fibrosis

DEFINITION: Congenital hepatic fibrosis is a disease characterized by the proliferation of fibrous tissue, cystic dilation of the small bile ducts, and hypoplasia of smaller portal vein radicles.

ANATOMIC FINDINGS

Bile Ducts
- Excess number of distorted terminal interlobular bile ducts

Portal Vein
- Hypoplasia of the smaller portal vein radicles

IMAGING

CT
Findings
- Tubular ectasia of the kidneys
- Periportal fibrosis
- Varices due to portal hypertension
- Cirrhosis

Utility
- CT is superior to ultrasound in showing cirrhosis and portal hypertension.

Ultrasound
Findings
- Tubular ectasia of the kidneys
- Periportal fibrosis
- Varices due to portal hypertension
- Cirrhosis

Utility
- Ultrasound is typically the first imaging test performed in pediartic patients with suspected biliary tract and hepatic pathology.

MRI and MR Cholangiopancreatography (MRCP)
Findings
- Tubular ectasia of the kidneys
- Periportal fibrosis with distortion of intrahepatic bile ducts
- Varices due to portal hypertension
- Cirrhosis

Utility
- MRCP is the best noninvasive imaging test in depicting the biliary abnormalities

DIAGNOSTIC PEARLS
- Congenital hepatic fibrosis is characterized by the proliferation of fibrous tissue, cystic dilation of the small bile ducts, and hypoplasia of the smaller portal vein radicles.
- Tubular ectasia of the kidneys resembling a medullary sponge kidney is commonly an associated abnormality.
- It is also associated with Caroli disease.

CLINICAL PRESENTATION
- Patients often exhibit variceal hemorrhage caused by portal hypertension.

DIFFERENTIAL DIAGNOSIS
- Biliary atresia
- Alagille syndrome
- Bile plug syndrome
- Byler syndrome

PATHOLOGY
- Congenital hepatic fibrosis is characterized by the proliferation of fibrous tissue, cystic dilation of the small bile ducts, and hypoplasia of the smaller portal vein radicles.
- Tubular ectasia of the kidneys resembling a medullary sponge kidney is commonly an associated abnormality.
- An autosomal-recessive inheritance pattern has been found.
- Caroli disease has also been associated with congenital hepatic fibrosis.

WHAT THE REFERRING PHYSICIAN NEEDS TO KNOW
- Tubular ectasia of the kidneys resembling a medullary sponge kidney is commonly an associated abnormality.
- It is also associated with Caroli disease.

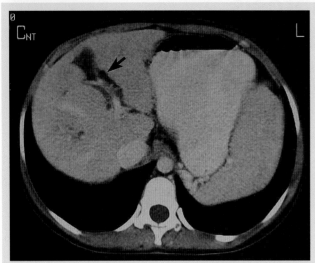

Figure 1. Axial CT images of a 13-year-old patient with periportal fibrosis and signs of portal hypertension. Characteristic periportal cuffing, believed to represent periportal fibrosis, may be clearly demonstrated with CT *(black arrow)*. Atrophy of the right liver is also noted.

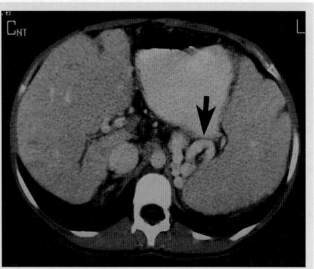

Figure 2. Axial CT images of a 13-year-old patient with periportal fibrosis and signs of portal hypertension. Perisplenic collaterals *(black arrow)* at the splenic hilum and splenomegaly are seen, indicators of portal hypertension.

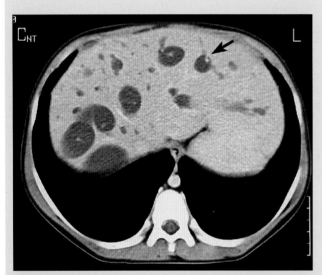

Figure 3. CT image of a 14-year-old patient with biopsy-proven congenital hepatic fibrosis with associated Caroli disease. Cystic and noncontinuous ductal dilation with characteristic central dot sign is seen *(black arrow)*.

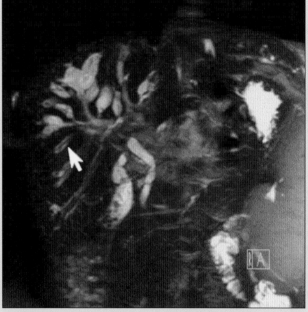

Figure 4. MRCP. Patient demonstrating diffuse periportal fibrosis with diffuse dilation of the intrahepatic bile ducts.

INCIDENCE/PREVALENCE AND EPIDEMIOLOGY

■ Congenital hepatic fibrosis may be sporadic.

Suggested Readings

Wanless IR: Anatomy and developmental anomalies of the liver. In Feldman M, Scharschmidt BF, Sleisenger MH (eds): *Gastrointestinal and Liver Disease*, 6th ed. Philadelphia, WB Saunders, 1998, pp 1055–1060.

Focal Inflammatory and Infectious Lesions of the Pediatric Liver

DEFINITION: Hepatic infectious and inflammatory lesions found in children.

IMAGING

Ultrasound
Findings
- Hypeochoic round lesion with well-defined mildly echogenic rim
- Distal acoustic enhancement
- Coarse clumpy debris and/or low-level echoes and/or fluid-debris level
- Intensely echogenic reflections with reverberation from intralesional gas

Utility
- Initial study obtained in pediatric patients with suspected hepatic disease

CT
Findings
- Low-attenuation hepatic mass
- Multiple, mixed-attenuation lesions
- Thrombus in the superior mesenteric vein
- Calcifications

Utility
- Contrast-enhanced MDCT is more sensitive than ultrasound in the depiction of focal hepatic disease.

CLINICAL PRESENTATION

- Chronic granulomatous disease (CGD) in children younger than 1 year causes pulmonary infections.
- Fever, right upper quadrant pain, chills, rigors, vomiting, malaise, and jaundice

DIFFERENTIAL DIAGNOSIS

- Hepatic abscess in the neonate
- Cat-scratch disease
- Chronic granulomatous disease

DIAGNOSTIC PEARLS

- Hepatic involvement of cat-scratch disease is typically associated with multiple, small, nodular lesions.
- Hepatic abscesses are pyogenic in 88%, amebic in 10%, and fungal in 2%.

PATHOLOGY

- Hepatic abscesses are often related to bacterial, fungal, or granulomatous infections.
- In infants, hepatic abscesses are associated with generalized sepsis or may be a sequela of umbilical line placement.
- In older children, sepsis is a common cause of abscesses; sepsis is also seen after trauma or in immunocompromised patients.
- Occasionally, pyogenic hepatic abscesses can result from perforated appendicitis.
- In children who are immunocompromised, fungal abscesses are the more common, usually caused by *Candida albicans* and *Aspergillus.*
- Cat-scratch disease is a self-limited, systemic infection with regional lymphadenopathy caused by *Bartonella henselae,* typically after a cat scratch.
- CGD is an inherited immune deficiency characterized by molecular defects that result in defective leukocytic activity, leading to recurrent infections.

INCIDENCE/PREVALENCE AND EPIDEMIOLOGY

- Amebic abscesses and hydatid cysts are common worldwide but occur infrequently in the general pediatric population in developed countries.
- CGD is most commonly inherited in an X-linked fashion and therefore occurs most commonly in boys.

WHAT THE REFERRING PHYSICIAN NEEDS TO KNOW

- Pyogenic bacterial hepatic abscesses require prompt diagnosis and treatment because they may be life threatening.
- Children with CGD develop recurrent infections, commonly with catalase-positive bacteria such as *Staphylococcus aureus* or fungi, including *Aspergillus.*

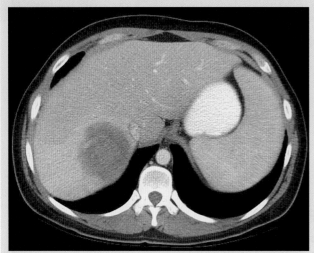

Figure 1. Chronic granulomatous disease. A low-attenuation hepatic abscess is seen in the dome of the right hepatic lobe in a teenage boy. Percutaneous drainage is unrewarding because there is little purulent material and because the abscess is mostly granuloma.

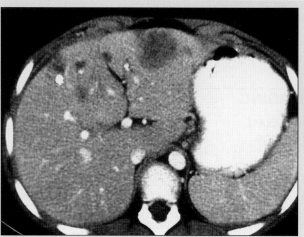

Figure 2. Chronic granulomatous disease. Multiple hepatic lesions are found on the CT scan of a 9-year-old boy. CT demonstrates calcifications from prior infections and low-attenuation masses from an active infection.

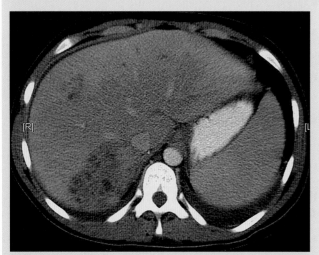

Figure 3. Pyogenic liver abscess. Multiple, mixed-attenuation lesions are seen in the liver of this 15-year-old girl with perforated appendicitis.

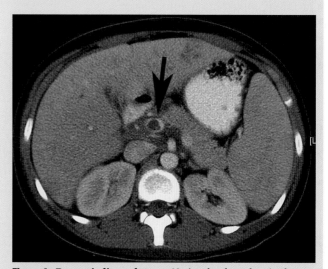

Figure 4. Pyogenic liver abscess. Notice the thrombus in the superior mesenteric vein *(arrow)* in the same child as in Figure 3.

Suggested Readings

Donnelly LF: CT imaging of immunocompromised children with acute abdominal symptoms. *AJR Am J Roentgenol* 167:909-913, 1996.

Kishimoto TK, Springer TA: Human leukocyte adhesion deficiency: Molecular basis for a defective immune response to infections of the skin. *Curr Probl Dermatol* 18:106-115, 1989.

Malech HL, Nauseef WM: Primary inherited defects in neutrophil function: Etiology and treatment. *Semin Hematol* 34:279-290, 1997.

Pennington DJ: Pulmonary disease in the immunocompromised child. *Thorac Imaging* 14:37-50, 1999.

Gaucher Disease Involving the Pediatric Liver

DEFINITION: Gaucher disease is a rare genetic disorder of glycolipid metabolism that leads to an abnormal accumulation of glucocerebroside in the cells of the reticuloendothelial system.

ANATOMIC FINDINGS

Liver
- Hepatomegaly

IMAGING

MRI
Findings
- Some children exhibit focal areas of low-intensity T1-weighted and high-intensity T2-weighted signal.

Utility
- Liver volumes are useful as an indicator of disease progression.
- They may correlate with changes in the bone marrow and development of avascular necrosis.

CT
Findings
- Distorted hepatic contour
- Peripheral parenchymal enhancement
- Relatively low-density central region surrounding the portal branches

Utility
- Liver volumes are useful as an indicator of disease progression.
- They may correlate with changes in the bone marrow and development of avascular necrosis.

Ultrasound
Findings
- Hepatomegaly with an abnormal echo architecture

Utility
- Liver volumes are useful as an indicator of disease progression.
- They may correlate with changes in the bone marrow and development of avascular necrosis.

CLINICAL PRESENTATION

- Rapidly fatal infantile form that is fatal during first 2 years of life (type 2): early onset of marked hepatosplenomegaly, severe progressive seizures, mental retardation, and spasticity

DIAGNOSTIC PEARLS

- Hepatomegaly may be the only liver imaging abnormality.
- Some children exhibit focal areas of low-intensity T1-weighted and high-intensity T2-weighted signal on MRI.
- Liver volumes are useful as an indicator of disease progression.

- Juvenile form that presents at ages 2-6 years (type 3): mild hepatosplenomegaly and neurologic involvement. Patients survive into adolescence.

DIFFERENTIAL DIAGNOSIS

- Niemann-Pick disease
- Glycogen storage disease
- Histiocytosis X
- Mucopolysaccharidoses

PATHOLOGY

- Gaucher disease is a rare genetic disorder of glycolipid metabolism that leads to an abnormal accumulation of glucocerebroside in the cells of the reticuloendothelial system.

INCIDENCE/PREVALENCE AND EPIDEMIOLOGY

- Rare autosomal recessive disorder common among Ashkenazi Jews
- More common in males than females

Suggested Readings

Hill SC, Damaska BM, Ling A, et al: Gaucher disease: Abdominal MR imaging findings in 46 patients. *Radiology* 184:561-566, 1992.
Terk MR, Esplin J, Lee K, et al: MR imaging of patients with type 1 Gaucher's disease: Relationship between bone and visceral changes. *AJR Am J Roentgenol* 165:599-604, 1995.

WHAT THE REFERRING PHYSICIAN NEEDS TO KNOW
- Hepatomegaly may be the only liver imaging abnormality.
- Liver volumes are useful as an indicator of disease progression.

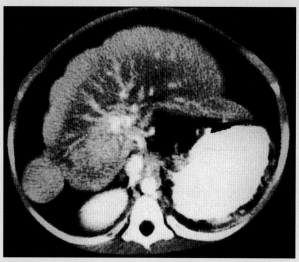

Figure 1. Gaucher disease. CT scan through the liver of a 9-year-old boy reveals distorted hepatic contour, peripheral parenchymal enhancement, and a relatively low-density central region surrounding the portal branches. The patient died within a few days of this CT study. At autopsy, the central portion of the liver was replaced with fibrosis.

Hepatic Cysts (Pediatric Liver)

DEFINITION: Cysts within the liver.

IMAGING

Ultrasound
Findings
- These lesions are smoothly marginated and anechoic and demonstrate acoustic enhancement posteriorly.

Utility
- Lesions may be discovered on antenatal ultrasound.

CT
Findings
- These lesions are well marginated, have an attenuation of <20 HU, and do not demonstrate contrast enhancement.

Utility
- CT is an excellent means of detecting cysts, but it employs ionizing radiation.

MRI
Findings
- These lesions are well marginated, have low signal intensity on T1-weighted images, high signal intensity on T2-weighted images, and do not demonstrate contrast enhancement.

Utility
- MRI superbly depicts hepatic disease.

CLINICAL PRESENTATION

- Lesions are almost always asymptomatic and are discovered incidentally.
- When large, they may cause symptoms.
- Right upper quadrant pain
- Weight loss
- Right upper quadrant mass

DIAGNOSTIC PEARLS

- Cystic structure within the liver

DIFFERENTIAL DIAGNOSIS

- Choledochal cysts
- Gastrointestinal duplications
- Hepatoblastoma
- Mesenchymal hamartoma
- Urachal abnormalities
- Omental and mesenteric cysts
- Pancreatic pseudocyst
- Vascular malformation

PATHOLOGY

- Hepatic cysts are thought to represent a growth arrest and dilation of the biliary tract.
- Support exists for a theory of vascular insult, leading to necrosis and cyst formation.

INCIDENCE/PREVALENCE AND EPIDEMIOLOGY

- Hepatic cysts are quite commonly seen incidentally in patients older than age 40 years on cross-sectional imaging examinations.

Suggested Readings

Avni EF, Rypens F, Donner D, et al: Hepatic cysts and hyperechogenicities: Perinatal assessment and unifying theory on their origin. *Pediatr Radiol* 24:569-572, 1994.

WHAT THE REFERRING PHYSICIAN NEEDS TO KNOW

- Hepatic cysts may be detected prenatally, but a precise diagnosis may be impossible until after birth.
- Differential diagnosis for peripheral lesions includes cystic hepatoblastoma, mesenchymal hamartoma, and vascular malformation.
- Differential diagnosis for a subhepatic location includes a choledochal cyst, pancreatic pseudocyst, alimentary duplication, mesenteric cyst, and urachal cyst.

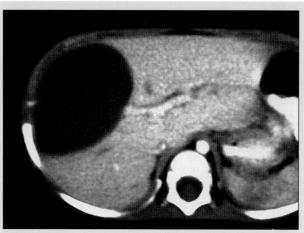

Figure 1. Hepatic cyst. A simple liver cyst in a 6-month-old infant was initially detected on prenatal ultrasound. Continued enlargement led to additional imaging and surgical resection.

Pediatric Polycystic Renal and Hepatic Disease

DEFINITION: Infantile polycystic kidney disease is an autosomal-recessive disorder, characterized by multiple cysts in the kidneys, that is most often fatal.

ANATOMIC FINDINGS

Kidney
- Multiple cysts within the kidneys
- Multiple cysts within the liver

IMAGING

CT
Findings
- Innumerable, small renal cysts replace and enlarge the kidneys.
- Hepatic and pancreatic cysts may be present as well.

Utility
- Ultrasound and MRI are preferred in pediatric patients because CT uses ionizing radiation.

Ultrasound
Findings
- Innumerable, small renal cysts replace and enlarge the kidneys.
- Hepatic and pancreatic cysts may be present as well.

Utility
- Is the initial imaging test ordered in pediatric patients with suspected renal and hepatic disease.

MRI
Findings
- Innumerable, small renal cysts replace and enlarge the kidneys.
- Hepatic and pancreatic cysts may be present as well.

Utility
- Very sensitive in depicting hepatic, renal, and pancreatic cysts

CLINICAL PRESENTATION

- Some patients develop hepatic fibrosis and portal hypertension.
- Hepatomegaly
- Pain
- Jaundice

DIAGNOSTIC PEARLS

- In adult-type (autosomal-dominant) polycystic kidney disease, hepatic cysts develop in one third of patients.
- In infantile polycystic kidney disease, some patients develop hepatic fibrosis and portal hypertension.
- In infantile polycystic kidney disease, some patients show multiple hepatic cysts at autopsy.

DIFFERENTIAL DIAGNOSIS

- von Meyenberg complexes
- Dilated bile ducts
- Caroli disease

PATHOLOGY

- Infantile polycystic kidney disease is an autosomal-recessive disorder that is most often fatal.
- In others, multiple hepatic and pancreatic cysts have been observed at autopsy.

INCIDENCE/PREVALENCE AND EPIDEMIOLOGY

- In adult-type (autosomal-dominant) polycystic kidney disease, hepatic cysts develop in one third of patients.
- In polycystic kidney disease, 25%-33% of patients have liver cysts.
- In polycystic liver disease, 50% of patients have polycystic kidney disease.

Suggested Readings

Wanless IR: Anatomy and developmental anomalies of the liver. In Feldman M, Scharschmidt BF, Sleisenger MH (eds): *Gastrointestinal and Liver Disease*, 6th ed. Philadelphia, WB Saunders, 1998, pp 1055-1060.

WHAT THE REFERRING PHYSICIAN NEEDS TO KNOW
- In adult-type (autosomal-dominant) polycystic kidney disease, hepatic cysts develop in one third of patients.
- In infantile polycystic kidney disease, some patients develop hepatic fibrosis and portal hypertension.
- Multiple hepatic and pancreatic cysts have been observed at autopsy.

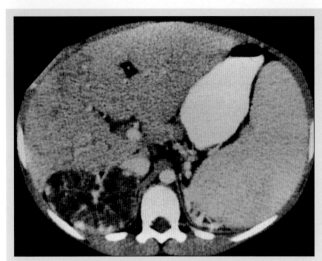

Figure 1. **Autosomal-dominant polycystic kidney disease.** CT scan through the upper abdomen reveals multiple, small renal cysts.

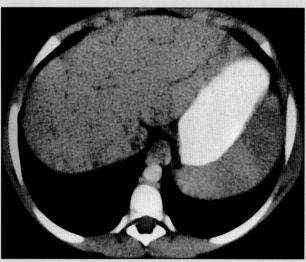

Figure 2. **Autosomal-dominant polycystic hepatic and kidney disease.** Numerous, small renal cysts are seen better on a lower section (see Fig. 1).

Primary Benign Pediatric Hepatic Neoplasms

DEFINITION: Primary benign pediatric hepatic neoplasms are hepatic tumors in which cells do not invade the surrounding tissues and do not metastasize to other parts of the body.

IMAGING

Ultrasound
Findings
- Infantile hemangioendothelioma produces well-circumscribed, hypoechoic lesions on sonography, some with finely stippled calcifications.
- Epithelioid hemangioendothelioma ultrasound characterics are nonspecific; they may be hypoechoic, isoechoic, or hyperechoic, with or without internal calcifications.
- Hepatic arteriovenous malformations (AVMs) appear as a cluster of enlarged, tortuous vessels in one liver lobe.
- On Doppler studies, these vessels show increased venous pulsatility and decreased arterial resistive indices.
- Intrahepatic portosystemic shunts show communication of the hepatic and portal vein branches through tubular, anechoic structures.
- A portosystemic shunt may show a pulsatile biphasic or triphasic spectral pattern in the portal vein or its branches.
- Absence of the portal vein may be detected by the presence of only the hepatic artery and common bile duct.

Utility
- Doppler evaluation is useful for the documentation of vascular communication and the evaluation of the shunt ratio in portosystemic shunts.
- Ultrasound can characterize mesenchymal hamartomas well by delineating their cystic and septate nature and solid components.

CT
Findings
- Infantile hemangioendothelioma appears hypodense compared with the normal hepatic parenchyma in noncontrast scans.
- After contrast injection, centripetal enhancement is seen, with the periphery of a lesion enhancing first.
- Large lesions may appear heterogeneous with various enhancement patterns.

DIAGNOSTIC PEARLS
- Hepatic vascular lesions demonstrate variable appearances on ultrasound, Doppler, CT scan, and MRI studies.
- Hepatic adenomas are solitary lesions that, although usually asymptomatic, are prone to acute hemorrhage.
- Mesenchymal hamartomas, focal nodular hyperplasia, and lymphoproliferative disorders are other benign hepatic neoplasms.

- Epithelioid hemangioendothelioma is hypodense relative to the normal hepatic parenchyma on non–contrast-enhanced CT.
- After contrast injection, peripheral enhancement is seen, followed by uniform enhancement that is isodense to the hepatic parenchyma.
- AVMs demonstrate intense homogeneous enhancement with contrast administration during the arterial or early portal-venous phases, followed by rapid clearing.
- Mesenchymal hamartomas show little septal enhancement after contrast administration; but with a soft-tissue component, enhancement may be inhomogeneous.

Utility
- Cross-sectional imaging with CT or MRI provides better delineation of the course of extrahepatic portosystemic shunt.
- Contrast-enhanced CT better delineates the relationship of mesenchymal hamartomas to adjacent structures.

MRI
Findings
- Infantile hemangioendothelioma appears as a well-defined, spherical lesion that is T1-hypointense and vividly T2-hyperintense relative to the liver.
- Intratumoral flow voids related to increased vascular shunting may be present.

WHAT THE REFERRING PHYSICIAN NEEDS TO KNOW
- Hepatic vascular lesions demonstrate variable appearances on ultrasound, Doppler, CT scan, and MRI studies.
- Ultrasound and CT scans characterize mesenchymal hamartomas well by delineating the cystic and septate nature and solid components.
- Hepatic adenomas are solitary lesions that, although usually asymptomatic, are prone to acute hemorrhage.
- Lymphoproliferative disorder is most commonly seen after solid organ transplantation, but it also occurs after stem cell transplantation.

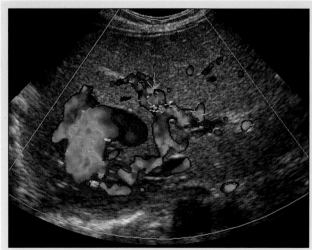

Figure 1. Color-flow Doppler ultrasound of the posterior right hepatic lobe in an infant reveals a large arteriovenous malformation, with direct communication between the right hepatic vein and the hepatic artery.

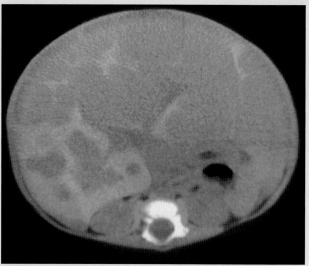

Figure 2. **Multifocal hemangioendothelioma of the liver in a 2-week-old girl with hepatomegaly.** Noncontrast CT of the abdomen demonstrates multiple, low-attenuation lesions within both lobes of the liver.

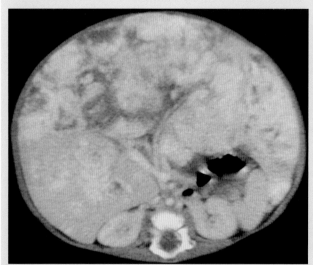

Figure 3. **Multifocal hemangioendothelioma of the liver in a 2-week-old girl with hepatomegaly.** After the administration of intravenous contrast material, dense peripheral enhancement of these lesions is seen (see Fig. 2).

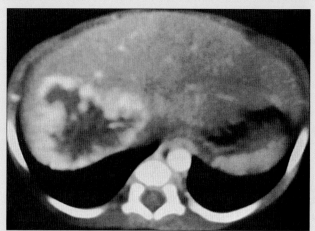

Figure 4. **Hemangioendothelioma in a newborn. This newborn had congestive heart failure, thrombocytopenia, and hepatomegaly.** After a bolus administration of contrast material, dense, peripheral enhancement of the mass is seen, which has frond-like extensions into the surrounding liver parenchyma. Notice the large caliber of the aorta.

- Epithelioid hemangioendothelioma demonstrates decreased T1-signals relative to the normal hepatic parenchyma with peripheral enhancement after intravenous gadolinium administration.
- Epithelioid hemangioendothelioma may be heterogeneous on T2-weighted sequences.
- On contrast-enhanced MRI, AVMs lack delayed contrast enhancement around the tortuous vessels commonly seen with hemangiomas.
- Mesenchymal hamartomas show little septal enhancement after contrast administration; but with a soft-tissue component, enhancement may be inhomogeneous.
- Cystic components of mesenchymal hamartoma demonstrate inconsistent signal patterns corresponding to the variable content of proteinaceous fluid.

Utility
- MRI may depict tumor characteristics of epithelioid hemangioendothelioma better than CT.
- MRI is particularly useful for differentiating hepatic AVM from hepatic hemangioma.

CLINICAL PRESENTATION

- Infantile hepatic hemangioendotheliomas are demonstrated in young infants as an abdominal mass caused by hepatomegaly along with other associated symptoms.
- In the neonatal period, hepatic AVMs cause congestive heart failure, anemia, hepatomegaly, and portal hypertension.
- In infants, AVMs are solitary, and imaging findings show overlap with those seen in a solitary hepatic hemangioma.
- In infants and young children, hepatic arterioportal fistulas commonly cause portal hypertension, along with ascites, malabsorption, and gastrointestinal bleeding.
- Mesenchymal hamartoma is large at presentation, typically characterized by a large, asymptomatic abdominal mass and normal serum α-fetoprotein levels.
- Adenomas are solitary lesions associated with normal serum α-fetoprotein levels, usually found incidentally but are prone to acute hemorrhage.
- Lymphoproliferative disorder is most commonly seen after solid organ transplantation, but it also occurs in children after stem cell transplantation.

DIFFERENTIAL DIAGNOSIS

- Hepatic abscess
- Hepatic infarction
- Malignant primary hepatic neoplasms
- Hepatic metastases
- Focal fatty deposition

PATHOLOGY

- Infantile hepatic hemangioendothelioma is a proliferative, predominantly endothelial cell, hepatic neoplasm.

- Epithelioid hemangioendothelioma consists of epithelioid and dendritic cells, the center of which is predominantly fibrous stroma.
- AVM is an abnormality of blood vessels, with direct shunting of blood between the arterial and venous channels.
- Intrahepatic portosystemic shunts are communications between the branches of the portal and hepatic veins and are probably sequelae of absent venous sinusoids.
- Extrahepatic portosystemic shunts include a congenital absence of the portal vein and the side-to-side communication between the portal veins and the inferior vena cava.
- Mesenchymal hamartoma is predominantly cystic, but tumors with a large solid component occasionally occur.
- Lymphoproliferative disorder results from T-cell dysfunction and abnormal proliferation of Epstein-Barr virus–infected B cells.

INCIDENCE/PREVALENCE AND EPIDEMIOLOGY

- Infantile hemangioendothelioma comprises 12% of all pediatric liver tumors and is the most common hepatic mass in infancy, occurring from 2-6 months of age and affecting girls more frequently than boys.
- Epithelioid hemangioendotheliomas occur after the second decade of life.
- Cutaneous hemangiomas and hemangiomas of other organs are seen in approximately 50% of children with these tumors.
- Mesenchymal hamartoma of the liver is rare, with most patients exhibiting the abnormality before 2 years of age.
- Hepatic adenomas, which are unusual tumors, are encountered frequently in children with a predisposing systemic disease or teenage girls taking oral contraceptive pills.
- Focal nodular hyperplasia is the second most common benign, solid hepatic neoplasm; it occurs in adults but is rare in children.

Suggested Readings

Akahoshi T, Nishizaki T, Wakasugi K, et al: Portal-systemic encephalopathy due to a congenital extrahepatic portosystemic shunt: Three cases and literature review. *Hepatogastroenterology* 47:1113-1116, 2000.

Barnhart DC, Hirschl RB, Garver KA, et al: Conservative management of mesenchymal hamartoma of the liver. *J Pediatr Surg* 32:1495-1498, 1997.

Burrows PE, Dubois J, Kassarjian A: Pediatric hepatic vascular anomalies. *Pediatr Radiol* 31:533-545, 2001.

Buscarini E, Buscarini L, Civardi G, et al: Hepatic vascular malformations in hereditary hemorrhagic telangiectasia: Imaging findings. *AJR Am J Roentgenol* 163:1105-1110, 1994.

Dachman AH, Lichtenstein JE, Friedman AC, Hartman DS: Infantile hemangioendothelioma of the liver: A radiologic-pathologic correlation. *AJR Am J Roentgenol* 140:1091-1096, 1983.

Donnelly LF: CT imaging of immunocompromised children with acute abdominal symptoms. *AJR* 167:909-913, 1996.

Donnelly LF, Bisset G 3rd: Pediatric hepatic imaging. *Radiol Clin North Am* 36:413-427, 1998.

Donnelly LF, Frush DP, Marshall KW, White KS: Lymphoproliferative disorders: CT findings in immunocompromised children. *AJR Am J Roentgenol* 171:725-731, 1998.

Fulcher AS, Sterling RK: Hepatic neoplasms: Computed tomography and magnetic resonance features. *J Clin Gastroenterol* 34:463-471, 2002.

Furui S, Itai Y, Ohtomo K, et al: Hepatic epithelioid hemangioendothelioma: Report of five cases. *Radiology* 171:63-68, 1989.

Hung CH, Changchien CS, Lu SN, et al: Sonographic features of hepatic adenomas with pathologic correlation. *Abdom Imaging* 26:500-506, 2001.

Icher-De Bouyn C, Leclere J, Raimondo G, et al: Hepatic focal nodular hyperplasia in children previously treated for a solid tumor: Incidence, risk factors and outcome. *Cancer* 97:3107-3113, 2003.

Keslar PJ, Buck JL, Selby DM: From the archives of AFIP. Infantile hemangioendothelioma of the liver revisited. *RadioGraphics* 13:657-670, 1993.

Lauffer JM, Zimmermann A, Krahenbuhl L, et al: Epithelioid hemangioendothelioma of the liver. A rare hepatic tumor. *Cancer* 78:2318-2327, 1996.

Lee PJ: Glycogen storage disease type I: Pathophysiology of liver adenomas. *Eur J Pediatr* 161(Suppl):46-49, 2002.

Miller JH, Greenspan BS: Integrated imaging of hepatic tumors in childhood. Part 2. Congenital, reparative and inflammatory. *Radiology* 154:91-100, 1985.

Mulliken JB, Glowacki J: Hemangiomas and vascular malformations in infants and children: A classification based on endothelial characteristics. *Plast Reconstr Surg* 69:412-422, 1982.

Pobiel RS, Bisset G 3rd: Pictorial essay: Imaging of liver tumors in the infant and child. *Pediatr Radiol* 25:495-506, 1999.

Ros PR, Goodman ZD, Ishak KG, et al: Mesenchymal hamartoma of the liver: Radiologic-pathologic correlation. *Radiology* 158:619-624, 1986.

Srouji MN, Chatten J, Schulman WM, et al: Mesenchymal hamartoma of the liver in infants. *Cancer* 42:2483-2487, 1978.

Van Beers B, Roche A, Mathieu D, et al: Epithelioid hemangioendothelioma of the liver: MR and CT findings. *J Comput Assist Tomogr* 16:420-424, 1992.

von Schweinitz D, Gluer S, Mildenberger H: Liver tumors in neonates and very young infants: Diagnostic pitfalls and therapeutic problems. *Eur J Pediatr Surg* 5:72-76, 1995.

Weiss SW, Enzinger FM: Epithelioid hemangioendothelioma: A vascular tumor often mistaken for a carcinoma. *Cancer* 50:970-981, 1982.

Primary Malignant Pediatric Hepatic Neoplasms

DEFINITION: Primary malignant neoplasms of the liver.

IMAGING

Ultrasound
Findings
- Hepatoblastoma appears as a well-circumscribed, predominantly echogenic, solid mass.
- Calcifications are apparent in one third of patients and are characterized by punctate heterogeneous hyperechoic areas with posterior shadowing.
- Hepatocellular carcinomas (HCCs) are typically hypoechoic to isoechoic compared with the normal hepatic parenchyma.
- When the tumor is infiltrative, subtle disruption of the normal liver echotexture may be seen.
- Undifferentiated embryonal sarcoma varies in appearance, from a septate, cystic mass to a heterogeneous, predominantly solid lesion.
- Solid lesions may demonstrate high-level echoes with acoustic shadowing from calcifications.

Utility
- Ultrasound is usually the initial imaging test obtained in pediatric patients with suspected hepatic pathology.

CT
Findings
- Hepatoblastoma appears as a large, hypoattenuating, well-defined mass with homogeneous enhancement after intravenous contrast administration.
- Calcifications are punctate and delicate in epithelial-type tumors but are often extensive and coarse in mixed-type tumors.
- HCC produces a solitary mass, an infiltrative tumor, or multiple, confluent low-attenuating to isoattenuating masses relative to the normal hepatic parenchyma.
- Tumors may be hyperattenuating with contrast-enhanced CT.

DIAGNOSTIC PEARLS

- Calcifications are uncommon, but hemorrhage and necrosis are frequently seen.
- Undifferentiated embryonal sarcomas are hypoattenuating on non–contrast-enhanced or contrast-enhanced images with enhancement of the internal septa and fibrous capsules after contrast administration.

Utility
- CT better defines calcifications than ultrasound or MRI.
- Contrast-enhanced CT and MRI readily depict invasion, encasement, or thrombosis of the main portal vein or the hepatic artery.

MRI
Findings
- Hepatoblastoma appears as a well-defined hepatic mass that is hypointense on T1-weighted images and hyperintense on T2-weighted images.
- When necrosis or hemorrhage exists within the tumor, regions of increased T1-weighted signal may be seen.
- HCCs appear isointense to hypointense relative to the normal hepatic parenchyma on T1-weighted studies and moderately hyperintense on T2-weighted images.

WHAT THE REFERRING PHYSICIAN NEEDS TO KNOW
- Imaging serves to characterize the lesion and define the extent of the disease relative to the segmental anatomy, vascular structures, and biliary system.
- Follow-up imaging is necessary for assessing tumor response to treatment protocols and determining potential resectability.
- Most pediatric malignant liver tumors require complete resection or transplantation as a prerequisite for cure.
- Hepatoblastoma appears as a well-defined solid mass, with homogeneous enhancement after contrast administration.
- Imaging findings for HCC are nonspecific, with variable appearance of this tumor on ultrasound, CT, and MRI.
- With hepatic angiosarcoma, radiographically, no clear features are seen to differentiate malignant from benign vascular tumors.

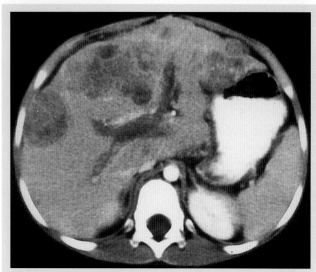

Figure 1. Multifocal hepatoblastoma. Contrast-enhanced CT demonstrates multiple low-attenuation hepatic masses and thrombosis of the portal vein in a 1-year-old child.

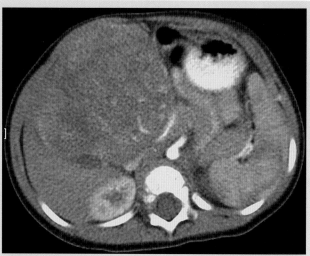

Figure 2. Hepatoblastoma. A 3-year-old boy with an abdominal mass. Bolus-enhanced CT demonstrates a low-density, well-marginated mass in the right lobe of the liver.

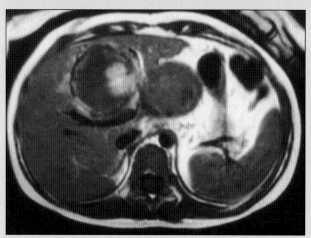

Figure 3. Undifferentiated embryonal sarcoma. Axial T1-weighted MRI through the upper abdomen in an 8-year-old girl demonstrates a bilobed mass arising from the left hepatic lobe.

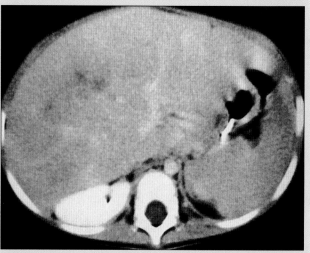

Figure 4. Hepatosarcoma. Dynamic, bolus-enhanced CT image reveals a large low-density liver mass arising in the right lobe and extending into the medial segment of the left lobe. Delayed scan.

- Mixed-signal-intensity lesions are seen in the setting of hemorrhage, necrosis, or fatty metaplasia.
- On MRI, undifferentiated embryonal sarcomas appear heterogeneous; the tumors appear hypointense on T1-weighted images and hyperintense on T2-weighted images.
- The fibrous pseudocapsule and internal septations appear hypointense on T1-weighted and T2-weighted sequences.

Utility

- Contrast-enhanced CT and MRI readily depict invasion, encasement, or thrombosis of the main portal vein or the hepatic artery.

CLINICAL PRESENTATION

- Hepatoblastoma produces a painless abdominal mass, but weight loss, anorexia, abdominal pain, and jaundice may be present.
- Serum α-fetoprotein levels are elevated in more than 90% of children with hepatoblastoma.
- HCC frequently leads to abdominal fullness associated with pain or discomfort, weight loss, and fatigue.
- Most common clinical finding on physical examination is hepatomegaly with elevated serum α-fetoprotein levels on presentation.

- Undifferentiated embryonal sarcoma is characterized by a large abdominal mass, although pain, fever, jaundice, and weight loss have been reported.
- Pediatric hepatic angiosarcoma produces an abdominal mass associated with jaundice, abdominal pain, vomiting, fever, tachypnea, dyspnea, or anemia.
- It is unresectable at presentation, and metastatic disease, particularly to the lungs, is a common early occurrence.

DIFFERENTIAL DIAGNOSIS

- Hepatic abscess
- Hepatic infarction
- Benign hepatic neoplasms
- Hepatic metastases
- Focal fatty deposition

PATHOLOGY

- Hepatoblastomas are embryonal tumors derived from pluripotent stem cells with the capability of differentiating into hepatocytes and biliary epithelial cells.
- Histologically, these tumors are classified as epithelial, mixed (i.e., epithelial and mesenchymal), or anaplastic type.
- Histologic features of HCC in children are similar to those in adults, with tumor cells that closely resemble hepatocytes.
- The classic trabecular pattern and fibrolamellar variants are the two most common types of HCC in children.
- Undifferentiated embryonal sarcoma consists histologically of undifferentiated spindle cells that resemble embryonal cells with a myxoid stroma.
- Pediatric hepatic angiosarcomas produce hypercellular whorls of sarcomatous cells or kaposiform spindle cells, in addition to features of adult angiosarcoma.

INCIDENCE/PREVALENCE AND EPIDEMIOLOGY

- Primary neoplasms of the liver comprise only 0.5%-2% of all childhood malignancies but are the most common primary gastrointestinal malignancies.
- Hepatoblastoma, the most common pediatric hepatic malignancy, accounts for 1% of all pediatric malignancies.
- Hepatoblastoma occurs in infants and children younger than age 3 years, with a male-to-female ratio of approximately 3:2.
- HCC is rare in childhood (0.5% of all pediatric malignancies) but is the second most common primary hepatic tumor of childhood.
- HCC has a bimodal age distribution, with first peak at age 4-5 years and second at age 12-14 years.
- Undifferentiated embryonal sarcoma occurs almost exclusively in the pediatric population, occurring in children between ages 6 and 10 years.

- Hepatic angiosarcoma is rare, with the mean age of presentation of 40 months and with a female-to-male ratio of approximately 2:1.

Suggested Readings

Awan S, Davenport M, Portmann B, Howard ER: Angiosarcoma of the liver in children. *J Pediatr Surg* 31:1729-1732, 1996.

Bisogno G, Pilz T, Perilongo G, et al: Undifferentiated sarcoma of the liver in childhood: A curable disease. *Cancer* 94:252-257, 2002.

Bulterys M, Goodman MT, Smith MA, et al: *Cancer Incidence and Survival Among Children and Adolescents: United States SEER Program 1975-1995*. Bethesda, MD, 1999, National Cancer Institute. National Cancer Institute SEER Program, NIH publication no. 99-4649.

Chen JC, Chen CC, Chen WJ, et al: Hepatocellular carcinoma in children: Clinical review and comparison with adult cases. *J Pediatr Surg* 33:1350-1354, 1998.

Czauderna P, Mackinlay G, Perilongo G, et al: Hepatocellular carcinoma in children: Results of the first prospective study of the International Society of Pediatric Oncology Group. *J Clin Oncol* 20:2798-2804, 2002.

Czauderna P, Otte JB, Aronson DC, et al: For the Childhood Liver Tumour Strategy Group of the International Society of Paediatric Oncology (SIOPEL): Guidelines for surgical treatment of hepatoblastoma in the modern era—Recommendations from the Childhood Liver Tumour Strategy Group of the International Society of Paediatric Oncology (SIOPEL). *Eur J Cancer* 41:1031-1036, 2005.

Dehner LP, Ishak KG: Vascular tumors of the liver in infants and children. A study of 30 cases and review of the literature. *Arch Pathol* 92:101-111, 1971.

Di Bisceglie AM, Rustgi VK, Hoofnagle JH, et al: NIH conference. Hepatocellular carcinoma. *Ann Intern Med* 108:390-401, 1988.

Dimashkieh HH, Mo JQ, Wyatt-Ashmead J, Collins MH: Pediatric hepatic angiosarcoma: Case report and review of the literature. *Pediatr Dev Pathol* 7:527-532, 2004.

Donnelly LF, Bisset GS III: Pediatric hepatic imaging. *Radiol Clin North Am* 36:413-427, 1998.

Ducreux M, Elias D, Rougier P, et al: Treatment of hepatocellular carcinoma in the presence of liver cirrhosis. *J Chir (Paris)* 132:279-286, 1995.

Emre S, McKenna GJ: Liver tumor in children. *Pediatr Transplant* 8:632-638, 2004.

Feusner J, Plaschkes J: Hepatoblastoma and low birth weight: A trend or chance observation? *Med Pediatr Oncol* 39:508-509, 2002.

Franco LM, Krishnamurthy V, Bali D, et al: Hepatocellular carcinoma in glycogen storage disease type Ia: A case series. *J Inherit Metab Dis* 28:153-162, 2005.

Gauthier F, Valayer J, Thai BL, et al: Hepatoblastoma and hepatocarcinoma in children: Analysis of series of 29 cases. *J Pediatr Surg* 21:424-429, 1986.

Hartley AL, Birch JM, Kelsey AM, et al: Epidemiological and familial aspects of hepatoblastoma. *Med Pediatr Oncol* 18:103-119, 1990.

Helmberger TK, Ros PR, Mergo PJ, et al: Pediatric liver neoplasms: A radiologic-pathologic correlation. *Eur Radiol* 9:1339-1347, 1999.

Herzog CE, Andrassy RJ, Eftekhari F: Childhood cancers: Hepatoblastoma. *Oncologist* 5:445-453, 2000.

Ikeda H, Matsuyama S, Tanimura M: Association between hepatoblastoma and very low birth weight: A trend or a chance. *J Pediatr* 130:557–560, 1997, comments in *J Pediatr* 130:516–517, 1997; *J Pediatr* 132:750, 1998; *J Pediatr* 133:585-586, 1998.

Katzenstein HM, Krailo MD, Malogolowkin, et al: Fibrolamellar hepatocellular carcinoma in children and adolescents. *Cancer* 97:2006-2012, 2003.

Kew MC: Hepatocellular carcinoma with and without cirrhosis. *Gastroenterology* 97:136-139, 1989.

King DR, Ortega J, Campbell J, et al: The surgical management of children with incompletely resected hepatic cancer is facilitated by intensive chemotherapy. *J Pediatr Surg* 26:1074-1080, 1991.

Kirchner SG, Heller RM, Kasselberg AG, Greene HL: Infantile hepatic hemangioendothelioma with subsequent malignant degeneration. *Pediatr Radiol* 11:42-45, 1981.

Moore SW, Hesseling PB, Wessels G, et al: Hepatocellular carcinoma in children. *Pediatr Surg Int* 12:266-270, 1997.

Ni YH, Chang MH, Hsu HY, et al: Hepatocellular carcinoma in childhood. Clinical manifestations and prognosis. *Cancer* 68:1737-1741, 1991.

Psatha EA, Semelka RC, Fordham L, et al: Undifferentiated (embryonal) sarcoma of the liver (USL): MRI findings including dynamic gadolinium enhancement. *Magn Reson Imaging* 22:897-900, 2004.

Saab S, Yao F: Fibrolamellar hepatocellular carcinoma. Case reports and a review of the literature. *Dig Dis Sci* 41:1981-1985, 1996.

Sanz N, de Mingo L, Florez F, Rollan V: Rhabdomyosarcoma of the biliary tree. *Pediatr Surg Int* 12:200-201, 1997.

Schnater JM, Kohler SE, Lamers WH, et al: Where do we stand with hepatoblastoma? A review. *Cancer* 98:668-678, 2003.

Tiao GM, Bobey N, Allen S, et al: The current management of hepatoblastoma: A combination of chemotherapy, conventional resection, and liver transplantation. *J Pediatr* 146:204-211, 2005.

Acinar Cell Carcinoma

DEFINITION: Exocrine pancreatic neoplasm, more common in men than women, which demonstrates a well-circumscribed, nodular mass with areas of necrosis.

ANATOMIC FINDINGS

Pancreas
- Mass can be cystic or have mixed solid and cystic components.

IMAGING

Ultrasound
Findings
- Mass is usually cystic or has mixed solid and cystic components.

Utility
- Ultrasound is the initial imaging modality of choice for the evaluation of the pediatric pancreas.
- Pancreas is better seen sonographically in children than in adults.

CT
Findings
- Hemorrhagic and cystic areas with heterogeneous enhancement

Utility
- CT is useful when ultrasound is not diagnostic because of overlying bowel gas.
- CT is reserved for defining the anatomic detail and extent of the disease and for evaluating trauma and assessing distant complications of pancreatic disease.

CLINICAL PRESENTATION

- Symptoms related to local tumor expansion or metastases
- Increased serum lipase and amylase
- Polyarthropathy
- Skin lesions resembling erythema nodosum

DIAGNOSTIC PEARLS

- Acinar cell carcinoma produces a well-circumscribed, nodular mass with areas of necrosis, which can be found anywhere in the pancreas.
- Sonographically, the mass is usually cystic or has mixed solid and cystic components.
- CT imaging demonstrates hemorrhagic and cystic areas with heterogeneous enhancement.

DIFFERENTIAL DIAGNOSIS

- Pancreatic adenocarcinoma
- Nonfunctioning islet cell tumor
- Solid or papillary epithelial neoplasm
- Oncocytic tumor of pancreas

PATHOLOGY

- Acinar cell carcinoma is an exocrine pancreatic adenocarcinoma that produces a well-circumscribed, nodular mass with areas of necrosis.
- It can occur anywhere in the pancreas.
- Metastases are commonly present at the time of diagnosis.

INCIDENCE/PREVALENCE AND EPIDEMIOLOGY

- Tumors of the pediatric pancreas are rare.
- In the pediatric population, the most common exocrine tumors are pancreatoblastoma and adenocarcinoma.
- Acinar cell carcinoma can develop during childhood or adulthood and is seen more commonly in male patients than female patients.

WHAT THE REFERRING PHYSICIAN NEEDS TO KNOW
- Metastases are commonly present at the time of diagnosis.

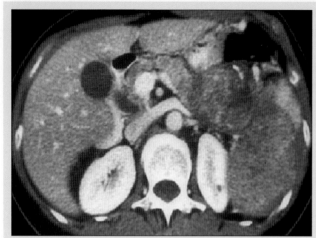

Figure 1. CT scan of a 14-year-old girl shows acinar cell carcinoma of the pancreatic tail invading the splenic hilum via the splenorenal ligament.

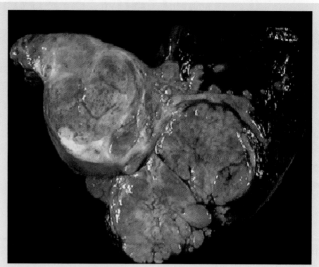

Figure 2. Gross pathologic specimen of this tumor.

Suggested Readings

Berrocal T, Prieto C, Pastor I, et al: Sonography of pancreatic disease in infants and children. *RadioGraphics* 15:301-313, 1995.

Johnson PR, Spitz L: Cysts and tumors of the pancreas. *Semin Pediatr Surg* 9:209-215, 2000.

Nijs E, Callahan MJ, Taylor GA: Disorders of the pediatric pancreas: Imaging features. *Pediatr Radiol* 35:358-373, 2004.

Vaughn DD, Jabra AA, Fishman EK: Pancreatic disease in children and young adults: Evaluation with CT. *RadioGraphics* 18:1171-1187, 1998.

Beckwith-Wiedemann Syndrome

DEFINITION: A rare disorder characterized by the classic triad of omphalocele, macroglossia, and gigantism and is associated with various degrees of visceromegaly.

IMAGING

Ultrasound
Findings
- Fetal macrosomia and anterior abdominal wall defects, most commonly omphalocele, hepatomegaly, nephromegaly, and macroglossia

Utility
- Prenatal ultrasound is used.
- Because of increased risk of intra-abdominal malignancies, routine abdominal ultrasounds are recommended.
- Routine ultrasound is performed every 4 months until the age of 7 or 8 years.

MRI
Findings
- Diffuse enlargement of the pancreas, which has normal signal intensity.

Utility
- MRI is preferred to CT since it does not use ionizing radiation.

CLINICAL PRESENTATION

- The classic triad of Beckwith-Wiedemann syndrome is omphalocele, macroglossia, and gigantism.
- Patients may demonstrate hemihypertrophy and various degrees of visceromegaly of the kidneys, liver, pancreas, and adrenal glands.
- It is associated with a high risk of neonatal hypoglycemia.
- Hypoglycemia often occurs in the first few days of life; if severe enough, it may cause mental retardation.

DIFFERENTIAL DIAGNOSIS

- Hepatoblastoma
- Hemihypertrophy

DIAGNOSTIC PEARLS

- Axial-view turbo T2-weighted MRI shows diffuse enlargement of the pancreas, which has normal signal intensity.
- The classic triad of Beckwith-Wiedemann syndrome is omphalocele, macroglossia, and gigantism.
- Patients may demonstrate hemihypertrophy and various degrees of visceromegaly of the kidneys, liver, pancreas, and adrenal glands.

PATHOLOGY

- Beckwith-Wiedemann syndrome can be familial, with autosomal-dominant inheritance, variable expressivity, and reduced penetrance; most cases are sporadic.
- It is a rare disorder characterized by the classic triad of omphalocele, macroglossia, gigantism and is associated with various degrees of visceromegaly.
- Beckwith-Wiedemann syndrome may demonstrate hemihypertrophy and visceromegaly of the kidneys, liver, pancreas, and adrenal glands.
- Associated malignancies include Wilms tumor and pancreatoblastoma.

INCIDENCE/PREVALENCE AND EPIDEMIOLOGY

- An uncommon autosomal-dominant overgrowth syndrome with reduced penetrance and variable expressivity related to short arm of chromosome 11
- Occurs in 1:13,700 to 1:14,300 live births
- Male-to-female occurrence is 1:1.

Suggested Readings

Choyke PL, Siegel MJ, Craft AW, et al: Screening for Wilms tumor in children with Beckwith-Wiedemann syndrome or idiopathic hemihypertrophy. *Med Pediatr Oncol* 32:196-200, 1999.

Fremond B, Poulain P, Odent S, et al: Prenatal detection of a congenital pancreatic cyst and Beckwith-Wiedemann syndrome. *Prenat Diagn* 17:276-280, 1997.

Nijs E, Callahan MJ, Taylor GA: Disorders of the pediatric pancreas: Imaging features. *Pediatr Radiol* 35:358-373, 2004.

WHAT THE REFERRING PHYSICIAN NEEDS TO KNOW

- Patients are at increased risk for developing malignancies.
- Beckwith-Wiedemann syndrome is associated with a high risk of neonatal hypoglycemia.
- Long-term prognosis depends on the occurrence of neoplasms, which are usually intra-abdominal in location.
- Routine abdominal ultrasounds are recommended every 4 months until 7 or 8 years of age because of the increased risk of intra-abdominal malignancies.

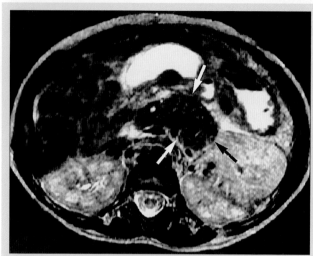

Figure 1. Pancreatic enlargement in Beckwith-Wiedemann syndrome. Axial-view turbo T2-weighted MRI shows diffuse enlargement of the pancreas *(arrows),* which has normal signal intensity, in a 19-month-old girl with Beckwith-Wiedemann syndrome being monitored for hepatoblastoma.

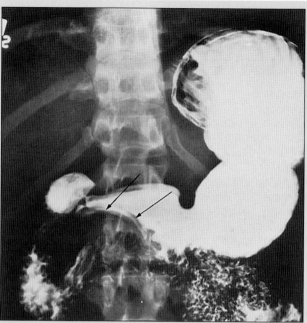

Figure 2. Impression on the greater curvature of the stomach that simulated pancreatic enlargement. *(From Keats TE, Anderson MW:* Atlas of Normal Roentgen Variants That May Simulate Disease, *8th ed. St. Louis, Mosby, 2007.)*

Pancreatoblastoma

DEFINITION: Pancreatoblastoma, also known as infantile carcinoma of the pancreas, is the most common pancreatic neoplasm of childhood.

IMAGING

Ultrasound
Findings
- Well-demarcated, predominantly hypoechoic mass is seen that may have central areas of low echogenicity.
- Mass is solid and can be multilobulated.

Utility
- Ultrasound is the initial imaging modality of choice for the evaluation of the pediatric pancreas.
- Pancreas is better seen sonographically in children than in adults.
- Ultrasound is noninvasive, uses no ionizing radiation, and is performed in all age groups without sedation.

CT
Findings
- Focal mass with attenuation generally lower than the liver is seen.
- Mass may contain areas of low attenuation with mild, heterogeneous contrast enhancement.
- Usually large and well defined, the mass may be lobulated.
- Metastases to the liver tend to be hypodense and may contain areas of central necrosis.
- Vascular encasement of the mesenteric vessels and inferior vena cava may develop.
- Calcifications can be present, which may make the differentiation from neuroblastoma difficult.

Utility
- Pediatric pancreas is well evaluated on abdominal CT.
- Modality is useful when ultrasound is not diagnostic because of overlying bowel gas.
- CT needs intravenous and oral administration of contrast and possible sedation of young patients.
- MRI and CT can show direct invasion of the adjacent structures, such as the spleen, left kidney, left adrenal gland, and omentum.

DIAGNOSTIC PEARLS
- Pancreatoblastoma produces a well-demarcated, predominantly hypoechoic mass and may have central areas of low echogenicity.
- Mass may contain areas of low attenuation, and mild heterogeneous contrast enhancement is seen.
- MRI features are suggestive but not specific, with variable signal intensity on T1-weighted images and high signal intensity on T2-weighted images.

MRI
Findings
- Features are suggestive but not specific, with variable signal intensity on T1-weighted images and high signal intensity on T2-weighted images.
- Mass usually demonstrates enhancement after contrast administration.

Utility
- MRI and CT can show direct invasion of the adjacent structures, such as the spleen, left kidney, left adrenal gland, and omentum.

CLINICAL PRESENTATION
- Patients exhibit abdominal distention or a large, palpable abdominal mass.
- Mass may be associated with nonspecific symptoms: failure to thrive, epigastric pain, anorexia, vomiting, diarrhea, and weight loss.
- Obstructive jaundice may be present.
- Serum α-fetoprotein level is elevated in 25%-55% of patients, and the tumor may secrete adrenocorticotropic hormone.

WHAT THE REFERRING PHYSICIAN NEEDS TO KNOW
- Pancreatoblastoma is often misdiagnosed as hepatoblastoma or neuroblastoma.
- This tumor is associated with Beckwith-Wiedemann syndrome.
- Given the nonspecific imaging findings of pancreatoblastoma, the diagnosis is established by percutaneous biopsy.
- Treatment consists of surgical excision and chemotherapy administered for metastatic disease.
- Radiation therapy is used for local recurrence or incomplete resection.
- Although some patients are cured with excision alone, recurrence has been described in up to 60% of patients.

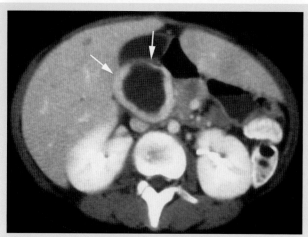

Figure 1. Pancreatoblastoma. CT demonstrates a large well-defined mass in the head of the pancreas *(arrows)* of a young boy with pancreatoblastoma.

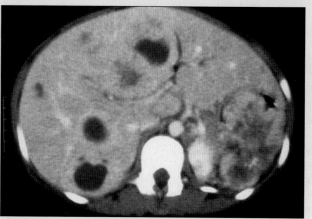

Figure 2. Pancreatoblastoma. CT scan through the liver demonstrates multiple heterogeneous masses within the hepatic parenchyma, consistent with metastatic disease.

DIFFERENTIAL DIAGNOSIS

- Hepatoblastoma
- Neuroblastoma

PATHOLOGY

- Infantile carcinoma of the pancreas is a rare epithelial tumor.
- Pancreatic head is a common location, but the mass can be located anywhere in the pancreas.
- Mass may be exophytic or may entirely replace the pancreas.
- Mass is large at the time of presentation: diameter of 7-18 cm, usually solitary, well defined, and surrounded by fibrous capsule.
- Metastasis is rare at the time of presentation; the mass is common in the liver and may occur in regional lymph nodes, lungs, and, rarely, bone.
- Local invasion of the bowel and peritoneal cavity can also occur.
- When metastatic disease is present, the prognosis is typically poor.

INCIDENCE/PREVALENCE AND EPIDEMIOLOGY

- Pancreatoblastoma is the most common pancreatic neoplasm of childhood.
- It has a 2:1 male-to-female ratio.

- Mean age at diagnosis is 4 years, but it can develop any time from the newborn period to adulthood.
- Increased incidence in East Asia has been found.

Suggested Readings

Enriquez G, Vazquez E, Aso C, et al: Pediatric pancreas: An overview. *Eur Radiol* 8:1236-1244, 1998.

Herman TE, Siegel MJ: CT of the pancreas in children. *AJR Am J Roentgenol* 157:375-379, 1991.

Johnson PR, Spitz L: Cysts and tumors of the pancreas. *Semin Pediatr Surg* 9:209-215, 2000.

Nijs E, Callahan MJ, Taylor GA: Disorders of the pediatric pancreas: Imaging features. *Pediatr Radiol* 35:358-373, 2004.

Roebuck DJ, Yuen MK, Wong YC, et al: Imaging features of pancreatoblastoma. *Pediatr Radiol* 31:501-506, 2001.

Shorter NA, Glick RD, Klimstra DS, et al: Malignant pancreatic tumors in childhood and adolescence: The Memorial Sloan-Kettering experience, 1967 to present. *J Pediatr Surg* 37:887-892, 2002.

Vaughn DD, Jabra AA, Fishman EK: Pancreatic disease in children and young adults: Evaluation with CT. *RadioGraphics* 18:1171-1187, 1998.

Shwachman-Diamond Syndrome

DEFINITION: Shwachman-Diamond syndrome is the second most common cause of exocrine pancreatic insufficiency in childhood after cystic fibrosis.

IMAGING

Ultrasound
Findings
- Diffusely increased echogenicity caused by fat deposition

Utility
- Ultrasound is the initial imaging modality of choice for the evaluation of the pediatric pancreas.
- Pancreas is better seen sonographically in children than in adults.
- Ultrasound is noninvasive, uses no ionizing radiation, and is performed in all age groups without sedation.

CT
Findings
- CT demonstrates fatty replacement of the pancreas.

Utility
- Pediatric pancreas is well evaluated on abdominal CT.
- Modality is useful when ultrasound is not diagnostic because of overlying bowel gas.
- CT needs intravenous and oral administration of contrast and possible sedation of young patients.

CLINICAL PRESENTATION

- Clinical spectrum ranges from mild to near-complete absence of exocrine function.
- Steatorrhea during infancy may occur.
- Diarrhea and failure to thrive may be seen.
- Stunted growth is the most constant clinical feature.
- Clinical condition of patients tends to improve with age.
- Patients may demonstrate hepatomegaly or splenomegaly, which may be caused by infection or malnutrition.
- Recurrent respiratory and skin infections secondary to bone marrow hypoplasia
- Dwarfism due to metaphyseal dysostosis

DIFFERENTIAL DIAGNOSIS

- Cystic fibrosis

DIAGNOSTIC PEARLS

- Fatty replacement of the pancreas is the primary imaging finding, and it is universal.
- Sonographic evaluation of the pancreas demonstrates diffusely increased echogenicity as a result of fat deposition.
- Pancreatic calcifications and cysts are not associated with Shwachman-Diamond syndrome, which distinguishes this disease from cystic fibrosis.

PATHOLOGY

- Autosomal-recessive inheritance has been found.
- Patients have exocrine pancreatic insufficiency, with a normal sweat test result.
- Pathologically, fatty infiltration of pancreas with reduction of acini is seen, but the islets and ducts are preserved.
- Initially, the pancreas may be enlarged, but the size later becomes normal or slightly smaller.

INCIDENCE/PREVALENCE AND EPIDEMIOLOGY

- Shwachman-Diamond syndrome is the second most common cause of exocrine pancreatic insufficiency in childhood after cystic fibrosis.

Suggested Readings

Berrocal T, Simon MJ, al-Assir I, et al: Shwachman-Diamond syndrome: Clinical, radiological and sonographic findings. *Pediatr Radiol* 25:356-359, 1995.

Bom EP, van der Sande FM, Tjon RT, et al: Shwachman syndrome: CT and MR diagnosis. *J Comput Assist Tomogr* 17:474-476, 1993.

Enriquez G, Vazquez E, Aso C, et al: Pediatric pancreas: An overview. *Eur Radiol* 8:1236-1244, 1998.

Herman TE, Siegel MJ: CT of the pancreas in children. *AJR Am J Roentgenol* 157:375-379, 1991.

Vaughn DD, Jabra AA, Fishman EK: Pancreatic disease in children and young adults: Evaluation with CT. *RadioGraphics* 18:1171-1187, 1998.

WHAT THE REFERRING PHYSICIAN NEEDS TO KNOW

- Fatty replacement of the pancreatic parenchyma suggests a pancreatic disorder, such as cystic fibrosis or Shwachman-Diamond syndrome.
- Patients have exocrine pancreatic insufficiency, with a normal sweat test result, allowing it to be distinguished from cystic fibrosis.
- Clinical condition of patients with Shwachman-Diamond syndrome tends to improve with age.

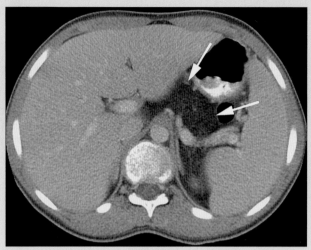

Figure 1. **Shwachman-Diamond syndrome.** CT shows the loss of pancreatic parenchyma from atrophy and infiltration of the pancreas by fat *(arrows)* in a young boy with Shwachman-Diamond syndrome.

Von Hippel-Lindau Disease in Pediatric Patients

DEFINITION: Von Hippel-Lindau disease is an autosomal-dominant disease with the classic triad of retinal angiomatosis, cerebellar hemangioblastomas, and cysts of various organs.

ANATOMIC FINDINGS

Pancreatic Body
- Small cystic lesions

Pancreatic Tail
- Small cystic lesions

Kidney
- Small cystic lesions

IMAGING

Ultrasound
Findings
- Multiple cystic areas in kidneys and pancreas

Utility
- Ultrasound is the initial imaging modality of choice for the evaluation of the pediatric pancreas.
- Pancreas is better seen sonographically in children than in adults.
- Ultrasound is noninvasive, uses no ionizing radiation, and is performed in all age groups without sedation.

CT
Findings
- Numerous, small cysts within the pancreas and kidney

Utility
- Pediatric pancreas is well evaluated on abdominal CT.
- Modality is useful when ultrasound is not diagnostic because of overlying bowel gas.
- CT needs intravenous and oral administration of contrast and possible sedation of young patients.

DIAGNOSTIC PEARLS

- Von Hippel-Lindau disease produces numerous, small cysts within the pancreas and kidney.
- Classic triad of the disease includes retinal angiomatosis, cerebellar hemangioblastomas, and cysts of various organs.

MRI
Findings
- Numerous, small cysts within the pancreas and kidney that have low signal intensity on T1-weighted images and high signal intensity on T2-weighted images

Utility
- MRI shows exquisite soft-tissue discrimination without using ionizing radiation.
- It may require sedation in pediatric patients.
- MRI is useful for patients who usually need multiple follow-up examinations to exclude malignant degeneration of the cystic lesions.

CLINICAL PRESENTATION

- Von Hippel-Lindau disease usually becomes clinically apparent in the second or third decade of life.
- Classic triad includes retinal angiomatosis, cerebellar hemangioblastomas, and cysts of various organs.
- Pancreatic lesions can be the only abdominal manifestation of von Hippel-Lindau disease and is found incidentally.
- Renal cysts, the most common abdominal lesion, are seen in 76% of patients; they are single to innumerable and simulate polycystic kidney disease.

WHAT THE REFERRING PHYSICIAN NEEDS TO KNOW

- Diabetes has been described in patients with extensive cystic replacement of the pancreas.
- Other differential possibilities for pancreatic cysts include autosomal-dominant polycystic renal disease and cystic fibrosis.
- Pancreatic carcinoma has been described in families with von Hippel-Lindau disease and may be a source of mortality in some families.
- With early diagnosis, surveillance for associated malignancies may begin, and genetic counseling can be instituted.
- Some investigators recommend screening CT or MRI starting in the second decade of life.

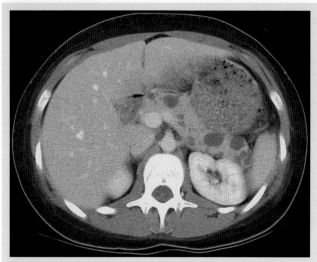

Figure 1. Pancreatic cysts in von Hippel-Lindau disease. The CT scan demonstrates numerous, small cysts within the pancreas in a young woman with von Hippel-Lindau disease.

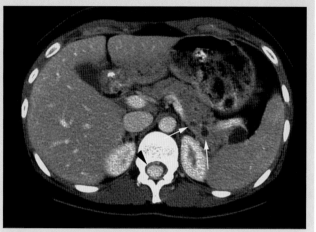

Figure 2. Von Hippel-Lindau disease. CT scan through the pancreas demonstrates small cysts within the tail of the pancreas *(arrows)* in a young woman with von Hippel-Lindau disease.

DIFFERENTIAL DIAGNOSIS

- Polycystic renal disease (pediatric liver)
- Cystic fibrosis

PATHOLOGY

- Von Hippel-Lindau disease is an autosomal-dominant disorder with variable penetrance and variable delayed expressivity.
- Pancreatic lesions can range from the typical simple pancreatic cyst to cystic replacement of pancreas; pancreatic calcifications are uncommon.
- Other lesions involving pancreas include nonfunctioning islet cell tumors, hemangioblastomas, serous cystadenoma, and adenocarcinoma of the ampulla of Vater.
- Pancreatic carcinoma has been described in families with von Hippel-Lindau disease and may be a source of mortality in some families.
- Common lesions of the central nervous system in the disease include cerebellar hemangioblastomas and retinal angiomas.
- Extrapancreatic manifestations include cysts originating in the liver, omentum, mesentery, spleen, adrenals, and epididymis.
- Other solid lesions can include liver hemangiomas, paragangliomas, polycythemia, and pheochromocytomas.

INCIDENCE/PREVALENCE AND EPIDEMIOLOGY

- Variable penetrance (80%-100%) and variable delayed expressivity
- Age of clinical presentation: second or third decade of life
- Male-to-female ratio of 1:1

Suggested Readings

Fill WL, Lamiell JM, Polk NO: The radiographic manifestations of von Hippel–Lindau disease. *Radiology* 133:289-295, 1979.

Herman TE, Siegel MJ: CT of the pancreas in children. *AJR Am J Roentgenol* 157:375-379, 1991.

Hough DM, Stephens DH, Johnson CD, Binkovitz LA: Pancreatic lesions in von Hippel–Lindau disease: Prevalence, clinical significance, and CT findings. *AJR Am J Roentgenol* 162:1091-1094, 1994.

Johnson PR, Spitz L: Cysts and tumors of the pancreas. *Semin Pediatr Surg* 9:209-215, 2000.

Levine E, Collins DL, Horton WA, Schimke RN: CT screening of the abdomen in von Hippel–Lindau disease. *AJR Am J Roentgenol* 139:505-510, 1982.

Nijs E, Callahan MJ, Taylor GA: Disorders of the pediatric pancreas: Imaging features. *Pediatr Radiol* 35:358-373, 2004.

Vaughn DD, Jabra AA, Fishman EK: Pancreatic disease in children and young adults: Evaluation with CT. *RadioGraphics* 18:1171-1187, 1998.

Splenic Variants

DEFINITION: Splenules are areas of normal splenic tissue separate from the main spleen, whereas splenosis is splenic pulp scattered intraperitoneally, usually after traumatic rupture or splenectomy.

ANATOMIC FINDINGS

Spleen
- Splenules are well-circumscribed, round, oval, or triangular and are homogeneous with and without enhancement.
- Usually found in splenorenal or gastrosplenic ligament
- Splenules are typically located near the main splenic hilum anteriorly or posteriorly.

Peritoneum
- Splenosis may occur anywhere in the peritoneum but most commonly on the serosal surface of the small bowel.
- It appears as multiple soft-tissue masses with imaging characteristics typical of normal splenic tissue.
- Masses may be too numerous to count and range in size from 1 mm to 5 cm.

IMAGING

CT
Findings
- Arterial supply to the splenules from splenic artery may be visible.

Utility
- CT may show volume averaging with the surrounding fat such that subcentimeter splenules may be more hypodense than the main spleen.

Nuclear Medicine
Findings
- Splenic tissue identified extrinsic to spleen

Utility
- Nuclear scintigraphy may confirm the diagnosis of splenosis.

DIAGNOSTIC PEARLS
- Splenules are well-circumscribed, round, oval, or triangular and are homogeneous with and without enhancement, usually near the main splenic hilum.
- Splenosis produces multiple soft-tissue masses with imaging characteristics typical of normal splenic tissue, commonly near the small bowel serosal surface.

CLINICAL PRESENTATION
- Splenosis is usually asymptomatic, but complications have been described.
- Abdominal pain may occur.
- Most splenules are asymptomatic

DIFFERENTIAL DIAGNOSIS
- Lymphoma (musculoskeletal)
- Lymphadenopathy and neoplasms of the mesentery
- Peritoneal carcinomatosis
- Endometriosis

PATHOLOGY
- Splenules are congenital and form from mesenchymal cells that fail to fuse with the rest of the splenic mesenchyme.
- Splenules are areas of normal splenic tissue separate from the main spleen, also known as an accessory spleen, supernumerary spleen, or splenunculum.

WHAT THE REFERRING PHYSICIAN NEEDS TO KNOW
- Splenules need to be removed if the patient is undergoing a therapeutic splenectomy for a hematologic disease.
- Splenules may resemble lymphadenopathy or a neoplasm if situated near the greater curve of the stomach, left adrenal, or pancreatic tail.
- Splenosis may be mistaken for lymphoma, peritoneal carcinomatosis, or endometriosis.
- Nuclear scintigraphy may confirm the diagnosis of splenosis.

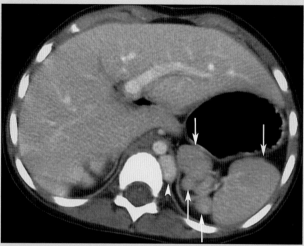

Figure 1. Normal splenules. In this contrast-enhanced CT scan of an 18-year-old girl with abdominal pain, two splenules are seen at the hilar surface *(arrows)*. They are 2.0 to 2.3 cm in the greatest dimension. The splenules have the same attenuation as the normal spleen on this 5-mm axial-view contrast-enhanced CT image.

■ Splenosis occurs when the splenic capsule is disrupted, scattering pulp intraperitoneally, usually after traumatic rupture or splenectomy.

■ Splenosis masses have a blood supply donated by local tissue, and they lack a capsule.

INCIDENCE/PREVALENCE AND EPIDEMIOLOGY

■ Splenules are seen in 10%-30% of people in CT scan, surgical, or autopsy series.

Suggested Readings

Brancatelli G, Vilgrain V, Zappa M, Lagalla R: Case 80: Splenosis. *Radiology* 234:728-732, 2005.

Brewster DC: Report of two cases and review of the literature. *Am J Surg* 126:14-19, 1973.

Dodds WJ, Taylor AJ, Erickson SJ, et al: Radiologic imaging of splenic anomalies. *AJR Am J Roentgenol* 155:805-810, 1990.

Freeman JL, Jafri SZ, Roberts JL, et al: CT of congenital and acquired abnormalities of the spleen. *RadioGraphics* 13:597-610, 1993.

Splenogonadal Fusion (Pediatric Spleen)

DEFINITION: Developmental fusion of splenic and gonadal anlage, with descent of splenic tissue with the gonad.

IMAGING

Ultrasound with Color Doppler
Findings
- Well-encapsulated, homogeneous extratesticular mass that is isoechoic with the normal testicle
- Nonhyperemic mass attached to the testicle

Utility
- Ectopic splenic tissue attached to the testicle mimics duplication of the testicle.

Nuclear Medicine
Findings
- Focus of uptake into the left side of the scrotum

Utility
- Technetium-99m–sulfur colloid scan can help characterize the soft-tissue mass within the testicle.

CLINICAL PRESENTATION

- Male children typically exhibit a painless testicular mass.

DIFFERENTIAL DIAGNOSIS

- Testicular masses
- Inguinal hernia
- Scrotal hematoma

DIAGNOSTIC PEARLS

- Well-encapsulated, homogeneous nonhyperemic extratesticular mass that is isoechoic with the normal testicle
- Nonhyperemic mass attached to the testicle
- Focus of uptake

PATHOLOGY

- During development, fusion of splenic anlage and gonadal anlage may occur as a result of their close developmental relationship.
- Portion of splenic tissue separates from the main spleen and descends with the gonad, resulting in this abnormality.

INCIDENCE/PREVALENCE AND EPIDEMIOLOGY

- This is a very rare developmental anomaly.

Suggested Readings

Cirillo RL Jr, Coley BD, Binkovitz LA, Jayanthi RV: Sonographic findings in splenogonadal fusion. *Pediatr Radiol* 29:73-75, 1999.
Sty JR, Conway JJ: The spleen: Development and functional evaluation. *Semin Nucl Med* 15:276-298, 1985.

WHAT THE REFERRING PHYSICIAN NEEDS TO KNOW
- Ectopic splenic tissue can be confirmed with nuclear colloid scintigraphy.
- Splenogonadal fusion should be considered preoperatively in the evaluation of scrotal masses to avoid an unnecessary orchiectomy.

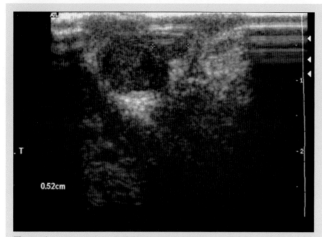

Figure 1. Splenogonadal fusion in a 4-year-old boy. Ultrasound demonstrates a 5-mm nodular lesion adjacent to the left testicle.

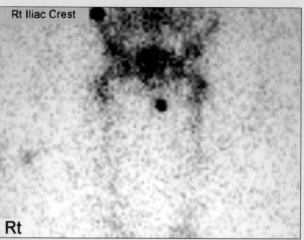

Figure 2. Splenogonadal fusion in a 4-year-old boy. Technetium-99m–sulfur colloid scan of the pelvis demonstrates a focus of uptake onto the left side of the scrotum.

Exstrophy of the Bladder (Pediatric)

DEFINITION: Failure of closure of anterior abdominal wall at the ventral end of the cloacal membrane produces an anterior herniation of the bladder, bladder neck, and urethra.

IMAGING

Ultrasound
Findings
- Prenatally, persistent nonvisualization of the bladder with normal-appearing kidneys and normal amniotic fluid volume should raise suspicion.
- Soft-tissue mass in the lower abdominal wall represents an exstrophic bladder.
- Additional findings include low insertion of the umbilical cord, small phallus, epispadias in male patients, and splaying of the iliac crests.

Utility
- Ultrasound is useful in the renal postnatal depiction of associated anomalies and complications.

CLINICAL PRESENTATION

- May be associated with omphalocele, gastrointestinal obstruction, imperforate anus, bilateral inguinal hernias, and ventral defect of infraumbilical abdominal wall

PATHOLOGY

- Bladder exstrophy results from failure of closure of the anterior abdominal wall at the ventral end of the cloacal membrane.
- This defect produces an anterior herniation of the bladder, bladder neck, and urethra.
- Malformation of the external genitalia is seen.
- Epispadias and a small phallus are seen in male patients.

DIAGNOSTIC PEARLS

- Prenatal ultrasound shows persistent nonvisualization of the bladder with normal-appearing kidneys and a normal volume of amniotic fluid.
- Soft-tissue mass in lower abdominal wall represents an exstrophic bladder.
- Additional findings include low insertion of the umbilical cord, small phallus, epispadias in male patients, and splaying of the iliac crests.

- Open urethral plate and labial separation are seen in female patients.
- Other associated anomalies include cleft palate, neural tube defects, cardiovascular and musculoskeletal abnormalities, and preterm birth.

INCIDENCE/PREVALENCE AND EPIDEMIOLOGY

- Exstrophy of the bladder is a rare congenital anomaly.
- Incidence is approximately 2 cases per 100,000 live births.
- Epidemiologic studies suggest equal male-to-female ratio.
- Higher incidence exists among white patients compared with nonwhite patients (e.g., Blacks, Hispanics, Asians).

Suggested Readings

Gearhart JP: Complete repair of bladder exstrophy in the newborn: Complications and management. *J Urol 165* (Pt 2):2431-2433, 2001.
Gearhart JP, Ben-Chaim J, Jeffs RD, Sanders RC: Criteria for the prenatal diagnosis of classic bladder exstrophy. *Obstet Gynecol* 85:961-964, 1995.

WHAT THE REFERRING PHYSICIAN NEEDS TO KNOW
- Bladder exstrophy results from failure of the closure of the anterior abdominal wall at the ventral end of the cloacal membrane.
- This defect produces an anterior herniation of the bladder, bladder neck, and urethra.
- Malformation of external genitalia is seen.
- Prenatal ultrasound shows persistent nonvisualization of the bladder with normal-appearing kidneys and a normal volume of amniotic fluid.
- Repair is usually staged.
- Findings suggest greater success when bladder closure is performed early.

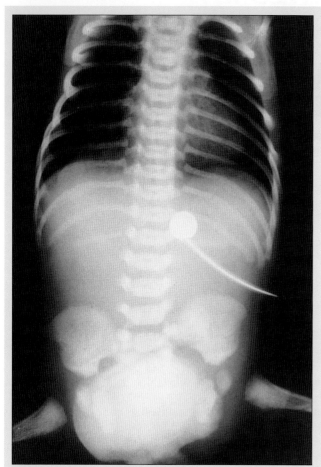

Figure 1. Plain radiograph of a neonate with bladder exstrophy demonstrates the soft-tissue mass effect of the exposed bladder, the wide diastasis of the symphysis pubis, and the posterior rotation of the acetabula. (*From Grosfeld JL, O'Neill JA, Colon AG, et al (eds):* Pediatric Surgery, *6th ed. St. Louis, Mosby, 1998.*)

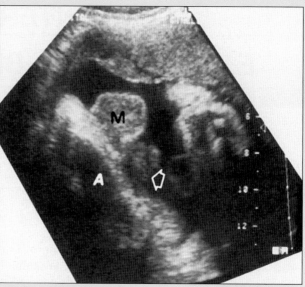

Figure 2. Bladder exstrophy, sagittal midline view. A large bulge can be seen related to the exstrophy (M). The cord insertion *(arrow)* is directly superior to the mass. (*A*, Abdomen.) (*From Sanders RC, Blackmon LR, Hogge WA, et al (eds):* Structural Fetal Abnormalities: The Total Picture, *2nd ed. St. Louis, Mosby, 2002.*)

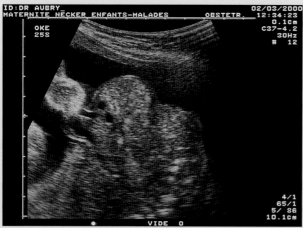

Figure 3. Bladder exstrophy. Note the abnormal appearance of the anterior abdominal wall, the absence of vesical image, and the low-lying fetal insertion of the umbilical cord, at 25 weeks. (*From James DK, Steer PJ, Weiner CP, et al (eds):* High Risk Pregnancy: Management Options, *3rd ed. Philadelphia, WB Saunders, 2005.*)

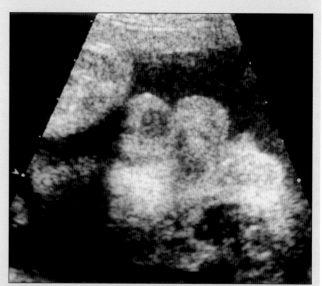

Figure 4. Fetal ultrasonography showing a low-set umbilical insertion, no evidence of bladder filling, normal kidneys, and a protuberance of tissue from the lower abdomen *(arrow)*. The scrotum may be seen below the tissue protuberance. This pattern is typical of classic bladder exstrophy. (*From Wein AJ, Kavoussi LR, Novick AC, et al (eds):* Campbell-Walsh Urology, *9th ed. Philadelphia, WB Saunders, 2007.*)

Langer JC: Abdominal wall defects. *World J Surg* 27:117-124, 2003.

Lee EH, Shim JY: New sonographic finding for the prenatal diagnosis of bladder exstrophy: A case report. *Ultrasound Obstet Gynecol* 21:498-500, 2003.

Mitchell ME: Bladder exstrophy repair: Complete primary repair of exstrophy. *Urology* 65:5-8, 2005.

Nelson CP, Bloom DA, Dunn RL, Wei JT: Bladder exstrophy in the newborn: A snapshot of contemporary practice patterns. *Urology* 66:411-415, 2005.

Nelson CP, Dunn RL, Wei JT: Contemporary epidemiology of bladder exstrophy in the United States. *J Urol* 173:1728-1731, 2005.

Wilcox DT, Chitty LS: Non-visualisations of the fetal bladder: Aetiology and management. *Prenat Diagn* 21:977-983, 2001.

Lymphadenopathy and Neoplasms of the Mesentery in the Pediatric Patient

DEFINITION: Focal or multiple masses within the abdominal mesentery.

IMAGING

CT

Findings

- CT pediatric standard for mesenteric lymphadenopathy is a short axis greater than 8 mm.
- Findings of mesenteric adenitis include lymphadenopathy anterior to the right psoas muscle and in the small-bowel mesentery.
- Affected lymph nodes are seen throughout the mesentery, from the root to the periphery.
- Associated inflammatory bowel changes are not necessary for adenopathy to be present.
- In lymphoma, the nodes tend to start as small and discrete but can coalesce, forming a soft-tissue mass.
- Nodes demonstrate soft-tissue attenuation with homogeneous enhancement, although peripheral enhancement has been described.
- Nodes that demonstrate a central low attenuation with peripheral enhancement are more consistent with an inflammatory process than a neoplastic one.

Utility

- CT is the most sensitive imaging modality for the evaluation of the morphologic features and size of abdominal lymph nodes.

Ultrasound

Findings

- Short-axis diameter greater than 4 mm and long-axis diameter greater than 10 mm

Utility

- Size can be underestimated because of obscuration by bowel gas, the limited field of view, and operator dependence.
- Echogenicity of the node is not sensitive for distinguishing normal nodes from lymphadenopathy.

CLINICAL PRESENTATION

- Mesenteric adenitis is characterized by benign inflammation of mesenteric lymph nodes.
- Patients tend to have acute, chronic, or recurrent abdominal pain, with no evidence of other abnormalities.

DIAGNOSTIC PEARLS

- CT pediatric standard for mesenteric lymphadenopathy is a short axis greater than 8 mm.
- Ultrasound standard is a short-axis diameter greater than 4 mm and a long-axis diameter greater than 10 mm.
- Different diseases may have different lymph node appearances.

- Additional findings might include nausea, vomiting, diarrhea, right lower quadrant pain and tenderness, fever, and leukocytosis.
- Mesenteric adenitis can be difficult to differentiate from acute appendicitis because of the similarities in clinical presentation.

DIFFERENTIAL DIAGNOSIS

- Splenic variants (pediatric spleen)
- Mesenteric cyst
- Omental cyst
- Gastrointestinal stromal tumor
- Mesenteric hemorrhage
- Mesenteric panniculitis

PATHOLOGY

- Focal masses within the abdominal mesentery may be lymphomas, mesenteric cysts, desmoids, teratomas, or lipomas; multiple masses usually represent lymphadenopathy.
- Desmoid tumors can be seen in patients with a history of Gardner syndrome or those with a history of prior surgery or trauma.
- Infectious or inflammatory lymphadenopathy in the pediatric population may result from tuberculosis, cat-scratch disease, fungal infection, or sarcoidosis.
- Mesenteric lymphadenopathy is commonly seen in patients with Crohn disease and tuberculosis.

WHAT THE REFERRING PHYSICIAN NEEDS TO KNOW

- CT is most sensitive imaging modality for the evaluation of abdominal lymph nodes.
- CT pediatric standard for mesenteric lymphadenopathy is a short axis greater than 8 mm.
- Ultrasound standard is a short-axis diameter greater than 4 mm and a long-axis diameter greater than 10 mm.
- Different diseases may have different lymph node appearances.

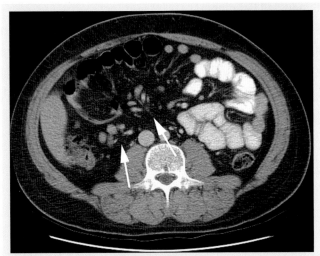

Figure 1. Mesenteric adenitis. Transverse CT image of a 13-year-old boy with abdominal pain demonstrates enlarged lymph nodes scattered along the mesentery *(arrows)*. The appendix was normal (not demonstrated).

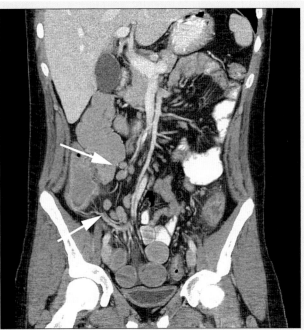

Figure 2. Crohn disease. The coronal reformatted image of 17-year-old boy with a history of Crohn disease demonstrates lymphadenopathy along the mesentery *(arrows)*.

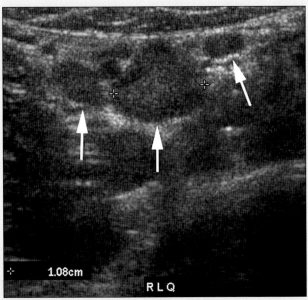

Figure 3. Mesenteric adenitis: ultrasound features. Sonographic evaluation of a 12-year-old boy with abdominal pain demonstrates lymphadenopathy in the right and left lower quadrants *(arrows)*. The appendix was normal (not shown).

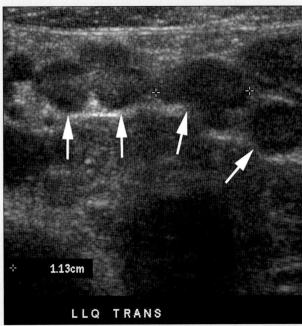

Figure 4. Mesenteric adenitis: ultrasound features. Sonographic evaluation of a 12-year-old boy with abdominal pain demonstrates lymphadenopathy in the right and left lower quadrants *(arrows)*. The appendix was normal (not shown).

- Malignant lymphadenopathy commonly results from lymphoma, lymphoproliferative disorders, and metastatic disease.
- Additional differential considerations for mesenteric masses include a solitary inflammatory or neoplastic lymph node or inflammatory pseudotumor.

INCIDENCE/PREVALENCE AND EPIDEMIOLOGY

- Solid masses of mesentery are rare in pediatric populations.

Suggested Readings

Grossman M, Shiramizu B: Evaluation of lymphadenopathy in children. *Curr Opin Pediatr* 6:68-76, 1994.

Karmazyn B, Werner EA, Rejaie B, Applegate KE: Mesenteric lymph nodes in children: What is normal? *Pediatr Radiol* 35:774-777, 2005.

Lucey BC, Stuhlfaut JW, Soto JA: Mesenteric lymph nodes seen at imaging: Causes and significance. *RadioGraphics* 25:351-365, 2005.

Sivit CJ, Newman KD, Chandra RS: Visualization of enlarged mesenteric lymph nodes at US examination: Clinical significance. *Pediatr Radiol* 23:471-475, 1993.

Watanabe M, Ishii E, Hirowatari Y, et al: Evaluation of abdominal lymphadenopathy in children by ultrasonography. *Pediatr Radiol* 27:860-864, 1997.

Zarewych ZM, Donnelly LF, Frush DP, Bisset GS 3rd: Imaging of pediatric mesenteric abnormalities. *Pediatr Radiol* 29:711-719, 1999.

Pediatric Omental and Mesenteric Cysts

DEFINITION: Rare intra-abdominal cystic masses that are usually grouped together.

IMAGING

Ultrasound
Findings
- Large, intra-abdominal cystic mass, usually with thin septations, is seen.
- Internal debris may be seen, consistent with hemorrhage or infection.

Utility
- Ultrasound is the initial imaging modality of choice.

CT
Findings
- Large, low-attenuation mass with very thin or indiscernible wall is seen.
- Lesion may be multiseptate and have fine mural calcifications.
- Mesenteric cyst tends to be surrounded by bowel loops.
- Omental cyst tends to compress the bowel posteriorly.

Utility
- CT is helpful in demonstrating that this mass does not arise from the kidneys, ovaries, or pancreas.

MRI
Findings
- Cystic lesion with high signal intensity on T2-weighted images and low signal intensity on T1-weighted images

Utility
- MRI can show the complete extent of these cysts without using ionizing radiation.

Radiography
Findings
- Homogeneous, water-density mass that displaces the bowel loops
- Nonspecific findings

Utility
- Radiographs and barium studies are often nondiagnostic.

CLINICAL PRESENTATION

- Patients with both types of lesions can be asymptomatic at the time of diagnosis.

DIAGNOSTIC PEARLS

- Ultrasound demonstrates a large intra-abdominal cystic mass, usually with thin septations.
- CT demonstrates a large low-attenuation mass with a very thin or indiscernible wall.
- Radiographs demonstrate a homogeneous, water-density mass that displaces the bowel loops.

- Some patients may exhibit findings of abdominal distention or report a *pulling sensation* in the abdomen.
- Patients may also exhibit findings of an acute abdomen.
- Omental and mesenteric cysts are probably related to bowel obstruction from a volvulus, mass effect, or from infection or hemorrhage into the lesion.
- Cyst torsion or rupture may occur, producing similar symptoms.
- Rarely, patients may develop respiratory, hepatic, or renal compromise from the mass effect.

DIFFERENTIAL DIAGNOSIS

- Appendiceal mucocele
- Hepatic cysts
- Widening of the duodenal sweep
- Omental adenopathy
- Mesenteric adenopathy
- Mesenteric and omental cystic tumors

PATHOLOGY

- Omental and mesenteric cysts are thought to have a common origin in the abnormal lymphatics that lack a normal connection to the central lymphatic system.
- Cysts tend to be multiseptate, mobile, and thin walled.
- Mesenteric cysts are most commonly found within the mesentery of the small bowel.
- They occur anywhere along the gastrointestinal tract from the duodenum to the rectum.
- Similarly, they can be attached to the peritoneal lining of the abdominal cavity.
- Within the mesentery, these cysts can extend from the base of the mesentery into the retroperitoneum.

WHAT THE REFERRING PHYSICIAN NEEDS TO KNOW
- Ultrasound is the imaging modality of choice.
- It demonstrates a large, intra-abdominal cystic mass, usually with thin septations.
- CT demonstrates a large, low-attenuation mass with a very thin or indiscernible wall.
- Treatment involves surgical resection to prevent torsion, bleeding, or infection and usually results in resolution of symptoms.
- Complete excision is recommended to prevent recurrence.

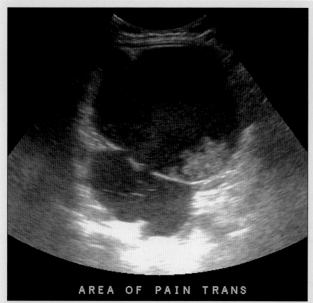

Figure 1. Mesenteric cyst. Transverse ultrasound image demonstrates a multiloculated cystic mass in the epigastric region with internal debris. The pancreas could not be visualized on this examination.

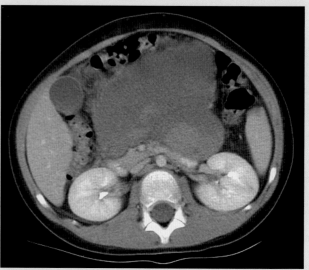

Figure 2. Mesenteric cyst. CT image demonstrates a large, mostly low-attenuation mass inferior to the normal pancreas. High-attenuation material within the cyst is consistent with internal hemorrhage.

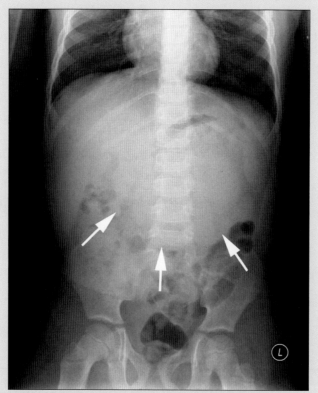

Figure 3. Mesenteric cyst. The supine radiograph of an 8-year-old boy with gradually worsening abdominal pain demonstrates a soft-tissue density in the epigastrium *(arrows)* that is causing a mass effect, displacing the small and large bowel inferiorly and the stomach superiorly.

INCIDENCE/PREVALENCE AND EPIDEMIOLOGY

- Approximately 75% of mesenteric cysts are found in young adults or children older than age 10 years.
- Omental cysts are seen in children, with 68% occurring in patients younger than 10 years.

Suggested Readings

Cain WC, Kennedy S, Evans N, et al: Renal failure as a result of mesenteric cyst. *J Pediatr Surg* 39:1440-1443, 2004.

Egozi EI, Ricketts RR: Mesenteric and omental cysts in children. *Am Surg* 63:287-290, 1997.

Mahaffey SM, Ryckman FC, Martin LW: Clinical aspects of abdominal masses in children. *Semin Roentgenol* 23:161-174, 1988.

Srivatsa KM, Brown RS: Mesenteric cysts. *Arch Dis Child* 75:272, 1996.

Uramatsu M, Saida Y, Nagao J, et al: Omental cyst: Report of a case. *Surg Today* 31:1104-1106, 2001.

Zarewych ZM, Donnelly LF, Frush DP, Bisset GS 3rd. Imaging of pediatric mesenteric abnormalities. *Pediatr Radiol* 29:711-719, 1999.

Cantrell Pentalogy

DEFINITION: Cantrell pentalogy is composed of two major abnormalities: ectopia cordis and midline thoracoabdominal wall defect and abnormalities of tissues between these two areas.

ANATOMIC FINDINGS

Abdominal Wall
- Anterior abdominal wall defect, usually an omphalocele

Heart
- Structural heart defect, such as atrial septal defect, ventricular septal defect, or Fallot tetralogy

IMAGING

Ultrasound
Findings
- Omphalocele, ectopic cordis, and congenital heart disease

Utility
- Diagnosis of Cantrell pentalogy is usually made by prenatal ultrasound.

Radiography
Findings
- Thoracic abnormalities are also evident, including pulmonary hypoplasia and rib anomalies.

Utility
- Postnatally, chest radiographs demonstrate abnormal positioning of the heart, usually with dextrorotation.

CT
Findings
- Omphalocele, ectopic cordis, and congenital heart disease
- Thoracic abnormalities are also evident, including pulmonary hypoplasia and rib anomalies.

Utility
- CT is useful in the preoperative evaluation of the thoracic cavity before repair of the ectopia cordis.
- CT angiography can define the cardiovascular anatomy, the degree of diaphragmatic deficiency, and the degree of transdiaphragmatic herniation of the bowel or liver.

DIAGNOSTIC PEARLS

- Ectopia cordis
- Midline thoracoabdominal wall defect
- Structural heart defect

MRI
Findings
- Omphalocele, ectopic cordis, and congenital heart disease
- Thoracic abnormalities are also evident, including pulmonary hypoplasia and rib anomalies.

Utility
- MRI can define the cardiovascular anatomy, the degree of diaphragmatic deficiency, and the degree of transdiaphragmatic herniation of the bowel or liver.

CLINICAL PRESENTATION

- Clinically, patients generally exhibit dyspnea and cyanosis.
- Newborns have an anterior abdominal wall defect, usually an omphalocele.
- Anterior abdominal wall defect (omphalocele) and structural heart defect (atrial septal defect, ventricular septal defect, Fallot tetralogy) may be seen.
- Anterior abdominal wall defect, paired with short or cleft sternum, gives the appearance of high epigastrium filled by the heart.

PATHOLOGY

- Cantrell pentalogy is composed of two major abnormalities—ectopia cordis and a midline thoracoabdominal wall defect.
- It is associated with abnormalities of tissues between these two areas, with defects of the lower sternum, diaphragmatic pericardium, and anterior diaphragm.
- The cause is unclear, but a genetic component may be involved.

WHAT THE REFERRING PHYSICIAN NEEDS TO KNOW
- Treatment of Cantrell pentalogy involves the closure of the thoracoabdominal wall defect, but success with corrective surgery has been limited.
- Postoperative complications include increased intrathoracic and intra-abdominal pressures, which can result in respiratory and cardiovascular compromise.
- Most patients die a few days after birth.

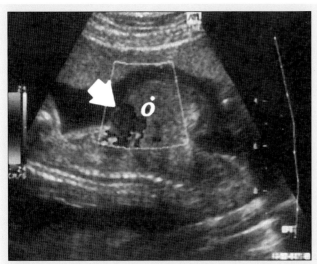

Figure 1. In addition to the omphalocele (O), the heart lies in the abdominal wall *(arrow)*. Color-flow Doppler shows flow in the heart.

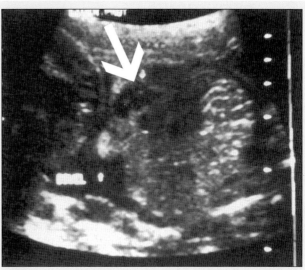

Figure 2. Cardiac chambers *(arrow)* are visualized here outside the thoracic cage. Bowel is also seen below the heart.

- Other associated abnormalities include cleft lip and palate and limb anomalies.
- The prognosis depends on the severity of the cardiac anomalies and on the severity of any other associated abnormalities.

INCIDENCE/PREVALENCE AND EPIDEMIOLOGY

- This is a sporadic and very rare abnormality.

Suggested Readings

Correa-Rivas MS, Matos-Llovet I, Garcia-Fragoso L: Pentalogy of Cantrell: A case report with pathologic findings. *Pediatr Dev Pathol* 7:649-652, 2004.

Oka T, Shiraishi I, Iwasaki N, et al: Usefulness of helical CT angiography and MRI in the diagnosis and treatment of pentalogy of Cantrell. *J Pediatr* 142:84, 2003.

Vazquez-Jimenez JF, Muehler EG, Daebritz S, et al: Cantrell's syndrome: A challenge to the surgeon. *Ann Thorac Surg* 65:1178-1185, 1998.

Prune-Belly Syndrome

DEFINITION: Prune-belly syndrome consists of abdominal wall muscle laxity, bilateral undescended testes, and urologic abnormalities.

ANATOMIC FINDINGS

Kidneys
- Varying degrees of renal dysplasia
- Kidneys possibly dysmorphic or demonstrating cystic changes

Ureters
- Dilated and tortuous bilaterally

Urinary Bladder
- Capacious, often with urachal remnant, including a urachal diverticulum or fistula

Urethra
- Possible urethral abnormalities, including urethral hypoplasia or atresia

IMAGING

Ultrasound
Findings
- Dilated, tortuous ureters
- Bilateral hydronephrosis
- Kidneys may be dysmorphic or demonstrate cystic changes.
- Bladder tends to be enlarged but does not appear trabeculated.
Utility
- The initial cross-sectional imaging examination obtained in neonates with prune-belly syndrome

Radiography
Findings
- Large, elongated bladder is seen, often with a urachal diverticulum or fistula.
- 85% of patients have vesicoureteral reflux, often bilateral, into dilated tortuous ureters.
- On voiding, the prostatic urethra is generally dilated, with tapering into the membranous urethra.
- Contrast medium can also reflux into the prostatic utricle.
- Large postvoid residual volumes of bladder are seen.

DIAGNOSTIC PEARLS
- Triad of abdominal wall muscle laxity, bilateral undescended testes, and urologic abnormalities
- Large, elongated bladder, often with a urachal diverticulum or fistula
- Vesicoureteral reflux, with dilated, tortuous ureters and hydronephrosis

Utility
- Voiding cystourethrography
- Very useful in the depiction of urinary tract abnormalities associated with this syndrome

CLINICAL PRESENTATION
- Wrinkled appearance of the skin overlying the anterior abdominal wall caused by muscular laxity
- Undescended testes
- Associated with malrotation, intestinal atresia, imperforate anus, and Hirschprung disease

PATHOLOGY
- Prune-belly syndrome is composed of abdominal wall muscle laxity, bilateral undescended testes, and urologic abnormalities.
- Cause of prune-belly syndrome is unknown.
- Theories include fetal insult resulting in poor abdominal muscle development and muscle atrophy from chronic intrauterine abdominal distention.
- Other anomalies associated with prune-belly syndrome involve musculoskeletal, cardiovascular, and gastrointestinal systems.
- Gastrointestinal anomalies include malrotation, imperforate anus, and Hirschsprung disease.
- Patients are prone to pulmonary infections and tend to develop scoliosis caused by abdominal muscle weakness.

WHAT THE REFERRING PHYSICIAN NEEDS TO KNOW
- With regard to the prognosis, two groups of patients have become apparent.
  - First group includes patients with significant genitourinary abnormalities, and tend to be stillborn or die shortly after birth.
  - Second group tends to have adequate renal function, although anatomic and functional abnormalities may be present.
- Many patients die within the first 2 years of life.
- Dilation of the urinary tract does not correlate with renal function.

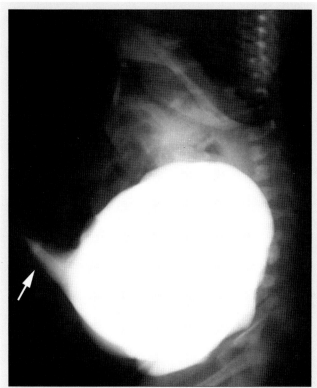

Figure 1. Prune-belly syndrome. Lateral view of the abdomen from a voiding cystourethrogram demonstrates a capacious bladder with a patent urachus *(arrow)*.

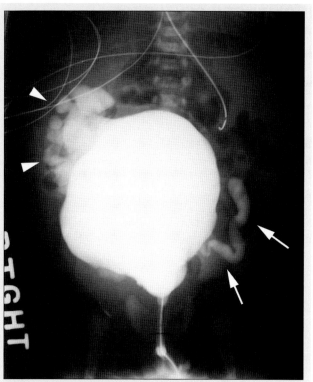

Figure 2. Prune-belly syndrome. Anteroposterior view of the abdomen during a voiding cystourethrogram demonstrates an enlarged, capacious bladder with reflux into the left ureter *(arrows)* and into the right renal collecting system, with right pelvocaliectasis *(arrowheads)*.

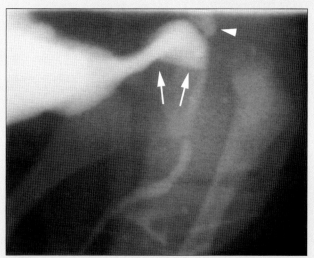

Figure 3. Prune-belly syndrome. Oblique view of the urethra during a voiding cystourethrogram demonstrates a dilated prostatic urethra that tapers into the membranous urethra *(arrows)*. Contrast medium refluxes into the prostatic utricle *(arrowhead)*.

INCIDENCE/PREVALENCE AND EPIDEMIOLOGY

- Prune-belly syndrome occurs almost exclusively in boys.
- In the familial form, prune-belly syndrome is slightly more common in girls (28% of patients, compared with 5% in the nonfamilial form).

Suggested Readings

Berrocal T, Lopez-Pereira P, Arjonilla A, Gutierrez J: Anomalies of the distal ureter, bladder, and urethra in children: Embryologic, radiologic, and pathologic features. *RadioGraphics* 22:1139-1164, 2002.

Denes FT, Arap MA, Giron AM, et al: Comprehensive surgical treatment of prune belly syndrome: 17 years' experience with 32 patients. *Urology* 64:789-793, discussion 793-784, 2004.

Levin TL, Soghier L, Blitman NM, et al: Megacystis-microcolon-intestinal hypoperistalsis and prune belly: Overlapping syndromes. *Pediatr Radiol* 34:995-998, 2004.

Noh PH, Cooper CS, Winkler AC, et al: Prognostic factors for long-term renal function in boys with the prune-belly syndrome. *J Urol* 162:1399-1401, 1999.

Ramasamy R, Haviland M, Woodard JR, Barone JG: Patterns of inheritance in familial prune belly syndrome. *Urology* 65:1227, 2005.

Common Clinical Problems

Abdominal Aortic Disease

DEFINITION: Rupture, dissection, aneurysm of the abdominal aorta.

IMAGING

CT
Findings
- Intimal flap is seen in an abdominal aortic dissection.
- Draped aorta sign: The posterior wall of the aorta cannot be identified and is closely applied to the spine.
- High-attenuation crescent sign is attributed to hemorrhage in the mural thrombus or aneurysmal wall.
- Focal discontinuity of intimal calcification is seen.
- Atherosclerotic walls of the aneurysms enhance and are perfused by the vasa vasorum.
- Aortic wall necrotic areas reveal nonenhancing focal areas of low density.
- Direct signs of rupture include retroperitoneal hematoma and frank extravasation of intravenous contrast.

Utility
- Multidetector CT is the imaging procedure of choice for patients with suspected aneurysm dissection and rupture.
- Unenhanced images are initially obtained to search for hyperdense blood as well as signs of impending rupture.

CLINICAL PRESENTATION

- The clinical triad of symptoms of a ruptured aortic aneurysm include abdominal pain, pulsatile mass, and hypotension.
- Almost one third of patients do not have this classic presentation and are usually misdiagnosed as having renal colic and diverticulitis.

DIFFERENTIAL DIAGNOSIS

- Renal colic
- Diverticulitis
- Pancreatitis

DIAGNOSTIC PEARLS

- Intimal flap is seen in aortic dissection.
- Draped aorta sign is seen.
- Direct signs of rupture include retroperitoneal hematoma and frank extravasation of intravenous contrast.
- The crescent sign indicates intramural hemorrhage.

- Mesenteric ischemia
- Appendicitis
- Epiploic appendagitis
- Degenerative disease of the spine
- Compression fracture of the spine

PATHOLOGY

- Aneurysms have a strong hereditary component.
- May be due to atherosclerosis, infection, or cystic media necrosis
- May be due to inflammation of the media and adventitia

INCIDENCE/PREVALENCE AND EPIDEMIOLOGY

- Abdominal aorta disease should be considered in elderly men who are smokers because they run a higher risk of rupture.

Suggested Readings

Bhalla S, Menias CO, Heiken JP: CT of acute abdominal aortic disorders. *Radiol Clin North Am* 41:1153-1170, 2003.

Coulman CH, Rubin GD: Acute aortic abnormalities. *Semin Roentgenol* 36:148-164, 2001.

Iezzi R, Cotroneo AR, Filippone A, et al: Multidetector CT in abdominal aortic aneurysm treated with endovascular repair: Are unenhanced and delayed phase enhanced images effective for endoleak detection? *Radiology* 241:915-921, 2006.

WHAT THE REFERRING PHYSICIAN NEEDS TO KNOW

- CT is the imaging procedure of choice for patients with suspected aneurysm dissection and rupture.
- Unenhanced images are initially obtained to search for hyperdense blood associated with signs of impending rupture.
- Direct signs of rupture include a retroperitoneal hematoma and frank extravasation of intravenous contrast.

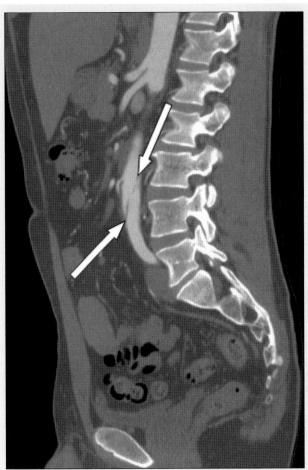

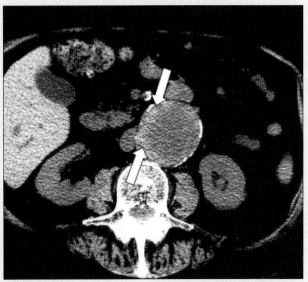

Figure 2. **The crescent sign of impending aortic rupture.** An aneurysmal infrarenal aorta, photographed at narrow window width, shows a hyperdense thrombus *(arrows)*, which is associated with an increased incidence of rupture.

Figure 1. **Dissection of the infrarenal abdominal aorta.** The sagittal reformatted image shows the intimal flap *(arrows)* in this normal-caliber aorta.

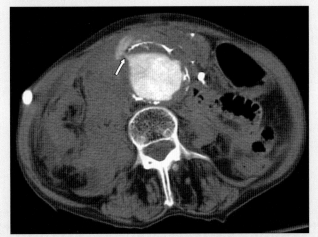

Figure 3. **Active rupture of an abdominal aortic aneurysm: CT findings.** Contrast *(arrow)* is actively extravasating from the right anterolateral aspect of the aorta. Notice the hemorrhage into the surrounding intraperitoneal, retroperitoneal, subperitoneal, and extraperitoneal spaces.

Bowel Obstruction

DEFINITION: Obstruction of the small and large bowels.

ANATOMIC FINDINGS

- Causes of small bowel obstruction: adhesions (49%), hernias (30%), neoplasm (15%), others (6%)
- Causes of large bowel obstruction: carcinoma (55%), volvulus (11%), diverticulitis (9%), extrinsic cancer (8%), adhesions (4%), impaction (3%), hernia (2%)

IMAGING

CT
Findings

- Delineation of the transition zone between the dilated and the decompressed bowel; the adhesion has a beak-like narrowing.
- Incarcerated or closed-loop obstruction exhibits as a loop-shaped, fluid-filled structure, causing the proximal segments to dilate with gas and fluid.
- Mesenteric vessels have radial distribution because they become stretched and converge toward a U- or C-shaped loop.
- Obstructing mass is seen.
- Two adjacent and collapsed round, oval, or triangular segments typically represent afferent and efferent entry points of the torsion site.
- When ischemia develops, the bowel wall may thicken and have a *target* appearance caused by submucosal edema.
- Mesentery becomes hazy in appearance, and ascites may develop in cases of ischemia, typically associated with a closed-loop obstruction.

Utility

- Multidetector CT (MDCT) has replaced conventional contrast studies because it can more reliably determine the site, cause, and degree of obstruction.
- MDCT is used for internal and external hernias, neoplasms, gallstone ileus, enteroenteric intussusception, and afferent-loop obstruction after the Billroth II operation.
- With high-grade obstruction of small bowel, CT has a reported sensitivity of 90%-99%.
- CT is less accurate in patients with low-grade obstruction.
- MDCT is very helpful in differentiating simple from closed-loop obstruction.

DIAGNOSTIC PEARLS

- On CT scan, the hallmark of bowel obstruction is the delineation of the transition zone between the dilated and the decompressed bowel.
- If no mass, hernia, intussusception, abscess, or inflammatory thickening is present, then adhesion is the most likely diagnosis.
- Incarcerated or closed-loop obstruction is characterized by a loop-shaped, fluid-filled structure causing the proximal segments to dilate with gas and fluid.

Radiography
Findings

- Dilated gut is outlined by air.
- Air-fluid levels are present on upright or decubitus radiographs.
- *String-of-pearls* sign is seen.
- If the obstructed loops are completely filled with fluid, the obstruction may be difficult to diagnose.

Utility

- Plain radiographs are often normal or misleading in patients with bowel obstruction.

CLINICAL PRESENTATION

- Abdominal distention
- Nausea and vomiting
- Abdominal pain
- Hernia

DIFFERENTIAL DIAGNOSIS

- Appendicitis
- Diverticulitis
- Mesenteric ischemia
- Epiploic appendagitis

WHAT THE REFERRING PHYSICIAN NEEDS TO KNOW

- MDCT has replaced conventional contrast studies because it can more reliably answer several questions.
- Differentiating between a simple and a closed-loop obstruction is important.
- Simple obstructions are treated conservatively, whereas a closed-loop obstruction requires prompt surgical intervention.
- CT hallmark of bowel obstruction is the delineation of the transition zone between the dilated and the decompressed bowel.

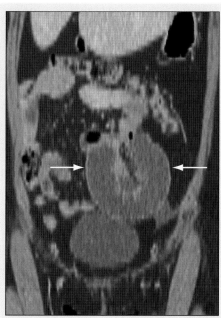

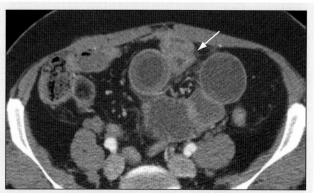

Figure 2. Closed-loop small-bowel obstruction. The corresponding axial image (see Fig. 1) shows the dilated loops converging toward the obstructing point *(arrow)*, where the loops have normal caliber as they exit and leave the internal hernia.

Figure 1. Closed-loop small-bowel obstruction. The coronal reformatted image shows an isolated, dilated, C-shaped small bowel loop *(arrows)*.

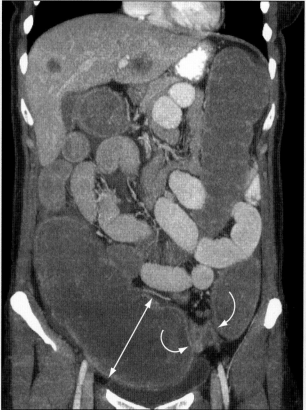

Figure 3. Carcinoma of the sigmoid colon causing large-bowel obstruction. The coronal reformatted image shows the obstructing sigmoid mass *(curved arrows)*. The cecum is dilated *(double-headed arrow)*, and liver metastases are present.

PATHOLOGY

- If no mass, hernia, intussusception, abscess, or inflammatory thickening is present, then adhesion is the most likely diagnosis.
- Fluid and hemorrhage may collect in the mesentery, bowel wall, and lumen of the involved segment.
- Differentiation should be made between a simple and a closed-loop obstruction.
- Incarcerated or closed-loop obstruction is characterized by a loop-shaped, fluid-filled structure, causing the proximal segments to dilate with gas and fluid.

INCIDENCE/PREVALENCE AND EPIDEMIOLOGY

- Obstruction of the small and large bowels accounts for approximately 20% of acute abdominal surgical conditions.

Suggested Readings

Aufort S, Charra L, Lesnik A, et al: Multidetector CT of bowel obstruction: Value of post-processing. *Eur Radiol* 15:2323-2329, 2005.
Hayanga AJ, Bass-Wilkins K, Bulkley GB: Current management of small-bowel obstruction. *Adv Surg* 39:1-33, 2005.
Huang BY, Warshauer DM: Adult intussusception: Diagnosis and clinical relevance. *Radiol Clin North Am* 41:1137-1152, 2003.
Jaffe TA, Martin LC, Thomas J, et al: Small-bowel obstruction: Coronal reformations from isotropic voxels at 16-section multi-detector row CT. *Radiology* 238:135-142, 2006.
Lassandro F, Romano S, Ragozzino A, et al: Role of helical CT in diagnosis of gallstone ileus and related conditions. *AJR Am J Roentgenol* 185:1159-1165, 2005.
Macari M, Megibow A: Imaging of suspected acute small bowel obstruction. *Semin Roentgenol* 36:108-117, 2001.
Mak SY, Roach SC, Sukumar SA: Small bowel obstruction: Computed tomography features and pitfalls. *Curr Probl Diagn Radiol* 35:65-74, 2006.
Mathieu D, Luciani A: Internal abdominal herniations. *AJR Am J Roentgenol* 183:397-404, 2004.
Nicolaou S, Kai B, Ho S, et al: Imaging of acute small-bowel obstruction. *AJR Am J Roentgenol* 185:1036-1044, 2005.
Petrovic B, Nikolaidis P, Hammond NA, et al: Identification of adhesions on CT in small-bowel obstruction. *Emerg Radiol* 12:88-93, 2006.
Yaghmai V, Nikolaidis P, Hammond NA, et al: Multidetector-row computed tomography diagnosis of small bowel obstruction: Can coronal reformations replace axial images? *Emerg Radiol* 13:69-72, 2006.
Zalcman M, Sy M, Donckier D, et al: Helical CT signs in the diagnosis of intestinal ischemia in small-bowel obstruction. *AJR Am J Roentgenol* 175:1601-1607, 2000.

Epiploic Appendagitis

DEFINITION: Epiploic appendagitis occurs when an epiploic appendage of the colon develops inflammation, torsion, or ischemia.

IMAGING

CT

Findings
- Inflamed appendage is demonstrated by a small, fat-attenuation mass with a hyperattenuating rim abutting the serosal surface of the colon.
- At center of the lesion, a small, round or linear, hyperdense focus is seen, probably representing vascular thrombosis.
- Mass effect is produced.
- Note of focal thickening of the adjacent bowel, infiltration of mesenteric fat, and focal thickening of the surrounding peritoneum

Utility
- Multidetector CT scan is diagnostic of this disorder and the single best imaging test for diagnosis.

CLINICAL PRESENTATION

- Sudden onset of severe abdominal pain.
- Physical examination is nonspecific and occasionally nondiagnostic.
- Epiploic appendagitis clinically simulates appendicitis and right- and left-sided diverticulitis.

DIFFERENTIAL DIAGNOSIS

- Appendicitis
- Diverticulitis
- Omental infarction

PATHOLOGY

- Epiploic appendagitis occurs when an epiploic appendage of the colon develops inflammation, torsion, or ischemia.

DIAGNOSTIC PEARLS

- Inflamed appendage is demonstrated by a small, fat-attenuation mass with a hyperattenuating rim abutting the serosal surface of the colon.
- At the center of the lesion is a small, round or linear, hyperdense focus, probably representing vascular thrombosis.
- It produces a mass effect, with focal thickening of the adjacent bowel, infiltration of the mesenteric fat, and focal thickening of the peritoneum.

- It is usually a self-limited disorder that does not require specific therapy.

INCIDENCE/PREVALENCE AND EPIDEMIOLOGY

- Is responsible for fewer than 1% of cases of acute abdomen.
- Occurs more commonly in obese patients.

Suggested Readings

Pereira JM, Sirlin CB, Pinto PS, et al: CT and MR imaging of extrahepatic fatty masses of the abdomen and pelvis: Techniques, diagnosis, differential diagnosis, and pitfalls. *RadioGraphics* 25:69-85, 2005.

Pickhardt PJ, Bhalla S: Unusual nonneoplastic peritoneal and subperitoneal conditions: CT findings. *RadioGraphics* 25:719-730, 2005.

Singh AK, Gervais DA, Hahn PF, et al: Acute epiploic appendagitis and its mimics. *RadioGraphics* 25:1521-1534, 2005.

WHAT THE REFERRING PHYSICIAN NEEDS TO KNOW

- Multidetector CT scans are diagnostic.
- Inflamed appendage exhibits as a small, fat-attenuation mass with a hyperattenuating rim abutting the serosal surface of the colon.
- Surgery may be avoided because epiploic appendagitis is a self-limited disorder.

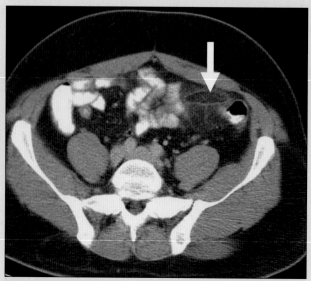

Figure 1. Epiploic appendagitis. CT shows an elliptical fat-density structure *(arrow),* the epiploic appendage, surrounded by increased attenuation in the pericolic fat.

Infectious Enterocolitides

DEFINITION: Infection of the bowel.

IMAGING

CT

Findings

- Nonspecific mural thickening is seen in more severe cases of infection.
- In pseudomembranous colitis, mural thickening averages 15-20 mm, with a target or halo pattern caused by submucosal edema.
- Contrast caught between the thick haustra may simulate a deep ulceration and produce an accordion-like appearance.
- In patients with AIDS, infections such as cryptosporidiosis and cytomegalovirus produce gut wall thickening, submucosal edema, and increased mucosal enhancement.
- Neutropenic enterocolitis CT features are nonspecific.
- Segmental mural thickening of the cecum, intramural regions of edema or necrosis, pericolic fluid, and perienteric stranding are seen.
- In advanced cases, pneumatosis intestinalis and frank perforation may develop.

Utility

- Multidetector CT is useful in showing the extent of involvement, complications, and response to therapy.

CLINICAL PRESENTATION

- Diarrhea
- Blood in stool
- Abdominal pain
- Tenesmus
- In atypical cases, colicky abdominal pain rather than diarrhea may be the predominant symptom.

DIFFERENTIAL DIAGNOSIS

- Ulcerative colitis
- Crohn disease
- Radiation enterocolitis

DIAGNOSTIC PEARLS

- Most cases are self-limited and do not require imaging.
- Normal findings are seen in most cases.
- Nonspecific mural thickening are seen in more severe cases of infection.

- Ischemic enterocolitis
- Behçet disease

PATHOLOGY

- In pseudomembranous colitis, potent antibiotics disrupt the normal bacterial flora of the colon, resulting in overgrowth of *Clostridium difficile.*
- Release of enterotoxins causes mucosal inflammation and pseudomembranous development, consisting of mucus and inflammatory debris.
- Neutropenic enterocolitis is an acute inflammatory, necrotizing process affecting the cecum, terminal ileum, or appendix of immunocompromised and neutropenic patients.

INCIDENCE/PREVALENCE AND EPIDEMIOLOGY

- Gastroenteritis and infectious enterocolitides are responsible for almost 70% of emergency department visits prompted by abdominal pain.

Suggested Readings

Thoeni RF, Cello JP: CT imaging of colitis. *Radiology* 240:623-638, 2006.

WHAT THE REFERRING PHYSICIAN NEEDS TO KNOW

- Most cases are self-limited and do not require imaging.
- Normal findings are seen in most cases.
- Nonspecific mural thickening is seen in more severe cases of infection.
- In pseudomembranous colitis, mural thickening averages 15-20 mm, with target or halo pattern caused by submucosal edema.
- Neutropenic enterocolitis CT features are nonspecific.

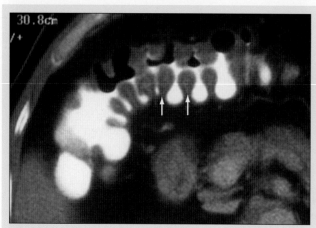

Figure 1. Pseudomembranous colitis. The haustra of the transverse colon have a thickened appearance *(arrows)* simulating an accordion. This nonspecific finding of colitis must always be correlated with the clinical picture.

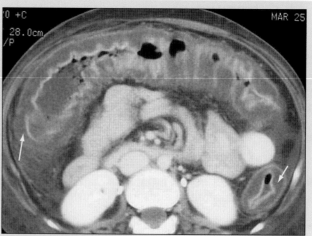

Figure 2. Cytomegalovirus colitis in a patient with AIDS. The scan shows marked mural thickening of the colon with increased enhancement of the mucosa and severe submucosal edema *(arrows)*. Mural stratification of the colon can be seen in many infectious colitides.

Inflammatory Bowel Disease

DEFINITION: Disease characterized by bowel inflammation, which includes Crohn disease and ulcerative colitis.

ANATOMIC FINDINGS

Bowel

- Crohn disease active inflammatory subtype: aphthae to deep ulcers, minimal fold thickening or distortion to marked wall thickening, nodular lymphoid hyperplasia, and obstruction caused by spasm
- Crohn disease, fibrostenotic subtype: stenosis, decrease in the luminal diameter, prestenotic dilation, minimal wall thickening, no bowel wall edema, and loss of mural stratification
- Crohn disease, fistulizing or perforating subtype: deep fissuring ulcers, sinus tracts, fistulas, and an associated inflammatory mass
- Crohn disease reparative or regenerative subtype: mucosal atrophy, regenerative polyps, and minimal decrease in lumen diameter, with no mural edema
- Early changes in ulcerative colitis: haustral thickening or loss, inflammatory polyps, crypt abscess, ulcers, confluent, contiguous, and circumferential disease
- Chronic changes in ulcerative colitis: haustral loss, luminal narrowing, loss of rectal valves, widened presacral space, postinflammatory pseudopolyps, and backwash ileitis
- Common findings (to both inflammatory bowel diseases): mural thickening and narrowed lumen

Mesentery

- Crohn disease: Increased mesenteric vascularity (*comb* sign) is an indicator of disease activity.
- Complications of Crohn disease include abscess, phlegmon, fibrofatty proliferation, and perianal disease.
- Common findings include increased lymph node size and number.

IMAGING

CT

Findings

- In obstruction, submucosal edema is seen as mural stratification and the *target* sign.
- In obstruction with loss of mural stratification, transmural fibrosis may be present (requires surgery).

DIAGNOSTIC PEARLS

- Crohn colitis (early findings): shallow to deep to confluent ulcerations, skip lesions, segmental distribution, a *cobblestone* appearance, and asymmetric involvement
- Ulcerative colitis (acute findings): mucosal granularity, mucosal stippling, *collar-button* ulcers, confluent, contiguous, and circumferential disease
- *Target* appearance and *comb* sign

- Ulcerative colitis causes mural thickening less than 1.5 cm; a *target* appearance in chronic cases represents submucosal fat (chronic); perirectal and presacral fat is increased.
- Crohn disease causes mural thickening greater than 2 cm; homogeneous density of wall, mesenteric changes, and perianal disease are seen.

Utility

- CT is the preferred means of establishing the diagnosis and guiding percutaneous drainage in abscesses of Crohn disease.
- It is also used to assess the status of the bowel wall and to detect early perforation in a toxic megacolon of fulminant ulcerative colitis.

MRI

Findings

- MR enteroclysis provides sufficient resolution to detect early lesions of Crohn disease.
- *Cobblestoning* exhibits as patchy, sharply demarcated areas of high signal intensity along the affected small bowel segments.
- Bowel wall thickening, usually ranging from 1-2 cm, is the most consistent feature of Crohn disease on MRI.
- Mural stratification: on central low T1-signal surrounded by a thin enhancing inner layer, thicker low-enhancing intermediate layer, and thin, strongly enhancing outer layer
- Sinus tracts and fistulas are demonstrated by high signal intensity of fluid content on true-FISP and HASTE images.

WHAT THE REFERRING PHYSICIAN NEEDS TO KNOW

- Although rare, emergencies such as bowel obstruction and abscess formation may occur with Crohn disease.
- Fulminant colitis, toxic megacolon, and perforation develop with ulcerative colitis.
- Differential diagnosis includes ulceration, amebiasis, ischemia, tuberculosis, *Strongyloides* infection, lymphogranuloma venereum, actinomycosis, and schistosomiasis colitis cystica profunda.
- Differential diagnosis for small-bowel disease includes *Yersinia* infection, Behçet disease, pseudomembranous enterocolitis, and tuberculosis.

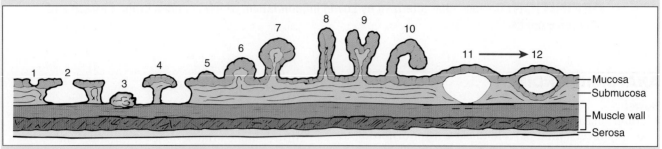

Figure 1. Spectrum of mucosal abnormalities in ulcerative colitis. 1, Punctate mucosal ulcer-crypt abscess; 2, *collar-button* ulcer; 3, polypoid accumulation of granulation tissue; 4, mucosal remnant forming inflammatory pseudopolyp; 5 and 6, sessile mucosal polyps (similar morphologic features to those seen in hyperplasia, adenoma, and carcinoma); 7, pedunculated polyp (typically hyperplastic or low-grade adenomas); 8, 9, and 10, postinflammatory pseudopolyps of various configurations; 11, mucosal remnant bridging area of active undermining ulceration; 12, mucosal bridge in quiescent state with previously denuded surfaces covered with new epithelium. (*From Lichtenstein JE: Radiologic-pathologic correlation of inflammatory bowel disease.* Radiol Clin North Am *25:324, 1987.*)

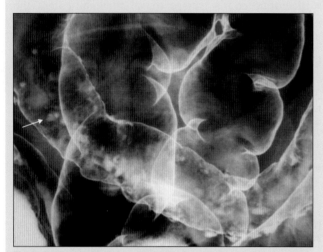

Figure 2. Crohn disease: aphthoid ulcerations. Double-contrast barium enema demonstrates aphthoid lesions *(arrow)* of varying sizes in the transverse colon.

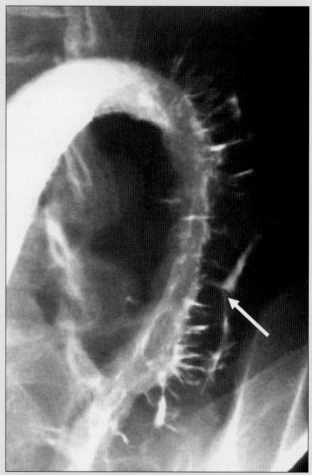

Figure 3. Crohn disease: deep ulcerations. Multiple deep ulcerations are identified in the descending colon. They communicate with a paracolic sinus tract *(arrow)*.

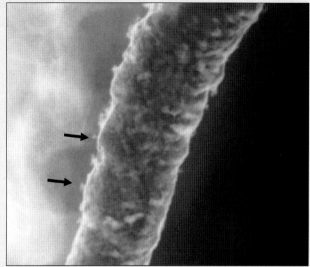

Figure 4. Ulcerative colitis: **collar-button ulcers.** Spot film of the splenic flexure shows multiple flask-like ulcers *(arrows)* with a flat base. The ulceration is limited to the layers superficial to the muscularis propria.

- Enhancing mesenteric lymph nodes are highly suggestive of active Crohn disease.
- Ulcerative colitis causes mural stratification and thickening and abnormal hypointensity of mucosal and submucosal layers on T1-weighted and T2-weighted images.

Utility
- MRI helps confirm the diagnosis and localize lesions; it assesses their severity, extent, and inflammatory activity and identifies extraintestinal complications that may require surgical intervention.
- MR enteroclysis is an emerging diagnostic tool that combines the advantages of conventional enteroclysis and MRI.
- Adequate distention of the bowel lumen is very important because collapsed bowel loops can hide lesions or mimic an abnormality.
- T2-weighted half-Fourier RARE or HASTE and T1-weighted gadolinium-enhanced spoiled gradient-echo images are important sequences.
- True-FISP sequence is particularly good for obtaining information about mural and extraintestinal complications.
- MR fluoroscopy is particular useful in the distinction of a high-grade from a low-grade obstruction.
- MR fluoroscopic images can be reviewed in a cine loop format to obtain functional information concerning a bowel obstruction.

Radiography
Findings
- Ulcerative colitis, barium enema acute findings: mucosal granularity, mucosal stippling, *collar-button* ulcers, and confluent, contiguous, circumferential disease
- Crohn colitis, early findings in barium enema: shallow to deep to confluent ulcerations, skip lesions, segmental distribution, *cobblestone* appearance, and asymmetric involvement

- Crohn colitis, late findings in barium enema: fissures, fistulas, haustral loss, sacculations, postinflammatory pseudopolyps, and intramural abscess strictures

Utility
- Barium studies are being replaced by CT, MRI, video capsule, and colonoscopy in the evaluation of inflammatory bowel disease.

Ultrasound with Doppler
Findings
- Ulcerative colitis: moderately thick, hypoechoic wall, typical wall stratification maintained, loss of haustration, and absent peristaltic motion
- Crohn colitis: clearly thickened and hypoechoic wall, loss of typical wall stratification in chronic disease, loss of haustration, diminished compressibility, and absent peristaltic motion
- Crohn colitis: increased blood flow of superior mesenteric artery with a decreased resistive index

Utility
- CT and MRI more fully depict the mural and extramural findings in patients with inflammatory bowel disease.

CLINICAL PRESENTATION

- Patients experience chronic symptoms punctuated by periodic exacerbations.
- Ulcerative colitis causes diarrhea, abdominal pain, rectal bleeding, weight loss, and tenesmus, as well as vomiting, fever, and constipation.
- Ulcerative colitis also causes fever, prostration, dehydration, and postural hypotension in most severe cases; the abdomen may be protuberant because of colonic atony and distention.

- Abdominal tenderness over the colon and absent bowel sounds are ominous signs suggesting a toxic megacolon or early perforation.
- Ulcerative colitis leads to uveitis and iritis, episcleritis, conjunctivitis, erythema nodosum, cutaneous vasculitis, stomatitis, pyoderma gangrenosum, and anemia.
- Crohn disease causes rectal bleeding, diarrhea, and abdominal pain, which may be colicky, in the lower abdomen, relieved by defecation or, if more severe, simulating appendicitis.
- Abdominal tenderness and distention, pronounced wasting, emaciation, and intra-abdominal mass are more frequently found in Crohn disease than in ulcerative colitis.

DIFFERENTIAL DIAGNOSIS

- Intestinal ischemia
- Peritoneal carcinomatosis
- Mural thickening of the gut from ischemia, infection, radiation

PATHOLOGY

- Primary etiologic agent or the cause of ulcerative colitis and Crohn disease is still unknown.
- Participation of genetic, environmental, neural, hormonal, infectious, immunologic, and psychological factors in pathogenesis is well established.
- Patients with ulcerative colitis have abnormal mucin production, which may permit various intraluminal bacterial products and toxins to attack the mucosa.
- In ulcerative colitis, the enteric nervous system and nerves containing substance P and vasoactive intestinal polypeptide become straight, thick, and highly immunoreactive.
- In vitro studies have demonstrated that levels of several prostaglandin species are significantly elevated in the mucosa in Crohn colitis and ulcerative colitis.
- Other immunologic evidence suggests failure of suppressor cell generation coupled with the hyperactive state of helper T cells in patients with inflammatory bowel disease.
- Active inflammatory subtype of Crohn disease is characterized by focal inflammation, a transmural inflammatory reaction with lymphoid aggregates, and granuloma formation.

INCIDENCE/PREVALENCE AND EPIDEMIOLOGY

- Ulcerative colitis worldwide prevalence is 35-100 cases/100,000 population; annual incidence is 2-10 cases/100,000 population.
- Ulcerative colitis bimodal age distribution: The peak is 15-25 years; a smaller peak occurs at 50-80 years.
- Ulcerative colitis risk factors include a family history (30-100 times the risk), white, Jewish (2-4 times the risk), lives in a developed country, urban dweller, single, oral contraceptive use, and a nonsmoker.
- Crohn disease worldwide prevalence is 10-70 cases/100,000 population; the annual incidence is 0.6-6.3 cases/100,000 population.
- Crohn disease bimodal age distribution: The peak is at 15-25 years; a smaller peak occurs at 50-80 years.
- True emergencies are uncommon but are associated with high rates of morbidity and mortality.
- Ulcerative colitis is often associated with autoimmune disorders, sacroiliitis, ankylosing spondylitis, enteropathic oligoarthritis, and anterior uveitis.

Suggested Readings

Bernstein CN, Rawsthorne P, Cheang M, et al: A population-based case-control study of potential risk factors for IBD. *Am J Gastroenterol* 101:993-1002, 2006.

Bernstein CN, Wajda A, Svenson LW, et al: The epidemiology of inflammatory bowel disease in Canada: A population-based study. *Am J Gastroenterol* 101:1559-1568, 2006.

Green C, Elliott L, Beaudoin C, et al: A population-based ecologic study of inflammatory bowel disease: Searching for etiologic clues. *Am J Epidemiol* 164:615-623, 2006.

Hong SS, Kim AY, Byun JH, et al: MDCT of small bowel disease: Value of 3D imaging. *AJR Am J Roentgenol* 187:1212-1221, 2006.

Horton KM, Fishman EK: The current status of multidetector row CT and three-dimensional imaging of the small bowel. *Radiol Clin North Am* 41:199-212, 2003.

Maglinte DDT, Gourtsoyiannis N, Rex D, et al: Classification of small bowel Crohn's subtypes based on multimodality imaging. *Radiol Clin North Am* 41:285-303, 2003.

Munkholm P, Binder V: Clinical features and natural history of Crohn's disease. In Sartor RB, Sandborn WJ (eds): *Kirsner's Inflammatory Bowel Diseases*, 6th ed. Edinburgh, Saunders, 2004, pp 289-300.

Patak MA, Mortele KJ, Ros PR: Multidetector row CT of the small bowel. *Radiol Clin North Am* 43:1063-1077, 2005.

Riddell RH: Pathology of idiopathic inflammatory bowel disease. In Sartor RB, Sandborn WJ (eds): *Kirsner's Inflammatory Bowel Diseases*, 6th ed. Edinburgh, Saunders, 2004, pp 399-424.

Thoeni RF, Cello JP: CT imaging of colitis. *Radiology* 240:623-638, 2006.

Intestinal Ischemia

DEFINITION: Vascular insufficiency of the gut after hypoperfusion, arterial or venous occlusion, or thrombosis.

IMAGING

CT
Findings
- Mural thickening
- Submucosal edema possibly causing a target or halo appearance
- Focal pneumatosis or thrombus in the superior mesenteric artery or vein
- Air in bowel wall, mesentery, and portal venous system
- Colonic ischemia revealing segmental thickening of the colon with scalloped, irregular margins caused by submucosal edema

Utility
- Findings are dependent on the cause, chronicity, and severity.
- CT plays an important role in identifying early changes of ischemia.
- Rapid intravenous contrast administration is required to optimize vascular opacification and to assess the superior mesenteric artery and vein patency.
- CT angiography and MR angiography can show stenoses and thromboses in the mesenteric vasculature.

CLINICAL PRESENTATION

- Patients complain of acute abdominal pain.
- Intestinal ischemia has a broad range of symptoms that make clinical diagnosis difficult.
- Blood in stool, diarrhea, and ileus
- Weight loss, abdominal distention, nausea and vomiting
- Symptoms typically out of proportion to physical findings

DIFFERENTIAL DIAGNOSIS

- Inflammatory bowel disease
- Infectious enterocolitis
- Bowel obstruction
- Ileus

DIAGNOSTIC PEARLS

- Mural thickening of the gut, with or without submucosal edema
- Focal pneumatosis or thrombus in the superior mesenteric artery or vein
- Air in the bowel wall, mesentery, and portal venous system
- Segmental thickening of the colon, with scalloped, irregular margins

- Gastrointestinal hemorrhage
- Behçet disease
- Radiation enterocolitis

PATHOLOGY

- Major causes of intestinal ischemia include hypoperfusion and arterial or venous occlusion or thrombosis.
- Colonic ischemia usually results from hypoperfusion or hypotension.

INCIDENCE/PREVALENCE AND EPIDEMIOLOGY

- Intestinal ischemia is associated with coronary artery disease, peripheral vascular disease, arteritis, hypotension, dehydration, and cardiac decompensation.

Suggested Readings

Chou CK, Wu RH, Mak CW, et al: Clinical significance of poor CT enhancement of the thickened small-bowel wall in patients with acute abdominal pain. *AJR Am J Roentgenol* 186:491-498, 2006.

Macari M, Balthazar EJ: CT of bowel wall thickening: Significance and pitfalls of interpretation. *AJR Am J Roentgenol* 176:1105-1116, 2001.

Macari M, Chandarana H, Balthazar E, et al: Intestinal ischemia versus intramural hemorrhage: CT evaluation. *AJR Am J Roentgenol* 180:177-184, 2003.

Rha SE, Ha HK, Lee SH, et al: CT and MR imaging findings of bowel ischemia from various primary causes. *RadioGraphics* 20:29-42, 2000.

WHAT THE REFERRING PHYSICIAN NEEDS TO KNOW

- CT is far more sensitive than radiography in detecting pneumatosis and portal venous gas.
- Air in the bowel wall, mesentery, and portal venous system has grave prognostic implications for patients with an ischemic bowel.

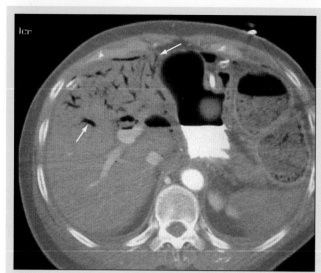

Figure 1. CT features of intestinal infarction with pneumatosis intestinalis and portal venous gas. CT scan at the level of the liver shows portal venous gas, primarily in the left lobe *(arrows)*.

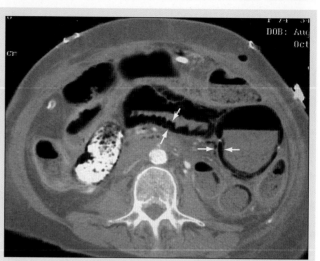

Figure 2. CT features of intestinal infarction with pneumatosis intestinalis and portal venous gas. CT scan obtained more caudally shows extensive pneumatosis intestinalis *(arrows)*.

Mesenteric Adenitis

DEFINITION: Benign inflammation of the ileocolic lymph nodes.

IMAGING

CT
Findings
- Mesenteric lymph nodes are enlarged (> 5 mm), with possible change in the surrounding mesentery.
- Appendix is normal, and the adjacent ileum and cecum may be thickened.

Utility
- CT is quite sensitive in depicting these nodes provided there is sufficient fat in the ileocolic mesentery.

Ultrasound
Findings
- Spherical hypoechoic masses contrasted by the echogenic fat of the ileocolic mesentery

Utility
- Ultrasound is often the initial examination obtained in pediatric patients with abdominal pain.

CLINICAL PRESENTATION

- Simulates appendicitis clinically
- Right lower quadrant pain
- Tenderness to abdominal palpation
- Fever

DIFFERENTIAL DIAGNOSIS

- Appendicitis (pediatric)
- Crohn disease
- Epiploic appendagitis
- Omental infarction
- Lymphoma

DIAGNOSTIC PEARLS

- Mesenteric lymph nodes are enlarged (> 5 mm).
- Inflammatory changes are seen in surrounding mesentery.
- Appendix is normal, and the adjacent colon and ileum may be thickened.

PATHOLOGY

- *Yersinia enterocolitica*, *Yersinia pseudotuberculosis*, and *Helicobacter jejuni* are the most commonly implicated organisms.
- Benign inflammation of ileocolic lymph nodes can cause mesenteric adenitis.

INCIDENCE/PREVALENCE AND EPIDEMIOLOGY

- Prominent lymph nodes are seen in a variety of infectious, inflammatory, and malignant abdominal disorders.

Suggested Readings

Coulier B: Segmental omental infarction in childhood: A typical case diagnosed by CT allowing successful conservative treatment. *Pediatr Radiol* 36:141-143, 2006.
Singh AK, Gervais DA, Lee P, et al: Omental infarct: CT imaging features. *Abdom Imaging* (Epub ahead of print), 2006.

WHAT THE REFERRING PHYSICIAN NEEDS TO KNOW

- Mesenteric lymph nodes are enlarged (>5 mm), and a possible change may be seen in the surrounding mesentery.
- *Y. enterocolitica*, *Y. pseudotuberculosis*, and *H. jejuni* are the most commonly implicated organisms.

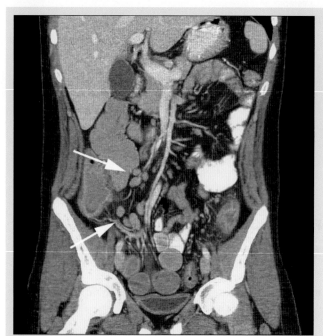

Figure 1. Mesenteric adenitis: multidetector CT features. Coronal reformats show multiple, borderline, enlarged lymph nodes *(arrows)* in the ileocolic mesentery.

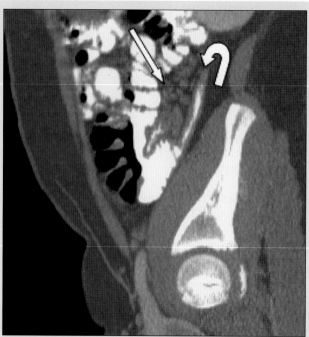

Figure 2. Mesenteric adenitis: multidetector CT features. Sagittal reformats show multiple, borderline, enlarged lymph nodes *(arrow)* in the ileocolic mesentery. Notice that the luminal contrast material refluxes into a normal-sized appendix *(curved arrow)*.

Omental Infarction

DEFINITION: Portions of the greater omentum undergo torsion or spontaneous venous thrombosis, or both, which leads to severe abdominal pain with exquisite point tenderness.

IMAGING

CT
Findings
- Region of increased attenuation is seen within the greater omentum in the involved segment.
- Size of the omental abnormality is typically larger in omental infarction and torsion than in epiploic appendagitis.

Utility
- The most reliable noninvasive imaging test

CLINICAL PRESENTATION

- Severe abdominal pain associated with exquisite point tenderness

DIFFERENTIAL DIAGNOSIS

- Appendicitis
- Acute cholecystitis
- Primary neoplasms of the omentum
- Epiploic appendagitis
- Omental infection

PATHOLOGY

- Portions of the greater omentum undergo torsion or spontaneous venous thrombosis, or both.

DIAGNOSTIC PEARLS

- CT demonstrates a region of increased attenuation within the greater omentum in the involved segment.
- It usually occurs in right upper or lower quadrants.
- Size of the anomaly is typically larger in omental torsion and infarction than in epiploic appendagitis.

INCIDENCE/PREVALENCE AND EPIDEMIOLOGY

- Omental infarction is an uncommon disorder.
- It occurs more commonly in obese patients.

Suggested Readings

Coulier B: Segmental omental infarction in childhood: A typical case diagnosed by CT allowing successful conservative treatment. *Pediatr Radiol* 36:141-143, 2006.

Singh AK, Gervais DA, Lee P, et al: Omental infarct: CT imaging features. *Abdom Imaging*: (Epub ahead of print), 2006.

WHAT THE REFERRING PHYSICIAN NEEDS TO KNOW

- Omental infarction usually occurs in right lower quadrant, where it clinically simulates acute appendicitis.
- It may occur in the right upper quadrant, where it simulates acute cholecystitis.
- This disorder is usually self-limited but may require surgery in some patients.

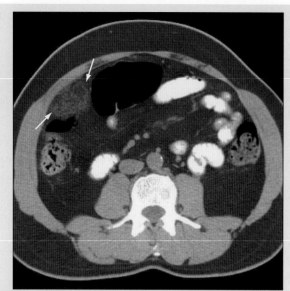

Figure 1. Focal torsion-infarction of the greater omentum: pathologic and multidetector CT (MDCT) findings. Axial image of a patient shows the focal increased attenuation *(arrows)* of the omental fat, typical of this disorder, caused by omental ischemia resulting from venous thrombosis.

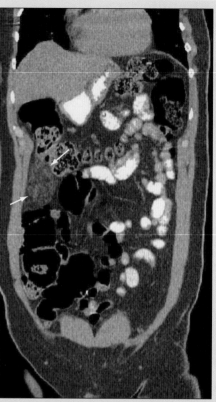

Figure 2. Focal torsion-infarction of the greater omentum: pathologic and MDCT findings. Coronal image of a patient shows the focal increased attenuation *(arrows)* of the omental fat, typical of this disorder, caused by omental ischemia resulting from venous thrombosis.

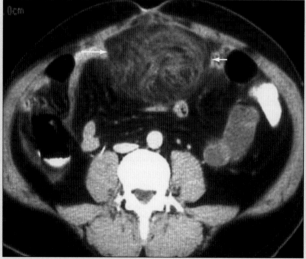

Figure 3. Focal torsion-infarction of the greater omentum: pathologic and MDCT findings. Axial scan in a patient shows torsion of the greater omentum *(arrows)* anterior to the transverse colon.

Perforation

DEFINITION: Perforation of the gastrointestinal tract as a catastrophic complication of various disease entities.

IMAGING

CT

Findings
- Pneumoperitoneum
- Loculated fluid and gas
- Focal mesenteric or omental infiltration
- Focal enhancement of the parietal peritoneum
- Extravasated intraluminal contrast material

Utility
- Multidetector CT is ideal for evaluating patients with signs of peritonitis.
- It can detect pneumoperitoneum that may be overlooked on chest or abdominal radiography.
- Detection of the perforation site may be assisted with the use of oral and intravenous contrast.

CLINICAL PRESENTATION

- Abdominal pain
- Peritonitis
- Sepsis
- Shoulder pain

DIFFERENTIAL DIAGNOSIS

- Colonic interposition
- Subdiaphragmatic fat simulating pneumoperitoneum
- Mach effect of rib superimposed

PATHOLOGY

- Gastrointestinal perforation indicates a catastrophic complication of peptic ulcer disease, diverticulitis, severe intestinal inflammation, infarction, trauma, neoplasm, or closed-loop obstruction.

DIAGNOSTIC PEARLS

- Pneumoperitoneum
- Loculated fluid and gas
- Focal mesenteric or omental infiltration
- Focal enhancement of the parietal peritoneum

INCIDENCE/PREVALENCE AND EPIDEMIOLOGY

- Free intraperitoneal perforation occurs in less than 1% of patients with diverticulitis.
- Perforation occurs in up to 10% of patients with appendicitis.

Suggested Readings

Grassi R, Romano S, Pinto A, et al: Gastro-duodenal perforations: Conventional plain film, US and CT findings in 166 consecutive patients. *Eur J Radiol* 50:30-36, 2004.

Hainaux B, Agneessens E, Bertinotti R, et al: Accuracy of MDCT in predicting site of gastrointestinal tract perforation. *AJR Am J Roentgenol* 187:1179-1183, 2006.

Rubesin SE, Levine MS: Radiologic diagnosis of gastrointestinal perforation. *Radiol Clin North Am* 41:1095-1116, 2003.

WHAT THE REFERRING PHYSICIAN NEEDS TO KNOW

- Multidetector CT is ideal for evaluating patients with suspected perforation.

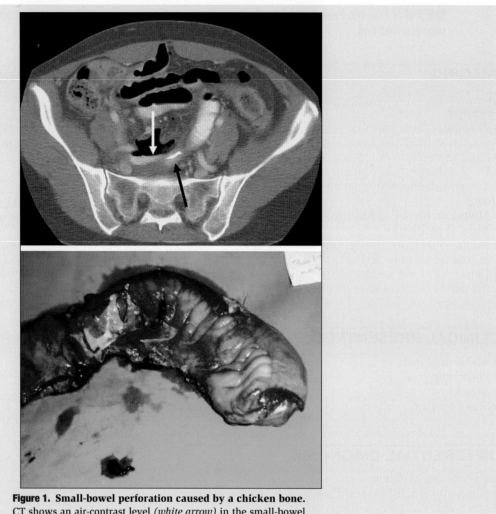

Figure 1. Small-bowel perforation caused by a chicken bone.
CT shows an air-contrast level *(white arrow)* in the small-bowel
mesentery caused by perforation by a chicken bone *(black arrow)*.

Renal Colic

DEFINITION: Acute flank pain in patients suspected of having acute ureteral obstruction from an impacted stone.

IMAGING

CT
Findings
- Calcifications are seen within the course of the ureter, with ureteral wall edema.
- Secondary signs include hydronephrosis, hydroureter, perinephric stranding, and periureteric stranding.
- Differential attenuation of the normal and affected kidney is greater than 5 HU.
- Infected right kidney is enlarged and edematous, and it may have a diminished, striated nephrogram.

Utility
- Multidetector CT has positive and negative predictive values greater than 95% for the diagnosis of obstructing urinary calculi.
- It is used to reveal the cause of flank pain in 25% of patients without ureterolithiasis.
- It can also accurately determine the site and size of ureteral calculi.
- If the initial scan result is negative or inconclusive for the detection of obstructing calculi, a contrast-enhanced scan can be obtained.

CLINICAL PRESENTATION

- Acute flank pain
- Hematuria
- Chills and fever
- Back pain
- Dysuria

DIFFERENTIAL DIAGNOSIS

- Abdominal aorta disease
- Appendicitis
- Diverticulitis
- Spinal compression fracture
- Testicular or ovarian torsion
- Pyelonephritis
- Renal abscess
- Renal neoplasm

DIAGNOSTIC PEARLS

- Calcifications within the course of the ureter, with ureteral wall edema
- Hydronephrosis, hydroureter, perinephric stranding, and periureteric stranding
- Differential attenuation of normal and affected kidney greater than 5 HU

- Ureteritis
- Renal vein thrombosis
- Renal artery thrombosis
- Renal infarct
- Splenic infarct

PATHOLOGY

- Presumptively, recent stone passage is diagnosed when hydroureteronephrosis and perinephric and periureteric stranding are present without a calculus.

INCIDENCE/PREVALENCE AND EPIDEMIOLOGY

- Renal colic accounts for 2.9% of the overall causes of acute abdomen.

Suggested Readings

Amilineni V, Lackner DF, Morse WS, et al: Contrast-enhanced CT for acute flank pain caused by acute renal artery occlusion. *AJR Am J Roentgenol* 174:105-106, 2000.

Hoppe H, Studer R, Kessler TM, et al: Alternate or additional findings to stone disease on unenhanced computerized tomography for acute flank pain can impact management. *J Urol* 175:1725-1730, 2006.

Kluner C, Hein PA, Gralla O, et al: Does ultra-low-dose CT with a radiation dose equivalent to that of KUB suffice to detect renal and ureteral calculi? *J Comput Assist Tomogr* 30:44-50, 2006.

Langer JE: Computed tomography and ultrasonography of acute renal abnormalities. *Semin Roentgenol* 36:99-108, 2001.

WHAT THE REFERRING PHYSICIAN NEEDS TO KNOW
- Pitfalls still remain in the ability of multidetector CT (MDCT) to diagnose renal colic.
- Lack of intravenous contrast limits the ability of MDCT to diagnose other acute renal abnormalities.
- If the initial scan is negative or inconclusive, contrast-enhanced scans can be obtained to search for other causes of the pain.

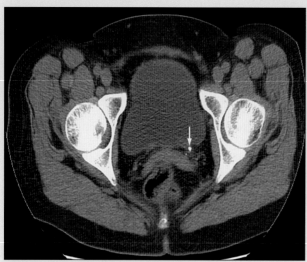

Figure 1. Ureterolithiasis: CT features. A 2-mm stone *(arrow)* is lodged at the left ureteropelvic junction.

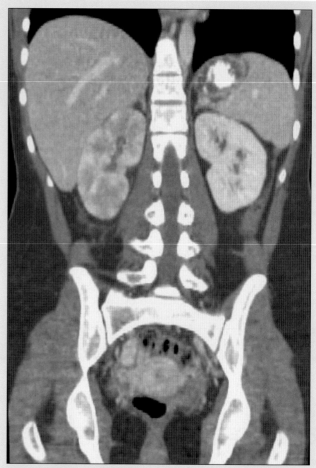

Figure 2. Pyelonephritis: MDCT features. The infected right kidney is enlarged and edematous, and it produces a diminished, striated nephrogram on this coronal reformatted image.

Abdominal Sepsis

DEFINITION: Abdominal infections result from the contiguous spread of bacteria from the gut, biliary tract, or genitourinary system.

IMAGING

CT

Findings

- Initially, abscesses appear as a mass of soft-tissue attenuation; with maturation, the lesion has a low-attenuation center with an enhancing rim.
- Small gas bubbles or air-fluid levels are present in 40%-50% of patients.
- Abscesses tend to be round or oval.
- If adjacent to a solid organ, masses may develop a lentiform or crescentic configuration.
- Abscesses also displace the surrounding structures and obliterate or thicken the adjacent fascial planes.

Utility

- Inflammatory changes are seen in contiguous mesenteric or omental fat.
- CT provides the most accurate imaging examination for the diagnosis of intra-abdominal abscesses.
- CT-directed percutaneous drainage is the preferred means of treating these abscesses.

CLINICAL PRESENTATION

- Patients with an abdominal abscess or peritonitis can have an acute abdomen.
- Sudden onset of severe abdominal pain may occur, requiring emergency medical or surgical treatment.
- Peritonitis
- Abdominal pain
- Nausea and vomiting
- Chills and fever
- Leukocytosis

DIFFERENTIAL DIAGNOSIS

- Intestinal ischemia
- Bowel obstruction
- Renal infarction
- Splenic infarction

PATHOLOGY

- Abdominal infections most commonly result from the contiguous spread of bacteria from the gut, biliary tract, or genitourinary system.

DIAGNOSTIC PEARLS

- Initially, abscesses appear as a mass of soft-tissue attenuation caused by the influx of the inflammatory cells.
- With maturation, the abscess undergoes central liquefaction necrosis, and a highly vascularized peripheral connective tissue develops.
- Abscesses tend to be round or oval, or they may adapt to a crescentic or lentiform configuration.

- Infections are typically polymicrobial in nature and include both aerobic and anaerobic organisms.
- Initially, abscesses appear as a mass of soft-tissue attenuation caused by the influx of the inflammatory cells.
- With maturation, the abscess undergoes central liquefaction necrosis, and a highly vascularized peripheral connective tissue develops.
- Abscesses may be round, oval, lentiform, or crescentic in shape.

INCIDENCE/PREVALENCE AND EPIDEMIOLOGY

- Intra-abdominal abscess occurs in up to 15%-20% of patients who have had major abdominal surgery.
- Perforation of the gut and cholangitis are other common sources of abdominal sepsis.

Suggested Readings

Federle MP: CT of the acute (emergency) abdomen. *Eur Radiol* 15(Suppl 4):D100-D104, 2005.
Gore RM, Miller FH, Pereles FS, et al: Helical CT in the evaluation of the acute abdomen. *AJR Am J Roentgenol* 174:901-913, 2000.
Marincek B: Nontraumatic abdominal emergencies. Acute abdominal pain: Diagnostic strategies. *Eur Radiol* 12:2136-2150, 2002.

WHAT THE REFERRING PHYSICIAN NEEDS TO KNOW

- CT provides the most accurate imaging examination for the diagnosis of intra-abdominal abscesses.

Angiodysplasia and Arteriovenous Malformations of the Colon

DEFINITION: Angiodysplasia is degenerative vascular ectasia associated with aging and aortic valve disease.

IMAGING

Nuclear Medicine
Findings
- Bleeding into the colonic lumen

Utility
- Radionuclide imaging has become accepted as the most sensitive, noninvasive study for detecting active gastrointestinal hemorrhage.
- Technetium-99m–labeled red blood cell imaging is the method of choice because it allows the monitoring of patients over a prolonged period.

Interventional Radiology
Findings
- Bleeding into the colonic lumen
- Dilation of the feeding arteries
- Slow emptying of densely opacified, dilated, tortuous intramural veins
- Early filling of the draining veins

Utility
- Arteriography is the diagnostic procedure of choice in patients with massive lower gastrointestinal hemorrhage.
- Bleeding rate must exceed 0.5 mL/min to locate the site of the hemorrhage.
- Scintigraphic studies should be performed before angiography to document active bleeding.

CT
Findings
- Bleeding into the colonic lumen

Utility
- Utility of multidetector CT (MDCT) in the diagnosis of active and occult sources of gastrointestinal hemorrhage has become accepted.

DIAGNOSTIC PEARLS

- Bleeding into the colonic lumen
- Dilation of the feeding arteries
- Slow emptying of densely opacified, dilated, and tortuous intramural veins
- Early filling of the draining veins

- Coronal and sagittal re-formations are helpful in demonstrating the origin of the hemorrhage.
- Unenhanced MDCT scan is initially obtained to reveal intraluminal blood followed by contrast injection and scanning.

CLINICAL PRESENTATION

- Hematochezia, which is the passage of bright-red or maroon blood, bloody diarrhea, or blood mixed with formed stool
- Occult blood, found only by testing stool with a chemical reagent
- Symptoms of blood loss such as dyspnea, dizziness, or shock
- History of inflammatory bowel disease or hematochezia, suggesting lower gastrointestinal bleeding

DIFFERENTIAL DIAGNOSIS

- Diverticulosis of the colon
- Inflammatory bowel disease
- Ischemic colitis
- Infectious colitis
- Radiation colitis
- Colonic neoplasm

WHAT THE REFERRING PHYSICIAN NEEDS TO KNOW

- Colonoscopy is used for the diagnosis of acute lower gastrointestinal bleeding.
- When bleeding cannot be identified and controlled, MDCT or arteriography may help localize the bleeding source.
- Bleeding stops spontaneously in more than 90% of patients, but the chance of recurrence is up to 85%.
- Endoscopic ablation is replacing right hemicolectomy as the treatment of choice for patients with colonic angiodysplasia.
- Abnormal vessels often preclude successful pharmacotherapy with intra-arterial vasopressin.
- Angiodysplasia and arteriovenous malformations can be treated by embolization.

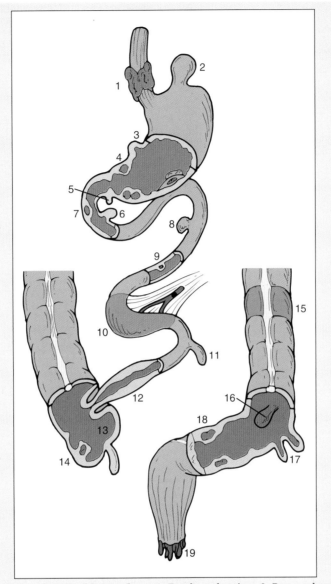

Figure 1. Common causes of acute gastrointestinal hemorrhage. 1. Esophageal varices. 2. Paraesophageal hernia. 3. Gastric ulcer and gastritis. 4. Gastric carcinoma. 5. Duodenal ulcer and duodenitis. 6. Duodenal diverticulum. 7. Duodenal neoplasm. 8. Duplication of the bowel. 9. Small-bowel tumor. 10. Mesenteric vascular disease. 11. Meckel diverticulum. 12. Crohn disease. 13. Intussusception. 14. Angiodysplasia. 15. Ulcerative, ischemic, and infectious colitis. 16. Colon polyp. 17. Diverticulosis. 18. Colon cancer. 19. Anal fissure, hemorrhoids, and tumor. (*From Beyer D, Modder U:* Diagnostic Imaging of the Acute Abdomen. *Berlin, Springer-Verlag, 1988, p 310.*)

PATHOLOGY

- One theory suggests that partial, intermittent obstruction of the submucosal veins as they penetrate the colon leads to tortousity and ectasia.
- With time, the arteriole-capillary-venule unit dilates, producing small arteriovenous communications.
- Bleeding primarily occurs from dilated capillaries and venules and tends to be moderate and intermittent.
- Episodes usually occur in the right side of the colon, presumably because of the greater tension of the cecal wall compared with the remainder of the colon.

INCIDENCE/PREVALENCE AND EPIDEMIOLOGY

- Angiodysplasia occurs in 0.83% of healthy, asymptomatic people.
- Colonic angioma or arteriovenous malformation makes up an incidence of 5.7% by disease cause of severe colonic bleeding.
- Acute, massive lower gastrointestinal bleeding has an incidence of 20-27 episodes per 100,000 persons annually.
- Angiodysplasia is a degenerative vascular ectasia associated with aging and aortic valve disease.

Suggested Readings

Howarth DM: The role of nuclear medicine in the detection of acute gastrointestinal bleeding. *Semin Nucl Med* 36:133-146, 2006.

Lin S, Rockey DC: Obscure gastrointestinal bleeding. *Gastroenterol Clin North Am* 34:679-698, 2005.

Manning-Dimmitt LL, Dimmitt SG, Wilson GR: Diagnosis of gastrointestinal bleeding in adults. *Am Fam Physician* 71:1339-1346, 2005.

Maurer AH: Gastrointestinal bleeding. In Murray IP, Ell PJ (eds): *Nuclear Medicine in Clinical Diagnosis and Treatment*. New York, Churchill Livingstone, 1994, pp 47-54.

Mallory-Weiss Tears

DEFINITION: Mallory-Weiss tears are esophageal tears caused by severe coughing, retching, or vomiting, which may cause upper gastrointestinal bleeding.

ANATOMIC FINDINGS

Esophagus
- Bleeding into the lumen
- Linear collection of barium in the distal esophagus just above the gastrointestinal junction

IMAGING

Nuclear Medicine
Findings
- Bleeding into the esophageal lumen

Utility
- Radionuclide imaging has become accepted as the most sensitive, noninvasive study for detecting active gastrointestinal hemorrhage.
- Technetium-99m–labeled red blood cell imaging is the method of choice because it allows the monitoring of patients over a prolonged period.

Interventional Radiology
Findings
- Bleeding into the esophageal lumen

Utility
- Angiography should be performed in patients with a brisk upper gastrointestinal hemorrhage if endoscopy is inconclusive in anticipation of transcatheterization.
- Bleeding rate must exceed 0.5 mL/min to locate the site of the hemorrhage.
- Scintigraphic studies should be performed before angiography to document active bleeding.

CT
Findings
- Bleeding into the esophageal lumen

Utility
- Utility of multidetector CT (MDCT) in the diagnosis of active and occult sources of gastrointestinal hemorrhage has become accepted.
- Coronal and sagittal re-formations are helpful in demonstrating the origin of the hemorrhage.

DIAGNOSTIC PEARLS

- Intraluminal presence of blood above the ligament of Treitz is seen.
- Esophagus as a source of the bleeding is identified through endoscopy, angiography, and red blood cell scan.

- Unenhanced MDCT scan is initially obtained to reveal intraluminal blood followed by contrast injection and scanning.

Radiography
Findings
- Linear collection of barium in the distal esophagus just above the gastroesophageal junction

Utility
- Barium studies have primarily been replaced by upper gastrointestinal endoscopy in patients with suspected tears.

CLINICAL PRESENTATION

- Patients exhibit excruciating epigastric and left-sided chest pain radiating to the back.
- Proximal lesions tend to cause hematemesis or melena.
- Hematochezia in massive hemorrhage of more than 1000 mL is seen.
- Symptoms of blood loss such as dyspnea, dizziness, or shock can occur.
- Aspiration of gastric contents with a nasogastric tube may reveal blood, which is diagnostic of an upper gastrointestinal bleeding source.

DIFFERENTIAL DIAGNOSIS

- Tuberculous esophagitis
- *Candida* esophagitis
- Linear ulcer

WHAT THE REFERRING PHYSICIAN NEEDS TO KNOW

- Most patients (75%-80%) are successfully treated with bed rest, sedation, antibiotics, and vigorous fluid and blood replacement.
- Endoscopy is the next therapeutic approach, with injection of sclerosant-hemostatic agents or coagulation with a heater or laser probe.
- If conservative measures and endoscopy fail to staunch the hemorrhage, diagnostic and therapeutic angiography is indicated.

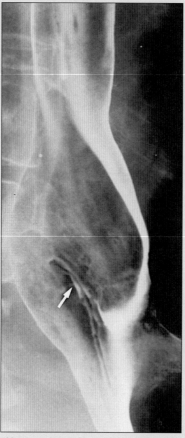

Figure 1. Mallory-Weiss tear. A linear collection of barium *(arrow)* is visible in the distal esophagus just above the gastroesophageal junction. Although a linear ulcer from reflux esophagitis could produce a similar appearance, the correct diagnosis was suggested by the clinical history. *(Courtesy of Harvey M. Goldstein, MD, San Antonio, TX.)*

- Crohn esophagitis
- Reflux esophagitis

PATHOLOGY

- Mallory-Weiss esophageal tears are caused by severe coughing, retching, or vomiting, particularly in alcoholic patients.
- Typically, the lower third of the esophagus ruptures along the left posterolateral wall, usually in a longitudinal direction.

INCIDENCE/PREVALENCE AND EPIDEMIOLOGY

- Mallory-Weiss tear makes up 5% incidence by disease cause of upper gastrointestinal hemorrhage.

Suggested Readings

Howarth DM: The role of nuclear medicine in the detection of acute gastrointestinal bleeding. *Semin Nucl Med* 36:133-146, 2006.

Lin S, Rockey DC: Obscure gastrointestinal bleeding. *Gastroenterol Clin North Am* 34:679-698, 2005.

Manning-Dimmitt LL, Dimmitt SG, Wilson GR: Diagnosis of gastrointestinal bleeding in adults. *Am Fam Physician* 71:1339-1346, 2005.

Maurer AH: Gastrointestinal bleeding. In Murray IP, Ell PJ (eds): *Nuclear Medicine in Clinical Diagnosis and Treatment*. New York, Churchill Livingstone, 1994, pp 47-54.

Small Bowel Hemorrhage

DEFINITION: Small bowel hemorrhage can be caused by ulcerations (usually ischemic), diverticula (e.g., Meckel diverticulum), neoplasm, angiodysplasia, varices, enteritis, and aortoenteric fistula.

IMAGING

Nuclear Medicine
Findings
- Bleeding into the small bowel lumen

Utility
- Radionuclide imaging has become accepted as the most sensitive, noninvasive study for detecting active gastrointestinal hemorrhage.
- Technetium-99m–labeled red blood cell imaging is the method of choice because it allows monitoring of patients over a prolonged period.

CT
Findings
- Bleeding into the small bowel lumen

Utility
- Utility of multidetector CT (MDCT) in the diagnosis of active and occult sources of gastrointestinal hemorrhage has become accepted.
- Coronal and sagittal re-formations are helpful in demonstrating the origin of the hemorrhage.
- Unenhanced MDCT scan is initially obtained to reveal intraluminal blood followed by contrast injection and scanning.

Interventional Radiology
Findings
- Bleeding into the small bowel lumen

Utility
- Arteriography is the diagnostic procedure of choice in patients with massive lower gastrointestinal hemorrhage.
- Bleeding rate must exceed 0.5 mL/min to locate the site of the hemorrhage.
- Scintigraphic studies should be performed before angiography to document active bleeding.

CLINICAL PRESENTATION

- Lower gastrointestinal bleeding more commonly produces hematochezia.
- Symptoms of blood loss such as dyspnea, dizziness, or shock may be seen.

DIAGNOSTIC PEARLS

- Intraluminal presence of blood below the ligament of Treitz is seen.
- Small bowel as source of bleeding is identified through angiography and red blood cell scan.

- Massive hemorrhage is less common from lesions distal to the ligament of Treitz.

DIFFERENTIAL DIAGNOSIS

- Small bowel ischemia
- Primary and metastatic small bowel neoplasms
- Crohn's disease
- Infectious or inflammatory enteritis

PATHOLOGY

- Common causes include ulcerations (usually ischemic), diverticula (e.g., Meckel diverticulum), neoplasm, angiodysplasia, varices, enteritis, and aortoenteric fistula.

INCIDENCE/PREVALENCE AND EPIDEMIOLOGY

- Almost 30% of lower gastrointestinal hemorrhages originate in the small bowel.

Suggested Readings

Howarth DM: The role of nuclear medicine in the detection of acute gastrointestinal bleeding. *Semin Nucl Med* 36:133-146, 2006.
Lin S, Rockey DC: Obscure gastrointestinal bleeding. *Gastroenterol Clin North Am* 34:679-698, 2005.
Manning-Dimmitt LL, Dimmitt SG, Wilson GR: Diagnosis of gastrointestinal bleeding in adults. *Am Fam Physician* 71:1339-1346, 2005.
Maurer AH: Gastrointestinal bleeding. In Murray IP, Ell PJ (eds): *Nuclear Medicine in Clinical Diagnosis and Treatment.* New York, Churchill Livingstone, 1994, pp 47-54.

WHAT THE REFERRING PHYSICIAN NEEDS TO KNOW

- Most episodes of upper or lower gastrointestinal hemorrhage resolve spontaneously.
- Vasopressin is a safe and dependable vasoconstrictor of mesenteric circulation.
- Surgery is indicated when a neoplasm, diverticulum, or aortoenteric fistula is found and when embolization cannot be performed safely.
- Embolization can be performed only when bleeding artery is superselectively catheterized near the vasa recta of the bleeding site.

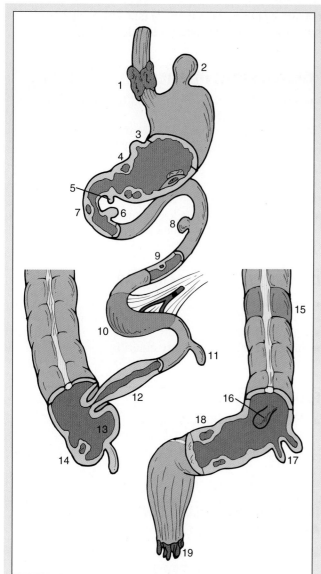

Figure 1. Common causes of acute gastrointestinal hemorrhage. 1. Esophageal varices. 2. Paraesophageal hernia. 3. Gastric ulcer and gastritis. 4. Gastric carcinoma. 5. Duodenal ulcer and duodenitis. 6. Duodenal diverticulum. 7. Duodenal neoplasm. 8. Duplication of the bowel. 9. Small bowel tumor. 10. Mesenteric vascular disease. 11. Meckel diverticulum. 12. Crohn disease. 13. Intussusception. 14. Angiodysplasia. 15. Ulcerative, ischemic, and infectious colitis. 16. Colon polyp. 17. Diverticulosis. 18. Colon cancer. 19. Anal fissure, hemorrhoids, and tumor. (*From Beyer D, Modder U:* Diagnostic Imaging of the Acute Abdomen. *Berlin, Springer-Verlag, 1988, p 310.*)

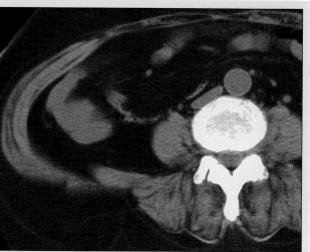

Figure 2. Ileal hemorrhage demonstrated on MDCT and confirmed angiographically. Transverse unenhanced CT image shows fluid-filled small bowel loops without high attenuation in the right lower quadrant of the abdomen. (*From Yoon W, Jeong YY, Shin SS, et al: Acute massive gastrointestinal bleeding: Detection and localization with arterial phase multi-detector row helical CT.* Radiology 239:160-167, 2006.)

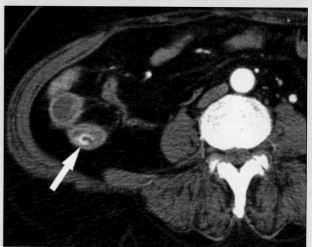

Figure 3. Ileal hemorrhage demonstrated on MDCT and confirmed angiographically. Same level, transverse arterial-phase multidetector row CT image demonstrates a jet of extravasated contrast material *(arrow)* in the small bowel lumen. (*From Yoon W, Jeong YY, Shin SS, et al: Acute massive gastrointestinal bleeding: Detection and localization with arterial phase multi-detector row helical CT.* Radiology 239:160-167, 2006.)

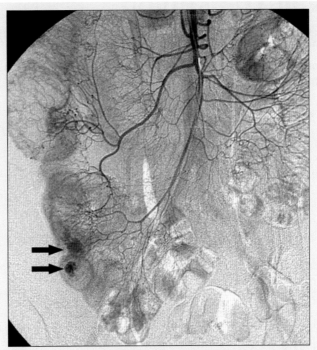

Figure 4. **Ileal hemorrhage demonstrated on multidetector CT and confirmed angiographically.** Corresponding posteroanterior-superior mesenteric arteriogram reveals active bleeding *(arrows)* in the distal ileum. *(From Yoon W, Jeong YY, Shin SS, et al: Acute massive gastrointestinal bleeding: Detection and localization with arterial phase multi-detector row helical CT. Radiology 239:160-167, 2006.)*

Bowel Wall Thickening

DEFINITION: Thickening of the bowel wall secondary to bowel injury, which may be the result of infection, inflammation, ischemia, radiation, vasculitis, or hemorrhage.

IMAGING

CT

Findings
- Bowel wall thickening is usually circumferential.
- Injury to the bowel is seen.

Utility
- Non–contrast-enhanced scan is used because the bowel loops are not opacified with contrast on a trauma CT study.
- Bowel wall thickening is diagnosed only when it is seen in the same loop of the bowel on two contiguous CT slices.

CLINICAL PRESENTATION

- Abdominal pain
- Diarrhea
- Blood in stool
- Bowel obstruction

DIFFERENTIAL DIAGNOSIS

- Mesenteric ischemia
- Infection
- Inflammatory bowel disease
- Intramural hemorrhage
- Neoplasm
- Postradiation change
- Trauma
- Low protein states
- Portal hypertension

DIAGNOSTIC PEARLS

- Bowel wall thickening is usually circumferential in a trauma patient.
- Finding of an unopacified loop of the bowel demonstrating a normal, paper-thin wall on the anterior surface of the loop precludes the circumferential area of wall thickening.
- Bowel wall thickening must be seen in the same loop of the bowel on two contiguous CT slices.

PATHOLOGY

- Bowel wall thickening is seen in an injury to the bowel wall.

INCIDENCE/PREVALENCE AND EPIDEMIOLOGY

- Trauma is the leading cause of death in Americans younger than 40 years of age.
- Trauma is the third leading cause of death overall.

Suggested Readings

Allen GS, Moore FA, Cox CSJ, et al: Hollow viscus injury and blunt trauma. *J Trauma* 45:69-77, 1998.

Cripps N, Cooper G: Intestinal injury mechanisms after blunt abdominal impact. *Ann R Coll Surg Engl* 79:115-120, 1997.

Halvorsen RA Jr, McCormick VD, Evans SJ: Computed tomography of abdominal trauma: A step by step approach. *Emerg Radiol* 1:283-291, 1994.

WHAT THE REFERRING PHYSICIAN NEEDS TO KNOW

- Bowel wall thickening is usually circumferential in a trauma patient.
- Intraluminal gas in the normal unopacified loop of the bowel showing thin walls often precludes circumferential thickening.
- Bowel wall thickening must be seen in the same loop of the bowel on two contiguous CT slices.

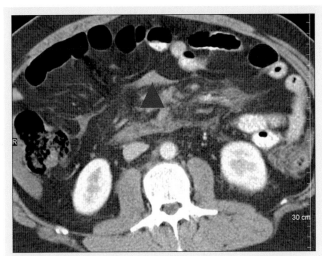

Figure 1. Intramesenteric hematoma with circumferential bowel wall thickening. A 37-year-old man was assessed after a motor-vehicle collision. Hematoma and a triangular fluid collection *(arrowhead)* are identified in the interloop mesentery along with jejunal wall thickening. Multiple mesenteric rents, a mesenteric hematoma, and a long segment of devascularized jejunum were found at laparotomy.

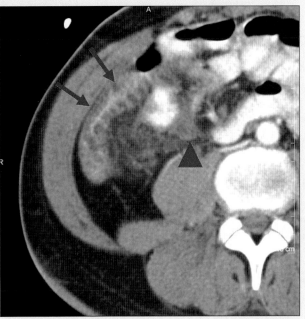

Figure 2. Intramesenteric triangular hematoma with adjacent bowel wall thickening. A 34-year-old female pedestrian was struck by an automobile. Small-bowel wall thickening *(arrows)* was identified adjacent to a mesenteric hematoma *(arrowhead)*. Exploratory laparotomy revealed a hematoma and a rent in the mesentery of the distal ileum, resulting in a 12-cm segment of the devascularized ileum that was resected.

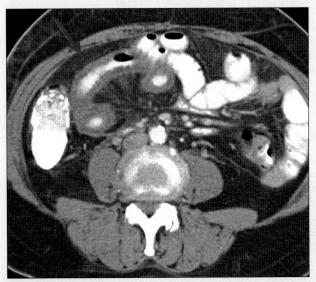

Figure 3. Intramesenteric triangular hematoma with adjacent bowel wall thickening. A 60-year-old woman was evaluated after a motor-vehicle collision. Mesenteric stranding at the root of the superior mesenteric artery branches leads to a segment of the small bowel (seen here) with marked wall thickening *(arrow)*. Exploratory laparotomy revealed a mesenteric defect and an ischemic 20-cm segment of the middle ileum.

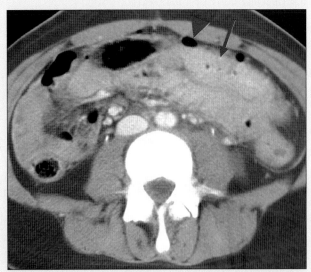

Figure 4. Small-bowel wall thickening with adjacent gas. A 16-year-old girl was evaluated after a high-speed motor-vehicle collision and partial ejection. Imaging showed small-bowel wall thickening *(arrow)* with adjacent foci of free intraperitoneal air *(arrowhead)*. A transmural jejunal injury 30 cm distal to the ligament of Treitz was found at laparotomy.

Intraperitoneal Fluid

DEFINITION: Fluid in the peritoneal cavity may be blood, bile, tumor, bowel contents, urine, or serum.

ANATOMIC FINDINGS

- Fluid in the supramesocolic space typically is first seen in Morison pouch.
- Fluid in the inframesocolic space is first identified in the pouch of Douglas or cul-de-sac.

IMAGING

CT
Findings
- Fluid caught between the leaves of the mesentery produces a V-shaped or triangular fluid, with the apex of the triangle pointing toward the mesenteric root.
- Matted loops of bowel resulting from blood extend between the loops of the bowel if the blood is isodense with bowel contents.
- Clotted blood (> 45 HU) is denser than serous blood (30-45 HU), which is denser than urine or bile.
- Sentinel clot (clotted blood adjacent to injury) helps localize the site of the bleeding.
- Active extravasation is visualized as an area of increased attenuation approximating arterial enhancement at the same level and at the same time.
- Vigorous arterial bleeding can sometimes appear as higher density than adjacent arterial enhancement and can occasionally be mistaken for bone.

Utility
- Contrast-enhanced CT is used.
- Trace amount of fluid seen on fewer than three slices seems likely to be physiologic.
- Matted appearance is nonspecific and can occasionally be seen in the normal unopacified bowel.
- Clotted blood is usually found adjacent to the bleeding site, and serous blood is found at a more remote location.
- When the hematoma is identified, images are scrutinized for evidence of active arterial bleeding (i.e., active extravasation).
- Fluid seen only adjacent to the bowel or caught between the leaves of the mesentery likely results from bowel injury.
- Fluid in large amounts seen throughout the abdomen is likely from solid organ injury such as splenic or hepatic laceration.

DIAGNOSTIC PEARLS

- Fluid caught between the leaves of the mesentery produces a V-shaped or triangular fluid, with the apex of the triangle pointing toward the mesenteric root.
- Clotted blood (> 45 HU) is denser than serous blood (30-45 HU), which is denser than urine or bile.
- Active extravasation is visualized as an area of increased attenuation approximating arterial enhancement at the same level and at the same time.
- Fluid with an attenuation less than −10 to −15 HU may represent chyle.

Ultrasound
Findings
- Anechoic or hypoechoic fluid
- Benign ascites conforms to adjacent organs.
- Malignant or infected ascites exhibits more of a mass effect.

Utility
- Ultrasound is very sensitive in the detection of small amounts of fluid in Morison pouch, pouch of Douglas, and cul-de-sac.

CLINICAL PRESENTATION

- Abdominal distention
- Abdominal mass
- Bowel obstruction
- Intraperitoneal fluid may be seen in cases of blunt-force abdominal trauma.

DIFFERENTIAL DIAGNOSIS

- Hepatic dysfunction
- Cardiac dysfunction
- Ischemia of the bowel
- Cirrhosis
- Trauma
- Infectious enterocolitides
- Inflammatory enterocolitides

WHAT THE REFERRING PHYSICIAN NEEDS TO KNOW

- Upper abdominal solid organ injuries initially bleed into the major peritoneal space adjacent to the organ.
- Identification of the sentinel clot is useful in determining the site of the bleeding.
- Fluid seen only adjacent to bowel or caught between the leaves of the mesentery likely results from bowel injury.
- Fluid in large amounts seen throughout the abdomen is likely from solid organ injury such as splenic or hepatic laceration.
- Active extravasation is considered an indication for embolization or surgery.

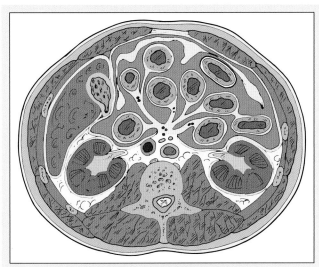

Figure 1. Mesenteric fluid or interloop fluid. Diagram of the mid-abdomen shows leaves of mesentery forming boundaries of the triangular-shaped interloop peritoneal spaces.

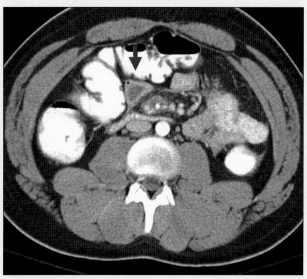

Figure 2. Mesenteric hematoma. A 20-year-old man was evaluated after a gunshot wound to the abdomen. A triangular hematoma *(arrow)* is identified at the mesenteric root, and the intramesenteric high-attenuation fluid is consistent with hematoma. Two jejunal enterotomies were observed and repaired at laparotomy. A mesenteric hematoma was also confirmed.

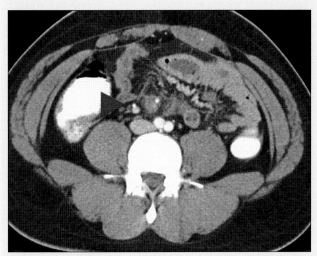

Figure 3. Mesenteric hematoma. A 20-year-old man was evaluated after a gunshot wound to the abdomen. A triangular hematoma *(arrowhead)* is identified at the mesenteric root, and the intramesenteric high-attenuation fluid is consistent with hematoma. Two jejunal enterotomies were observed and repaired at laparotomy. A mesenteric hematoma was also confirmed.

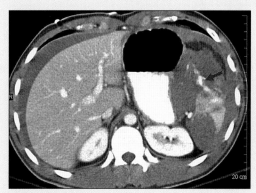

Figure 4. Splenic vascular injury. A 23-year-old man was assessed after a collision between a bicycle and a car. CT scan demonstrates multiple foci of high attenuation *(arrow)* similar to the aorta within a splenic laceration, indicating vascular injury. The patient was initially managed by transcatheter embolization but subsequently experienced delayed splenic rupture and underwent emergent splenectomy.

PATHOLOGY

■ Peritoneal fluid detected in trauma patient may have a traumatic or nontraumatic origin.
■ Intraperitoneal fluid from trauma may be blood from a solid organ, bowel, or mesentery or from bowel contents, bile, or urine.
■ If the patient has ascites from a comorbid condition such as cirrhosis, differentiating ascites from dilute blood is often difficult.

Suggested Readings

Halvorsen RA: MDCT of abdominal trauma. In Bae KT, Costello P, Saini S, Rubin GD (eds): *MDCT: A Practical Approach.* New York, Springer, 2006.
Jeffrey RB Jr, Cardoza JD, Olcott EW: Detection of active intraabdominal hemorrhage: Value of dynamic contrast-enhanced CT. *AJR Am J Roentgenol* 156:725-729, 1991.
Sivit CJ, Peclet MH, Taylor GA: Life-threatening intraperitoneal bleeding: Demonstration with CT. *Radiology* 171:430, 1989.

Index

Note: Page numbers followed by *f* indicate figures.

A

AAA. *See* Abdominal aortic aneurysm (AAA)
Abdomen, in Gaucher disease, 630, 631f
Abdominal aorta
  atherosclerotic changes, 11f
  dissection, 954, 955f
  extrinsic compression, in median arcuate ligament
    syndrome, 8f–9f
  rupture, 954, 955f
Abdominal aortic aneurysm (AAA), 954, 955f
  calcification, 23
Abdominal masses, pediatric (neonatal), 806, 807f
Abdominal sepsis, 977
Abdominal wall
  calcifications in, 23
  fluid collections, 789, 790f
  hernias, 791, 792f
  metastases to, 794, 795f
  neoplasms, 794, 795f
Abetalipoproteinemia, 299, 319, 320f
Abscess
  abdominal, 474, 475f, 977
  abdominal wall, 789, 790f
  amebic, of liver, 411f, 606, 607f
  appendiceal, 475f, 869, 871f
    percutaneous drainage, complications of, 473f
  catheter drainage of, 473f
  with colonic diverticulitis, 385, 386f–387f
  crypt, 403
  diverticular, 475f
  hepatic
    amebic, 411f, 606, 607f
    bacterial (pyogenic), 610, 611f
    pediatric, 909, 910f
    percutaneous drainage, complications of, 473f
  pancreatic, 701f
  percutaneous drainage, complications of, 472, 473f
  peripouch, with ileoanal pouch, 361, 363f
  pouch of Douglas, 775, 777f
  presacral, 475f
  psoas muscle, 475f
  splenic, 761, 762f
Accessory spleen, 730, 731f, 767f
Achalasia
  primary, esophagus in, 44, 45f
  secondary, 45f
    esophagus in, 113, 114f
Acinar cell carcinoma, 925, 926f
Actinomycosis
  colonic, 407
  in HIV-infected (AIDS) patients, small-bowel
    involvement in, 296, 297f
Adenitis, mesenteric, 969, 970f
  in pediatric patient, 942, 943f
Adenocarcinoma
  in Barrett esophagus, 104, 105f
  colonic, 425, 426f
  esophageal, 104, 105f
  gastric, mucinous, 222, 223f
  jejunal, 331, 332f
  pancreatic ductal, 707, 708f
Adenomas
  bile duct, 564, 565f
  biliary, 481
  cystic, appendiceal, 400
  esophageal, 98, 99f
  hepatocellular, 573, 574f, 919
  of small bowel, 325, 326f
  villous
    colonic, 422, 423f
    of small bowel, 325
Adhesions, colonic, 458
AIDS. *See* HIV-infected (AIDS) patients

Alagille syndrome, 891
Amebiasis
  colonic involvement in, 410, 411f
  pathology of, 608f
Amiodarone, hepatotoxicity, 650, 651f
Amyloidosis
  gastric involvement in, 277, 278f
  hepatic involvement in, 625
  of small bowel, 626f
Ancylostomiasis, of small bowel, 284
Aneurysm
  celiac artery, 16f, 351, 352f
  celiac axis, 352f
  gastroduodenal artery, 351
  hepatic artery, 16f, 351, 686, 687f
  large, in lipomatous hepatic tumor, 577
  pancreatic artery, 351
  portal venous, 678
  splanchnic artery, 351, 352f
  splanchnic vein, 678
  splenic artery, 686, 687f
  superior mesenteric artery, 16f, 351
  umbilical vein, 679f
  visceral artery, 15, 16f, 686, 687f
Angiodysplasia, colonic, 431, 978, 979f
Angiomyolipoma, hepatic, 577, 578f
Angiosarcoma, hepatic, 583, 584f
  pediatric, 922–923
Anisakiasis
  colonic involvement in, 410
  of small bowel, 284
Annular pancreas, 692, 693f–694f, 849, 850f
Anorectum, vascular lesions, 467, 468f
Antral gastritis, 174, 175f
Antral pad sign, 265
Antral-pyloric fold, hypertrophied, with antral
  gastritis, 174, 175f
Anus, imperforate, 821, 822f–823f
Aortic arch
  double, 846, 847f
  right, 846, 847f
Aphthoid ulcers, in gastric Crohn disease, 185, 186f
Appendiceal abscess, 869, 871f
Appendiceal carcinoid, 402
Appendicitis, 393–396
  pediatric, 869, 870f
Appendicoliths, 23
Appendix
  cystadenocarcinoma, 400, 401f
  cystadenoma, 400
  mucocele, 397, 398f, 400
Areae gastricae
  in atrophic gastritis, 183, 184f
  enlarged, in *Helicobacter pylori* gastritis, 176, 177f
Arteriovenous malformations (AVMs)
  colonic, 978
  hepatic, 917, 918f
Aryepiglottic folds
  neurofibroma, 36, 37f
  retention cysts, 36
Arytenoid cartilage, retention cyst, 37f
Ascariasis
  biliary tract involvement in, 535, 536f, 772, 773f
  colonic involvement in, 410, 411f
  intestinal, pediatric, 890f
  of small bowel, 284, 285f
Ascites, 21, 22f, 778, 779f
  biliary, 546, 547f, 553f
  cerebrospinal fluid, 778
  chylous, 778
  fetal, 826, 837
  hemorrhagic, 780
  signs of, 21
  transudative, 779f, 780

Asplenia, 732, 733f
Atherosclerosis, of splanchnic arteries, 10, 11f
Atrophic gastritis, 183, 184f
Avastin, hepatotoxicity, 650
AVMs. *See* Arteriovenous malformations (AVMs)
Azathioprine, hepatotoxicity, 650

B

Babygram, in meconium peritonitis, 827f
Backwash ileitis, 403, 404f
Bacterial infections
  colonic, 407, 408f
  ileal, 287, 288f
  of small bowel, 287, 288f
Barium, hanging drop of. *See also* Stalactite
  on hyperplastic polyp, 204, 205f
Barrett esophagus, 55, 56f
  adenocarcinoma in, 104, 105f
  long-segment, 55
  short-segment, 55
BDH. *See* Bile duct hamartoma (BDH)
Beak appearance, of colonic volvulus, 458
Beaklike appearance, of diffuse esophageal spasm,
  46
Beckwith-Wiedemann syndrome
  and omphalocele, 837
  pancreatic involvement in, 927, 928f
Behçet disease, 84, 344
Benign gastric emphysema, 277, 278f
Bezoars
  gastric, 267, 268f
    soap bubble appearance, 209
  small-bowel, 379
Bile, milk of calcium, 522, 523f
Bile duct hamartoma (BDH), 566, 567f
Bile ducts
  adenomas, 564, 565f
  calculi, 486, 487f
  in familial adenomatous polyposis syndrome, 446
  gas in, 18
  intrahepatic
    cystadenocarcinoma, 524, 525f
    cystadenoma, 524, 525f
    paucity of, 891, 892f–894f
  in recurrent pyogenic cholangitis, 544, 545f
  strictures, 549, 550f
  surgical injury to, 546
Bile leak, postoperative, 546, 547f, 550f, 553f
Bile peritonitis, 547f
Bile plug syndrome, 895
Biliary atresia, 896, 897f–898f, 905, 906f
Biliary-enteric fistula, 18
Biliary sludge, 507, 508f
Biliary tract
  calculi, 23, 24f
  infection/disease spread through, 772, 773f
  inflammation, 478, 479f
  neoplasia, 481, 482f–483f
  parasitic infestations, 535, 536f
Biloma, 546, 547f, 689f
Bird beak esophagus, in secondary achalasia, 113,
  114f
Bird's claw appearance, in schistosomiasis, 620
Blood vessels. *See also* Vasculature; *specific vessel*
  calcifications in, 23, 24f
Bochdalek hernia, 796, 797f
  neonatal, 813, 814f
Boerhaave syndrome, 130f
Bowel, malignant neoplasm of, 5f
Bowel gas, abnormal, in neonate, 809, 810f
Bowel obstruction, 956, 957f
  neonatal, 809, 810f